Handbook of
Cosmetic Science
and Technology

Handbook of
Cosmetic Science
and Technology

edited by

André O. Barel
Free University of Brussels
Brussels, Belgium

Marc Paye
Colgate-Palmolive Research and Development, Inc.
Milmort, Belgium

Howard I. Maibach
University of California at San Francisco School of Medicine
San Francisco, California

MARCEL DEKKER, INC.   NEW YORK · BASEL

ISBN: 0-8247-0292-1

This book is printed on acid-free paper.

Headquarters
Marcel Dekker, Inc.
270 Madison Avenue, New York, NY 10016
tel: 212-696-9000; fax: 212-685-4540

Eastern Hemisphere Distribution
Marcel Dekker AG
Hutgasse 4, Postfach 812, CH-4001 Basel, Switzerland
tel: 41-61-261-8482; fax: 41-61-261-8896

World Wide Web
http://www.dekker.com

The publisher offers discounts on this book when ordered in bulk quantities. For more information,
write to Special Sales/Professional Marketing at the headquarters address above.

PRINTED IN THE UNITED STATES OF AMERICA

Preface

Cosmetic composition and formulation are becoming increasingly complex, and cosmetic ingredients more sophisticated and functional, while laws and regulations impose more constraints on the cosmetic scientist and manufacturer. The *Handbook of Cosmetic Science and Technology* reviews in a single volume the multiple facets of the cosmetic field and provides the reader with an easy-to-access information source.

This handbook covers topics as varied as the physiology of the potential targets of cosmetics, safety, legal and regulatory considerations throughout the world, cosmetic ingredients, vehicles and finished products, and new delivery systems, as well as microbiology and safety and efficacy testing.

To achieve our goal, we, the editors, requested the contributions of expert scientists from academic dermatology and dermato-cosmetics, the cosmetics industry, ingredients and raw materials producers, and regulatory agencies. Because cosmetology is universal, while having some regional specificity, those authors were selected on a broad geographical basis, with some coming from the United States, Europe, Japan, and Australia. They share in their chapters not only their experience and knowledge but also new information and their expert views regarding the future. We thank the authors for their high dedication, which permitted us to make this handbook a review of the state of the art in cosmetology in the new millennium. The staff of Marcel Dekker, Inc., played a great role in the production of the handbook, ensuring on a day-to-day basis the contact between the editors and the authors. Our thanks especially go to Sandra Beberman, Jane Roh, and Moraima Suarez for their constant and excellent help.

Finally, we encourage our readership to send us their comments and suggestions on what should be modified or considered in future editions.

André O. Barel
Marc Paye
Howard I. Maibach

Contents

Part 6   COSMETIC PRODUCTS

Skincare Products

Haircare Products

Other Cosmetic Products

Contributors

Albert Zorko Abram, B.Sc. Soltec Research Pty Ltd., Rowville, Victoria, Australia

Josette André, M.D. Faculty of Medicine, Free University of Brussels, and Department of Dermatology, Hôpital Saint-Pierre, Brussels, Belgium

John E. Bailey, Ph.D. Office of Cosmetics and Colors, Center for Food Safety and Applied Nutrition (CFSAN), U.S. Food and Drug Administration, Washington, D.C.

Robert Baran, M.D. Nail Disease Center, Cannes, France

André O. Barel, Ph.D. Faculty of Physical Education and Physiotherapy, Free University of Brussels, Brussels, Belgium

John Barr, Ph.D. Pharmaceutical Sciences, Advanced Polymer Systems, Redwood City, California

Saqib J. Bashir, B.Sc.(Hons), M.B., Ch.B. Department of Dermatology, University of California at San Francisco School of Medicine, San Francisco, California

Enzo Berardesca, M.D. Department of Dermatology, University of Pavia, Pavia, Italy

Janet M. Blakely, B.Sc.(Hons) Life Sciences Group, Science and Technology, Dow Corning S.A., Brussels, Belgium

Leon H. Bruner, D.V.M., Ph.D. Gillette Medical Evaluation Laboratory, The Gillette Company, Needham, Massachusetts

Stephan Buchmann, Ph.D. Department of Pharmaceutical Technology, Spirig Pharma AG, Egerkingen, Switzerland

Ai-Lean Chew, M.B.Ch.B. Department of Dermatology, University of California at San Francisco School of Medicine, San Francisco, California

William J. Cunningham, M.D. CU-TECH, Mountain Lakes, New Jersey

Rodger D. Curren, Ph.D. Institute for In Vitro Sciences, Inc., Gaithersburg, Maryland

Anton C. de Groot, M.D., Ph.D. Department of Dermatology, Carolus Hospital, 's-Hertogenbosch, The Netherlands

Michel J. Devleeschouwer, Ph.D. Laboratory of Microbiology and Hygiene, Institute of Pharmacy and Biocontaminants Unit, School of Public Health, Free University of Brussels, Brussels, Belgium

Ekong A. Ekong, Ph.D. Technology Division, Hercules Incorporated, Wilmington, Delaware

Joel J. Elias, Ph.D. Department of Anatomy, University of California at San Francisco School of Medicine, San Francisco, California

Peter Elsner, M.D. Department of Dermatology and Allergology, University of Jena, Jena, Germany

Howard Epstein, M.S. Product Development, The Andrew Jergens Company, Cincinnati, Ohio

Paquita E. Erazo-Majewicz, Ph.D. Aqualon Division, Hercules Incorporated, Wilmington, Delaware

Spiros A. Fotinos, B.Sc.(Pharm), B.Sc.(Chem) Corporate Research and Innovation, Lavipharm, Peania Attica, Greece

Bernard Gabard, Ph.D. Department of Biopharmacy, Spirig Pharma Ltd., Egerkingen, Switzerland

Abdul Gaffar, Ph.D. Advanced Technology, Corporate Technology, Department of Oral Care, Colgate-Palmolive Company, Piscataway, New Jersey

Joshua B. Ghaim, Ph.D. Product Development, Skin Care Global Technology, Colgate-Palmolive Company, Piscataway, New Jersey

An E. Goossens, B.Pharm., Ph.D. Department of Dermatology, University Hospital, Katholieke Universiteit Leuven, Leuven, Belgium

Gary Grove, Ph.D. Research and Development, KGL's Skin Study Center, Broomall, and cyberDERM, inc., Media, Pennsylvania

Mary Jo Grove, M.S. KGL's Skin Study Center, Broomall, and cyberDERM, inc., Media, Pennsylvania

Gary S. Hahn, M.D. Department of Pediatrics, University of California at San Diego School of Medicine, San Diego, and Board of Scientific Advisors, Cosmederm Technologies, LLC, La Jolla, California

Allen R. Halper Office of Cosmetics and Colors, Center for Food Safety and Applied Nutrition (CFSAN), U.S. Food and Drug Administration, Washington, D.C.

John W. Harbell, Ph.D. Institute for In Vitro Sciences, Inc., Gaithersburg, Maryland

Jorge Heller, Ph.D. Advanced Polymer Systems, Redwood City, California

Jocélia Jansen, Ph.D. Department of Pharmaceutical Sciences, State University of Ponta Grossa, Ponta Grossa, Paraná, Brazil

Joerg Kahre, Ph.D. VTP Department, Henkel KGaA, Düsseldorf, Germany

Daisuke Kaneko, Ph.D. Department of Product Development, AminoScience Laboratories, Ajinomoto Co., Inc., Kanagawa, Japan

Cees Korstanje, R.Ph., Ph.D. Biological Research Department, Yamanouchi Europe B.V., Leiderdorp, The Netherlands

Alois Kretz, M.D. Cosmetics, Roche Vitamins Europe Ltd., Basel, Switzerland

Hans Lautenschläger, Ph.D. Development & Consulting, Pulheim, Germany

Sabrina Lazzerini, M.D. Department of Dermatology, University of Pavia, Pavia, Italy

Stanley B. Levy, M.D. Department of Dermatology, University of North Carolina School of Medicine at Chapel Hill, Chapel Hill, North Carolina, and Medical Affairs, Revlon Research Center, Edison, New Jersey

Marie Lodén, Pharm.Sc., Dr.Med.Sc. Department of Dermatology, ACO HUD AB, Upplands Väsby, Sweden

John K. Lodge, Ph.D. School of Biological Sciences, University of Surrey, Guildford, Surrey, England

Kate Lusvardi, Ph.D. Aqualon Division, Hercules Incorporated, Wilmington, Delaware

Howard I. Maibach, M.D. Department of Dermatology, University of California at San Francisco School of Medicine, San Francisco, California

Mitsuteru Masuda, Ph.D. Life Science Research Center, Research and Development Headquarters, Lion Corporation, Tokyo, Japan

James K. Maurer, D.V.M., Ph.D.   Human and Environmental Safety Division, The Procter & Gamble Company, Cincinnati, Ohio

Mohand Melbouci, Ph.D.   Personal Care Department, Aqualon Division, Hercules Incorporated, Wilmington, Delaware

Bozena B. Michniak, Ph.D.   College of Pharmacy, University of South Carolina, Columbia, South Carolina

Stanley R. Milstein, Ph.D.   Office of Cosmetics and Colors, Center for Food Safety and Applied Nutrition (CFSAN), U.S. Food and Drug Administration, Washington, D.C.

Ulrich Moser, Ph.D.   Roche Vitamins Europe Ltd., Basel, Switzerland

Linda P. Oddo, B.S.   Hill Top Research, Inc., Scottsdale, Arizona

Louis Oldenhove de Guertechin, Ph.D.   Department of Advanced Technology, Colgate-Palmolive Research and Development, Inc., Milmort, Belgium

Rosemarie Osborne, Ph.D.   Human and Environmental Safety Division, The Procter & Gamble Company, Cincinnati, Ohio

Gisbert Otterstätter   Color Department, DRAGOCO Gerberding & Co. AG, Holzminden, Germany

Lester Packer, Ph.D.   Department of Molecular and Cellular Biology, University of California at Berkeley, Berkeley, California

Marc Paye, Ph.D.   Skin Research Division, Department of Advanced Technology, Colgate-Palmolive Research and Development, Inc., Milmort, Belgium

Alessandra Pelosi, M.D.   Department of Dermatology, University of Pavia, Pavia, Italy

Mary A. Perkins, A.Sc.   Human and Environmental Safety Division, The Procter & Gamble Company, Cincinnati, Ohio

Véronique Préat, Ph.D.   Unité de Pharmacie Galénique, Université Catholique de Louvain, Brussels, Belgium

Charles Reich, Ph.D.   Advanced Technology, Hair Care, Colgate-Palmolive Technology Center, Piscataway, New Jersey

Michael K. Robinson, Ph.D.   Department of Human and Environmental Safety Division, The Procter & Gamble Company, Cincinnati, Ohio

Perry Romanowski, B.S., M.S.   Research and Development, Alberto Culver Company, Melrose Park, Illinois

Kazutami Sakamoto, Ph.D. Applied Research Department, AminoScience Laboratories, Ajinomoto Co., Inc., Kanagawa, Japan

Claude Saliou, Pharm.D., Ph.D. Department of Molecular and Cell Biology, University of California at Berkeley, Berkeley, California

Subhash J. Saxena, Ph.D. Research and Development, Advanced Polymer Systems, Redwood City, California

Sibylle Schliemann-Willers, M.D. Department of Dermatology and Allergology, University of Jena, Jena, Germany

Mitchell L. Schlossman, B.A., F.A.I.C., F.S.C.C. Kobo Products, Inc., South Plainfield, New Jersey

Uwe Schönrock, Ph.D. Active Ingredient Research, Beiersdorf AG, Hamburg, Germany

Douglas Schoon, M.S. Research and Development, Creative Nail Design Inc., Vista, California

Jörg Schreiber, Ph.D. Research New Delivery Systems, Beiersdorf AG, Hamburg, Germany

Randy Schueller, B.S. Consumer Products Research and Development, Alberto Culver Company, Melrose Park, Illinois

Jørgen Serup, M.D., D.M.Sc. Department of Dermatological Research, Leo Pharmaceutical Products, Copenhagen, Denmark

Ghassan Shaker, M.B.Ch.B., D.Sc. Skinterface sprl, Tournai, Belgium

Kathy Shannon, B.S. Hill Top Research, Inc., Scottsdale, Arizona

F. Anthony Simion, Ph.D. Product Development, The Andrew Jergens Company, Cincinnati, Ohio

Françoise Siquet, Ph.D. Department of Microbiology, Colgate-Palmolive Technology Center, Milmort, Belgium

Klaus Stanzl, Ph.D. DRAGOCO Gerberding & Co. AG, Holzminden, Germany

Dean T. Su, Ph.D. Personal Care, Colgate-Palmolive Technology Center, Piscataway, New Jersey

Takamitsu Tamura, Ph.D. Material Science Research Center, Lion Corporation, Tokyo, Japan

Yoshimasa Tanaka, Ph.D.   Life Science Research Center, Lion Corporation, Tokyo, Japan

Roderick Peter John Tomlinson   Soltec Research Pty Ltd., Rowville, Victoria, Australia

Rita Vanbever, Ph.D.   Unité de Pharmacie Galénique, Université Catholique de Louvain, Brussels, Belgium

René Van Essche, D.V.M., M.B.A.   Institute of Pharmacy, Free University of Brussels, Brussels, Belgium

Dominique Van Neste, M.D., Ph.D.   Skinterface sprl, Tournai, Belgium

Jürgen Vollhardt, Ph.D.   Research and Development, Cosmetic Division, DRAGOCO Inc., Totowa, New Jersey

Elizabeth D. Volz, M.ChE.   Research and Development, Colgate-Palmolive Company, Piscataway, New Jersey

Stefan Udo Weber, M.D.   Department of Molecular and Cell Biology, University of California at Berkeley, Berkeley, California

Philip W. Wertz, Ph.D.   Dows Institute, University of Iowa, Iowa City, Iowa

Ronald C. Wester, Ph.D.   Department of Dermatology, University of California at San Francisco School of Medicine, San Francisco, California

Leszek J. Wolfram, Ph.D.   Independent Consultant, Stamford, Connecticut

Hongbo Zhai, M.D.   Department of Dermatology, University of California at San Francisco School of Medicine, San Francisco, California

Germaine Zocchi, Ph.D.   Department of Advanced Technology, Colgate-Palmolive Research and Development, Inc., Milmort, Belgium

Introduction

André O. Barel
Free University of Brussels, Brussels, Belgium

Marc Paye
Colgate-Palmolive Research and Development, Inc., Milmort, Belgium

Howard I. Maibach
University of California at San Francisco School of Medicine,
San Francisco, California

Although cosmetics for the purposes of beautifying, perfuming, cleansing, or for rituals have existed since the origin of civilization, only in the twentieth century has great progress been made in the diversification of products and functions, as well as in the safety and protection of the consumer.

Before 1938, cosmetics were not regulated as drugs, and cosmetology could often be considered a way to sell dreams rather than objective efficacy. Safety for consumers was also precarious at times. Subsequently, the Food and Drug Administration (FDA), through the Federal Food, Drug and Cosmetic Act, regulated cosmetics that were required to be safe for the consumer.

With industrialization, many new ingredients from several industries (oleo- and petrochemical, food, etc.) were used in the preparation of cosmetics, often introducing new functions and forms. For better control of these ingredients, U.S. laws have required ingredient classification and product labeling since 1966.

The latest innovation in the field of cosmetics is the development of active cosmetics. Currently, cosmetics are not only intended for the improvement of the appearance or odor of the consumer, but are also intended for the benefit of their target, whether it is the skin, the hair, the mucous membrane, or the tooth. With this functional approach, products became diversified and started to claim a multitude of actions on the body. Subsequently, the cosmetic market greatly expanded, becoming accessible to millions of consumers worldwide. The competitive environment also pushed manufacturers to promise more to consumers and to develop cosmetic products of better quality and higher efficacy. Today, many cosmetic products aim at hydrating the skin, reducing or slowing the signs of aged skin, or protecting the skin against the multitude of daily aggressions that it encounters. In order for cosmetic products to support these activities, raw materials became more efficacious, safe, bioavailable, and innovative, while remaining affordable. With the continuous improvement of the basic sciences and the development of new sciences (e.g., molecular biology), new sources for pure raw material have been found. Raw materials are not only produced from natural sources and highly purified, but can also be specifically synthesized or even produced from genetically manipulated microorganisms. However, the availability and use of these sophisticated and active ingredients are not always sufficient for them to be optimally delivered to their targets and to sustain their activity. The cosmetic vehicle is also crucial to obtain this effect, and the role of the formulator is to combine the right ingredient with the most appropriate vehicle.

Additional sciences also developed parallel to active cosmetology and contributed significantly to its rise; this is the case for biometric techniques, which have been developing for two decades now and allow a progressive and noninvasive investigation of many skin properties. Instruments and methods are now available to objectively evaluate and measure cutaneous elasticity, topography, hydration, turn-over rate, or even to see directly in vivo inside the skin through microscope evolution. The major innovations in the field are reported by the International Society of Bioengineering and the Skin. Guidelines for the appropriate usage of instrumental techniques and for the accurate measurement of skin function and properties are regularly published by expert groups such as the Standardization Group of the European Society of Contact Dermatitis or the European Group for Efficacy Measurement of Cosmetics and Other Topical Products (EEMCO). Today, any claimed effect of a cosmetic on the skin should find appropriate techniques for a clear demonstration.

For better protection of the consumer against misleading claims, national or federal laws prohibit false advertisement on cosmetic products. More recently, the Sixth Amendment of the European Directive on Cosmetic Products has required manufacturers to have a dossier with the proof of the claims made on their products readily available.

Finally, the recent evolution of cosmetic products and the constraints imposed on the cosmetic manufacturer have led cosmetology to largely increase its credibility before scientists, physicians, and consumers. Cosmetology has become a science based on a combination of various types of expertise, whether they are in chemistry, physics, biology, bioengineering, dermatology, microbiology, toxicology, or statistics, among others.

Because of this complexity in cosmetic science, it is not possible to cover in a useful manner all the aspects of cosmetology in only one book. Details of most of the aforementioned fields are covered in different volumes of the Cosmetic Science and Technology series. With the *Handbook of Cosmetic Science and Technology*, we aim to produce a useful guide and source of innovative ideas for the formulation of modern cosmetics. The esteemed contributors to the handbook review many of the major ingredients, major technologies, and up-to-date regulations throughout the world that the formulator needs to know. For more experienced scientists, recent innovations in ingredients and cosmetic vehicle forms are described, which should orient the type of products of tomorrow. Finally, the large overview of cosmetic formulations should serve the dermatologist who is faced with patients requesting recommendations for the most appropriate product for their skin type or who have specific intolerance to an ingredient. This should help them to better understand cosmetics.

For easier access to the information contained herewith, the handbook has been subdivided into nine parts, such including several chapters written by different authors. It may seem to some an excessive number of contributors, but we intentionally chose this format to guarantee that each subject is described by recognized experts in the field who are well aware of the latest developments in their topic. In addition, authors were selected worldwide. Indeed, cosmetology is universal, but there exists some regional specificity that should be addressed.

The first three parts present the reader with a series of generalities going from definitions of cosmetics, to a description of the anatomy and physiology of the body targets for cosmetics, to safety terminology, and finally to a description of the principles and mechanism of unwanted interactions of cosmetics with their target.

Part 4 covers cosmetic vehicles with a special emphasis on a few types of recently introduced delivery systems, such as cosmetic patches and iontophoresis. Part 5 describes cosmetic ingredients. For some categories of ingredients, the most useful information is a list of the ingredients they comprise, with a critical analysis of the advantages and disadvantages for each. For others, however, a good understanding is needed of the role of an ingredient in a product, its limitations, its mechanism of action, and its regulatory constraints.

Part 6, the largest section, is the core of the handbook and provides guidance to the formulation of skin cleansing products, skin care products, hair products, oral care products, and decorative products. Chapters 58 and 59 cover special cosmetics for infant and elderly consumers.

The last three parts of the handbook compare the cosmetic legislation in the United States, Europe, and Japan; briefly describe how to control the stability of cosmetic products; and give an overview on the clinical tests often performed for proving efficacy, tolerance, or perception of the products. These latter chapters, however, remain quite general, being more extensively covered in other, more specialized volumes.

Given the number of contributions and the need to publish them while they are still current, it has been a formidable challenge to edit the handbook; if we have succeeded, it is attributable to the dedication of the authors and the continuous follow-up made with the authors by Sandra Beberman and Jane Roh from Marcel Dekker, Inc. We thank all of them for making this enormous task easy, enjoyable, and mainly feasible.

In view of the evolution of cosmetology over these past years, and seeing where we are today, we would like to conclude this introduction with a question that came after reading these outstanding contributions: How will cosmetology continue to evolve without reaching and overlapping the pharmaceutical field in the future? There is still a margin, but this margin is becoming increasingly thinner. Has the time arrived to describe, after the ''functional'' or ''active'' cosmetology, the cosmetology of regulators?

Definition of Cosmetics

Stanley R. Milstein, John E. Bailey, and Allen R. Halper
Office of Cosmetics and Colors, Center for Food Safety and Applied Nutrition (CFSAN),
U.S. Food and Drug Administration, Washington, D.C.

INTRODUCTION

Cosmetics are a category of consumer products marketed worldwide, the purpose and functions of which are universal to people of all cultures. The 1998 global cosmetics and toiletries market was valued at $125.7 billion [1], including skincare, fragrance, haircare, personal hygiene, and makeup products. In the United States alone there are over 1400 domestic manufacturing and repacking establishments, which in the aggregate use more than 10,500 different cosmetic ingredients [2] and a corresponding number of fragrance ingredients to make over 25,000 product formulations [3]. Once considered luxuries by consumers of modest economic means, cosmetics and toiletries are seen today as necessities by growing numbers of consumers, regardless of their relative states of affluence [4]. Indeed, cosmetics are regarded not as mere pampered indulgences, but as key aids to maintaining and promoting better standards of personal hygiene and health. Yet, what are these products that we call *cosmetics*?

COSMETICS IN HISTORY

The word ''cosmetic'' is derived from the Greek *Kosm tikos*, meaning ''having the power to arrange, skilled in decorating giving *kosmein*, ''to adorn,'' and *kosmos*, ''order, harmony'' [5], but the true origin of cosmetics probably lies further still in antiquity, because early cave paintings of 30,000 years ago depict the use of body adornment (rudimentary cosmetics) in the rituals of mating and hunting [5].

Throughout the recorded history of man, cosmetics have been used with essentially the same three goals in mind, namely (1) to enhance personal appeal through decoration of the body, (2) to camouflage flaws in the integument, and (3) to alter or improve upon nature (6). Consider several historical vignettes showing the role of cosmetics down through the ages (4–6). Vases of alabaster and obsidian for cosmetics discovered by Flinders Petrie in 1914 illustrate that the ancient Egyptians were well versed in the use of eye and face paints, body oils, and ointments. Theophrastus (363–278 B.C.), a student of Aristotle, demonstrated considerable knowledge of the compounding of perfumes, and the Roman physician, Galen of Pergamon (130–200 A.D.), is said to have innovated that time-honored toiletry: cold cream (Cera Alba). Other people throughout the Middle East as well as the Orient were reported to have made extensive use of cosmetics. The Babylonians were said by Herodotus (490–420 B.C.) to be well practiced in the use of depilatories and the eye adornment, kohl, while Alexander the Great (356–323 B.C.) reported the use of unguents, incense, and other cosmetics by the countries of the Indo-Sumerian civilization. In Tudor England of the 1500s, sycophants of the Virgin Queen, Elizabeth I, adopted whatever cosmetic artifice and whimsy she chose to champion, whether by powdering their faces with the toxic lead paint, ceruse, to simulate the Queen's pale complexion, rouging their cheeks with red ochre, or dyeing their hair orange to simulate the Queen's once-abundant wavy red-gold hair, which she had inherited from her father, King Henry VIII. In the 17th century, the phrase "makeup" was first used to connote "cosmetics" by the poet Richard Cranshaw (1612–1649), while author and playwright Ben Johnson satirized women who "put on their faces" upon rising each morning before facing the world.

STATUTORY DEFINITION OF COSMETICS

Consumers possess a reasonable operational understanding of what a cosmetic does (i.e., its so-called function). The average consumer envisions a cosmetic to be a product such as lipstick, cold cream, facial foundation powder, nail polish, and other so-called decorative personal-care items of makeup, which are all designed to enhance superficial appearance and beautify the body. Frequently, the consumer will also equate the term "cosmetic" with "toiletry," at which point other topical preparations intended to cleanse and perfume the body are also included in the layperson's operational definition of the term.

Despite the increasingly systematic and objective science associated with the art, formulation, and manufacture of cosmetics, our operational understanding of costmetics has to the present date failed to produce a corresponding harmonized international statutory agreement concerning what a cosmetic is and what the legitimate functions of such a product ought to be before it ceases to be a bonafide cosmetic. In the United States, the statutory definition of cosmetic enacted in the 1938 Federal Food, Drug, and Cosmetic Act (hereinafter, the Act) is more far reaching than the lay definition and implicitly addresses intended use as much as it does beauty-enhancing attributes of a "cosmetic" [7].

The term "cosmetic" is defined in Section 201 (i) of the 1938 Food, Drug, and Cosmetic Act (FD&C Act) as:

> . . . 1) articles intended to be rubbed, poured, sprinkled, or sprayed on, introduced into, or otherwise applied to the human body or any part thereof for cleansing, beautifying, promoting attractiveness, or altering the appearance, and 2) articles intended for use as a component of any such articles; except that such term shall not include soap . . .

The Act thus views cosmetics as articles intended to be applied to the human body for cleansing, beautifying, promoting attractiveness, or altering the appearance. No mention is explicitly made in this denotation of whether achieving such improvements in beauty, attractiveness, or appearance can legitimately be accomplished by a cosmetic product through its efficacy in affecting the body's structure or functions. The implications of such efficacy are taken into account in the treatment of the term "drug" by the Statute (see the following).

The 13 subdivided cosmetic product categories currently recognized by the U.S. Food & Drug Administration (FDA) for the voluntary filing of cosmetic product ingredient composition statements are enumerated in Title 21 of the Code of Federal Regulations (c.f., 21 CFR 720.4); these are presented in Table 1. Here one can find all of the product categories that the consumer usually connotes with the terms "cosmetics & toiletries." Included in the definition of cosmetics are products intended to cleanse the body in the bath or shower, mask the various malodors of the oral, perigenital, and axillary regions of the human anatomy, adorn the face, eyes, hair, and extremities in fashionable topical "decorative" colors, alter the color and style of the scalp hair, and afford the integument conditioning against losses of moisture caused by changes in environmental conditions (i.e., sun, wind, relative humidity) [8]. Note that the Act includes in the definition of "cosmetic" any material intended for use as a component of a cosmetic product, so that an ingredient intended to be used in a cosmetic is also considered to be a cosmetic.

Soap products, consisting primarily of an alkali metal salt of free fatty acids, making no label claims other than cleansing of the human body, and labeled, sold, and represented only as soap are not considered cosmetics under the law (c.f., 21 CFR 701.20). However, detergent-based "beauty or body bars," so-called combination or combo-bars based on mixtures of soap and detergent(s), and those products containing other functional cosmetic ingredients (i.e., emollients, moisturizers, or botanical ingredients) that make product performance claims other than cleansing of the human body, are considered "cosmetics." Additionally, soaps that contain antimicrobial active ingredients and that make antibacterial or germ-killing efficacy claims are regulated under the FD&C Act as "over-the-counter" (OTC) drug products. If they make cosmetic claims as well they may also be regulated as cosmetics [8] (see the following).

Other authoritative treatises in cosmetic science such as those of Jellinek [9], Poucher [5], deNavarre [10], Balsam and Sagarin [11], and *Harry's* [12] discuss cosmetic product formulations in similar categories to those that have been adopted by regulation under authority of the Act in the United States. Jackson [13] also presents an excellent and up-to-date tabulation of the product types that could reasonably be considered, wholly or in part, cosmetics. These include, as he correctly notes, some topical OTC drug products among his count of 77 product types, in addition to those products that the FDA would consider bonafide cosmetics.

The Act also contains statutory provisions to regulate cosmetics in order to ensure that only products deemed safe for their intended use and properly labeled are legally offered for sale in the United States. Thus, various prohibited actions are defined in Section 301 of the Act that relate to the conditions under which cosmetics are deemed to be "adulterated" (Section 601) or "misbranded" (Section 602) under the Act. These regulatory provisions will be discussed in Chapter 62.

COSMETICS THAT ARE ALSO DRUGS: THE INTENDED USE DOCTRINE

All topical products are not necessarily cosmetics. Dermatologics, for example, are topical products generally regulated as drug products based on the therapeutic or medicinal purpose for which the product is marketed as well as its formulation, which includes one or more pharmacologically active ingredients. Section 201 (g)(1) of the FD&C Act defines the term "drug" as:

> . . . (A) articles recognized in the official United States Pharmacopoeia, official Homeopathic Pharmacopeia of the United States, or official National Formulary, or any supplement to any of them; and (B) articles intended for use in the diagnosis, cure, mitigation, treatment, or prevention of disease in man or other animals; and (C) articles (other than

TABLE 1 Cosmetic Product Categories (21 CFR 720.4)

Baby Products
Baby shampoos
Lotions, oils, powders, and creams
Other baby products

Bath Preparations
Bath capsules
Bath oils, tablets, and salts
Bubble baths
Other bath preparations

Eye makeup preparations
Eyebrow pencil
Eyeliner
Eye lotion
Eye makeup remover
Eye shadow
Mascara
Other eye makeup preparations

Fragrance Preparations
Colognes and toilet waters
Perfumes
Powders (dusting and talcum, excluding aftershave talc)
Sachets
Other fragrance preparations

Hair Preparations (Noncoloring)
Hair conditioners
Hair sprays (aerosol fixatives)
Hair straighteners
Permanent waves
Rinses (noncoloring)
Shampoos (noncoloring)
Tonics, dressings, and other hair grooming aids
Wave sets
Other hair preparations

Hair Coloring Preparations
Hair bleaches
Hair dyes and colors*
Hair lighteners with color
Hair tints
Hair rinses (coloring)
Hair shampoos (coloring)
Hair color sprays (aerosol)
Other hair coloring preparations

Makeup Preparations (Not Eye)
Blushers (all types)
Face powders
Foundations
Leg and body paints
Lipstick
Makeup bases
Makeup fixatives
Rouges
Other makeup preparations

Manicuring Preparations
Basecoats and undercoats
Cuticle softeners
Nail creams and lotions
Nail extenders
Nail polish and enamel
Nail polish and enamel removers
Other manicuring preparations

Oral Hygiene Products
Dentifrices (aerosols, liquids, pastes, and powders)
Mouthwashes and breath fresheners (liquids and sprays)
Other oral hygiene products

TABLE 1 Continued

Personal Cleanliness	
Bath soaps and detergents	Feminine hygiene deodorants
Deodorants (underarm)	Other personal cleanliness products
Douches	
Shaving Preparations	
Aftershave lotions	Shaving cream (aerosol, brushless, and
Beard softeners	lather) products
Men's talcum	Shaving soap (e.g., cakes, sticks)
Preshave lotions (all types)	Other shaving preparations
Skincare Preparations (Creams, Lotions,	
Powders, and Sprays)	
Body and hand (excluding shaving	Foot powders and sprays
preparations)	Night
Cleansing (cold creams, cleansing lotions,	Paste masks (mud packs)
liquids, and pads)	Skin fresheners
Depilatories	Other skincare preparations
Face and neck (excluding shaving	
preparations)	
Suntan Preparations	
Indoor tanning preparations	
Suntan gels, creams, and liquids	
Other suntan preparations	

* All types requiring caution statement and patch test.

food) intended to affect the structure or any function of the body of man or other animals; and (D) articles specified in clause (A), (B), or (C); but does not include devices or their components, parts, or accessories.

The so-called Doctrine of Intended Use of an FDA-regulated product generally will govern how it is to be regulated [14]; the maxim frequently cited here that embodies this doctrine is "You are what you claim." The most recent comprehensive discussion of intended use may be found in Section II.E of the August 1996 Annex to the "Nicotine in Cigarettes and Smokeless Tobacco Jurisdictional Determination" document issued by FDA [15].

Prior to enactment of the 1938 Act, a 1935 Senate report foreshadowed the direction that the Congress would later take in providing that the manufacturer's intended use of the product should determine if it is to be regulated as a drug, cosmetic, or some other regulatory category [14]:

> The use to which the product is to be put will determine the category into which it will fall. If it is to be used only as a food it will come within the definition of food and none other. If it contains nutritive ingredients but is sold for drug use only, as clearly shown by the labeling and advertising, it will come within the definition of drug, but not that of food. If it is sold to be used both as a food and for the prevention or treatment of disease it would satisfy both definitions and be subject to the substantive requirements for both. The manufacturer of the article, through his representations in connection with its sale, can determine the use to which the article is put . . .

Thus, the definitions of drug and cosmetic are not mutually exclusive. A product may legally be a cosmetic, a drug, or both a drug and a cosmetic. Products that are cosmetics but are also intended to treat or prevent disease, or otherwise intended to affect the structure or any functions of the human body, are also considered drugs under the Act and must comply with both the drug and cosmetic provisions of the law [8].

Examples of products that are drugs as well as cosmetics are anticaries (fluoride) toothpastes, hormone creams, suntanning preparations containing a sunscreen active ingredient and either intended to protect against sunburn or make tanning claims [16], antiperspirants and/or deodorants, antibacterial detergent bars or soaps, and antidandruff shampoos. Most currently marketed cosmetics that are also drugs are OTC drugs. Several are new drugs for which safety and effectiveness had to be proven to FDA (i.e., in a New Drug Application or NDA) before they could be marketed [8]. A ''new drug'' is defined in Section 201 (p) of the Act as a drug that is not ''generally recognized as safe and effective'' (GRAS/E) by experts under the conditions of intended use or that has become so recognized but has not been used to a material extent or for a material time under such conditions.

It is relatively easy to market a cosmetic. Cosmetic products can be brought to market very quickly—a fact that is clearly reflected in the rapid pace with which innovations and changes occur in the cosmetic marketplace. No premarket approval (or mandatory manufacturing establishment, product, or ingredient registration) is required. No delays are thereby incurred by the marketer while waiting for FDA approval. Nor does FDA have a statutory mandate to monitor and regulate cosmetic performance advertising claims; the Agency's oversight responsibility in this area extends only to ensure that cosmetic product package labeling is not violative with respect to ''misbranding'' (i.e., that the product performance claims are not false or misleading) [8]. More about U.S. cosmetic regulations will be said in Chapter 62.

The regulatory requirements for drugs (which are beyond the scope of this chapter) are more extensive than the requirements applicable to cosmetics. For example, the Act requires that drug manufacturers register every year with the FDA and update their lists of all manufactured drugs twice annually (c.f., 21 CFR 207). Additionally, FDA drug labeling requirements and regulatory oversight of prescription drug advertising (FTC has regulatory oversight for OTC drug advertising [17,18]) are more stringent than for cosmetics. Finally, drugs must be manufactured in accordance with Current Good Manufacturing Practice (CGMP) regulations (c.f., 21 CFR 210-211) [8].

THE COSMETIC/DRUG DISTINCTION: THE ROLE OF THE INTENDED USE DOCTRINE IN FDA ASSIGNMENT OF REGULATORY CATEGORY AND TRADE CORRESPONDENCE

The regulatory category occupied by a product clearly has a great impact on the marketing of that product. Because the drug approval process required by the Act (see previous section) is rigorous, expensive, and time consuming, marketers of personal-care products would rather market their products as cosmetics than as drugs. Some topical personal-care products are formulated in a nearly identical manner, and it is the manufacturer of the topical product that frequently determines what the intended use of the product is, and whether it should be marketed as a cosmetic or as a drug by means of statements and other representations or performance claims made on product package labeling, collateral promotional literature, and advertising. In other circumstances, whether this is done intentionally for marketing reasons or is otherwise unintentional, the manufacturer's intended use may not be easy to discern, and it is not nearly as straightforward for FDA to determine the most appropriate regulatory category for the product. How, then, is FDA to determine whether such a product is a drug or a cosmetic?

It is the interpretation of what "intended use" means that has helped FDA to clarify how cosmetic products are distinguished from drugs. Needless to say it has also caused uncertainty, as topical cosmetic formulations have become more sophisticated and capable of delivering enhanced performance benefits to the consumer, or, viewed from the other end of the drug–cosmetic continuum, as dermatological drug products have been formulated with ever increasing degrees of cosmetic elegance. FDA's interpretation of cosmetic versus drug status for the various products that it regulates in the years since the enactment of the 1938 Act has been guided by several sources of information.

Labeling

Intended use is determined principally, but not solely, by the claims that are made on product labeling (i.e., all labels and other written, printed, or graphic matter either on or accompanying the product). "Puffery" claims [19] may draw upon the stylized artful imagery and "hope in a bottle" that have traditionally sold cosmetics from the dawn of the cosmetic marketing era, when the formulation of cosmetics was more art than science, to the present day. "Subjective" and "objective" claims (20) are those that can and should be substantiated, usually by focus-group panel interviews; home-placement tests, follow-up questionnaires, and phone interviews; or controlled-use medically supervised clinical studies, with or without the use of accompanying bioengineering instrument assessments of various skin, hair, eye, or nail condition paramters. The Agency has even, on occasion, determined "intended use" of a product based, in part, on statements made on behalf of the product by manufacturer sales associates at the point of sale, or on training and guidance provided to salespersons at the cosmetic counter.

Trade Correspondence

Early FDA guidance with respect to intended use commenced soon after passage of the 1938 Act, when the Agency issued a series of informal opinions, known as Trade Correspondence (TC), that applied the statute to specific questions and situations; some of the TCs are still relied on as support for FDA regulatory policy [21]. Such TCs were the basis for decisions setting Agency policy with respect to a cosmetic's intended use. TC-10, for example, notified marketers of cosmetic claims considered by the Agency to be "misbrandings" in that they are "false and misleading" [22], while TC-229 stated that the word "healthful" contained in the labeling of a tooth powder would trigger the drug provisions of the Act [23]. TC-26 held that a product's mechanism of action could be the basis of a cosmetic vs. drug intended-use determination, in that a deodorant powder inhibiting the normal physiological process of perspiration would be a drug (i.e., an antiperspirant-deodorant), but the same product merely serving as a "reodorant-deodorant" by absorbing the perspiration or masking the malodor would probably be a cosmetic [24]. TC-42 provided further clarification of the "affect the body" clause of Section 201 (g) of the Act, in stating that a topical product containing emollient ingredients whose claims to efficacy were through such temporary improvements in skin condition parameters as "softening" (or, by extrapolation, smoothing or moisturizing) would not necessarily be considered drugs [25]. TC-61, recently revoked in light of new science [16], served for many years as the "line in the sand" for distinguishing between products that referred to sunburn protection as drugs and those represented exclusively for the production of an even tan as cosmetics [26]. Other TCs have established that ordinary facial tissue for wiping purposes is not a cosmetic [27], that other appliances used as adjuncts to, or in combination with, bonafide cosmetic products, such as manicuring instruments [28], razors and razor blades [28], shaving brushes [29], toothbrushes [29], and toilet brushes [29] are not considered devices, and that cuticle removers [30] are cosmetics rather than drugs.

FDA Case Law

The most direct guidance has been provided by Agency enforcement actions involving cosmetics that were determined to be drugs. For example, case law from the 1960s established that promotional claims for the bovine serum albumin antiwrinkle products, Sudden Change (Hazel Bishop) and Line Away (Coty), taken in the overall context of product labeling, caused these products to be classified as drugs [31,32]. The court held that advertising claims for these products, which included claims such as "[n]ot a face lift, not a treatment," "[c]ontains . . . no hormones," "[y]ou'll feel a tingling sensation", "[n]ourishes the skin," '[t]ightens and goes to work on wrinkles''; "made in a pharmaceutical laboratory," "packaged under biologically aseptic conditions," "a face lift without surgery," and "it lifts puffs under the eyes," among others, established the respective vendor's intent that the article had physiological and therapeutic effects. It is important to note in these cases that, aside from the claims, there was no evidence that they exerted any real effects on the structure or function of the body. In a third court case in the early 1970s, claims that the bovine serum albumin–containing products, Magic Secret (Helene Curtis), is "pure protein" and "causes an astringent sensation" alone were considered appropriate for a cosmetic [33].

1980s Regulatory Letters

The next actions taken by FDA that served to define labeling claims that may cause a product to be classified as a drug occurred in the late 1980s. In the spring of 1987, FDA sent 23 Regulatory Letters [34] to companies that were again marketing antiwrinkle and antiaging topical skincare products with aggressive marketing claims, which were deemed by the Agency to be "daring" [35]. These products made claims such as "revitalizes by accelerating the rate of cellular renewal," "revitalizes skin cells and promotes the skin's natural repair process," "helps stimulate the natural production of structural proteins," "increases the proper uptake of oxygen and blood supply to the cells," "reverses facial aging," "restructures the deepest epidermal layers," "increases collagen production," and "provides vital nourishing supplements," among others. All of these claims, taken in the context of individual product labeling, were sufficient in the view of the Agency to establish intended use as a drug; indeed, it would be very difficult to use these terms and *not* trigger the structure or function definition of a drug. Again, in all of the products covered in this action, there was little expectation that they actually exerted an effect on the body outside of that which normally occurs from topical application of any conventional moisturizer. The Regulatory Letters issued by the Agency served as useful precedents of the legal rationale regarding product classification, and also provided very clear guidance to the Industry, as had been requested in a Citizen Petition [36] concerning what label claims could get a product into regulatory difficulty.

OTC Drug Monographs: Cosmetics That Contain Active Ingredients

FDA has clearly stated that determination of intended use goes beyond direct label statements. The history of use of the ingredient, its functionality in the product, and the consumer's perception all play a role in product classification. This is the case with products that contain drug active ingredients in their formulations but do not make explicitly stated claims about the drug effects of the active ingredient. Although there is no case law that addresses product classification based on presence of active ingredients alone, this issue has been addressed over the years in regulations for OTC drug products and other actions by the Agency.

FDA acknowledged in the Tentative Final Monograph for First Aid Antiseptic Drug Products, published August 16, 1991 (56 FR 33644), that antimicrobial soap products making cosmetic claims only are not subject to regulation as OTC drugs and should not be considered in a review of drug effectiveness. The Agency further established the policy that the presence of an antimicrobial ingredient does not, in and of itself, make a product a drug, provided that no drug claim (i.e., "kills germs," "antibacterial") is made. However, the level of antimicrobial ingredient in a cosmetic product, when such ingredient is intended only as part of a cosmetic preservative system, may not exceed the concentration provided for in the OTC Monograph. The Agency also noted in this rulemaking that the "intended use" of a product may be inferred from labeling, promotional material, advertising, and any other relevant factor, arguing that, based on case law, a manufacturers' subjective claims of intent may be pierced to find its actual intent on the basis of objective evidence.

Analogously, the Agency acknowledged in the Final Monograph for Topical Acne Drug Products, published in August, 1991 (56 FR 41008), that the final rule covers only the drug uses of the active ingredients and does not apply to the use of the same ingredients for non–drug effects in products intended solely as cosmetics.

FDA noted in the May 12, 1993 Tentative Final Monograph for OTC Sunscreen Drug Products (58 FR 28194) that a product may contain a sunscreen ingredient and be a cosmetic if it is not intended to protect against the sun and no claims are made about the ingredient. In these cases, the term sunscreen is not used, no SPF value is given, and the sunscreen ingredient is only mentioned in the product's labeling by its cosmetic name in the ingredient list in accordance with Agency regulations at 21 CFR 701.3. However, the presence of a sunscreen active ingredient in a product *intended* to protect from sun exposure makes the product a drug. Again, FDA noted that it is not bound by the manufacturer's subjective claims, but can find actual therapeutic intent on the basis of objective evidence. Such intent may be derived from labeling, promotional material, advertising, and any other relevant source, where "relevant source" can even include the consumer's intent in using the product. The Agency reaffirmed these views in the May 21, 1999 Final Monograph for OTC Sunscreen Drug Products (64 FR 27666) and codified them at 21 CFR 700.35, adding only the caveat that when a cosmetic product contains a sunscreen ingredient not intended to be used for therapeutic or physiological efficacy and uses the term "sunscreen" or similar sun protection terminology anywhere in its labeling, the term must be qualified by describing the cosmetic benefit provided by the sunscreen ingredient, and this statement must appear prominently and conspicuously at least once in the labeling, contiguous with the term "sunscreen" or other similar sun-protection terminology used in the labeling.

The Agency provided clear guidance in the February 3, 1994 Withdrawal of Advance Notice of Proposed Rulemaking for OTC Vaginal Drug Products (59 FR 5226) that the mere presence of a pharmacologically active ingredient in therapeutically active concentrations could make a product a drug, even in the absence of explicit drug claims, if the intended use would be implied because of the known or recognized drug effects of the ingredient (i.e., fluoride in a dentrifice or zinc pyrithione in a shampoo). Thus, although explicitly stated intended use is the primary factor in determining cosmetic vs. drug product category, the type and amount of ingredient(s) present in a product must be considered in determining its regulatory status, even if that product does not make explicit drug claims.

Finally, FDA noted in a Notice of Proposed Rulemaking concerning Cosmetic Products Containing Certain Hormone Ingredients that was published on September 9, 1993 (58 FR 47611), along with a final rule on Topically Applied Hormone-Containing Drug Products for Over-the-Counter Use (58 FR 47608), that "certain hormone-containing products not bearing drug claims could be cosmetics depending on the levels of hormones used and whether that level of use affects the structure or any function of the body . . .". It was noted that only these hormone ingredients present at a level below that which exerts an effect on the structure or function of the body would be acceptable for use in products marketed as cosmetics. However, if the hormone ingredient was present at physiologically active levels, then the product would be classified as a drug for regulatory purposes.

The Alpha Hydroxy Acid Situation

The alpha hydroxy acids (AHAs) have been hailed as the first examples of the new cosmeceuticals since their first appearance in the marketplace several years ago [37]. Through their promotional claims, AHAs promise skincare benefits that far exceed the humectant and moisturization attributes that were once associated with AHA salts such as sodium lactate as components of the skin's so-called natural moisturizing factor (NMF) in the cosmetics of the 1970s [38]. The scientific, clinical, and patent literature show that AHAs, as used today, probably function under at least certain conditions of formulation not only as traditional cosmetic moisturizers but as epidermal exfoliants and modulators of epidermal and dermal structure and function [39–42]. They are promoted in mass-marketed and salon-treatment products alike for treatment of a number of cosmetic (i.e., severe dry skin, tone/texture) and more significant dermatological (i.e., acneiform, photoaging, age spots) conditions [43, 44]. Manufacturers of these products have sought to market them directly to consumers as cosmetics or through phsician offices, salons, and professional estheticians [37, 45–47]. Although most marketers have artfully avoided making direct and impactful efficacy claims that might invite triggering the drug provisions of the Act [48], FDA is also cognizant that the addition of chemical exfoliants to cosmetics on such a wide scale is unprecedented [43], and 7 years of marketing history with such products may prove an inadequate and unreliable predictor of future adverse impacts on public health. Therefore, despite prior evaluations of AHA safety by the Cosmetic Ingredient Review (CIR) [49] and some more recent evaluations conducted by FDA [50] as well, the Agency has reserved its judgement concerning the appropriate regulatory category designation(s) for AHA skincare products and remains vigilant concerning the adequacy of the safety substantiation for AHAs, particularly with respect to potential chronic effects of AHAs on the sun sensitivity and photocarcinogenic responses of the skin [51].

SUMMARY: COSMECEUTICALS, COSMETIC THERAPEUTICS, AND OTHER PROPOSED DEFINITIONS

Topical products marketed in the United States are regulated under the Act, variously, as cosmetics, drugs, or OTC drug-cosmetics. There is no intermediate category that corresponds, for example, to the "quasi-drugs," defined under the Japanese Pharmaceutical Affairs Law [52]. Neither are there any provisions under the U.S. statute that would accomodate classes of topical skincare products with levels of efficacy that exceed those of traditional cosmetics but whose safety have not been as rigorously substantiated as traditional drugs. Reed [53] and Kligman [54] proposed that such high performance cosmetics be classified as "cosmeceuticals," despite the lack of legal standing of such a product category. Piacquadio [55] favors the term "cosmetic therapeutics" when referring to drugs and devices having known risk/benefit profiles and established efficacy for a cosmetic indication, pending or with FDA approval. Privat [56] suggested the categories "decorative and/or protective cosmetics" for those products that embellish by modifying (appearance, color, feel) or protecting the integument from external insults (i.e., UVR or bacteria), while reserving the term "remedial and/or active cosmetics" for those products that modify or correct the physiological state of the integument [e.g., stratum corneum (SC), epidermis, melanocytes, intercellular lipid layer, sudoral glands, hypodermis]. Morganti [57] coined the term "cosmetognosy" to denote the science that deals with the biological effects of cosmetics. Although these proposals each have varying degrees of merit, they, too have no regulatory standing in the United States under provisions of the 1938 FD&C Act.

ACKNOWLEDGMENT

We wish to acknowledge the assistance given by Ms. Beth Meyers, Technical Editor, Division of Programs and Policy Enforcement, Office of Cosmetics and Colors, FDA-CFSAN, in proofreading this manuscript and formatting Table 1.

DISCLAIMER

The views expressed herein are those of the authors and do not necessarily represent those of the FDA.

REFERENCES

1. Bucalo AJ. 1999 State of the Industry. Global Cosmet Ind, 1999; June: 32.
2. Wenninger JA, R. Canterbery R, McEwen GA Jr, eds. *CTFA International Cosmetic Ingredient Dictionary*. 8th ed., 1999.
3. FDA Compliance Program Guidance Manual 7329.001, pt. 1 at 1. August 1993.
4. McDonaugh EG. *Truth About Cosmetics*. Drug Markets, Inc. 1937: vii.
5. Butler H. Historical Background. In: Butler H, ed. *Poucher's Perfumes, Cosmetics and Soaps*, 9th ed. London: Chapman & Hall, 1993: 639–692.
6. Romm S. *The Changing Face of Beauty*. St. Louis: Mosby-Yearbook, Inc., 1992.

7. Yingling GL, Onel S. Cosmetic regulation revisited. In: Brady RP, Cooper RM, Silverman RS, eds. *Fundamentals of Law and Regulation*. Vol. 1. Washington, DC: FDLI, 1997: 321.
8. *FDA's Cosmetics Handbook*. Washington, D.C.: U.S. Government Printing Office, 1993: 1–3.
9. Jellinek JS. *Formulation and Function of Cosmetics*. New York: Wiley-Interscience, 1970.
10. deNavarre MG. *The Chemistry and Manufacture of Cosmetics*. 2nd ed. Vols. I–IV. Princeton: D. Van Nostrand Company, Inc., 1969.
11. Balsam MS, Sagarin E. *Cosmetics: Science and Technology*. Vols 1–3. New York: John Wiley and Sons, Inc., 1972.
12. Wilkinson JB, Moore RJ. *Harry's Cosmeticology. 7th ed*. New York: Chemical Publishing Co., Inc., 1982.
13. Jackson EM. Consumer products: cosmetics and topical over-the-counter drug products. In: Chengelis CP, Holson JF, Gad SC, eds. *Regulatory Toxicology*. New York: Raven Press, 1995: 105–121.
14. Yingling GL, Swit MA. Cosmetic regulations. In: Cooper RM. *Food and Drug Law*. Washington, D.C.: FDLI, 1991: 362.
15. The 'Intended Use' of a product is not determined only on the basis of promotional claims. In: *Nicotine in Cigarettes and Smokeless Tobacco is a Drug and These Products Are Nicotine Delivery Devices Under the Federal Food, Drug, and Cosmetic Act: Jurisdictional Determination*. U.S. Food & Drug Administration, Department of Health and Human Services, August 1996, Annex, Section II.E.
16. Final Rule for Over-the-Counter (OTC) Sunscreen Products for Human Use. 64 FR 27666 @ 27668. May 21, 1999.
17. Hobbs CO. The FDA and the Federal Trade Commission. In: Cooper RM. *Food and Drug Law*. Washington, D.C.: FDLI, 1991: 429–430, 452–456.
18. Memorandum of Understanding Between FTC and FDA. 36 FR 18539. 1971.
19. (a) McNamara SH. FDA Regulation of Cosmeceuticals. Cosmet Toilet 1997; *112*(3): 41–45. (b) FTC Deception Policy Statement. Letter to the Honorable John D. Dingell, Chairman, Committee on Energy and Commerce, U.S. House of Representatives, @ n42. October 14, 1983. (c) Feldman JP. Puffery in Advertising. Arent Fox Advertising Law (*http://www.arentfox.com*), June 1995. (d) Hobbs CO. Advertising for foods, veterinary products, and cosmetics. In: Brady RP, Cooper RM, Silverman RS, eds. Fundamentals of Law and Regulation. Vol. 7. Washington, D.C., 1997: 350. (e) Legal aspects of promotion strategy: advertising. In: Stern LW, Eovaldi TL. *Legal Aspects of Marketing Strategy: Antitrust and Consumer Protection Issues*. Englewood Cliffs: Prentice-Hall, Inc., 1984: 375–377.
20. (a) McNamara SH. Performance claims for skin care cosmetics. *Drug Cosmet Ind* 1985; October: 34. (b) Weinstein S, Weinstein C, Drozdenko R. A current and comprehensive skin-evaluation program. *Cosmet Technol*, 1982; April: 36. (c) Grove GL. Noninvasive methods for assessing moisturizers. In: Waggoner WC, ed. *Clinical Safety and Efficacy Testing of Cosmetics*. New York: Marcel Dekker, 1990: 121–148. (d) Smithies RH. Substantiating preformance claims. *Cosmet Toilet* 1984; *99*(3): 79–81, 84.
21. Kleinfeld VA, Dunn CW. Trade correspondence. In: *Federal Food, Drug, and Cosmetic Act. Judicial and Administrative Record (1938–1949)*. New York: Commerce Clearing House, Inc., 1949: 561.
22. TC-10, (in Ref. 21) August 2, 1939: 566.
23. TC-229, (in Ref. 21) April 11, 1940: 659.
24. TC-26, (in Ref. 21) February 9, 1940: 581.
25. TC-42, (in Ref. 21) February 12, 1940: 586.
26. TC-61, (in Ref. 21) February 15, 1940: 593.
27. TC-39, (in Ref. 21) February 9, 1940: 585.
28. TC-112, (in Ref. 21) February 29, 1940: 613.
29. TC-109, (in Ref. 21) February 29, 1940: 612.

30. TC-245, (in Ref. 21) April 25, 1940: 665.
31. *United States v. An Article . . . Line Away*, 284 F. Supp. 107 (D. Del. 1968); affirmed, 415 F. 2d 369 (3d Cir. 1969).
32. *United States v. An Article . . . Sudden Change*, 288 F. Supp. 29 (E.D.N.Y. 1968); reviewed 409 F.2d 734 (2d Cir. 1969).
33. *United States v. An Article . . . Magic Secret*, 331 F. Supp. 912 (D. MD 1971).
34. FDA Regulatory Letters No. 87-HFN 312-08 to 87-HFN 312-29 (April 17, 1987 to June 23, 1987).
35. McNamara SH. Performance claims for skin care cosmetics or how far may you go in claiming to provide eternal youthfulness. Food Drug Law J 1986; *41*:151–159.
36. Citizen petition of McCutcheon, Doyle, Brown & Emerson. Bio Advance, FDA Docket No. 87P-0006, (January 6, 1987).
37. (a) Godfrey-June J. The AHA phenomenon. Longevity 1993; Sept.: 36–39. (b) Jackson EM. AHA-type products proliferate in 1993. Cosmet Dermatol 1993; *6*(12):22, 24–26. (c) Kintish L. AHAs: today's fountain of youth? Soap/Cosmetics/Chemical Specialties 1994; Feb: 26–31.
38. (a) Harding CR, Bartolone J, Rawlings AV. Effects of Natural Moisturizing Factor and Lactic Acid Isomers on Skin Function. In: Loden M, Maibach HI, eds. *Dry Skin and Moisturizers: Chemistry and Function*. Boca Raton: CRC Press, 2000:229–241. (b) Middleton JD, Sodium Lactate as a Moisturizer. *Cosmet Toilet* 1978; *93*:85–86.
39. (a) Leyden JJ, Lavker RM, Grove G, Kaidbey K. Alpha hydroxy acids are more than moisturizers. J Geriatr Dermatol 1995 *3* (suppl. A): 33A–37A. (b) Van Scott EJ, Yu RJ. Actions of alpha hydroxy acids on skin compartments. J Geriatr Dermatol 1995; 3(suppl A): 19A–25A.
40. Smith WP. Hydroxy acids and skin aging. Soap/Cosmetics/Chemical Specialties 1993; *93*(9): 54, 56, 57–58, 76.
41. Smith WP. Hydroxy acids and skin aging. Cosmet Toilet 1994; *109*: 41–48.
42. Smith WP. Epidermal and dermal effects of topical lactic acid. 1996; J Am Acad Dermatol 35: 388–391.
43. Kurtzweil P. Alpha hydroxy acids for skin care. FDA Consumer 1998; March-April: 30–35.
44. Anonymous. Alpha hydroxy acids in cosmetics. FDA Backgrounder, BG 97-4, February 19, 1997.
45. Brody HJ. *Chemical Peeling and Resurfacing* (2nd ed.), St. Louis: Mosby-Year Book, Inc., 1997:90–100.
46. Draelos ZD. New Developments in Cosmetics and Skin Care Products. In: *Advances in Dermatology*. Vol. 12. St. Louis: Mosby-Year Book, Inc., 1997; 3–17.
47. (a) AHA '95 Preview: New Developments in Alpha Hydroxy Acids. Symposium and Live Patient Workshop, Jointly Sponsored by Cosmetic Peel Workshop and Medical Education Resources, Inc., Orlando, FL, December 3–4, 1994. (b) AHA '96 Preview: New Advances in AHAs and Skin Rejuvenation Techniques. Symposium and Live Patient Workshop, Jointly Sponsored by Medical Education Resources, Inc. and Herald Education & Research Foundation, San Diego, CA, December 2–3, 1995.
48. Yingling GL and Onel S. Cosmetic Regulation Revisited. In: RP Brady, RM Cooper, RS Silverman, eds, *Fundamentals of Law and Regulation*, Vol. 1, FDLI (Washington, DC), 1997: 341–342.
49. (a) Cosmetic Ingredient Review. Final Report: Safety Assessment of Glycolic Acid; Ammonium, Calcium, Potassium and Sodium Glycolate; Methyl, Ethyl, Propyl, and Butyl Glycolate; Lactic Acid; Ammonium, Calcium, Potassium, Sodium, and TEA-Lactate; Methyl, Ethyl, Propyl, and Butyl Lactate; and Lauryl, Myristyl, and Cetyl Lactate. Washington, D.C.: Cosmetic Ingredient Review, 1997. (b) Jackson, EM. CIR Expert Panel Releases AHA Report. Cosmet Dermatol 1997; *10*(7):37–39
50. Effects of Alpha Hydroxy Acids on Skin. Report Submitted by KRA Corporation (Silver Spring, MD) to the Office of Cosmetics and Colors, CFSAN, FDA, DHHS under Contract No. 223-94-2276. February 22, 1996.

51. (a) Kaidbey K. An Investigation of the Effects of Topical Treatment with an Alpha-Hydroxy Acid (AHA) on the Sensitivity of Human Skin to UV-Induced Damage (FDA Sponsored Study # 1). Philadelphia: Ivy Laboratories (KGL, Inc.), 1999. (b) Kaidbey K. An Investigation of the Effects of Topical Treatment with Alpha-Hydroxy Acid (AHA) on UVB-Induced Pyrimidine Dimers in Human Skin (FDA Sponsored Study #2). Philadelphia: Ivy Laboratories (KGL, Inc.), 1999.

52. Santucci LG, Rempe JM. Legislation and Safety Regulations for Cosmetics in the United States, Europe, and Japan'', Ref. 3, *op. cit.*, Chapter 20; 556–571.

53. Reed RE. The definition of 'cosmeceutical.' J Soc Cosmet Chemists 1962; *13*:103–106.

54. (a) Skin: the hot topics. Vogue 1988; October:417. (b) HAPPI, 1996; May:61. (c) Kligman AM. Why Cosmeceuticals? Cosmet Toilet 1993; *108*(8):37–38. (d) Waleski M. Reed coined 'cosmecutical.' Letter to the Editor. HAPPI 1996; August: 12.

55. Piacquadio D. Cosmetic therapeutic *vs.* cosmeceutical: which is it and why? AHA '95 Preview: New Developments in Alpha Hydroxy Acids. Symposium and Live Patient Workshop, Jointly Sponsored by Cosmetic Peel Workshop and Medical Education Resources, Inc., Orlando, FL, Dec. 3–4, 1994.

56. Privat Y. A new definition of cosmetology. In: Baran R, Maibach HI, eds. *Cosmetic Dermatology*. London: Martin Dunitz, Ltd., 1994: xiv–xv.

57. Morganti P-F. The cosmetic patch. A new frontier in cosmetic dermatology. Soap/Cosmetics/ Chemical Specialties 1996; *96*(2):48–50.

3

The Microscopic Structure of the Epidermis and Its Derivatives

Joel J. Elias
University of California at San Francisco School of Medicine,
San Francisco, California

A general review of the microscopic structure of the epidermis and those epidermal derivatives that are distributed widely over the skin and, therefore, may be of interest in considerations of mechanisms of percutaneous absorption, will be presented here. Both light and electron microscopic information will be discussed in order to give an integrated brief summary of the basic morphological picture.

The epithelial component of the skin, the epidermis, is classified histologically as a stratified squamous keratinizing epithelium. It is thickest on the palms and soles (Fig. 1) and thinner elsewhere on the body (Fig. 2). It lies on the connective tissue component of the skin, the dermis, in which are located the blood vessels and lymphatic vessels. Capillary loops in the dermis come to lie in close apposition to the underside of the epidermis. The epidermis, in common with other epithelia, is avascular. The living cells of the epidermis receive their nutrients by diffusion of substances from the underlying dermal capillaries through the basement membrane and then into the epithelium. Metabolic products of the cells enter the circulation by diffusion in the opposite direction.

As in the case of other epithelia, the epidermis lies on a basement membrane (basal lamina). This extracellular membrane, interposed between the basal cells of the epidermis and the connective tissue of the dermis, serves the important function of attaching the two tissues to each other. The point of contact of the epidermis with this structure is the basal cell membrane of the basal cells. Along this surface the basal cells show many hemidesmosomes, which increase the adherence of the basal cells (and therefore of the entire epidermis) to the basement membrane (and therefore to the dermis). In some locations, such as the renal glomerulus, the basal lamina has been shown to also play a role as a diffusion barrier to certain molecules.

The plane of contact between the epidermis and dermis is not straight but is an undulating surface, more so in some locations than others. Upward projections of connective tissue, the dermal papillae, alternate with complementary downgrowths of the epider-

This chapter is reproduced with permission from Bronaugh RL, Maibach HI, eds. Percutaneous Absorption: Mechanisms—Methodology—Drug Delivery. 2nd ed. New York: Marcel Dekker, Inc., 1989.

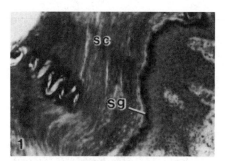

FIGURE 1   Thick epidermis from sole. The spiral channel through the extremely thick stratum corneum (sc) carries the secretion of a sweat gland to the surface. The stratum granulosum (sg) stands out clearly because its cells are filled with keratohyalin granules that stain intensely with hematoxylin. Hematoxylin and eosin. ×100.

mis. This serves to increase the surface area of contact between the two and presumably, therefore, the attachment.

Within the epidermis are found four different cell types with different functions and embryologic origins: keratinocytes, melanocytes, Langerhans cells, and Merkel cells. These will be considered in turn.

The keratinocytes are derived from the embryonic surface ectoderm and differentiate into the stratified epithelium. Dead cells are constantly sloughed from the upper surface of the epidermis and are replaced by new cells being generated from the deep layers. It is generally considered that the basal layer is the major source of cell renewal in the epidermis. Lavker and Sun (1982) distinguish two types of basal cells, a stem cell type and a type that helps anchor the epidermis to the dermis, and an actively dividing suprabasal cell population. The basal cells have desmosomes connecting them to surrounding cells and, as mentioned earlier, hemidesmosomes along the basal lamina surface. They have tonofilaments coursing through the cytoplasm and coming into close apposition to the desmosomes. These protein filaments are of the intermediate filament class and are made up principally of keratin. Basal cells have the usual cell organelles and free ribosomes, the site of synthesis of intracytoplasmic proteins.

As a result of the proliferation of cells from the deeper layers the cells move upward through the epidermis toward the surface. As they do, they undergo differentiative changes

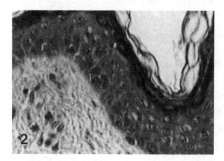

FIGURE 2   Thin epidermis. The strata spinosum, granulosum, and corneum are considerably thinner than in Figure 1. Hematoxylin and eosin. ×200.

which allowed microscopists to define various layers. The cells from the basal layer enter the stratum spinosum, a layer whose thickness varies according to the total thickness of the epidermis. The layer derives its name from the fact that, with light microscopic methods, the surface of the cell is studded with many spiny projections. These meet similar projections from adjacent cells and the structure was called an intercellular bridge by early light microscopists (Fig. 3). Electron microscopy showed that the so-called "intercellular bridges" were really desmosomes, and the light microscopic appearance is an indication of how tightly the cells are held to each other at these points. The number of tonofilaments increases in the spinous cells (prickle cells) and they aggregate into coarse bundles—the tonofibrils—which were recognizable to light microscopists using special stains.

Electron microscopy reveals the formation within the spinous cells of a specific secretory granule. These small, membrane-bound granules form from the Golgi apparatus and are the membrane-coating granules (MCG; lamellar bodies; Odland bodies). They contain lipids of varying types which have become increasingly characterized chemically (Grayson and Elias, 1982; Wertz and Downing, 1982).

As the cells of the stratum spinosum migrate into the next layer there appear in their cytoplasm large numbers of granules that stain intensely with hematoxylin. These are the keratohyalin granules and their presence characterizes the stratum granulosum. Electron microscopy shows that the granules are not membrane bound but are free in the cytoplasm. Histidine-rich proteins (Murozuka et al., 1979; Lynley and Dale, 1983) have been identified in the granules. The tonofilaments come to lie in close relationship to the keratohyalin granules. The membrane-coating granules are mainly in the upper part of the granular cell.

When observed by either light or electron microscopy there is an abrupt transformation of the granular cell to the cornified cell with a loss of cell organelles. In thick epidermis, the first cornified cells stain more intensely with eosin and this layer has been called the stratum lucidum. The interior of the cornified cell consists of the keratin filaments, which appear pale in the usual electron microscopic preparations, and interposed between them a dark osmiophilic material. The interfilamentous matrix material has been shown to have derivations from the keratohyalin granule and is thought to serve the function of aggregation of the keratin filaments in the cornified cell (Murozuka et al., 1979; Lynley and Dale, 1983).

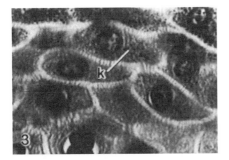

FIGURE 3 High power view of upper part of stratum spinosum and lower part of stratum granulosum. Note the many "intercellular bridges" (desmosomes) running between the cells, giving them a spiny appearance. When the cells move up into the stratum granulosum, keratohyalin granules (k) appear in their cytoplasm. Hematoxylin and eosin. ×1000.

In the uppermost cells of the granular layer the membrane-coating granules move toward the cell surface, their membrane fuses with the cell membrane and their lipid contents are discharged into the intercellular space. Thus, the intercellular space in the cornified layer is filled with lipid material which is generally thought to be the principal water permeability barrier of the epidermis (Grayson and Elias, 1982; Wertz and Downing, 1982). The stratum corneum has been compared to a brick wall, with the bricks representing the cornified cells, surrounded completely by mortar, representing the MCG material (Elias, 1984).

The cornified cell is further strengthened by the addition of protein to the inner surface of the cell membrane. Two proteins that have been identified in this process are involucrin (Banks-Schlegel and Green, 1981; Simon and Green, 1984) and keratolinin (Zettergren et al., 1984). A transglutaminase cross-linking of the soluble proteins results in their fusion to the inner cell membrane to form the tough outer cell envelope of the cornified cell. Desmosomes between the cells persist in the cornified layer.

It can be seen that formation of an outer structure (stratum corneum) which can resist abrasion from the outside world and serve as a water barrier for a land-dwelling animal has proven incompatible with the properties of living cells. The living epidermal cells, therefore, die by an extremely specialized differentiative process that results in their non-living remains having the properties that made life on land a successful venture for vertebrates.

Distributed among the keratinocytes of the basal layer are cells of a different embryologic origin and function, the melanocytes. In the embryo, cells of the neural crest migrate from their site of origin to the various parts of the skin and take up a position in the basal layer of the epidermis. They differentiate into melanocytes and extend long cytoplasmic processes between the keratinocytes in the deep layers of the epidermis. Because they contain the enzyme tyrosinase they are able to convert tyrosine to dihydroxyphenylalanine (dopa) and the latter to dopaquinone with the subsequent formation of the pigmented polymer melanin. The tyrosinase is synthesized in the rough endoplasmic reticulum and transferred to the Golgi body. From the latter organelle, vesicles with an internal periodic structure are formed which contain the tyrosinase. These are the melanosomes, the melanin-synthesizing apparatus of the cell. Melanin is formed within the melanosome, and as it accumulates the internal structure of the melanosome becomes obscured. Seen with the light microscope the pigmented melanosome appears as the small brown melanin granule. The melanin granules are then transferred from the melanocyte's cytoplasmic extensions to the keratinocytes, and become especially prominent in the basal keratinocyte's cytoplasm. In this position their ability to absorb ultraviolet radiation has a maximal effect in protecting the proliferating basal cell's DNA from the mutagenic effects of this radiation. Within the keratinocyte varying numbers of melanosomes are often contained within a single membrane-bound vesicle. The classic method of demonstrating melanocytes is the dopa test. Sections of skin are placed in a solution of dopa and only the melanocytes turn a dark brown color (Fig. 4).

Within the epidermis is another population of cells which were first demonstrated by Langerhans in 1868. By placing skin in a solution of gold chloride he showed that a number of cells in the epidermis, particularly in the stratum spinosum, turned black. The cytoplasmic extensions of the cell give them a dendritic appearance. For many decades the nature of this cell type was unknown, including whether it was a living, dead, or dying cell. Electron microscopy showed that it was a viable cell in appearance, lacked desmosomes, and possessed a very unusual cytoplasmic structure—the Birbeck granule.

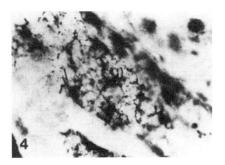

FIGURE 4   A thick section of the epidermis was made with the plane of section running parallel to the surface of the skin and including the deep layers of the epidermis. Dopa reaction shows whole melanocytes on surface view, illustrating their branching, dendritic nature. ×340.

With the development of methods for identifying cell membrane receptors and markers in immune system cells it was shown that Langerhans cells originate in the bone marrow. They are now thought to be derived from circulating blood monocytes, with which they share common marker characteristics. The monocytes migrate into the epidermis and differentiate into Langerhans cells. Considerable evidence shows that these dendritic cells capture cutaneous antigens and present them to lymphocytes in the initiation of an immune response. Their population in the epidermis is apparently constantly replenished by the bloodborne monocytes.

Finally, a fourth cell type, the Merkel cell, can be found in the epidermis. These appear to be epithelial cells and are found in the basal layer. A characteristic feature is the presence of many small, dense granules in their cytoplasm. Sensory nerve endings form expanded terminations in close apposition to the surface of Merkel cells.

Hair follicles begin their formation as a downgrowth of cells from the surface epidermis into the underlying connective tissue. The growth extends into the deep dermis and subcutaneous tissue and forms in the deepest part of the structure a mass of proliferative cells—the hair matrix. The cells of the outermost part of the hair follicle, the external root sheath, are continuous with the surface epidermis. The deepest part of the hair follicle is indented by a connective tissue structure, the hair papilla, which brings blood vessels close to the actively dividing hair matrix cells (Fig. 5). As the cells in the matrix divide the new cells are pushed upward toward the surface. Those moving up the center of the hair follicle will differentiate into the hair itself. The structure of the hair, from the center to the outer surface, consists of the medulla (when present), the cortex and the cuticle of the hair. The cortex forms the major part of the hair. These cells accumulate keratin to a very high degree. They do not die abruptly as in the case of the surface epidermis. Instead, the nucleus of the cell gradually becomes denser and more pyknotic and eventually disappears. Keratohyalin granules are not seen with the light microscope. Cells moving up from the matrix in the region between the hair and the external root sheath form the internal root sheath. Here, the cells adjacent to the hair form the cuticle of the internal root sheath. Next is Huxley's layer and, adjacent to the external root sheath, Henle's layer. These cells accumulate conspicuous trichohyalin granules in their cytoplasm in the deeper part of the internal root sheath. The cells of the internal root sheath disintegrate higher up in the hair follicle and disappear at about the level of the sebaceous gland. Thereafter, the hair is found in the central space of the hair follicle without a surrounding internal root sheath.

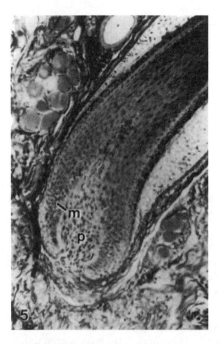

FIGURE 5   The connective tissue hair papilla (p) indents into the base of the hair follicle. The follicle cells in the hair matrix region (m) show many mitotic figures. Iron hematoxylin and aniline blue. ×150.

When viewed with the light microscope the hair follicle is surrounded by an exceedingly thick basement membrane called the glassy membrane. Scattered among the keratinocytes in the hair matrix are melanocytes which transfer pigment to the forming hair cells and give the hair color. Hair growth is cyclic, with each follicle having alternating periods of growth and rest.

About a third of the way down the hair follicle from the surface epidermis, the sebaceous glands connect to the hair follicle. The sebaceous alveoli consist of a rounded, solid mass of epithelial cells surrounded by a basement membrane. The outer cells proliferate and the newly formed cells are pushed into the interior of the sebaceous alveolus. As they move in this direction they accumulate a complex of lipids and lipidlike substances. As the lipids fill the cell it begins to die and the nucleus becomes more and more pyknotic. The cells eventually disintegrate, releasing their oily contents by way of a short duct into the space of the hair follicle (Fig. 6). This is the classic example of holocrine secretion where the entire gland cell becomes the secretion. In some scattered locations (e.g., nipple) sebaceous glands can be found independent of the hair follicle. In other areas their size relative to the hair follicle is very large (Fig. 7). Because the lipids are extracted in the usual histologic preparations the cells typically appear very pale.

The major type of sweat gland in the human, the eccrine sweat gland, is distributed over practically all parts of the body. It produces a watery secretion which is conveyed to the surface of the skin where its evaporation plays an important thermoregulatory role. The eccrine glands arise as tubular downgrowths from the surface epidermis independent of hair follicles. The tubule extends deep into the dermis or the subcutaneous tissue level where it becomes coiled. The eccrine gland, therefore, is a simple coiled tubular gland.

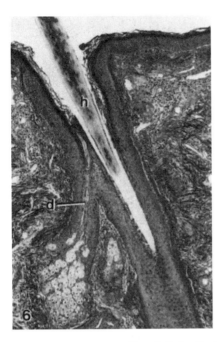

FIGURE 6   Upper part of hair follicle. The hair (h) is shown emerging from the follicle (the lower part of the hair passed out of the plane of section). The sebaceous gland is shown emptying its secretion by way of the duct (d) into the space of the follicle. Iron hematoxylin and aniline blue. ×50.

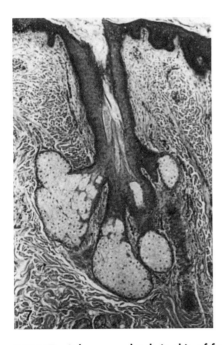

FIGURE 7   Sebaceous glands in skin of forehead. Hematoxylin and eosin. ×50.

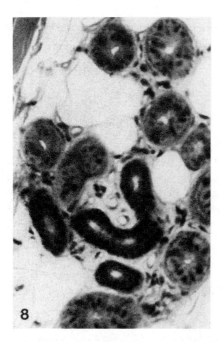

FIGURE 8   Section through a sweat gland. The pale structures are part of the secretory coiled tubule, the dark ones are part of the duct. Hematoxylin and eosin. ×250.

The coiled segment at the blind-ending terminus represents the secretory portion of the gland. This leads to the duct portion of the gland which is also coiled. The duct then ascends toward the surface. When it reaches the underside of the epidermis a spiralling channel through it conveys the secretion to the skin surface (Fig. 1). It is not understood how this channel remains patent in an epidermis whose keratinocytes are constantly proliferating and migrating.

When viewed with the light microscope the two parts of the gland can be easily distinguished from each other (Fig. 8). Compared to the duct, the secretory portion is wider, has a larger lumen, its epithelial lining cells appear pale and many myoepithelial cells are present. The latter are contractile cells that are part of the epithelium, lying within the basement membrane. Their contraction is thought to forcefully expel the secretion toward the skin surface. With the electron microscope, two types of epithelial lining cells are seen in the secretory portion. The so-called dark cells have an extensive contact with the lumen of the tubule and have secretory granules containing glycoprotein substances. The clear cells are distinguished by abundant glycogen in their cytoplasm. Continuous with the tubule lumen are many intercellular canaliculi between the clear cells. It is thought that the clear cells secrete a more or less isotonic solution via these channels into the lumen. The duct portion is lined by two layers of epithelial cells and lacks myoepithelial cells. It is thought that electrolytes are absorbed from the lumen here, making the sweat hypotonic by the time it reaches the surface of the skin.

ACKNOWLEDGMENTS

I would like to express my appreciation to Ms. Linda Prentice and Ms. Simona Ikeda for the photomicrographic work.

REFERENCES

1. S Banks-Schlegel, H Green. Involucrin synthesis and tissue assembly by keratinocytes in natural and cultured human epithelia. J Cell Biol 90:732–737, 1981.
2. PM Elias. Stratum corneum lipids in health and disease. In: Progress in Diseases of the Skin, Vol. 2, R. Fleischmajer, ed. Grune and Stratton, San Diego, 1984, pp. 1–19.
3. S Grayson, PM Elias. Isolation and lipid biochemical characterization of stratum corneum membrane complexes: implications for the cutaneous permeability barrier. J Invest Dermatol 78: 128–135, 1982.
4. RM Lavker, T Sun. Heterogeneity in epidermal basal keratinocytes: morphological and functional correlations. Science 215:1239–1241, 1982.
5. AM Lynley, BA Dale. The characterization of human epidermal filaggrin: a histidine-rich, keratin filament-aggregating protein. Biochim Biophys Acta 744:28–35, 1983.
6. T Murozuka, K Fukuyama, WL Epstein. Immunochemical comparison of histidine-rich protein in keratohyalin granules and cornified cells. Biochim Biophys Acta 579:334–345, 1979.
7. M Simon, H Green. Participation of membrane-associated proteins in the formation of the cross-linked envelope of the keratinocyte. Cell 36:827–834, 1984.
8. PW Wertz, DT Downing. Glycolipids in mammalian epidermis: structure and function in the water barrier. Science 217:1261–1262, 1982.
9. JG Zettergren, LL Peterson, KD Wuepper. Keratolinin: the soluble substrate of epidermal transglutaminase from human and bovine tissue. Proc Natl Acad Sci USA 81:238–242, 1984.

4

The Normal Nail

Josette André
Free University of Brussels and Hôpital Saint-Pierre, Brussels, Belgium

ANATOMY

The nail plate, also abbreviated to "nail," is a hard keratin plate, slightly convex in the longitudinal and transverse axes. It is set in the soft tissues of the dorsal digital extremity, from which it is separated by the periungual grooves (proximal, lateral, and distal) (Fig. 1) [1,2]. It stems from the nail matrix located in the proximal part of the nail apparatus. The nail plate and matrix are partly covered by a skin fold called the proximal nail fold. The lunula, also known as "half moon," is a whitish crescent visible at the proximal part of some nails and more specifically at those of the thumbs and big toes. It corresponds to the distal part of the matrix. From the latter, the nail plate grows towards the distal region, sliding along the nail bed to which it adheres closely and from which it only separates at the distal part, called hyponychium.

Two other structures deserve our attention:

1. The cuticle, which is the transparent horny layer of the proximal nail groove. It adheres to the nail surface and acts as a seal between the nail plate and the proximal nail fold.
2. The onychodermal band, which is "orangey," is located in the distal region of the nail. It can be partly blanched by pressure, thus exsanguinating the region. It provides a zone of rugged attachment of the nail-to-nail bed.

The upper surface of the nail plate is smooth and has discrete longitudinal ridges that become more obvious with age (Fig. 2). The under surface is corrugated with parallel longitudinal grooves that interdigitate with the opposite ones of the nail-bed surface, enhancing the adhesion of the nail plate to the nail bed.

HISTOLOGY

The nail plate is made up of parallel layers of keratinised, flat, and completely differentiated cells with no nucleus. Three zones can be identified at the distal part of the nail: the upper (or dorsal) nail plate which makes up one third of the nail; the lower (or ventral) nail plate which makes up two thirds of the nail; and the subungual keratin. The latter corresponds to the thick, dense, horny layer of the hyponychium (Fig. 3) [3,4].

29

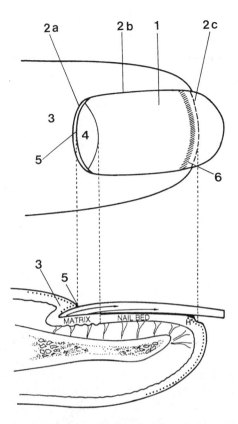

FIGURE 1   The normal nail. (1) nail plate, (2) nail grooves [(2a) proximal nail groove, (2b) lateral nail groove, (2c) distal nail groove], (3) proximal nail fold, (4) lunula, (5) cuticle, (6) onychodermal band, H, hyponychium, small dots, stratum granulosum.

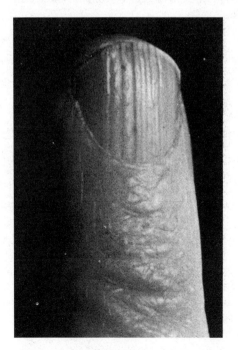

FIGURE 2   Obvious longitudinal ridges on the nail surface, as noticed in older people.

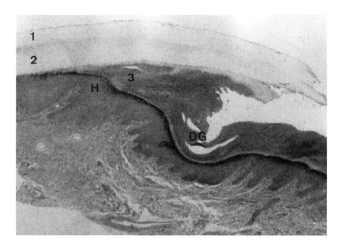

FIGURE 3 Longitudinal section of the distal part of the nail apparatus. (1) upper or dorsal nail plate, (2) lower or ventral nail plate, (3) subungual keratin. H, hyponychium; DG, distal groove.

In electron microscopy (Fig. 4) [5], the nail plate cells appear to be made of a regular weft of keratin filaments within an interfilamentous matrix. In the upper (or dorsal) nail plate, cells are flat, their cellular membranes are discreetly indented, and they are separated from each other by ampullar dilatations. At the surface, those cells are piled up like roof tiles, which gives the nail surface its smooth aspect. In the lower (or ventral) nail plate, cells are thicker, their cellular membranes are anfractuous, and they interpenetrate through extensions, making real anchoring knots that seem to be partly responsible for nail elasticity.

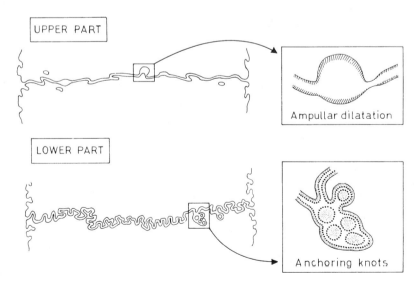

FIGURE 4 Schematic drawing of the cell membranes in the dorsal and ventral part of the nail plate, as observed in electron microscopic examination. (From Ref. 5.)

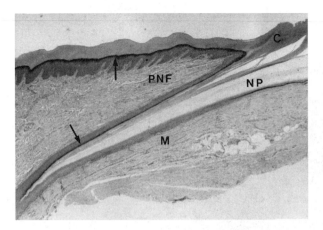

FIGURE 5 Longitudinal section of the proximal part of the nail apparatus. PNF, proximal nail fold; C, cuticle; NP, nail plate; M, matrix. A stratum granulosum (arrows) is present in the dorsal and ventral part of the proximal nail fold epithelium but absent in the matrix epithelium.

A longitudinal section of the nail apparatus enables us to visualize most characteristics of the other ungual structures (Fig. 1). From the proximal to the distal region, the following are identified:

- The proximal nail fold (Fig. 5). Its dorsal part is in continuity with the epidermis of the digit back. Its ventral part is a flat and rather thin epithelium that keratinizes with a stratum granulosum. The cuticle corresponds to the stratum corneum of the most distal part of the proximal nail fold, at the angle of the dorsal and ventral part.
- The nail matrix is a multilayered epithelium characterized by an abrupt keratinization without interposition of keratohyaline granules (Fig. 5). It gives birth to the nail plate: the proximal part of the matrix gives birth to its dorsal part and the distal part of the matrix gives birth to its ventral part. The epithelium of the matrix also contains melanocytes and Langerhans cells. Most melanocytes are dormant [6] and do not produce pigment. However, in dark-skinned individuals, longitudinal pigmented bands can be observed in nails. This racial physiological pigmentation is attributable to the activation of the matrix melanocytes and to the melanin incorporation in the nail plate (longitudinal melanonychia). It usually affects several nails and tends to become more frequent with aging; this can only be observed in 2.5% of 0- to 3-year-old black children but in 96% of blacks older than 50 years of age (Fig. 6) [7].
- The nail bed epithelium, like the one of the matrix, keratinizes abruptly. The stratum granulosum reappears only at the hyponychium, which represents the distal thickened part of the nail bed and is bordered by the distal groove and the digital pulp (Fig. 3). Melanocytes are rare in the nail bed.

The nail apparatus is strongly attached to the periosteum of the distal phalanx by thick collagen bundles. Elastic fibers are rare and eccrine sweat glands are absent.

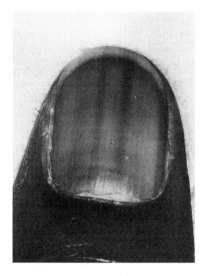

FIGURE 6   Multiple longitudinal melanonychia in an adult black patient.

PHYSICOCHEMISTRY

The nail is highly rich in keratins, specially in hard keratins which are close to those of hair and have a high content of disulfide linkage (cystine) [1,2]. The high sulfur-containing keratins play an important role in the nail toughness and presumably in its good barrier property as well.

Sulfur represents 10% of the nail's dry weight; calcium represents 0.1 to 0.2%. The latter, contrary to conventional wisdom, does not intervene in the nail toughness.

Lipid content (particularly cholesterol) is low in nails: from 0.1 to 1% compared with 10% in the stratum corneum of the skin. Water concentration varies from 7 to 12% (15–25% in the stratum corneum) but the nail is highly permeable to water: when its hydration level increases, it becomes flack and opaque and when its hydration level drops, it becomes dry and brittle.

Studies carried on nail permeability are important for the development of cosmetic and pharmaceutical products specifically devoted to nails [8]. As a permeation barrier, it has been shown that the nail plate reacts like a hydrogel membrane, unlike the epidermis which reacts like a lipophilic membrane.

The normal nail is hard, flexible, and elastic, which gives it good resistance to the microtraumatisms it undergoes daily. Those properties are attributable to the following factors: the regular arrangement and important adhesion of keratinocytes, the anchoring knots, the high-sulfur–containing keratins and the hydration level of the nail.

PHYSIOLOGY

The nail grows continuously. In 1 month, fingernails grow about 3 mm and toenails grow about 1 mm. A complete renewal therefore takes 4 to 6 months for normal fingernails whereas 12 to 18 months are needed for toenails [1,2].

The origin of nail plate production is still a debatable point. At least 80% of the nail plate is produced by the matrix, and the main source of nail plate production is the proximal part of the matrix. This probably explains why distal matrix surgery or nail bed surgery has a low potential for scarring compared with proximal matrix surgery [9]. Some studies suggest that the nailbed produces 20% of the nail plate, whereas others suggest that the nail bed hardly participates in the making of the nail plate [9,10].

The nail plays an important role in everyday life. It protects the distal phalanx from traumatisms it undergoes regularly. It plays a role in the sensitivity of the digital extremity and intervenes more specifically in the picking up of small objects such as needles. The nail allows scratching in case of itching and can be used as a means of attack or defense. Finally, the aesthetic importance of the nail should not be neglected.

AESTHETICS

For centuries the nail has played an important aesthetic role. Having clean nails is essential to looking well groomed and refined, and among women nails also need to be long and painted.

A "good-looking" nail has a smooth and shiny surface. It is transparent and adheres to its bed. Regarding the proximal groove, the cuticle has to be intact and thin. The distal and the lateral grooves have to be clean and the periungual tissues must be without hang-nails and sores. The free border has to be smooth; its shape can be round, pointed, oval, or square. Women often wear long fingernails cut oval, which makes fingers look longer and thinner. Yet, square nails are in fashion. Too-long nails can look unpleasant and can even be a nuisance.

Men wear short fingernails cut square. Both women and men have short toenails cut square. A normal nail structure and appropriate cosmetic care are necessary to obtain such "good-looking" nails.

REFERENCES

1. RPR Dawber, D de Berker, R Baran. Science of the nail apparatus. In: R Baran, RPR Dawber, eds. Diseases of the Nails and Their Management. 2d ed. Oxford: Blackwell Scientific Publications, 1994, pp. 1–34.
2. D de Berker. The normal nail. In: J André, ed. CD-ROM: Illustrated Nail Pathology. Diagnosis and Management. Antwerpen: Lasion Europe, 1995.
3. G Achten, J André, M Laporte. Nails in light and electron microscopy. Semin Dermatol 10: 54–64, 1991.
4. J André, M Laporte. Ungual histology in practice. In: J André, ed. CD-ROM: Illustrated Nail Pathology. Diagnosis and Management. Antwerpen: Lasion Europe, 1995.
5. D Parent, G Achten, F Stouffs-Vanhoof. Ultrastructure of the normal human nail. Am J Dermatopathol 7: 529–535, 1985.
6. Ch Perrin, JF Michiels, A Pisani, JP Ortonne. Anatomic distribution of melanocytes in normal nail unit. An immunohistochemical investigation. Am J Dermatopathol 19:462–467, 1997.
7. JJ Leyden, DA Spott, H Goldschmidt. Diffuse and banded melanin pigmentation in nails. Arch Dermatol 105:548–550, 1972.
8. Y Sun, J-C Liu, JCT Wang, P De Doncker. Nail penetration. Focus on topical delivery of antifungal drugs for onychomycosis treatment. In: RL Bronaugh, HI Maibach, eds. Percutaneous Absorption. Drugs-Cosmetics-Mechanisms-Methodology, 3rd ed. New York: Marcel Dekker, 1999, pp. 759–778.
9. D de Berker, B Mawhinney, L Sviland. Quantification of regional matrix nail production. Br J Dermatol 134:1083–1086, 1996.
10. M Johnson, S Shuster. Continuous formation of nail along the bed. Br J Dermatol 128:277–280, 1993.

5

Hair

Ghassan Shaker and Dominique Van Neste
Skinterface sprl, Tournai, Belgium

INTRODUCTION

Hair is a symbol of good looks and beauty in some areas of the human body. So much time, effort, and money are spent in caring for it, especially in the case of scalp hair. In some other areas, like the beard, daily care by shaving is necessary for the majority of males. In females, abundant scalp hair is very much welcomed, unlike leg hair, facial hair, and armpit (axillary) hair. Hair distribution in certain body regions is a secondary sex characteristic and starts to appear around puberty as the beard, moustache, and body hair in males, and pubic and axillary hair in both sexes.

The social meaning of hair is very important. So many old and present social and/ or religious practices deal with hair. Enforced shaving of scalp hair has long been used as a sign of punishment and in certain religious practices as a sign of obedience. The Romans completely shaved the scalps of prisoners, adulterers, and traitors. Scalping the warring enemies, which was long practiced by some primitive societies was meant to express victory and revenge [1].

Hair styling can serve as a form of expression. Rebellion of youth to the existing social order is often manifested as a change in appearance, and especially change of hair style, e.g., long hair on males, shaved hair (skinheads), and dyed hair (punks) [1].

Hair also plays a role as a distinguishing sign of one's ethnicity, varying from straight to curly in form and from dark to blond in color. There is also a difference in the amount of body hair between races. Hair is generally subject to so much interracial and interindividual variation that it can be said that, apart from the hair follicle, there is no organ in the human body that is morphologically so much variable as hair.

Although hair is not vital to human existence, it is greatly important to one's psychological equilibrium [2–4]. Psychological problems of hair loss occur in both sexes, and more among women because of the relevance of physical attractiveness [5]. Hair is closely related to physical attractiveness and the difference between male and female hair patterning provides a recognition phenomenon. In general, baldness leads to overestimation of age of affected males [1].

In addition to the aesthetic function of hair, it has more natural functions, which are becoming less important because of the anthropological evolution and technical progress of mankind. Scalp hair protects against certain environmental conditions like sun rays and cold. Body hair in man is very much reduced in comparison with other mammals, and many theories have been postulated to explain this fact; most are based on temperature and thermal regulation of the human body all along the course of the evolution of mankind. Nasal hair protects against dust and acts as an air filter. Axillary and perineal hair reduce the friction during body movement and also serve for the wider or prolonged dissemination of apocrine gland odor. Pubic hair is said to have some excitatory functions during sexual intercourse.

Innumerable are the cosmetic products intended for use in hair care to remove sebum and dirt and to improve the look, shininess, uniformity, softness, color, odor, and ease of comb of the hair, as well as deposition of conditioning molecules and reduction of static "fly-aways" (e.g., shampoos, conditioners, hair dyes, fixation sprays, gels, creams, etc.) There are also many products that have been marketed and used by people as anti–hair loss preparations and/or hair growth–promoting agents. Many have not stood the test of time. Ancient medical literature is full of pharmaceutical prescriptions and formulas to be used to treat hair loss or to promote hair growth. They are so diverse in source and nature that any attempt to categorize them seems useless.

In addition to scalp hair formulas, many other compounds are intended to remove or to assist the removal of hair from other parts of the body, e.g., preshave and aftershave preparations, depilatories, and so on. Other products aim to decrease the contrast of hair with the skin, making hair less visible, e.g., bleaching agents. Besides the variable efficacy of these products, consumers may develop many nonintended effects on the hair and skin such as hair damage, hair loss, skin irritation, and/or allergy and photoreactions attributable to some active ingredients and/or their additives. In order to understand hair production, it is necessary to revisit the embryogenesis and to have an idea about the structure and functional activity of the hair follicle. These aspects will now be briefly described.

THE HAIR FOLLICLE

Embryology

In the early stages of hair follicle development in human fetal skin, a simultaneous differentiation of some epidermal and dermal cells takes place between the second and third months of intrauterine life in some areas such as the eyebrows and chin, followed by other body regions in the fourth month. Histologically, it begins as a crowding of cells in the basal layer of the epidermis with a simultaneous aggregation of mesenchymal cells directly beneath the developing epithelial component. Cells in the basal layer elongate to form the hair peg, which grows obliquely downwards in an orientation characteristic for each body region. The broad tip of the hair peg will become slightly concave and carries before it the aggregated mesenchymal cells, which will become the dermal papilla. During the downward course of the hair peg, two swellings appear at the posterior side of the follicle. The upper swelling will form the sebaceous gland, whereas the lower will become the insertion site of the arrector pili muscle. In some body sites, such as the axilla, groin, skin of genitalia, and face, a third swelling is going to develop above the sebaceous gland bud and this will form the apocrine gland [6–8].

Hair follicle development proceeds in a cephalocaudal direction and is completed by the 22nd week of intrauterine life. These follicles progressively synthesize hair shafts (lanugo hair), which are visible at the cutaneous surface by the 28th week. The first hair coat of fine lanugo hair is shed in utero at about 1 month before birth at full term. The shedding course follows a cephalo caudal direction, which means that frontal hair follicles begin their second hair cycle while occipital hair follicles are still in their first hair cycle. The second coat of lanugo hair is going to shed from all areas during the first 3 to 4 months of life [6–8].

Histology

The hair follicle bulb is composed of a central dermal papilla and a surrounding hair matrix. It undergoes many changes according to the cyclical activity of the hair follicle in health and disease. At the level of attachment of the arrector pili muscle to the follicle is the bulge zone of the root sheaths. This is considered to be the stem cell site from which a new hair cycle is initiated. The hair shaft is enclosed in two sheaths, i.e., the inner root sheath and the outer root sheath. The inner root sheath consists of a cuticle layer on the inside (next to the cuticle layer of the hair cortex), Huxley's layer in the middle, and Henle's layer on the outside. The inner root sheath hardens before the presumptive hair within it, and it is consequently thought to control the definitive shape of the hair shaft [6–8].

The outer root sheath cells have a characteristic vacuolated aspect. This sheath is covered by the vitreous membrane. Next to this layer we can find the connective tissue sheath with its characteristic fibroblasts [6–8].

Cyclical Activity

Production of a hair segment by a hair follicle undergoes a cyclical rhythm. Activity (anagen) is followed by a relatively short transitional phase (catagen) and a resting phase (telogen) (Fig. 1). The duration of activity or anagen varies greatly with species, body region, season, age, and the type of hair (i.e., terminal or vellus).

In adult humans the activity of each follicle is independent of its neighbors (asynchronous). However, during the development of the human embryo as well as the early months of life, there is a more or less synchronous moult of scalp hairs. Each follicle goes through the hair cycle a variable number of times in the course of a lifetime. On average, at any one time about 13% of the scalp hair follicles are in telogen and only 1% or less are in catagen. Telogen ratio may count higher in certain stressful physical and/or mental conditions such as telogen effluvium and postpartum alopecia [6–8].

HAIR STRUCTURE

Postnatal hair may be divided into two broad categories: vellus hair, which is soft, unmedullated, occasionally pigmented, and seldom exceeds 2 cm in length; and terminal, which is longer, coarser, and often pigmented and medullated [8]. Before puberty, terminal hair is limited to the scalp, eyebrows, and eyelashes. After puberty, secondary sexual terminal hair is developed from vellus hair in response to androgens. The bulk of any hair segment is formed mainly by the cortex, which is surrounded by a cuticle and may also have a continuous or discontinuous core or medulla [8,9]. The medulla is usually found in thicker

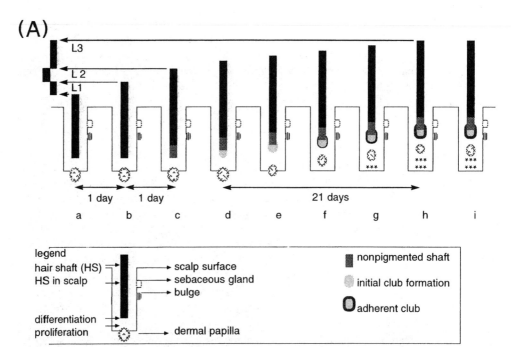

(A)

L3
L2
L1

1 day   1 day   21 days

a   b   c   d   e   f   g   h   i

legend
hair shaft (HS) → scalp surface
HS in scalp → sebaceous gland
→ bulge

differentiation
proliferation → dermal papilla

■ nonpigmented shaft
initial club formation
O adherent club

FIGURE 1   Schematic view of hair cycling of a human hair follicle. The latest steps of the hair-growth phase (anagen 6) during which hair is visible at the skin surface and growing are shown in (A) while the apparent rest phase of the hair cycle (telogen phase) is shown in (B) during which a new hair cycle can be initiated. The legend [between (A) and (B)] helps the reader to orient himself within the various components of the human hair follicle, which are essential to understanding growth and rest.

(A) *From growth to rest*: The same hair follicle is represented at various times (days) at the very end of the growth phase. At the skin surface, there is normal pigmented hair production (days a–b and b–c) representing the constant daily hair production (L1 and L2). Then, the pigmentation of the newly synthesized hair shaft (appearing at the bottom of the hair follicle) is decreased (c). This early event announces the regression of the impermanent portion of the hair follicle and is followed by terminal differentiation of cells in the proliferation compartment (d) and shrinkage of the dermal papilla (e). The latter starts an ascending movement together with the hair shaft (f–h; 21 days). This characterizes the catagen phase (d–h). The apparent elongation of the hair fiber (L3) reflects the outward migration of the hair shaft. What is left after disappearance of the epithelial cells from the impermanent portion of the hair follicle is, first, basement membranes, followed by dermal connective tissue usually referred to as streamers or stelae (***). The true resting stage begins when catagen is completed, i.e., when the dermal papilla abuts to the bottom of the permanent portion of the hair follicle. In the absence of physical interaction between dermal papilla and bulge the next cycle (see B) is definitely compromised. As from now no hair growth is observed at the surface (h–i).

(B)

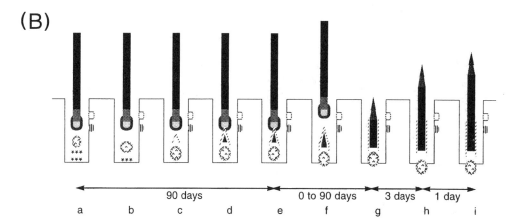

	90 days	0 to 90 days	3 days	1 day
a b	c d	e f	g	h i

FIGURE 1 Continued   (B) *From rest to growth:* During this stage, one notices absence of hair growth at the skin surface (a–g) but significant changes occur in the deeper parts of the hair follicle. The dermal papilla expands and attracts epithelial cells from the bulge (stem cell zone) in a downward movement (a–b). To create space, previously deposited materials have to be digested (a–b, ***). The epithelial cells then start differentiation in an orderly fashion starting with the inner root sheath (c) and the tip of the cuticle and hair cortex of the newly formed unpigmented hair fiber (d). The resting hair remains in the hair follicle for approximately 1 to 3 months (a–e), then the detached hair is shed (f). The shiny root end of the shed hair is the club. Before, during, or after hair shedding there may be replacement by a new hair shaft (e–f–g). Indeed, under physiological conditions, the follicle proceeds immediately or only slowly with new hair production (from f to g; maximum 90 days). Certain conditions are characterized by a much longer interval before regrowth is visible. Usually, a nonpigmented hair tip is seen first (h), followed by a thicker, more pigmented, and faster-growing hair fiber (i) depending on the many regulatory factors controlling the hair follicle. (Reproduced with permission from H.A.I.R. Technology [Skinterface sprl, Tournai, Belgium].)

hair, and its protein composition contains trichohyaline. Above the level of the epidermis some medullar cells dehydrate, forming air-filled vacuoles, which are responsible for the interrupted appearance of the medulla because of the reflection of light on these air-filled spaces. The mature cortex consists of closely packed spindle-shaped cells separated by intercellular lamella cementing the cells together. Within the cells most of the microfibrils are closely packed and oriented longitudinally [8,9].

The hair cuticle consists of five to 10 overlapping cell layers imbricated like roof tiles and aimed outwards (towards the distal end of the hair). The mature cells are thin scales consisting of dense keratin. Over the newly formed part of the hair the scale margins are intact, but as the hair emerges from the skin they break off progressively. The outer surface of each cuticular cell has a very clear A-layer, which is rich in high-sulfur protein; this layer protects the cuticular cells from premature breakdown caused by chemical and physical insults [8,9].

Keratins are a group of insoluble cystine-containing helicoidal protein complexes produced in the epithelial tissues of vertebrates. Because of the resistance of these protein complexes, hairs have been said to contain hard keratins as opposed to the soft keratins of desquamating tissues [9].

CLINICAL HAIR-GROWTH–EVALUATION METHODS

Subjective evaluation and personal satisfaction of people using hair-growth modulators and/or cosmetics on a wide scale are the most important factors for the survival of these products in the market. This evaluation will be based on whether they are perceived as efficacious, especially when the benefit is cosmetic in nature (acknowledging the massive placebo effect and the possible bias). Hence, before they reach the hands of consumers, safety and efficacy testing have to be performed according to the science, ethics, and rules of good clinical practice and medical research in order to adequately support the claims made to the patient and the consumer.

For an evaluation method to be considered valuable, it should provide information about the following variables: hair density, which is the number of hairs per unit area (usually number/cm^2); linear hair growth rate (LHGR) as millimeters per day; percentage of anagen growth phase (%A); hair diameter in micrometers; and time to hair regrowth after completion of telogen phase [10]. For many evaluation techniques, the methodology details are lacking as well as information about sensitivity and reproducibility usually required for clinical investigative techniques [11]. Much effort is needed for the standardization of evaluation methods in order to make it possible to compare different methods, or different results from different centers using the same method. For classification purposes these methods can be categorized as invasive, semi-invasive, and noninvasive.

Invasive methods

Biopsy

In addition to the ordinary vertical sectioning of skin biopsies which permits the study of longitudinal follicular sections, horizontal sectioning (parallel to the skin surface) of scalp biopsies offers further diagnostic opportunities. First described by Headington [12], it has been demonstrated that horizontal sectioning may provide a better diagnostic yield than vertical sectioning [13,14]. Horizontal sectioning allows the study of larger number of follicular structures. Inflammatory infiltrates are more easily seen and their relationship to the follicular structures is more obvious than in vertical sectioning. Fibrous tracts, which are often difficult to visualise on vertical sectioning, become much more apparent on horizontal sectioning. It is possible as well to distinguish vellus from terminal hairs, to identify the stages of all hairs in one section and to classify them into anagen, telogen or catagen follicles.

Semi-invasive Methods

Trichogram

The idea of estimating changes affecting hair growth by examining hair roots was first suggested by Van Scott et al. [15]. In order to examine hair root status necessary to diagnose hair disorders, at least 50 hairs should be plucked in order to reduce sampling errors. The roots are examined under a low-power microscope. The root morphology is stable and hairs can be kept for many weeks in dry packaging before analysis. Due to the relative values generated telogen/anagen (T/A) ratio, this technique is a relatively poor indicator of disease activity and/or disease severity in androgen-dependent alopecia in women [16]. In our center this method has been abandoned because it generates only relative values as compared with the method described in the following section.

Unit Area Trichogram

The unit area trichogram (UAT) is a technique in which all the hairs within a defined area (usually 60 mm²) are plucked and mounted onto double-sided tape attached to a glass slide. Optical microscopical examination of these slides estimate various hair variables as hair density, anagen%, hair length and hair diameter. The scalp area to be sampled should first be degreased (with an acetone/isopropanol mixture) and then delineated with a roller pen. All hairs contained in the area are epilated individually (one by one). Each hair is grasped at a uniform point above the scalp and the forceps are rotated to ensure firm grasp. Epilation should be performed rapidly in a single action in the direction of hair growth orientation, in order to minimize trauma to the roots [17].

The unit area trichogram is one of the rare exceptions to a strange general rule or law in trichology; indeed, most methods are promoted along with a new drug or a new cosmetic efficacy evaluation program. The exception in the unit area trichogram is that the method has been evaluated independently in terms of reproducibility and clinical relevance. Therefore, it could serve for comparative purposes. Most hair-growth variables estimated through unit area trichogram and the phototrichogram are comparable. However, the unit area trichogram has the advantage in that it can be used reliably in subjects in whom there is no contrast between hair and skin color [18].

Noninvasive Methods
Global Methods

Scoring Classification Systems   The patterns produced by the gradual process of scalp hair loss in male pattern baldness were first described by Hamilton in 1951. In 1975, Norwood proposed a modification of Hamilton's classification. In this modification he mentioned three patterns that referred to women. Finally, in 1977 Ludwig published the stages of female androgenetic alopecia in three patterns. For more details we refer the interested reader to the following references: Camacho F, Montagna W [19] and Ludwig E, Montagna W, Camacho F [20]. Although static by definition, such diagrams can be enriched by more gradual variations [8], an updated version of which appears in Figure 2, but these will only rarely match the continuum that one observes in the hair clinic.

Global Photography   Global photography apprehends all factors involved in hairiness at once and can be used for drug efficacy evaluation provided that adequate scalp preparation and hair style are maintained throughout the study. This is the most patient-friendly photographic method. This method is used in the clinic under standardized conditions of exposure [21]. Processing and rating have to be performed under controlled (i.e., blinded as to treatment and/or time) conditions. Trained raters could generate reproducible data.

Daily Collection of Shed Hair   The cyclic hair growth activity results in a daily shedding process in which telogen hairs are shed to be replaced by anagen hairs. The reported normal average daily loss of hair ranges somewhere between 40 to 180 hairs per day. In a study of 404 females without hair or scalp disease, lost hair was collected daily over 6 weeks in the aim of comparing two shampoos. Results showed mean hair loss rates ranging from 28 to 35 per day. No significant differences were noted in the mean daily hair loss rates during the 2-week baseline and the 4-week treatment period [22].

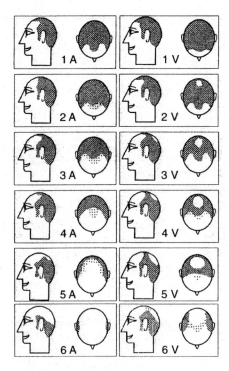

FIGURE 2 Scoring of androgen-dependent alopecia (ADA) in men. The present classification shows ADA patterns that affect the scalp of genetically susceptible male subjects after puberty. They are subdivided in six stages from mild to severe balding (1–6). The anterior pattern (A) indicates a backward progression of hair follicle miniaturization and deficient hair production with the ensuing bald appearance. The vertex type (V) indicates isolated regression occurring on the vertex but this is usually combined with the involvement of the frontal temporal areas. (Reproduced with permission from H.A.I.R. Technology [Skinterface sprl, Tournai, Belgium].)

Quantitating daily hair loss in women was assessed in another study of 234 women complaining of hair loss among which 89 had apparently normal hair density. They have found that subjects with normally dense hair (although complaining about hair loss) shed less than 50 hairs a day [16]. So the magic number of 100 so often referred to in textbooks and found in the lay press should be seriously revisited. Less than 50 hairs can be significantly abnormal in a patient having lost 50% of his hair. Further standardization studies are currently being run in our laboratory.

Hair Weight and Hair Count   The efficacy of hair-growth–promoting agents can be established by comparing the total hair mass (weight) and counts of grown hair in a small, carefully maintained area of the scalp [23,24]. A plastic sheet with a 1.2 cm^2 hole was placed over the selected site. All hairs within the square hole were pulled through it and hand clipped to 1 mm in length. The apparent advantage of this method is that it provides a global measurement of growth on a small sample size for the detection of drug effects and between treatment regimens (e.g., 2 vs. 5% minoxidil) [24]. One must be aware of the technical skills necessary to handle the samples in the proper way to avoid the loss of some hairs between the clinic and the laboratory. Again, as for many of these techniques, the methodological comparisons are lacking and there are no evaluations of the reproducibility and sensitivity usually required for laboratory evaluation methods because they were introduced on the occasion of drug evaluation protocols. The major limitation of this method is that it generates a global index of growth, the individual components of which cannot be analyzed separately.

Hair-Pull Test The hair-pull test is based on the idea that "gentle" pulling of the hair brings about the shedding of telogen hairs [16]. It is a very rough method and difficult to standardize because it is subject to so much interindividual variation among the investigators. Physically speaking, the pulling force is not uniformly distributed over the whole hair bundle, thereby creating variation in the pulling force from one hair to another. It seems to be useful only in acute and severe conditions, not in chronically evolving conditions like androgen-dependent alopecia.

Analytical Methods

Phototrichogram The basic principle of the phototrichogram (PTG) consists of taking a photograph of a certain area of the scalp in which the hair is cut in preparation for the photograph, and to repeat this photographic documentation after a certain time period. This period of time should be long enough to permit the evaluation of the growth of a hair segment (which is usually between 24-72 h). The growth is then evaluated by comparing the two pictures. Hairs that have grown are in anagen phase and those that have not are in telogen phase (Fig. 3).

The assessment is made on defined scalp sites considered representative of the condition. The data that can be generated from a PTG include the total number of hairs present in a certain surface area, which allows us to calculate hair density (N/cm²). Hair density is a quantitative element through which we can estimate the degree of hair loss.

Also from a PTG, we can determine the percentage of hairs in the growth phase

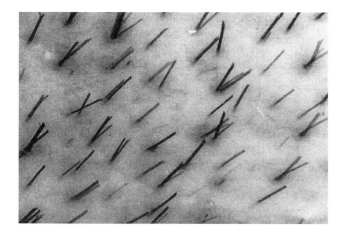

FIGURE 3 Day 2 picture of scalp hair (48 hrs after clipping short all scalp hairs from the photographed scalp site): long growing hairs represent follicles in anagen phase; shorter nongrowing hairs represent follicles in telogen.

(anagen%) and can calculate the LHGR. Meanwhile, the reliability of the evaluation of hair thickness has been the subject of detailed analysis. The most precise instrument used for hair-diameter evaluation remains the microscope.

One of the main advantages of the PTG is that first of all it is a patient-friendly method. Secondly it is a totally noninvasive method so it does not affect the natural process of hair growth/loss by itself. However, many patients are afraid of the idea of having their hair cut at one or more given scalp surface sites (area $\pm$ 1 cm^2 in our protocol). Most are reassured by the fact that this process cannot prevent them from enjoying a normal private and social life. Finally, PTG also permits the chronological follow-up of exactly the same area under the study, and this has been shown to bring about a lot of valuable information [25]. Some technical improvements have been introduced during the course of evolution of the PTG technique. For example, the application of a frontal window with a glass slide mounted on it has been considered a major improvement [26,27]. It reduces the curvature of the scalp and permits a better image clarity.

Some technical photography problems have been identified during the course of the evolution of the PTG, and a series of detailed analysis performed at our laboratory and clinic have pinpointed a number of them, including the primary enlargement factor (PEF), which is one of the factors responsible for the "visibility" of hair on a photograph [28]; the secondary enlargement factor (size of printouts); and the experience of technicians. A further improvement was the development of scalp immersion proxigraphy (SIP), which is routinely used at our hair clinic and permits a better diffusion of light through a medium of lower optic heterogeneity [29].

After comparison with UAT [18], weak points of the method have been considered with great care, and using photography in combination with hair-micrometry results in a valid method for global hair perception while allowing an analytical description of all variables intervening in hair-quality evaluation.

Variants of Phototrichogram

Video PTG   In this method, the photographic camera is replaced by a video camera equipped with specific lenses. In fact, recent reports in which this method has been used have been on Asians. In these subjects the contrast between hair and scalp seems favorable for the application of this method. Moreover, the reported low figures of hair density could possibly be racial in origin. However, we advise taking these factors into account in order to keep the biological variation as low as possible [30]. The recent introduction of cheap CCD cameras will certainly contribute to further developments in this field.

Traction PTG   This test is based on the fact that hairs that can be easily pulled from the scalp are in telogen and those resisting pull are in anagen [31]. This test has been performed on a surface area of 0.25 cm^2. Hairs present at this surface area are held gently between the thumb and index fingers and pulled repeatedly. Hairs that can be easily pulled are counted and their number is considered the number of telogen hairs. Those resisting pulling are clipped and counted, and their number represents the anagen hairs. Through this method, we can calculate the hair density per unit area as well as the anagen%.

It is necessary to evaluate this semi-invasive method more critically to define its reproducibility through the standardization of the pulling technique. Other comparative studies may be essential as well to estimate the sensitivity and specificity of this method, which as it stands today would be rated as flawed with many weak points (e.g., small surface area, lack of control on traction forces etc.).

REFERENCES

1. Van der Donk A. Psychological aspects of androgenetic alopecia. Thesis, University of Rotterdam, The Netherlands, 1992.
2. Passchier J. Quality of life issues in male pattern hair loss. Dermatology 1998; 197:217–218.
3. Girman CJ, Rhodes T, Lilly FRW, Guo SS, Siervogel RM, Patrick DL, Chumlea WC. Effects of self-perceived hair loss in a community sample of men. Dermatology 1998; 197:223–229.
4. Cash TF. The psychological effects of androgenetic alopecia in men. J Am Acad Dermatol 1992; 26:926–931.
5. Cash TF, Price VH, Savin RC. Psychological effects of androgenetic alopecia on women: comparison with balding men and with female control subjects. J Am Acad Dermatol 1993; 29:568–575.
6. Montagna W, Camacho F. The anatomy and development of hair, hair follicles, and the hair growth cycles. In: Camacho F, Montagna W, eds. Trichology: Diseases of the Pilosebaceous Follicle. Madrid: Aula Medica Group, 1997:1–27.
7. Messenger AG, Dawber RPR. The physiology and embryology of hair growth. In: Dawber R, ed. Diseases of the Hair and Scalp. 3rd ed. Oxford: Blackwell Science Ltd, 1997:1–22.
8. Dawber R, Van Neste D. Hair and Scalp Disorders. London: Martin Dunitz Ltd, 1995.
9. Zviak C. The Science of Hair Care. New York: Marcel Dekker, 1986.
10. Van Neste D. Hair growth evaluation in clinical dermatology. Dermatology 1993; 187:233–234.
11. Trancik RJ. Physical methods for human hair evaluation. In: Van Neste D, Randall VA, eds. Hair Research for the Next Millenium. Amsterdam: Elsevier, 1996: 84–85.
12. Headington JT. Transverse microscopic anatomy of human scalp. Arch Dermatol 1984; 120: 449–456.
13. Whiting DA. The value of horizontal sections of scalp biopsies. J Cut Aging Cosm Dermatol 1990; 1:165–173.
14. Whiting DA. Diagnostic and predictive value of horizontal sections of scalp biopsy specimens in male pattern androgenetic alopecia. J Am Acad Dermatol 1993; 28:755–763.
15. Van Scott EJ, Reinerston RP, Steinmuller R. The growing hair roots of human scalp and morphologic changes therein following amethopterin-therapy. J Invest Dermatol 1957; 29: 197–204.
16. Guarrera M, Semino MT, Rebora A. Quantitating hair loss in women: a critical approach. Dermatology 1997; 194:12–16.
17. Rushton DH. Chemical and morphological properties of scalp hair in normal and abnormal states. Ph. D. thesis, University of Wales, United Kingdom, 1988.
18. Rushton DH, de Brouwer B, De Coster W, Van Neste DJJ. Comparative evaluation of scalp hair by phototrichogram and unit area trichogram analysis within the same subjects. Acta Dermato Venereologica 1993; 73:150–153.
19. Camacho F, Montagna W. Current concept and classification. Male androgenetic alopecia. In: Camacho F, Montagna W, eds. Trichology. Madrid: Aula Medica Group, 1997: 325–342.
20. Ludwig E, Montagna W, Camacho F. Female androgenetic alopecia. In: Camacho F, Montagna W, eds. Trichology. Madrid: Aula Medica Group, 1997: 343–355.
21. Canfield D. Photographic documentation of hair growth in androgenetic alopecia. Dermatol Clin 1996; 14:713–721.
22. Kullavanijaya P, Gritiyarangsan P, Bisalbutra P, Kulthanan R, Cardin CW. Absence of effects of dimethicone and non-dimethicone containing shampoos on daily hair loss rates. J Soc Cosmet Chem 1992; 43:195–206.

23. Price VH, Menefee E. Quantitative estimation of hair growth. 1. Androgenetic alopecia in women: effect of minoxidil. J Invest Dermatol 1990; 95:683–687.

24. Price VH, Menefee E. Quantitative estimation of hair growth: comparative changes in weight and hair count with 5% and 2% minoxidil, placebo and no treatment. In: Van Neste D, Randall VA, eds. Hair Research for the Next Millenium. Amsterdam: Elsevier, 1996: 67–71.

25. Courtois M. The phototrichogram. In: Baran R, Maibach HI, eds. Cosmetic Dermatology. London: Martin Dunitz, 1994:397–400.

26. Barth JH. Measurement of hair growth. Clin Exp Dermatol 1986; 11:127–138.

27. Friedel J, Will F, Grosshans E. Le phototrichogramme. Adaptation, standardisation et application. Ann Dermatol Vénéréol 1989; 116:629–636.

28. Van Neste DJJ, de Brouwer B, De Coster W. The phototrichogram: analysis of some factors of variation. Skin Pharmacology 1994; 7:67–72.

29. Van Neste D, Dumortier M, de Brouwer B, De Coster W. Scalp immersion proxigraphy (SIP): an improved imaging technique for phototrichogram analysis. J Eur Acad Dermatol Venereol 1992; 1:187–191.

30. Hayashi S, Miayamoto I, Takeda K. Measurement of human hair growth by optical microscopy and image analysis. Brit J Dermatol 1991; 125:123–129.

31. Bouhanna P. Le tractiophototrichogramme, méthode d'appréciation objective d'une chute de cheveux. Ann Dermatol Venereol 1988; 115:759–764.

6

Safety Terminology

Ai-Lean Chew and Howard I. Maibach
University of California at San Francisco School of Medicine,
San Francisco, California

INTRODUCTION

One of the skin's primary physiological functions is to act as the body's first line of defense against exogenous agents. However, the skin should not be viewed as a flawless physicochemical barrier. Many low–molecular weight compounds are capable of penetrating this barrier. When toxic agents (such as irritants or allergens in cosmetic products) permeate it, the resulting adverse effects may cause considerable discomfort to the consumer. Even minor disturbances of the skin surface can produce discomfort, especially in the facial area which has an extensive network of sensory nerves. Moreover, because most cosmetics are applied to the highly permeable facial skin, the majority of reported cosmetic reactions occur in the face. Therefore, safety with regard to cosmetic products is a vital issue.

This chapter provides a brief summary of the safety terminology pertaining to cosmetic reactions, as well as an overture to the succeeding chapters. The reader is directed toward some in-depth reviews of each topic in the bibliography.

CONTACT DERMATITIS

This is a nonspecific term used to describe any inflammatory skin disease resulting from contact with an irritant or allergenic substance. Whatever the causative agent, the clinical features are similar: itching, redness, and skin lesions. It is also often used (inaccurately) as a synonym for allergic contact dermatitis (ACD).

IRRITANT CONTACT DERMATITIS (IRRITATION)

Irritant contact dermatitis (ICD) is a term given to a complex group of localized inflammatory reactions that follow nonimmunological damage to the skin. The inflammation may be the result of an acute toxic (usually chemical) insult to the skin, or of repeated and cumulative damage from weaker irritants (chemical or physical). There is no definite laboratory test for ICD—diagnosis is by clinical morphology, of course, and appropriate negative patch-test results.

Irritant

An irritant is any agent, physical or chemical, that is capable of producing cell damage if applied for sufficient time and in sufficient concentration. Irritants can produce a reaction in anyone, although individual susceptibility varies. The clinical reaction produced by irritants varies considerably.

Acute Irritant Contact Dermatitis

Acute ICD is the result of a single overwhelming exposure to a strong irritant or a series of brief physical or chemical contacts, leading to acute inflammation of the skin. The resultant clinical appearance is that of erythema, edema, pain, and sometimes vesiculation at the site of contact, usually associated with burning or stinging sensations.

Irritant Reaction

An irritant reaction is a transient noneczematous dermatitis characterized by erythema, chapping, or dryness, and resulting from exposure to less potent irritants. Repeated irritant reactions may lead to contact dermatitis.

Cumulative Irritant Contact Dermatitis

Cumulative irritant contact dermatitis or chronic ICD develops as a result of a series of repeated and damaging insults to the skin. The insults may be chemical or physical.

Delayed Acute Irritant Contact Dermatitis

Some chemicals produce acute irritation in a delayed manner so that the signs and symptoms of acute irritant dermatitis appear 12 to 24 hours or more after the original insult.

Subjective (Sensory) Irritation

This refers to sensations of burning, stinging, and itching that are experienced by certain susceptible individuals after contact with certain chemicals, although no visible inflammatory pathology can be seen. Examples of sensory irritants in cosmetics are lactic acid, salicylic acid, propylene glycol, and some benzoyl peroxide preparations.

ALLERGIC CONTACT DERMATITIS

ACD occurs when a substance comes into contact with skin that has undergone an acquired specific alteration in its reactivity as a result of prior exposure of the skin to the substance eliciting the dermatitis. The skin response of ACD is delayed, immunologically mediated (Type IV), and consists of varying degrees of erythema, edema, papules, and papulovesicles. Patch testing is the gold standard; it is imperative for proving ACD, determining the actual allergen, predictive testing, i.e., determining "safe" materials for the consumer, and exclusion of other diagnoses.

Allergen

Allergens are low–molecular-weight (<500–1000 Da) molecules capable of penetrating the skin and binding to skin proteins to form a number of different antigens that may stimulate an allergic response in an individual. Common allergens in cosmetic products are fragrances (e.g., cinnamic aldehyde) and preservatives (e.g., formaldehyde and formaldehyde donors).

PHOTOIRRITANT CONTACT DERMATITIS (PHOTOIRRITATION/PHOTOTOXICITY)

Photoirritant contact dermatitis (PICD) is a chemically induced nonimmunological skin irritation requiring light. This reaction will occur in all individuals exposed to the chemical–light combination. The clinical picture is that of erythema, edema, or vesiculation in sun-exposed areas, resembling an exaggerated sunburn. This may be followed by hyperpigmentation, or if the exposure is repeated, scaling and lichenification may occur. Bergapten, a component of bergamot oil, which used to be a popular ingredient in perfume, is a potent photoirritant that causes berloque dermatitis.

PHOTOALLERGIC CONTACT DERMATITIS

Photoallergic contact dermatitis (PACD) is an immunological response to a substance that requires the presence of light. The substance in the skin absorbs photons and is converted to a stable or unstable photoproduct, which binds to skin proteins to form an antigen, which then elicits a delayed hypersensitivity response. Examples of photoallergens present in cosmetics are musk ambrette and 6-methylcoumarin, which are present in fragrances. Photopatch testing is the diagnostic procedure for photoallergy.

CONTACT URTICARIA SYNDROME

Contact urticaria syndrome (CUS) represents a heterogeneous group of inflammatory reactions that appear, usually within a few minutes to an hour, after contact with the eliciting substance. Clinically, erythematous wheal-and-flare reactions are seen, and sensations of burning, stinging, or itching are experienced. These are transient, usually disappearing within a few hours. In its more severe forms, generalized urticaria or extracutaneous manifestations, such as asthma, nausea, abdominal cramps, and even anaphylactic shock, may occur. Diagnosis may be achieved by a variety of skin tests—the open test is the simplest of these and is the "first-line" test.

CUS may be divided into two categories on the basis of pathophysiological mechanisms: nonimmunological and immunological. There are also urticariogens that act by an uncertain mechanism.

Nonimmunological Contact Urticaria

Nonimmunological contact urticaria (NICU), which occurs without prior sensitization, is the most common class of CUS. The reaction usually remains localized. Examples of cosmetic substances known to produce NICU are preservatives (e.g., benzoic acid and sorbic acid) and fragrances (e.g., cinnamic aldehyde).

Immunological Contact Urticaria

Immunological contact urticaria (ICU) are immediate (Type I) allergic reactions in people who have previously been sensitized to the causative agent. ICU is IgE mediated and is more common in atopic individuals. Food substances are common causes of ICU.

ACNEGENICITY

This refers to the capacity of some agents to cause acne or aggravate existing acne lesions. This term may be subdivided to include comedogenicity and pustulogenicity.

Comedogenicity

This is the capability of an agent to cause hyperkeratinous impactions in the sebaceous follicle, or the formation of microcomedones, usually in a relatively short period of time.

Pustulogenicity

This refers to the capability of an agent to cause inflammatory papules and pustules, usually in a relatively short period of time.

SENSITIVE SKIN

This term is a neologism for consumers' feelings about their intolerance to a variety of topical agents, be it topical medicaments or cosmetics and toiletries. Individuals present with very similar complaints, such as burning, stinging or itching sensations, on contact with certain cosmetic products that most people do not seem to react to, sometimes accompanied by slight erythema or edema. They frequently complain of a ''tight feeling'' in their skin, secondary to associated dry skin. Sensitive skin describes the phenotype noted by the consumer; mechanisms include sensory irritation, suberythematous irritation, acute and cumulative irritation, contact urticaria, allergic contact dermatitis, as well as photoallergic and phototoxic contact dermatitis. Sensory irritation and suberythematous irritation are believed to be far more common than the remaining mechanisms.

Cosmetic Intolerance Syndrome

The term cosmetic intolerance syndrome (CIS) is applied to the multifactorial syndrome in which certain susceptible individuals are intolerant of a wide range of cosmetic products. CIS is thought to be caused by one or more underlying occult dermatological conditions, such as subjective irritation, objective irritation, allergic contact dermatitis, contact urticaria, or subtle manifestations of endogenous dermatological diseases, such as atopic eczema, psoriasis, and rosacea.

Status Cosmeticus

Status cosmeticus is a condition in which every cosmetic product applied to the face produces itching, burning or stinging, rendering the sufferer incapable of using any cosmetic product. The patient's history usually includes ''sensitivity'' to a wide range of products. This diagnosis is only declared after a full battery of tests have proved negative, and may be considered the extreme end of the spectrum of sensitive skin.

BIBLIOGRAPHY

Irritant Contact Dermatitis

Elsner P, Maibach HI, eds. Irritant Dermatitis: New Clinical and Experimental Aspects. Current Problems in Dermatology Series, Vol. 23, Basel; Karger, 1995.

Lammintausta K, Maibach HI. Irritant contact dermatitis. In: Moschella SL, Hurley HJ, eds. Dermatology, 3rd edition. Philadelphia; W.B. Saunders Company, 1992:425–432.

Van Der Valk PGM, Maibach HI. The Irritant Contact Dermatitis Syndrome. Boca Raton: CRC Press, 1996.

Wilkinson JD, Rycroft RJG. Contact dermatitis. In: Champion RH, Burton JL, Ebling FJG, eds. Rook/Wilkinson/Ebling Textbook of Dermatology, 5th edition. Oxford; Blackwell Scientific Publications, 1992:611.

Allergic Contact Dermatitis

Cronin E. Contact Dermatitis. Edinburgh; Churchill Livingstone, 1980.

Larsen WG, Maibach HI. Allergic contact dermatitis. In: Moschella SL, Hurley HJ, eds. Dermatology, 3rd edition. Philadelphia; W.B. Saunders Company, 1992; 17:391–424.

Rietschel RL, Fowler JF Jr, eds. Fisher's Contact Dermatitis, 4th edition. Williams & Baltimore; Williams and Wilkins, 1995.

Phototoxic/Photoallergic Contact Dermatitis

DeLeo VA, Maso MJ. In: Moschella SL, Hurley HJ, eds. Dermatology, 3rd edition. Philadelphia: W.B. Saunders Company, 1992:507.

Harber LC, Bickers DR, eds. In: Photosensitivity Diseases: Principles of Diagnosis and Treatment, 2nd edition. Ontario; BC Decker Inc. 1989.

Marzulli FN, Maibach HI. Photoirritation (phototoxicity, phototoxic dermatitis). In: Dermatotoxicology, 5th edition. Washington, DC: Taylor & Francis, 1996; 231–237.

Contact Urticaria Syndrome

Amin S, Lahti A, Maibach HI. Contact Urticaria Syndrome. Boca Raton: CRC Press, 1997.

Lahti A, Maibach HI. Contact Urticaria Syndrome. In: Moschella SL, Hurley HJ, eds. Dermatology, 3rd edition. Philadelphia; W.B. Saunders Company, 1992, 19:433.

Acnegenicity

Mills OH Jr, Berger RS. Defining the susceptibility of acne-prone and sensitive skin populations to extrinsic factors. Dermatologic Clinics, 1991; 9(1):93–98.

Sensitive Skin

Amin S, Engasser P, Maibach HI. Sensitive skin: what is it? In: Baran R, Maibach HI. Textbook of Cosmetic Dermatology, 2nd edition. London; Martin Dunitz Ltd, 1998; 343–349.

Fisher AA. Cosmetic actions and reactions: Therapeutic, irritant and allergic. Cutis 1980; 26:22–29.

Maibach HI, Engasser P. Management of cosmetic intolerance syndrome. Clin Dermatol 1988; 6(3): 102–107.

7

Principles and Practice of Percutaneous Absorption

Ronald C. Wester and Howard I. Maibach
*University of California at San Francisco School of Medicine,
San Francisco, California*

INTRODUCTION

Percutaneous absorption is a complex biological process. The skin is a multilayered bio-membrane that has certain absorption characteristics. If the skin were a simple membrane, absorption parameters could easily be measured, and these would be fairly constant provided there was no change in the chemistry of the membrane. However, skin is a dynamic tissue and as such its absorption parameters are susceptible to constant change. Many factors and skin conditions can rapidly change the absorption parameters. Additionally, skin is a living tissue and it will change through its own growth patterns, and this change will also be influenced by many factors. This chapter reviews some of the principles and technologies of percutaneous absorption for developers and users of cosmetics.

STEPS TO PERCUTANEOUS ABSORPTION

A cosmetic that comes in contact with human skin will be absorbed into and through the skin. The components of the cosmetic will respond to the chemical and physical laws of nature, which direct the absorption process. Examples of this are solubility, partition coefficients, and molecular weight. The skin presents a barrier, both physical structure and chemical composition. A cosmetic component will transverse from a lipophilic stratum corneum to a more progressively hydrophilic epidermis, dermis, and blood microcirculation.

Percutaneous absorption has been defined as a series of steps [1]. Table 1 lists our current knowledge of these steps. Step 1 is the vehicle containing the chemical(s) of interest. There is a partitioning of the chemical from the vehicle to the skin. This initiates a series of absorption and excretion kinetics that are influenced by a variety of factors, such as regional and individual variation. These factors moderate the absorption and excretion kinetics [2].

Once a chemical has been absorbed through the skin, it enters the systemic circulation of the body. Here, the pharmacokinetics of the chemical define body interactions. This is illustrated for [^{14}C]hydroquinone in vivo in man, where plasma radioactivity was measured ipsilaterally (next to the dose site) and contralaterally (in the opposite arm) after a topical dose. Thirty minutes after the dose, the hydroquinone has been absorbed through the skin and has reached a near-peak plasma concentration (Fig. 1) [3]. Figure 2 shows

TABLE 1   Steps to Percutaneous Absorption

Vehicle
Absorption kinetics
    Skin site of application
    Individual variation
    Skin condition
    Occlusion
    Drug concentration and surface area
    Multiple-dose application
    Time
Excretion kinetics
Effective cellular and tissue distribution
Substantivity (nonpenetrating surface adsorption)
Wash and rub resistance/decontamination
Volatility
Binding
Anatomical pathways
Cutaneous metabolism
Quantitative structure activity relationships
Decontamination
Dose accountability
Models

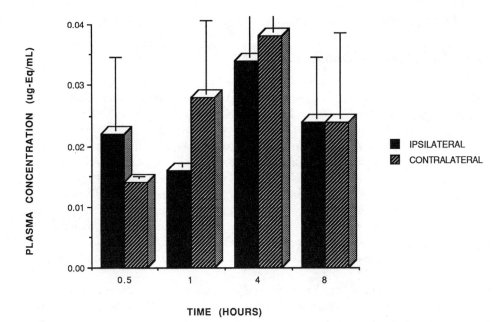

FIGURE 1   Plasma radioactivity is detected in human volunteers 30 minutes after [^{14}C]hydroquinone is applied to skin. Ipsilateral is blood taken near the site of dosing, and contralateral is from the other arm. Hydroquinone is rapidly absorbed into and through human skin.

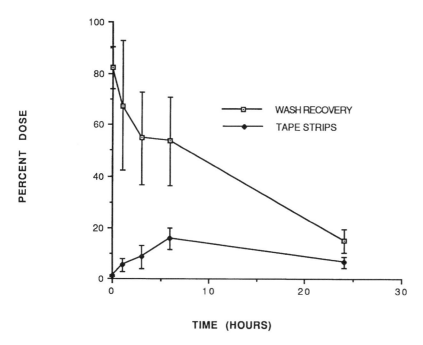

FIGURE 2 Hydroquinone is applied to human skin. Wash recovery with time decreases because hydroquinone is being absorbed into and through human skin. At the same time, tape strips of the skin surface show a rise in stratum-corneum content of hydroquinone. It is a dynamic process; hydroquinone disappears from the skin surface, appears and increases in the stratum corneum, and then appears in the blood.

hydroquinone disappearance from the surface of the skin (decreased wash recovery) and concurrent appearance in the stratum corneum (obtained from skin tape strips) [3]. As the cosmetic component transverses the skin, the chemical can be exposed to skin enzymes, which are capable of altering the chemical structure through metabolism [3].

METHODS FOR PERCUTANEOUS ABSORPTION

Ideally, information on the dermal absorption of a particular compound in humans is best obtained through studies performed on humans. However, because many compounds are potentially toxic, or it is not convenient to test them in humans, studies can be performed using other techniques. Percutaneous absorption has been measured by two major methods: (1) in vitro diffusion cell techniques, and (2) in vivo determinations, both of which generally use radiolabeled compounds. To ensure their applicability to the clinical situation, the relevance of studies using these techniques must constantly be challenged [4].

In vitro techniques involve placing a piece of human skin in a diffusion chamber containing a physiological receptor fluid. The compound under investigation is applied to one side of the skin. The compound is then assayed at regular intervals on the other side of the skin. The skin may be intact, dermatomed, or separated into epidermis and dermis; however, separating skin with heat will destroy skin viability. The advantages of the in vitro techniques are that they are easy to use and results are obtained quickly. Their major disadvantage is the limited relevance of the conditions present in the in vitro system to those found in humans.

Percutaneous absorption in vivo is usually determined by the indirect method of measuring radioactivity in excreta after the topical application of a labeled compound. In human studies, the plasma level of a topically applied compound is usually extremely low—often below assay detection. For this reason, tracer methodology is used. After the topical application of the radiolabeled compound, the total amount of radioactivity excreted in urine or in urine plus feces is determined. The amount of radioactivity retained in the body or excreted by a route not assayed (CO_2) is corrected for by determining the amount of radioactivity excreted after parenteral administration. Absorption represents the amount of radioactivity excreted, expressed as percentage of the applied dose. Percutaneous absorption can also be assessed by the ratio of the areas under the concentration-versus-time curves after the topical and intravenous administration of a radiolabeled component. The metabolism of a compound by the skin as it is absorbed will not be detected by this method. A biological response, such as vasoconstriction after the topical application of steroids, has also been used to assess dermal absorption in vivo [4].

An emerging method is that of skin tape stripping. After washing, consecutive stratum corneum tape strips exhibit a profile, such as that for estradiol (Fig. 3) in human stratum corneum. The first few strips have higher estradiol content because they contain residual surface estradiol. Tape stripping can show a profile of a cosmetic within skin

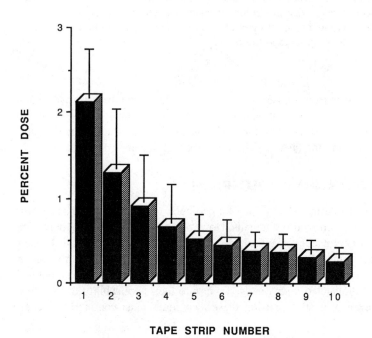

FIGURE 3   Estradiol is applied to human skin, then washed 24 hours after dosing. Tape strips (consecutive 1–10 in some areas) show a concentration pattern of estradiol through the stratum corneum.

over a time course. In addition, the chemical content of the tape strippings can be used to compare bioavailability of competing products. Proof can be obtained by using this technique to observe which products penetrate skin faster and deeper.

INDIVIDUAL AND REGIONAL VARIATION

In vivo and in vitro percutaneous absorption studies give data as mean absorption ± some standard deviation. Some of this variability is attributable to conduct of the study and is called *experimental error*. However, when viewing a set of absorption values it is quite clear that some people (as well as some rhesus monkeys) are low absorbers and some are high absorbers. This becomes evident with repeat studies. This is *individual variation*.

The first occupational disease in recorded history was scrotal cancer in chimney sweeps. The historical picture of a male worker holding a chimney brush and covered from head to toe with black soot is vivid. But why the scrotum? Percutaneous absorption in humans and animals varies depending on the area of the body on which the chemical resides. This is called *regional variation*. When a certain skin area is exposed, any effect of the chemical will be determined by how much is absorbed through the skin. Feldmann and Maibach [5–7] were the first to systemically explore the potential for regional variation in percutaneous absorption. The first absorption studies were performed on the ventral forearm because this site is convenient to use. However, skin exposure to chemicals exists over the entire body. The scrotum was the highest-absorbing skin site (scrotal cancer in chimney sweeps is the key). Skin absorption was lowest for the foot area, and highest around the head and face (Fig. 4). There are two major points. First, regional variation was confirmed with the different chemicals. Second, those skin areas that would be exposed to cosmetics—the head and face—were among the higher absorbing sites.

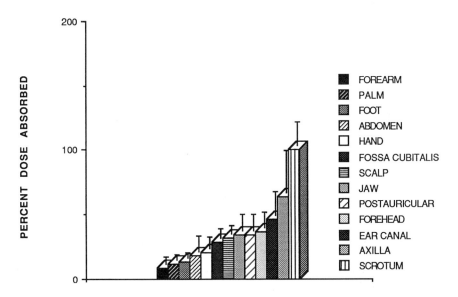

FIGURE 4 Percutaneous absorption of parathion from various parts of the body varies with region of the body.

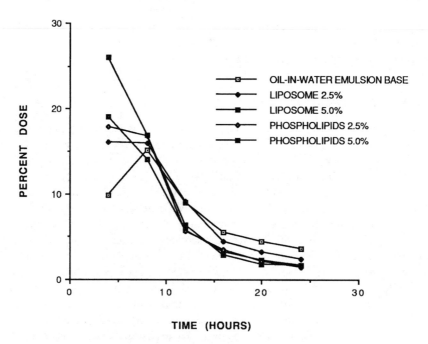

FIGURE 5 Lidocaine percutaneous absorption through human skin. Formulation determines the initial absorption.

VEHICLE INFLUENCE ON PERCUTANEOUS ABSORPTION

A cosmetic can be a single ingredient or a mixture of chemicals in a vehicle. The vehicle can have a great effect on skin absorption of the chemical(s). Lidocaine was applied to human skin in an in vitro absorption study. Figure 5 shows receptor fluid (circulating under the skin to collect absorbed lidocaine) accumulation with time. Initially the vehicle had a great influence on the partitioning of lidocaine into the skin. With time, the influence of the vehicle decreased and lidocaine absorption was constant for all vehicles. Interestingly, when the lidocaine content of epidermis and dermis was determined, there was more lidocaine retained by the oil-in-water (o/w) emulsion (Fig. 6). Vehicles can direct chemical distribution within skin and this can be validated with the proper experiment.

There is also an interesting vehicle effect for multiple dosing on skin. A multiple dose exceeds that predicted by absorption from single-dose administration (Fig. 7). The hypothesis is that the second and subsequent dosed vehicles ''reactivate/solubilize'' the initial chemical from skin binding and push the chemical further down into and through the skin [8].

SKIN CLEANSING AND DECONTAMINATION

Although decontamination of a chemical from the skin is commonly performed by washing with soap and water (because it is largely assumed that washing will remove the chemical), recent evidence suggests that the skin and the body are often unknowingly subjected to enhanced penetration and systemic absorption/toxicity because the decontamination procedure does not work or may actually enhance absorption [9].

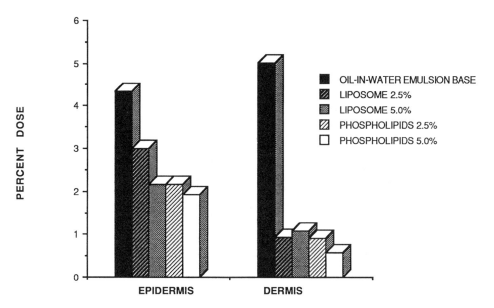

FIGURE 6 Distribution of lidocaine in human epidermis and dermis. Formulation determines the concentration within the skin component.

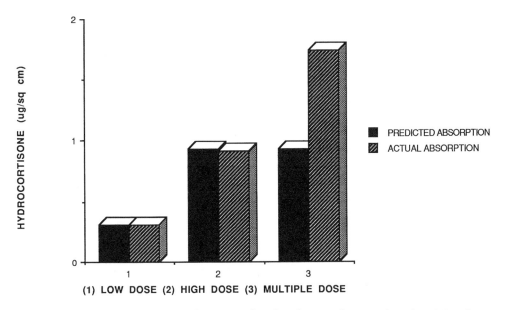

FIGURE 7 Hydrocortisone in cream base was dosed on human skin as a low dose (x) and a high dose (3x). When the low dose (x) was dosed three consecutive times (9 A.M., 1 P.M., 9 P.M.) totaling the high dose (3x), the absorption exceeded that predicted from the single high dose.

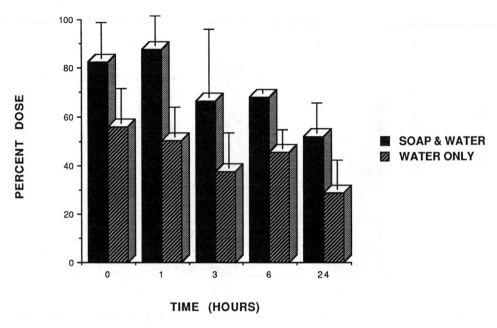

FIGURE 8 Skin decontamination of alachlor (lipophilic chemical) requires some soap to exceed removal by water only.

Figure 8 (alachlor) shows skin decontamination with soap and water or water only over a 24-hour dosing period, using the grid methodology. A series of 1 cm² areas are marked on the skin and each individual area is washed at a different time. Certain observations are made. First, the amount recovered decreased over time. This is because this is an in vivo system and percutaneous absorption is taking place, decreasing the amount of chemical on the skin surface. There also may be some loss attributable to skin desquamation. The second observation is that alachlor is more readily removed with soap-and-water wash than with water only. Alachlor is lipid soluble and needs the surfactant system for more successful decontamination [10].

Soap-and-water wash may not be the best method to cleanse skin. Soap and water will remove visible dirt and odor, but may not be a good skin cleanser. Figure 9 shows methylene bisphenyl isocyanate (MDI) (an industrial chemical) decontamination with water, soap and water, and some polyglycol and oil-based cleansers. Water and soap and water didn't work well but the polyglycol and oil-based cleansers did the job. The unknown question that remains is whether soap and water would then remove the polyglycol and oil-based cleansers [11].

COSMETIC PERCUTANEOUS ABSORPTION AND TOXICITY

The potential toxicity of cosmetics has in the past been dismissed as an event unlikely to occur. The argument was put forth that cosmetics did not contain ingredients that could prove harmful to the body. The argument went further to say that, because cosmetics were applied to skin with its barrier properties, the likelihood that a chemical would become systemically available was remote. The argument was proven false when carcinogens were

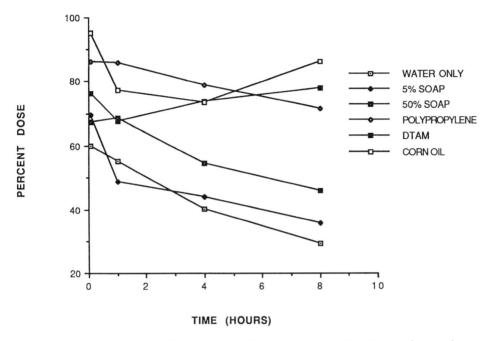

FIGURE 9 Methylene bisphenyl isocyanate (MDI) skin decontamination. Water alone and soap and water were relatively ineffective in removing MDI compared with the polypropylene-based decontaminants and corn oil.

shown to be present in cosmetics, and subsequent studies showed that these carcinogenic chemicals could be percutaneously absorbed [12].

Table 2 shows the relationship between percutaneous absorption and erythema for several oils used in cosmetics. The investigators attempted to correlate absorbability with erythema. The most-absorbed oil, isopropyl myristate, produced the most erythema. The lowest-absorbing oil, 2-hexyldecanoxyoctane, produced the least erythema. Absorbability and erythema for the other oils did not correlate [13]. The lesson to remember with percutaneous toxicity is that a toxic response requires both an inherent toxicity in the chemical and percutaneous absorption of the chemical. The degree of toxicity will depend on the contributions of both criteria.

In the rhesus monkey, the percutaneous absorption of safrole, a hepatocarcinogen,

TABLE 2 Relationship of Percutaneous Absorption and Erythema for Several Oils Used in Cosmetics

Absorbability (greatest to least)	Erythema
Isopropyl myristrate	++
Glycol tri(oleate)	−
n-Octadecane	±
Decanoxydecane	+
2-Hexyldecanoxyoctane	−

was 6.3% of applied dose. When the site of application was occluded, the percutaneous absorption doubled to 13.3%. Occlusion is a covering of the application site, either intentionally, as with a piece of plastic taped over the dosing site during experimentation, or unintentionally, as by putting on clothing after applying a cosmetic. The percutaneous absorption of cinnamic anthranilate was 26.1% of the applied dose, and this increased to 39.0% when the site of application was occluded. The percutaneous absorption of cinnamic alcohol with occlusion was 62.7%, and that of cinnamic acid with occlusion was 83.9% of the applied dose. Cinnamic acid and cinnamic aldehyde are agents that elicit contact urticaria [14], and cinnamic aldehyde is positive for both Draize and maximization methods [15,16].

In vivo human skin has the ability to metabolize chemicals. Figure 10 shows the metabolic profile of extracted human skin after pure hydroquinone had been dosed on the skin for 24 hours. The metabolic profile shows unchanged hydroquinone and its metabolite benzoquinone [3].

We have thus learned that common cosmetic ingredients can readily penetrate skin and become systemically available. If the cosmetic chemical has inherent toxicity, then that chemical will get into the body of a user and exert a toxic effect. Metabolically, the skin can also produce a more toxic compound.

The development of topical drug products requires testing for skin toxicology reactions. A variety of patch-test systems are available with which chemicals are applied to skin. A study was performed to determine the skin absorption of *p*-phenylenediamine (PPDA) from a variety of such systems. [^{14}C]PPDA (1% petrolatum UDP) was placed in a variety of patch-test systems at a concentration normalized to equal surface area (2 mg/

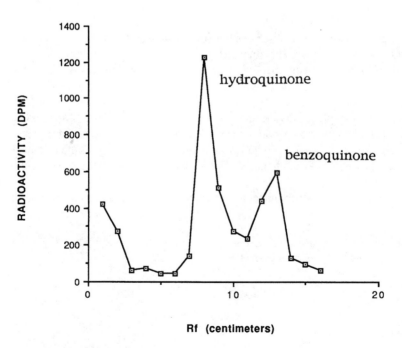

FIGURE 10   Hydroquinone dosed on viable skin was metabolically converted into the potential carcinogen benzoquinone within the human skin. The fate of a chemical within skin is more important than what is on the surface of skin.

TABLE 3 Percutaneous Absorption of *p*-Phenylenediamine (PPDA) from Patch-Test Systems

	Total load in chamber (mg)	Concentration in chamber (mg/mm²)	Absorption	
			Percent*	Total (mg)
Hill Top chamber	40	2	53.4 ± 20.6	21.4
Teflon (control)	16	2	48.6 ± 9.3	7.8
Small Finn chamber	16	2	29.8 ± 9.0	4.8
Large Finn chamber	24	2	23.1 ± 7.3	5.5
AL-test chamber	20	2	8.0 ± 0.8	1.6
Small Finn chamber with paper disc insert	16	2	34.1 + 19.8	5.5

* Each value is the mean + standard deviation for three guinea pigs.

mm²). Skin absorption was determined in the guinea pig by urinary excretion of ^{14}C. There was a sixfold difference in the range of skin absorption ($p < 0.02$). In decreasing order, the percentage skin absorption from the systems were 53.4 ± 20.6 (Hill Top chamber), 48.6 ± 9.3 (Teflon control patch), 23.1 + 7.3 (small Finn chamber), and 8.0 + 0.8 (AL-test chamber). Thus, the choice of patch system could produce a false-negative error if the system inhibits skin absorption, with a subsequent toxicology reaction (Table 3) [17].

COSMECEUTICS

The early concept of cosmetics was one of inert ingredients used as coloring or cover agents to enhance visual appearance. There was no concern with systemic toxicity because skin had barrier properites and it was assumed nothing would permeate across the skin. The line between cosmetics and pharmaceutics has become a gray area as more active agents are incorporated into cosmetics. These active agents are referred to as *cosmeceutics*. Hydroquinone when prescribed by a physician is a drug. Hydroquinone in a cosmetic as a lightening agent is not a drug. The only differentiation between the two preparations is the hydroquinone concentration in the preparation. However, applied concentration does not matter; what matters is how much of the hydroquinone gets into and through the skin. For hydroquinone, percutaneous absorption is 45% of the applied dose for a 24-hour application to in vivo human skin [3]. That is a lot of drug—or is it cosmetic, or cosmeceutic? The important point is that for active chemicals the bioavailability needs to be known to assess risk assessment.

Another example is α-tocopherol, or vitamin E [18]. The biological activities of vitamin E in cosmetics are supported by several studies of its percutaneous absorption. In data obtained in vitro on rat skin 6 hours after application of a 5% vitamin E alcohol solution, 38.6% of the applied dose was recovered in the viable epidermis and dermis. The amount detected in the horny layer was 7.12%, and the residual fraction persisting on the surface on the integument represented 54.3% of the applied dose. Both the alcohol and acetate forms of vitamin E are readily absorbed through the human scalp, and within 6 to 24 hours after treatment they concentrate in the dermis. These results substantiate the claim that vitamin E can be used as an active ingredient in cosmetology with the possibility of efficacy in the deeper structures of the skin. Table 4 summarizes the in vitro percutaneous absorption of vitamin E acetate into and through human skin. Each

TABLE 4 In Vitro Percutaneous Absorption of Vitamin E Acetate Into and Through Human Skin

	Percent dose absorbed		
Treatment	Receptor fluid	Skin content	Surface wash
Formula A			
Skin source 1	0.34	0.55	74.9
Skin source 2	0.39	0.66	75.6
Skin source 3	0.47	4.08	89.1
Skin source 4	1.30	0.96	110.0
Mean + SD	0.63 + 0.45*	1.56 + 1.69†	87.4 + 16.4
Formula B			
Skin source 1	0.24	0.38	—
Skin source 2	0.40	0.64	107.1
Skin source 3	0.41	4.80	98.1
Skin source 4	2.09	1.16	106.2
Mean + SD	0.78 + 0.87*	1.74 + 2.06†	103.8 + 5.0

* $p = 0.53$ (nonsignificant; paired t-test).
† $p = 0.42$ (nonsignificant; paired t-test).

formulation was tested in four different human skin sources. The percent dose absorbed for a 24-hour dosing period is given for receptor-fluid accumulation (absorbed), skin content, and surface wash (soap-and-water wash recovery after the 24-hour dosing period).

Table 4 also contains what is referred to as *material balance*. All of the applied dose is accounted for in the receptor fluid, skin content, and skin-surface wash. Total absorbed dose would be the sum of that in the receptor fluid plus that in the skin (content). This is an example of a complete in vitro percutaneous absorption study.

DISCUSSION

The concepts of cosmetics and of the skin have undergone changes in the last few decades. Cosmetics have evolved from being formulations of inert ingredients to containing ingredients that have some biological activity directed to living skin. This is sometimes referred to as cosmeceutics. The concept of skin has evolved from an impenetrable barrier to one where percutaneous absorption does occur. Risk assessment requires a knowledge of percutaneous absorption so that health is not jeopardized. This applies to any topically applied chemical, be it cosmetic, pharmaceutic, industrial, or environmental.

REFERENCES

1. Wester RC, Maibach HI. Cutaneous pharmacokinetics: 10 steps to percutaneous absorption. Drug Metab Rev 14:169–205, 1983.
2. Wester RC, Maibach HI. Percutaneous absorption of drugs. Clin Pharmacokin 23:253–266, 1992.
3. Wester RC, Melendres J, Hui X, Wester RM, Serranzana S, Zhai H, Quan D, Maibach HI. Human in vivo and in vitro hydroquinone topical bioavailability. J Toxicol Environ Health 54:301–317, 1998.

4. Wester RC, Maibach HI. Toxicokinetics: dermal exposure and absorption of toxicants. In: Bond J, ed. Comparative Toxicology, Vol. 1, General Principles. New York: Elsevier Sciences, 1997:99–114.

5. Feldmann RJ, Maibach HI. Percutaneous penetration of steroids in man. J Invest Dermatol 542:89–94, 1969.

6. Feldmann RJ, Maibach HI. Absorption of some organic compounds through the skin in man. J Invest Dermatol 54:399–404, 1970.

7. Feldmann RJ, Maibach HI. Percutaneous penetration of some pesticides and herbicides in man. Toxicol Appl Pharmacol 28:126–132, 1974.

8. Wester RC, Melendres J, Logan F, Maibach HI. Triple therapy: multiple dosing enhances hydrocortisone percutaneous absorption in vivo in humans. In: Smith E, Maibach HI, eds. Percutaneous Penetration Enhancers. Boca Raton: CRC Press, 1995:343–349.

9. Feldmann RJ, Maibach HI. Systemic absorption of pesticides through the skin of man. In: Occupational Exposure to Pesticides: Report to the Federal Working Group on Pest Management from the Task Group on Occupational Exposure to Pesticides. Appendix B, pp. 120–127.

10. Wester RC, Melendres J, Maibach HI. In vivo percutaneous absorption of alachlor in rhesus monkey. J Toxicol Environ Health 36:1–12, 1992.

11. Wester RC, Hui X, Landry T, Maibach HI. In vivo skin decontamination of metheylene bisphenyl isocyanate (MDI): soap and water ineffective compared to polypropylene glycol, polyglycol-based cleanser, and corn oil. Toxicol Sci 48:1–4, 1999.

12. Wester RC, Maibach HI. Comparative percutaneous absorption. In: Maibach HI, Boisits EK, eds. Neonatal Skin: Structure and Function. New York: Marcel Dekker, 1982:137–147.

13. Suzuki M, Asaba K, Komatsu H, Mockizuki M. Autoradiographic study on percutaneous absorption of several oils useful for cosmetics. J Soc Cosmet Chem 29:265–271, 1978.

14. von Krogh G, Maibach HI. The contact urticaria syndrome. In: Marzulli FN, Maibach HI, eds. Dermatotoxicology. Washington, D.C.: Hemisphere, 1983:301–322.

15. Marzulli FN, Maibach HI. Contact allergy: predictive testing in humans. In: Marzulli FN, Maibach HI, eds. Dermatotoxicology. Washington, D.C.: Hemisphere, 1983:279–299.

16. Marzulli FN, Maibach HI. Allergic contact dermatitis. In: Marzulli FN, Maibach HI, eds. Dermatotoxicology. Washington, D.C.: Taylor and Francis, 1996:143–146.

17. Kim HO, Wester RC, McMaster JA, Bucks DAW, Maibach HI. Skin absorption from patch test systems. Contact Dermat 17:178–180, 1987.

18. Wester RC, Maibach HI. Cosmetic percutaneous absorption. In: Baran R, Maibach HI, eds. Textbook of Cosmetic Dermatology. London: Martin Dunitz, 1998:75–83.

8

Principles and Mechanisms of Skin Irritation

Sibylle Schliemann-Willers and Peter Elsner
University of Jena, Jena, Germany

INTRODUCTION

In contrast to allergic contact dermatitis (ACD), irritant contact dermatitis (ICD) is the result of unspecified damage attributable to contact with chemical substances that cause an inflammatory reaction of the skin [1]. The clinical appearance of ICD is extremely variable. It is determined by the type of irritant and a dose-effect relationship [2]. The clinical morphology of acute irritant contact dermatitis as one side of the spectrum is characterized by erythema, edema, vesicles that may coalesce, bullae, and oozing. Necrosis and ulceration can be seen with corrosive materials. Clinical appearance of chronic ICD is dominated by redness, lichenification, excoriations, scaling, and hyperkeratosis.

Any site of skin may be affected. Most frequently the hands as human "tools" come into extensive contact with irritants, whereas most adverse reactions to cosmetics occur in the face because of the particular sensitivity of this skin region. Airborne ICD develops in uncovered skin areas, mostly in the face and especially the periorbital region after exposure to volatile irritants or vapor [3,4].

Despite their different pathogenesis, allergic and irritant contact dermatitis, particularly chronic conditions, show a remarkable similarity with respect to clinical appearance, histopathology [5,6], and immunohistology [7,8]. Therefore, ICD can be regarded as an exclusion diagnosis after negative patch testing. The histological pattern of chronic irritant contact dermatitis is characterized by hyper- and parakeratosis, spongiosis, exocytosis, moderate to marked acanthosis, and mononuclear perivascular infiltrates with increased mitotic activity [9,10].

MOLECULAR MECHANISMS OF SKIN IRRITANCY

As mentioned, striking clinical similarities exist between ICD and ACD, and even extensive immunostaining of biopsies does not allow discrimination between the two types of dermatitis [8].

In contrast to ACD, ICD lacks hapten-specific T-lymphocytes. The pathogenic pathway in the acute phases of ICD starts with the penetration of the irritant into the barrier, either activation or mild damage of keratinocytes, and release of mediators of inflammation with unspecific T-cell activation [11]. Epidermal keratinocytes play the crucial role in the inflammation of ICD; they can be induced to produce several cytokines and provoke a dose-dependent leukocyte attraction [12]. The upregulation of certain adhesion molecules like α6 integrin or CD 36 is independent from the stimulus and not cytokine induced [13,14]. A number of agents and cytokines themselves are capable of mediating cytokine production in keratinocytes. IL-1 and TNF-α play a role as inflammatory cytokines, IL-8 and IP-10 are known to act as chemotaxins, and IL-6, IL-7, IL-15, GM-CSF, and TGF-alpha can promote growth. Other cytokines, such as IL-10, IL-12, and IL-18, are known to regulate humoral versus cellular immunity [15]. It is controversial whether the cytokine profile induced by irritants differs from that induced by allergens [16]. In irritant reactions, TNF-alpha, IL-6, IL-1β, and IL-2 have been reported to be increased [17,18].

In subliminal contact to irritants, barrier function of the stratum corneum and not the keratinocyte is the main target of the insulting stimulus. Damage of the lipid barrier of the stratum corneum is associated with loss of cohesion of corneocytes and desquamation with increase of transepidermal water loss (TEWL). This is one triggering stimulus for lipid synthesis and it promotes barrier restoration [19]. Nevertheless, recent studies show that the concept of TEWL increase after sodium lauryl sulfate (SLS) being directly related to a delipidizing effect of surfactants on the stratum corneum cannot be kept up without limitation. Fartasch et al. showed that SLS exposure for 24 hours causes damage in the deeper nucleated cells of the epidermis, leaving the lamellar arrangements of lipids intact. This means that the hypothetical model of SLS-induced irritation is mainly modulated by keratinocytes rather than the stratum corneum [20].

The stratum corneum influences epidermal proliferation after contact to irritants by increasing the mitotic activity of basal keratinocytes and in this way enhancing the epidermal turnover [21,22]. Disruption of the stratum corneum can even stimulate cytokine production itself and in this way promote the inflammatory skin reaction, as shown by Wood et al. [23]. They found an increase of TNF-α, various interleukins, and granulocyte-macrophage colony-stimulating factor (GM-CSF).

Recently it has been shown that chemically different irritants induce differences in the response in the epidermis during the first 24 hours with respect to cytokine expression, indicating different "starting points" for the inflammatory response that results in the same irritant response clinically after 48 hours. Nonanionic acid, but not SLS, induced an increase in m-RNA expression for IL-6, whereas m-RNA expression for GM-CSF was increased after SLS [24]. Forsey et al. saw a proliferation of keratinocytes after 48 hours of exposure, and apoptosis of keratinocytes after 24 and 48 hours of exposure to SLS. In contrast, nonanionic acid decreased keratinocyte proliferation after 24 hours of exposure and epidermal cell apoptosis after only 6 hours of exposure [25]. In conclusion, it becomes clear that the concept of skin irritation is complicated and we are only beginning to understand the underlying molecular mechanisms.

FACTORS PREDISPOSING TO CUTANEOUS IRRITATION

The skin of different individuals differs in susceptibility to irritation in a remarkable manner, and a number of individual factors influencing development of irritant dermatitis that have been identified include age, genetic background, anatomical region exposed, and pre-existing skin disease.

Although experimental studies did not support sex differences of irritant reactivity [26,27], females turned out to be at risk in some epidemiological studies [28,29]. It is probable that increased exposure to irritants at home, caring for children under the age of 4 years, lack of dishwashing machine [30], and preference for high-risk occupations contribute to the higher incidence of ICD in females [27]. The most established individual risk factor, out of several studies about occupational hand eczema, is probably atopic dermatitis [28,31–33]. On the other hand, experimental studies concerning the reactivity of atopics and nonatopics to standard irritants have given contradictory results [34,35] and, as shown in a Swedish study, about 25% of the atopics in extreme-risk occupations, such as hairdressers and nursing assistants, did not develop hand eczema [36]. Age is as well related to irritant susceptibility insofar as irritant reactivity declines with increasing age. This is true not only for acute but also for cumulative irritant dermatitis [37,38]. Fair skin, especially skin type I, is supposed to be the most reactive to all types of irritants, and black skin is the most resistant [39,40].

Clinical manifestation of ICD is also influenced by type and concentration of irritant, solubility, vehicle, and length of exposure [41], as well as temperature and mechanical stress. During the winter months, low humidity and low temperature decrease the water content of the stratum corneum and increase irritant reactivity [42,43].

EPIDEMIOLOGY

Population-based data on the incidence and prevalence of ICD are rare, but there is agreement that incidence of ICD is higher than that of ACD in general. The figures on the incidence of ICD vary considerably, depending on the study population. Most data stem from studies about occupational hand dermatoses, and in this an overview is given about the important findings of these studies. In general, it can be assumed that nonoccupational contact dermatitis attributable to all causes is more frequent in comparison to occupational contact dermatitis [29].

Coenraads and Smit reviewed international prevalence studies for eczema attributable to all causes conducted with general populations in different countries (England, The Netherlands, Norway, Sweden, the United States) and found point prevalence rates of 1.7 to 6.3%, and 1- to 3-year period prevalence rates of 6.2 to 10.6% [44].

An extensive study of Meding on hand eczema in Gothenburg, Sweden, included 20,000 individuals randomly selected from the population register [28]. She estimated a 1-year period prevalence of hand eczema of 11% attributable to all causes, and a point prevalence of 5.4%. ICD contributed to 35% of the cases, whereas 22% were diagnosed as atopic hand dermatitis and 19% as ACD. In a multicenter epidemiological study on contact dermatitis in Italy by GIRDCA (Gruppo Italiano Ricerca Dermatiti da Contatto e Ambientali) 42,839 patients with contact dermatitis underwent patch testing. In accordance with the findings of Meding, nonoccupational as well as occupational ICD affected women in a higher percentage compared with males [28,29]. In Heidelberg, Germany, a retrospective study of 190 cases of hand dermatitis revealed 27% as ICD, 15,8% as ACD, and the majority (40%) as being of atopic origin with 10% various other diseases [45].

Shenefelt studied the frequency of visits by university students to campus prepaid–health-plan dermatologists for irritant and allergic contact dermatitis compared with other types of dermatitis and skin problems. In contrast to other studies, he found slightly more cases of allergic (3.1% of all first visits) than irritant contact dermatitis (2.3%) [46].

Reports on adverse reactions to cosmetics, including those with only subjective perceptions without morphological signs, are more frequent than assumed. In a questionnaire carried out in Thuringia, eastern Germany, even 36% of 208 persons reported adverse cutaneous reactions against cosmetics, 75% of them being female [47]. Nevertheless, it must be emphasized that this includes, in addition to allergic contact dermatitis, dermatoses as seborrheic dermatitis, perioral dermatitis, rosacea and psoriasis, which cannot be separated by the unexperienced. Higher incidence in females was confirmed by several studies [48]. Most untoward reactions caused by cosmetics occur on the face, including the periorbital area [49].

In a study by Broeckx et al., 5.9% of a test population of 5202 patients with possible contact dermatitis had adverse reactions to cosmetics. Patch testing classified only 1.46% as irritant reactions whereas 3.0% could be classified as ACD. More than 50% of the cases of irritation were attributable to soaps and shampoos [50]. In Sweden, the top-ranking products causing adverse effects, as reported by the Swedish Medical Products Agency, were moisturizers, haircare products, and nail products [48].

In other studies, the incidence of cosmetic intolerance varied between 2 and 8.3%, depending on the test population [49,51,52]. In a large multicenter prospective study on reactions caused by cosmetics, Eiermann et al. found irritancy to account for only 16% of 487 cases of contact dermatitis caused by cosmetics. Of 8093 patients tested for contact dermatitis, 487 cases (6%) were diagnosed as contact dermatitis caused by cosmetics [53]. Since most consumers just stop using cosmetics when experiencing mild irritant or adverse reactions and seldom consult a physician, it can be assumed that mild irritant reactions to cosmetic products are underestimated [54].

CLINICAL TYPES OF IRRITANT CONTACT DERMATITIS

According to the highly variable clinical picture, several different forms of ICD have been defined. The following types of irritation have been described [55,56]:

- Acute ICD
- Delayed acute ICD
- Irritant reaction
- Cumulative ICD
- Traumiterative ICD
- Exsiccation eczematid
- Traumatic ICD
- Pustular and acneiform ICD
- Nonerythematous
- Sensory irritation

Acute ICD

Acute ICD is caused by contact to a potent irritant. Substances that cause necrosis are called corrosive and include acids and alkaline solutions. Contact is often accidental at the workplace. Cosmetics are unlikely to cause this type of ICD because they do not contain primary irritants in sufficient concentrations.

Symptoms and clinical signs of acute ICD develop with a short delay of minutes to hours after exposure, depending on the type of irritant, concentration, and intensity of contact. Characteristically the reaction quickly reaches its peak and then starts to heal; this is called "decrescendo phenomenon." Symptoms include burning rather than itching, stinging, and soreness of the skin, and are accompanied by clinical signs such as erythema, edema, bullae, and even necrosis. Lesions are usually restricted to the area that came into contact, and sharply demarcated borders are an important sign of acute ICD. Nevertheless, clinical appearance of acute ICD can be highly variable and sometimes may even be indistinguishable from the allergic type. In particular, combination of irritant and allergic contact dermatitis can be troublesome. Prognosis of acute ICD is good if irritant contact is avoided.

Delayed Acute ICD

For some chemicals, such as anthralin, it is typical to produce a delayed acute ICD. Visible inflammation is not seen until 8 to 24 hours or more after exposure [57]. Clinical picture and symptoms are similar to acute ICD. Other substances that cause delayed acute ICD include dithranol, tretinoin, and benzalkonium chloride. Irritation to tretinoin can develop after a few days and results in a mild to fiery redness followed by desquamation, or large flakes of stratum corneum accompanied by burning rather than itching. Irritant patch-test reactions to benzalkonium chloride may be papular and increase with time, thus resembling allergic patch-test reactions [58]. Tetraethylene glycol diacrylate caused delayed skin irritation after 12 to 36 hours in several workers in a plant manufacturing acrylated chemicals [59].

Irritant Reaction

Irritants may produce cutaneous reactions that do not meet the clinical definition of a ''dermatitis.'' Irritant reaction is therefore a subclinical form of irritant dermatitis and is characterized by a monomorphic rather than polymorphic picture. This may include one or more of the following clinical signs: dryness, scaling, redness, vesicles, pustules, and erosions [60]. Irritant reactions often occur after intense water contact and in individuals exposed to wet work, such as hairdressers or metal workers, particularly during their first months of training. It often starts under rings worn on the finger or in the interdigital area, and may spread over the dorsum of the fingers and to the hands and forearms. Frequently, the condition heals spontaneously, resulting in hardening of the skin, but it can progress to cumulative ICD in some cases.

Cumulative ICD

Cumulative ICD is the most common type of ICD [55]. In contrast to acute ICD that can be caused by single contact to a potent irritant, cumulative ICD is the result of multiple subthreshold damage to the skin when time is too short for restoration of skin-barrier function [61]. Clinical symptoms develop after the damage has exceeded a certain manifestation threshold, which is individually determined and can vary within one individual at different times. Typically, cumulative ICD is linked to exposure of several weak irritants and water contact rather than to repeated exposure to a single potent irritant. Because the link between exposure and disease is often not obvious to the patient, diagnosis may be considerably delayed, and it is important to rule out an allergic cause. Symptoms include itching and pain caused by cracking of the hyperkeratotic skin. The clinical picture is dominated by dryness, erythema, lichenification, hyperkeratosis, and chapping. Xerotic dermatitis is the most frequent type of cumulative toxic dermatitis [62]. Vesicles are less frequent in comparison to allergic and atopic types [28]; however, diagnosis is often complicated by the combination of irritation and atopy, irritation and allergy, or even all three. Lesions are less sharply demarcated in contrast to acute ICD.

Prognosis of chronic cumulative ICD is rather doubtful [63,64]. Some investigators suggest that the repair capacity of the skin may enter a self-perpetuating cycle [61].

Traumiterative ICD

This term is often used similarly to cumulative ICD [55,60]. Clinically, the two types are very similar as well. According to Malten and den Arend, traumiterative ICD is a result of too-early repetition of just one type of load, whereas cumulative ICD results from too-early repetition of different types of exposures [2].

Exsiccation Eczematid

Exsiccation eczematid is a subtype of ICD that mainly develops on the extremities. It is often attributable to frequent bathing and showering as well as extensive use of soaps and cleansing products. It often affects elderly people with low sebum levels of the stratum corneum. Low humidity during the winter months and failure to remoisturize the skin contribute to the condition. The clinical picture is typical, with dryness, ichthyosiform scaling, and fissuring. Patients often suffer from intense itching.

Traumatic ICD

Traumatic ICD may develop after acute skin traumas such as burns, lacerations, and acute ICD. The skin does not heal as expected, but ICD with erythema, vesicles and/or papulovesicles, and scaling appears. The clinical course resembles that of nummular dermatitis [55].

Pustular and Acneiform ICD

Pustular and acneiform ICD may result from contact to irritants such as mineral oils, tars, greases, some metals, croton oil, and naphthalenes. Pustules are sterile and transient. The syndrome must be considered in conditions in which acneiform lesions develop outside typical acne age. Patients with seborrhoea, macroporous skin, and prior acne vulgaris are predisposed along with atopics.

Nonerythematous ICD

Nonerythematous ICD is an early stage of skin irritation that lacks visible inflammation but is characterized by changes in the function of the stratum corneum that can be measured by noninvasive bioengineering techniques [55,65].

Sensory Irritation

Sensory irritation is characterized by subjective symptoms without morphological changes. Predisposed individuals complain of stinging, burning, tightness, itching, or even painful sensations that occur immediately or after contact. Those individuals with hyperirritable skin often report adverse reactions to cosmetic products with most reactions occurring on the face. Fisher defined the term ''status cosmeticus,'' which describes a condition in patients who try a lot of cosmetics and complain of being unable to tolerate any of them [66]. Lactic acid serves as a model irritant for diagnosis of so called ''stingers'' when it is applied in a 5% aqueous solution on the nasolabial fold after induction of sweating in a sauna [67]. Other chemicals that cause immediate-type stinging after seconds or minutes include chloroform and methanol (1:1) and 95% ethanol. A number of substances that have been systematically studied by Frosch and Kligman may also cause delayed-type stinging [67,68]. Several investigators tried to determine parameters that characterize those individuals with sensitive skin, a term that still lacks a unique definition [69,70]. It could be shown that individuals who were identified as having sensitive skin by their own assessment have altered baseline biophysical parameters, showing decreased capacitance values, increased transepidermal water loss, and higher pH values accompanied by lower sebum levels [70]. Possible explanations for hyperirritability (other than diminished barrier function) that have been discussed are heightened neurosensory input attributable to altered nerve endings, more neurotransmitter release, unique central information processing or slower neurotransmitter removal, and enhanced immune responsiveness [69,71]. It is not clear whether having sensitive skin is an acquired or inherited condition; most probably it can be both. As in other forms of ICD, seasonal variability in stinging with a tendency to more intense responses during winter has been observed [72]. Detailed recommendations for formulation of skincare products for sensitive skin have been given by Draelos [69].

REFERENCES

1. Mathias CGT, Maibach HI. Dermatotoxicology monographs I. cutaneous irritation: factors influencing the response to irritants. Clin Toxicol 1978; 13:333–346.
2. Malten KE, den Arend JA. Irritant contact dermatitis. Traumiterative and cumulative impairment by cosmetics, climate, and other daily loads. Derm Beruf Umwelt 1985; 4:125–132.
3. Dooms-Goossens AE, Debusschere KM, Gevers DM, Dupre KM, Degref HJ, Loncke JP, Snauwaert JE. Contact dermatitis caused by airborne agents. A review and case reports. J Am Acad Dermatol 1986; 15:1–10.
4. Lachapelle JM. Industrial airborne irritant or allergic contact dermatitis. Contact Dermatitis 1986; 14:137–145.
5. Brand CU, Hunziker T, Braathen LR. Studies on human skin lymph containing Langerhans cells from sodium lauryl sulphate contact dermatitis. J Invest Dermatol 1992; 5:109s–110s.
6. Brand CU, Hunziker T, Limat A, et al. Large increase of Langerhans cells in human skin lymph derived from irritant contact dermatitis. Br J Dermatol 1993; 2:184–188.
7. Medenica M, Rostenberg A Jr. A comparative light and electron microscopic study of primary irritant contact dermatitis and allergic contact dermatitis. J Invest Dermatol 1971; 4:259–271.
8. Brasch J, Burgard J, Sterry W. Common pathogenetic pathways in allergic and irritant contact dermatitis. J Invest Dermatol 1992; 2:166–170.
9. Cohen LM, Skopicki DK, Harrist DJ, Clark WH. Noninfectious vesiculobullous and vesiculopustular diseases. In: Elder D, Elenitsas R, Jaworsky C, Johnson B, eds. Lever's Histopathology of the Skin. (8th ed.) Philadelphia: Lippincott-Raven, 1997:209–252.
10. Le TK, Schalkwijk J, van de Kerkhof PC, van Haelst U, van der Valk PG. A histological and immunhistochemical study on chronic irritant contact dermatitis. Am J Contact Dermat 1998; 9:23–28.
11. Berardesca E, Distante F. Mechanisms of skin irritation. In: Elsner P, Maibach HI, eds. Irritant Dermatitis: New Clinical and Experimental Aspects. Current Problems in Dermatology. Basel: Karger, 1995: 1–8.
12. Nickoloff BJ, Naidu Y. Perturbation of epidermal barrier function correlates with initiation of cytokine cascade in human skin. J Am Acad Dermatol 1994; 30:535–546.

13. Willis CM, Stephens CJ, Wilkinson JD. Epidermal damage induced by irritants in man: a light and electron microscopic study. J Invest Dermatol 1989; 93:695–699.
14. Jung K, Imhof BA, Linse R, Wollina U, Neumann C. Adhesion molecules in atopic dermatitis: upregulation of α6 integrin expression in spontaneous lesional skin as well as in atopen, antigen and irritative induced patch test reactions. Int Arch Allergy Immunol 1997; 113:495–504.
15. Corsini E, Galli CL. Cytokines and irritant contact dermatitis. Toxicol Lett 1998; 28:277–282.
16. Kalish RS. T cells and other leukocytes as mediators of irritant contact dermatitis. In: Beltrani VS, ed. Immunology and Allergy Clinics of North America. Contact Dermatitis. Irritant and Allergic. Philadelphia: W.B. Saunders Company 1997:407–415.
17. Larsen CG, Ternowitz T, Larsen FG, Zachariae CO, Thestrup-Pedersen K. ETAF/interleukin-1 and epidermal lymphocyte chemotactic factor in epidermis overlying an irritant patch test. Contact Dermatitis 1989; 20:335–340.
18. Hunziker T, Brand CU, Kapp A, Waelti ER, Braathen LR. Increased levels of inflammatory cytokines in human skin lymph derived from sodium lauryl sulphate-induced contact dermatitis. Br J Dermatol 1992; 127:254–257.
19. Grubauer G, Elias PM, Feingold KR: Transepidermal water loss: the signal for recovery of barrier structure and function. J Lipid Res 1989; 30:323–333.
20. Fartasch M, Schnetz E, Diepgen TL. Characterization of detergent-induced barrier alterations—effect of barrier cream on irritation. J Invest Dermatol Symp Proceed 1998; 3:121–127.
21. Fisher LB, Maibach HI. Effects of some irritants on human epidermal mitosis. Contact Dermatitis 1975; 1:273–276.
22. Wilhelm KP, Saunders JC, Maibach HI. Increased stratum corneum turnover induced by subclinical irritant dermatitis. Br J Dermatol 1990; 122:793–798.
23. Wood LC, Jackson SM, Elias PM, Grunfeld C, Feingold KR. Cutaneous barrier perturbation stimulates cytokine production in the epidermis of mice. J Clin Invest 1992; 90:482–487.
24. Grängsjö A, Leijon-Kuligowski A, Törmä H, Roomans GM, Lindberg M. Different pathways in irritant contact eczema? Early differences in the epidermal elemental content and expression of cytokines after application of 2 different irritants. Contact Dermatitis 1996; 35:355–360.
25. Forsey RJ, Shahidullah H, Sands C, McVittie E, Aldridge RD, Hunter JA, Howie SE. Epidermal Langerhans cell apoptosis is induced in vivo by nonanionic acid but not by sodium lauryl sulphate. Br J Dermatol 1998; 139:453–461.
26. Bjornberg A. Skin reactions to primary irritants in men and women. Acta Derm Venereol (Stockh) 1975; 55:191–194.
27. Hogan DJ, Dannaker CJ, Maibach HI. The prognosis of contact dermatitis. J Am Acad Dermatol 1990; 23:300–307.
28. Meding B. Epidemiology of hand eczema in an industrial city. Acta Derm Venereol Suppl (Stockh) 1990; 153:1–43.
29. Sertoli A, Francalanci S, Acciai MC, Gola M. Epidemiological survey of contact dermatitis in Italy (1984–1993) by GIRDCA (Gruppo Italiano Ricera Dermatiti da Contatto e Ambientali). Am J Contact Dermat 1999; 10:18–30.
30. Nilsson E. Individual and environmental risk factors for hand eczema in hospital workers. Acta Derm Venereol (Stockh) (Suppl) 1986; 128:1–63.
31. Wilhelm KP, Maibach HI. Factors predisposing to cutaneous irritation. Dermatol Clin 1990; 8:17–22.
32. Coenraads PJ, Diepgen TL. Risk for hand eczema in employees with past or present atopic dermatitis. Int Arch Occup Environ Health 1998; 71:7–13.
33. Berndt U, Hinnen U, Iliev D, Elsner P. Role of the atopy score and of single atopic features as risk factors for development of hand eczema in trainee metal workers. Br J Dermatol 1999; 140:922–924.

34. Gallacher G, Maibach HI. Is atopic dermatitis a predisposing factor for experimental acute irritant contact dermatitis? Contact Dermatitis 1998; 38:1–4.
35. Basketter DA, Miettinen J, Lahti A. Acute irritant reactivity to sodium lauryl sulfate in atopics and non-atopics. Contact Dermatitis 1998; 38:253–257.
36. Rysted I. Work-related hand eczema in atopics. Contact Dermatitis 1985; 12:164–171.
37. Suter-Widmer J, Elsner P. Age and irritation. In: van der Valk PGM, Maibach HI, eds. The Irritant Contact Dermatitis Syndrome. Boca Raton: CRC Press, 1994: 257–261.
38. Schwindt DA, Wilhelm KP, Miller DL, Maibach HI. Cumulative irritation in older and younger skin: a comparison. Acta Derm Venereol 1998; 78:279–283.
39. Lammintausta K, Maibach HI, Wilson D. Susceptibility to cumulative and acute contact dermatitis. Contact Dermatitis 1988; 19:84–90.
40. Maibach HI, Berardesca E. Racial and skin color differences in skin sensitivity: implications for skin care products. Cosmet Toilet 1990; 105:35–36.
41. Dahl MV. Chronic, irritant contact dermatitis: mechanisms, variables, and differentiation from other forms of contact dermatitis. Adv Dermatol 1988; 3:261–275.
42. Mozzanica N. Pathogenetic aspects of allergic and irritant contact dermatitis. Clin Dermatol 1992; 10:115–121.
43. Uter W, Gefeller O, Schwanitz HJ. An epidemiological study of the influence of season (cold and dry air) on the occurrence of irritant skin changes of the hands. Br J Dermatol 1998; 138: 266–272.
44. Coenraads PJ, Smit J. Epidemiology. In: Rycroft RJG, Menné T, Frosch PJ, eds. Textbook of Contact Dermatitis. (2nd ed.) Berlin: Springer, 1995:133–150.
45. Kühner-Piplack B. Klinik und Differentialdiagnose des Handekzems. Eine retrospektive Studie am Krankengut der Universitäts-Hautklinik Heidelberg 1982–1985. Thesis, Ruprecht-Karls-University, Heidelberg, Germany.
46. Shenefelt PD. Descriptive epidemiology of contact dermatitis in a university student population. Am J Contact Dermat 1996; 7:88–93.
47. Röpcke F. Auswertung zur Umfrage ''Epidemiologie von Kosmetika-Unverträglichkeiten— eine bevölkerungsbasierte Studie.'' 1999, unpublished data.
48. Berne B, Bostrom A, Grahnen AF, Tammela M. Adverse effects of cosmetics and toiletries reported to the Swedish Medical Products Agency 1989–1994. Contact Dermatitis 1996; 34: 359–362.
49. Adams RM, Maibach HI. A 5-year study of cosmetic reactions. J Am Acad Dermatol 1985; 13:1062–1069.
50. Broeckx W, Blondeel A, Dooms-Goossens A, Achten G. Cosmetic intolerance. Contact Dermatitis 1987; 16:189–194.
51. Skog E. Incidence of cosmetic dermatitis. Contact Dermatitis 1980; 6:449–451.
52. Romaguera C, Camarasa JMG, Alomar A, Grimalt F. Patch tests with allergens related to cosmetics. Contact Dermatitis 1983; 9:167–168.
53. Eiermann HJ, Larsen W, Maibach HI, Taylor JS. Prospective study of cosmetic reactions: 1977–1980. J Am Acad Dermatol 1982; 6:909–917.
54. Amin S, Engasser PG, Maibach HI. Adverse cosmetic reactions. In: Baran R, Maibach HI, eds. Textbook of Cosmetic Dermatology. 2nd ed. London: Martin Dunitz Ltd., 1998:709–746.
55. Lammintausta K, Maibach HI. Contact dermatitis due to irritation: General principles, etiology, and histology. In: Adams RM, ed. Occupational skin disease. Philadelphia: WB Saunders Company, 1990:1–15.
56. Berardesca E, Distante F. Mechanisms of skin irritation. In: Elsner P, Maibach HI, eds. Irritant dermatitis. New clinical and experimental aspects. Basel: Karger 1995:1–8.
57. Malten KE, den Arend JA, Wiggers RE. Delayed iritation: hexanediol diacrylate and butanediol diacrylate. Contact Dermatitis 1979; 3:178–184.
58. Bruynzeel DP, van Ketel WG, Scheper RJ, von Blomberg-van der Flier BME. Delayed time

course of irritation by sodium lauryl sulfate: observations on threshold reactions. Contact Dermatitis 1982; 8:236–239.

59. Nethercott JR, Gupta S, Rosen C, Enders LJ, Pilger CW. Tetraethylene glycol diacrylate. A cause of delayed cutaneous irritant reaction and allergic contact dermatitis. J Occup Med 1984; 26:513–516.

60. Frosch PJ. Cutaneous irritation. In: Rycroft RJG, Menné T, Frosch PJ, eds. Textbook of Contact Dermatitis. 2nd ed. Berlin: Springer, 1995:28–61.

61. Malten KE. Thoughts on irritant contact dermatitis. Contact Dermatitis 1981; 7:238–247.

62. Eichmann A, Amgwerd D. Toxische Kontaktdermatitis. Schweiz Rundsch Med Prax 1992; 19:615–617.

63. Keczkes K, Bhate SM, Wyatt EH. The outcome of primary irritant hand dermatitis. Br J Dermatol 1983; 109:665–668.

64. Elsner P, Baxmann F, Liehr HM. Metal working fluid dermatitis: A comparative follow-up study in patients with irritant and non-irritant dermatitis. In: Elsner P, Maibach HI, eds. Irritant Dermatitis: New Clinical and Experimental Aspects. Basel: Karger, 1995:77–86.

65. Van der Valk PGM, Maibach HI. Do topical corticosteroids modulate skin irritation in human beings? Assessment by transepidermal water loss and visual scoring. J Am Acad Dermatol 1989; 21:519–522.

66. Fisher AA. Cosmetic actions and reactions: therapeutic, irritant and allergic. Cutis 1980; 26: 22–29.

67. Frosch PJ, Kligman AM. A method for appraising the stinging capacity of topically applied substances. J Soc Cosm Chem 1977; 28:197–209.

68. Parrish JA, Pathak MA, Fitzpatrick TB. Facial irritation due to sunscreen products. Letter to the editor. Arch Dermatol 1975; 111:525.

69. Draelos ZD. Sensitive skin: perceptions, evaluation, and treatment. Am J Contact Dermat 1997; 8:67–78.

70. Seidenari S, Francomano M, Mantovani L. Baseline biophysical parameters in subjects with sensitive skin. Contact Dermatitis 1999; 38:311–315.

71. Muizzudin N, Marenus KD, Maes DH. Factors defining sensitive skin and its treatment. Am J Contact Dermat 1998; 9:170–175.

72. Leyden JJ. Risk assessment of products used on skin. Am J Contact Dermat 1993; 4:158–162.

9

Allergy and Hypoallergenic Products

An E. Goossens
University Hospital, Katholieke Universiteit Leuven, Leuven, Belgium

INTRODUCTION

The assessment and detection of the number of contact allergic reactions to cosmetics are not simple. Generally, a consumer who has a problem with cosmetics will consult a doctor only if he or she does not recognize the cause to be a particular cosmetic product or if the dermatitis persists when the suspect product has been replaced by another, determined by trial and error. Consequently, only a small proportion of the population with cosmetic intolerance problems is ever seen by a dermatologist. Moreover, cosmetic reactions may present in unusual clinical forms, which may evoke an erroneous diagnosis [1–3].

In general, adverse effects are underreported [4], certainly to the cosmetics industry which obtains its most reliable information in this regard mainly from the relatively few dermatologists who concentrate on cosmetic-intolerance problems and from reports in the literature which are, almost by definition, out of date. Sometimes beauticians and consumers report adverse reactions, but in most cases this kind of information is difficult to objectify unless it is verified by a dermatologist.

Application of cosmetic products to the skin may cause irritant, phototoxic, contact, and photocontact allergic reactions as well as contact urticaria. It is generally agreed that most skin-adverse reactions to cosmetic products are irritant in nature and that people with "sensitive skin," as indicated by conditions like atopic dermatitis, rosacea, or seborrheic dermatitis, are particularly liable to develop such reactions. However, contact allergic reactions attract much more attention and thus tend to be overestimated [4]. Indeed, the identification of the cosmetic allergen is by no means a simple task. It demands special skills and interest on the part of the dermatologist, even though the labeling of all cosmetic ingredients, which is now obligatory also in Europe, is facilitating that task. Moreover, there are many factors involved in the sensitization to a specific cosmetic product, all of which have to be taken into account when one seeks an allergen [1,2] (see the following section).

FACTORS CONTRIBUTING TO CONTACT ALLERGIC REACTIONS TO A COSMETIC PRODUCT

Frequency of Use

One may expect frequently used products to cause more skin reactions than more exclusive products simply because more people are exposed to them. This alone does not imply anything about the quality of these products (the same thing may be said about individual cosmetic ingredients).

Composition

The complexity of a formula can be either positive or negative as far as its allergenicity is concerned. One of the principles of creating "hypoallergenic" cosmetics and perfumes is simplicity of formula. The fewer the constituents, the easier it is to identify the offending substance should difficulties arise, and the less danger there is of synergism. The more ingredients there are, the more chance there is of sensitization by one of them. However, some investigators recommend placing upper limits on concentrations rather than advising against the use of any particular ingredient. They may also suggest more complex formulas [5].

Preservatives are needed in water-based or other easily contaminated products and are common cosmetic allergens. It seems that it is very difficult to combine potent antimicrobial and antifungal properties with low allergenicity. Indeed, it is very difficult to restrict the biological activity of a substance to a single domain.

Concentration of Ingredients

Although the use of low concentrations does not assure complete safety, the incidence of sensitization induction is, indeed, a function of the concentration of the allergen, at least to some extent. Cases of allergy to the preservative agent (chloro)methylisothiazolinone illustrate this problem very well. At first, when a 50 ppm concentration of this agent was allowed for use in cosmetic products in the European Community and when this concentration was actually used in some products, there were "epidemics" of contact allergic reactions to it [6]. Of late, the frequency of positive reactions has been diminishing considerably, not only because its use is declining and primarily limited to "rinse-off" products [3] but also because its usage concentration has been reduced to 15 to 7.5 ppm (as the manufacturers recommended). Of course, once a patient has become sensitized, even low concentrations can trigger a reaction.

Purity of Ingredients

It is impossible to refine raw materials to absolute purity. More or less strict quality control of raw materials and finished products has long been general practice in modern cosmetic manufacturing. However, one can never rule out the sensitizing potential of impurities in these materials [5].

The Common Use of Cosmetic Ingredients in Pharmaceuticals

Patients easily become sensitized to topical pharmaceutical products which, unlike cosmetics, are most often used on diseased skin. Once sensitization has occurred, however, they may react to cosmetics containing the same ingredients [5].

The Role of Cross-Sensitivity

Chemically related substances are likely to induce cross-reactions and contact eczematous lesions may be maintained in this way. This is especially the case with perfume ingredients, which often cross-react with each other, but applies to all other cosmetic ingredients as well.

Penetration-Enhancing Substances

The chemical environment can substantially affect the sensitizing potential of individual chemicals. For example, emulsifiers and solvents enhance skin penetration and thereby contact sensitization. Penetration-enhancing agents can also be the root of false-negative patch-test reactions; the cosmetic product itself may be clearly allergenic (or irritant) although the individual ingredients, abstracted from the environment of the product and tested separately, may not cause a reaction.

Application Site

Some areas of the skin, like the eyelids, are particularly prone to contact dermatitis reactions. A cream applied to the entire face such as a facecare product, along with hair products may cause an allergic reaction only on the eyelids. Moreover, "ectopic dermatitis" [caused by the transfer of the allergen by the hand, as often occurs with tosylamide/formaldehyde (= para-toluenesulfonamideformaldehyde) resin, the allergen in nail polish], "airborne" contact dermatitis (e.g., caused by perfumes) [7], as well as "connubial" dermatitis (caused by products used by the partner) [8] often occur only on "sensitive" skin areas such as the eyelids, the lips, and the neck.

Moreover, the penetration potential of cosmetics is heightened in certain "occluded" areas, such as the body folds (axillary, inguinal) and the anogenital region, which also increases the risk of contact sensitization. In the body folds, the allergenic reactions tend to persist for weeks after the initial contact with the allergen. This may be partly attributable to residual contamination of clothing as well as the increased penetration of the allergen, which is certainly assisted by occlusion and friction [9]. Indeed, a reservoir may be formed from which the allergen is subsequently released.

Condition of the Skin

Application on damaged skin, where the skin barrier is impaired, enhances the penetration of substances and thus increases the risk of an allergic reaction. This is the case with bodycare products used to alleviate dry, atopic skin and with barrier creams for protecting the hands, which often suffer from irritancy problems (e.g., dryness, cracking). Sometimes, the allergic reaction may be limited to certain areas of the skin (areas already affected react more readily to another application of the same allergen) and may even present an unusual clinical picture that does not immediately suggest contact dermatitis. Indeed, contact allergic reactions to preservative agents on the face may present as a lymphocytic infiltrate or even have a lupus erythematous–like picture [3,10].

Contact Time

In the world of cosmetics, a distinction is now being made between leave-on products, which remain on the skin for several hours (e.g., face- and bodycare products and makeup), and rinse-off products, which are removed almost immediately.

The division between these two kinds of products is not always relevant to the sensitization process because a thin film can remain on the skin and be sufficient to allow ingredients to penetrate. This occurs, for example, with moist toilet paper (with mainly preservatives as the allergens) and makeup removers.

Frequency of Application and Cumulative Effects

Daily use or use several times a day of cosmetics may cause ingredients to accumulate in the skin and thus increase the risk of adverse reactions. In fact, the concentration of an ingredient may be too low to induce sensitivity in a single product but may reach critical levels in the skin if several products containing it are used consecutively. This may be the case for people who are loyal to the same brand of, e.g., day and night creams, foundations, and cleansing products, because a manufacturer will often use the same pre-servative system for all of its products. This should be taken into consideration by compa-nies that use biologically active ingredients such as preservative agents, emulsifiers, anti-oxidants, and perfumes, because it might well account for many of the adverse reactions to these particular substances. In our experience, intense users of cosmetics are more prone to cosmetic dermatitis than others.

CORRELATIONS WITH THE LOCATION OF THE LESIONS

Like many other contact allergens, cosmetics can reach the skin in several different ways [1,2]: by direct application; by airborne exposure to vapors, droplets, or particles that are released into the atmosphere and then settle on the skin [7]; by contact with people (part-ners, friends, coworkers) who transmit allergens to cause "connubial" or "consort" der-matitis [8]; by transfer from other sites on the body, often the hands, to more sensitive areas such as the mouth or the eyelids (ectopic dermatitis); and by exposure to the sun with photoallergens.

The most common sources of cosmetic allergens applied directly to the body are listed in Table 1.

THE NATURE OF COSMETIC ALLERGENS

Fragrance Ingredients

Fragrance ingredients are the most frequent culprits in cosmetic allergies [11–15]. Katsarar et al., who investigated the results of patch testing over a 12-year period, found an increas-ing trend in sensitivity to fragrance compounds, which reflects the effectiveness of the advertising of perfumed products [16]. Common features of a fragrance contact dermatitis are localization in the axillae, localization on the face (including the eyelids) and neck, and well-circumscribed patches in areas of dabbing-on perfumes (wrists, behind the ears) and hand eczema or its aggravation. Airborne or connubial contact dermatitis should be considered as well.

Other less frequent adverse reactions to fragrances are photocontact dermatitis, con-tact urticaria, irritation, and pigmentation disorders [17].

Sensitization is most often induced by highly perfumed products, such as toilet wa-ters, aftershave lotions, and deodorants, the last of which have recently been shown to contain well-known allergens such as cinnamic aldehyde and iso-eugenol [18].

TABLE 1 Cosmetic and Cosmetic-Related Dermatitis Caused by Direct Application of the Allergen

Area of dermatitis	Cosmetics that may contain allergens
Face in general	Facial skincare products (creams, lotions, masks), sunscreen products, makeup (foundations, blushes, powders), cleansers (lotions, emulsions), and cosmetic appliances (sponges), perfumed products (after-shave lotion)
Forehead	Haircare products (dyes, shampoos)
Eyebrows	Eyebrow pencil, depilatory tweezers
Upper eyelids	Eye makeup (eye shadow, eye pencils, mascara), eyelash curlers
Lower eyelids	Eye makeup
Nostrils	Perfumed handkerchiefs
Lips, mouth, and perioral area	Lipstick, lip pencils, dental products (toothpaste, mouthwash), depilatories
Neck and retroauricular area	Perfumes, toilet waters, haircare products
Head	Haircare products (hair dyes, permanent-wave solutions, bleaches, shampoo ingredients), cosmetic appliances (metal combs, hairpins)
Ears	Haircare products, perfume
Trunk/upper chest, arms, wrists (elbow flexures)	Bodycare products, sunscreens and self-tanning products, cleansers, depilatories
Axillae	Deodorants, antiperspirants, depilatories
Anogenital areas	Deodorants, moist toilet paper, perfumed pads, depilatories
Hands	Handcare products, barrier creams, all cosmetic products that come in contact with the hands
Feet	Footcare products, antiperspirants

As reported in the literature, the fragrance mix remains the best screening agent for contact allergy to perfumes because it detects some 70 to 80% of all perfume allergies [19,20]. However, additional perfume-allergy markers are certainly needed.

Preservatives

Preservatives are second in frequency to fragrance ingredients; they are important allergens in cleansers, skincare products, and makeup [12,21]. However, within this class important shifts have occurred over the years.

The methyl(chloro)isothiazolinone mixture was commonly used in the 1980s and was then a frequent cause of contact allergies. This frequency has declined considerably in recent years [3,12]. Since then, formaldehyde and its releasers—particularly methyldibromoglutaronitrile (=dibromodicyanobutane) as used in a mixture with phenoxyethanol, better known as EUXYL K400—did gain in importance in this regard [12,21–25], although the frequency of positive reactions observed seems to be influenced by the patch-test concentration [24,25].

The spectrum of the allergenic preservatives also varies from country to country. For example, in contrast to continental Europe where reactions to methyl(chloro)isothiazolinone and more recently methyldibromoglutaronitrile have been the most frequent, [12,13,21,26], in the United Kingdom formaldehyde and its releasers have always been much more important, particularly as concerns quaternium-15 [21] although its incidence seems to have recently slightly decreased [27]. Parabens are rare causes of cosmetic dermatitis. When a paraben allergy does occur, the sensitization source is most often a topical pharmaceutical product, although its presence in other products can be sensitizing as well [28]. Recently, we observed such a case (data on file): a young lady, after having previously been sensitized to mefenesin in a rubefacient, presented with an acute contact dermatitis on the face at the first application of a new cosmetic cream containing chlorphenesin, which was used as a preservative agent. Apparently it is a potential sensitizing agent [29] and probably cross-reacts with mefenesin, which is used in pharmaceuticals.

Antioxidants

Antioxidants form only a minor group of cosmetic allergens. Examples are propyl gallate, which may cross-react with other gallates and are also used as food additives, and t-butyl hydroquinone, a well-known allergen in the United Kingdom but not in continental Europe [21].

"Active" or Category-Specific Ingredients

With regard to "active" or category-specific ingredients, in contrast to de Groot [3] we found an increase of the number of reactions to oxidative hair dyes (PPD and related compounds) during the period 1991–1996 compared with the period 1985–1990 [12,13]. According to one cosmetic manufacturer (personal communication, L'Oréal, 1997), the use of such hair dyes has more than doubled in recent years. However, the replacement since 1987 of PPD-hydrochloride by PPD-base—a more appropriate screening agent for PPD-allergy—may also have influenced the incidence [30]. They are important causes of professional dermatitis in hairdressers, who also often react to allergens in bleaches (persulfates, also causes of contact urticaria), permanent-wave solutions (primarily glycerylmonothioglycolate, which may provoke cross-sensitivity to ammoniumthioglycolate), and sometimes shampoos (e.g., cocamidopropylbetaine and formaldehyde) [31,32]. Sodium pyrosulfite (or metabisulfite), present in oxidative hair dyes (data on file), was recently also found to be a professional allergen.

Tosylamide/formaldehyde (=toluenesulfonamide formaldehyde) resin is considered an important allergen [4] and is the cause of "ectopic" dermatitis attributable to nail lacquer, which may also contain epoxy and (meth)acrylate compounds [3]. It often gives rise to confusing clinical pictures and may mimic professional dermatitis [33].

(Meth)acrylates are also causes of reactions to artificial nail preparations, more recently to gel formulations, in both manicurists and their clients [34].

Moreover, some more recently introduced "natural" ingredients may induce contact-allergic reactions. Some examples are butcher broom (*Ruscus aculateus*), which is also a potential allergen in topical pharmaceutical products [35], hydrocotyl (asiaticoside) [36], and dexpanthenol [37]. Farnesol, a well-known perfume ingredient and cross-reacting agent to balsam of Peru, has become a potential allergen in deodorants in which it is used for its bacteriostatic properties [38].

Some sunscreen agents such as benzophenone-3, which may also cause contact urticaria, and dibenzoylmethane derivatives have been recognized in the past as being important allergens [3,21,39–41]. Indeed, isopropyldibenzoylmethane was even withdrawn for this reason [3]. Methylbenzylidene camphor, cinnamates, and phenylbenzimidazole sulfonic acid are only occasional, sometimes even rare, causes of cosmetic reactions. The use of para-aminobenzoic acid (PABA) and its derivatives has decreased considerably. Contact allergic reactions to them were generally related to their chemical relationship to para-amino compounds [42], although they were also important photosensitizers [39].

In our experience [12,13,21], the contribution of sunscreens to cosmetic allergy is relatively small despite the increase in their use because of media attention being given to the carcinogenic and accelerated skin-aging effects of sunlight. The low rate of allergic reactions observed may well be because a contact allergy or a photoallergy to sunscreen products is often not recognized, since a differential diagnosis with a primary sun intolerance is not always obvious. Furthermore, the patch-test concentrations generally used might be too low [43], in part because of the risk of irritancy.

Excipients and Emulsifiers

Many excipients and emulsifiers are common ingredients to topical pharmaceutical and cosmetic products, the former being likely to induce sensitization. Typical examples are wool alcohols, fatty alcohols (e.g., cetyl alcohol), and propylene glycol [13]. They may also be sensitizing in cosmetics, as is the case with maleated soybean oil [44]. Emulsifiers in particular have long been regarded as irritants, but their sensitization capacities should not be overlooked. It is imperative, of course, that patch testing be properly performed to avoid irritancy and that the relevance of the positive reactions be determined. This is certainly the case for cocamidopropylbetaine, an amphoteric tenside mainly present in hair-and skin-cleansing products. Whether the compound itself or cocamidopropyl dimethylamine, an amido-amine, or dimethylaminopropylamine (both intermediates from the synthesis) are the actual sensitizers is still a matter of discussion [45,46]. It is also not clear whether cocamidopropyl-PG-dimonium chloride phosphate (phospholipid PTC) [47], a new allergen in skincare products, can cross-react with cocamidopropylbetaine.

Coloring Agents

Coloring agents other than hair dyes have rarely been reported as cosmetic allergens. However, with the increased use of cosmetic tattoos (e.g., eye and lip makeup), more treatment-resistant skin lesions might develop in the future [48].

DIAGNOSING COSMETIC ALLERGY

Taking the history of the patient and noting the clinical symptoms and localization of the lesions are critical. Allergen identification for a patient with a possible contact allergy to cosmetics is performed by means of patch testing with the standard series, specific cosmetic-test series, the product itself, and all its ingredients. We can only find the allergens we look for. For skin tests with cosmetic products the patients supply themselves, there are several guidelines [49]. Not only patch and photopatch tests but also semiopen tests, usage tests, or repeated open application tests (ROATs) may need to be performed to obtain a correct diagnosis.

HYPOALLERGENIC PRODUCTS

Most of the cosmetic industry is making a great effort to commercialize products that are the safest possible. Some manufacturers market cosmetics containing raw materials having a "low" sensitization index or a high degree of purity, or from which certain components have been eliminated [5,50] (generally perfume ingredients). Sometimes "active" preservative agents are also omitted, and immunologically inert physical agents are being used more often in sunscreens rather than chemical ultraviolet (UV) absorbants.

Statements such as "recommended by dermatologists," "allergy-tested," or "hypoallergenic" have been put on packaging by manufacturers to distinguish their products from those of their competitors. Although there are several ways to reduce allergenicity [3], there are no governmentally mandated standards or industry requirements [51].

The latest trend is target marketing to people with hypersensitive skin—an often-used term for the shadowy zone between normal and pathological skin. These would be people with increased neurosensitivity (e.g., atopics), heightened immune responsiveness (e.g., atopic and contact allergic individuals), or a defective skin barrier, i.e., people with irritable skin such as atopics or those suffering from seborrheic dermatitis [52] or rosacea. This means that part of the cosmetic industry is moving more into the area of pathological skin and that certain products are in fact becoming drugs, often called cosmeceuticals. This has caused a great deal of regulatory concern [53,54] both in the United States and the European Union because it suggests some middle category between cosmetics and drugs that does not yet legally exist. In Japan, however, these products fall in the category of "quasidrugs."

The meaning of most such claims used nowadays is unclear both for the dermatologist [50–52] and the consumer, the latter being convinced that hypersensitive skin is allergic skin. It is the dermatologist's task to diagnose the skin condition and to provide specific advice about the products that can safely be used. All such problems must be approached individually, not at least the contact allergic types because people sensitive to specific ingredients must avoid products containing them. Therefore, ingredient labeling, which is also now required in Europe, can be of tremendous help. Providing the allergic patient with a limited list of cosmetics that can be used is practical and effective [55].

CONCLUSION

The identification of cosmetic allergens is challenging because of the extreme complexity of the problem. This applies not only for the dermatologist who is trying to identify the culprit and advise his patient but also certainly for cosmetic manufacturers, who are extremely concerned about assuring the innocuousness of their products. Precise, current, and rapid information about adverse reactions to cosmetic products is critical in product design. Apparently, premarketing studies are unable to identify all the pitfalls. Therefore, the fruitful communication that is developing between dermatologists and cosmetic manufacturers must be encouraged. Sensitivity to cosmetics can never be totally avoided, but its incidence can be substantially reduced.

REFERENCES

1. Dooms-Goossens A. Contact allergy to cosmetics. Cosmetics & Toiletries 1993; 108:43–46.
2. Dooms-Goossens A. Cosmetics as causes of allergic contact dermatitis. Cutis 1993; 52:316–320.
3. de Groot AC. Fatal attractiveness: the shady side of cosmetics. Clin Dermatol 1998; 16:167–179.
4. Berne B, Boström A, Grahnén AF, Tammela M. Adverse effects of cosmetics and toiletries

reported to the Swedish medical products agency 1989–1994. Contact Dermatitis 1996; 34: 359–362.

5. Dooms-Goossens A. Reducing sensitizing potential by pharmaceutical and cosmetic design. J Am Acad Dermatol 1984; 10:547–553.

6. Pasche E, Hunziker N. Sensitization to Kathon CG in Geneva and Switzerland. Contact Dermatitis 1989; 20:115–119.

7. Dooms-Goossens AE, Debusschere KM, Gevers DM, Dupré KM, Degreef H, Loncke JP, Snauwaert JE. Contact dermatitis caused by airborne agents. J Am Acad Dermatol 1989; 15: 1–10.

8. Morren M-A, Rodrigues R, Dooms-Goossens A, Degreef H. Connubial contact dermatitis. Eur J Dermatol 1992; 2:219–223.

9. Dooms-Goossens A, Dupré K, Borghijs A, Swinnen C, Dooms M, Degreef H. Zinc ricinoleate: sensitizer in deodorants. Contact Dermatitis 1987; 16:292–293.

10. Morren M-A, Dooms-Goossens A, Delabie J, Dewolf-Peeters C, Mariën K, Degreef H. Contact allergy to isothiazolinone derivatives. Dermatologica 1992; 198:260–264.

11. Adams RM, Maibach HI. A five-year study of cosmetic reactions. J Am Acad Dermatol 1985; 13:1062–1069.

12. Goossens A, Merckx L. l'Allergie de contact aux cosmétiques. Allergie et Immunologie 1997; 29:300–303.

13. Dooms-Goossens A, Kerre S, Drieghe J, Bossuyt L, Degreef H. Cosmetic products and their allergens. Eur J Dermatol 1992; 2:465–468.

14. Berne B, Lundin A, Enander Malmros P. Side effects of cosmetics and toiletries in relation to use: a retrospective study in a Swedish population. Eur J Dermatol 1994; 4:189–193.

15. de Groot AC, Nater JP, van der Lende R, Rijcken B. Adverse effects of cosmetics: a retrospective study in the general population. Int J Cosm Science 1987; 9:255–259.

16. Katsarar A, Kalogeromitros D, Armenaka M, Koufou V, Davou E, Koumantaki E. Trends in the results of patch testing to standard allergens over the period 1984–1995. Contact Dermatitis 1997; 37:245–246.

17. de Groot AC, Frosch PJ. Adverse reaction to fragrances. Contact Dermatitis 1997; 36: 57–86.

18. Rastogi SC, Johansen JD, Frosch P, Menné T, Bruze M, Lepoittevin J-P, Dreier B, Andersen KE, White IR. Deodorants on the European market: quantitative chemical analysis of 21 fragrances. Contact Dermatitis 1998; 38:29–35.

19. Johansen JD, Menné T. The fragrance mix and its constituents: a 14-year material. Contact Dermatitis 1995; 32:18–23.

20. Frosch PJ, Pilz B, Andersen KE, Burrows D, Camarasa JG, Dooms-Goossens A, Ducombs G, Fuchs T, Hannuksela M, Lachapelle J-M, Lahti A, Maibach HI, Menné T, Rycroft RJG, Shaw S, Wahlberg JE, White IR, Wilkinson JD. Patch testing with fragrances: results of a multicenter study of the European Environmental and Contact Dermatitis Research Group with 48 frequently used constituents of perfumes. Contact Dermatitis 1995; 33:333–342.

21. Goossens A, Beck M, Haneke E, McFadden J, Nolting S, Durupt G, Ries G. Cutaneous reactions to cosmetic allergens. Contact Dermatitis 1999; 40:112–113.

22. de Groot AC, de Cock PAJJM, Coenraads PJ, van Ginkel CJW, Jagtman BA, van Joost T, van der Kley AMJ, Meinardi MMHM, Smeenk G, van der Valk PGM, van der Walle HB, Weyland JW. Methyldibromoglutaronitrile is an important contact allergen in the Netherlands. Contact Dermatitis 1996; 34:118–120.

23. Okkerse A, Geursen-Reitsma AM, Van Joost T. Contact allergy to methyldibromoglutaronitrile and certain other preservatives. Contact Dermatitis 1996; 34:151–152.

24. Corazza M, Mantovani L, Roveggio C, Virgili A. Frequency of sensitization to Euxyl K400 in 889 cases. Contact Dermatitis 1993; 28:298–299.

25. Tosti A, Vincenzi C, Trevisi P, Guerra L, Euxyl K400: incidence of sensitization, patch test concentration and vehicle. Contact Dermatitis 1995; 33:193–195.

26. Perrenoud D, Birchner A, Hunziker T, Suter H, Bruckner-Tuderman L, Stäger J, Thürlimann W, Schmid P, Suard A, Hunziker N. Frequency of sensitization to 13 common preservatives in Switzerland. Contact Dermatitis 1994; 30:276–279.

27. Jacobs M-C, White IR, Rycroft RJG, Taub N. Patch testing with preservatives at St. John's from 1982–1993. Contact Dermatitis 1995; 33:247–254.

28. Verhaeghe I, Dooms-Goossens A. Multiple sources of allergic contact dermatitis from parabens. Contact Dermatitis 1997; 36:269–270.

29. Wakelin SH, White IR. Dermatitis from Chlorphenesin in a facial cosmetic. Contact Dermatitis 1997; 37:138–139.

30. Dooms-Goossens A, Scheper RJ, Andersen KE, Burrows D, Camarasa JG, Frosch PJ, Lahti A, Wilkinson J. Comparative patch testing with PPD-base and PPD-dihydrochloride: human and animal data compiled by the European Environmental Contact Dermatitis Research Group. In: Frosch PJ, Dooms-Goossens A, Lachapelle J-M, Rycroft RJG, eds. Current Topics in Contact Dermatitis. Berlin, Heidelberg: Springer-Verlag, 1989:281–285.

31. Frosch PJ, Burrows D, Camarasa JG, Dooms-Goossens A, Ducombs G, Lahti A, Menné T, Rycroft RJG, Shaw S, White IR, Wilkinson JD. Allergic reactions to a hairdressers' series: results from 9 European centers. Contact Dermatitis 1993; 28:180–183.

32. Holness DL, Nethercott JR. Epicutaneous testing results in hairdressers. Am J Contact Dermatitis 1990; 1:224–234.

33. Liden C, Berg M, Färm G, Wrangsjö K. Nail varnish allergy with far-reaching consequences. Br J Derm 1993; 128:57–62.

34. Kanerva L, Lauerma A, Estlander T, Alanko K, Henriks-Eckerman ML, Jolanki R. Occupational allergic contact dermatitis caused by photobonded sculptured nail and a review of (meth)acrylates in nail cosmetics. Am J Contact Dermatitis 1996; 7:109–115.

35. Landa N, Aguirre A, Goday J, Ratón JA, Díaz-Pérez JL. Allergic contact dermatitis from a vasoconstrictor cream. Contact Dermatitis 1990; 22:290–291.

36. Santucci B, Picardo M, Cristando A. Contact dermatitis to Centelase®. Contact Dermatitis 1985; 13:39.

37. Stables GI, Wilkinson SM. Allergic contact dermatitis to panthenol. Contact Dermatitis 1998; 38:236–237.

38. Goossens A, Merckx L. Allergic contact dermatitis from farnesol in a deodorant. Contact Dermatitis 1997; 37:179–180.

39. Gonçalo M, Ruas E, Figueiredo A, Gonçalo S. Contact and photocontact sensitivity to sunscreens. Contact Dermatitis 1995; 33:278–280.

40. Berne B, Ros A-M. 7 years experience of photopatch testing with sunscreen allergens in Sweden. Contact Dermatitis 1998; 38:61–64.

41. Schauder S, Ippen H. Photoallergische and allergisches Kontaktekzem durch dibenzoylmethanverbindungen und andere lichtschutzfilter. Hautarzt 1988; 39:435–440.

42. Theeuwes M, Degreef H, Dooms-Goossens A. Para-aminobenzoic acid (PABA) and sunscreen allergy. Am J Contact Dermatitis 1992; 3:206–207.

43. Ricci C, Vaccari S, Cavalli M, Vincenzi C. Contact sensitization to sunscreens. Am J Contact Dermatitis 1997; 8:165–166.

44. Dooms-Goossens A, Buyse L, Stals H. Maleated soybean oil, a new cosmetic allergen. Contact Dermatitis 1995; 32:49–51.

45. Pigatto PD, Bigardi AS, Cusano F. Contact dermatitis to cocamidopropyl betaine is caused by residual amines: relevance, clinical characteristics and review of the literature. Am J Contact Dermatitis 1995; 6:13–16.

46. Fowler JF, Fowler LM, Hunter JE. Allergy to cocamidopropyl betaine may be due amidoamine: a patch and product use test study. Contact Dermatitis 1997; 37:276–281.

47. Lorenzi S, Placucci F, Vincenzi C, Tosti A. Contact sensitisation to cocamido-propyl-PG-dimonium chloride phosphate in a cosmetic cream; Contact Dermatitis 1996; 34:149–150.

48. Duke D, Urioste SS, Dover JS, Andersen RR. A reaction to a red lip cosmetic tattoo. J Am Acad Dermatol 1998; 39:488–490.

49. Dooms-Goossens A. Testing without a kit. In: Guin JD, ed. Handbook of Contact Dermatitis. New-York: McGraw-Hill, 1995:63–74.

50. Dooms-Goossens A. Hypo-allergenic products. J Appl Cosmetol 1985; 3:153–172.

51. Draelos ZD, Rietschel RL. Hypoallergenicity and the dermatologist's perception. J Am Acad Dermatol 1996; 35:248–251.

52. Draelos ZD. Sensitive skin: perceptions, evaluation, and treatment. Am J Contact Dermatitis 1997; 8:67–78.

53. Barker MO. Cosmetic industry. If the regulators don't get you, your competitors will. Am J Contact Dermatitis 1997; 8:49–51.

54. Jackson EM. Science of cosmetics. Lawyers, regulations, and cosmetic claims. Am J Contact Dermatitis 1997; 8:243–246.

55. Goossens A, Drieghe J. Computer applications in contact allergy. Contact Dermatitis 1998; 38:51–52.

10

Dermatological Problems Linked to Perfumes

Anton C. de Groot
Carolus Hospital, 's-Hertogenbosch, The Netherlands

INTRODUCTION

Perfumes are so much a part of our culture that we take them for granted. However, if they were suddenly taken from us, society would suffer immeasurably. We do pay a price for their service, and part of that concerns dermatological and other medical reactions. Adverse reactions to fragrances in perfumes and in fragranced cosmetic products include allergic contact dermatitis, irritant contact dermatitis, photosensitivity, immediate contact reactions (contact urticaria), pigmented contact dermatitis [1] and (worsening of) respiratory problems [2]. In this chapter, the issue of allergic contact reactions is discussed. (For a full review of side effects of fragrances [and essential oils] see Ref. 3.) A recent book on beneficial and adverse reactions to fragrances also provides valuable information [4]. The history of fragrances has been well described [5,6].

ALLERGIC CONTACT DERMATITIS FROM FRAGRANCES
Epidemiology

Considering the extensive use of fragrances, the frequency of contact allergy to them is relatively small. In absolute numbers, however, fragrance allergy is common. In a group of 90 student nurses, 12 (13%) were shown to be fragrance allergic [7]. In a group of 1609 adult subjects, 196 (12%) reported cosmetic reactions in the preceding 5 years. Sixty-nine of these (35% of the reactors and 4.3% of the total population) attributed their reactions to products primarily used for their smell (deodorants, aftershaves, perfumes) [8]. In 567 unselected individuals aged 15 to 69 years, 6 (1.1%) were shown to be allergic to fragrances as evidenced by a positive patch test reaction to the fragrance mix (vide infra) [9].

In dermatitis patients seen by dermatologists, the prevalence of contact allergy to fragrances is between 6 and 14%; only nickel allergy occurs more frequently. When tested with 10 popular perfumes, 6.9% of female eczema patients proved to be allergic to them [10] and 3.2 to 4.2% were allergic to fragrances from perfumes present in various cosmetic products [11]. In cosmetics causing contact allergic reactions, perfumes account for up to 18% and deodorants/antiperspirants for up to 17% of all cases. When patients with suspected allergic cosmetic dermatitis are investigated, fragrances are identified as the most frequent allergens, not only in perfumes, aftershaves, and deodorants, but also in other cosmetic products not primarily used for their smell [12–15].

Patients allergic to fragrances are usually adult individuals of either sex. They mainly become allergic by the use of cosmetics and personal-care products; occupational contact with fragrances is seldom important, not even in workers in the cosmetics industry [3].

Clinical Picture of Contact Allergy to Fragrances

Contact allergy to fragrances usually causes dermatitis of the hands, face, and/or armpits [16–18], the latter site being explained by contact allergy to deodorants and fragranced antiperspirants. In the face, the skin behind the ears and neck is exposed to high concentrations of fragrances in perfumes and aftershaves. Microtraumata from shaving facilitates (photo)contact allergy to aftershave fragrances. The sensitive skin of the eyelids is particularly susceptible to developing allergic contact dermatitis to fragrances in skincare products, decorative cosmetics, and cleansing preparations, as well as from fragrances spread through the air (airborne contact dermatitis) [19]. Most reactions are mild and are characterized by erythema (redness) only with some swelling of the eyelids. More acute lesions with papules, vesicles, and oozing may sometimes be observed. Dermatitis attributable to perfumes or toilet water tends to be "streaky." In some cases, the eruption resembles other skin diseases such as nummular eczema, seborrhoeic dermatitis, sycosis barbae, or lupus erythematosus [20]. Lesions in the skin folds may be mistaken for atopic dermatitis. Psoriasis of the face may be induced or worsened by allergic contact dermatitis from fragrances. Hand eczema is also common in fragrance-sensitive patients [17,18]. However, fragrances are rarely the sole cause of hand eczema. Usually, patients first have irritant dermatitis or atopic dermatitis, which is later complicated by contact allergy to products used for treatment (fragranced topical drugs) or prevention (hand creams and lotions) of hand dermatitis, or to other perfumed products in the household, recreation, or work environment.

The Causative Products

Patients appear to become sensitized to fragrances especially by the use of deodorant sprays and/or perfumes, and to a lesser degree by cleansing agents, deodorant sticks, or hand lotions [21]. Thereafter, new rashes may appear or are worsened by contact with other fragranced products: cosmetics, toiletries, oral hygiene products, household products, industrial contacts (e.g., cutting fluids, electroplating fluids, paints, rubber, plastics, additives in air-conditioning water), paper and paper products, laundered fabrics and clothes, topical drugs, and fragrances used as spices in foods and drinks [22]. By their ubiquitous use, virtually everyone is in daily contact with fragrance materials, which are very hard to completely avoid [3].

The Fragrance Allergens

Over 100 fragrances have been identified as allergens [3]. Most reactions are caused by the eight fragrances in the perfume mix (vide infra), and of these oak moss, isoeugenol, and cinnamic aldehyde (cinnamal) are the main sensitizers. Other fragrances (and essential

TABLE 1 Fragrances and Essential Oils That May
Cause Contact Allergy in >1% of Patch-Tested
Dermatitis Patients

α-amylcinnamic aldehyde	jasmine absolute
benzyl salicylate	jasmine synthetic
cananga oil	lilial
cinnamic alcohol	majantol
cinnamic aldehyde	methoxycitronellal
citral	methyl heptine carbonate
coumarin	methyl salicylate
dehydro-isoeugenol	musk ambrette
(in ylang-ylang oil)	narcissus oil
dihydrocoumarin	oak moss absolute
eugenol	oil of bergamot
geraniol	patchouli oil
geranium oil	rose oil
hydroabietyl alcohol	sandalwood oil
hydroxycitronellal	sandela
isobornyl cyclohexanol	santalol
(synthetic sandalwood)	ylang-ylang oil
isoeugenol	

Source: Refs. 3, 22.

oils used as fragrances) that cause contact allergy more than occasionally (>1% positive patch-test reactions in dermatitis patients routinely tested) are listed in Table 1.

The Diagnosis of Contact Allergy to Fragrances

Contact allergy to a particular product or chemical is established by means of patch testing. A perfume may contain as many as 200 or more individual ingredients. This makes the diagnosis of perfume allergy by patch-test procedures complicated. The fragrance mix, or perfume mix, was introduced as a screening tool for fragrance sensitivity in the late 1970s. It contains eight commonly used fragrances: α-amylcinnamic aldehyde, cinnamic alcohol, cinnamic aldehyde (cinnamal), eugenol, geraniol, hydroxycitronellal, isoeugenol, and oak moss absolute. It is estimated that this mix detects 70 to 80% of all cases of fragrance sensitivity [23]; this may be an overestimation because it was positive in only 57% of patients who were allergic to popular commercial fragrances [10]. The response rate to the fragrance mix in dermatological patients nowadays ranges worldwide from 6 to 14% [3,24]; only nickel sulphate yields more positive reactions.

In the United States, cinnamic aldehyde is routinely tested and scores 2.4% positive reactions [24]. In cases of suspected allergic cosmetic dermatitis, patients' personal products are always tested and may give positive patch-test reactions, proving that the patient is allergic to that product [18]. In addition, many investigators test (a series of) additional fragrances.

The fragrance mix is an extremely useful tool for the detection of cases of contact allergy to fragrances, but unfortunately is far from ideal: it misses 20 to 30% of relevant reactions or more, and may cause both false positive (i.e., a "positive" patch test reaction in a non–fragrance-allergic individual) and false negative (i.e., no patch test reaction in an individual who is actually allergic to one or more of the ingredients of the mix) reactions [25].

Another useful test in cases of doubt (e.g., with weakly positive patch-test reactions that are difficult to interpret) is the repeated open application test (ROAT). The suspected allergen, which may be both an individual fragrance or scented product, is applied to the elbow flexure twice daily for a maximum of 14 days. A positive reaction confirms the existence of contact allergy and makes relevance of the reaction (vide infra) more likely.

The Relevance of Positive Patch Test Reactions to the Fragrance Mix

The finding of a positive reaction to the fragrance mix should be followed by a search for its relevance, i.e., if fragrance allergy is the cause of the patient's current or previous complaints or if it at least contributes to it. Often, however, correlation with the clinical picture is lacking and many patients can tolerate perfumes and fragranced products without problem [11]. This sometimes may be explained by irritant (false positive) patch-test reactions to the mix. Alternative explanations include the absence of relevant allergens in those products or a concentration too low to elicit clinically visible allergic contact reactions.

It is assumed that between 50 and 65% of all positive patch-test reactions to the mix are relevant, although this is sometimes hard to prove [24,26]. Nevertheless, there is a highly significant association between the occurrence of self-reported visible skin symptoms to scented products earlier in life and a positive patch test to the fragrance mix, and most fragrance-sensitive patients are aware that the use of scented products may cause skin problems [27].

In perfume-mix–allergic patients with concomitant positive reactions to perfumes or scented products used by them, interpretation of the reaction as relevant is highly likely. In such patients the incriminated cosmetics very often contain fragrances present in the mix, and thus the fragrance mix appears to be a good reflection of actual exposure [18]. Indeed, one or more of the ingredients of the mix are present in nearly all deodorants [28], popular prestige perfumes [10], perfumes used in the formulation of other cosmetic products [11], and natural-ingredient–based cosmetics [29], often in levels high enough to cause allergic reactions [30,31]. Thus, fragrance allergens are ubiquitous and virtually impossible to avoid if perfumed cosmetics are used.

CONCLUSIONS

Contact allergy to fragrance materials is common in both eczema patients and in the general population. Allergic contact dermatitis caused by perfumes and scented cosmetics is usually located in the face (including the eyelids), on the hands, and in the axillae. Patients appear to become sensitized to fragrances especially by the use of deodorant sprays and/ or perfumes, and to a lesser degree by cleansing agents, deodorant sticks, or hand lotions. Thereafter, new rashes may appear or be worsened by contact with other fragranced products: cosmetics, toiletries, oral-hygiene products, household products, industrial contacts, paper and paper products, laundered fabrics and clothes, topical drugs, and fragrances used as flavors in foods and drinks.

Over 100 fragrances have been identified as allergens. The diagnosis of fragrance allergy is established by positive patch-test reactions to the fragrance mix (a mixture of eight commonly used fragrances) and/or to the patients' personal perfumes or scented products. Most reactions to the mix are relevant, i.e., fragrance allergy is the cause of the patient's current or previous complaints, and most fragrance-sensitive patients are aware that the use of scented products may cause skin problems. One or more of the ingredients of the mix are present in nearly all deodorants, perfumes, and scented cosmetics, often in levels high enough to cause allergic reactions. Industry is advised to pay special attention to the safety evaluation of fragrance materials, notably those used in perfumes and deodorants.

REFERENCES

1. Ebihara T, Nakayama H. Pigmented contact dermatitis. Clin Dermatol 1997; 15:593–599.
2. De Groot AC, Frosch PJ. Fragrances as a cause of contact dermatitis in cosmetics: clinical aspects and epidemiological data. In: Frosch PJ, Johansen JD, White IR, eds. Fragrances. Beneficial and Adverse Effects. Berlin: Springer-Verlag, 1998:66–75.
3. De Groot AC, Frosch PJ. Adverse reactions to fragrances. A clinical review. Contact Dermatitis 1997; 36:57–86.
4. Frosch PJ, Johansen JD, White IR, eds. Fragrances. Beneficial and Adverse Effects. Berlin: Springer-Verlag, 1998.
5. Guin JD. History, manufacture, and cutaneous reactions to perfumes. In: Frost P, Horwitz SW, eds. Principles of Cosmetics for the Dermatologist. St Louis: The CV Mosby Company, 1982: 111–129.
6. Scheinman PL. Allergic contact dermatitis to fragrance: a review. Am J Contact Dermatitis 1996; 7:65–76.
7. Guin JD, Berry VK. Perfume sensitivity in adult females. A study of contact sensitivity to a perfume mix in two groups of student nurses. J Am Acad Dermatol 1980; 3:299–302.
8. De Groot AC, Nater JP, van der Lende R, Rijcken B. Adverse effects of cosmetics: a retrospective study in the general population. Int J Cosm Science 1987; 9:255–259.
9. Nielsen NH, Menné T. Allergic contact sensitization in an unselected Danish population. Acta Derm Venereol (Stockh) 1992; 72:456–460.
10. Johansen JD, Rastogi SC, Menné T. Contact allergy to popular perfumes; assessed by patch test, use test and chemical analysis. Br J Dermatol 1996; 135:419–422.
11. Johansen JD, Rastogi SC, Andersen KE, Menné T. Content and reactivity to product perfumes in fragrance mix positive and negative eczema patients. A study of perfumes used in toiletries and skin-care products. Contact Dermatitis 1997; 36:291–296.
12. Adams RM, Maibach HI. A five-year study of cosmetic reactions. J Am Acad Dermatol 1985; 13:1062–1069.
13. De Groot AC, Bruynzeel DP, Bos JD, van Joost Th, Jagtman BA, Weyland JW. The allergens in cosmetics. Arch Dermatol 1988; 124:1525–1529.
14. Berne B, Boström Å, Grahnén AF, Tammela M. Adverse effects of cosmetics and toiletries reported to the Swedish Medical Product Agency 1989–1994. Contact Dermatitis 1996; 34: 359–362.
15. Dooms-Goossens A, Kerre S, Drieghe J, Bossuyt L, Degreef H. Cosmetic products and their allergens. Eur J Dermatol 1992; 2:465–468.
16. Larsen W, Nakayama H, Lindberg M, Fisher T, Elsner P, Burrows D, Jordan W, Shaw S, Wilkinson J, Marks J Jr, Sugawara M, Nethercott J. Fragrance contact dermatitis. A worldwide multicenter investigation (Part I). Am J Contact Dermatitis 1996; 7:77–83.
17. Santucci B, Cristaudo A, Cannistraci C, Picardo M. Contact dermatitis to fragrances. Contact Dermatitis 1987; 16:93–95.
18. Johansen JD, Rastogi SC, Menné T. Exposure to selected fragrance materials. A case study of fragrance-mix-positive eczema patients. Contact Dermatitis 1996; 34:106–110.
19. Dooms-Goossens A. Cosmetics as causes of allergic contact dermatitis. Cutis 1993; 52:316–320.

20. Meynadier J-M, Raison-Peyron N, Meunier L, Meynadier J. Allergie aux parfums. Rev fr Allergol 1997; 37:641–650.
21. Johansen JD, Andersen TF, Kjøller M, Veien N, Avnstorp C, Andersen KE, Menné T. Identification of risk products for fragrance contact allergy: a case-referent study based on patients' histories. Am J Contact Dermatitis 1998; 9:80–87.
22. Larsen WG, Nethercott JR. Fragrances. Clin Dermatol 1997; 15:499–504.
23. Larsen WG. Perfume dermatitis. J Am Acad Dermatol 1985; 12:1–9.
24. Marks JG Jr, Belsito DV, DeLeo VA, Fowler JF Jr, Fransway AF, Maibach HI, Mathias CGT, Nethercott JR, Rietschel RL, Sheretz EF, Storrs FJ, Taylor JS. North American Contact Dermatitis Group patch test results for the detection of delayed-type hypersensitivity to topical allergens. J Am Acad Dermatol 1998; 38:911–918.
25. De Groot AC, van der Kley AMJ, Bruynzeel DP, Meinardi MMHM, Smeenk G, van Joost Th, Pavel S. Frequency of false-negative reactions to the fragrance mix. Contact Dermatitis 1993; 28:139–140.
26. Frosch PJ, Pilz B, Burrows D, Camarasa JG, Lachapelle J-M, Lahti A, Menné T, Wilkinson JD. Testing with the fragrance mix—is the addition of sorbitan sesquioleate to the constituents useful? Contact Dermatitis 1995; 32:266–272.
27. Johansen JD, Andersen TF, Veien N, Avnstorp C, Andersen KE, Menné T. Patch testing with markers of fragrance contact allergy. Do clinical tests correspond to patients' self-reported problems? Acta Derm Venereol (Stockh) 1997; 77:149–153.
28. Rastogi SC, Johansen JD, Frosch PJ, Menné T, Bruze M, Lepoittevin JP, Dreier B, Andersen KE, White IR. Deodorants on the European market: quantitative chemical analysis of 21 fragrances. Contact Dermatitis 1998; 38:29–35.
29. Rastogi S, Johansen JD, Menné T. Natural ingredients based cosmetics. Content of selected fragrance sensitizers. Contact Dermatitis 1996; 34:423–426.
30. Johansen JD, Andersen KE, Menné T. Quantitative aspects of isoeugenol contact allergy assessed by use and patch tests. Contact Dermatitis 1996; 34:414–418.
31. Johansen JD, Andersen KE, Rastogi SC, Menné T. Threshold responses in cinnamic-aldehyde-sensitive subjects: results and methodological aspects. Contact Dermatitis 1996; 34:165–171.

11

In Vitro Tests for Skin Irritation

Michael K. Robinson, Rosemarie Osborne, and Mary A. Perkins
The Procter & Gamble Company, Cincinnati, Ohio

INTRODUCTION

The manufacture, transport, and marketing of chemicals and finished products requires the prior toxicological evaluation and assessment of skin corrosivity and skin irritation that might result from intended or accidental skin exposure. Traditionally, animal testing procedures have provided the data needed to assess the more severe forms of skin toxicity, an assessment requiring extrapolation of the data from the animal species to humans [1]. Current regulations may require animal test data before permission is granted for the manufacture, transport, or marketing of chemicals [2], as well as for the formulations that contain them [3].

In recent years, animal testing for dermatotoxic effects has come under increasing scrutiny and criticism from animal-rights activists for being inhumane and unnecessary. Legislation is pending that would restrict the marketing of products containing ingredients that have been tested on animals [4]. The often conflicting needs to protect worker and consumer safety, comply with regulatory statutes, and reduce animal testing procedures has led to a significant effort within industry, government, and academia to develop alternative testing methods for assessing the skin corrosion and irritation hazard of chemicals and product formulations without reliance on animal test procedures [5].

A recent example for which regulatory requirements have been coupled to the pressing need for alternative methods development is in the evaluation of skin corrosion. United States and international regulations require that chemicals be properly classified, labeled, packaged, and transported on the basis of their potential to damage or destroy tissue, including the speed with which such tissue-destructive reactions occur [2,6]. The most common animal testing methods used over the years for the evaluation of chemical corrosion potential are all based on the original method by Draize [7]. We, as well as other laboratories, have been active in the development of alternative procedures for skin-corrosion testing [8–11]. Recently, several test methods have been evaluated in an international validation program [12]. Certain of these methods should provide short-term and cost-effective alternatives to the Draize procedure, at the same time providing experimental systems for developing a better mechanistic understanding of the process of skin corrosion [8].

Skin irritation, by definition, is a less severe response than corrosion, but can span a range of responses from near corrosive at one extreme to weak cumulative or neurosensory responses at the other. The development of alternatives for skin irritation testing has lagged behind that of skin corrosion testing, likely because of the greater urgency of developing alternatives for the more severe skin responses and because of the range of responses encompassed within the "skin irritation" umbrella. Currently, the irritation hazard potential of chemicals is often determined through use of the same Draize procedure used for corrosion testing, the difference being mainly in the length of chemical exposure, with results used to determine labeling requirements for chemicals and products according to European Commission (EC) directives [2,3]. For noncorrosive chemicals, there has been a recent effort to develop and promote the use of clinical patch testing methods for a more relevant assessment of chemical skin irritation potential than that provided by the rabbit test [13–16]. This approach has not yet been extended to the testing of product formulations, although the European Cosmetic, Toiletry and Perfumery Association (COLIPA) has recently issued guidelines for skin-compatibility testing of cosmetic formulations in man [17]. The major problem of human testing for skin irritation or compatibility is the extended duration and relatively high cost of this clinical testing. In vitro skin irritation test methods could be used to rank chemicals or formulations for skin irritation potential, even at the low end of the irritation spectrum [18,19]. These methods (and others under development elsewhere) might provide for short-term, cost-effective approaches for screening chemicals and product formulations of interest, so that only those with satisfactory skin irritation profiles would undergo longer and more costly clinical evaluations.

This chapter will provide a brief summary of the developmental status of in vitro skin irritation test methods. It includes a brief description and update on the current validation status of skin corrosion tests. Then, it summarizes ongoing efforts in our laboratory, and the work of others, towards development of a battery of skin irritation tests that might predict varying degrees of skin irritation potential of chemicals and formulations, including many with relatively mild clinical skin irritation properties.

SKIN CORROSION TESTING

Assay Systems

Screening of chemicals for skin corrosion properties in vitro has followed three general formats. These include 1) changes in electrical conductance across intact skin (rat or human), 2) breaching of noncellular biobarriers, and 3) cellular cytotoxicity in skin or epidermal equivalent cell culture systems. Each of these systems has been subject to intra- and interlaboratory development, evaluation, and validation.

Skin corrosivity has been distinguished from skin irritation in two important ways. First, corrosive skin reactions generally occur soon after chemical exposure and are irreversible. Second, it is thought that the major processes leading to chemical corrosivity are more commonly physicochemical in nature rather than the result of inflammatory biological events [11], although inflammation is a common consequence of skin corrosion.

Initial efforts to develop a screening test for skin corrosivity examined the effects of chemical exposure on barrier function of skin through assessment of changes in the resistance of the exposed skin to transmission of electric current [20]. This test method, called transcutaneous electrical resistance (TER), was based on early studies of the electrical resistance properties of skin [21] and has been developed as a corrosivity assay over the past 15 years using either rat or human skin [9,11,20,22–26]. In the TER assay, full-thickness skin is stretched over a hollow tube opening with the stratum corneum side exposed to the lumen. Test materials are applied to the skin surface for varying periods of time while the skin is immersed in buffer. After chemical exposure, the electrical resistance of the skin is measured. TER values empirically established as corrosion thresholds have been set at 4 K ohms for rat skin and 11 K ohms for human skin [9,11]. The current validation status of this assay is described in the following section.

The biobarrier destruction assay approach for corrosivity testing is exemplified by the commercial Corrositex® assay system manufactured by In Vitro International (Irvine, CA). Like the TER assay, the premise here is physicochemical destruction of a barrier by direct chemical action of a test material. Instead of intact stratum corneum, the Corrositex® assay relies on a macromolecular protein matrix as the barrier. Chemicals that breach this barrier come into contact with an underlying chemical detection system (CDS). A color change indicates penetration of the test material into the CDS. The speed with which the color change occurs after application of the chemical to the biobarrier is proportional to the severity of corrosive action. A summary of results on 75 chemicals and detergent-based formulations has been published [10], as well as a recent study on the corrosivity of organosilicon compounds [27]. An update of the current validation status of this assay is provided in the following section.

A variety of cell-based biological assay systems have been developed over the past 10 years to investigate the dermatotoxic effects of chemicals and product formulations on the skin. These have included simple submerged cell cultures, submerged cell cocultures incorporating more than a single cell type, and, more recently, the development of full-thickness skin and epidermal equivalent systems. The latter are characterized by stratified epidermal cell layers and a multilayered stratum corneum. The full-thickness culture systems also have different types of cellular and macromolecular matrices serving as a dermal element. These systems have undergone extensive development and evaluation in various academic and commercial laboratories [28–38]. We have recently reviewed features of many of the submerged and skin/epidermal equivalent cell systems [39,40]. A few of these systems have been used to develop skin corrosion screening assays [8,27]. A review of the current validation status of those assays is presented in the following section.

Validation Status

In the early 1990s a program was initiated under the auspices of the European Center for the Validation of Alternative Methods (ECVAM) to develop and validate alternative methods for the assessment of skin corrosion. This program focused on three assay systems, the TER, Corrositex®, and Skin^2® systems. The Skin^2 system was a commercial "skin equivalent" culture system, manufactured by Advanced Tissue Sciences (La Jolla, CA) and comprising human neonatal foreskin–derived dermal fibroblasts in a collagen matrix grown on nylon mesh and seeded with human neonatal foreskin–derived epidermal keratinocytes to form a stratified and cornified epidermal component. A prevalidation study was completed with these three assay systems in seven different laboratories to assess intralaboratory and interlaboratory consistency as well as overall sensitivity and specificity of the assays in identifying known corrosive and noncorrosive chemicals. The results of the prevalidation study were published in 1995 [41]. All three tests performed well, and no firm conclusions could be drawn as to the superiority or inferiority of one test versus the others. Individual tests had specific problems that warranted further study. These problems included relatively low specificity (TER), a high number of incompatible chemicals (Corrositex), and an inferior interlaboratory consistency profile (Skin^2). It was recommended that effort be made to address these individual deficiencies and that each assay be further evaluated in a future validation study.

The formal ECVAM-sponsored skin corrosivity validation study began in early 1995 and was completed in October 1997 with the submission of the study findings [12]. In addition to the assays included in the prevalidation work (TER, Corrositex, and Skin^2), the validation study included a second commercially available skin equivalent culture construct, Episkin® (Chaponost, France). Each assay was evaluated by three independent test laboratories, and each laboratory evaluated only one of the four assays. Hence, 12 laboratories participated in the validation study. A total of 60 corrosive and noncorrosive chemicals from a variety of chemical classes (including organic and inorganic acids and bases, neutral organics, phenols, inorganic salts, electrophiles, and soaps/surfactants) were tested [42].

All four assay systems showed acceptable intralaboratory and interlaboratory reproducibility, and all but Corrositex were applicable to the testing of all the selected chemicals. Two of the assays, TER and Episkin met the first of two major objectives of the validation study. They were capable of distinguishing corrosive from noncorrosive chemicals with acceptable rates of under- or overprediction. Only the Episkin assay system met the second major objective of the study, the ability to distinguish between known R35 (United Nations packing group I) and R34 (UN packing group II/III) chemicals across all of the chemical classes. Only 60% of the test chemicals could be adequately evaluated by the Corrositex assay. For this reason, it did not meet the criteria for a validated replacement test, although it might be valid for certain chemical classes. The Skin^2 assay system showed high specificity (100% of noncorrosive chemicals were properly identified) but low sensitivity (only 43% of corrosive chemicals were correctly identified). It also performed poorly with respect to distinguishing known R35 and R34 chemicals. Only 35% of the assays conducted on these chemicals resulted in proper classification. Previously, both the Skin^2 and Corrositex assays had received exemptions from the U.S. Department of Transportation as valid alternatives to assess skin corrosivity based on more limited evaluation. It is not certain what effect the recent ECVAM-sponsored study will have on the exemption status of these assays, although for the Skin^2 assay it is a moot point given that this culture system is no longer commercially available.

SKIN IRRITATION TESTING

Our Experience

Introduction

As previously indicated, development of in vitro methods to assess skin irritation is complicated by the fact that skin irritation encompasses a range of clinical responses from near corrosive at one extreme to very mild (perhaps sensory only) skin responses at the other. Hence, we believe that test methods and prediction models will need to be optimized for different categories of test materials or formulations and for anticipated ranges of irritation severity. That is the approach we have taken in developing in vitro skin irritation test methods for several chemical and product categories [32,39,40].

Methods

Cell Cultures. The culture system used in our studies was a stratified epidermal culture with a stratum corneum obtained from MatTek Corp. (EpiDerm® No. EPI-100; Ashland, MA). These cultures were composed of a multilayered and differentiated epidermis and multilayered stratum corneum seeded onto a permeable transwell filter. On arrival, the cultures were placed at 4°C until used for experiments (within 24 h). Before treatment, the cultures were aseptically transferred to 6-well culture plates containing assay medium.

Treatments. Test materials were reagent grade chemicals from Sigma Chemical Co. (St. Louis, MO), Aldrich Chemical Co. (Milwaukee, WI), or The Procter & Gamble Co. (Cincinnati, OH). Test-product formulations were obtained from The Procter & Gamble Co. Application of test materials to skin-equivalent cultures was as previously described [32].

MTT Viability Assay. The MTT assay is a colorimetric method of determining cell viability based on reduction of the yellow tetrazolium salt 3-[4,5-dimethylthiazol-2-yl] 2,5-diphenyl tetrazolium bromide (Sigma Chemical Co., St. Louis, MO) to a purple formazan dye by mitochondrial succinate dehydrogenase in viable cells [43]. This assay was performed as previously described [8].

Enzyme-Release Assay. At the end of the test material and control treatment exposures, the assay medium from under each treated or control skin culture was collected in plastic vials and immediately analyzed for lactate dehydrogenase (LDH) and aspartate-aminotransferase (AST) enzymes. The enzymes, LDH and AST, were analyzed using a colorimetric method performed with a Hitachi 717 autoanalyser with commercial test kits (Boehringer Mannheim Corp., Indianapolis, IN).

Interleukin-1α Assay. Assay medium was recovered from treated and control skin cultures (EPI-100) and stored at -20°C until analyzed. Interleukin-1α (IL-1α) was assayed with a specific enzyme-linked immunoassay kit (Quantikine; R&D Systems, Inc., Minneapolis, MN).

Results

In vitro methods for screening product formulations for mild to moderate irritation potential can aid selection of formulations for further clinical evaluation. Our approach has been to directly compare in vitro assay endpoints to in vivo human skin responses using historic or concurrent skin-response data for products and ingredients including surfactants, cosmetics, antiperspirants, and deodorants. For the in vitro studies we evaluated the cornified human epidermal skin cultures (EpiDerm, MatTek, EPI-100) dosing neat or diluted test substances to the stratum corneum surface of the skin cultures. The in vitro endpoints included the MTT metabolism assay of cell viability, enzyme release (lactate dehydrogenase and aspartate aminotransferase), and inflammatory cytokine (IL-1α) release.

We have been able to rank order chemicals (surfactants), product formulations and control materials in the in vitro and clinical studies to determine the value of the EpiDerm assay system in providing a clinically relevant ordering of irritancy potential. Whereas the details of these results are presented elsewhere [19], Table 1 provides a summary of results to date. The in vitro rank ordering has been highly predictive of both surfactant and formulation irritancy. Surfactants (anionic, nonionic, and amphoteric) were tested in vivo using three repeat 24-hour exposures under occluded patch, and cumulative erythema grades were determined for each material. The in vitro irritancy was assessed using the MTT cytotoxicity assay. With the exception of one nonionic surfactant, the rank ordering of irritation was the same for the in vivo and in vitro tests. For antiperspirants/deodorants, the clinical irritation data were derived from home-use study diaries. The in vitro data included MTT, enzyme-release, and IL-1α assays. All showed good correlation with the human data, but the IL-1α assay showed the greatest correlation along the entire range of irritation. For cosmetics, the clinical data were derived from cumulative irritation tests where benchmark materials (0.05% and 0.1% sodium lauryl sulfate [SLS]) were included as high-irritant controls. The cumulative irritation indices for different cosmetic formula-

TABLE 1 Rank Ordering of Irritation Within Chemical or Product Classes[a]

Material/product class	Test substance	Potency rank order	
		In vivo[b]	In vitro[c]
Surfactants	.01% SLS	1	1
	.02% AE[d]/A	2	3
	.02% AE/B	3	4
	.02% AE/C	4	5
	0.6% Nonionic A	5	6
	0.2% Amphoteric	6	7
	0.6% Nonionic B	7	2
Antiperspirants/	GD-2F[e]	1	1
deodorants	GD-2M	1	2
	GSOC	3	3
	GDF	3	5
	GSO	5	6
	HER	6	4
	HEU	7	6
Cosmetics/controls	0.1% SLS	1	1
	COS-4[f]	2	2
	0.05% SLS	3	3
	COS-3	4	4
	COS-2	5	6
	COS-1	6	5

[a] Irritation rank ordering: 1 = most irritating or cytotoxic, 7 = least irritating or cytotoxic.
[b] In vivo data were obtained from three repeat 24-hour exposure patch tests (surfactants), from home-use study diaries (antiperspirants/deodorants), or from cumulative irritation patch tests (cosmetics).
[c] Surfactants were tested in vitro by the MTT assay and antiperspirants/deodorants and cosmetics were tested by the IL-1α assay.
[d] Alkyl ethoxylate.
[e] Product codes (antiperspirants/deodorants); tested in vitro as is.
[f] Product codes (cosmetics); tested in vitro as is.
Source: Ref. 39.

tions were compared with the in vitro test data. Again, the IL-1α assays provide the best correlation with the human data across the entire range of clinical irritation responses.

Other Literature

A number of other laboratories have used various constructs of skin cultures to examine the in vitro irritation potential of chemicals and formulations. The developers of the EpiDerm cultures examined dose-response profiles to surfactants and surfactant-containing formulations, and found a good correlation between residual cell viability measures and clinical irritation profiles [44]. Later testing of chemical irritants and allergens showed a comparable irritant response profile regardless of whether cytotoxicity or cytokine release was measured. However, cytokine release in response to contact allergens occurred at noncytotoxic doses and was thought to provide additional mechanistic and perhaps a predictive application for these cultures [45]. Recently, the EpiDerm system has been used by a group from Unilever (Sharnbrook, U.K.) to examine the cytotoxicity patterns of mixed surfactants [46]. They found that, in vitro as in vivo, mixtures of surfactants produce less irritation than expected based on the irritation properties of the individual components of the mixture, a phenomenon known as antagonism.

A group from Leiden University (Leiden, The Netherlands) has been developing and applying their own unique skin-culture system to the assessment of skin irritation responses. They have used a system comprising epidermal keratinocytes seeded on de-epidermized dermis (RE-DED) and have tested various skin irritants [34,36]. This group confirmed the ability of the RE-DED system to effectively assess skin irritation potential of the anionic surfactant sodium lauryl sulfate [36]. They also showed that in vitro skin irritation patterns for oleic acid were different in submerged keratinocyte cultures versus the RE-DED system [34]. In the latter, higher doses were required because of the requirement for the chemical to penetrate the barrier. Of course, the irritation potential of acids and bases can also be underestimated in submerged cultures because of the buffering effects of the culture media [32,39,40].

Quite recently, another group of researchers (Lyon, France) have used skin-equivalent culture systems to examine the irritation potential of cosmetic product formulations. Testing cosmetic formulations of various types (creams, lotions, oils, mascaras), they observed a good correlation between in vitro indices of irritation and previously known Draize irritation indices [47,48]. Like our group, they have used viability, enzyme release, and IL-1α release to profile in vitro skin irritation. All of the above results point to the utility of skin-equivalent culture systems to detect skin irritation responses in vitro in a manner consistent with the clinical skin irritation properties of the chemicals. They offer opportunities for the further development of valid alternative test methods.

DISCUSSION

It has been important to validate the relevance of in vitro skin irritation endpoints to in vivo toxicity by confirming the presence of these endpoints in skin models representing various levels of skin organization, from intact skin to isolated cell cultures. The initial response of human cells to chemical irritants is cell damage, ranging from subtle perturbations or biochemical changes to cell death. As a response to damage, skin cells release inflammatory mediators and cytokines to initiate a local inflammation response, resulting in the visual hallmark of erythema and edema attributable to increased blood flow and leakage of plasma from blood vessels [32,49,50].

The isolated keratinocyte culture represents the simplest of the test systems for evaluating skin irritancy in vitro. For test materials compatible with the aqueous culture medium, there has been an excellent correlation shown between human irritation potential and in vitro cytotoxicity over several orders of magnitude [32]. However, many types of chemicals (particularly acids, alkalis, and oxidants) are incompatible with the assay system. For acids and alkalis, the buffering capacity of the medium will interfere with their evaluation if pH is a key factor in their in vivo irritancy. Formulations are also difficult to test in vitro because, from a pharmacokinetic standpoint, conditions of exposure of viable keratinocytes to key irritant components of the formulation may be quite different in the culture system versus intact skin. Lastly, skin irritation can sometimes be overpredicted in these submerged cultures because they bypass the need for chemicals to penetrate a stratum corneum barrier [34].

In the late 1980s, cultured human-skin models were developed to provide a hopeful therapeutic approach to skin transplantation. An offshoot of this technology was to provide skin-equivalent culture systems for dermatotoxicity testing. Although clearly not the same as intact skin, these cultures provided a three-dimensional model of skin with the major structural components intact. The availability of cornified versions of these culture systems has provided for a major advance in development and validation of in vitro skin corrosion and irritation test methods. Although still lacking key cellular elements, these culture systems have very similar structural features as intact skin, including many of the same structural proteins, although they are generally more permeable than intact skin. The major advantage of these cultures is the ability to test anything that can be applied to and tested on intact human skin, including highly toxic materials. Validation testing has verified the ability of at least certain constructs to predict the corrosive potential of chemicals of different classes [12].

Use of these cultures for testing milder materials (e.g., cosmetics) provides a tool for early screening of new product formulations in a time- and cost-effective manner prior to more costly clinical evaluations. They also provide a means to investigate mechanisms of skin irritation. Our early efforts using cornified culture systems to screen and rank order the mild to moderate skin irritation potential of product ingredients and formulations have been highly successful [18,19]. It is well known that the irritation potential of any material in vivo is a function of both concentration and time of exposure. The in vitro testing of materials that are relatively mild after acute testing, and produce clinical irritation only after chronic or repeated exposure, is complicated by the limited duration of exposure possible in vitro. In the development of more sensitive in vitro methods, we are looking to extend the duration of exposure as much as the cultures will allow and/or use noncornified culture systems. Clearly, any increase in permeability of the culture systems versus intact skin (often viewed as a negative property for many applications) can be a benefit for the skin irritation assessment of relatively mild chemicals or product formulations. In addition, skin irritation responses in epidermal skin equivalents, with and without dermal components, are being investigated.

Although the development of one skin-equivalent culture system and the TER assay have achieved validation status under the recent ECVAM recommendation, the same is not true for skin irritation assessment. An ECVAM task force recently summarized the status of alternative methods for skin irritation testing [51]. A major recommendation was to continue development of reconstituted human-skin models and preliminary prediction models for their use in predictive skin irritation testing. In addition, it was noted that ethical human-skin testing procedures are being developed for skin irritation hazard assessment [13–16,52] and deserve consideration in the hierarchical scheme of skin irritation testing [51].

Many issues remain unanswered in the future development of cell-based in vitro assays for skin toxicity. Continued interlaboratory validation is needed to enhance acceptance into the regulatory evaluation and approval process. Further refinement and development of irritation testing methods will enhance the utility of the models for screening purposes. Included is the development of ''flanker'' models that contain additional epidermal cell types such as melanocytes or Langerhans cells. For example, MatTek (Ashland, MA) has developed a melanocyte containing epidermal model (MelanoDerm®) and is investigating its use in UVB-protection studies [53]. Finally, the increased reliance on these models for toxicity testing and irritation screening has also created concerns over their long-term commercial supply. Increased use of high-quality culture systems and continued efforts to validate methods using these cultures may help in this process and thus ensure future access to this important technology.

NOTE ADDED IN PROOF

In the months since the submission of this chapter, several advances have occurred in the field of in vitro skin corrosion and irritation testing. In addition to the TER and Episkin assays, a second skin construct, EpiDerm, has now completed successful 'catch-up' validation [54,55] and has been endorsed by ECVAM as an alternative skin corrosivity test [56]. Also, the noncellular corrosion assay, Corrositex, was cited by the U.S. Interagency Coordinating Committee on the Validation of Alternative Methods (ICCVAM) as equivalent to the Draize test for predicting corrosivity and noncorrosivity for specified chemical classes (acids and bases) [57]. In the European Union, a new test method on skin corrosion (including the rat skin TER and human skin model assays) has just been incorporated into Annex V of Directive 67/548/EEC [58], and a draft guideline on in vitro tests for skin corrosion is under consideration by the Organization for Economic Cooperation and Development (OECD) member countries. In regard to in vitro skin irritation test methods, efforts are currently underway to identify potential in vitro acute skin irritation test methods and evaluate them through rigorous prevalidation and validation studies [59].

REFERENCES

1. OECD guideline for testing of chemicals. Guideline No. 404. Acute dermal irritation/corrosion 1992.
2. EEC. Annex I to Commission Directive 91/325/EEC of 1st March 1991 adapting to technical progress for the twelfth time Council Directive 67/548/EEC on the approximation of the laws, regulations and administrative provision relating to the classification, packaging and labeling of dangerous substances. Off J Eur Comm 1991; L180:34.
3. EEC. Council Directive of 7 June 1988 on the approximation of the laws, regulations and administrative provisions of the Member States relating to the classification, packaging and labeling of dangerous preparations. Off J Eur Comm 1988; L18:14.
4. EEC. Council Directive 93/35/EEC of 14 June 1993 amending for the 6th time Directive 76/768/EEC on the approximation of the laws of the Member States relating to cosmetic products. Off J Eur Comm 1993; L15:32.

5. Rougier A, Goldberg AM, Maibach HI, eds. In Vitro Skin Toxicology. New York: Mary Ann Liebert, Inc., 1994.
6. Department of Transportation. Method of testing corrosion to the skin. 1991; Title 49, Appendix A: Code of Federal Regulations.
7. Draize JH, Woodard G, Calvery HO. Methods for the study of irritation and toxicity of substances applied topically to the skin and mucous membranes. J Pharm Exp Therap 1944; 82: 377–390.
8. Perkins MA, Osborne R, Johnson GR. Development of an in vitro method for skin corrosion testing. Fundam Appl Toxicol 1996; 31:9–18.
9. Whittle E, Barratt MD, Carter JA, Basketter DA, Chamberlain M. Skin corrosivity potential of fatty acids: in vitro rat and human skin testing and QSAR studies. Toxicol In Vitro 1996; 10:95–100.
10. Gordon VC, Harvell JD, Maibach HI. Dermal corrosion, the CORROSITEX® system: a DOT accepted method to predict corrosivity potential of test materials. In: Rougier A, Goldberg AM, Maibach HI, eds. In Vitro Skin Toxicology. New York: Mary Ann Liebert, 1994:37–45.
11. Lewis RW, Botham PA. Measurement of transcutaneous electrical resistance to assess the skin corrosivity potential of chemicals. In: Rougier A, Goldberg AM, Maibach HI, eds. In Vitro Skin Toxicology. New York: Mary Ann Liebert, 1994:161–169.
12. Fentem JH, Archer GEB, Balls M, Botham PA, Curren RD, Earl LK, Esdaile DJ, Holzhütter HG, Liebsch M. The ECVAM international validation study on in vitro tests for skin corrosivity. 2. Results and evaluation by the management team. Toxicol In Vitro 1998; 12:483–524.
13. Basketter DA, Whittle E, Griffiths HA, York M. The identification and classification of skin irritation hazard by a human patch test. Food Chem Toxicol 1994; 32:769–775.
14. York M, Griffiths HA, Whittle E, Basketter DA. Evaluation of a human patch test for the identification and classification of skin irritation potential. Contact Dermatitis 1996; 34:204–212.
15. Griffiths HA, Wilhelm KP, Robinson MK, Wang XM, McFadden J, York M, Basketter DA. Interlaboratory evaluation of a human patch test for the identification of skin irritation potential/hazard. Food Chem Toxicol 1997; 35:255–260.
16. Robinson MK, Perkins MA, Basketter DA. Application of a 4-h human patch test method for comparative and investigative assessment of skin irritation. Contact Dermatitis 1998; 38:194–202.
17. Walker AP, Basketter DA, Baverel M, Diembeck W, Matthies W, Mougin D, Paye M, Rothlisberger R, Dupuis J. Test guidelines for assessment of skin compatibility of cosmetic finished products in man. Food Chem Toxicol 1996; 34:651–660.
18. Perkins MA, Osborne R, Robinson MK, Rana F, Ghassemi A, Hall B. Comparison of in vitro and in vivo human skin responses to consumer products and ingredients with a range of irritancy potential. Fundam Appl Toxicol 1996; 30(abstr):168–169.
19. Perkins MA, Osborne R, Rana F, Ghassemi A, Robinson MK. Comparison of in vitro and in vivo human skin responses to consumer products and ingredients with a range of irritancy potential. Toxicological Sciences 1999; 48:218–229.
20. Oliver GJ, Pemberton MA, Rhodes C. An in vitro skin corrosivity test—modifications and validation. Food Chem Toxicol 1986; 24:507–512.
21. Blank IH, Finesinger JE. Electrical resistance of the skin. Arch Neurol Psychiat 1964; 56: 544–557.
22. Oliver GJ, Pemberton MA. An in vitro epidermal slice technique for identifying chemicals with potential for severe cutaneous effects. Food Chem Toxicol 1985; 23:229–232.
23. Oliver GJA, Pemberton MA, Rhodes C. An in vitro model for identifying skin-corrosive chemicals: I. Initial validation. Toxicol In Vitro 1988; 2:7–18.
24. Barlow A, Hirst R, Pemberton MA, Rigden A, Hall TJ, Oliver G-JA, Botham PA. Refinement

of an in vitro test for the identification of skin corrosive chemicals. Toxicol Methods 1991; 1:106–115.

25. Botham PA, Hall TJ, Dennett R, McCall JC, Basketter DA, Whittle E, Cheeseman M, Esdaile DJ, Gardner J. The skin corrosivity test in vitro: results of an interlaboratory trial. Toxicol In Vitro 1992; 6:191–194.

26. Basketter DA, Whittle E, Chamberlain M. Identification of irritation and corrosion hazards to skin: an alternative strategy to animal testing. Food Chem Toxicol 1994; 32:539–542.

27. Cassidy SL, Stanton ES. In vitro skin irritation and corrosivity studies on organosilicon compounds. J Toxicol Cutan Ocul Toxicol 1996; 15:355–367.

28. Harvell J, Bason MM, Maibach HI. In vitro skin irritation assays: relevance to human skin. J Toxicol Clin Toxicol 1992; 30:359–369.

29. Harvell J, Maibach HI. In vitro dermal toxicity tests: validation aspects. Cosmet Toiletries 1992; 107:31–34.

30. Harvell JD, Maibach HI. Validation of in vitro skin irritation assays using human in vivo data. In Vitro Toxicol 1992; 5:235–239.

31. Harvell JD, Tsai YC, Maibach HI, Gay R, Gordon VC, Miller K, Munn GC. An in vivo correlation with three in vitro assays to assess skin irritation potential. J Toxicol-Cutan Ocul Toxicol 1994; 13:171–183.

32. Osborne R, Perkins MA. An approach for development of alternative test methods based on mechanisms of skin irritation. Food Chem Toxicol 1994; 32:133–142.

33. Rheins LA, Edwards SM, Miao O, Donnelly TA. Skin(2^{TM}): an in vitro model to assess cutaneous immunotoxicity. Toxicol In Vitro 1994; 8:1007–1014.

34. Boelsma E, Tanojo H, Bodde HE, Ponec M. Assessment of the potential irritancy of oleic acid on human skin: evaluation in vitro and in vivo. Toxicol In Vitro 1996; 10:729–742.

35. Ponec M. The use of in vitro skin recombinants to evaluate cutaneous toxicity. In: Rougier A, Goldberg AM, Maibach HI, eds. In Vitro Skin Toxicology. New York: Mary Ann Liebert, Inc., 1994:107–116.

36. Ponec M, Kempenaar J. Use of human skin recombinants as an in vitro model for testing the irritation potential of cutaneous irritants. Skin Pharmacol 1995; 8:49–59.

37. Lawrence JN. Application of in vitro human skin models to dermal irritancy: a brief overview and future prospects. Toxicol In Vitro 1997; 11:305–312.

38. Rosdy M, Bertino B, Butet V, Gibbs S, Ponec M, Darmon M. Retinoic acid inhibits epidermal differentiation when applied topically on the stratum corneum of epidermis formed in vitro by human keratinocytes grown on defined medium. In Vitro Toxicol 1997; 10:39–47.

39. Robinson MK, Perkins MA, Osborne R. Comparative studies on cultured human skin models for irritation testing. In: van Zutphen LFM, Balls M, eds. Animal Alternatives, Welfare and Ethics. Amsterdam: Elsevier, 1997:1123–1134.

40. Perkins MA, Robinson MK, Osborne R. Alternative methods in dermatotoxicology. In: Marzulli FN, Maibach HI, eds. Dermatotoxicology Methods. Washington, DC: Taylor & Francis, 1998:319–336.

41. Botham PA, Chamberlain M, Barratt MD, Curren RD, Esdaile DJ, Gardner JR, Gordon VC, Hildebrand B, Lewis RW, Liebsch M, Logemann P, Osborne R, Ponec M, Regnier JF, Steiling W, Walker AP, Balls M. A prevalidation study on in vitro skin corrosivity testing. The report and recommendations of ECVAM workshop 6. ATLA-Altern Lab Anim 1995; 23:219–255.

42. Barratt MD, Brantom PG, Fentem JH, Gerner I, Walker AP, Worth AP. The ECVAM international validation study on in vitro tests for skin corrosivity. 1. Selection and distribution of the test chemicals. Toxicol In Vitro 1998; 12:471–482.

43. Mossman T. Rapid colorimetric assay for cellular growth and survival: applications to proliferation and cytotoxicity assays. J Immunol Methods 1983; 65:55–63.

44. Cannon CL, Neal PJ, Southee JA, Kubilus J, Klausner M. New epidermal model for dermal irritancy testing. Toxicol In Vitro 1994; 8:889–891.

45. Kubilus J, Cannon C, Neal P, Sennott H, Klausner M. Response of the EpiDerm skin model to topically applied irritants and allergens. In Vitro Toxicol 1996; 9:157–166.
46. Holland G, Earl LK, Hall-Manning TJ. Assessment of the skin irritation effect of mixed surfactants using the 4 hour human patch test and EpiDerm EPI-100 in vitro skin model. Proceedings of 38th International Detergency Conference 1998:81–85.
47. Augustin C, Collombel C, Damour O. Use of dermal equivalent and skin equivalent models for identifying phototoxic compounds in vitro. Photodermatol Photoimmunol Photomedicine 1997; 13:27–36.
48. Augustin C, Collombel C, Damour O. Use of dermal equivalent and skin equivalent models for in vitro cutaneous irritation testing of cosmetic products: comparison with in vivo human data. J Toxicol Cutan Ocul Toxicol 1998; 17:5–17.
49. Willis CM. The histopathology of irritant contact dermatitis. In: van der Valk PGM, Maibach HI, eds. The Irritant Contact Dermatitis Syndrome. Boca Raton: CRC Press, 1996:291–303.
50. Thestrup-Pedersen K, Halkier-Sorensen L. Mechanisms of irritant contact dermatitis. In: van der Valk PGM, Maibach HI, eds. The Irritant Contact Dermatitis Syndrome. Boca Raton: CRC Press, 1996:305–309.
51. Botham PA, Earl LK, Fentem JH, Roguet R, Johannes JM. Alternative methods for skin irritation testing: the current state. ATLA Altern Lab Anim 1998; 26:195–211.
52. Basketter DA, Chamberlain M, Griffiths HA, Rowson M, Whittle E, York M. The classification of skin irritants by human patch test. Food Chem Toxicol 1997; 35:845–852.
53. Kubilus J, Neal PJ, Klausner M. Initial characterization of an epidermal model containing functional melanocytes. J Invest Dermatol 1995; 104(abstr):616.
54. Balls M, Fentem JH. The validation and acceptance of alternatives to animal testing. Toxicology In Vitro 1999; 13:837–846.
55. Liebsch M, Traue D, Barrabas C, Spielmann H, Uphill P, Wilkins S, Wiemann C, Kaufmann T, Remmele M, Holzhütter HG. The ECVAM prevalidation study on the use of EpiDerm for skin corrosivity testing. ATLA Altern Lab Anim 2000; 28:371–401.
56. ECVAM. Statement on the application of the Epiderm® human skin model for skin corrosivity testing. ATLA-Altern Lab Anim 2000; 28:365–366.
57. Scala R, Fentem JH, Chen J, Derelanko MJ, Green S, Harbell J, Kohrman KA, Sauder DN, Stegeman J. Corrositex®: An in vitro test method for assessing dermal corrosivity potential of chemicals. 1999; URL:http://iccvam.niehs.nih.gov/corprep.htm.
58. EEC. Annex I to Commission Directive 2000/33/EC adapting to technical progress for the 27th time Council Directive 67/548/EEC on the approximation of laws, regulations and administrative provisions relating to the classification, packaging and labeling of dangerous substances. Official Journal of the European Communities 2000; L136:91–97.
59. Fentem JH, Botham PA, Earl LK, Roguet R, van de Sandt JJM. Prevalidation of in vitro tests for acute skin irritation. In: Clark DG, Lisansky SG, Macmillan R, eds. Alternatives to Animal Testing. II. Proceedings of the Second International Scientific Conference Organised by the European Cosmetic Industry. Newbury, U.K.: CPL Press, 1999:228–231.

12

In Vivo Irritation

Saqib J. Bashir and Howard I. Maibach
*University of California at San Francisco School of Medicine,
San Francisco, California*

INTRODUCTION

Irritant Dermatitis

Skin irritation is a localized nonimmunologically mediated inflammatory process. It may manifest objectively with skin changes such as erythema, edema, and vesiculation, or subjectively with the complaints of burning, stinging, or itching, with no detectable visible or microscopic changes. Several forms of objective irritation exist (see Table 1). Acute irritant dermatitis may follow a single, usually accidental, exposure to a potent irritant and generally heals soon after exposure. An irritant reaction may be seen in individuals such as hairdressers and wet-work performing employees, who are more extensively and regularly exposed to irritants. Repeated irritant reactions may develop into a contact dermatitis, which generally has a good prognosis. Other forms of irritant dermatitis include delayed acute irritant contact dermatitis, which occurs when there is a delay between exposure and inflammation, and cumulative irritant dermatitis, which is the most common form of irritant contact dermatitis. After exposure, an acute irritant dermatitis is not seen but invisible skin changes occur, which eventually lead to an irritant dermatitis when exposure reaches a threshold point. This may follow days, weeks, or years of exposure [1]. These various forms require specialized models to predict their occurrence after exposure to specific products.

Need for Models

Prevention of skin irritation is important for both the consumer who will suffer from it and for the industry, which needs a licensable and marketable product. Accurate prediction of the irritation potential of industrial, pharmaceutical, and cosmetic materials is therefore necessary for the consumer health and safety and for product development. Presently, animal models fulfill licensing criteria for regulatory bodies. In the European Union, animal testing for cosmetics was to be banned in 1998; however, the deadline was extended to June 30, 2000 because scientifically validated models were not available. Until alternative models can be substituted, in vivo models provide a means by which a cosmetic can be

TABLE 1 Classification of Irritant Dermatitis

Classification	Features	Clinical picture
Acute irritant dermatitis	Single exposure Strong irritant Individual predisposition considered generally unimportant	Reaction usually restricted to exposed area, appears within minutes Erythema, edema, blisters, bullae, pustules, later eschar formation Symptoms include burning, stinging, and pain Possible secondary infection Good prognosis
Irritant reaction	Follows repeated acute skin irritation Often occupational; hairdressers, wet workers	Repeated irritant reactions may develop into contact dermatitis Good prognosis
Cumulative irritant dermatitis	Repeated exposure required Initial exposures cause invisible damage Exposure may be weeks, months, or years until dermatitis develops Individual variation is seen	Initially subject may experience stinging or burning Eventually erythema, edema, or scaling appears Variable prognosis
Delayed acute irritant contact dermatitis	Latent period of 12–24 hours between exposure and dermatitis	Clinically similar to acute irritant dermatitis Good prognosis
Subclinical irritation	Irritation detectable by bioengineering methods prior to development of irritant dermatitis	
Subjective irritation	Subject complains of irritant symptoms with no clinically visible irritation	Perceived burning, stinging, or itching
Traumatic irritant dermatitis	Follows acute skin trauma, e.g., burn or laceration	Incomplete healing, followed by erythema, vesicles, vesicopapules, and scaling; may later resemble nummular (coin-shaped) dermatitis.
Pustular and acneiform dermatitis	Caused by metals, oils, greases, tar, asphalt, chlorinated napthalenes, polyhalogenated naphthalenes, cosmetics	Develops over weeks to months Variable prognosis
Friction dermatitis	Caused by friction trauma	Sometimes seen on hands and knees

tested on living skin, at various sites, and under conditions that should closely mimic the intended human use.

Many aspects of irritation have been described, ranging from the visible erythema and edema to molecular mediators such as interleukins and prostaglandins. Therefore, a variety of in vivo and in vitro approaches to experimental assay are possible. However, no model assays inflammation in its entirety. Each model is limited by our ability to interpret and extrapolate of the features of inflammation to the desired context. Therefore, predicting human responses based on data from nonhuman models requires particular care.

Various human experimental models have been proposed, providing irritant data for the relevant species. Human models allow the substance to be tested in the manner that the general public will use it; e.g., wash testing (see the following section) attempts to mimic the consumer's use of soaps and other surfactants. Also, humans are able to provide subjective data on the degree of irritation caused by the product. However, human studies are also limited by pitfalls in interpretation, and by the fear of applying new substances to human skin before their irritant potential has been evaluated.

ANIMAL MODELS

Draize Rabbit Models

The Draize model [2] and its modifications are commonly used to assay skin irritation using albino rabbits. Various governmental agencies have adopted these methods as standard test procedure. The procedure adopted in the U.S. Federal Hazardous Substance Act (FHSA) is described in Tables 2 and 3 [3,4,5]. Table 4 compares this method some other modifications of the Draize model.

Draize used this scoring system to calculate the primary irritation index (PII). This is calculated by averaging the erythema scores and the edema scores of all sites (abraded and nonabraded). These two averages are then added together to give the PII value. A value of less than 2 was considered nonirritating, 2 to 5 mildly irritating, and greater than 5 severely irritating. A value of 5 defines an irritant by Consumer Product Safety Commission (CPSC) standards. Subsequent laboratory and clinical experience has shown the value judgments (i.e., non-, mild, and severely irritating) proposed in 1944 requires clinical judgment and perspective, and should not be viewed in an absolute sense. Many materials irritating to the rabbit may be well tolerated by human skin.

TABLE 2   Draize-FHSA Model

Number of animals	6 albino rabbits (clipped)
Test sites	2×1 inch^2 sites on dorsum
	One site intact, the other abraded, e.g., with hypodermic needle
Test materials	Applied undiluted to both test sites
	Liquids: 0.5 mL
	Solids/semisolids: 0.5g
Occlusion	1 inch^2 surgical gauze over each test site
	Rubberized cloth over entire trunk
Occlusion period	24 hours
Assessment	24 and 72 hours
	Visual scoring system

TABLE 3   Draize-FHSA Scoring System

	Score
Erythema and eschar formation	0
No erythema	
Very slight erythema (barely perceptible)	1
Well-defined erythema	2
Moderate to severe erythema	3
Severe erythema (beet redness) to slight eschar formation (injuries in depth)	4
Edema formation	
No edema	0
Very slight edema (barely perceptible)	1
Slight edema (edges of area well defined by definite raising)	2
Moderate edema (raised >1 mm)	3
Severe edema (raised >1 mm and extending beyond the area of exposure)	4

Source: Ref. 4.

Although the Draize scoring system does not include vesiculation, ulceration, and severe eschar formation, all of the Draize-type tests are used to evaluate corrosion as well as irritation. When severe and potentially irreversible reactions occur, the test sites are further observed on days 7 and 14, or later if necessary.

Modifications to the Draize assay have attempted to improve its prediction of human experience. The model is criticized for inadequately differentiating between mild and moderate irritants. However, it serves well in hazard identification, often overpredicting the severity of human skin reactions [5]. Therefore, Draize assays continue to be recommended by regulatory bodies for drugs and industrial chemicals.

Cumulative Irritation Assays

Several assays study the effects of cumulative exposure to a potential irritant. Justice et al. [6] administered seven applications of surfactant solutions at 10-minute intervals to the clipped dorsum of albino mice. The test site was occluded with a rubber dam to prevent evaporation and the skin was examined microscopically for epidermal erosion.

Frosch et al. [7] described the guinea pig repeat irritation test (RIT) to evaluate protective creams against the chemical irritants sodium lauryl sulfate (SLS), sodium hydroxide (NaOH), and toluene. The irritants were applied daily for 2 weeks to shaved back skin of young guinea pigs. Barrier creams were applied to the test animals 2 hours before and immediately after exposure to the irritant. Control animals were treated with the irritant only. Erythema was measured visually, and by bioengineering methods: laser doppler flowmetry and transepidermal water loss. One barrier cream was effective against SLS and toluene, whereas the other tested was not. In a follow-up study, another allegedly protective cream failed to inhibit irritation caused by SLS and toluene and exaggerated irritation to NaOH, contrary to its recommended use [8]. The RIT is proposed as an animal model to test the efficacy of barrier creams, and a human version, described below, has also been proposed.

TABLE 4 Examples of Modified Draize Irritation Method

	Draize	FHSA	DOT	FIFRA	OECD
Number of animals	3	6	6	6	6
Abrasion/intact	Both	Both	Intact	2 of each	Intact
Dose liquids	0.5 mL undiluted	0.5 mL undiluted	0.5 mL	0.5 mL undiluted	0.5 mL
Dose solids in solvent	0.5 g	0.5 g moistened	0.5 g moistened	0.5 g	0.5 g
Exposure period (h)	24	24	4	4	4
Examination (h)	24, 72	24, 72	4, 48	0.5, 1, 24, 48, 72	0.5, 1, 24, 48, 72
Removal of test materials	Not specified	Not specified	Skin washed	Skin wiped	Skin washed
Excluded from testing	—	—	—	Toxic materials pH $\leq$2 or $\geq$11.5	Toxic materials pH $\leq$2 or $\geq$11.5

Abbreviations: FHSA, Federal Hazardous Substance Act; DOT, Department of Transportation; FIFRA, Federal Insecticide, Fungicide and Rodenticide Act; OECD, Organization for Economic Cooperation and Development.
Source: Ref. 4.

Repeat application patch tests have been developed to rank the irritant potential of products. Putative irritants are applied to the same site for 3 to 21 days, under occlusion. The degree of occlusion influences percutaneous penetration, which may in turn influence the sensitivity of the test. Patches used vary from Draize-type gauze dressings to metal chambers. Therefore, a reference irritant material is often included in the test to facilitate interpretation of the results. Various animal species have also been used, such as the guinea pig and the rabbit [9,10]. Wahlberg measured skinfold thickness with Harpenden calipers to assess the edema-producing capacity of chemicals in guinea pigs. This model showed clear dose-response relationships and discriminating power, except for acids and alkalis where no change in skinfold thickness was found.

Open application assays are also used for repeat irritation testing. Marzulli and Maibach [11] described a cumulative irritation assay in rabbits that uses open applications and control reference compounds. The test substances are applied 16 times over a 3-week period and the results are measured with a visual score for erythema and skin thickness measurements. These two parameters correlated highly. A significant correlation was also shown between the scores of 60 test substances in the rabbit and in man, suggesting that the rabbit assay is a powerful predictive model.

Anderson et al. [12] used an open application procedure in guinea pigs to rank weak irritants. A baseline response to SLS solution was obtained after 3 applications per day for 3 days to a 1 cm^2 test area. This baseline is used to compare other irritants, of which trichloroethane was the most irritant, similar to 2% SLS. Histology showed a mononuclear dermal inflammatory response.

Immersion Assay

The guinea pig immersion assay was developed to assess the irritant potential of aqueous surfactant–based solutions, but might be extended to other occupational settings such as aqueous cutting fluids. Restrained guinea pigs are immersed in the test solution while maintaining their head above water. The possibility of systemic absorption of a lethal dose restricts the study to products of limited toxic potential. Therefore, the test concentration is usually limited to 10%.

Ten guinea pigs are placed immersed in a 40°C solution for 4 hours daily for three days. A comparison group is immersed in a reference solution. Twenty-four hours after the final immersion, the animals' flanks are shaved and evaluated for erythema, edema, and fissures [13,14,15,16]. Gupta et al. [17] concomitantly tested the dermatotoxic effects of detergents in guinea pigs and humans, using the immersion test and the patch test, respectively. Epidermal erosion and a 40 to 60% increase in the histamine content of the guinea pig skin was found, in addition to a positive patch test reaction in seven of eight subjects.

Mouse Ear Model

Uttley and Van Abbe [18] applied undiluted shampoos to one ear of mice daily for four days, visually quantifying the degree of inflammation as vessel dilatation, erythema, and edema. Patrick and Maibach [19] measured ear thickness to quantify the inflammatory response to surfactant–based products and other chemicals. This allowed quantification of dose-response relationships and comparison of chemicals. Inoue et al. [20] used this model to compare the mechanism of mustard oil–induced skin inflammation to the mechanism of capsaicin-induced inflammation. Mice were pretreated with various receptor antagonists, such as 5-HT$_2$, H$_1$, and tachykinin antagonists, showing that the tachykinin NK1 receptor was an important mediator of inflammation induced by mustard oil. The mouse models provide simplicity and objective measurements. Relevance for man requires elucidation.

Other Methods

Several other assays of skin irritation have been suggested. Humphrey [21] quantified the amount of Evans blue dye recovered from rat skin after exposure to skin irritants. Trush et al. [22] used myeloperoxidase in polymorphonuclear leukocytes as a biomarker for cutaneous inflammation.

HUMAN MODELS

Human models for skin irritation testing are species relevant, thereby eliminating the precarious extrapolation of animal and in vitro data to the human setting. As the required test area is small, several products or concentrations can be tested simultaneously and compared. Inclusion of a reference irritant substance facilitates interpretation of the irritant potential of the test substances. Prior animal or in vitro studies, depending on model relevance and regulatory issue, can be used to exclude particularly toxic substances or concentrations before human exposure.

Single-Application Patch Testing

The National Academy of Sciences (NAS) [23] outlined a single-application patch test procedure determining skin irritation in humans. Occlusive patches may be applied to the intrascapular region of the back or the volar surface of the forearms, using a relatively nonocclusive tape for new or volatile materials. More occlusive tapes or chambers generally increase the severity of the responses. A reference material is included in each battery of patches.

The exposure time may vary to suit the study. NAS suggests a 4-hour exposure period, although it may be desirable to test new or volatile materials for 30 minutes to 1 hour. Studies longer than 24 hours have been performed. Skin responses are evaluated 30 minutes to 1 hour after removal of the patch, using the animal Draize scale (Table 2) or similar. Kligman and Wooding [24] described statistical analysis on test data to calculate the IT50 (time to produce imitation in 50% of the subjects) and the ID50 (dose required to produce irritation in 50% of the subjects after a 24-hour exposure).

Robinson et al. [25] suggested a 4-hour patch test as an alternative to animal testing. Assessing erythema by visual scoring, they tested a variety of irritants on Caucasians and Asians. A relative ranking of irritancy was obtained using 20% SLS as a benchmark. Taking this model further, McFadden et al. [26] investigated the threshold of skin irritation in the six different skin types. Again using SLS as a benchmark, they defined the skin irritant threshold as the lowest concentration of SLS that would produce skin irritation under the 4-hour occluded patch conditions. They found no significant difference in irritation between the skin types.

Cumulative Irritation Testing

Lanman et al. [27] and Phillips et al. [9] described a cumulative irritation assay, which has become known as the ''21-day'' cumulative irritation assay. The purpose of the test was to screen new formulas before marketing. A 1 inch square of Webril was saturated with liquid of 0.5 g of viscous substances and applied to the surface of the pad to be applied to the skin. The patch was applied to the upper back and sealed with occlusive tape. The patch is removed after 24 hours, and then reapplied after examination of the test site. This is repeated for 21 days and the IT50 can then be calculated. Note that the interpretation of the data is best done by comparing the data to an internal standard for which human clinical experience exists.

Modifications have been made to this method. The chamber scarification test (see the following) was developed to predict the effect of repeated applications of a potential irritant to damaged skin, rather than healthy skin. The cumulative patch test described above had failed to predict adverse reactions to skin damaged by acne or shaving, or sensitive areas such as the face [28].

Wigger-Alberti et al. [29] compared two cumulative models by testing skin reaction to metalworking fluids (MWF). Irritation was assessed by visual scoring, transepidermal water loss, and chromametry. In the first method, MWF were applied with Finn Chambers on the volunteers' midback, removed after 1 day of exposure, and reapplied for a further 2 days. In the second method, cumulative irritant contact dermatitis was induced using a repetitive irritation test for 2 weeks (omitting weekends) for 6 hours per day. The 3-day model was preferred because of its shorter duration and better discrimination of irritancy. For low-irritancy materials in which discrimination is not defined with visual and palpatory scores, bioengineering methods (i.e., transepidermal water loss) may be helpful.

The Chamber Scarification Test

This test was developed [30,31] to test the irritant potential of products on damaged skin. Six to eight 1 mm sites on the volar forearm were scratched eight times with a 30-gauge needle without causing bleeding. Four scratches were parallel and the other four are perpendicular to these. Duhring chambers, containing 0.1 g of test material (ointments, creams, or powders), were then placed over the test sites. For liquids, a fitted pad saturated (0.1 mL) may be used. Chambers containing fresh materials are reapplied daily for 3 days. the sites are evaluated by visual scoring 30 minutes after removal of the final set of chambers. A scarification index may be calculated if both normal and scarified skin are tested to reflect the relative degree of irritation between compromised and intact skin; this is the score of scarified sites divided by the score of intact sites. However, the relationship of this assay to routine use of substances on damaged skin remains to be established. Another compromised skin model, the arm immersion model of compromised skin, is described in the following immersion tests section.

The Soap Chamber Test

Frosch & Kligman [32] proposed a model to compare the potential of bar soaps to cause "chapping." Standard patch testing was able to predict erythema, but unable to predict the dryness, flaking, and fissuring seen clinically. In this method, Duhring chambers fitted with Webril pads were used to apply 0.1 mL of an 8% soap solution to the human forearm. The chambers were secured with porous tape, and applied for 24 hours on day 1. On days 2 to 5, fresh patches were applied for 6 hours. The skin is examined daily before patch application and on day 8, the final study day. No patches are applied after day 5. Applications were discontinued if severe erythema was noted at any point. Reactions were scored on a visual scale of erythema, scaling, and fissures. This test correlated well with skin-washing procedures, but tended to overpredict the irritancy of some substances [33].

Immersion Tests

These tests of soaps and detergents were developed in order to improve irritancy prediction by mimicking consumer use. Kooyman & Snyder [34] describe a method in which soap solutions of up to 3% are prepared in troughs. The temperature was maintained at 105°F while subjects immersed one hand and forearm in each trough, comparing different products (or concentrations). The exposure period ranged from 10 to 15 minutes, three times each day for 5 days, or until irritation was observed in both arms. The antecubital fossa was the first site to show irritation, followed by the hands [6,34]. Therefore, antecubital wash tests (see the following) and hand immersion assays were developed [5].

Clarys et al. [35] used a 30-minute/4-day immersion protocol to investigate the effects of temperature as well as anionic character on the degree of irritation caused by detergents. The irritation was quantified by assessment of the stratum corneum barrier function (transepidermal water loss), skin redness (a* color parameter), and skin dryness (capacitance method). Although both detergents tested significantly affected the integrity of the skin, higher anionic content and temperature, respectively, increased the irritant response.

Allenby et al. [36] describe the arm immersion model of compromised skin, which is designed to test the irritant or allergic potential of substances on damaged skin. Such skin may show an increased response, which may be negligible or undetectable in normal skin. The test subject immersed one forearm in a solution of 0.5% sodium dodecyl sulfate for 10 minutes, twice daily until the degree of erythema reached 1 to 1+ on visual scale. This degree of damage corresponded to a morning's wet domestic work. Patch tests of various irritants were applied to the dorsal and volar aspects of both the pretreated and untreated forearms, and also to the back. Each irritant produced a greater degree of reaction on the compromised skin.

Wash Tests

Hannuksela and Hannuksela [37] compared the irritant effects of a detergent in use testing and patch testing. In this study of atopic and nonatopic medical students, each subject washed the outer aspect of the one forearm with liquid detergent for 1 minute, twice daily for 1 week. Concurrently, a 48-hour chamber patch test of five concentrations of the same detergent was performed on the upper back. The irritant response was quantified by bioengineering techniques: transepidermal water loss, electrical capacitance, and skin blood flow. In the wash test, atopics and nonatopics developed irritant contact dermatitis equally, whereas atopics reacted more readily to the detergent in chamber tests. The disadvantage of the chamber test is that, under occlusion, the detergent can cause stronger irritation than it would in normal use [38]. Although the wash test simulates normal use of the product being tested, its drawback is a lack of standard guidelines for performing the test. Charbonnier et al. [39] included squamometry in their analysis of a hand-washing model of subclinical irritant dermatitis with SLS solutions. Squamometry showed a significant difference between 0.1 and 0.75% SLS solutions whereas visual, subjective, capacitance, transepidermal water loss, and chromametry methods were unable to make the distinction. Charbonnier suggests squamometry as an adjunct to the other bioengineering methods.

Frosch [33] describes an antecubital washing test to evaluate toilet soaps, using two washing procedures per day. Simple visual scoring of the reaction (erythema and edema) allows products to be compared. This comparison can be in terms of average score, or number of washes required to produce an effect.

Assessing Protective Barriers

Zhai et al. [40] proposed a model to evaluate skin protective materials. Ten subjects were exposed to the irritants SLS and ammonium hydroxide (in urea), and Rhus allergen. The occluded test sites were on each forearm, with one control site on each. The irritant response was assessed visually using a 10-point scale, which included vesiculation and maceration unlike standard Draize scales. The scores were statistically analyzed for non-parametric data. Of the barrier creams studied, paraffin wax in cetyl alcohol was found to be the most effective in preventing irritation.

Wigger-Alberti and Elsner [41] investigated the potential of petrolatum to prevent epidermal barrier disruption induced by various irritants in a repetitive irritation test. White petrolatum was applied to the backs of 20 human subjects who were exposed to SLS, NaOH, toluene, and lactic acid. Irritation was assessed by transepidermal water loss and colorimetry in addition to visual scoring. It was concluded that petrolatum was an effective barrier cream against SLS, NaOH, and lactic acid, and moderately effective against toluene.

Frosch et al. [42] adapted the guinea pig RIT previously described for use in humans. Two barrier creams were evaluated for their ability to prevent irritation to SLS. In this repetitive model, the irritant was applied to the ventral forearm, using a glass cup, for 30 minutes daily for 2 weeks. One arm of each subject was pretreated with a barrier cream. As in the animal model, erythema was assessed by visual scoring, laser doppler flow, and transepidermal water loss. Skin color was also measured by colorimetry (La* value). The barrier cream decreased skin irritation to SLS, the most differentiating parameter being transepidermal water loss and the least differentiating being colorimetry.

Bioengineering Methods in Model Development

Many of the models previously described do not use the modern bioengineering techniques available, and therefore data based on these models may be imprecise. Despite the investigations skill, subjective assessment of erythema, edema, and other visual parameters may lead to confounding by inter and intraobserver variation. Although the eye may be more sensitive than current spectroscopy and chromametric techniques, the reproducibility and increased statistical power of such data may provide greater benefit. A combination of techniques, such as transepidermal water loss, capacitance, ultrasound, laser doppler flowmetry, spectroscopy, and chromametric analysis, in addition to skilled observation may increase the precision of the test. Andersen and Maibach [43] compared various bioengineering techniques, finding that clinically indistinguishable reactions induced significantly different changes in barrier function and vascular status. An outline of many of these techniques is provided by Patil et al. [5].

REFERENCES

1. Weltfriend S, Bason M, Lammintausta K, Maibach HI. Irritant dermatitis (irritation). In: Marzulli FN, Maibach HI, eds. Dermatotoxicology. 5th ed. Washington, D.C.: Taylor Francis, 1996.
2. Draize TH, Woodland G, Calvery HO. Methods for the study of irritation and toxicity of substances applied to the skin and mucous membranes. J Pharmacol Exp Ther 1944; 82:377–390.
3. Code of Federal Regulations. Office of the Federal Registrar, National Archive of Records. General Services Administration, 1985, title 16, parts 1500.40–1500.42.
4. Patrick E, Maibach HI. Comparison of the time course, dose response and mediators of chemically induced skin irritation in three species. In: Frosch PJ et al., eds. Current Topics in Contact Dermatitis. New York: Springer-Verlag, 1989:399–402.
5. Patil SM, Patrick E, Maibach HI. Animal, human and in vitro test methods for predicting skin irritation. In: Marzulli FN, Maibach HI, eds. Dermatotoxicology Methods: The Laboratory Worker's Vade Mecum. Washington, D.C.: Taylor & Francis, 1998:89–104.
6. Justice JD, Travers JJ, Vinson LJ. The correlation between animal tests and human tests in assessing product mildness. Proc Scientific Section Toilet Goods Assoc 1961; 35:12–17.
7. Frosch PJ, Schulze-Dirks A, Hoffmann M, Axthelm I, Kurte A. Efficacy of skin barrier creams (I). The repetitive irritation test (RIT) in the guinea pig. Contact Derm 1993a; 28(2):94–100.
8. Frosch PJ, Schulze-Dirks A, Hoffmann M, Axthelm I. Efficacy of skin barrier creams (II). Ineffectiveness of a popular ''skin protector'' against various irritants in the repetitive irritation test in the guinea pig. Contact Derm 1993; 29(2):74–77.
9. Phillips L, Steinberg M, Maibach HI, Akers WA. A comparison of rabbit and human skin responses to certain irritants. Toxicol Appl Pharmacol 1972; 21:369–382.
10. Wahlberg JE. Measurement of skin fold thickness in the guinea pig. Assessment of edema-inducing capacity of cutting fluids acids, alkalis, formalin and dimethyl sulfoxide. Contact Derm, 1993; 28:141–145.
11. Marzulli FN, Maibach HI. The rabbit as a model for evaluating skin irritants: a comparison of results obtained on animals and man using repeated skin exposure. Food Cosmet Toxicol 1975; 13:533–540.
12. Anderson C, Sundberg K, Groth O. Animal model for assessment of skin irritancy. Contact Derm 1986; 15:143–151.
13. Opdyke DL, Burnett CM. Practical problems in the evaluation of the safety of cosmetics. Proc Scientific Section Toilet Goods Assoc 1965; 44:3–4.
14. Calandra J. Comments on the guinea pig immersion test. CTFA Cosmet J 1971; 3(3):47.
15. Opdyke DL. The guinea pig immersion test—a 20 year appraisal. CTFA Cosmet J 1971; 3(3):46–47.
16. MacMillan FSK, Ram RR, Elvers WB. A comparison of the skin irritation produced by cosmetic ingredients and formulations in the rabbit, guinea pig, beagle dog to that observed in the human. In: Maibach HI, ed. Animal Models in Dermatology. Edinburgh: Churchill Livingstone, 1975:12–22.
17. Gupta BN, Mathur AK, Srivastava AK, Singh S, Singh A, Chandra SV. Dermal exposure to detergents. Veterinary Human Toxicol 1992; 34(5):405–407.
18. Uttley M, Van Abbe NJ. Primary irritation of the skin: mouse ear test and human patch test procedures. J Soc Cosmet Chem 1973; 24:217–227.
19. Patrick E, Maibach HI. A novel predictive assay in mice. Toxicologist 1987; 7:84.
20. Inoue H, Asaka T, Nagata N, Koshihara Y. Mechanism of mustard oil–induced skin inflammation in mice. Eur J Pharmacol 1997; 333(2,3):231–240.
21. Humphrey DM. Measurement of cutaneous microvascular exudates using Evans blue. Biotechnic Histochem 1993; 68(6):342–349.

22. Trush MA, Egner PA, Kensler TW. Myeloperoxidase as a biomarker of skin irritation and inflammation. Food Chem Toxicol 1994; 32(2):143–147.

23. National Academy of Sciences. Committee for the Revision of NAS Publication 1138. Principles and Procedures for Evaluating the Toxicity of Household Substances. Washington, D.C.: National Academy of Sciences, 1977:23–59.

24. Kligman AM, Wooding WM. A method for the measurement and evaluation of irritants on human skin. J Invest Dermatol 1967; 49:78–94.

25. Robinson MK, Perkins MA, Basketter DA. Application of a 4-h human patch test method for comparative and investigative assessment of skin irritation. Contact Derm 1998; 38(4):194–202.

26. McFadden JP, Wakelin SH, Basketter DA. Acute irritation thresholds in subjects with type I–type VI skin. Contact Derm 1998; 38(3):147–149.

27. Lanman BM, Elvers WB, Howard CS. The role of human patch testing in a product development program. In: Proc. Joint Conference on Cosmetic Sciences. Washington, D.C.: Toilet Goods Association, 1968:135–145.

28. Battista CW, Rieger MM. Some problems of predictive testing. J Soc Cosmet Chem 1971; 22:349–359.

29. Wigger-Alberti W, Hinnen U, Elsner P. Predictive testing of metalworking fluids: a comparison of 2 cumulative human irritation models and correlation with epidemiological data. Contact Derm 1997; 36(1):14–20.

30. Frosch PJ, Kligman AM. The chamber scarification test for irritancy. Contact Derm 1976; 2:314–324.

31. Frosch PJ, Kligman AM. The chamber scarification test for testing the irritancy of topically applied substances. In: Drill VA, Lazar P, eds. Cutaneous Toxicity. New York: Academic Press, 1977:150.

32. Frosch PJ, Kligman AM. The soap chamber test. A new method for assessing the irritancy of soaps. J Am Acad Dermatol 1979; 1(1):35–41.

33. Frosch PJ. The irritancy of soap and detergent bars. In: Frost P, Howitz SN, eds. Principles of Cosmetics for the Dermatologist. St. Louis: C. V. Mosby, 1982:5–12.

34. Kooyman DJ, Snyder FH. The test for mildness of soaps. Arch Dermatol Syphilol 1942; 46:846–855.

35. Clarys P, Manou I, Barel AO. Influence of temperature on irritation in the hand/forearm immersion test. Contact Derm 1997; 36(5):240–243.

36. Allenby CF, Basketter DA, Dickens A, Barnes EG, Brough HC. An arm immersion model of compromised skin (I). Influence on irritation reactions. Contact Derm 1993; 28(2):84–88.

37. Hannuksela A, Hannuksela M. Irritant effects of a detergent in wash, chamber and repeated open application tests. Contact Derm 1996; 34(2):134–137.

38. Van der Valk PG, Maibach HI. Post-application occlusion substantially increases the irritant response of the skin to repeated short-term sodium lauryl sulfate (SLS) exposure. Contact Derm 1989; 21(5):335–338.

39. Charbonnier V, Morrison Jr BM, Paye M, Maibach HI. Open application assay in investigation of subclinical dermatitis induced by sodium lauryl sulfate (SLS) in man: advantage of squamometry. Skin Res Technol 1998; 4:244–250.

40. Zhai H, Willard P, Maibach HI. Evaluating skin-protective materials against contact irritants and allergens. An in vivo screening human model. Contact Derm 1998; 38(3):155–158.

41. Wigger-Alberti W, Elsner P. Petrolatum prevents irritation in a human cumulative exposure model in vivo. Dermatology 1997; 194(3):247–250.

42. Frosch PJ, Schulze-Dirks A, Hoffmann M, Axthelm I, Kurte A. Efficacy of skin barrier creams (I). The repetitive irritation test (RIT) in the guinea pig. Contact Derm 1993; 28(2):94–100.

43. Andersen PH, Maibach HI. Skin irritation in man: a comparative bioengineering study using improved reflectance spectroscopy. Contact Derm 1995; 33(5):315–322.

13

Eye Irritation Testing

Leon H. Bruner
Gillette Medical Evaluation Laboratory, The Gillette Company, Needham, Massachusetts

Rodger D. Curren and John W. Harbell
Institute for In Vitro Sciences, Inc., Gaithersburg, Maryland

Rosemarie Osborne and James K. Maurer
The Procter & Gamble Company, Cincinnati, Ohio

INTRODUCTION

The eye is the sensory organ that captures visible light energy and converts it into neural impulses that give rise to vision, our most important sense. Because of its external location, the eye is constantly exposed. It can be damaged by drying, natural environmental contaminants, and micro-organisms. It is also vulnerable to injury induced by a variety of traumatic insults, including chemical exposure.

Accidental eye exposure to chemicals or consumer products occurs at home and in the workplace. Therefore, developers of consumer goods and chemicals must perform ocular safety assessments in order to prevent dangerous products from reaching the market and to correctly advise consumers and workers on the safety of the materials they use [1–3].

Data from animal tests have been used to make eye safety assessments since the 1940s. These tests use the albino rabbit as the animal model and a systematic numerical scoring system for quantifying the irritation response [4]. Although the in vivo eye irritation tests provide important and useful information, they are not without faults. Thus, there is great interest in developing alternative methods that will allow toxicologists to make accurate ocular safety assessments without using animals. Accomplishing such a goal is a great challenge.

This chapter will review the state of the art in developing nonanimal methods for the Draize eye irritation test. It will describe the anatomical and physiological features of the anterior eye relevant to ocular safety testing and development of alternative assay systems. The work that has been done to develop alternative methods will be reviewed. The chapter closes with a discussion of how alternative methods may be used in the safety assessment process and the areas where additional research is needed in order to provide more reliable tests for the future.

HUMAN OCULAR ANATOMY

The eyeball is a fibrovascular spheroid globe suspended in a bony orbit by numerous ligaments and extrinsic muscles [5,6]. The globe is lightproof except for the transparent corneal surface. Only the anterior aspect of the eyeball is exposed to the environment. The rest is protected behind the eyelids and bony orbital rim.

The eyeball has three coats that are further divided into subparts. The outer coat is the transparent cornea and the gray-white sclera that provides the primary supporting framework of the globe. The middle coat is the uvea that contains the choroid, ciliary body, and iris. The inner coat is the retina, the neural photoreceptive tissue in the eye.

The majority of the nonretinal structures perform secondary functions that aid the primary photoreception process. These include focusing images on the retina (cornea and lens), regulating the amount of light entering the eye (iris), providing nutrients to ocular tissues (vasculature, aqueous humor, vitreous humor, and lachrymal or tear system), moving the eyes (extrinsic musculature), and protection (somatosensory nerves and eyelids).

Outer Coat

Cornea and Precorneal Tear Film

The cornea is the transparent anterior surface of the eye where light passes to the retina (Fig. 1). Because the cornea is the main refractive surface of the eye, it also plays a key role in focusing images on the photoreceptor surface. A clear, properly shaped cornea is therefore critical for normal vision. Its exposed location makes it particularly vulnerable to injury, and any scarring that occurs may lead to opacities or shape changes that permanently impair vision.

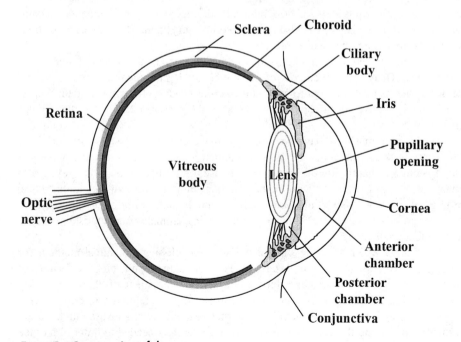

FIGURE 1 Cross section of the eye.

Precorneal Tear Film. The anterior surface of the cornea is covered by the precorneal tear film. This outer film is important for proper corneal function. It hydrates the anterior cornea and provides a smooth, continuous surface that enhances its optical properties. The tear film comprises an anterior lipid layer, with an aqueous and mucin-containing layer underneath. The lipid layer slows the evaporation of the aqueous layer, and provides a smooth, regular optical surface. The mucin wets the microvilli of the corneal epithelial cells and must be intact for the precorneal tear film to form and remain on the corneal surface.

Cornea. The cornea has three layers: the epithelium with its basement membrane, the stroma or substantia propria, and the endothelium with its basement membrane (Fig. 2).

Epithelium. In humans, the corneal epithelium is approximately 50 to 90 μm thick and covers the entire stromal surface. It is a stratified, nonkeratinized epithelium of five to six cell layers. The outermost epithelium has two to three layers of squamous cells. The midzone or wing cell layer consists of two to three layers of polyhedral cells, and the bottom-most or basal cell layer is a single layer of cells. The epithelial cells regenerate in the basal layer, and become progressively flatter as they migrate toward the surface. Epithelial stem cells reside in the basal cell layer in the more peripheral cornea (limbus), whereas transient amplifying cells lie over the cornea. The limbus is 5 to 10 cell layers thick, and overlies a rather loose and highly vascular connective tissue clearly distinct from the dense and avascular corneal stroma. It contains melanocytes and Langerhans cells, and marks the boundary of the cornea with the bulbar conjunctiva. Squamous surface

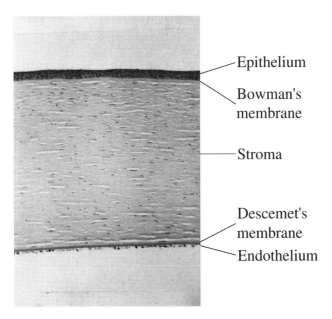

Epithelium

Bowman's membrane

Stroma

Descemet's membrane

Endothelium

FIGURE 2 Cross section of human cornea showing from top to bottom the epithelium, Bowman's membrane, stroma, Descemet's membrane, and endothelium (H&E stain, 200× magnification). (Courtesy of I. Cree, Moorefield's Eye Hospital, London, England.)

cells are shed from the surface of the cornea after approximately 7 days. Directly below the basal cell layer is the basement membrane.

Stroma. The stroma constitutes approximately 90% of the corneal thickness. Its anterior portion, Bowman's layer, is an acellular region lying just under the epithelial basement membrane. It is more resistant to deformation, trauma, passage of foreign bodies, or infecting organisms than the other layers. Once damaged, its architecture may not be restored, leading to abnormalities in corneal thickness and optical properties that could result in permanent vision deficit. The remainder of the stroma is composed of collagen fibrils gathered together in lamellae that run in parallel with the corneal surface. The fibrils within a lamella are highly organized and are surrounded by a glycosaminoglycan matrix. Corneal glycosaminoglycans are 60% keratin sulfate, and 40% chondroitin sulfates. These act as anions and bind cations and water. The posterior surface of the stroma is lined with the loosely attached Descemet's layer that is the basement membrane for the endothelial cells. Scattered throughout the lamellae are long, flat fibroblast-like cells called keratocytes. These cells have long processes that extend to adjacent cells. There are also a few neutrophils and macrophages that migrate through the stroma. Branches of the ophthalmic branch of the fifth (trigeminal) cranial nerve, which are primarily sensory, run through the anterior third of the corneal stroma and associate with the epithelium.

Endothelium. The endothelium is a single layer resting on Descemet's layer. The endothelium originates from the neural crest and therefore is not a true endothelium. The apical surface is in contact with the aqueous humor of the anterior chamber. The cells are tightly bound to each other with desmosomes. The endothelium serves the important function of maintaining the dehydration (deturgescence) that is also required to maintain corneal clarity (see the following section).

Sclera

The sclera is a dense, fibrous, collagenous structure that makes up the gray-white part of the globe. Like the cornea, it has three layers. The outermost layer is the episclera. The episclera is a vascularized connective tissue that merges with the scleral stroma and extends connective tissue bundles into the fascia surrounding the globe. The major layer of the sclera is the stroma. The stroma lies in the middle and is composed of irregularly arranged bundles of collagen fibrils. The irregular size and arrangement of these fibrils leads to the white color of the majority of the eyeball. The inner surface of the sclera is the lamina fuscia, which lies interior to the scleral stroma. It contains fine collagen fibers that form the connection between the choroid and sclera. The anterior external scleral surface of the stroma is covered by the conjunctiva. The conjunctiva is a transparent mucous membrane that covers the externally exposed scleral surface (bulbar conjunctiva) as well as the inner surface of the eyelids (palpebral conjunctiva). The conjunctival epithelium is continuous with the corneal epithelium and the lachrymal drainage system. The conjunctiva contains many blood vessels, nerves, conjunctival glands, and inflammatory cells. Small blood vessels are present throughout. They are usually not visible, but dilate and become leaky during inflammation. The nerves transmit pain responses and mediate neurogenic vasodilatation and tearing. The conjunctival glands provide moisture and secrete the constituents of the precorneal tear film.

Anterior Chamber, Posterior Chamber, and Aqueous Humor

Between the rear surface of the cornea and the front surface of the lens capsule is a fluid-filled chamber (Fig. 1). This chamber is divided into anterior and posterior regions by the iris. These chambers are connected through the pupillary opening. The anterior chamber lies in front of the iris and the posterior chamber lies behind the iris and in front of the lens capsule.

The Middle Coat.   The middle coat of the eye is the uvea. It consists of the choroid, the ciliary body, and the iris (Fig. 1). The choroid is a blood vessel–rich layer that provides blood to the retinal pigmented epithelium and outer half of the adjacent sensory retina. The ciliary body secretes the aqueous humor that fills the anterior and posterior chambers and contains the smooth muscle that alters the lens shape as needed for near and far vision. The iris is a diaphragm that lies in front of the lens and ciliary body. Contraction of iris circular or radial muscles leads to closing or opening of the pupil, respectively, which regulates the amount of light entering the eye.

The Inner Coat.   The inner coat of the eye is the retina. This layer contains the neurosensory cells that transmit light-induced signals to the brain for visual interpretation. The two major parts of the retina are the inner sensory layer and the outer pigmented epithelium. The sensory layer lies between the pigmented epithelium on the outside and the vitreous humor on the inside. It is stratified into several sublayers containing the different photoreceptor and accessory cells involved with sensing and processing the light projected onto the retinal surface. The pigmented epithelium is only one layer thick and lies between the sensory epithelium and choroid. Readers interested in more details on ocular anatomy, physiology, and biochemistry should consult recent texts on the subject [7–11].

ROUTINE IN VIVO OCULAR IRRITATION TESTING

The need for ocular safety testing became clear early in the 1930s when an untested eyelash product containing p-phenylene diamine was marketed in the United States. Use of this and similar products led to sensitization of the external ocular structures, corneal ulceration, vision loss, and at least one fatality [12]. These events resulted in passage in the United States of the Food, Drug and Cosmetic Act of 1938, which required that materials sold to consumers be safe.

In response to the need for test methods to assess ocular safety, in vivo assays were developed and put into use. One of the earliest reported experimental animal procedures was devised by Friedenwald to assess the effects of acids and bases on the eye [13]. This was the first time the effects of test materials on the cornea, conjunctiva, and iris were separately recorded. Subsequently, Carpenter and Smyth [14] studied many materials and primarily recorded their effects on the cornea. Draize et al. [4] improved the test by standardizing Friedenwald's method and simplifying the scoring system. Subsequently, the Draize procedure and modifications of it have become the standard for assessing the irritancy potential of test materials for more than 50 years. The data are also used by toxicologists to assure that chemicals and consumer products (1) can be made safely in factories, (2) are safe for their intended use and any foreseeable misuse, (3) are appropriately labeled, and (4) meet regulatory safety testing requirements [15].

The Draize Eye-Irritation Test

The standard Draize eye-irritation test uses either three or six albino rabbits. Statistical studies conducted to determine the effect of reducing the number of animals used in a single study from six to three showed that a three-animal test provides eye-irritation classification similar to that obtained by using six rabbits [16,17]. Standard Draize eye-irritation test protocols normally require that 100 μL of a test material is placed in the lower cul-de-sac of one eye, and the eyelids are held shut for a brief period of time. The untreated contralateral eye is used as the control. The eyes are sometimes rinsed after treatment to determine the effect of irrigation on the extent of irritation or to remove test substances trapped within the cul-de-sac.

Generally the eyes are examined using a pen light and graded by a technician for irritation on days 1, 2, 3, 4, and 7 after dosing and weekly thereafter. However, times at which the eyes are examined for irritation after dosing may vary because of differences in government regulations and preferences of different toxicologists. In some cases, the eyes are examined at time points earlier than day 1 (e.g., 1h, 3h). Similarly the maximum period allowed to determine recovery may vary (e.g., 3–5 weeks). Eyes are generally not examined once they have returned to normal. Examinations are sometimes augmented by fluorescein staining and slit-lamp examinations to better assess corneal changes. A grading scale has been proposed based on examinations with a slit lamp [18].

The Draize test uses a systematic numeric grading system to quantify the eye irritation response (Table 1). Changes associated with the cornea, conjunctiva, and iris are assessed by using a pen light. Scores are assigned for the various changes. The scores for the cornea, conjunctiva, and iris are weighted such that changes associated with the cornea are given the most weight, with the maximum score for the cornea being 80 out of a total possible score of 110. A test substance's potential to cause ocular irritation is then determined by assessing the individual animal scores, the maximum average score (highest mean group score during the study), and days to recovery. In general, innocuous or slightly irritating materials tend to affect only the conjunctiva, and the eye recovers in 1 to 2 days; mildly to moderately irritating materials affect the conjunctiva and cornea, and the eye recovers in days to weeks; and moderately to severely irritating materials affect the cornea, iris, and conjunctiva, and the eye recovers in weeks or not at all. These results are often further classified according to various regulatory classification schemes in use around the world. The interested reader should consult Chan and Hayes [19] for a summary of regulatory considerations.

Although the Draize eye-irritation test and slight variations of it have remained the standard procedure for determining ocular-irritation responses, the use of this test has not continued without significant criticism. The sensitivity and relevance of the Draize test have been questioned because the dose given is greater than the volume of the conjunctival cul-de-sac of the rabbit eye (30 μl) [20], thereby considerably exceeding the dose received in human accidental eye exposure [21,22]. Additionally, the in vivo tests have been criticized for their subjectivity [23], lack of repeatability [24,25], overprediction of human responses [26–28], and by animal welfare advocates because they require the use of animals [29]. Therefore, efforts have been made to develop and validate significantly modified in vivo test protocols as well as develop in vitro tests to reduce and perhaps ultimately eliminate the use of animals in ocular-irritation testing.

Modifications of the In Vivo Eye-Irritation Test

The Low-Volume Eye Test

In the early 1980s, modifications made in the amount of test material dosed and site of application resulted in a refined version of the classical Draize test, called the low-volume eye test (LVET). The LVET has been reported to be less stressful to rabbits and more predictive of human ocular irritancy potential than the standard Draize procedure

TABLE 1   Scale of Weighted Scores for Grading the Severity of Ocular Lesions

Ocular effects	Grade
Cornea	
(A) Opacity-degree of density (area that is most dense is taken for reading)	
Scattered or diffuse area—details of iris clearly visible	1
Easily discernible translucent areas, details of iris clearly visible	2
Opalescent areas, no details of iris visible, size of pupil barely discernible	3
Opaque, iris invisible	4
(B) Area of cornea involved	
One quarter (or less) but not zero	1
Greater than one quarter—less than one half	2
Greater than one half—less than three quarters	3
Greater than three quarters—up to whole area	4
Total maximum* = 80	
Iris	
(A) Values	
Fold above normal, congestion, swelling, circumcorneal injection (any one or all of these or combination of any thereof), iris still reacting to light (sluggish reaction is positive)	1
No reaction to light, hemorrhage; gross destruction (any one or all of these)	2
Total maximum** = 10	
Conjunctivae	
(A) Redness (refers to palpebral conjunctivae only)	
Vessels definitely injected above normal	1
More diffuse, deeper crimson red, individual vessels not easily discernible	2
Diffuse beefy red	3
(B) Chemosis	
Any swelling above normal (includes nictitating membrane)	1
Obvious swelling with partial eversion of the lids	2
Swelling with lids about half closed	3
Swelling with lids about half closed to completely closed	4
(C) Discharge	
Any amount different from normal (does not include small amounts observed in inner canthus of normal animals)	1
Discharge with moistening of the lids and hairs just adjacent to the lids	2
Discharge with moistening of the lids and considerable area around the eye	3
Total maximum† = 20	

* Score = A $\times$ B $\times$ 5.
** Score = A $\times$ 5.
† Score (A + B + C) $\times$ 2.
Note: The maximum total score is the sum of the total maximum scores obtained for the cornea, iris, and conjunctivae.
Source: Ref. 4.

[26,27,30,31]. The LVET differs from the standard Draize eye-irritation test in three ways: (1) the volume of test substance applied is 10 μL instead of 100 μL; (2) the test substance is placed directly on the corneal surface instead of into the lower conjunctival cul-de-sac; and (3) the eyes are not held shut after the test substance is applied. This method of application and the dose applied much more closely simulates accidental human exposures [32]. Normally either three or six rabbits are used per test substance. Statistical studies similar to those conducted for the Draize test indicate that results from three rabbits provide eye-irritation classification similar to that obtained from studies using six rabbits, so that animal use in this test can be minimized [33].

Objective Measurements of Eye Injury

In addition to the LVET, other modifications have been made to the in vivo test. Most of these changes have been made in an attempt to minimize variability. Because the subjective nature of the grading is thought to be a major source of variability, work has been done to eliminate as much as possible the subjective components of the test. Some of the methods evaluated include assessing corneal thickness [34–36], water content [36,37], permeability [38–40], and surface area damaged using fluorescein, wound healing, and exfoliative cytology [41]. Objective measurements of conjunctivitis have included assessments of capillary permeability [36,37], redness, and exfoliative cytology [41]. Others have attempted to assess the utility of measuring intraocular pressure [42] and protein content of the aqueous humor [36,37]. None of these methods is in routine use.

REPLACING THE ANIMAL TEST WITH IN VITRO METHODS
Introduction

There are strong social, political, ethical, and scientific arguments for the development and use of nonanimal methods as alternatives to the Draize eye-irritation test. Alternative methods currently under investigation use a diverse set of human and animal cells, tissues, and biochemical reagents, and measure a diverse set of endpoints thought to be associated with eye-irritation responses in vivo. Few of these tests, however, attempt to model the entire eye. Instead, they usually model subparts of the larger, more complex eye-irritation response. Figure 3 shows this reductionist relationship across the spectrum of available

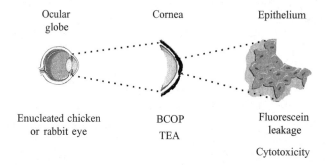

Ocular globe   Cornea   Epithelium

Enucleated chicken or rabbit eye   BCOP   Fluorescein leakage

TEA

Cytotoxicity

FIGURE 3   A diagram illustrating how in vitro assays have been developed to model different parts of the eye-irritation response. In the development of in vitro tests, the eye is in effect reduced to component parts. The tests developed model different parts of the eye-irritation response and allows studies on mechanisms of action. The first reduction step from the intact animal uses isolated whole eyes obtained from the abattoir. Examples include the chicken enucleated eye test and the isolated rabbit eye test. The next level of reduction is represented by tests that use isolated corneas and 3-dimensional tissue constructs. Examples include the bovine cornea opacity and permeability test (BCOP) and the topical application assays (TEA), respectively. The final level of reduction represents tests based on cell cultures containing single cell types. Examples of tests in this category include the fluorescein leakage test and other cytotoxicity tests.

in vitro methods. These methods use (1) isolated whole eyes, (2) isolated corneas, (3) multilayer (3-dimensional) single- and multicell systems, and (4) single-cell culture systems. Representatives of each of these levels will now be reviewed.

Isolated Whole Eyes

At the first stage of reduction, in vitro tests use isolated whole eyes usually obtained from an abattoir. Examples of such tests include the Isolated Rabbit Eye Test (IRE) [43–45] and the Chicken Enucleated Eye Test (CEET) [45–47]. In these model systems, test substances are applied directly to the cornea of an isolated eye for short time periods (usually around 10 sec). Subsequently, several measurements are made to estimate the severity of the resulting injury. These measurements are generally similar to those that can be made in the whole animal, including corneal opacity, corneal swelling, and fluorescein retention. Histopathological examination of the injured tissue can also be conducted. Both isolated eye models have generally performed quite well in identifying severely irritating materials; in fact, the IRE is accepted by regulatory agencies in the United Kingdom for the classification of severely irritating materials, as is the CEET in the Netherlands. Both test methods are compatible with solid and liquid test articles.

Isolated Cornea Models

The substrate used at the next level of reduction is isolated corneas (Fig. 3). The most common source of corneas for these studies is bovine eyes obtained from the abattoir. These corneas are used in an assay called the bovine cornea opacity and permeability (BCOP) test [45,48]. In this assay, test materials are applied directly to the anterior surface of corneas mounted in the center of a dual-sided organ culture chamber. After the designated exposure time, the test substance is washed away and the resulting corneal opacity and changes in epithelial barrier function, evaluated by increased permeability to fluorescein, are measured. An advantage of this model is that the corneal opacity can be measured quantitatively with a photometer because the organ chamber has transparent glass covers on each end. As with the isolated whole eye, it has been shown that assessment of histopathological changes provides additional useful information [49,50].

Multilayer (3-Dimensional) Cultures

The next level of reduction is represented by artificial 3-dimensional tissues constructed from human cells. These tissues are of two types: one is designed to model the corneal epithelium, whereas the second attempts to reconstruct the cornea in vitro.

Dermal and Corneal Epithelium Models. Because the corneal epithelium provides an important barrier function and the epithelial surface is normally the first part of the eye to contact a potentially hazardous material, several in vitro models have been developed to assess the effects of chemicals on epithelial cells. These models are generally reconstructed from human epidermal or corneal cells (either primary or immortalized cultures), which are seeded onto a specialized substrate. Under the appropriate conditions the epithelial cells stratify vertically and differentiate into 3-dimensional, nonkeratinized structures. Test material is placed directly on this substrate and injury is assessed by monitoring changes in the construct's barrier property, the release of cytokines, or cytotoxicity. For example, an immortalized human cornea cell line (10.014 pRSV-T) has been grown on cell culture inserts at an air-liquid interface so that the cultures form an epithelium containing four to six cell layers [51–53]. Test substances are applied to the epithelial surface for brief periods (up to 5 min) in dose-response experiments. Endpoints measured include the barrier function of the epithelium using transepithelial permeability to fluorescein and electrical resistance, along with cell viability [54]. Results from this model, called HCE-T, correlate with historical rabbit-eye data for water-soluble ingredients and surfactant-based personal care products [52]. Others have reported that early (1 h) release of the cytokine interleukin 1-α is a predictive marker for surfactant responses in another human corneal epithelial cell line, CEPI 17 c1.4 [55]. Interleukin 8 appears to be a late (24 h) marker of response, although the bulk of the IL-8 response appears secondary to the release of IL-1α. Taken together, this work shows the potential utility of human cornea epithelial cells to assess effects of test substances on epithelial barrier function, viability, and inflammation, as well as to evaluate specific biochemical and molecular mechanisms of these responses.

Other models have been constructed using primary human epidermal cells rather than immortalized cell lines. Several tissues of this type are available commercially. Currently available substrates include EpiOcular [56] (MatTek Corporation, Ashland, MA) and SkinEthic cultures [57,58] (SkinEthic, Nice, France). In these assays, test substances are applied to the surface of the cultures for a specified period of time. Then, the test substance is washed away and viability of the cells is measured by using one of several vital dyes [57–61]. The release of various cytokines is also measured. These models have been shown capable of differentiating degrees of irritancy between mild test substances. Another advantage of these systems is that they have proven useful for assessing both water-soluble and water-insoluble consumer products, cosmetics, and ingredients [56,59,62].

Human Cornea Models. The development of human corneal cultures analogous to 3-dimensional human skin cultures that are used to evaluate skin irritation [63,64] is now an active area of research. Martin et al. [65] have reported on trilaminar substrates developed from early passage human corneal epithelial, stroma, and endothelial cells. Endpoints evaluated in this model include barrier function, cytotoxicity, and release of the inflammatory mediators PGE_2 and LTB_4. Development of immortalized human cornea cell lines and their incorporation into trilaminar corneal models have also been reported by Griffith and coworkers [66,67]. Functional and biochemical analysis of these cultures indicate the presence of differentiation markers and other properties similar to those found in intact human corneas. In initial characterization, cultures treated with model surfactants elicit responses similar to those observed in vivo.

Single-Cell Culture Systems, Isolated Single Cells

At the last step in the reductionist scheme are assays that use monolayer cell cultures derived from epithelial cells of eyes or other organs such as the skin. The study of interactions between test substances and single cells and monolayer cultures of various types was one of the earliest approaches evaluated for eye-irritation tests in vitro. The most commonly used endpoint is assessment of direct cytotoxicity after a short-term exposure to test articles. Examples of methods in this category include the neutral red uptake test [62,68–71], the neutral red release test [72,73], and the red blood cell lysis test [62,70,74,75]. In addition, the real-time effects of a test material on the metabolic rate of cultured cells can be assessed by using the Cytosensor microphysiometer (Molecular Devices Corp., Menlo Park, CA) [62,69,70,76–78]. The Fluorescein Leakage Test is another cytotoxicity assay that measures the capacity of a test substance to damage the barrier function normally associated with epithelial cells. With this assay, confluent monolayer cultures of renal epithelial cells are treated with test material. After exposure the change in the capacity of the epithelial cells to block fluorescein passage is measured [62,70,79–81]. Additional information on these tests may be found in an extensive review of assays based on single-cell cultures published by U.S. Interagency Regulatory Alternatives Group (IRAG) [82,83].

Other Test Systems

There are several in vitro tests that have been evaluated extensively as alternatives for eye-irritation testing that do not fit entirely within the reductionist scheme just described. The most significant tests in this category are the chorioallantoic membrane (CAM) assays. Use of the CAM of the chicken egg as a substrate for in vitro testing was first described by Luepke et al. [84], who reasoned that the highly vascularized CAM might be an acceptable surrogate for conjunctival tissue. To this end, they developed a model called the hen's egg test–CAM (HET–CAM). In this procedure, test substances are placed directly on the CAM exposed directly underneath the air cell. The resulting hemorrhage, coagulation, and lysis appearing on the CAM are measured at defined timepoints after the test article is applied. Results from this test are accepted by regulatory agencies in Germany as adequate for identifying severe irritants. A complementary test called the CAM vascular assay (CAMVA) has also been developed [85,86]. The CAMVA differs from the HET–CAM in several ways, including the site of the egg shell that is opened (side of the egg instead of the air cell), the endpoint measured (changes in characteristics of the CAM vasculature), and the dosing scheme (serially diluted test substances instead of a single test concentration). Both the HET–CAM and the CAMVA assay are reviewed in detail in the U.S. IRAG evaluations [87]. Results from evaluation of this test in several international validation studies have been reported [62,88–90].

Practical Use of In Vitro Tests for Eye-Irritation Testing

The effort to develop and validate nonanimal test methods has significantly increased the use of these tests for assessing eye safety. Experience gained from this work has shown that the methods provide information useful for safety assessments, but the conduct and interpretation of results from in vitro tests are more complex than for standard in vivo testing. Therefore, considerable care and planning need to be undertaken before beginning a study in order to obtain reliable results. Given the increased complexity associated with in vitro testing, we have found that the use of the new methods is greatly facilitated by the establishment of a standard framework that contains four elements. These include 1) a well-defined process that specifies the steps to follow during the conduct of an eye safety assessment of a test article, 2) protocols and standard operating procedures (SOPs) that define all the tests used within the eye safety assessment process, 3) prediction models that guide the interpretation of results obtained from in vitro and other test methods, and 4) a summary document that provides practical guidance to toxicologists on how to conduct the overall process. The important aspects of each of these elements will now be reviewed.

Process for the Assessment of Test Materials in Nonanimal Methods

A clearly defined testing process is the central element in a nonanimal testing framework. These processes usually take the form of flow charts showing the key decision points, data-gathering procedures, and test methods that may be conducted during a safety assessment. An example suitable for eye-irritation testing is shown in Figure 4. The process begins with the entry of a test substance into a safety assessment program. The first step in the process involves gathering as much previously existing information as possible about the material. The information obtained should include all available toxicity data on the test article, such as in vivo and in vitro data, human clinical data, supplier information, results from quantitative structure activity relationship (QSAR) analyses, physical-chemical data, marketplace experiences, and data on consumer habits and practices. In the case of completely new chemicals or formulations, information on similar materials should be gathered. Once these data are obtained, they must be assessed to determine if it is possible to complete the safety assessment without further testing. At this point, three decisions are possible: 1) market the product because the pre-existing data are considered adequate to support the product safety without further testing, 2) terminate or reformulate because the pre-existing data indicate the article is not safe for intended use, or 3) conduct additional testing because more data are necessary in order to complete the assessment. When the third decision is made, the next step in the process is to evaluate the article in an appropriate in vitro test(s). When the testing is complete, the results are passed through the algorithms of the prediction model so that a toxicity prediction can be obtained. The toxicity prediction is then considered along with the previously existing results. At this point it is again necessary to ask whether the test article is considered safe for intended use. If the answer is no, then reformulation or termination are the available options. If the answer is yes, it is necessary to decide whether human tolerance testing is necessary. Such studies may be needed, for example, to develop data for marketing claims support. If there is no need for human tolerance testing, then the safety assessment is completed.

Protocols and SOPs

Each safety assessment process contains several different tests. In order to facilitate the generation of reliable data from these tests, it is essential that all factors important to their conduct are clearly documented. It is therefore important that protocols and SOPs be provided for each test used in the safety assessment process. Adequate protocols and SOPs will contain at least four key elements. First, each SOP must have a detailed step-by-step description of how to conduct a test. Enough details need to be provided such that any appropriately trained and competent laboratory technician need use only this document as the guide to conduct the assay. Secondly, the SOP must indicate the steps used to define the final endpoint of the assay and the number of replicates necessary. Any data transformation or algorithms applied to the data should be clearly documented and consistently applied. Thirdly, the protocol should specify the positive and negative controls to be performed concurrently with each assay and the acceptable ranges for the resulting responses. Assays where the positive or negative controls values fall outside of those specified ranges would be considered invalid and should be repeated. Finally, the protocol must specifically describe the prediction model used to guide the interpretation of results.

Prediction Models

In order to use an in vitro test method in the safety assessment process, it must be possible to convert the in vitro results into a meaningful prediction of toxicity. The tool that is used to make this conversion is the prediction model [25,91]. A prediction model is considered adequate when it defines four elements. These elements include 1) a definition of the specific purpose(s) for which the alternative method is to be used, 2) a definition of all the possible results that may be obtained from an alternative method (inputs), 3) an algo-

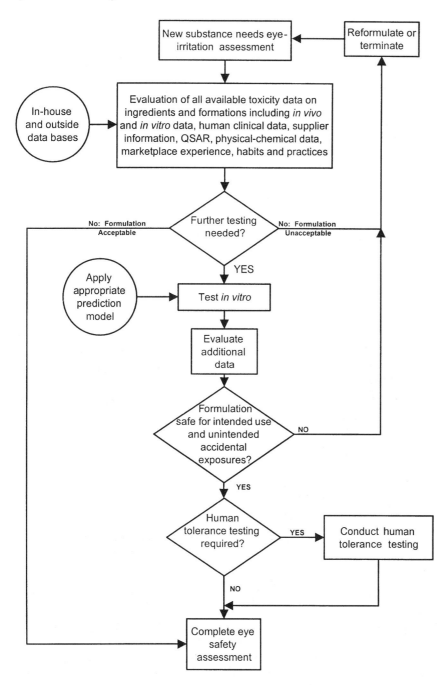

FIGURE 4 Typical eye-irritation assessment process using nonanimal test methods.

rithm that defines how to convert each alternative method result into a prediction of the in vivo toxicity endpoint (outputs), and 4) an indication of the accuracy and precision of outputs obtained from the model. An example of a prediction model for the Cytosensor microphysiometer is given in Figure 5. This figure shows the relationship between the in vitro test result (abscissa) and the predicted in vivo eye-irritation score (ordinate). The regression line fit to the data is shown running through the center of the data set and the upper 95% prediction interval is shown running through the upper periphery of the data. This model is useful when the test articles are surfactant-containing liquids.

Summary Document

The last element included in a nonanimal testing framework is a summary document. The purpose of this document is to advise toxicologists on the practical aspects of completing a safety assessment using the process previously described. These documents provide guidance on the test methods available for given classes of test substances, advice on

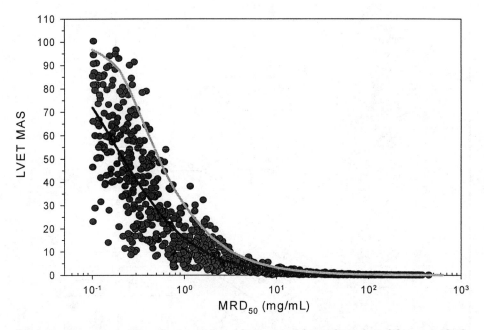

FIGURE 5 Cytosensor Microphysiometer prediction model. Prediction models are tools that allow the conversion of results from nonanimal tests into predictions of toxicity in vivo. The in vitro scores from the Cytosensor Microphysiometer are shown on the abscissa and the predicted in vivo scores, in terms of the low-volume eye-irritation test maximum average score (LVET MAS), are shown on the ordinate. The regression line running through the center of the data was derived by comparing the actual LVET MAS with corresponding data obtained from the same test substances evaluated in the Cytosensor Microphysiometer. Computer modeling was then used to simulate the data points shown in the plot and to generate the upper 95% confidence interval for predicting the LVET MAS from a cytosensor score (line running through the upper-right side of the data set). Models like the one depicted can be used to convert Cytosensor Microphysiometer scores into predictions of the LVET MAS with the indicated confidence as long as the test substance belongs to the same class as was used to develop the model. (From Ref. 25.)

which test should be used with different types of test substances, and an indication of the most appropriate prediction model to use with the test substance(s) being evaluated. Finally, these documents provide a wide range of relevant information on the technical aspects of the safety testing process (see the following) and names of individuals within the organization who can provide advice. All of this information is placed in a readily available location so that toxicologists can use the reference material easily.

Practical Considerations in the Conduct of Eye-Safety Assessments Without Animal Testing

In addition to establishing a framework for the practical conduct of eye-safety programs, it is also important to address several important technical issues that need to be considered when conducting in vitro tests. These matters have considerable influence on the choice of nonanimal tests to be used and the interpretation of the results. The matters that need to be considered include (1) the physical characteristics of the test article, (2) the expected toxicity of the test article, (3) the level of resolution required from the testing, and (4) resources available for a safety program.

Physical Characteristics of the Test Article. One of the most important considerations in the conduct of an in vitro test is the compatibility of the test article with the in vitro test being conducted. There are two general forms of in vitro tests: dilution-based tests where the target cells are completely immersed in growth medium, and topical application tests where the target cell surface is available for direct application of the test material (Table 2). For in vitro tests of the first type, it is necessary to serially dilute the test substance into a water-based cell culture medium and then apply the diluted test articles to the target cells. Dilution-based tests are particularly well suited for screening large numbers of water-soluble test substances quickly at a relatively low cost. The dilution-based tests also appear to have an increased capacity to distinguish between different degrees of mildness compared with the topical application tests [92].

Despite these advantages, the dilution of test articles in cell culture media results in technical problems that need to be considered before the procedure is used. First, because water-insoluble test substances cannot be diluted easily in aqueous cell culture media, it is generally unwise to evaluate water-insoluble substances in dilution-based tests. Second, when diluting test substances it is important to note that the dilution process can

TABLE 2 **Dilution-Based and Topical Application–Based Assays: Examples of Dilution-Based and Topical Application–Based Assays Are Shown. Dilution-Based Tests Are More Suited for Test Substances That Are Water Soluble. Topical Application–Based Tests Have the Advantage That Dilution of Test Substance Is Not Required, Which Alleviates Technical Problems That Can Arise After Dilution. See Text for Details.**

Dilution-based tests	Topical application–based tests
Cytosensor microphysiometer	Bovine corneal opacity and permeability assay
Fluorescein leakage test	Chicken enucleated eye test
Neutral red release test	Corneal and dermal 3-dimensional culture-based tests
Neutral red uptake test	Hen's egg test-chorioallantoic membrane (HET-CAM)
Red blood cell lysis test	Isolated rabbit eye test
Chorioallantoic membrane vascular assay (CAMVA)	

TABLE 3 Advantages and Disadvantages of Dilution-Based Assays. See Text for Details.

Advantages of dilution-based tests	Disadvantages of dilution-based tests
Rapid to execute	Cannot be used easily with water insoluble test substances
Most are machine scored	Dilution may mask toxicity of neat test substances
Generally very cost effective	The physical form of the test substance is changed
Work well with surfactants	Buffering may affect test substance toxicity
Often differentiate between mild test substances	Test substance may react with the diluent

significantly change the physical-chemical characteristics of a test substance. For example, the structure of complex emulsions can be changed dramatically by dilution in cell culture media. Crossing the critical micelle concentrations (CMC) for surfactants can change the toxicity observed. Dilution often changes the pH of a test article. If the irritant properties of a test substance in vivo are dependent on any factors such as physical form, micelle dissolution/formation, or pH, then the dilution of a test article may result in unreliable predictions from the in vitro test.

Topical application assays have a considerable advantage over dilution-based tests in that they are suitable for testing both water-soluble and insoluble test substances. Also, test articles can be assessed in exactly the same form as they were tested in vivo, thereby alleviating the technical concerns associated with dilution. Problems associated with topical application–based tests usually arise from the source and/or complexity of the target substrate. The use of abattoir-derived tissues may introduce variability into the results obtained from tests like IRE, CEET, and BCOP because of the random source of the animals. Also, because of the difficulties in producing large amounts of consistent substrate, the production of the 3-dimensional culture systems has most commonly been undertaken by commercial suppliers. These substrates therefore tend to be considerably more expensive than abattoir-derived tissues. It is necessary to carefully monitor the quality of commercial substrates to assure a consistent product. Withdrawal of product by several commercial suppliers in the past has also been a problem. The advantages and disadvantages of dilution- and topical application–based tests are summarized in Tables 3 and 4.

TABLE 4 Advantages and Disadvantages of Topical Application Assays. See Text for Details.

Advantages of topical application tests	Disadvantages of topical application tests
Material is tested in the same form as in vivo.	Test substrate is often expensive.
Exposure of the target tissue independent of solubility.	Exposure times may be inconveniently long.
In some models, exposure time can be selected to match expected in vivo exposure.	

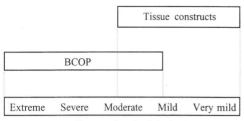

FIGURE 6   A diagram illustrating the relative sensitivity of the bovine cornea opacity and permeability test (BCOP) and 3-dimensional tissue constructs across the eye-irritation scale. Tissue constructs are most effective at the milder end and isolated eye and BCOP appear to be more suited for testing stronger irritants.

Toxicity Expected and Resolution Required.   Another consideration in the choice of which in vitro test to use in a given situation is the expected level of toxicity possessed by the test material. Ocular toxicity ranges from very slight irritation to full corrosive destruction of eye tissues. Given this diversity of response it has been found that the results from single in vitro tests are incapable of reliably predicting irritation across the entire range of response. Experience has shown that the choice of in vitro assays must therefore balance between the resolution obtained from a test and its dynamic range. Topical application assays based on tissue constructs provide poorer resolution for more aggressive test articles that can kill cell cultures within a few seconds. In contrast, the bovine cornea does not resolve very mild products without excessively long exposures [49]. However, it has the robustness to discriminate at the medium to high end of the eye-irritation response [48]. Therefore, it is best to use tissue construct models if the expected irritancy of the test article is low to moderate. Models like the BCOP, IRE, and CEET are more appropriate for test substances thought to be of moderate or greater irritancy (Fig. 6).

Resources Available.   The choice of which test to use also depends to some extent on the resources available for a given project. As previously noted, the cost of the different test methods varies considerably depending on the time required, the need for proprietary commercial substrates, and the equipment needed to conduct the test. It is often wise to use cheaper, less precise methods when large numbers of test substances need to be screened. Once the most promising candidates are identified, a limited number of definitive studies can be carried out using more definitive nonanimal tests that might involve more time and cost.

LOOKING TO THE FUTURE: WHERE DO WE GO FROM HERE?

Considerable progress has been made in the development of nonanimal methods for eye-irritation testing. These tests are increasingly used by industrial toxicologists in conjunction with previously existing in vivo data on benchmark formulations to help complete eye safety assessments of finished products. This progress has made it possible, for example, to support the elimination of in vivo eye-irritation testing of cosmetic finished products.

Despite the success with finished product testing, the progress observed with testing chemicals has been much more limited. The results of two large international validation studies illustrate the problems encountered. The first study, sponsored by the British Home Office and the European Commission through the European Centre for the Validation of Alternative Methods (ECVAM), evaluated nine in vitro methods using a set of 60 chemicals of known eye-irritation potential. The results from this study showed none of the tests could adequately predict eye-irritation responses of chemicals [70]. The second study, sponsored by the European Cosmetic Toiletry and Perfumery Association (COLIPA), evaluated 10 in vitro methods. The results were the same: current in vitro methods did not adequately predict the eye-irritation response of single chemicals [62].

Likewise, results from smaller studies on in vitro eye-irritation tests have not provided significant evidence that current nonanimal methods can fully replace the Draize eye-irritation test. In Germany, a study of the HET–CAM and the Neutral Red Uptake Test did not show that these assays could replace the in vivo eye-irritation test [88,89]. The results from the Japanese Ministry of Health and Welfare and the Japanese Cosmetic Industry Association suggested that several cytotoxicity tests were useful for testing a range of surfactant solutions, but more data would be needed to extend conclusions beyond this class of test substances [93].

Considerable analysis of the data from these validation studies has now been conducted in order to determine why the in vitro methods have been found insufficient for testing chemicals. The first major review of results from these efforts took place during an international workshop on nonanimal eye-irritation test methods in Brighton, United Kingdom [94]. The workshop panelists concluded that there are two likely explanations for the outcome: 1) the mechanistic understanding of current nonanimal methods has not been fully established, and 2) there are several parts of the eye-injury response that current in vitro tests do not assess. In addition to the Brighton Workshop, an ECVAM Task Force on eye-irritation testing reviewed the results of recently completed validation studies and made recommendations on the way forward [3]. The authors of the report concluded that further refinement of current methods might improve them for use as screening tests. However, because current in vitro tests cannot yet replace animal tests for assessing chemical irritancy, there is a need for additional research leading to improved understanding of eye-irritation mechanisms.

Mechanistic Basis for the Development of Nonanimal Replacements for the Draize Eye-Irritation Test

Attempts to validate a nonanimal replacement for the in vivo eye-irritation test have principally been by correlative analyses using information derived from the Draize scoring scheme. As can be seen in Table 1, the assessment of the eye-irritation response scoring is based on subjective visual observations made by a technician aided with a pen light. This approach to the measurement of in vivo eye-irritation responses does not provide insight into the primary and secondary pathophysiological responses occurring in the cornea, iris, or conjunctiva after chemical injury [15,95–98]. The subjective observations used in the Draize scoring scheme also provide little information on the differences in the underlying pathological changes associated with scores obtained across the time-course of an eye-irritation test [15,95–100]. For example, a high score occurring very early in an eye-irritation test is more likely reflective of the primary damage caused by a chemical, whereas a high score occurring later in a study more likely reflects secondary inflammatory responses developing in response to the primary injury. Overall, these observations suggest that the scoring system used in the current in vivo eye-irritation test may not provide enough information about the critical cellular and molecular changes involved in ocular injury and repair to be used as the basis for developing adequately predictive nonanimal tests.

In order to address this shortcoming it has been proposed that more data must be obtained on the pathophysiological processes underlying chemical-induced eye-irritation responses [99]. The new information needs to be derived from additional in vivo testing of a panel of test substances covering relevant chemical classes and the appropriate range of eye-irritation response. Where possible, these studies should include test substances for which there is human eye-irritation data so that alternative methods can be developed to predict human responses [101]. The information derived from the new in vivo studies would characterize the key cellular and molecular events and extent of variability occurring with the ocular irritation response and serve as the basis for the development mechanism–based replacement tests [15,95–100]. Preliminary work suggests that two areas of research are likely to be most beneficial. These include studies to (1) characterize the pathological changes associated with the initial eye injury caused by chemical, and (2) characterize changes in the expression of cytokines and other extracellular factors associated with inflammation and corneal repair.

Characterizing the Pathological Changes Associated with Initial Eye Injury

Differences in extent of the initial tissue injury after chemical exposure has been hypothesized to be one of the primary factors that determine the responses and ultimately the final outcome of an ocular irritation response [15,96–100]. Results from studies of a broad sampling of surfactants support this premise [15,95–100,102–104]. Light microscopy [15,97,99] and in vivo confocal microscopy [95,96,102] studies in rats and rabbits show there are differences in the extent of ocular injury induced by surfactants of known irritancy occurring as early as 3 hours after treatment. Collectively, these studies indicate that slight irritants affect only the superficial corneal epithelium, mild and moderate irritants affect the epithelium and superficial stroma, and severe irritants affect the epithelium, deep stroma, and at times the endothelium. Additional work suggests that the extent of surfactant-induced injury correlates with cell death [98] and that the extent of the primary injury correlates with subsequent responses and the eventual outcome in rats [97] and rabbits [100].

Overall, these results suggest that prediction models for mechanism-based in vitro tests could be developed based on measurements of the extent of injury and, perhaps more specifically, on measures of cell death in the cornea after chemical treatment in vivo [98,100]. Such an approach would require that replacement tests assess the area and depth of injury in multilayered in vitro substrates that contain at least a stratified epithelium and keratocyte-laden stroma [98]. Examples of appropriate substrates for such studies include isolated whole eye and isolated cornea models, or perhaps 3-dimensional corneal models like those previously described [98].

Characterizing Changes in Expression of Cytokines and Other Extracellular Factors

Changes in the expression and/or levels of biomarkers, cytokines, and other extracellular factors associated with the different stages of chemically induced eye injury have also been proposed as possible endpoints for mechanism-based replacement [15,96,97,105]. For example, Sotozono et al. [106] have observed that the production of IL-1α and IL-6 reflect the severity of alkali burns on the cornea. Shams et al. [107] have shown that levels of corneal IL-1 correlate with severity of inflammation. Planck et al. [108] have proposed that cytokine signatures characterized by varying patterns of expression of biological factors occur with different types of corneal injury. In this regard, their studies in rats have indicated IL-6 induction occurs with alkali burns and incisional trauma of the cornea, whereas IL-1β induction occurs with alkali burns but not incisional trauma. Further, differences in mRNA expression for different chemokines were observed in mouse corneas infected with HSV-1 versus traumatic injury [109]. Finally, a more recent study has indicated that differences in expression of corneal IL-1α, IL-1β, and IL-6 levels are observed after surfactant-induced injury in rats with the magnitude of the differences reflecting the extent of injury observed [105].

Other Endpoints Worthy of Consideration

In addition to studies of pathology and inflammatory mediator release associated with chemical injury, there are other areas of research that may be of interest. First, it may be useful to examine other early events occurring after exposure of the eye to chemicals. Studies could explore the interaction of chemicals with cell membranes that lead to acute damage of the eye tissue and activation of ocular nerves. Approaches that may be useful for such work include quantitative structure-activity relationship approaches and neurophysiological models of the eye [110]. After the initial chemical trauma, various physiological responses in addition to inflammatory mediator release take place in the intermediate stages of the response depending on the extent of the initial damage and the modulating influence of nerve activation. Therefore studies on the physiological effects of chemicals on isolated eyes may prove useful. In the later stages of the reaction, the inflammation subsides and the eye returns to a quiet state. Of critical importance is whether or not the eye returns to the normal pre-exposure state or whether there is scarring of the cornea that can lead to vision deficit or, in the worst case, loss of sight. Therefore, the biological responses related to recovery need to be studied. As these areas are evaluated in ongoing research programs sponsored by industry and relevant governmental agencies, the new knowledge gained may be directly applied to the development of mechanism-based assays that may be validated by interested parties.

CONCLUSION

Nonanimal test methods are now routinely used by industrial toxicologists to assess the safety of certain test articles [111]. These tests are most useful when conducted as part of a larger process that uses significant amounts of other supporting information. No single test or battery of tests can yet completely replace the need for animals in ocular safety testing. If complete elimination of animal use in eye safety assessment is to be achieved, a better understanding of the mechanisms by which chemicals cause eye irritation will be needed. The areas of research needed have been outlined in considerable detail and proposals have been made for the conduct of the research. The application of recent progress in tissue-culture techniques, cellular and molecular biology, and analytical cytometric techniques will greatly facilitate the conduct of this research and lead us closer to our ultimate goal of eliminating the need for animals in ocular safety testing.

ACKNOWLEDGEMENT

We wish to acknowledge Janet Smith for her assistance in preparation of this manuscript.

REFERENCES

1. Grant WM. Toxicology of the Eye. Effects on the eyes and visual system from chemicals, drugs, metals and minerals, plants, toxins and venoms; also systemic side effects from eye medications. 3rd ed. Springfield: Charles C. Thomas, 1986.
2. Bruner LH. Ocular irritation. In: Frazier JM, ed. In Vitro Toxicity Testing. Applications to Safety Evaluation. New York: Marcel Dekker, Inc.:1992:149–190.
3. Balls M, Berg N, Curren RD, deSilva O, Earl LK, Esdaile DJ, Fentem JH, Liebsch M, Ohno Y, Prinsen MK, Spielmann H, Worth AP. Eye irritation testing: the way forward. Report and recommendations of ECVAM Workshop 32. Alternatives to Laboratory Animals 1999; 27:53–77.
4. Draize JH, Woodard G, Calvery HO. Methods for the study of irritation and toxicity of substances applied topically to the skin and mucous membranes. J Pharmacol Exp Ther 1944; 82:377–390.
5. Prince JH, Diesem CD, Eglitis, I, Ruskell GL. Anatomy and Histology of the Eye and Orbit in Domestic Animals. Springfield: Charles C. Thomas, 1960.
6. Copenhaver WM, Kelly DE, Wood RL. The organs of special senses. In: Bailey FR, ed. Bailey's Textbook of Histology. 17th ed. Baltimore: Williams & Wilkins, 1983: 731–765.
7. Newell FW. Ophthalmology Principles and Concepts, 6th ed. St. Louis: Mosby, 1986.
8. Wikehart DR. Biochemistry of the Eye. Boston: Butterworth-Heinemann, 1994.
9. Krachmer JH, Mannis MJ, Holland EJ. Cornea. St. Louis: Mosby, 1997.
10. Kaufman HE, Barron BA, McDonald MB. The Cornea. 2d ed. Boston: Butterworth-Heinemann, 1998.
11. Nishida T. Corneal Healing Responses to Injuries and Refractive Surgeries. Hague: Kugler Publications, 1998.
12. McCally AW, Farmer AG, Loomis, EC. Corneal ulceration following use of lash lure. JAMA 1933; 101:1560–1561.
13. Friedenwald JS, Hughes WF, Herrmann H. Acid-base tolerance of the cornea. Arch Ophthalmol 1944; 31:279–283.
14. Carpenter CP, Smyth HF. Chemical burns of the rabbit cornea. Am J Ophthalmol 1946; 29: 1363–1372.
15. Maurer JK, Parker RD. Light microscopic comparison of surfactant-induced eye irritation in rabbits and rats at 3 hours and recovery/day 35. Toxicol Pathol 1996; 24:403–411.
16. DeSousa DJ, Rouse AA, Smolon WJ. Statistical consequences of reducing the number of rabbits utilised in eye irritation testing: data on 67 petrochemicals. Toxicol Appl Pharmacol 1984; 76:234–242.
17. Talsma DM, Leach CL, Hatoum NS, Gibbons RD, Roger J-C, Garvin PJ. Reducing the number of rabbits in the Draize eye irritancy test: a statistical analysis of 155 studies conducted over 6 years. Fund Appl Toxicol 1988; 10:146–153.
18. Hackett RB, McDonald TO. Eye irritation. In: Marzulli FN, Maibach HI, eds. Dermatotoxicology, Fourth Edition. New York: Hemisphere Pub. Corp., 1991:749–815.
19. Chan PK, Hayes AW. Acute toxicity and eye Irritancy. In: Hayes AW, ed. Principles and Methods of Toxicology. New York: Raven Press, 1994:579–648.
20. Edelhauser HF, Ubels JL. Models and methods for testing toxicity with tear fluid, cornea, conjunctiva. In: Hockwin O, ed. Manual of Oculotoxicity Testing of Drugs. New York: Gustav Fischer Verlag, 1992:195–218.
21. Swanston DW. Assessment of the validity of animal techniques in eye irritation testing. Food Chem Toxicol 1985; 23:169–173.

22. Daston GP, Freeberg FE. Ocular irritation testing. In: Hobson DW, ed. Dermal and Ocular Toxicology. Fundamentals and Methods. Ann Arbor: CRC Press, 1991:509–540.
23. Heywood R, James RW. Towards objectivity in the assessment of eye irritation. J Soc Cosmet Chem 1978; 29:25–29.
24. Weil CS, Scala RA. Study of intra- and interlaboratory variability in the results of rabbit eye and skin irritation tests. Toxicol Appl Pharmacol 1971; 19:276–360.
25. Bruner LH, Carr GJ, Chamberlain M, Curren RD. Validation of alternative methods for toxicity testing. Toxicol In Vitro 1996; 10:479–501.
26. Freeberg FE, Hooker DT, Griffith JF. Correlation of animal eye data with human experience for household products. J Toxicol Cut Ocular Toxicol 1986; 5:115–123.
27. Freeberg FE, Nixon GA, Reer PJ, Weaver JE, Bruce RD, Griffith JF, Sanders III LW. Human and rabbit eye responses to chemical insult. Fund Appl Toxicol 1986; 7:626–634.
28. Marzulli FN, Simon ME. Eye irritation from topically applied drugs and cosmetics: preclinical studies. Am J Optom Arch Am Acad Optom 1971; 48:61–79.
29. Rowan AN. The future of animals in research and training. The search for alternatives. Fundam Appl Toxicol 1984; 4:508–516.
30. Cormier EM, Hunter JE, Billhimer W, May J, Farage MA. Correlation of animal eye data with human experience for household products. J Toxicol Cut Ocular Toxicol 1995; 14:197–205.
31. Freeberg FE, Griffith JF, Bruce RD, Bay PHS. Correlation of animal test methods with human experience for household products. J Toxicol Cut Ocular Toxicol 1984; 3:53–64.
32. Griffith JF, Nixon GA, Bruce RD, Reer PJ, Bannan EA. Dose-response studies with chemical irritants in the albino rabbit eye as a basis for selecting optimum testing conditions for predicting hazard to the human eye. Toxicol Appl Pharmacol 1980; 55:501–513.
33. Bruner LH, Parker RD, Bruce RD. Reducing the number of rabbits in the low-volume eye test. Fundam Appl Toxicol 1992; 19:330–335.
34. Burton ABD. A method for the objective assessment of eye irritation. Food Cosmet Toxicol 1972; 10:209–217.
35. Kennah HE, Hignet S, Laux PE, Dorko JD, Barrow CS. An objective procedure for quantitating eye irritation based upon changes of corneal thickness. Fund Appl Toxicol 1989; 12:258–268.
36. Conquet P, Durand G, Laillier J, Plazonnet B. Evaluation of ocular irritation in the rabbit: objective versus subjective assessment. Toxicol Appl Pharmacol 1977; 39:129–139.
37. Laillier J, Plazonnet B, LeDourarec JC. Evaluation of ocular irritation in the rabbit: development of an objective method of studying eye irritation. Proc Eur Soc Toxicol 1975; 17:336–350.
38. Green K, Tonjum A. Influence of various agents on corneal permeability. Am J Ophthalmol 1971; 72:897–905.
39. Etter JC, Wildhaber A. Biopharmaceutical test of ocular irritation in the mouse. Food Chem Toxicol 1985; 23:321–323.
40. Maurice D, Singh T. A permeability test for acute corneal toxicity. Toxicol Lett 1986; 31:125–130.
41. Walberg J. Exfoliative cytology as a refinement of the Draize eye irritancy test. Toxicol Lett 1983; 18:49–55.
42. Walton RM, Heywood R. Applanation tonometry in the assessment of eye irritation. J Soc Cosmet Chem 1978; 29:365–368.
43. Burton ABD, York M, Lawrence RS. The in vitro assessment of severe eye irritants. Food Cosmetics Toxicol 1981; 19:471–480.
44. Whittle E, Basketter D, York M. Findings of an inter-laboratory trial of the enucleated eye method as an alternative eye irritation test. Toxic Meth 1992; (2):30–41.
45. Chamberlain M, Gad SC, Gautheron P, Prinsen MK. IRAG Working Group 1: organotypic

models for the assessment/prediction of ocular irritation. Food Chem Toxicol 1997; 35:23–37.

46. Prinsen MK, Koëter HBWM. Justification of the enucleated eye test with eyes from slaughter-house animals as an alternative to the Draize eye irritation test with rabbits. Food Chem Toxicol 1993; 31:69–76.

47. Prinsen MK. The chicken enucleated eye test (CEET): a practical (pre)screen for the assessment of eye irritation/corrosion potential of test materials. Food Chem Toxicol 1996; 34:291–296.

48. Gautheron P, Dukic M, Alix D, Sina JF. Bovine corneal opacity and permeability test: an in vitro assay of ocular irritancy. Fund Appl Toxicol 1992; 18:442–449.

49. Bruner LH, Evans MG, McPherson JP, Southee JA, Williamson PS. Investigation of ingredient interactions in cosmetic formulations using isolated bovine corneas. Toxic In Vitro 1998; 12:669–690.

50. Harbell JW, Raabe HA, Evans MG, Curren RD. Histopathology associated with opacity and permeability changes in bovine corneas in vitro. Toxicol Sci 1999; 48(1-S):336–337.

51. Kruszewski FH, Walker TL, Ward SL, Dipasquale LC. Progress in the use of human ocular tissues for in vitro alternative methods. Comments Toxicol 1995; 5:203–224.

52. Kruszewski FH, Walker TL, DiPasquale LC. Evaluation of a human corneal epithelial cell line as an in vitro model for assessing ocular irritation. Fund Appl Toxicol 1997; 36:130–140.

53. Kruszewski FH. New directions in in vitro eye irritation testing. Proceedings of the Toxicology Forum Annual Winter Meeting, February 2–5, 1998. The Toxicology Forum, Washington, D.C., 1998.

54. Ward SL, Walker TL, Dimitrijevich SL. Evaluation of chemically induced toxicity using an in vitro model of human corneal epithelium. Toxicol In Vitro 1997; 11:121–139.

55. Faquet B, Buiatti-Tcheng M, Tromvoukis Y, Offord EA, Leclaire L. Cytokines production after treatment with surfactants in a human corneal epithelial cell line. Invest Ophthalmol Vis Sci 1997; 38:S866.

56. Stern M, Klausner M, Alvarado R, Renskers K, Dickens M. Evaluation of the EpiOcular™ tissue model as an alternative to the Draize eye irritation test. Toxicol In Vitro 1998; 12:455–461.

57. Doucet O, Lanvin M, Zastrow L. Comparison of three in vitro methods for the assessment of the eye irritation potential of formulated products. In Vitro & Molec Toxicol 1999; (12):63–76.

58. Doucet O, Lanvin M, Zastrow L. A new in vitro human epithelial model for assessing the eye irritation potential of formulated cosmetic products. In Vitro & Molec Toxicol 1998; (11):273–283.

59. Osborne R, Perkins MA, Roberts DA. Development and intralaboratory evaluation of an in vitro human cell-based test to aid ocular irritancy assessments. Fund Appl Toxicol 1995; 28:139–153.

60. Southee JA, McPherson JP, Osborne R, Carr GJ, Rasmussen E. The performance of the tissue equivalent assay using the skin2 ZK1200 model in the COLIPA international validation study on alternatives to the Draize eye irritation test. Toxicol In Vitro 1999; 13:355–373.

61. Curren RD, Sina JF, Feder P, Kruszewski FH, Osborne RM, Regnier J-F. Interagency regulatory alternatives group (IRAG) working group 5: other assays. Food Chem Toxicol 1997; 35:127–158.

62. Brantom PG, Bruner LH, Chamberlain M, de Silva O, Dupuis J, Earl LK, Lovell DP, Pape WJW, Uttley M, Bagley DM, Baker FW, Bracher M, Courtellemont P, Declercq L, Freeman S, Steiling W, Walker AP, Carr GJ, Dami N, Thomas G, Harbell J, Jones PA, Pfannenbecker U, Southee JA, Tcheng M, Argembeaux H, Castelli D, Clothier R, Esdaile DJ, Itigaki H, Jung K, Kasai Y, Kojima H, Kristen U, Larnicol M, Lewis RW, Marenus K, Moreno O,

Peterson A, Rasmussen ES, Robles C, Stern M. A summary report of the COLIPA international validation study on alternatives to the Draize rabbit eye irritation test. Toxicol In Vitro 1997; 11:141–179.

63. Botham PA, Earl LK, Fentem JH, Roguet R, van de Sandt JJM. Alternative methods for skin irritation testing: the current status. ATLA 1998; 26:195–211.

64. Robinson MK, Osborne R, Perkins MA. Chapter 11 of this volume.

65. Martin KM, Bernhofer LP, Stott CW. Preliminary evaluation of a three dimensional corneal construct as an in vitro model for ocular irritation. In Vitro Toxicol 1993; 7:164.

66. Griffith CM. Future directions in in vitro testing: human corneal cell lines and reconstructed corneal equivalents. Proceedings of the Toxicology Forum Annual Winter Meeting, February 2–5, 1998. The Toxicology Forum, Washington, D.C., 1998.

67. Griffith M, Osborne R, Munger Xiong X, Doillon CJ, Laycock NLC, Hakim M, Song Y, Watsley MA. Functional human corneal equivalents constructed from all lines. Science 1999; 286:2169–2172.

68. Borenfreund E, Puerner JA. Toxicity determined in vitro by morphological alterations and neutral red absorption. Toxicol Lett 1985; 24:119–124.

69. Bruner LH, Kain JD, Roberts D, Parker RD. Evaluation of seven in vitro alternatives for ocular safety testing. Fund Appl Toxicol 1991; 17:136–149.

70. Balls M, Botham PA, Bruner LH, Spielmann H. The EC/HO international validation study on alternatives to the Draize eye irritation test. Toxicol In Vitro 1995; 9:871–929.

71. Jones PA, Bracher M, Marenus K, Kojima H. Performance of the neutral red uptake assay in the COLIPA validation study on alternatives to the rabbit eye irritation test. Toxicol In Vitro 1999; 13:335–342.

72. Reader SJ, Blackwell V, O'Hara R, Clothier RH, Griffin G, Balls M. A vital dye release method for assessing the short term cytotoxic effects of chemicals and formulations. ATLA 1989; 17:28–37.

73. Courtellemont P, Hebert P, Biesse JP, Castelli D, Friteau L, Serrano J, Robles C. Relevance and reliability of the predisafe assay in the COLIPA eye irritation validation programme (phase 1). Toxicol In Vitro 1999; 13:305–312.

74. Pape WJW, Pfannenbecker U, Hoppe U. Validation of the red blood cell test system as an in vitro assay for the rapid screening of irritation potential of surfactants. Mol Toxicol 1987; 1:525–536.

75. Pape WJW, Pfannenbecker U, Argembeaux H, Bracher M, Esdaile DJ, Hagino S, Kasai Y, Lewis RW. COLIPA validation project on in vitro eye irritation tests for cosmetic ingredients and finished products (phase 1): the red blood cell test for the estimation of acute eye irritation potentials. Present status. Toxicol In Vitro 1999; 13:343–354.

76. Bruner LH, Kercso KM, Owicki JC, Parce JW, Muir VC. Testing ocular irritancy in vitro with a cellular biosensor. Toxicol In Vitro 1991; 5:277–284.

77. Cartoux P, Rougier A, Dossou KG, Cottin M. The silicon microphysiometer for testing ocular toxicity in vitro. Toxicol In Vitro 1993; 7:465–469.

78. Harbell JW, Osborne R, Carr GJ, Peterson A. Assessment of the cytosensor microphysiometer assay in the COLIPA in vitro eye irritation validation study. Toxicol In Vitro 1999; 13:313–323.

79. Tchao R. Trans-epithelial permeability of fluorescein in vitro as an assay to determine eye irritants. In: Goldberg AM, ed. Alternative Methods in Toxicology. Vol 6. New York: Mary Ann Liebert, 1988:271–283.

80. Shaw AJ, Clothier RH, Balls M. Loss of trans-epithelial impermeability of a confluent monolayer of Madin-Darby canine kidney (MDCK) cells as a determinant of ocular irritancy potential. Alternatives to Laboratory Animals 1990; 18:145–151.

81. Zanvit A, Meunier P-A, Clothier R, Ward R, Buiatti-Tcheng M. Ocular toxicity assessment of cosmetics formulations and ingredients: fluorescein leakage test. Toxicol In Vitro 1999; 13:385–391.

82. Botham P, Osborne R, Atkinson K, Carr G, Cottin M, van Buskirk RG. Cell function-based assays (for eye irritation testing). Interagency regulatory alternatives group (IRAG) working group 3. Food Chemi Toxicol 1997; 35:67–77.

83. Harbell JW, Koontz SW, Lewis RW, Lovell D, Acosta D. Interagency regulatory alternatives group (IRAG) working group 4: cell cytotoxicity assays. Food Chem Toxicol 1997; 35:79–126.

84. Luepke NP. Hen's egg chorioallantoic membrane test for irritation potential. Food Chem Toxicol 1985; 23:287–291.

85. Bagley DM, Waters D, Kong BM. Development of a 10-day chorioallantoic membrane vascular assay as an alternative to the Draize rabbit eye irritation test. Food Chem Toxicol 1994; 32:1155–1160.

86. Bagley DM, Cerven D, Harbell J. Assessment of the chorioallantoic membrane vascular assay (CAMVA) in the COLIPA in vitro eye irritation validation study. Toxicol In Vitro 1999; 13:285–293.

87. Spielmann H, Liebsch M, Moldenhauer F, Holzhutter H-G, Bagley DM, Lipman JM, Pape WJW, Miltenburger H, deSilva O, Hofer H, Steiling W. Interagency regulatory alternatives group (IRAG) working group 4: cam-based assays. Food Chem Toxicol 1997; 35:39–66.

88. Spielmann H, Kalweit S, Liebsch M, Wirnsberger T, Gerner I, Bertram-Neis E, Kranser K, Kreiling R, Miltenberger HG, Pape WS, Steiling W. Validation study of alternatives to the Draize eye irritation test in Germany: cytotoxicity testing and HET-CAM test with 136 industrial chemicals. Toxicology in Vitro 1993; 7:505–510.

89. Spielmann H, Liebsch M, Kalweit S. Results of a validation study in Germany on two in vitro alternatives to the Draize eye irritation test, the HET-CAM test and the 3T3-NRU cytotoxicity test. Alternatives to Laboratory Animals 1996; 24:741–858.

90. Steiling W, Bracher M, Courtellemont P, de Silva O. The HET-CAM, a useful in vitro assay for assessing the eye irritation properties of cosmetic formulations and ingredients. Toxicol In Vitro 1999; 13:375–384.

91. Bruner LH, Carr G, Chamberlain M, Curren R. No prediction model, no validation study. ATLA 1996; 24:139–142.

92. Grabarz R, Sharma R, Dressler W, Harbell J, Raabe H, Curren R. Successful use of a battery of in vitro tests to screen for ocular safety before human trials. COLIPA Symposium on Alternatives to Animal Testing, In: Alternatives to Animal Testing II. Clark DG, Lisansky SG, Macmillan R, eds. CPL Press, Newbury, Berkshire, UK, 1999:192.

93. Ohno Y, Kaneko T, Kobayashi T. First-phase interlaboratory validation of the in vitro eye irritation tests for cosmetic ingredients. I. Overview, organization and results of the validation study. Alternatives to Animals Testing and Experimentation. 1995; 3:123–136.

94. Bruner LH, de Silva O, Earl LK, Easty DL, Pape W, Spielmann H. Report on the COLIPA Workshop on Mechanisms of Eye Irritation. Alternatives to Laboratory Animals 1998; 26:811–820.

95. Jester JV, Maurer JK, Petroll WM, Wilkie DA, Parker RD, Cavanagh HD. Application of in vivo confocal microscopy to the understanding of surfactant-induced ocular irritation. Toxicol Pathol 1996; 24:412–428.

96. Maurer JK, Li HF, Petroll WM, Parker RD, Cavanagh HD, Jester JV. Confocal microscopic characterization of initial corneal changes of surfactant-induced eye irritation in the rabbit. Toxicol Appl Pharmacol 1997; 143:291–300.

97. Maurer JK, Parker RD, Carr GJ. Ocular irritation: microscopic changes occurring over time in the rat with surfactants of known irritancy. Toxicol Pathol 1998; 26:217–225.

98. Jester JV, Li HF, Petroll WM, Parker RD, Cavanagh HD, Carr GJ, Smith B, Maurer JK. Area and depth of surfactant induced corneal injury correlates with cell death. Invest Ophthalmol Vis Sci 1998; 39:922–936.

99. Maurer JK, Parker RD, Carr GJ. Ocular irritation: pathological changes occurring in the rat with surfactants of unknown irritancy. Toxicol Pathol 1998; 26:226–233.

100. Jester JV, Petroll WM, Bean J, Parker RD, Carr GJ, Cavanagh HD, Maurer JK. Area and depth of surfactant-induced corneal injury predicts extent of subsequent ocular responses. Invest Ophthalmol Vis Sci 1998; 39(13):2610–2625.

101. National Institute of Environmental Health Sciences. Validation of test materials. In: Validation and Regulatory Acceptance of Toxicological Test Methods. A Report of the ad hoc Interagency Coordinating Committee on the Validation of Alternative Methods, NIH Publication No. 97-398 1, NIEHS, Research Triangle Park, NC, 1997, pp. 9–25.

102. Maurer JK, Parker RD, Petroll WM, Carr GJ, Cavanagh HD, Jester JV. Quantitative measurement of acute corneal injury occurring in rabbits with surfactants of different type and irritancy. Toxicol Appl Pharmacol 1999; 158:61–70.

103. Maurer JK. Pathobiology of surfactant-induced eye irritation. In: The Toxicology Forum, Washington, D.C., February 1998, pp. 222–234.

104. Maurer JK, Jester JV. Use of in vivo confocal microscopy to understand the pathology of accidental ocular irritation. Toxicol Pathol 1999; 27:44–47.

105. Maurer JK, Parker RD, Carr GJ. Differences in corneal cytokine levels with surfactant-induced ocular irritation in rats. J Toxicol Cut Ocul Toxicol 2000; 19:3–20.

106. Sotozono C, He J, Matsumoto Y, Masakazu K, Imanishi J, Kinoshita S. Cytokine expression in alkali-burned cornea. Curr Eye Res 1997; 16:670–676.

107. Shams NBK, Reddy CV, Watanabe K, Elgebaly SA, Hanninen LA, Kenyon KR. Increased interleukin-1 activity in the injured vitamin-A-deficient cornea. Cornea 1994; 13:156–166.

108. Planck SR, Rich LF, Ansel JC, Huang XN, Rosenbaum JT. Trauma and alkali burns induce distinct patterns of cytokine gene expression in the rat cornea. Ocul Immunol Inflamm 1997; 5:95–100.

109. Su Y-H, Yan X-T, Oakes JE, Lausch RN. Protective antibody therapy is associated with reduced chemokine transcripts in herpes simplex virus type I corneal infection. J Virol 1997; 70:1277–1281.

110. Belmonte C, Garcia-Hirschfeld J, Gallar J. Neurobiology of Ocular Pain. Progress in Retinal and Eye Research 1997; 16(1):117–156.

111. Anonymous. Guidelines for the Safety Assessment of a Cosmetic Product. Brussels: The European Cosmetic Toiletry and Perfumery Association, 1997.

14

Main Cosmetic Vehicles

Stephan Buchmann
Spirig Pharma AG, Egerkingen, Switzerland

INTRODUCTION

The aim of this chapter is to treat the topic of cosmetic vehicles in a conceptual way. It is not the purpose to present a lot of formulations or types of vehicles that are used for all the different cosmetic products and sites of application. Neither will the topic be presented in a comprehensive way, because of its complexity. There are many good examples of formulation compositions described in cosmetic literature and brochures of companies offering cosmetic excipients. In this chapter an overview of various selected aspects is given that should be taken into account when cosmetic preparations are to be formulated. The critical issues for formulation development will be pointed out.

FUNCTION OF VEHICLES

Direct Intrinsic Effect

The term vehicle is used in pharmaceutics as well as in cosmetics in the area of formulation. In general, this term implies differentiation between active and inactive principles. The active principle is embedded into a matrix, the vehicle. With the aid of the vehicle the active principle is delivered to the application site or to the target organ, respectively, where the desired effect is achieved. As a matter of fact, however, when dermatological and cosmetical preparations are applied, sharp differentiation between active and inactive principle is generally not possible because of the so-called vehicle effect.

The aim of application of both a pharmaceutical preparation as well as a cosmetic topical care product is to achieve a desired effect. Pharmaceutical preparations are effective because of a pharmacologically active compound delivered with the aid of a vehicle, whereas cosmetic formulations are not allowed to contain such compounds. Nevertheless, an effect is also achieved by a cosmetic preparation—not any systemic or central or curative effect—but a caring or preventing effect mainly on skin, hair, or nails. This effect may be achieved either by cosmetically active ingredients or by the vehicle itself on the site of application, i.e., on the skin in most cases. In contrast to pharmaceutics, in cosmetics the vehicle is of greater importance.

Depending on the composition, a vehicle is used to exert mainly five types of effects on the skin, briefly described in following sections.

Cleansing

The most common and probably oldest use of cosmetic preparations is to clean the human body. In our modern time and society, not just soap but a variety of sophisticated cosmetic cleansing products are available.

Decoration

Decoration serves to produce a pleasing appearance by minimizing facial defects of color or shape and unobtrusively enhancing and directing attention toward better points [1]. Decorative cosmetic preparations are not the main object of this chapter on vehicles, although similar principles have to be considered for decorative cosmetic preparations.

Care

Probably more cosmetic preparations are applied to care for the outermost organs of the body, i.e., skin, hair, and nails, than to decorate these organs. Care of skin, hair, and nails and improvement of their state is an important function of an applied cosmetic product. Application of an appropriate vehicle may be fully sufficient for care of the body.

Hydration

The state of dry skin may be treated by applying a cosmetic product. In this case the skin is hydrated by application of an appropriate vehicle containing specific components that are able to reduce the transepidermal water loss. This results in an increase in water in the stratum corneum and a smoother surface of the skin.

Protection

A further important function of cosmetic vehicles is to build up a protective layer against external potentially damaging factors that could come into contact with the body. Especially in recent years the protective and preventive function of vehicles has become increasingly important, because of an increase of various external harmful factors or at least higher awareness about them (e.g., air pollution, UV radiation).

Delivery of Actives

From a stringent medicinal and legal point of view, a cosmetic preparation must not contain any (pharmacologically) active substance or ingredient that treats or prevents disease or alters the structure or function of the human body [2]. That means just the vehicle is effective directly at the site of application. This is in contrast to pharmaceutical vehicles, which in principle should serve as pure vehicles delivering active substances to the target organ and showing no effect on the body. However, in reality there are no such distinct but floating boundaries. Therefore, cosmetic vehicles can also be considered as means containing cosmetic actives that are applied to the outermost layer of the body. Furthermore, many cosmetically used substances are bifunctional: first they constitute the vehicle structure and second they show a positive effect on the skin status when applied.

Carrying Actives to Target (Targeting)

Going even one step further, cosmetic vehicles can also be considered and used as carriers for cosmetic actives which, after application, are carried and delivered to the specified target sites, i.e., to legally allowed targets in deeper regions of skin. However, this is only allowed if no systemic, physiological, or pharmacological effect is achieved and the product has shown to be safe.

Delivering active substances to these targets requires the right concentration of actives in the formulation to achieve the optimal release rate and desired distribution of active substances between the vehicle and the target site. That means the vehicle should penetrate (superficially) into the stratum corneum and release the active substance at the optimal rate (immediate or sustained for depot effect) at the target site where the desired effect is achieved.

CLASSIFICATION SYSTEMS OF VEHICLES

There are many types of classification systems based on various principles described in the literature. But one has to be aware that cosmetic preparations are rather complex systems. Most of the various classification systems are unsatisfactory and it is difficult to set up a comprehensive system. In most cases, it is problematic to make clear distinctions for classifying the vehicles in a proper and unambigous way. This is because of various possible points of view and characterization criteria used. The state of matter, e.g., depends on temperature, and therefore a lipid-based vehicle might exist either in liquid or semisolid form.

A few systems are discussed in this chapter. For modern formulation development the physicochemically based systems have been found to be the most useful and practical for understanding and explanation of formulation issues.

Appearance

The most obvious and simple classification may be performed according to the appearance of the preparations or vehicles, respectively. Based on the macroscopic physical state of matter, three types of preparations are distinguished: liquid, semisolid, and solid forms. This classification is not of great interest for rational formulation design and development. However, for many practical issues it is quite useful, e.g., for manufacturing, packaging, and application on the body.

A further classification system is based on state of matter and optical discrimination, be it macroscopically or microscopically. That means vehicles can be classified into monophasic, isotropic systems on one hand and into anisotropic heterophasic systems on the other. For example, the term ''solution'' is commonly used to describe a liquid form with isotropic appearance. However, solutions also occur in solid form, so-called solid solutions. With regard to macroscopic appearance, colloidal systems (e.g., mixed micellar solutions, microemulsions) are also isotropic, whereas e.g., coarse dispersions belong to the anisotropic systems. Unlike solutions, most cosmetic vehicles are anisotropic, heterophasic systems (mixtures). Thus, a more sophisticated system is needed to describe and classify the heterogeneity of possible vehicle forms in a satisfactory way (see Table 1).

Application, Use

Classification of vehicles may also be performed as a function of their use and application site, i.e., preparations used for the following:

TABLE 1 **Junginger's Physical-Chemical Classification System**

System	Brief description (examples)
Liquid systems	
Monophasic systems	
Aqueous solutions	Molecular disperse systems of solute in solvent (water, alcohol); liquid, transparent
Alcoholic, alcoholic-aqueous solutions	
Oily systems	Solutions based on (mixtures of) liquid lipids as solvent, e.g., oils for massage
Micellar systems	Solubilisates of low soluble substances due to aggregation formation of surfactants in solution
Microemulsions	Optically isotropic liquid: gel composed of water, lipid, and surfactant in distinct ratio
Multiphasic liquid systems	
O/W emulsions	Internal lipid phase dispersed in the external (continuous) aqueous phase stabilized by surfactants
W/O emulsions	Internal aqueous phase dispersed in the external (continuous) lipid phase stabilized by surfactants
Suspensions	Solid particles dispersed in a liquid phase
Aerosols	
Semisolid systems	
Water-free systems, ointments	
Apolar systems, hydrocarbon gels	Petrolatum
Polar systems	
Polar systems without surfactants	
Lipogels	E.g., hydrogenated vegetable oils
Oleogels	Colloidal silica in oils
Polyethylene glycol gels	
Polar systems with surfactants	
W/O absorption bases	Simple ointment (British Pharmacopoeia 1993): emulsifying system (cetostearyl alcohol, wool fat) in paraffin-petrolatum base
O/W absorption bases	Cetomacrogol emulsifying ointment (British Pharmacopoeia 1993): cetomacrogol 600, cetostearyl alcohol in paraffin-petrolatum base
Water-containing systems	
Monophasic systems: hydrogels	
Hydrogels with anorganic gelating agents	Colloidal silica in water (high concentration, labile gel structure)
Hydrogels with organic gelating agents	Hydroxyethylcellulose gel
	Polyacrylate gel
Multiphasic water-containing systems: creams	
O/W creams	
W/O creams	
Amphiphilic systems	
Amphiphilic systems with crystalline gel matrix	*
Amphiphilic systems with liquid crystalline gel matrix	*
Liposomes	Phospholipid vesicles in aqueous medium
Niosomes	Nonionic surfactant vesicles (analogous to liposomes) in aqueous medium
High-concentrated suspensions, pastes	
Powders	

* See discussion on mesophases, p. 161.
Source: Modified from Ref. 3.

- hairs, e.g., shampoo, depilatory agents, hair colorant
- nails, e.g., polish, lacquer
- mouth, e.g., toothpaste, lipstick, lip-protection stick
- skin, e.g., moisturizing product, body lotion, aftershave, deodorant, antiperspirant, sunscreen

It is obvious that for the different application sites and modes different vehicles and forms with appropriate characteristics are needed. On the other hand, different types of vehicles may also be used for the same purpose, e.g., an aqueous-alcoholic solution or a balm for application after shaving.

Physical Chemical

In the development of cosmetic care products, a practical physical-chemical classification system that describes the principal properties and structural matrix of vehicles is preferred. Of course, there is no perfect and comprehensive classification system. A good example

TABLE 2 Definitions of Selected Vehicle Systems

Systems	
Aerosol	Dispersion of liquid or solid in gas.
Colloidal	Colloidal systems are dispersions with particle size range of 1–500 nm. They may be classified into the following three groups: 1. Lyophilic colloids: particles interact with the dispersion medium (e.g., gelatin) 2. Lyophobic colloids: composed of materials that have little attraction (e.g., gold in water) 3. Association colloids: amphiphiles or surfactive agents aggregated to micelles [4].
Dispersion	Dispersed systems consist of particulate matter (dispersed phase) distributed throughout a continuous, or dispersion, medium [5].
Emulsion	According to IUPAC (International Union of Pure and Applied Chemistry), emulsion is defined as liquid droplets and/or fluid crystals dispersed in a liquid. The dispersed phase is also called the internal phase, in contrast to the external or continuous phase. If the internal phase is lipophilic, e.g., vegetable oil or paraffin oil, and dispersed in the external hydrophilic aqueous phase, an emulsion of type O/W is obtained. On the other hand, there are W/O emulsions with the hydrophilic aqueous phase dispersed in the continuous lipophilic phase. For formation and stabilization of emulsions, emulsifiers are required. Emulsions may show liquid or semisolid consistency. Further related aspects are treated in p. 151.
Foam	Dispersion of gas in liquid phase, i.e., structure of air pockets enclosed within thin films of liquid, stabilized by a foaming agent [6].
Gel	A gel is a solid or semisolid system of at least two constituents, consisting of a condensed mass enclosing and interpenetrated by a liquid [7].
Solution	A true solution is defined as a mixture of two or more components that form a homogeneous molecular dispersion, a one-phase system [8].
Suspension	A suspension is a coarse dispersion in which insoluble solid particles are dispersed in a liquid medium [9].

of a physical chemical system is described by Junginger [3] and slightly modified in Table 1. Although not comprehensive, such a system is a useful tool for rational formulation design and development, in particular when controlled and targeted delivery of active principles has to be achieved. Such a vehicle classification system is also a practical basis for production, use, and understanding of cosmetic vehicles. However, the boundaries between the different classes are flexible, and changing with the state of art and science. More important than pure classification of a cosmetic vehicle is its exact characterization, based on physical, chemical, and biological principles that may eventually lead to a variety of classification possibilities.

In a physical chemical classification system, various characterization criteria are used for classification of the vehicles:

- Polarity: hydrophilicity, lipophilicity
- State of matter: solid, semisolid, liquid, gaseous
- Size/dimensions of particulates dispersed in the mixtures (dispersions)
    true solution, molecular dispersion: particle size <1 nm
    colloidal dispersion: particle size 1 nm–500 nm
    coarse dispersion: particle size >500 nm
- Solubility characteristics
- Rheology, viscosity
- Composition: physical chemical characteristics of the main vehicle components
    waterfree, oily
    aqueous
    hydrophilic, nonaqueous solvents

For clarification of the terminology, a selection of definitions or descriptions of the major systems is given in Table 2. (See also Refs. 4–9.)

DESCRIPTION AND DEFINITION OF MAIN VEHICLES

Solutions

The term "solution" may be used in a narrow sense, describing true solutions (molecular dispersions; see Table 2), or in a broader sense, also comprising colloidal solutions, i.e., more or less transparent liquids, e.g., micellar solutions and vesicular systems (media containing liposomes, niosomes).

In general, true solutions used in cosmetics are either based on aqueous, or aqueous-alcoholic, media or on inert oily vehicles. Most organic solvents cannot be used because of their local or systemic toxicity, which causes skin irritation or permeation across the skin barrier into the body, respectively. Although good solvents for lipophilic substances, oils may not be used in every case because of their grassy characteristic, low acceptance, and exclusion for hairy application sites. However, for special applications oils are preferred, e.g., for massage. "Massage oils" contain essential oils and fragrances, compounds that are easily dissolved in the oily vehicle because of their lipophilic properties.

Prerequisite for solution formulation is a sufficiently high solubility of the solute in the solvent. Classical examples for solutions used in cosmetics are "eau de parfums" and "eau de toilettes." In order to enable solubilization of the lipophilic fragrances, alcohol or aqueous-alcoholic solutions are prepared. The addition of alcohol to water, or other suitable hydrophilic but less polar solvents (e.g., glycerol, polyethylene glycol), decreases the polarity of the solvent and thus increases the solubility of the lipophilic solutes. Frequently, a solute is more soluble in a mixture of solvents than in one solvent alone. This phenomenon is known as cosolvency, and the solvents that in combination increase the solubility of the solute are called cosolvents [10].

Another classical example is preparations for mouthwashes. They usually contain essential oils or liquid plant extracts like peppermint or myrrh extract, which are kept in solution by the added ethanol (ca. 70%). When used for application, these concentrates are diluted with water. Then turbidity occurs because of overstepping saturation solubility. In order to prevent turbidity, solubilizing agents (surfactants, e.g., PEG-40 hydrogenated castor oil) may be added. The solubilization effect is attributed to aggregation formation of surfactants when in solution. In aqueous solutions surfactants form micelles, small aggregates, when the concentration of the surfactant exceeds the critical micelle concentration (CMC) [11]. With the aid of those micelles, the solubility of low soluble, apolar compounds may be increased because of an association or incorporation of the apolar compounds with the apolar region of the micelle. Thus, solubilization or formation of micelles is a favorable means for formulation of solutions.

Finally, salt formation or adjustment of pH also results in improved solubility of originally low soluble, ionizable solutes. Thus, e.g., addition of sodium hydroxide may be used to improve the solubility of hyaluronic acid or preservatives such as sorbic or benzoic acid. Accordingly, appropriate acids, e.g., lactic acid and citric acid, may be added when solubility of a basic substance must be increased. Although not the main type of formulation used in cosmetics, solutions have the following advantages:

1. They remain physically stable (if true solution and not oversaturated),
2. Are easily prepared: simple mixing, under heating if necessary,
3. Are transparent, clear, and have a "clean" appearance, and
4. Are especially suitable for rinsing and cleaning body surfaces.

However, it must be kept in mind that many compounds are chemically less stable when in a dissolved state.

In summary, whenever a solution has to be formulated, the optimal solvent must be selected, that (1) guarantees sufficient solubility and stability for the solute(s), and (2) is acceptable and safe for application to the body. Solubility may be improved by (1) adaptation of the solvent's polarity with regard to the solute, (2) salt formation/pH adjustment (ionizable compounds), (3) using mixtures of suitable solvents and cosolvents, and (4) solubilization with the aid of surfactants.

Emulsions: Lotions and Creams

Out of the range of cosmetic care products, the emulsion is the form that is probably the most used. For reasons of skin feeling, consumer appeal, and ease of application, emulsions are preferred to waterless oils and lipids along with gels. The main components of emulsions are lipids (lipophilic compounds) and water (and/or hydrophilic compounds). These two immiscible phases are allowed to remain in a metastable mixed state by an amphiphilic component, an emulsifier. This biphasic system may be regarded in analogy to the skin or even to the skin cells, which, simply put, consist of lipophilic and hydrophilic components. Emulsions can either be of the water-in-oil (w/o) or oil-in-water (o/w) types. Showing very similar structural principles, both lotions and creams are discussed in this chapter. If emulsions are liquid, they are generally called lotions. Creams are emulsions occurring in semisolid form. Under gravitation, creams do not flow out through the orifice of reversed containers because of the heavier consistency in comparison with lotions.

Emulsions are prepared by dispersion of the internal in the external phase. For this energy-consuming process, emulsifiers that decrease the interfacial tension between the two immiscible phases are required. Emulsifiers are not only used for formation but also for stabilizing emulsions. Emulsions are metastable systems and the two phases tend to separate because of coalescence, i.e., when the dispersed droplets fuse. This process may be slowed by the addition of appropriate emulsifiers, which are ionic or anionic surfactants. The emulsifiers are thought to be located at the interfaces between the two phases, the hydrophilic part of the molecule in contact with the water phase and the lipophilic domain of the emulsifier contacting/touching the lipid phase. Large molecules may even dig into the lyophilic phase and serve as stabilizing anchors. Being adsorbed at the interfaces, the emulsifying substances form a film—monomolecular or multimolecular, depending on the substances' structures—that stabilizes the emulsion [12]. The addition of viscosity-increasing substances further results in an improved consistency and consequently more stable emulsions.

Except for the emulsifiers, the following types of ingredients are usually added to cosmetic emulsions:

- *Emollients*: They improve the sensory properties of the emulsions. Addition of an emollient results in better spreading when the emulsion is applied to the skin. Examples: isopropyl myristate, silicon oils.
- *Moisturizers and humectants*: They increase and control the hydration state of the skin. Examples: glycerol, urea.
- *Viscosity-increasing agents* are added to increase the viscosity of the external phase, if desired. Examples: xanthan gum, cellulose esters.
- *Active substances* such as UV sunscreens and vitamins.
- *Preservatives* to prevent microbial growth, particularly in o/w emulsions.
- *Perfumes and coloring agents* for aesthetic purposes.

Oil-in-Water Emulsions

The high acceptance of o/w emulsions is based on the following reasons:

- They feel light and not greasy when applied.
- They show good skin spreadability and penetration and an active hydration effect by the external water phase.
- They cause a cooling effect because of the evaporation of the external aqueous phase.

However, o/w emulsions show a lower effect in preventing dry skin in comparison with w/o emulsions. A typical o/w emulsion is composed as follows:

1. Lipid(s) + lipophilic thickening agent (optional, e.g., microcrystalline wax)   10–40%
2. Emulsifier system with optimal HLB-value (approx. 9–10 [13])   5%
3. Co-emulsifier (e.g., cetostearyl alcohol, behenyl alcohol)   2%
4. Preservatives (antimicrobial, antioxidants)   q.s.
5. Water + hydrophilic thickening agent (optional, e.g., carbomer) ad 100%

Depending on the desired product effect, different types of lipids may be used for formulation. Addition of nonpolar, occluding lipids (e.g., paraffin oil) improves retention of moisture in the skin but lowers spreading on the skin. A good spreading effect is achieved by formation of a low-viscosity emulsion containing polar oils that show a high spreading coefficient (e.g., macadamia nut oil, wheat germ oil, isostearyl neopentanoate) [14].

Selection of the lipophilic ingredients and the excipients of the water phase determine the emulsifier system to be used and additional adjuvants, e.g., viscosity-increasing thickening agents. There is no universal emulsifier system, and a huge variety of combinations might be used. Today, complex emulgator systems that consist of one or more surfactants and a cosurfactant are commonly used. That means at least two surfactants with different HLB-values are combined. For example, steareth-21 (HLB = 15.5) may be combined with PEG-5-glyceryl stearate (HLB = 8.7). The latter emulsifier is especially suitable when nonpolar oils are to be incorporated. In recent years selected polymeric excipients have been used for emulsion stabilization, e.g., crosslinked and linear polyacrylates, polyacrylamides, and derivates of cellulose.

In selecting a co-emulsifier, the following general guidelines apply:

- For the same fatty residue, the viscosity decreases if the degree of ethoxylation increases.
- For the same degree of ethoxylation, the viscosity increases if the fatty carbon chain length increases [14].

The degree of viscosity (consistency) of o/w emulsions depends on various factors [15]:

- Volume ratio of internal to external phase: increasing lipid percentage results in higher viscosity, but not necessarily in a semisolid cream.
- Type of lipid: incorporation of high melting lipophilic compounds, e.g., solid paraffin and petrolatum, may result in soft semisolid o/w creams.
- Presence of thickening agents in the lipid phase: addition of cetostearyl alcohol generally results in (''hard'') semisolid creams.
- Presence of thickening agents in the external aqueous phase: the ultimate mean to increase the consistency of a thin o/w emulsion. Addition of hydrocolloids, e.g., carbomers or hydropropyl guar (Jaguar 8600, Rhodia Inc., Cranbury, NJ), is the most efficient method to increase the viscosity of o/w emulsions. However, depending on the properties of the added polymer, the skin feeling of the emulsion may become negatively influenced because of the stickiness.

An interesting phenomenon is the occurrance of liquid crystal structures (mesophases) in emulsions under certain conditions. This has been investigated and has become of interest more and more during the last 10 to 20 years. This subject is treated on p. 161.

Water-in-Oil Emulsions

Water-in-oil (w/o) emulsions may still be regarded as heavy, greasy, and sticky although during recent years great progress has been achieved in the preparation of pleasant w/o emulsions. Therefore, the w/o emulsion type is not only the basis for water-resistant sun protection, baby creams, or night creams, but also for protective day creams. This is because during recent years better excipients have become available. The advantages of w/o emulsions are:

- Close resemblance to the natural protective lipid layer in the stratum corneum
- Efficient skin protection attributable to formation of a continuous layer of lipids on skin after application
- Sustained moisturization because on skin a continuous semiocclusive barrier is formed that reduces evaporation of skin water and that in addition actively releases the incorporated water from the internal phase, generally several times more efficient than o/w emulsions
- Improved penetration into the lipophilic stratum corneum coupled with improved carrier function of lipophilic active substances, and even of hydrophilic substances incorporated in the internal aqueous phase
- Lowered risk of microbial growth
- Liquid at very low temperatures (beneficial for winter sport products)

A typical w/o emulsion is composed as follows:

1.	Lipid component	20%
2.	Lipophilic thickening agent (e.g., wax, optional)	1%
3.	Emulsifier system with optimal HLB-value (3–8)	7–10%
4.	Preservatives (antimicrobial, antioxidants)	q.s.
5.	$MgSO_4 \cdot 7H_2O$	0.5%
6.	Water (+ hydrophilic thickening agent, optional) ad	100%

In order to avoid the heavy feel of w/o emulsions, appropriate excipients must be selected to get products with well-accepted sensory properties. This heavy feel of w/o emulsions is directly related to the spreading characteristics of the external oil phase. Therefore, polar oils with a high spreading coefficient [16] are preferably used, e.g., macadamia nut oil, isopropyl isostearate, isostearyl neopentanoate. Addition of low-viscosity silicone fluids or volatile cyclomethicone also improves the spreading effect. The physicochemical nature of the lipid components not only determines the spreading on the skin, the degree of occlusivity, and skin protection, but also influences the selection of the emulsifier system. Therefore, choosing an optimal emulsifier system is crucial. For example, glyceryl sorbitan unsaturated fatty acid ester (Arlacel 481) and glyceryl sorbitan saturated fatty acid ester (Arlacel 986) are better suited to emulsify apolar lipids, whereas more hydrophilic emulsifyers like the analogous ethoxylated sorbitan fatty acid esters (Arlacel 581, saturated, and Arlacel 582, unsaturated) or fatty acid esters of polyols (Arlacel 1689, saturated, and 1690, unsaturated) are designed for more polar lipids. A combination of PEG-7-hydrated castor oil and polyglyceryl-3-diisostearate may also be used. Skin feel may be improved by causing thixotropic behavior of the product, which is achieved by addition of a thixotropic agent or by reduction of the emulsifier content.

Multiple Emulsions

Multiple emulsions are triphasic systems or emulsions of emulsions. That means there is a primary emulsion dispersed in an external phase, e.g., water-in-oil-in-water (w/o/w). The dispersed phase in the resulting system contains smaller droplets having the same composition as the external phase [17]. The inner aqueous phase is separated from the outer aqueous phase by the oil phase, and therefore the composition of the two aqueous phases may be different, at least after preparation and for a certain storage time. Preparation and stabilization of multiple emulsions is a challenging task. They may either be prepared by a two-step method or by the relatively new one-step process "Partial Phase

Solu-Inversion Technology PPSIT" [18]. The two-step method includes preparation of the primary emulsion, which thereafter is dispersed in the external phase. In the PPSIT the lipid and electrolyte-containing water phase are heated and mixed above the phase inversion temperature (PIT), where the hydrophilic emulsifier forms w/o emulsions. By cooling down, a w/o/w system occurs at the PIT for a short time period. Then the system is immediately fixed by salting out and forming a lamellar matrix structure based on the emulsifier [19]. The advantage of w/o/w emulsions is that they comprise both the light feeling and positive sensory characteristics of o/w-emulsions and the skin hydration effect of w/o-emulsions.

Gels

Gels are dispersed systems, originally liquids (solutions) that have a certain consistency useful and practical for topical application. In contrast to emulsions, gels generally do not comprise two immiscible phases of opposite lyophilicity. Therefore, the polarity and solubility characteristics of the incorporated substances are either hydrophilic—in hydrogels—or lipophilic—in lipogels (or oleogels). The consistency of gels is caused by gelling (thickening) agents, usually polymers, building a three-dimensional network. Intermolecular forces bind the solvent molecules to the polymeric network, and thus the reduced mobility of these molecules results in a structured system with increased viscosity. Pure gels are transparent and clear or at least opalescent. Transparency is only achieved if all ingredients are dissolved or occur at least in colloidal form, i.e., the size of particles is in the submicron range. Transparency in particular is an attractive property of gels. Gel products have positive aesthetic characteristics and are thus becoming more and more popular in cosmetic care products today. Gels can also serve as the basis for more complex formulations:

- Solid particles can be incorporated, resulting in stabilized suspensions
- Incorporation of oily lipids results in so-called hydrolipid dispersions or quasi-emulsions (see p. 156).

Hydrogels

Hydrogels are hydrophilic, consisting mainly (85–95%) of water or an aqueous-alcoholic mixture and the gelling agent. The latter is usually an organic polymeric compound such as polyacrylic acid (Carbopol), sodium carboxy methylcellulose, or nonionic cellulose-ethers. Hydrogels have to be preserved against microbial growth.

After application, hydrogels show a cooling effect caused by evaporation of the solvent. They are easily applicable and humidify instantaneously, but if applied over a long time they desiccate the skin. For that reason, humectants such as glycerol may be added. After evaporation, the polymer residue may cause a sticky or "tearing" feel on the skin if inappropriate thickening agents have been used. Careful selection and testing of the needed adjuvants is therefore recommended.

Hydrophobic Gels

Lipogels or oleogels are obtained by adding a suitable thickening agent to an oil or liquid lipid. For example, colloidal silica may be used for that reason. A special type of hydrophobic gels is silicone-based systems.

Hydrolipid Dispersions

Hydrolipid dispersions are a special type of emulsion and are therefore treated separately in this chapter. They are disperse systems with a hydrophilic continuous phase and a lipophilic internal phase. The concentration of lipids lies between 2 and 20%. In principle, such a system is thermodynamically unstable. For stabilization, suitable large polymers are added, which are hydrated lyophilic colloids in the aqueous medium. Because of their molecular structure these polymeric emulsifiers are able to form mono- to multilamellar films at the interfaces and hence stabilize the emulsion. Typical examples are acrylates/C10-30alkyl acrylate crosspolymers. These polymers must have a sufficient surface activity that enables them to interact between the two different phases, resulting in a "quasi-emulsion," alternatively called balm, costabilized by hydroxypropyl methylcellulose or polyacrylate. The dispersed oil droplets may show a relatively large size of 20 to 50 μm, but such a quasiemulsion remains stable [20]. The great advantage of hydrolipid-dispersions is their lack of conventional emulsifiers, surfactants with skin irritation potential.

Microemulsions

According to the definition of Danielsson and Lindman [21], a microemulsion is defined as a system of water, oil, and amphiphile, which is a single optically isotropic and thermodynamically stable liquid solution. "This definition should be widened, however, to include metastable states, spontaneous emulsions of long-lived kinetic stability [22]." The term microemulsion may be a misnomer, because microemulsions consist of large or "swollen" micelles containing the internal phase, much like that found in a solubilized solution [23]. Microemulsions contain oil droplets in a water phase or water droplets in oil with diameters of about 10 to 200 nm. Therefore they appear as isotropic, optically clear liquid or gel-like systems. Unlike micellar solubilized systems, microemulsions may not be thermodynamically stable; nevertheless, they are more stable than ordinary emulsions. They are a type of ternary system composed from water, lipid, and surfactant mixture in a distinct ratio. The latter is usually a surfactant, such as Brij 96 [polyoxyethylene (10) oleyl ether] combined with a cosurfactant such as propylene glycol or ethylene glycol. Microemulsions may be used to incorporate or dissolve active substances and have been found to improve skin penetration and permeation [24].

The disadvantage of microemulsions is their rather high concentration of surfactants, which is a risk for increased skin irritation and sensitization. Nevertheless, modern microemulsion formulation is based on alkyl polyglycosides which are regarded to be milder than conventional nonionic surfactants with polyoxyethylene chains.

Nanoemulsions and Nanoparticles

During the last years, special dispersion formulations have been developed and described that contain ultra small particles used as carriers for active substances. The particles have a size in the range of 10 to a few hundred nanometers. This group of formulations shows a large heterogeneity and very often various terms or trade names have been created naming the same or similar systems. Generally the particles are dispersed in an aqueous medium.

For example, solid lipid nanoparticles possess a solid matrix composed of physiological lipids or lipoids with a mean diameter in the range of approximately 50 to 1000 nm

[25]. Active substances may be incorporated into these lipid nanoparticles serving as carriers, provided that the active substances are released after application on the skin.

Alternatively, the core of nanoparticles may either be a liquid lipid functioning as carrier or a lipophilic agent being directly effective, e.g., an emollient or occlusive agent. For stabilization, a monolayer of surfactants surrounding/covering the lipid droplet is used, e.g., phospholipids combined with a selected cosurfactant in a defined ratio [26,27]. Instead of a lipid, lipophilic active substances may be incorporated, e.g., vitamin A or E, UV filters, fragrances, etc. This type of nanoparticle is thought to be relatively insensitive toward the presence of additional surfactants in contrast to liposomes; therefore they can be mixed with conventional emulsions and the size of the nanoparticles remains in the submicron range.

Suspensions

Strictly considered, suspensions are not just vehicles but products consisting of particles, generally actives or functional excipients, that are dispersed in a liquid or semisolid medium that functions as a vehicle. Nevertheless, a suspension is also a type of formulation that may be used for application on the skin and to deliver substances to a target. In this way, a suspension can be regarded as a vehicle entity affecting the application site. Examples are sun-protection products or pearlescent nail lacquers containing pigments.

In suspension, sedimentation of unsoluble particles may happen because of difference in density. In order to guarantee a homogeneous product when applied, the particles must be redispersible by shaking before use. Alternatively, sedimentation must be hindered or at least reduced during storage. This is achieved by reduction of particle size and/or by increasing the viscosity of the vehicle, ideally creating a thixotropic system. The vehicle effect of the suspension on the skin is primarily caused by the liquid or semisolid phase of the vehicle comparable to solutions and emulsions.

Sticks

A stick is a solid delivery vehicle cast in an elongated form. By rubbing a stick onto skin, a variety of cosmetic ingredients can be delivered, such as fragrances, coloring agents, and emollients. In particular, sticks are ideally suited to deliver insoluble substances, e.g., pigments. The most popular cosmetic sticks are lipsticks and antiperspirant/deodorant sticks.

There are mainly three basic vehicle types of sticks:

1. Mixture of waxes (e.g., beeswax, carnauba) and oils (e.g., mineral, castor oil) that are cast into solid form, containing dissolved or undissolved active ingredients
2. Hydrophilic or aqueous sticks: solutions based on aqueous, propylene glycol, alcohol mixtures, solidified usually by sodium stearate, containing, e.g., aluminium chlorohydrate as antiperspirant
3. Matrix consisting of a high-boiling volatile silicone (e.g., cyclomethicone) gelled by fatty alcohol (e.g., stearyl alcohol)

In recent years, clear sticks have become popular. As a gelling agent, dibenzylidene sorbitol is used in propylene glycol or other related polyols [28].

FUNCTIONAL DESIGN, COMPOSITION, AND RESULTING EFFECT

There is no universal cosmetic vehicle available that can simply be mixed with an active cosmetic substance to get the cosmetic care product of choice, nor is there a general principle that could be observed to perform development of such a product. But a cosmetic care product has to be developed and whenever this is the case, various issues and aspects have to be considered and many problems must be solved step-by-step. Although formulation (galenical development) of cosmetic products is still rather empirical today, a rational approach is suggested. This section discusses the main issues that are to be considered when a functionally designed cosmetic product is being developed.

Target Profile

First, a clear target profile of the product must be defined. This includes the following:

1. Site of application. Depending on the site, certain forms may not be adequate, e.g., a w/o cream is not at all suitable for application on hair.
2. Area of application. A sticky, greasy cream cannot be applied on the whole body surface.
3. Target site. For example, the uppermost layer of stratum corneum or viable epidermis.
4. Sensory properties. For example, foaming shampoo or a light, smooth, low-viscosity cream.
5. Optical aspect. Clear, transparent, or milky, mono- or multiphasic.
6. State of matter. Liquid, semisolid, or solid.
7. Basic type of form. Solution or emulsion.
8. Active substances. Selected vegetable oil, vitamins, UV screen.
9. Storage stability and conditions.
10. Packaging.
11. Comparable, competitor products.

Selection of Vehicle Type

The type of vehicle may already be determined by the product target profile. If various types are possible, the most suitable should be selected. The following selection criteria are important: function or desired effect of the vehicle on the skin, ease of formulation feasibility, and physical and chemical stability. Furthermore, solubility, polarity, saturation solubility, vehicle interactions, and formation of mesophases are subjects to be considered when dealing with development and selection of vehicles. These topics are discussed later.

True Solution Versus Disperse System

Whenever the target of an active substance lies in deeper regions of the skin or even in skin cells, the substance must be present in molecular form for successful and efficient delivery, i.e., it must be dissolved in the vehicle or it must be able to dissolve, at least, after application. In other words, dissolution of a substance is a prerequisite for its delivery to a biological viable target (e.g., cell, enzyme). It is only in the dissolved state that fast and efficient penetration and transport into the deeper skin layers and cells is possible.

Thus, the first goal in formulation development is to dissolve the active substance in the vehicle. Therefore, the vehicle should be an ideal solvent for the active substance. If a substance cannot be dissolved in the vehicle—this may happen because of low solubility properties or stability reasons—then the substance has to be incorporated in particulate form; the smaller the size, the better. Fine particles in the order of 1 μm can be delivered onto or even into the uppermost layers of the skin, as close as possible to the target site. There they may dissolve, faster or slower, depending on their solubility in the skin. In vehicle systems containing particulate matter, homogeneous distribution of the undissolved substances must be guaranteed.

In summary, if the first goal—dissolution of active substance in the vehicle—is not achieved, the first alternative in formulation development must be targeted: the substance to be delivered must occur in particulate form as fine as possible. This is the prerequisite for fast and efficient delivery of unsoluble matter into the skin close to the target site.

Polarity

In order to achieve dissolution of a substance (solute), the adequate vehicle (solvent) has to be selected. The solubility of a substance is attributable in large measure to the polarity of the solvent, and it generally depends on chemical, electrical, and structural effects that lead to mutual interactions between the solute and solvent [29]. Polar solvents dissolve ionic solutes and other polar substances, whereas nonpolar substances are dissolved in nonpolar, lipophilic solvents. Solubility properties determine the selection of the appropriate vehicle for both, for solid as well as for liquid substances. Only nonpolar liquids are mutually completely miscible and thus can be used to make a nonpolar liquid vehicle. Accordingly, the same is true for polar liquids (e.g., water and alcohol).

Solubility characteristics of a compound used in formulation is one of the most important factors to be considered. Solubility data can be found in the literature; very often they are delivered by suppliers of the substances or they must be determined experimentally. In formulation the solubility parameter δ, according to Hildebrand and Scott [30], is a useful tool for selection of appropriate solvents. The more alike the δ-values of the compounds, the greater is their mutual solubility. A list of solubility parameters of cosmetic ingredients is given in Ref. 31. Very apolar substances have a low δ-value, and water has the highest value [23]. A rule of thumb states that mutual solubility is given if the difference between the two specific δ-values is at maximum 2 units $(cal/cm^3)^{-2}$.

Particularly in cosmetic formulation, where oils and lipids play a dominating role, polarity of oils is a factor to be considered. According to ICI Surfactants [16], the polarity may also be expressed by the polarity index based on the surface tension between the oil and water. Another interesting and simple characterization method is based on the bathochromic effect of a suitable dye dissolved in oils. The absorption maximum in the visible light—and therefore the color—of a nil-red-oil solution depends on the polarity of the oil; the higher the absorption maximum, the more polar is the oil or oil mixture [32].

In conclusion, if a monophasic system has to be formulated, only substances with mutual solubility can be combined. In contrast, if multiphasic systems such as emulsions and suspensions are made, the phase-forming components must be mutually insoluble. Nevertheless, preparation and solubilization of multiphasic systems require the addition of amphiphilic substances (emulsifiers in emulsions, surfactants for wetting and repulsing the particles in suspensions). In emulsions, polar as well as nonpolar substances can be dissolved in the hydrophilic or lipophilic phase, respectively. This is one reason for the popularity of emulsions.

Saturation, Supersaturation

Theoretically, a solute can be dissolved in a solvent up to the saturation solubility. Beyond this concentration, precipitation of the solute or phase separation usually occurs. Some substances are able to remain transiently in solution above saturation solubility. This phenomenon is known as supersaturation, a metastable condition. Supersaturated solutions can be caused to return to saturation equilibrium by triggers such as agitation, scratching the wall of containers, or addition of seeding crystals.

The driving force for delivery of substances, i.e., release from vehicle and penetration into skin, is thermodynamic activity, which is maximal at saturation concentration [33]. Consequently, in order to achieve maximal penetration rate into the skin, a substance must be dissolved in a vehicle at saturation concentration. Moreover, saturated or supersaturated systems are necessary, but not the only prerequisites for optimal topical delivery. For example, the skin—vehicle partition coefficient of the solute also plays a role. The partition coefficient may be raised because of the vehicle—skin interaction yielding in increased skin penetration. In conclusion, achieving the highest possible concentration in the dissolved state is the second goal to be aimed for in formulation development if delivery into the skin is targeted.

Vehicle Interactions

Sun-protection products are a good example of showing interactions between vehicle, active substance, and the skin. The absorption of UV radiation not only depends on the molecular structure and concentration of the protecting agent, but on the solvent as well. Also, water resistancy may be influenced by selection and composition of the vehicle.

Vehicle components may penetrate into the stratum corneum and interact with the stratum corneum lipids. This may result in disturbance of their lamellar structures and increased and faster penetration of compounds in the stratum corneum. Alternatively, presence of vehicle components in the stratum corneum may cause a depot effect for certain compounds.

Substantivity

The term substantivity describes adherence properties of materials to keratinous substrates in the upper skin layers, in particular regarding deposition and retention capacity when in contact with water, which could deplete the material [34]. High substantivity is especially important for sun protection products. It is primarily a function of the physicochemical properties of the active molecules but may also be influenced by the vehicle. For example, addition of film-forming, skin-adherent polymeric substances to the vehicle may increase retention of sunscreens in the skin and thus result in an improved water-resistant product. Another means is creating formulations that contain phospholipids, enabling the formation of vesicular, liposomal structures in the vehicle or in the upper layers of stratum corneum and thus yielding in a depot effect.

An interesting model to assess substantivity has been presented by Ref. 34. The investigators used human callus to simulate and quantify solute sorption to human skin, which was found to be more suitable than octanol or animal keratin. However, water resistancy still has to be determined in vivo to know the true quality of the product.

Mesophases

Not only the type of vehicle, e.g., solution or o/w emulsion, but also occurrence and type of mesophases (liquid crystal structures) determine the properties and behavior of a vehicle. At certain concentrations and combinations of specific emulsifying agents in liquids, associations may be formed, resulting in liquid crystal structures, also called mesomorphic state or mesophase. The mesophase shows anisotropy and is thermodynamically stable. Different types of mesophases have been described: middle phase (hexagonal), cubic phase, and neat phase (lamellar).

Fatty amphiphiles (e.g., long chain alcohols, acids, monoglycerides) that are dispersed in water in the presence of a high hydrophilic-lipophilic balance (HLB) surfactant form lamellar phases. They are able to swell at an elevated temperature close to the melting point of the hydrocarbon chain. These swollen lamellar liquid crystalline phases can incorporate significant quantities of water. The hydrocarbon chains are liquid-like, i.e., disordered. If the temperature decreases, the lamellar liquid crystalline phases of fatty amphiphiles are transformed to so-called lamellar crystalline gel network phases, which build complex gel networks. Such networks not only stabilize creams and lotions, but also control their consistency because of their viscoelastic properties. Such mesophases provide the following advantages to emulsions:

1. Increased stability
2. Prolonged hydration properties
3. Controlled release of active ingredient
4. Easy to formulate
5. Well-liked skin feel [35]

Metamorphosis of Vehicles

Most vehicles undergo considerable changes during and after application to the skin because of mechanical stress when spread over the surface and/or evaporation of volatile ingredients. Mechanical stress and skin temperature may influence the viscosity of the vehicle and consequently the release rate of active ingredients. Uptake of water from the skin may alter the composition of the vehicle. All these factors may also cause phase inversion or phase separation. And last but not least, as a consequence of these alterations the thermodynamic activity of an active ingredient within its vehicle will change as well. Thus, by controlling or changing the thermodynamic activity, release of a substance from the vehicle and penetration into the skin can be modulated. For example, if after application the volatile component of the vehicle, being an excellent solvent of the active substance, evaporates, saturation concentration of the active in the remaining vehicle or even supersaturation may be achieved. This results either in improved release and delivery as previously mentioned (see Section 5.2.3) or in precipitation and deposition of the active substance. Another interesting example is given by an optimally composed sun-protecting o/w-emulsion; after application the emulsion has transformed to the w/o type because of water evaporation and the mechanical stress caused by spreading. The remaining lipophilic protective film yields in improved water resistance.

In conclusion, the optimally designed and developed vehicle not only demonstrates excellent properties after manufacturing and storage, but also after application and metamorphosis at the application site.

Rheology

The term rheology describes the flow characteristics of liquids and the deformation of solids. Viscosity is an expression of the resistance of a fluid to flow. Rheological properties are crucial for liquid and semiliquid cosmetic formulations because they determine the product's properties meaningful in mixing and flow when produced, filled into containers and removed before use, as well as sensory properties when applied, such as consistency, spreadability, and smoothness. Furthermore, the rheology of a product may also affect the physical stability and the biological availability of the product [36].

Regarding rheological characteristics, there are two main types of systems: Newtonian and non-Newtonian. The former show constant viscosity when stressed, i.e., the rate of shear (flow velocity) is directly proportional to the shearing stress, e.g., water, mineral oil, etc. In non-Newtonian systems (most cosmetic products), however, viscosity changes with varying stress, i.e., viscosity depends on the degree of shearing stress, resulting either in plastic, pseudoplastic, or dilatant flow or in thixothropy, characteristics that are not discussed in depth here although they are of practical significance. An ideal topical product, e.g., shows optimal thixotropic properties; it does not flow out of a tube's orifice unless slightly pressed, and when on the skin it does not immediately flow and drop off unless easily spread over the application area, where under a certain stress it becomes more fluid because of the thixotropy. The rheological properties of semisolid products are determined first for general characterization in the development phase and second for quality-control reasons after manufacturing. There are various instrumental methods used to measure rheology or viscosity. Today, apparatus based on rotation or oscillation are commonly used for non-Newtonian systems.

In order to adjust the rheology of products, various means and excipients are available. If the viscosity has to be increased, addition of viscosity increasing agents is needed. Addition or increase in concentration of electrolytes may influence viscosity. Many systems, e.g., polyacrylates, are sensitive to the presence of ions and the viscosity is reduced.

In particular, emulsions are susceptible to rheological issues. Various factors determine the rheological properties of emulsions, such as viscosity of internal and external phases, phase volume ratio, particle size distribution, type and concentration of emulsifying system, and viscosity-modifying agents. However, this topic is too complex to be treated comprehensively in this context. It is further discussed in a review by Sherman [37]. It is important to realize that small changes in concentrations or ratio of certain ingredients may result in drastic changes of the rheological characteristics. Emulsified products may undergo a wide variety of shear stresses during either preparation or use. Thus, an emulsion formulation should be robust enough to resist external factors that could modify its rheological properties or the product should be designed so that change in rheology results in a desired effect.

Preservation

Antimicrobials

Most cosmetic care products must be protected against microbial growth. Not only for the protection of consumers against infection but also for stability reasons. Growth of microorganisms might result in degradation of ingredients and consequently in deterioration of physical and chemical stability. In general, presence of water in the vehicle as well as other ingredients susceptible to microbial metabolism require adequate preservation.

There are various ways to protect a product against microbial growth:

1. Addition of an antimicrobial agent, which is common practice
2. Sterile or aseptic production and filling into packaging material, preventing microbial contamination during storage and usage
3. Reduced water activity, i.e., controlling growth of spoilage microorganisms by reducing the available amount of water in cosmetic preparations [38]

It is not only mandatory to add antimicrobials but also to test their efficacy after manufacturing and after storage until the expiration date. Nowadays performance of the preservative efficacy test (PET), also known as the challenge test, is state of the art [39]. Today more and more in-use tests are performed to simulate the usage by the consumer and to show efficacious protection against microbial growth after contamination.

Addition of preservatives to complex, multiphasic systems, in particular, is a critical formulation issue for the following reasons:

1. Many preservatives interact with other components of the vehicle, e.g., with emulsifyers, resulting in change of viscosity or in phase separation in the worst case.
2. Depending on the physicochemical characteristics, preservatives are distributed between the different phases which might result in too-low effective concentration in the aqueous phase.
3. Adsorption of the preservatives to polymers in the formulation and/or packaging material; complexation or micellization might also result in too-low antimicrobial activity.

In conclusion, it is not sufficient to add a preservative at recommended concentration. To protect the vehicle sufficiently, a properly designed preservative system is required that must be tested in the formulation regarding efficacy and safety. It is a great formulation challenge to achieve sufficient protection against microbial growth in the product, especially as many antimicrobials are discredited because of their irritation and sensitization potential.

Antioxidants

Protection against oxidation may also be a formulation issue although not so relevant as antimicrobial efficacy. It is achieved by addition of antioxidants or by manufacturing and storing in an inert atmosphere. In particular, modern formulations containing oxidation-sensitive compounds, such as certain vitamins and vegetable oils with unsaturated fatty acid derivatives, must be sufficiently protected against oxygen.

Development Strategy and Rationale

Having considered the aforementioned issues, formulation development is preferably conducted according to a suitable, rational procedure. The complex formulation development process may be represented symbolically by the ''magic formulation triangle'' (Fig. 1), showing the mutual interaction and dependency of the following:

1. Feasibility of preparation or formulation of the active substance(s) in the vehicle
2. Stability (chemical and physical) of the product, and
3. Effectivity or activity of the product when applied.

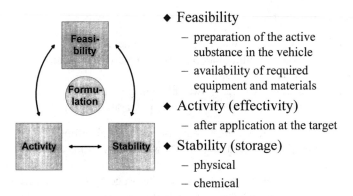

- ◆ Feasibility
  - – preparation of the active substance in the vehicle
  - – availability of required equipment and materials
- ◆ Activity (effectivity)
  - – after application at the target
- ◆ Stability (storage)
  - – physical
  - – chemical

FIGURE 1   Magic triangle of formulation: mutual interaction and dependency.

First, the feasibility of preparation and formulation has to be checked. For example, if a low–water-soluble compound should be dissolved in an aqueous vehicle, solubility-enhancing studies are performed. Or if an emulsion is desired, it has to be checked whether the phases can be emulsified with the selected emulsifying system.

After having prepared the desired formulation, both stability and effect must be assessed, preferably more or less in parallel. It does not make any sense to have a stable but ineffective product, or to develop a very effective system that remains stable for a few days or that contains an ingredient that is irritating or sensitizing. Such a product cannot be marketed. For example, if a relatively unstable active substance (e.g., ascorbic acid) must be delivered in dissolved form to be effective or bioavailable at the target site, then a suitable vehicle with good solvent properties must be used. However, the chemical stability of compounds is generally lower when in solution. Therefore, not every suitable solvent can be used as a vehicle, but an optimum has to be found, a vehicle enabling both, keeping the active to remain dissolved and in a chemically stable state.

Having in mind those three cornerstones of the formulation triangle, formulation development to find the right vehicle is performed stepwise, addressing the following issues:

1. Objective, definition of target profile (See p. 158.)
2. Preformulation investigation: determination of physicochemical properties of (active) substances to be formulated, such as solubility data, partition coefficient, dissociation constant, pH, crystal morphology, particle size distribution, and assessment of their stability and incompatibility
3. Selection of appropriate excipients to be used for formulation
4. Based on the outcome of these three working steps the feasibility of preparation is checked and modifications are made if necessary, all of these together to prepare the next step
5. Formulation screening on a small-scale basis with as many as possible and feasible variations in composition, excipients, preparation methods, and so on
6. Selection of the best formulations and preparation methods from the screening program for technical scaling-up as well as for confirmation and validation of the results obtained with the formulations. The selection of the formulations is based on criteria such as physical stability or absence of precipitation in solu-

tion, no sedimentation or phase separation or recrystallization in multiphasic systems; chemical stability or degradation, respectively; preservative efficacy test (PET); biological assessment, e.g., skin-hydration effect, sun-protecting effect, and antioxidant or radical scavenger effect in cells; and

7. Safety evaluation in human beings with formulation chosen for introduction into market.

PREPARATION METHODS

It is not the intention to present a review on preparation methods and equipment for the manufacturing of cosmetic vehicles and products in this chapter. But it is common sense that the preparation method may influence a product's quality. Thus, not only the composition but also the way of preparation should be in the scope of development and preparation work. There are many types and variations of mixing, dispersion, emulsification, and size-reduction equipment that can be used to prepare vehicles that are used in cosmetics. For example, size reduction of the internal phase droplets in an emulsion depends on the mechanical principle of the used equipment, and best results are achieved with a valve homogenizer. In every case the goal is to get a homogeneous product of specified and reproducible quality. Only with a product of specified and constant quality a reproducible effect can be achieved when applied. Standard, basic operations are dissolution, blending and mixing, dispersion and homogenization, and size reduction, which may all be associated by energy transfer involving cooling or heating.

It is of paramount importance that in early development phases preparation is performed under well-defined and known conditions, otherwise scaling-up and reproducibility of product quality becomes a risky task. Closely related with the preparation method is testing and characterization of the product. This is treated in the following section.

CHARACTERIZATION

Physical Characterization

Appearance

Assessment and description of appearance is one of the easiest, most practical, and nevertheless powerful tests. It may be performed macroscopically, describing color, clearness, transparency, turbidity, and state of matter. In addition, microscopic investigation is recommended; taking microphotographs is useful for documentation.

Rheology

Rheological properties (viscosity, consistency) are important characteristics of most types of cosmetic care products because they have an impact on preparation, packaging, storage, application, and delivery of actives. Thus these properties should be assessed for characterization and quality control of the product.

Most disperse systems and thus cosmetic care products show Non-Newtonian flow behavior, namely pseudoplastic, plastic, or dilatant behavior. A wide variety of techniques and methods have been developed to measure viscosity properties. These procedures can be classified as either absolute or relative. The absolute either directly or indirectly measures specific components of shear stress and shear rate to define an appropriate rheological function. Methods used for absolute viscosity measurements are flow through a tube, rotational methods, or surface viscosity methods. Methods used for relative viscosity measurement are those using orifice viscometers, falling balls, or plungers. Such instruments, although they do not measure stress or shear rate, offer valuable quality-control tests for relative comparison between different materials [40]. Apparatus based on rotational or even oscillating principles to assess viscoelastic properties is state of the art.

pH

Measurement of pH value (concentration of hydrogen ions) in aqueous vehicles (solutions, suspensions, o/w emulsions, gels) is a valuable control mean. First of all, if possible, a pH value in the physiological range is generally targeted, ideally similar to that of the skin or the specific application site, in order to prevent irritation. Many reactions and processes depend on pH, e.g., efficacy of antimicrobial preservatives, stability and degradation of substances, and solubility. Thus, pH measurement is a ''must'' and it is easily performed with the available measurement systems.

Homogeneity

In many cases, at a first step homogeneity may be assessed visibly; precipitation in a solution or distinct phase separation in an emulsion is easily detected. Nontransparent, multiphasic systems are more difficult to check. In these cases, microscopic investigation of representative samples is suggested along with quantitative assays regarding active ingredients (uniformity of content).

Droplet or Particle Size and Distribution

The physical stability of colloidal systems as well as emulsions or suspensions partially depends on the particle size. In particular, preparations containing small particles with identical electrical charge are more resistant to flocculation and sedimentation than systems containing larger or uncharged entities. Similarly, reduced particle size is an indicator of improved kinetic stability of emulsions or suspensions. For that reason, determination of particle size and size distribution is an important characterization method. Various optical methods are available; A minireview is given in Ref. 41 and a selection is listed as follows:

1. Perhaps the most commonly used method today is based on laser diffraction, suitable to measure solid particles and also dispersed droplets under special conditions, size range 1 to 600 μm.
2. Dynamic light scattering (DLS), also known as photon correlation spectroscopy (PCS), is used for measuring micelles, liposomes, and submicron suspensions (size range 0.003 to 3 μm).
3. Optical or electron microscopy are further methods of choice.

Chemical Characterization

Besides physical characterization, chemically based investigations are indispensable to assess the quality of a product. It is well known that the quality and composition of a vehicle can influence the chemical stability of ingredients. Many reactions, such as ester hydrolysis or other degradations, may be enhanced or sustained by change in pH, presence of catalytic or stabilizing agents, respectively. Thus, development and optimal selection of the best vehicle is supported by chemical stability investigations.

Biological Characterization

Further important assessment methods are based on biological tests. This is to evaluate and validate the desired targeted effects in vivo after application of the product. Examples include hydration of the skin, protection against sun radiation, and protection against skin irritating substances during work. This subject is treated in other chapters of this textbook.

Sensory Assessment

The sensory assessment is a useful tool for product and concept development and for quality control in the cosmetic industry. Although a very subjective and liable method, valuable data is obtained if sensory assessment is conducted in a systematic way. Terms like pick up, consistency, peaking, cushion, absorption, smoothness, stickiness, tackiness, oiliness, and greasy are used. An interesting paper on that subject has been published by Busch and Gassenmeier [42].

Barry and coworkers carried out sensory testing on topical preparations and established rheological methods for use as control procedures to maintain uniform skin feel and spreadability [43]. The consistency of a material can be assessed by using three attributes: smoothness, thinness, and warmth [44].

REFERENCES

1. Wilkinson JB, Moore RJ, eds. Harry's Cosmeticology. New York: Chemical Publishing, 1982.
2. Rieger MM. Cosmetics and their relation to drugs. In: Swarbrick J, Boylan JC, eds. Encyclopedia of Pharmaceutical Technology, Vol. 3. New York: Marcel Dekker, 1990:361–373.
3. Junginger HE. Systematik der dermatika—kolloidchemischer aufbau. In: Niedner R, Ziegenmeyer J, eds. Dermatika. Stuttgart: Wissenschaftliche Verlagsgesellschaft mbH, 1992:476.
4. Martin A, Bustamante P, Chun AHC. Physical Pharmacy. Philadelphia: Lea & Febiger, 1993: 393–396.
5. Martin A, Bustamante P, Chun AHC. Physical Pharmacy. Philadelphia: Lea & Febiger, 1993: 393.
6. Martin A, Bustamante P, Chun AHC. Physical Pharmacy. Philadelphia: Lea & Febiger, 1993: 386.
7. Martin A, Bustamante P, Chun AHC. Physical Pharmacy. Philadelphia: Lea & Febiger, 1993: 496.
8. Martin A, Bustamante P, Chun AHC. Physical Pharmacy. Philadelphia: Lea & Febiger, 1993: 101.
9. Martin A, Bustamante P, Chun AHC. Physical Pharmacy. Philadelphia: Lea & Febiger, 1993: 477.
10. Martin A, Bustamante P, Chun AHC. Physical Pharmacy. Philadelphia: Lea & Febiger, 1993: 234.
11. Martin A, Bustamante P, Chun AHC. Physical Pharmacy. Philadelphia: Lea & Febiger, 1993: 396.
12. Martin A, Bustamante P, Chun AHC. Physical Pharmacy. Philadelphia: Lea & Febiger, 1993: 488.
13. Martin A, Bustamante P, Chun AHC. Physical Pharmacy. Philadelphia: Lea & Febiger, 1993: 490.
14. ICI Surfactants, brochure 41-1E. Personal Care. Middlesbrough, Cleveland, United Kingdom, 1996.
15. Herzog B, Marquart D, Müller S, Pedrussio R, Sucker H. Einfluss von zusammensetzung und phasenverhältnis auf die konsistenz von cremes. Pharm Ind 1998; 60:713–721.

16. ICI Surfactants, brochure 42-4E. Personal Care, emulsifiers for water in oil emulsions. Middlesbrough, Cleveland, United Kingdom, 1996:5.

17. Rosoff M. Specialized pharmaceutical emulsions. In: Liebermann HA, Rieger MM, Banker GS, eds. Pharmaceutical Dosage Forms: Disperse Systems, Vol. 3. New York: Marcel Dekker, 1998:11.

18. Gohla SH, Nielsen J. Partial phase solu-inversion technology (PPSIT). Seifen Oele Fette Wachse J 1995; 121:707–713.

19. Kutz G, Friess S. Moderne Verfahren zur Herstellung von halbfesten und flüssigen Emulsionen—eine aktuelle Uebersicht. Seifen Oele Fette Wachse J 1998; 124:308–313.

20. Daniels R. Neue anwendungsformen bei sonnenschutzmitteln. Apotheken Journal. 1997; 19(5):22–28.

21. Danielsson L, Lindman B. Colloids Surfaces 1981; 3:391.

22. Rosoff M. Specialized pharmaceutical emulsions. In: Liebermann HA, Rieger MM, Banker GS, eds. Pharmaceutical Dosage Forms: Disperse Systems, Vol. 3. New York: Marcel Dekker, 1998:20.

23. Martin A, Bustamante P, Chun AHC. Physical Pharmacy. Philadelphia: Lea & Febiger, 1993: 495.

24. Martin A, Bustamante P, Chun AHC. Physical Pharmacy. Philadelphia: Lea & Febiger, 1993: 496.

25. Müller RH, Weyhers H, zur Mühlen A, Dingler A, Mehnert W. Solid lipid nanoparticles—ein neuartiger Wirkstoff-carrier für Kosmetika und Pharmazeutika. Pharm Ind 1997; 59:423–427.

26. Zülli F, Suter F. Preparation and properties of small nanoparticles for skin and hair care. Seifen Oele Fette Wachse J 1997; 123:880–885.

27. Herzog B, Sommer K, Baschong W, Röding J. Nanotopes™: a surfactant resistant carrier system. Seifen Oele Fette Wachse J 1998; 124:614–623.

28. Schueller R, Romanowsky P. Gels and sticks. Cosmet Toilet Mag 1998; 113:43–46.

29. Martin A, Bustamante P, Chun AHC. Physical Pharmacy. Philadelphia: Lea & Febiger, 1993: 215.

30. Hildebrand JR, Scott RL. Solubility of Nonelectrolytes. New York: Dover, 1964; (Chap. 23).

31. Vaughan CD. Using solubility parameters in cosmetics formulation. J Soc Cosmet Chem 1985; 36:319–333.

32. Dietz Th. Solvatochromie von Nilrot. Parfümerie und Kosmetik 1999; 80:44–49.

33. Flynn GL, Weiner ND. Topical and transdermal delivery—provinces of realism. In: Gurny R, Teubner A, eds. Dermal and Transdermal Drug Delivery. Stuttgart: Wissenschaftliche Verlagsgesellschaft mbH, 1993:44.

34. Hagedorn-Leweke U, Lippold BC. Accumulation of sunscreens and other compounds in keratinous substrates. Eur J Pharmaceutics Biopharmaceutics 1998; 46:215–221.

35. Loll P. Liquid crystals in cosmetic emulsions. Reprint RP 94-93E. ICI Europe Limited, Everberg, B, 1993.

36. Martin A, Bustamante P, Chun AHC. Physical Pharmacy. Philadelphia: Lea & Febiger, 1993: 457.

37. Sherman P. Rheology of Emulsions. Oxford: Pergamon Press, 1963.

38. Enigl DC, Sorrells KM. Water activity and self-preserving formulas. In: Kabara JJ, Orth DS, eds. Preservative-Free and Self-Preserving Cosmetics and Drugs. New York: Marcel Dekker, 1997:45.

39. Sabourin JR. A Perspective on Preservation for the New Millennium, Cosmetics and Toiletries Manufacture Worldwide. Hemel Hempstead, United Kingdom: Aston Publishing Group, 1999: 50–59.

40. Hanna SA. Quality assurance. In: Liebermann HA, Rieger MM, Banker GS, eds. Pharmaceutical Dosage Forms: Disperse Systems, Vol. 3. New York: Marcel Dekker, 1998:460.

41. Haskell RJ. Characterization of submicron systems via optical methods. J Pharm Sci 1998; 87:125–129.
42. Busch P, Gassenmeier Th. Sensory assessment in the cosmetic field. Parfümerie und Kosmetik 1997; 7/8:16–21.
43a. Barry BW, Grace AJ. J Pharm Sci 1971; 60:1198, J Pharm Sci 1972; 61:335.
43b. Barry BW, Meyer MC. J Pharm Sci 1973; 62:1349.
44. Martin A, Bustamante P, Chun AHC. Physical Pharmacy. Philadelphia: Lea & Febiger, 1993: 471.

15

Encapsulation to Deliver Topical Actives

Jocélia Jansen
*State University of Ponta Grossa, Ponta Grossa,
Paraná, Brazil*

Howard I. Maibach
*University of California at San Francisco School of Medicine,
San Francisco, California*

INTRODUCTION

Cosmetic technology is constantly developing raw materials and formulation with active ingredients. The new surfactant molecules, the search for original active substances and efficient combinations, and the design of novel vehicles or carriers has led to the implementation of new cosmetic systems in contrast to the classic forms such as creams or gels.

The achievements of recent extensive research has resulted in the development of controlled delivery systems. Some of these systems have been extensively investigated for their therapeutic potential while simultaneously being examined for their possible cosmetic uses. One objective in the design of novel drug delivery systems is controlled delivery of the active to its site of action at an appropriate rate. Novel polymers and surfactants in different forms, sizes, and shapes can aid in this goal. Encapsulation techniques are used in pharmaceuticals, cosmetics, veterinary application, food, copying systems, laundry products, agricultural uses, pigments, and other less well-known uses to control the delivery of encapsulated agents as well as to protect those agents from environmental degradation.

DESIGN ASPECTS OF A VECTOR

Microparticles

Microencapsulation is a process by which very thin coatings of inert natural or synthetic polymeric materials are deposited around microsized particles of solids or droplets of liquids. Products thus formed are known as microparticles, covering two types of forms: microcapsules, micrometric reservoir systems, and microspheres, micrometric matrix systems (Fig. 1).

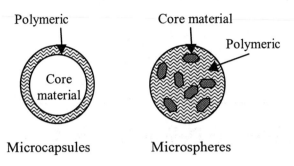

FIGURE 1   Schematic representation of microparticles.

These systems consist of two major parts. The inner part is the core material containing one or more active ingredients. These active ingredients may be solids, liquids, or gases. The outer part is the coating material that is usually of a high–molecular weight polymer or a combination of such polymers. The coating material can be chosen from a variety of natural and synthetic polymers. The coating material must be nonreactive to the core material, preferably biodegradable, and nontoxic. Other components, such as plasticizers and surfactants, may also be added.

Initially, microparticles were produced mainly in sizes ranging from 5 μm to as much as 2 mm, but around 1980 a second generation of products of much smaller dimensions was developed. This includes nanoparticles from 10 to 1000 nm in diameter [1], as well as 1 to 10 μm microspheres, overlapping in size with nonsolid microstructures such as liposomes. Commercial microparticles typically have a diameter between 1 and 1000 μm and contain 10 to 90 wt% core. Most capsule shell materials are organic polymers, but fat and waxes are also used. Various types of physical structures of the product of microencapsulation such as mononuclear spheres, multinuclear spheres, multinuclear irregular particles, and so on can be obtained depending on the manufacturing process.

Recently, a polymeric system consisting of porous microspheres named Microsponge has been developed (Microsponge System [2]; Advanced Polymer System Inc., Redwood City, CA). These systems are made by suspension polymerization and typically consist of cross-linked polystyrene or polymethacrylates.

No encapsulation process developed to date is able to produce the full range of capsules desired by potential capsule users. The methods, which are significantly relevant to the production of microparticles used in pharmaceutical products and cosmetics, are shown in Table 1. Many techniques have been proposed for the production of microparticles, and it was suggested [9] that more than 200 methods could be identified in the literature. A thorough description of the formation of microparticles are given by several reviews [4,6,10,11].

Nanoparticles

Nanoparticles can generally be defined as submicron (<1μm) colloidal systems, but are not necessarily made of polymers (biodegradable or not). According to the process used for the preparation of nanoparticles, nanocapsules or nanospheres can be obtained. Nanocapsules are vesicular systems in which the drug is confined to a cavity surrounded by a

TABLE 1 Microencapsulation Methods

Type	Reference
Coacervation-phase separation procedures using aqueous vehicles	3
Coacervation-phase separation procedures using nonaqueous vehicles	4
Interfacial polymerization	5
In situ polymerization	6
Polymer-polymer incompatibility	3
Spray drying, spray congealing, spray embedding, and spray polymerization	4
Droplet extrusion	7
	8

unique polymeric membrane; nanospheres are matrix systems in which the drug is dispersed throughout the particles.

Several methods have been developed for preparing nanoparticles. They can be classified in two main categories according to whether the formation of nanoparticles requires a polymerization reaction (Table 2) or whether it is achieved from a macromolecule or a preformed polymer (Table 3). De Vringer and Ronde [25] proposed a water-in-oil (w/o) cream containing nanoparticles of solid paraffin to obtain a topical dermatological product with a high degree of occlusivity combined with attractive cosmetic properties. Kim et al. [26] reported the encapsulation of fat vitamin series in nanospheres prepared with soybean lecithin coated with a nonionic surfactant. Müller [27,28] believes that the solid lipid nanoparticles (SLN) appear as an attractive carrier system for cosmetic ingredients—unloaded and loaded. In the case of unloaded particles, the SLN themselves represent the active ingredient, e.g., when made from skin-carrying lipids. Alternatively, the SLN can be blended with special lipids, e.g., ceramides. Finally, good reviews with methods of preparation for nanoparticles can be found in the literature, such those by Kreuter [12] and Couvreur et al. [29].

Multiple Emulsions

Multiple emulsions are emulsions in which the dispersion phase contains another dispersion phase. Thus, a water-in-oil-in-water (w/o/w) emulsion is a system in which the globules of water are dispersed in globules of oil, and the oil globules are themselves dispersed

TABLE 2 Nanoparticles Obtained by Polymerization of a Monomer

Type	Reference
Nanospheres	
Poly(methylmethacrylate) and Polyalkyl-cyanoacrilate nanoparticles	12
Polyalkylcyanoacrylate nanospheres	13
Nanocapsules	
Polyalkylcyanoacrylate nanocapsules	14, 15

TABLE 3 Nanoparticles Obtained by Dispersion of Preformed Macromolecules

Type	Reference
Nanospheres prepared by emulsification	
Solution emulsification	16
Phase inversion	17
Self-emulsification	18
Nanospheres of synthetic polymers	19, 20, 21
Nanospheres of natural polymers	21
Nanospheres prepared by desalvation	
Nanospheres of synthetic polymers	22
Nanospheres of natural polymers	23, 24
Nanocapsules	14, 22

in an aqueous environment. A parallel arrangement exists in oil-in-water-in-oil (o/w/o) type of multiple emulsions in which an internal oily phase is dispersed in aqueous globules, which are themselves dispersed within an external oily phase (Fig. 2).

Multiple emulsions, first described by Seifriz in 1925, have recently been studied in detail. The operational technique plays an even more important role in the production of multiple emulsions than in the production of simple emulsions [30–35]. Multiple emulsions have been prepared in two main modes: one-step and two-step emulsification.

One-step emulsification is prepared by forming w/o emulsion with a large excess of relatively hydrophobic emulsifier and a small amount of hydrophilic emulsifier followed by heat treating the emulsion until, at least in part, it will invert. At a proper temperature, and with the right hydrophilic lipophilic balance (HLB) of the emulsifiers, w/o/w emulsion can be found in the system. In most recent studies, multiple emulsions are prepared in a two-step emulsification process by two sets of emulsifiers: a hydrophobic emulsifier I (for the w/o emulsion) and a hydrophilic emulsifier II (for the oil-in-water (o/w) emulsion). The primary emulsion is prepared under high shear conditions (ultrasonification, homogenization), whereas the secondary emulsification step is carried out without any severe mixing (an excess of mixing can rupture the drops, resulting in a simple emulsion).

The composition of the multiple emulsions is of significant importance, because the different surfactants along with the nature and concentration of the oil phase will affect the stability of the double emulsion. Parameters such as HLB, oil phase volume, and the

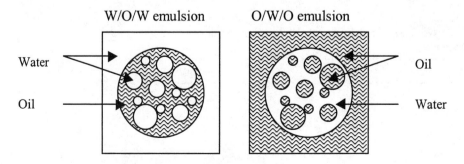

FIGURE 2 Schematic representation of multiple emulsions.

nature of the entrapped materials have been discussed and optimized. Several reviews and studies include Florence and Whitehill [36–38], Matsumoto et al. [39,40] and Frenkel [41–43].

Microemulsions

Miocroemulsions are stable dispersions in the form of spherical droplets whose diameter is in the range of 10 to 100 nm. They are composed of oil, water, and usually surfactant and cosurfactant. These systems show structural similarity to micelles and inverse micelles, resulting in o/w or w/o microemulsions, respectively. They are highly dynamic systems showing fluctuating surfaces caused by forming and deforming processes.

The main characteristics of microemulsions are the low viscosity associated with a Newtonian-type flow, a transparent or translucid appearance, and isotropic and thermodynamic stability within a specific temperature setting. Certain microemulsions may thus be obtained without heating, simply by mixing the components as long as they are in a liquid state. One of the conditions for microemulsion formation is a very small, rather than a transient negative, interfacial tension (44). This is rarely achieved by the use of a single surfactant, usually necessitating the addition of a cosurfactant. The presence of a short chain alcohol, e.g., can reduce the interfacial tension from about 10 mN/m to a value less than 10^{-2}mN/m. Exceptions to this rule are provided by nonionic surfactants which, at their phase inversion temperature, also exhibit very low interfacial tensions.

A microemulsion is usually created by the establishment of pseudoternary diagram for which a ratio of surfactant/cosurfactant is fixed, representing a sole constituent. The establishment of a ternary diagram is generally accomplished for locating the microemulsion or the microemulsion zones by titration. Using a specific ratio of surfactant/cosurfactant, various combinations of oil and surfactant/cosurfactant are produced. The water is added drop by drop. After the addition of each drop, the mixture is stirred and examined through a crossed polarized filter. The appearance (transparence, opalescence, isotropy) is recorded, along with a number of phases. In this way, an approximate delineation of the boundaries can be obtained in which it is possible to refine through the production of compositions point by point beginning with the four basic components.

Nanoemulsions (Submicron Emulsions)

Emulsions are heterogeneous systems in which one immiscible liquid is dispersed as droplets in another liquid. Such a system is thermodynamically unstable and is kinetically stabilized by the addition of one further component or mixture of components that exhibits emulsifying properties. Depending on the nature of the diverse components of the emulsifying agents, various types of emulsions can result from the mixture of immiscible liquids. The main characteristic of nanoemulsions or submicron emulsions is the droplet size, which must be inferior to 1μm.

Emulsions prepared by use of conventional apparatus, e.g., electric mixers and mechanical stirrers, show large droplet sizes and wide particle distribution. The techniques usually used to prepare submicron emulsions involve the use of ultrasound, evaporation of solvent (45), two-stage homogenizer [46,47], and the microfluidizer [48,49]. The nanoemulsion preparation process involves the following steps:

1. Three approaches can be used to incorporate the drug and/or the emulsifiers in the aqueous or oil phase. The most common is to dissolve the water-soluble

ingredients in the aqueous phase and the oil-soluble ingredients in the oil phase. The second approach, which is used in fat emulsion preparations [46], involves the dissolution of an aqueous-insoluble emulsifier in alcohol, the dispersion of the alcohol solution in water, and the evaporation and total removal of the alcohol until a fine dispersion of the alcohol solution of the emulsifer in the aqueous phase is reached. The third, which is mainly used for amphotericin B incorporation into an emulsion, involves the preparation of a liposome-like dispersion. The drugs and phospholipids are first dissolved in methanol, dichloromethane, chloroform, or a combination of these organic solvents, and then filtered into a round-bottom flask. The drug-phospholipid complex is deposited into a thin film by evaporation of the organic solvent under reduced pressure. After sonication with the aqueous phase, a liposome-like dispersion is formed in the aqueous phase. The filtered oil phase and the aqueous phase are heated separately to 70°C and then combined by magnetic stirring.

2. The oil and aqueous phases are emulsified with a high-shear mixer at 70 to 80°C.
3. The resulting coarse emulsion (1–5μm) is then rapidly cooled and homogenized into a fine monodispersed emulsion.

Vesicles

Bangham [50] clearly shows that the dispersion of natural phospholipids in aqueous solutions leads to the formation of "closed vesicles structures," which morphologically resemble cells. Since 1975 [51], vesicles have been prepared from surfactants. In 1986, the first commercial product incorporating liposomes identical to those described by Bangham appeared on the market (Capture). At the same time, a synthetic one made by nonionic surfactants [52] was also launched (Niosomes). Several different compositions, for scientific, economic and business reasons, prevailed in cosmetic vesicles. None of them really resembles the liposomes we have seen in medical applications. These main groups include: (1) liposomes made from soya phospholipids; (2) sphingosomes, i.e., liposomes made from sphingolipids, and (3) nonionic surfactant vesicles (niosomes) which are a proprietary product of L'Óréal and other synthetic amphiphiles. In the 1990s, transfersomes, i.e., lipid vesicles containing large fractions of fatty acids, were introduced. Transfersomes [53–55] consist of a mixture of a lipidic agent with a surfactant. Consequently, their bilayers are much more elastic than those of most liposomes.

This chapter focuses on nonionic surfactant vesicles and transfersomes. Nonionic surfactant vesicles (NSVs or niosomes) consist of one or more nonionic surfactant bilayers enclosing an aqueous space. NSVs consisting of one bilayer are designed as small unila-

TABLE 4 Vesicles Preparation Methods

Method	Reference
Sonication	56, 58, 60
Ether injection	56
Handshaking	56
Reversed phase evaporation	61
Method as described by Handjani-Vila	52

mellar vesicles (SUVs) or large unilamellar vesicles (LUVs). Vesicles with more bilayers are called multilamellar vesicles.

Niosomes can be prepared from various classes of nonionic surfactants, e.g., polyglycerol alkyl ethers [52,56], glucosyl dialkyl ethers [57], crown ethers, and polyoxyethylene alkyl ethers and esters [58]. The preparation methods used should be chosen according to the use of niosomes, because the preparation methods influence the number of bilayers, size, size distribution, entrapment efficiency of the aqueous phase, and membrane permeability of the vesicles [56,59]. NSVs can be formed using the same methods that are used for the preparation of liposomes (Table 4).

PROPERTIES OF A VECTOR

Microparticles

Microencapsulation has been applied to solve problems in the development of pharmaceutical dosage forms as well as in cosmetics for several purposes. These include the conversion of liquids to solids, separation of incompatible components in dosage form, taste masking, reduction of gastrointestinal irritation, protection of the core materials against atmospheric deterioration, and enhancement of stability and controlled-release of active ingredients.

For drug follicular targeting, microspheres were envisaged mainly as site-specific drug delivery systems because they present several advantages: 1) good stability of the microspheres when applied on the skin, 2) easy preparation of microspheres with a defined size in a narrow size distribution, 3) protection of the active incorporated, 4) controlled release of the active in the hair follicles from the microspheres, and 5) the possibility of incorporating either lipophilic or hydrophilic actives into the microspheres [62]. Concerning the microsponge system, each microsphere is composed of thousands of small beads wrapped together to form a microscopic sphere capable of binding, suspending, or entrapping a range of substances. The outer surface is porous, allowing the controlled flow. Microsponges can be incorporated into gels, creams, liquids, powders, or other formulations, and can release ingredients depending on their temperature, moisture, friction, volatility of the entrapped ingredient, or time.

Nanoparticles

Nanoparticles are attractive delivery systems. In most cases the advantages are 1) the solid matrix gives flexibility to modify the drug release profile, 2) the relatively slow degradation allows long release times, and 3) the protection of incorporated compounds against chemical degradation. Drug release from colloidal carriers is dependent on both the type of carrier and the loading mechanisms involved.

Nanospheres

Release from nanospheres may be different according to the drug-entrapment mechanism involved. When the drug is superficially adsorbed, the release mechanism can be described as a partitioning process (rapid and total release if sink conditions are met). When the drug is entrapped within the matrix, diffusion plus bioerosion will be involved with a biodegradable carrier, whereas diffusion will be the only mechanism if the carrier is not biodegradable. From this, it can be inferred that entrapment within the matrix of nanospheres may lead to sustained release, the rate of which may be related to the rate of biodegradation of the polymer.

Nanocapsules

Release from nanocapsules is related to partitioning processes within immiscible phases. The equilibrium between the carrier (loaded drug) and the dispersing aqueous medium (free drug) is dependent both on the partition coefficient of the molecule between the oily and the aqueous phases and on the volume ratio of these two phases. This means that the amount released is directly related to the dilution of the carrier and that the release is practically instantaneous when sink conditions exist. Diffusion of the drug through the polymeric wall of nanocapsules does not seem to be a rate-limiting step [63]. Coating the polymeric wall with an outer layer of phospholipids can advantageously reduce drug leakage from nanocapsules.

Multiple Emulsions

Double emulsions are an excellent and exciting potential system for slow or controlled release of active entrapped compounds. The fact that the inner w/o emulsion serves as a large confined reservoir of water is a very attractive property for dissolving it in significant amounts of water-soluble drugs. The oil membrane seems to serve as good transport barrier for the confined ionized and/or nonionized water-soluble drugs. The two amphiphilic interfaces are yet an additional barrier. The possibility to manipulate transport and release characteristics of the formulations seems to be feasible. However, despite 20 years of research, no pharmaceutical preparation using the multiple emulsion technology exists in the marketplace. It seems that the main reasons are the droplet instability and the uncontrolled release.

Although the release of the encapsulated active substance is complicated, because of the existence of different mechanisms, the multiple emulsion's behavior after application to the skin appears to be relatively simple because it is similar to the behavior observed with simple emulsions.

Microemulsions

Miocroemulsions are effective vehicle systems for dermal as well as for transdermal drug delivery because of their high drug-loading capacity of their colloidal structure. Furthermore, thermodynamic stability and simple preparation process favor them to be considered as vehicles for skin applications.

Several workers have reported studies in which the lipophilicity of the drug has been increased to enhance its solubility in the dispersed oil droplets. In this way, a reservoir of the drug is produced and a sustained-release effect is achieved as the drug continuously transfers from the oil droplets to the continuous phase to replace drug release from the microemulsion.

Nanoemulsions

Nanoemulsions have been gaining more and more attention in the last few years, mainly as vehicles for the intravenous administration of lipophilic drugs. In the skin, the patents claimed that these systems could penetrate through the skin to a greater extent compared with usual topical compositions. Nanoemulsions are so strongly compressed that they become ultralight and, like vesicular systems constitute a new form that could prove extremely fruitful for the release of substances.

Vesicles

Vesicles appear to be promising transdermal drug-delivery systems. The major advantages of topical vesicle drug formulations are:

- hydrophilic, lipophilic, as well as amphiphilic substances can be encapsulated in the vesicles
- for the lipophilic and amphiphilic drugs the liposomes serve as "organic" solvent and as a result, higher local drug concentrations can be applied
- the vesicles can act as depot, releasing their drug content slowly and controlled
- systemic effect of a dermal active compound can be reduced and the systemic effect of a transdermal drug can be increased depending on the vesicle composition
- the vesicles may serve as penetration enhancer
- the vesicles can interact with the skin because of the amphiphilic character of the bilayer
- liposomes are biocompatible and biodegradable and have a low toxicity and lack antigenicity status as well
- vesicle formulations are cosmetically accepted

There are also some disadvantages of vesicles as drug carriers:

- low encapsulation efficiencies for lipophilic or amphiphilic drugs
- no drug release from the vesicle
- low–molecular weight drugs can leak out of the vesicle
- instability of vesicles during shelf life
- sterilization of liposome formulations

DERMATOLOGICAL AND COSMETIC USES OF ENCAPSULATION

Microparticles

In recent years, numerous vectors have been proposed and used in topical formulations as drug-carrier vehicles. It has been claimed that these drug vehicles can improve and control the drug release from conventional topical formulations. Although the application of these colloidal particles in dermatology is of great interest, there are few articles about the characteristics of these vehicles for topical formulations and most of the background is based on different patents.

Miocroparticles can serve as a drug reservoir in skin products. Rolland et al. [62] investigated in vitro and in vivo the role of 50:50 poly (DL-lactic-co-glycolic acid) microspheres as particulate carriers to improve the therapeutic index of adaptalene. The percutaneous penetration pathway of the microspheres was shown to be dependent on their mean diameter. Thus, after topical application onto hairless rat or human skin, adaptalene-loaded microspheres (5 μm diameter) were specifically targeted to the follicular ducts and did not penetrate via the stratum corneum. A reduction of either the applied dose (0.01%) or the frequency of administration (every day) was shown to give pharmacological results in the animal model comparable to a daily administration of 0.1% free adaptalene-containing aqueous gel.

Egg albumin microspheres of size 222 ± 25 µm, containing a vitamin A (15.7 ± 0.8%), were used to prepare o/w creams. The *in vitro* and *in vivo* drug release of a microencapsulated vitamin A cream was studied and compared with a nonmicroencapsulated vitamin A cream. The *in vitro* study showed that, during the first 3 hours, the microspheres could remain on the surface of the skin, and as a consequence, were able to prolong the release of vitamin A. The relative bioavailability of the microencapsulated formulation was 78.2 ± 7.3% [64].

Mizushima [65] reported that lipid microspheres containing prostaglandin E_1 (PGE_1), delivered preferentially to specific lesion sites, increased local action and prevented systemic side effects. Sakakibara et al. [66] evaluated the potential of topical application of lipid microspheres containing PGE_1 to treat ischemic ulcers. Nine of the 10 patients responded to the treatment, and at the sixth month of follow-up six patients had healed ulcers and recurrence was noted in three patients.

Skin absorption of benzoyl peroxide from a topical lotion containing freely dispersed drug was compared with that from the same lotion in which the drug was entrapped in a controlled-release styrene-divinylbenzene polymer system (Microsponge). The studies done by Wester et al. [67] showed the following: 1) *in vivo*, less benzoyl peroxide was absorbed through rhesus monkey skin from the polymeric system, 2) reduced skin irritation in cumulative irritancy studies on rabbits and human, and 3) when the experimental formulations were evaluated for antimicrobial activity in vivo, their efficiency was in line with that of conventional products.

A formulation containing 0.1% tretinoin was tested on 360 patients during 12 weeks for antiacne efficacy in a multicenter, double-blind, placebo-controlled study. Compared with placebo, statistically significant greater reductions in inflammatory, noninflammatory, and the total number of lesions were obtained with the entrapped retinoic acid formulation [68]. Encapsulation of deet in liposphere microdispersion resulted in improved efficacy and reduced dermal absorption. Deet-containing liposphere (10%) were effective against mosquitoes for at least 3.5 hours. The deet absorption through skin from these formulations was a third of that from alcoholic solution for the same concentration [69].

Nanoparticles

Although cosmetic applications of nanoparticles proliferate (numerous patents have been granted), publications, studies, or reports on the skin after topical application have been rare. The incorporation of active substances in the nanospheres attempt to modulate the release of the substances in the skin. When nanocapsules are concerned, the active substances are usually of lipophilic nature, and they can be composed of an oily compound or dispersion. Here again the objective is to control the release of the actives because the molecule is protected. The release profile of the actives depends on the nature of the constituents.

Recently, Lancôme launched a cosmetic product containing nanocapsules of vitamin E (Primordiale). They claim that the vitamin is widely distributed throughout the outer layers of the skin in the form of a gradient. The effectiveness of vitamin E protection when it is incorporated into nanoparticles has been shown in vivo. Dingler et al. [70] reported that the incorporation of vitamin E into solid lipid nanoparticles enhances the stability. The ultrafine particles possess an adhesive effect. This leads to a formation of fine adhesive film on the skin leading to occlusion and subsequent hydration. Hydration of the skin promotes penetration of actives and enhances their cosmetic efficiency. In another publication of the same research group [71], drug release of encapsulated material as well as nonencapsulated material was measured by tape stripping assay. The drug (RMAD 95) was released into the skin at approximately 53%, whereas the control (RMAD 95/isopropanol) was at 31%.

Immobilization of nanoparticles (polyamide) on the skin for prolonged periods of time has been proved feasible [72]. It has been shown to be dependent on formulation because particle retention was increased from 40% up to 98% when embedding the particles into a emulsion. Particle size, surface charge, and payload determine the properties of the nanoparticles and their application. Zülli et al. [73] encapsulated Uvinil T 150 (UV-B filter) into lipid nanoparticles. They observed an almost one-hundredfold higher affinity of Uvinil T to hair from positively charged particles compared with negatively charged particles. The same group also showed the application of a gel containing nanoparticles loaded with vitamin A and E derivatives enhances the skin humidity compared with controls.

In a 1997 patent, De Vringer [74] showed that the size of particles can change the occlusion factor. Lipoid microparticles are greatly inferior to solid lipoid nanoparticles in their occlusive effect, and the addition of solid lipoid microparticles in a cream lowers the cream's occlusivity, whereas the addition of solid lipoid nanoparticles in a cream raises the cream's occlusivity. Nanospheres containing beta carotene and a blend of UV-A and UV-B sun filters were prepared by Olivier-Terras [75]. The results clearly show the synergistic effect resulting from the combination of nanospheres and filters. They obtained with this formulation better bioavailability, better efficacy, and lastly a synergy that possesses an inhibitory effect on tyrosinase as a result of the cinnamic nature of the UV-B screening agents.

The effect of poly (methylmethacrylate) and poly (butylcyanoacrylate) nanoparticles on the permeation of methanol and octanol through hairless mouse skin was reported by Cappel and Kreuter [76]. Nanoparticles increase the permeability of methanol through hairless mouse skin and the permeability of lipophilic octanol is either unaffected by nanoparticles or decreases as a function of nanoparticle concentration depending on the lipophilicity of the polymer material. The potential use of nanoparticles as an ophthalmic drug-delivery system has been shown in numerous studies for either hydrophobic or hydrophilic drugs [77–79]. Despite the promising in vivo results, many issues must be resolved before an ophthalmic product can be developed using this technology.

Tobio et al. [80] encapsulated a model protein antigen, tetanus toxoid, into PLA-PEG nanoparticles and evaluated the potential of these colloidal carriers for the transport of proteins through the nasal mucous. The results showed that PLA-PEG nanoparticles have a great potential for delivery of proteins, either to the lymphatic system or to the blood circulation, after nasal administration. Regarding the mode of action of nanoparticles, one might hypothesize that they are associated with the skin surface, facilitating drug transport by changing the vehicle/stratum corneum partition coefficient.

Multiple Emulsions

The first commercial use of a w/o/w type multiple emulsion is Unique Moisturizing by Lancaster, which was marketed in 1991. Cosmetic application of multiple emulsions have been reported in the patents issued for their composition. One example of an application is perfume encapsulated in the internal phase; very small amounts of it are released over a long period of time. The patents show that multiple emulsions are recommended for all kinds of cosmetic applications: sunscreens, makeup removers, cleansers, and nutritive, hydrating, and cooling products. Kamperman and Sallis [81] show that a highly charged small water-soluble molecule such as phosphocitrate can be presented in the form of a liposome or multiple emulsion and be capable of exerting a positive action against dystrophic calcification. In a rat calcergy model, both vehicles effectively reduced the formation of induced subcutaneous calcified plaques at doses for which the phosphocitrate salt alone was inactive. Three emulsions type (w/o/w, o/w, and w/o) containing a water-soluble molecule (glucose) were obtained with the same formula [82,83]. The release of glucose from the o/w emulsion was the fastest, and the w/o emulsion was the slowest, whereas the release obtained from the w/o/w emulsion was intermediate. The w/o/w emulsion showed some tendency toward steady state during the first 3 to 12 hours and the flux was found to be 1.7 times greater than that from the w/o emulsion.

In vivo release of 2.5% lidocaine hydrochloride from simple and multiple emulsion systems was compared with that from aqueous and micellar solution, and anesthetic effects such as duration of action and tolerability were also compared. The double emulsions showed a longer duration of action, less eye irritation, and improved efficacy compared with aqueous solutions [44].

Microemulsions

Over the last 15 years, many studies have been performed with the percutaneous absorption of various actives carried by microemulsions. There are numerous cosmetic products in the form of microemulsions. These products range from body care to facial and hair treatments. They include bath oils, body-thinning products, fixatives for hair, hardeners for nails, hydrating products, antiwrinkle products, seborrhea preventive products, and antiaging serums marketed principally in Europe, the United States, and Japan. In biopharmaceutics, microemulsions were used to solubilize drugs and to improve systemic and topical drug availability.

Gasco et al. [84] ascertained concentrations of timolol in aqueous humor after multiple instillation in rabbit eyes. The microemulsion, a solution of the ion-pair, and a solution of timolol alone was used. The bioavailability of timolol from the microemulsion and the ion-pair solution was higher than that obtained from timolol alone. Transport of glucose across human cadaver skin was shown [85] using microemulsions containing up to 68% water. A thirtyfold enhancement of the glucose transport was achieved. The enhancing effect for drugs contained in microemulsions in comparison to a cream gel formulation consisting of the same components was shown by Ziegnmeyer and Führer [86]. The in vitro permeation across skin membranes as well as the in vivo penetration of tetracycline hydrochloride was higher from a microemulsion than from conventional systems. Thus is can be shown that in addition to the composition, the structure of each of the typically applied vehicles may play a dominant role in the process of penetration.

Février [87] has reported in vitro experiments designed to simulate the percutaneous penetration of tyrosine when administered using an o/w microemulsion composed of a betaine derivative as surfactant, benzyl alcohol, hexadecane, and water. The release of radiolabeled tyrosine from this vehicle was compared with that from a liquid-crystal system and an emulsion using a diffusion cell equipped with rat skin. Both the microemulsion and liquid-crystal formulation enhanced the penetration of tyrosine through the epidermis when compared with the emulsion. However, cutaneous irritation studies showed a strongly irritant effect from the liquid-crystal formulation but none from the microemulsion.

The penetration of the hydrophilic diphenhydramine hydrochloride from a w/o microemulsion into human skin under ex vivo conditions was studied by Schmalfuß et al. [88]. Modifications of the vehicle components clarified the extent to which it is possible to control the penetration of a hydrophilic drug incorporated in a microemulsion system. A standard microemulsion showed an accumulation of penetrated drug in the dermis, indicating a potential after high absorption rate. Incorporation of cholesterol into the system leads to an even higher penetration rate and a shifting of the concentration profile further towards the epidermis. The addition of oleic acid had no effect.

Wallin et al. [89] showed that high concentrations of lidocaine base included in a microemulsion produced peripheral nerve block of long duration, compared with solutions as a consequence of slow release of lidocaine. The effect of polysorbate 80 concentration on the permeation of propanolol incorporated into micelles of polysorbate 80 in water, o/w microemulsions of isopropyl myristate-polysorbate 80-sorbitol water, and o/w emulsions of isopropyl myristate-polysorbate 80-sorbitan monooleate-water has been investigated by use of an artificial double-layer membrane, composed of a barrier foil and a lipid barrier, in Franz-type diffusion cells [90]. For each system, the apparent permeability coefficient of propanolol decreased with increasing polysorbate 80 concentration. Moreover, for a given polysorbate 80 concentration, the apparent permeability coefficient of propanolol increased when the system was changed from emulsion to a microemulsion and then to a solubilized system because of the increasing interfacial area of total disperse phase.

Microemulsions may exert irritative effects, often by their high content of surfactants. It is possible to overcome this problem by the use of physiologically compatible nonionic and polymeric surfactants. The irritation potential of the formulation depends strongly on its structure. Because of an equilibrium between microemulsions and liquid crystals, when brought into contact microemulsions may dissolve skin structures that are organized in liquid crystalline form. Thus, an irritation is produced. Deduced from this, the nature of the system formed during the penetration process and the residue remaining on the skin surface are of importance in this regard.

Acute and cumulative tests were performed on human subjects in vivo with lecithin microemulsion gels using as comparison a unilamellar soybean lecithin liposome preparation and the solvent isopropyl palmitate [91]. The study showed a very low acute and a low cumulative irritancy potential for the soybean lecithin microemulsion gel. In general, microemulsions undergo structural changes after an application to the skin because of the penetration and/or evaporation of constituents and under occlusion by the uptake of water from the skin surface. The formed substances and their penetration behavior finally influences the effectiveness of the systems for dermal drug transport.

Nanoemulsions

Many formulations of nanoemulsion are available in patents. Recently, Lancôme launched a nanoemulsion rich in ceramides, Re-source. The scientific studies, however, are orientated mainly in the parenteral use of these formulations. Amselem and Friedman [92] indicated that the actives incorporated in submicron emulsions (diameter between 100–300 nm) can penetrate through the skin to a greater extent compared with the usual topical compositions. Improved efficacy of different steroidal and nonsteroidal anti-inflammatory drugs and local anesthetics has been observed.

Anselem and Zwoznik [93] determined drug penetration through the skin, local tissue (muscle and joint), and plasma levels of ketoprofen and diclofenac after topical administration in submicron emulsion (SME) creams compared with peroral administration. Compared with peroral drugs, SME-diclofenac and SME-ketoprofen showed sixty- to eightyfold more drug in muscle tissue, about ninefold more drug in joints, and four- to sixfold less drug in plasma. The improved skin penetrative properties of the solvent-free SME delivery makes this topical carrier very promising to achieve increased transcutaneous penetration of lipophilic drugs and site specificity.

Diazepam was formulated in various regular topical creams and SMEs of different composition [94]. The different formulations were applied topically on mice. The efficacy of diazepam applied topically in emulsions strongly depends on the oil droplet size and, to a lesser degree, on the formulation and oil type. The SMEs as vehicles for transdermal delivery of diazepam generate significant systemic activity of the drug as compared with regular creams or ointments. Transdermal delivery of diazepam via SME is effective, and the activity may reach the range of parenteral delivery. A single application of diazepam in SME cream to mice skin provides pronounced transdermal drug delivery and prolonged protective activity up to 6 hours.

Using a nanoemulsion composed of lanolin, polyethylene glycol ether of lanolin's alcohol and water [95], the investigators showed the transdermal delivery of a number of pharmaceutically active ingredients (testosterone, ibuprofen, 5-fluorouracil, verapamil hydrochloride, metronidazole, vincristine sulphate, fentanyl citrate) across isolated stratum corneum. The studies indicated that nanoemulsions derived from lanolin and its derivatives are capable of being developed into useful drug-delivery systems.

Vesicles

The effectiveness of vesicles has been investigated by several research groups (Table 5). Liposomes in particular have received considerable attention [103]. In several studies the diffusion of a drug was facilitated or achieved certain selectivity into human and nonhuman skin by vesicle encapsulation. Other studies show that the influence of vesicles on drug transport is negligible. The conflicting results can be understood in terms of vesicle characteristics or in terms of protocol of investigation. Special surface characteristics of vesicle hydration and electrostatic forces, in addition to Van der Waals, can govern the short and long range of repulsive or attractive forces between vesicles and biological media.

The particle sizes, the physical state (liquid or gel) of the bilayers, the number of bilayers, the electrostatic nature of drugs and vesicles, and the stability of the vesicles face to face with biofluids in different ranges of pHs, temperatures, and degrees of dehydration can also play an important role in the phenomenon. An important contribution to the understanding of the interactions between vesicles and human skin was made by Junginger and his group [100,104]. They used freeze fracture electron microscopy and small-angle radiograph scattering to study the effects that vesicle formulations have on the stratum corneum. They identified two types of liposome-skin interactions: 1) adsorption and fusion of loaded vesicles on the surface of the skin leading to increased thermodynamic activity and enhanced penetration of lipophilic drugs, and 2) interaction of the vesicles within the deeper layers of the stratum corneum promoting impaired barrier function of

TABLE 5 Effect of Vesicles on the Permeation of Drugs Through the Skin

Reference	Year	Drug	Type of vesicle	Results
96	1995	Retinyl palmitate	NSV	Augmentation of the retention of hydrophobic substances in stratum corneum
97	1998	Gap junction	Transferosomes	Protein transported across the intact murine skin and processed immunologically
98	1998	Estradiol	Transferosomes	Augmentation of the flux in 8-fold
99	1998	Cu, Zn-superoxide dismutase	Transferosomes	Reduced local inflammation
55	1998	Insulin	Transferosomes	Transported into the body between the intact skin with a bioefficiency of at least 50% of subcutaneous penetration-enhancing effect
100	1994	Estradiol	NSV	
101	1996	Lidocaine	NSV	The flux was not influenced by the encapsulation
102	1998	Levonorgestrel	Niosomes	Penetration-enhancing effect

these strata for the drug. Recent approaches in modulating delivery through the skin are the design of two novel vesicular carriers: the ethosomes and the transferosomes. The ethosomes are soft phospholipid vesicles; their size can be modulated from tens of nanometers to microns. These vesicular systems have been found to be very efficient for enhanced delivery of molecules with different physical-chemical characteristics to/through the skin. They can be modulated to permit enhancement into the skin strata as far as the deep dermis or to facilitate transdermal delivery of lipophilic and hydrophilic molecules [105].

Transferosomes have been shown to be versatile carriers for the local and systemic delivery of various steroids, proteins and hydrophilic macromolecules [106]. The mechanism proposed by the investigator for transferosomes is that they are highly deformable, thus facilitating their rapid pentration through the intercellular lipids of the stratum corneum. The osmotic gradient, caused by the difference in water concentrations between the skin surface and skin interior, has been proposed as the major driving force for transferosome penetration [54].

THE FUTURE OF ENCAPSULATION

What can we expect from encapsulation in the future? Trying to predict what the future will be is not easy. When one addresses future developments in the field of encapsulation, one has to realize that, at present time, application-oriented research is mainly focused to solve problems. If the number of published articles on encapsulation (liposomes, nanoparticles, microparticles, microemulsions, multiple emulsions, and nanoemulsions) under the heading of drug therapy is a reliable indicator of the state of knowledge, then the field has made progress over the last two decades. Between 1975 and 1980, the Medline Data

Base registered about 20 articles per year with the term "liposomes" in their title in the domain of drug therapy. This number has grown to over 100 per year. Because many of these publications dealt directly with new experimental data, we must conclude that our experience has expanded dramatically.

The skin has been "in the picture" since Mezei and his collaborators reported around 1980 on their early work on the liposomal delivery of drugs. Through the efforts of the cosmetic industry, liposomal formulations and nanoparticle formulations on the skin have definitively been an economic success. However, many unanswered questions remain. Molecular biology has provided us with tools to identify and build genetic materials that can be used for the treatment of hereditary diseases. Developing a carrier for gene therapy is one of the main challenges that the encapsulation field faces today. With respect to gene therapy for the skin, both molecular biology and encapsulation technology are in their debut, and much progress may and should be made in the coming years.

Again, what will the future bring us? We have already indicated where, on the basis of our present knowledge, encapsulation in many vectors offer a rational advantage as active carrier systems to the skin. Therefore, efforts should be made to obtain a better understanding concerning the mechanisms of formulations of these systems at the molecular and supramolecular level. This could lead to new formulation processes and could open new prospects in the area of active delivery by means of encapsulated systems. The field will develop in a more useful fashion when appropriate well-controlled biological and percutaneous penetration studies accompany the advances in chemistry.

REFERENCES

1. Kreuter J. Evaluation of nanoparticles as drug-delivery systems. I. Preparation methods. Pharm Acta Helv 1983; 58:196–201.
2. Won R. U.S. Patent 4,690,825. 1987.
3. Bakan J. Microencapsulation using coacervation/phase separation techniques. In: Controlled Release Technologies: Methods, Theory and Applications, Vol. 2. Boca Raton: CRC press, 1980:83–105.
4. Deasy P. Microencapsulation and Related Drug Processes. New York: Marcel Dekker, 1984.
5. Chang TMS. Artificial Kidney, Artificial Liver and Artificial Cells. New York: Plenum Press, 1978.
6. Thies C. A survey of microencapsulation processes. In: Benita S, ed. Microencapsulation, Methods and Industrial Applications. New York: Marcel Dekker, 1996:1–9.
7. Lim F, Moss RD. Microencapsulation of living cells and tissues. J Pharm Sci 1981; 70:351–356.
8. Matsumoto S, Kabayashi H, Takashima Y. Production of monodispersed capsules. J Microencaps 1986; 3:25–31.
9. Finch CA. Ullman's Encyclopedia of Industrial Chemistry. Vol. A 16. 5th ed. New York: VCH Publishers, 1990:575–588.
10. Kondo A. Microcapsule Processing and Technology. New York: Marcel Dekker, 1979.
11. Jacobs IC, Mason NS: Polymeric delivery systems. In: Elnolkaly MA, Piatt DM, Charpentier BA, eds. ACS Symposium Series 520. Washington, D.C.: American Chemical Society, 1993:1–17.
12. Kreuter J. Nanoparticles—preparation and applications. In: Donbrow M, ed. Microcapsules and Nanoparticles in Medicine and Pharmacy. Boca Raton: CRC Press, 1992:125–148.
13. Couvreur P, Kante B, Rolland M. Polycyanoacrylate nanocapsules as potential lysosomotric carriers: preparation morphological and sorptive properties. J Pharm Pharmacol 1979; 31:331–338.

14. Al Khoury FN, Roblot-/Treupel L, Fessi H. Development of new process for the manufacture of poly-isobutylcyanoacrylate nanocapsules. Int J Pharm 1986; 28:125–132.
15. Rollot JM, Couvreur P, Roblot-Treupel L, Puisieux F. Physicochemical and morphological characterization of polyisobutyl cyanoacrylate nanocapsules. J Pharm Sci 1986; 75(4):361.
16. Aleony D, Wittcoff H. U.S. Patent 2, 899, 397, 1959.
17. Cooper W. U.S. Patent 3, 009, 891, 1961.
18. Judd P. Brit. Patent 1, 142, 375, 1969.
19. Gurny R, Peppas NA, Harrington DD, Banker GS. Development of biodegradable lactices for controlled release of potent drugs. Drug Dev Ind Pharm 1981; 7:1–12.
20. Rhone-Poulenc Rorer. Fr Patent 2, 660, 556, 1990.
21. Kramer PA. Albumin microspheres as vehicles for achieving specificity in drug delivery. J Pharm Sci 1974; 63:1646–1652.
22. Fessi H, Devissaguet JP, Puisieux F, Thies C. Fr Patent 8, 618, 446, 1986.
23. Marty JJ, Oppenheim RC, Speiser PP. Nanoparticles—a new colloidal drug delivery system. Pharm Acta Helv 1978; 53:17–24.
24. Stainmesse S, Fessi H, Devissaguet JP, Puisieux F. 1st add to Fr Patent 8, 618, 446, 1988.
25. De Vringer T, de Ronde HAG. Preparation and structure of a water-in-oil cream containing lipid nanoparticles. J Pharm Sci 1995; 84(4):466–472.
26. Kim SY, Lee YM, Lee SI. Preparation and evaluation of in vitro stability of lipid nanospheres containing vitamin A and vitamin E for cosmetic application. Proc Intl Symp Cont Rel Bioact Mater 24. 1997:483–484.
27. Müller RH. Particulate systems for the controlled delivery of active compounds in pharmaceutics and cosmetics. In: Diederichs JE, Müller RH, eds. Future strategies for drug delivery with particulate systems. Stuttgart: CRC Press, 1998:73–90.
28. Müller RH, Mehnert W, Dingler A, Runge SA, zur Mühlen A, Freitas C. Solid lipid nanoparticles (SLN™, Lipopearls™). Proc Intl Symp Cont Rel Bioact Mater 24, 1997; 923–924.
29. Couvreur P, Coarraze G, Devissaguet JP, Puisieux F. Nanoparticles: preparation and characterization. In: Benita S, ed. Microencapsulation, Methods and Industrial Applications. New York: Marcel Dekker, 1996:183–211.
30. Matsumoto S, Kita Y, Yonezava D. An attempt at preparing water-in-oil-in-water multiple phase emulsion. J Colloid Interf Sci 1976; 57:353–361.
31. Matsumoto S, Sherman P. A preliminary study of w/o/w emulsions with a view to possible food applications. J Texture Studies 1981; 12:243–257.
32. Matsumoto S. Development of w/o/w type dispersion during phase inversion of concentrated w/o emulsions. J Colloid Interf Sci 1983; 94:362–368.
33. Kavaliunas DR, Franck SG. Liquid crystal stabilization of multiple emulsion. J Colloid Interf Sci 1978; 66:586–588.
34. Magdassi S, Frenkel M, Garti N. On the factors affecting the yield of preparation and stability of multiple emulsions. J Dispersion Sci Technol 1984; 5:49–59.
35. De Luca M. Les emulsions multiples H/L/H. Obtention, validation, et liberation. Thèse de l'Université de Paris XI, Paris, 1991.
36. Florence AT, Whitehill D. Some features of breakdown in w/o/w multiple emulsions. J Colloid Interf Sci 1981; 79:243–256.
37. Florence AT, Whitehill D. The formulation and stability of multiple emulsions. Int J Pharm 1982; 11:277–308.
38. Florence AT, Whitehill D. Stability and stabilization of w/o/w multiple emulsions. In: Shah DO, ed. Macro and micro emulsions, theory and applications. Washington, D.C.: American Chemical Society, 1985:359–380.
39. Matsumoto S, Inoue T, Khoda M, Ikurak K. Water permeability of oil layers in w/o/w emulsion under osmotic pressure gradients. J Colloid Interf Sci 1980; 77:555–563.
40. Matsumoto S, Koh J, Michura A. Preparation of w/o/w emulsions in edible form on the basis of phase inversion technique. J Dispos Sci Technol 1985; 6:507–521.

41. Frenkel M, Schwartz R, Garti N. Multiple emulsions. I. Stability inversion, apparent and weighed HLB. J. Colloid Interf Sci 1983; 94:174–178.

42. Csóka I, Erõs I. Stability of multiple emulsions. I. Determination of factors influencing multiple drop breakdown. Int J Pharm 1997; 156:119–123.

43. Opawale FO, Burgess DJ. Influence of interfacial rheological properties of mixed emulsifier films on the stability of w/o/w emulsions. J Pharm Pharmacol 1998; 50:965–973.

44. Garti N, Aserin A. Pharmaceutical emulsions, double emulsions and microemulsions. In: Benita S, ed. Microencapsulation, Methods and Industrial Applications. New York: Marcel Dekker, 1996:412–534.

45. Yu W, Tabosa do Egito ES, Barrat G, Fessi H, Devissaguet JP, Puisieux F. A novel approach to the preparation of injectable emulsions by a spontaneous emulsification process. Int J Pharm 1993; 89:139–146.

46. Hansrani PK, Davis SS, Groves MJ. The preparation and properties of sterile intravenous emulsions. J Parenter Sci Technol 1983; 37:145–150.

47. Yalabik-Kas HS, Erylmaz S, Hincal AA. Formation, stability and toxicity studies of intravenous fat emulsions. STP Pharm 1985; 1:12–19.

48. Washington C, Davis SS. The production of parenteral feeding emulsions by microfluidizer. Int J Pharm 1988; 169–176.

49. Lidgate DM, Fu RC, Fleitman JS. Using a microfluidizer to manufacture parenteral emulsions. Pharm Technol 1990; 14:30–33.

50. Bangham AD, Standish MM, Watkins JC. Diffusion of univalent ions across the lamellae of swollen phospholipids. J Mol Biol 1965; 13:238–252.

51. Gebicki JM, Hicks M. Preparation and properties of vesicle enclosed by fatty acid membranes. Chem Phys Lipids 1975; 16:142–160.

52. Handjani-Vila RM, Ribier A, Rondot B, Valenberghe G. Dispersions of lamellar phases of non-ionic lipids in cosmetic products. Int J Cosmet Sci 1979; 1:303–314.

53. Planas ME, Gonzalez P, Rodriguez L. Non invasive percutaneous induction of topical analgesia by a new type of drug carriers and prolongation of the local pain-insensitivity by analgesic liposomes. Anesth Analg 1992; 95:614–621.

54. Cevc G, Glume G. Lipid vesicles penetrate into the skin owing to the transdermal osmotic gradients and hydration force. Bioch Biophys Acta 1992; 1104:226–232.

55. Cerc G, Gebauer D, Stieber J, Schätzlein A, Blume G. Ultraflexible vesicles, transfersomes, have an extremely low pore penetration resistance and transport therapeutic amounts of insulin across the intact mammalian skin. Bioch Biophys Acta 1998; 1368:201–215.

56. Baillie AJ, Florence AT, Hume LR, Muirhead GT, Rogerson A. The preparation and properties of niosome non-ionic surfactant vesicles. J Pharm Pharmacol 1985; 37:863–868.

57. Van Hal DA, Bowstra JA, Junginger HE. Preparation and characterization of new dermal dosage form for antipsoriatic drug, dithranol, based on non ionic surfactant vesicles. Eur J Pharm Biopharm 1992; 38:47.

58. Hofland HEJ, Bowstra JA, Ponec M, Boddé HE, Spies F, Verhoef JC, Junginger HE. Interactions of non-ionic surfactant vesicles with cultured keratinocytes and human skin in vitro. J Control Rel 1991; 16:155–168.

59. Hofland HEJ, Bowstra JA, Verhoef JC, Buckton G, Chowdry BZ, Ponec M, Junginger HE. Safety aspects of non-ionic surfactant vesicles. A toxicity study related to the physiochemical characteristics of non ionic surfactants. J Pharmacol 1992; 44:287–294.

60. Carafa M, Al Haique F, Coviello T, Murtas E, Riccieri FM, Lucania G, Torrisi MR. Preparation and properties of new unilamellar non-ionic/ ionic surfactant vesicles. Int J Pharm 1998; 160:51–59.

61. Kiwada H, Nimura H, Fujisali Y, Yamada S, Kato Y. Application of synthetic alkyl glycoside vesicles as drug carriers. (1) Preparation and physical properties. Chem Pharm Bull 1985; 33:753–759.

62. Rolland A, Wagner N, Chatelus A, Shroot B, Schaefer H. Site-specific drug delivery to

pilosebaceous structures using polymeric microspheres. Pharm Res 1993; 10(12):1738–1744.

63. Ammoury N, Dubrasquet M, Fessi H. Indomethacin-loaded poly (d,l-lactide) nanocapsules: protection from gastrointestinal ulcerations and anti-inflammatory activity evaluation in rats. Clin Mat 1993; 13:121–127.

64. Torrado S, Torrado JJ, Cadorniga R. Topical application of albumin microspheres containing vitamin A. Drug release and availability. Int J Pharm 1992;86: 147–152.

65. Mizushima Y. Lipid microspheres as novel drug carriers. Drug Exp Clin Res 1985; 11:595–600.

66. Sakakibara Y, Jikuya T, Mitsui T. Application of lipid microspheres containing prostaglandin E1 ointment to peripheral ischemic ulcers. Dermatology 1997; 195:252–257.

67. Wester RC, Rajesh P, Nacht S, Leyden J, Melendres J, Maibach HI. Controlled release of benzoyl peroxide from a porous microsphere polymeric system can reduce topical irritancy. J Am Acad Dermat 1991; 24(5):720–726.

68. Embil K, Natch S. The Microsponge® delivery system (MDS): a topical delivery system with reduced irritancy incorporating multiple triggering mechanisms for the release of actives. J Microencaps 1996; 13(5):575–588.

69. Domb AJ, Marlinsky A, Maniar M, Teomim L. Insect repellent formulations of n,n-diethyl-m-toluamide (deet) in a liposphere system: efficacy of skin uptake. J Am Mosquito Control Ass 1995; 11(1):29–34.

70. Dingler A, Hildebrand G, Niehus H, Müller RH. Cosmetic anti-aging formulation based on vitamin E–loaded solid lipid nanoparticles. Proc Intl Symp Cont Rel Bioact Mater 25. 1998:433–434.

71. Müller RH, Dingler A, Hildebrand G, Gohla S. Development of cosmetic products based on solid lipid nanoparticles (SLN). Proc Intl Symp Cont Rel Bioact Mater 25. 1998:238–239.

72. Deniau N, Ponchel G, Bonze F, Meybeck A, Duchene D. Immobilization of particulate systems on the skin by the mean of emulsions. Dru Dev Ind Pharm 1993; 19(13):1521–1540.

73. Zülli F, Suter F, Birman M. Cationic nanoparticles: a new system for the delivery of lipophilic UV-filters to hair. Drug Cosmet Ind 1996; 4:46–48.

74. De Vringer T. U.S. Patent 5, 667, 800, 1997.

75. Olivier-Terras J. U.S Patent 5, 554, 374, 1996.

76. Cappel MJ, Kreuter J. Effect of nanoparticles on transdermal drug delivery. J Microencaps 1991; 8(3):369–374.

77. Calvo P, Vila-Jato JL, Alonso MJ. Comparative in vitro evaluation of several colloidal systems, nanoparticles, nanocapsules, and nanoemulsions, as ocular drug carriers. J Pharm Sci 1996; 85(5):530–536.

78. Calvo P, Alonso MJ, Vila-Jato JL, Robinson JR. Improved ocular bioavailability of indomethacin by novel ocular drug carriers. J Pharm Pharmacol 1996; 48:1147–1152.

79. Heussler LM, Sirbart D, Hoffman M. Maincent P. Poly (ε- caprolactone) nanocapsules in carteolol ophthalmic delivery. Pharm Res 1993; 10(3):386–390.

80. Tobio M, Greef R, Sánchez A, Langer R, Alonso MJ. Stealth PLA-PEG nanoparticles as protein carriers for nasal administration. Pharm Res 1998; 15(2):270–275.

81. Kamperman H, Sallis JD. Liposome and multiple emulsion formulations augment the anticalcifying efficacy of phosphocitrate in a cutaneous calcergy model. J Pharm Pharmacol 1995; 47:802–807.

82. Ferreira LAM, Seiller M, Grossiord JL, Marty JP, Wepierre J. Vehicle influence on in vitro release of glucose: w/o, w/o/w and o/w systems compared. J Cont Rel 1995; 33:349–356.

83. Ferreira LAM, Doucet J, Seiller M, Grossiord JL, Marty JP, Wepierre J. In vitro percutaneous absorption of metronidazole and glucose: comparison of o/w, w/o/w and o/w systems. Int J Pharm 1995; 121: 169–179.

84. Gasco MR, Gallarate M, Trotta M, Bauchiero L, Gremmo E, Chiappero O. Microemulsions

as topical delivery vehicles: ocular administration of timolol. J Pharm Biom Anal 1989; 7(4): 433–434.

85. Osborne DW, Ward AJI, O'Neill KJ. Microemulsions as topical drug delivery vehicles: invitro transdermal studies of a hydrophilic model drug. J Pharm Pharmacol 1991; 43:451–455.

86. Ziegnmeyer J, Führer C. Mikroemulsionen als topishe arzneiform. Acta Pharm Technol 1980; 26(4):273–275.

87. Février F. Formulation de microemulsion cosmetiques. Nouv Dermatol 1991; 10:84–87.

88. Schmalfuß U, Neubert R, Wohlrab W. Modification of drug penetration into human skin using microemulsions. J Cont Rel 1997; 46:279–285.

89. Wallin R, Dyhre H, Björkman S, Fyge A, Engström S, Renck H. Prolongation of lidocaine induced regional anaesthesia by a slow release microemulsion formulation. Proc Intl Symp Cont Rel Bioact Mater 24. 1997:555–556.

90. Kristis G, Niopas I. A study on the in vitro percutaneous absorption of propanolol from dispersed systems. J Pharm Pharmacol 1998; 50:413–418.

91. Dreher F, Walde P, Luisi PL, Elsner P. Human skin irritation studies of a lecithin microemulsion gel and of lecithin liposomes. Skin Pharmacol 1996; 9:124–129.

92. Amselem S, Friedman D. U.S. Patent 5, 662, 932, 1997.

93. Amselem S, Zwoznik E. Enhanced skin penetration and site specificity of ketoprofen and diclorofenac formulated in submicron emulsion topical creams. Pharm Sci, 1998;(suppl):65.

94. Schwarz JS, Weisspapir MR, Friedman DL. Enhanced transdermal delivery of diazepam by submicrom emulsion (SME) creams. Pharm Res 1995; 12(5):687–692.

95. Flockart IR, Steel I, Kitchen G. Nanoemulsions derived from lanolin show promising drug delivery properties. J Pharm Pharmacol 1998; 50(suppl):141.

96. Guénin EP, Zatz J. Skin permeation of retinyl palmitate from vesicles. J Soc Cosmet Chem 1995; 46:261–270.

97. Paul A, Cevc G, Bachawat BK. Transdermal immunisation with an integral membrane component, gap junction protein, by means of ultradeformable drug carriers, transfersomes. Vaccine 1998; 16(2/3):188–195.

98. El Maghraby GMM, Williams AC, Barry BW. Optimization of deformable vesicles for epidermal delivery of oestradiol. J Pharmacol 1998; 50 (suppl):146.

99. Simões SI, Marins MBF, Cruz MEM, Cevc G. Anti-inflammatory effects of Cu, Zn-superoxide dismutase in liposomes, transfersomes or micelles in the acute murine ear edema model. Perspec Percutan Penetration 1997; 5b:50.

100. Hofland HEJ, Van der Geest R, Bodde HE, Junginger HE, Bowstra JA. Estradiol permeation from non-ionic surfactant vesicles through human stratum corneum in vitro. Pharm Res 1994; 11(5):659–664.

101. Van Hal DA, Jeremiasse E, de Vringer T, Junginger HE, Bowstra JA. Encapsulation of lidocaine base and hydrochloride into non-ionic surfactant vesicles (NSVs) and diffusion through stratum corneum in vitro. Eur J Pharm Sci 1996; 4:147–157.

102. Vora B, Khopade AJ, Jain NK. Proniosome based transdermal delivery of levanorgestrel for effective contraception. J Cont Rel 1998; 54:149–165.

103. Bowstra JA, Junginger HE. Non-ionic surfactant vesicles (niosomes) for oral and transdermal administration of drugs. In: Puisieux F, Couvreur P, Dellatre J, Devissaguet JP, eds. Lipsomes, New Systems and New Trends in Their Applications. 1995:101–121.

104. Hofland HEJ, Bowstra JA, Bodde HE, Spies F, Junginger HE. Interactions between liposomes and human stratum corneum in vitro: freeze fracture electron microscopic visualization and small angle x-ray scattering studies. Br J Dermatol 1995; 132:853–866.

105. Touitou E, Alkabes M, Dayan N, Eliaz N. Ethosomes: novel vesicular carriers for enhanced skin delivery. Pharm Res 1997; 14(11):(Suppl):305.

106. Cevc G. Material transport across permeability barriers by means of lipid vesicles. In: Powsky RL ed. Handbook of Physics of Biological Systems, vol. I, Elsevier Science. Ch. 9, 1995: 441–466.

16

Encapsulation Using Porous Microspheres

Jorge Heller, Subhash J. Saxena, and John Barr
Advanced Polymer Systems, Redwood City, California

INTRODUCTION

Encapsulation can be broadly defined as the formation of small, spherical particles that incorporate an active agent. The first commercial application of encapsulation was by the National Cash Register Company, who developed an improved copying paper using two dyes that were coated with a clay. When these capsules were ruptured by the application of pressure, a colored imprint was produced. This successful application triggered other uses in agriculture, pharmaceuticals, oil industries, food industries, and consumer products [1].

Because such spherical particles are very small, usually in the range of several to about 20 microns, the process of forming such particles is referred to as microencapsulation. However, we need to distinguish between microcapsules and microspheres. Microcapsules have a core containing the active agent surrounded by a membrane, whereas microspheres are solid particles that contain an active agent homogeneously dispersed within the solid matrix. Microspheres can be either solid or porous. These three types are shown schematically in Figure 1.

Release of agents incorporated into microcapsules can occur either abruptly, as in the National Cash Register Company product, or the ''scratch and sniff'' product manufactured by the 3M Company, where the outer membrane is ruptured by the application of pressure or can occur in a controlled manner by diffusion of the active agent from the core through the outer rate-limiting membrane. In the latter case, if the thermodynamic activity of the drug in the core reemains constant and the drug is removed rapidly from the aqueous environment surrounding the microcapsule, constant release kinetics, referred to as zero order, are obtained. No such products have been applied to the cosmetics and cosmeceutical field, but have been extensively investigated in controlled-release applications, particularly in contraception [2] and narcotic addiction [3].

Agents incorporated into microspheres are released by kinetics that are typical of matrix systems and follow $t^{1/2}$ kinetics as predicted by the Higuchi equation [4]. Thus, initial release rate is rapid and then declines as the thickness of the drug-depleted layer increases. Studies of release kinetics from biodegradable porous microspheres indicate that release kinetics similar to that noted for matrix-type microspheres are obtained [5].

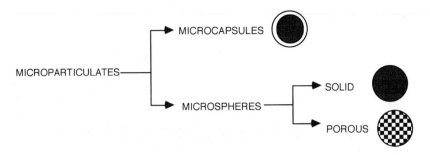

FIGURE 1 Schematic representation of various microparticulates.

Other than liposomes, which are covered in Chapter 17, only one type of micro-particulate has found important applications in cosmetics and skincare technology, and these are porous microspheres. This chapter will cover the application of porous micro-spheres in cosmetics and skincare applications.

POROUS MICROSPHERES

Preparation

A special kind of porous microsphere is a patented [6,7], highly cross-linked polymer sphere having a size that can vary from about 3 to 3000 microns. The porous spheres are produced by an aqueous suspension of polymerization of monomer pairs consisting of a vinyl and a divinyl monomer, e.g., methyl methacrylate (the vinyl monomer) and ethylene glycol dimethacrylate (the divinyl monomer), or styrene and divinylbenzene. The divinyl monomer functions as a cross-linker, and because it is used in concentrations as high as 50 to 60%, the copolymer is a very highly cross-linked material. As a consequence of their chemical structure and the high cross-link density, the micrpsheres are totally inert and do not degrade in the body, nor do they dissolve or swell, when exposed to any organic solvent. They have been found to be stable between pH 1 and 11 and at temperatures as high as 135°C.

To prepare the copolymer, the vinyl and divinyl monomers, initiator, suspending agent (emulsifier), and a porogen, which produces the porous structure, are dispersed in water and the copolymerization started by thermally activating the initiator. The porogen must be miscible with the monomers and function as a precipitant for the polymer. Polymer particle size is controlled by the size of the suspended monomer droplets, which in turn is a function of the nature and amount of the suspending agent and the shear induced by the stirring process. When all variables are carefully controlled, a uniform batch of parti-cles having the desired size and the desired porosity can be obtained. Typically, the surface area of such porous microspheres can be varied between 20 to 500 m^2/g and the pore volume can be varied from 0.1 to 3.4 cm^3/g.

A scanning electron micrograph of a porous microsphere magnified 5000 times is shown in Figure 2. A view of the interior, in this case magnified 6000 times and obtained by freeze fracture, is shown in Figure 3. As can be seen, the internal structure comprises small polymer particles enclosed in a porous membrane. The porosity of the microspheres

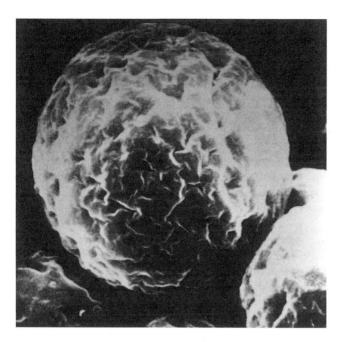

FIGURE 2 Electron scanning micrograph of porous microsphere. Magnification 5000×.

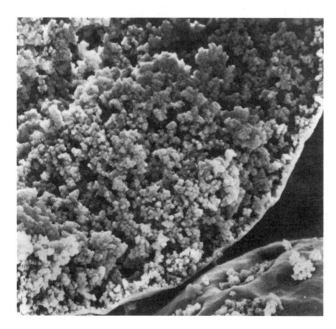

FIGURE 3 Freeze fracture micrograph of a single porous microsphere. Magnification 6000×.

is attributable to the interstitial volumes between the polymer particles, and because the membrane that surrounds the solid polymer particles is porous, the interstitial volume is open to the outside.

Loading of Active Agents

These can be incorporated by two different procedures. In one procedure, referred to as the one-step procedure, the active agent functions as the porogen and is incorporated during the polymerization process. However, this method has some limitations because the active agent has to satisfy the requirements of a porogen, it must be stable towards free radicals generated during the copolymerization process, and it must not inhibit the copolymerization process. For this reason, a procedure where porous microspheres are produced first, and subsequently loaded with the active agent, is more generally applicable. Such a process is known as the two-step procedure.

Loading is achieved by stirring empty porous microspheres in a solution of the active agent, which diffuses into the microsphere particles. The solvent is then evaporated to obtain microspheres with the active agent loaded within the pores. If the agent is soluble in the polymer, some may partition into the matrix. Should a high loading be desired, or if the active agent is only sparingly soluble in the solvent, the process can be repeated a number of times. Clearly, using such a procedure, some of the active agent will also be found on the outside of the microspheres particles.

The incorporation of an active agent into these microspheres can be investigated by environmental scanning electron microscopy (ESEM). This method has the advantage over conventional scanning electron microscopy (SEM) in that no metallic coating is required and samples can be analyzed at ambient pressures in a water vapor. Samples are sprinkled lightly onto a metallic stub, 1 cm in diameter, bearing conductive double-sided adhesive tape, and then analyzed using a Phillips XL30 ESEM FEG instrument operated with greater than 99% relative humidity [Davies, M., and Patel, N., private communication]. Using this procedure, a good visualization of the microspheres and any free drug, if present, can be achieved.

Such a visualization method is important because loading efficiency depends on the nature of the active agent, primarily its solubility and the partition coefficient between the microspheres and the solvent used in the entrapment procedure. Both lipophilic and hydrophilic materials can be loaded into such microspheres, and range from water to petrolatum to silicone oil. Extensive studies have shown that the active agent is not bound to the microspheres and can be completely extracted.

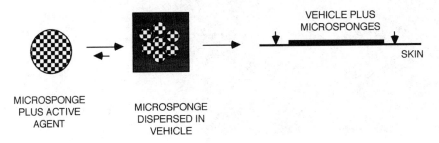

FIGURE 4 **Schematic representation of controlled release of active agent from porous microspheres dispersed in a vehicle.**

Release of Active Agents

Although porous microspheres can function in a limited way as a sustained-release delivery vehicle, they are best viewed as a reservoir. However, the combination of microspheres with incorporated active agents dispersed in a vehicle can function as a controlled-release device if a vehicle in which the drug is only poorly soluble is chosen. When such a formulation is applied to the skin, only that amount of the drug dissolved in the vehicle is presented to the skin. Then, as the drug diffuses from the vehicle into the skin, the saturation concentration of the drug in the vehicle is maintained by diffusion of drug from the microspheres into the vehicle. This process is shown schematically in Figure 4.

APPLICATIONS

Porous microspheres have been used in two major applications. One application takes advantage of the high porosity of the microspheres to entrap liquid materials, such as silicone oil, to convert a liquid into a free-flowing powder. This allows significant formulation flexibility, and a babywipe product has been developed where silicone in porous microspheres has been formulated in an aqueous medium.

In the other application, microspheres with incorporated active agents are dispersed in a suitable vehicle for topical applications. As already discussed, when active agents that are normally skin irritants are used and a vehicle in which the active agent is only poorly soluble is chosen, a significant reduction of irritation, when compared with ordinary formulation, is noted. Such a reduction in irritancy will be illustrated with two products, one incorporating benzoyl peroxide and the other incorporating *trans*-retinoic acid (RA).

Benzoyl Peroxide

Benzoyl peroxide (BPO) is clinically effective in acne, primarily because of its bactericidal activity against *Proprionibacterium acnes* and possibly also through its mild keratolytic effects [8–10]. The main site of pharmacological action is the pilosebaceous canal [11]. BPO penetrates through the follicular opening, probably by dissolving into sebaceous lipids, and then exerts its antimicrobial activity [12]. Skin irritation is a common side effect and a dose relation seems to exist between efficacy and irritation [13]. Thus, a controlled-release formulation would clearly be advantageous.

In vitro release kinetics were determined by applying formulations to silastic membranes mounted in static diffusion cells, and by using excised human skin. Release of BPO from two formualtions applied to a silastic membrane, one incorporating free BPO and one incorporating BPO entrapped in porous microspheres is shown in Figure 5. Initial release of BPO dispersed in the vehicle shows good linearity, but with further release would decline, as expected for $t^{1/2}$ kinetics. The calculated flux for the initial release is 0.09 mg/cm^2/h. The release of BPO entrapped in the porous microspheres shows a discontinuity. Initial flux is about 0.1 mg/cm^2/h, very close to the release from BPO dispersed in the vehicle, followed by a slower release with a flux of 0.04 mg/cm^2/h. These data indicate that not all BPO has been entrapped in the porous microspheres, and that the formulation contains some free BPO. Initial release is attributable to release of the free BPO, followed by the release of entrapped BPO.

The topical irritancy of a BPO controlled-release formulation has been determined in rabbits, in rhesus monkeys, and in human volunteers [14] using formulations with BPO dispersed in a vehicle and BPO entrapped in porous microspheres dispersed in a vehicle.

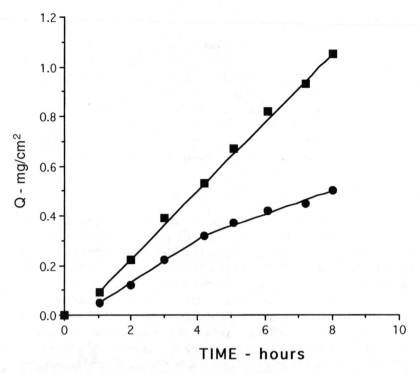

FIGURE 5   Release of BPO dispersed in vehicle (■) abd BPO entrapped in porous microspheres and dispersed in vehicle (●). Results are the average of two determinations. Formulations applied to silastic membrane. Receiving fluid 1:1 mixture of water and acetone. (From Ref. 14.)

Cumulative 14-day irritancy scores in human volunteers are shown in Figure 6 and Table 1. In this study involving 29 patients, total irritaancy of four commercial products, three containing free BPO and one containing entrapped BPO at the BPO concentrations shown, were compared. Clearly, the entrapped BPO product is significantly less irritating. A 12-week human trial, comparing the efficacy of entrapped BPO formulations at various concentrations, a placebo formulation and a free BPO formulation has also been carried out. The total reduction of inflammatory lesions shown in Figure 7 and the total reduction of noninflammatory lesions shown in Figure 8 clearly shows that the entrapped BPO is as efficacious as the free BPO. These results support evidence also obtained independently, that most, if not all, BPO entrapped in the porous microspheres is released.

Retinoic Acid

All *trans*-RA is a highly effective topical treatment for acne vulgaris. However, cutaneous irritation reduces patient compliance, and thus clinical effectiveness. A gel formulation with 0.1% RA entrapped in a porous microsphere has been developed and a single-center, double-blind, positive-controlled, randomized Phase I study carried out. The formulation with entrapped RA was designated as 0.1% TMG (tretinoin microsphere gel), and the one with free RA was designated 0.1% RA cream. Either study formulation was assigned to be applied to the right side of a subject's face on a randomized basis, the alternate formula-

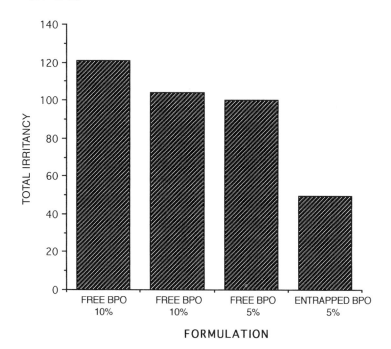

FIGURE 6 Fourteen-day cumulative irritancy test on BPO formulations in human volunteers comparing three commercial products containing BPO dispersed in a vehicle and one commercial formulation containing BPO entrapped in porous microspheres at BPO concentrations shown.

tion to the left side of the face. The dose for each formulation was 0.1 g, which was applied to the cheek areas once daily for up to 14 days. The subjects were evaluated daily by an expert grader for dryness and erythema. Results of subjects' self-assessment are shown in Table 2 and in Figure 9. Clearly, a formulation with RA entrapped in porous microspheres resulted in a statistically significant preference for the TMG formulation,

TABLE 1 14-day Cumulative Irritancy in Human Volunteers

Formulation	% Total subjects with postive response	Cumulative response index*
2.5% BPO		
Commercial product	36	1.04 (1)
Entrapped BPO	12	0.24 (2)
Vehicle	0	0.0 (3)
10% BPO		
Commercial product	52	2.59 (4)
Entrapped BPO	24	1.64 (5)
Vehicle	0	0.0 (6)

* Duncan's Multiple Range tests showed significant difference ($p < 0.05$) between (1) and (2), (1) and (3), (4) and (6), (5) and (6), but no significant difference ($p > 0.05$) between (2) and (3).
Source: Ref. 14.

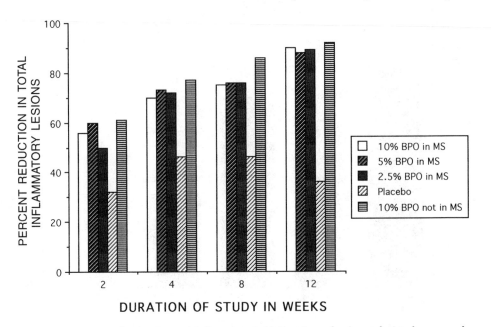

FIGURE 7   Percent reduction in total inflammatory lesions (papules/pustules) in human volunteers at 2, 4, 8, and 12 weeks, using the formulations shown.

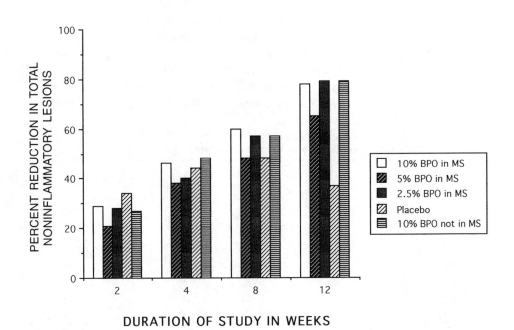

FIGURE 8   Percent reduction in total noninflammatory lesions (open and closed comedones) in human volunteers at 2, 4, 8, and 12 weeks, using the formulations shown.

TABLE 2 Subject Self-Assessment

	0.1% TMG*	0.1% RA cream	p Value
Number who prefer	23	2	
Preference score†	1.88	0.10	0.0002

* TMG is Retin-A® Micro Cream 0.1%.
† Preference score perceived as less burning and/or stinging graded on a scale from 0 (no difference) to 4 (maximal difference).

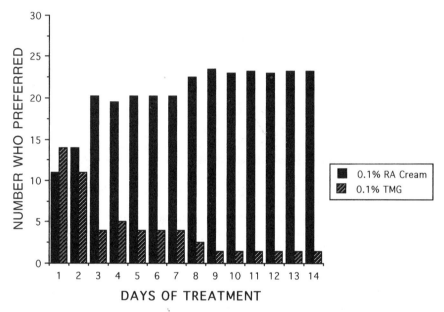

FIGURE 9 Daily self-assessment of preference for mildness. Single-center, double-blind, randomized, half-face study comprising 25 adult Caucasian women selected for having sensitive skin. 0.1% TMG is retinoic acid entrapped in porous microspheres and 0.1% RA cream in a commercial formulation. 0.1% TMG and 0.1% RA cream applied to corresponding side of subject's face, once a day for up to 14 days by a blinded technician.

which was perceived as causing less burning and stinging. In an independent, controlled multicenter trial, this TMG formulation has also proven effective for the treatment of acne and is now commercially available.

CONCLUSIONS

Porous microspheres are highly cross-linked and highly porous copolymers, which have found extensive use in the skincare arena. The nature of the polymer allows the loading of a wide range of chemical entities with subsequent release dependent on the vehicle into which the porous microspheres has been dispersed. This polymer has found widespread acceptance as a means of reducing irritation without decreasing efficacy when used appropriately.

REFERENCES

1. Luzzi, L. A. (1970). Microencapsulation. J. Pharm. Sci. 59:1367–1376.
2. Beck, L. R., and Tice, T. R. (1983). Poly(lactic) and poly(lactic acid-*co*-glycolic acid) contraceptive delivery systems. In Mishell, D. R. (ed.), Long-Acting Steroid Contraception. New York: Raven Press, 175–199.
3. Nuwayser, E. S., Gay, M. H., DeRoo, D. J., and Blaskovich, P. D. (1988). Sustained release injectable naltrexone microcapsules. Proc. Intern. Symp. Control Rel. Bioact. Mater. 15:201–202.
4. Higuchi, T. (1961). Rates of release of medicamenets from ointment bases containing drugs in suspension. J. Pharm. Sci. 50:874–875.
5. Sato, T., Kanke, M., Schroeder, H. G., and DeLuca, P. (1988). Porous biodegradable microspheres for controlled drug delivery. I. Assesssssment of processing conditions and solvent removal techniques. Pharm. Res. 5:21–30.
6. Won, R. Method for delivering an active ingredient by controlled time release utilizing a novel delivery vehicle which can be prepared by process utilizing the active ingredient as a porogen. U.S. Patent 4,690,825. September 1, 1987.
7. Won, R. Two step method for preparation of controlled release formulations. U.S. Patent 5,145,675, September 8, 1992.
8. Nacht, S. (1983). Comparative activity of benzoyl peroxide and hexachlorophene. In vivo studies against *Proprionibacterium acnes* in humans. Arch. Dermatol. 119:577–579.
9. Fulton, J. E., and Bradley, S. (1976). The choice of vitamin A, erythromycin and benzoyl peroxide for the topical treatment of acne. Cutis 17:560–564.
10. Kligman, A. M., Leyden, J. J., and Stewart, R. (1977). New uses of benzoyl peroxide: a broad spectrum antimicrobial agent. Int. J. Dermatol. 16:413–417.
11. Nacht, S. (1981). Methods to assess the transepidermal and intrafollicular penetration of anti-acne agents. In: Proceedings of the 1980 Research and Scientific Development Conference, New York, pp. 88–91.
12. Leyden, J. J. Topical antibiotics and topical antimcrobial agents in acne therapy. In: Julin, L. A., Rossman, H., and Strauss, H. (eds.), Symposium in Lund, Uppsala, Sweden: Uppland Grafisker AB. 1980:151–164.
13. Fulton, J. E., and Bradley, S. (1974). Studies on the mechanism of action of topical benzoyl peroxide in acne vulgaris. J. Cuta. Pathol. 1:191–194.
14. Wester, R. C., Patel, R., Nacht, S., Leyden, J., Melendres, J., and Maibach, H. (1991). Controlled release of benzoyl peroxide from a porous microsphere polymeric system can reduce topical irritancy. J. Am. Acad. Dermatol. 24:720–726.

17

Liposomes

Hans Lautenschläger
Development & Consulting, Pulheim, Germany

INTRODUCTION

Publications about and patents on liposomes, along with their different chemical components, preparation, and use in skincare products have often been reviewed [1–4]. The reviews do not need any additional comments. Of interest are general questions, such as why liposomes should be used in cosmetics, which functionalities are expected from them, and which advantages they do provide compared with alternative formulations.

The properties of the widely used main component of liposomes, phosphatidylcholine, play a key role for answering these questions. Other compounds such as niotensides and ceramides, which are naturally predestinated for the preparation of liposomes, are less important today. Niotensides do not offer superior claims, and ceramides are not available in sufficient quantities and qualities at convenient prices.

PHOSPHATIDYLCHOLINE

Looking at the horny layer, which is the barrier against external materials, phospholipids and phosphatidylcholine in particular play a minor role. The lipid bilayers contain only traces of phospholipids, and the main components are free fatty acids, cholesterol, triglycerides, hydrocarbons, and ceramides. But looking deeper into the living part of the epidermis, phosphatidylcholine is usually found as the most important constituent of all biological membranes, especially of plasma cell membranes. Over and above that phosphatidylcholine is the source of phosphocholine to transform ceramides to sphingomyelins. In this context, phosphatidylcholine stands for living tissues whereas the increase of ceramides in the cells means that their death by apoptosis is soon ahead (Fig. 1).

Human phosphatidylcholine and phosphatidylcholine of vegetable origin show a fatty acid composition, which is dominated by unsaturated fatty acids. The fatty acid content of soy phosphatidylcholine, which is readily available and mostly used in cosmetic formulas, is characterized by a ratio of linoleic acid up to 70% of the total fatty acids. Consequently, soy phosphatidylcholine has a very low phase-transition temperature of below 0°C in water-containing systems. This may be the reason for its ability to fluidize the lipid bilayers of the horny layer, which can be measured by an increase of the transepidermal water loss (TEWL) after application for a short while. The slight increase of TEWL

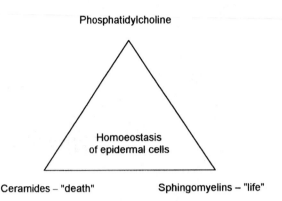

FIGURE 1 Homoeostasis of epidermal cells.

coincides with the penetration of phosphatidylcholine and active agents, which are coformulated with phosphatidylcholine. Because of its high content of linoleic acid and penetration capability, soy phosphatidylcholine delivers linoleic acid very effectively into the skin, and antiacne properties have been shown as a result [5].

By adhering very strongly to surfaces containing proteins like keratin, phosphatidylcholine shows conditioning and softening effects, which are known from the beginning of skincare products' development. So, e.g., shampoos were formulated in the past very often with egg yolk to soften hair and prevent it from becoming charged with static electricity. Egg yolk is very rich in lecithin. The main compound of egg lecithin is phosphatidylcholine.

In a given mixture it is not relevant in which form the phosphatidylcholine is incorporated. However, when phosphatidylcholine is formulated, it is practically inevitable that bilayer-containing systems like liposomes will occur, because this is the most natural form of the material. For example, phosphatidylcholine swollen by water transforms spontaneously to liposomes when "disturbed" by little amounts of salts or watersoluble organic compounds, like urea. On the other hand, it has been known for a long time that horny layer pretreated by phosphatidylcholine can be penetrated much more easily by nonencapsulated materials. So liposomes are not really needed to turn out the functionalities of phosphatidylcholine, but they are very convenient because the handling of pure phosphatidylcholine requires a lot of experience and sometimes patience as well.

Because phosphatidylcholine is known as a penetration enhancer, this property is usually associated with liposomes. Liposomes are the vesicles said to transport cosmetic agents better into the horny layer. That is true and, moreover, the conditioning effect causes the horny layer to become a depot for these agents. Measurements of systemically active pharmaceuticals revealed that an increase of penetration is not synonymous with an increase of permeation. Actually, permeation of active agents is often slowed by phosphatidylcholine in such a way that a high permeation peak in the beginning of the application is prevented. Instead, a more continuous permeation takes place out of the horny layer depot into the living part of the body over a longer period of time. This property makes phosphatidylcholine and liposomes very attractive for the application of vitamins, provitamins, and other substances influencing the regenerating ability of the living epidermis.

CH$_2$-O-CO-(CH$_2$)$_n$-CH$_3$

|

CH-O-CO-(CH$_2$)$_n$-CH$_3$

|⁻ ⁺

CH$_2$-O-PO$_2$-O-CH$_2$-CH$_2$-N(CH$_3$)$_3$

FIGURE 2 Hydrogenated phosphatidylcholine (n = 14,16).

On the other hand, liposomes consisting of unsaturated phosphatidylcholine have to be used with caution in barrier creams because they do not strengthen the natural barrier function of the skin with the exception of its indirect effect of supporting the formation of ceramide I. Ceramide I is known for containing linoleic acid and for being one of the most important barrier-activating substances. Instead of unsaturated phosphatidylcholine, a fully hydrogenated phosphatidylcholine (Fig. 2) should be selected for products designed for skin protection.

Hydrogenated phosphatidylcholine stabilizes the normal TEWL similarly to ceramides when the horny layer is attacked by hydrophilic or lipophilic chemicals [6]. Table 1 shows a summary of the properties of unsaturated and hydrogenated phosphatidylcholine. Hydrogenated phosphatidylcholine is synonymous with hydrogenated soy phosphatidylcholine, which contains mainly stearic and palmitic acid, and semisynthetic compounds like dipalmitoylphosphatidylcholine (DPPC) and distearoylphosphatidylcholine (DSPC). Because of their special properties it can make sense to combine unsaturated with saturated phosphatidylcholine in one and the same cosmetic or dermatological product.

TABLE 1 Properties of Phosphatidylcholines

Parameter	Soy phosphatidylcholine	Hydrogenated soy phosphatidylcholine
Skin barrier function	Penetration enhancement; conditioning the horny layer	Stabilizing the barrier function; conditioning the horny layer
Barrier compatibility	Yes, slightly enhancing TEWL	Yes, stabilizing normal TEWL
Phase transition temperature (aqueous system)	Below 0°C	50–60°C
Fatty acid composition	Unsaturated fatty acids: predominantly linoleic acid, oleic acid	Saturated fatty acids: predominantly stearic and palmitic acid
Solubility	Soluble in triglycerides, alcohols, water (lamellar)	Insoluble in triglycerides, alcohols, and water
Toxicity	CIR-report [7]; anticomedogen	CIR-report [7]
Dispersing ability	Hydrophilic and lipophilic compounds	Hydrophilic and lipophilic compounds

Abbreviations: TEWL, transepidermal water loss; CIR, Cosmetic Ingredient Review.

LIPOSOMES

Liposomes are spherical vesicles whose membranes consist of one (unilamellar) or more (oligolamellar, multilamellar) bilayers of phosphatidylcholine. Sometimes, especially in patents, reference is made not about liposomes but about ''vesicles with an internal aqueous phase.'' The vesicles can differ in size (diameter about 15–3500 nm) and shape (single and fused particles). At a given chemical composition, these parameters strongly depend on the process of preparation. Very often the preparations are metastable. That means the state of free enthalpy is not in an equilibrium with the environment. As a result the vesicles change their lamellarity, size, size distribution, and shape with time. For example, small vesicles tend to form larger ones and large vesicles smaller ones. Fortunately this is mostly not critical for quality because the properties of the phosphatidylcholine, which the vesicles are based on, remain unchanged as a rule. Nevertheless the stability seems to be best in a range of about 100 to 300 nm. That is the case of pure aqueous dispersions of highly enriched (80–100%) soy phosphatidylcholine.

In a complete formulation together with further ingredients, other influences like compatibility, concentration of salts, amphiphilics, and lipophilics play an important role. Therefore, it is often very difficult to prove the existence of liposomes, e.g., in a gel phase or a creamy matrix. However, this is more a marketing problem than a problem of effectiveness of the formulation. Today we can assume that the effectiveness of phosphatidylcholine is based more on the total chemical composition of the cosmetic product and less on the existence or nonexistence of the added liposomes. This may seem curious, but is in fact the reality.

Of course, formulations are very effective in particular when consisting of pure liposomal dispersions bearing lipophilic additives in the membrane spheres and/or hydrophilics in the internal and external aqueous phases within the range of their bearing capacity. In this respect, there has been an intensive search to increase the encapsulation capacity of liposomes for lipids because consumers are used to applying lipid-rich creams. Efforts were made to add emulsifier to the liposomal dispersions to stabilize higher amounts of lipids. Formulators now know that the compatibility of liposomes with regard to emulsifiers is generally limited, more or less. On the other hand, additional emulsifiers have a weakening effect on the barrier affinity of phosphatidylcholine. They cause the phosphatidylcholine and the lipids to be more easily removed from the skin while washing. In this respect there is only one rational consideration: to make use of nanoemulsions consisting of phosphatidylcholine and lipids instead of liposomes. Nanoemulsions are a consequence of the observation that oil droplets can fuse with liposomes when the capacity of bilayers for lipids is exhausted [8]. Further increasing the lipid/phosphatidylcholine ratio and using high-pressure homogenizers lead to nanoemulsions. Nanoemulsions consist of emulsion-like oil droplets surrounded by a monolayer of phosphatidylcholine. The advantage of nanoemulsions is that they allow formulations to tolerate more lipids and remain stable. Also, additional emulsifiers are not needed.

Liposomal dispersions based on unsaturated phosphatidylcholine are lacking in stability against oxidation. Like linoleic esters and linoleic glycerides, these dispersions have to be stabilized by antioxidants. Thinking naturally, a complex of Vitamin C and E (respectively, their derivatives like acetates and palmitates) can be used with success. In some cases, phosphatidylcholine and urea seem to stabilize each other [9,10]. Moreover, agents that are able to mask traces of radical-forming ions of heavy metals, like iron, can be added. Such additives are chelators like citrates, phosphonates, or EDTA. Alternatively, the unsaturated phosphatidylcholine can be substituted by a saturated one like DPPC or hydrogenated soy phosphatidylcholine, which should be favored with regard to its price. Because of the higher phase-transition temperature, liposomal dispersions based on hydrogenated material are more sophisticated in their preparation and are reserved for pharmacological applications as a rule. An interesting new development in the field of cosmetic compositions with hydrogenated soy phosphatidylcholine is the Derma Membrane Structure (DMS)-technology [11]. DMS stands for cream bases (technically the creams are gels) containing hydrogenated soy phosphatidylcholine, sebum-compatible medium chain triglycerides (MCT), shea butter, and squalane. In addition to liposomal dispersions and nanoemulsions, DMS is a third way to formulate phosphatidylcholine with hydrophilic and lipophilic compounds free of further emulsifiers (Fig. 3). DMS is water- and sweatproof and therefore suitable for skin protection and sun creams without using silicones or mineral oil additives. It can easily be transformed into other final products by stirring at room temperature together with liquid lipids and/or aqueous phases.

As previously mentioned, DMS is predestined for skin protection, but by addition of nanoemulsions and/or liposomal dispersions DMS can easily be enriched by unsaturated phosphatidylcholine containing esterified linoleic acid. The resulting products are creamy, stable, and anticomedogenic. The effect of pure DMS basic creams on skin moisturizing, smoothing, and tightening are still significant several days after finishing the application.

Liposomes, nanoemulsions, and DMS have to be preserved. This may be a problem, because phosphatidylcholine (lecithin) inactivates most of the conventional preservatives [12]. On the other hand, preservatives should not be penetrated in the skin to prevent irritation and sensitization. Therefore, glycols like propyleneglycol, glycerol, butyleneglycol, pentyleneglycol, hexyleneglycol, sorbitol, and their mixtures are the compounds of choice. These polyols show a moisturizing effect at the same time.

One of the reasons to substitute phosphatidylcholine by polyglycerols and other synthetic derivatives at the beginning of the liposomal developments was its hydrolytic instability in aqueous preparations for longer periods of time and at higher temperatures. In fact phosphatidylcholine, like other glycerides, is attacked by water to form lysophosphatidylcholine and free fatty acids. But the cleavage of the glyceride bond occurs mainly at a pH greater than 7, so formulations in the range of pH 5.5 to 7 are sufficiently stable

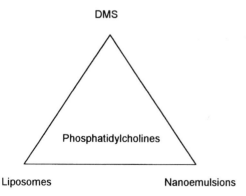

DMS

Phosphatidylcholines

Liposomes   Nanoemulsions

FIGURE 3 Formulations with phosphatidylcholine free of further emulsifiers.

for most purposes. It is possible that hydrolysis depends on the amount of additional surface active compounds. That is another reason to use liposomal dispersions without additional emulsifiers.

AVAILABILITY

As previously mentioned, liposomal dispersions are a very comfortable method to use to work phosphatidylcholine into cosmetic formulations to obtain its superior spectrum of multifunctionality. Preliposomal fluid phases up to 20% phosphatidylcholine and more are commercially available [13]. Also, there are references to the use of instant liposomes in combination with carbohydrates as dry powders [1]. An interesting consideration is bath oils, which form in situ liposomal dispersions free of additional emulsifiers [14]. These compositions are based on mixtures of phosphatidylcholine, triglycerides, and alcohol. By pouring the mixtures into water, liposomes are spontaneously formed. These liposomes strongly tend to adhere to the skin surface. Numerous other methods for preparing liposomes have been described [1].

APPLICATIONS

Today, most of the experts working in the field of liposomal dispersions agree that liposomes do not penetrate as intact vesicles into the skin or permeate through the skin. Liposomes are believed to be deformed and transformed into fragments as a rule. Therefore size, shape, and lamallarity are not so relevant for the application, but for the chemical composition of the total formulation.

The multifunctional properties of phosphatidylcholines lead to a number of different applications. So, formulations with unsaturated phosphatidylcholine are preferred to support skin regeneration, antiaging, acne preventing, and penetrating other active agents like vitamins and their derivatives into the skin. Formulations with hydrogenated phosphatidylcholine may be used for skin and sun protection, but it should be emphasized that in this

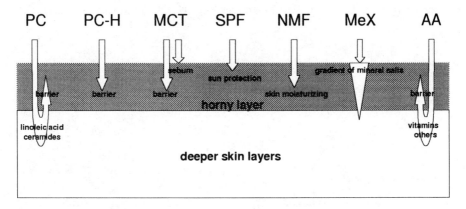

FIGURE 4 Main components of "natural" formulations.

TABLE 2 Phosphatidylcholine-Containing Formulations

Parameter	Liposomes	Nanoemulsions	DMS	Conventional emulsions
Phosphatidylcholine	++	+	Used as additive	(+)
Phosphatidylcholine hydrogenated	Rarely used	+	++	Rarely used
Lipophilic ingredients	Limited	+	+	+
Hydrophilic ingredients	+	+	+	+
Amphiphilic ingredients	Limited	Limited	+	+
Auxiliary compounds	As few as possible	As few as possible	Rarely used	++
Preparation (usual)	Usual and high pressure homogenizers	High pressure homogenizer	High pressure homogenizer	Phase conversion method
Physical stability	(+)	+	+	+
Chemical stability	Depending on pH	Depending on pH	Depending on pH	Depending on pH
Preservation	Glycols	Glycols	Glycols	Glycols
Penetration	++	+	+	(+)
Skin protection	−	(+)	++	(+)
Convenient particle size	(Unsaturated PC) 100–300 nm	50–200 nm	Not detectable	Usual droplets
Cosmetic applications	Antiaging, regeneration	Versatile	Skin protection, sun protection	Versatile
Prevention of skin diseases	++	++	++	(+)

Abbreviations: DMS, derma membrane structure; PC, phosphatidylcholine.

respect nanoemulsions and DMS are still more convenient. The main components of choice to prepare "natural" formulations, which are compatible with horny layer, sebum constituents, and their functions are illustrated in Figure 4. About the role of mineral salts see Ref. 15.

THE FUTURE OF LIPOSOMAL PREPARATIONS

Liposomal dispersions have proved not only to be innovative and effective cosmetic ingredients, but also to be a very convenient form to work with phosphatidylcholine. In dermatology, they will be used with success for preventing and treating several skin diseases. Complementary formulations are established where liposomal dispersions come up against limiting factors. Table 2 shows liposomal and complementary formulations in a direct comparison.

Generally, liposomes, nanoemulsions, and DMS are more compatible with the skin structure than conventional emulsions usually applied. Compatible means that formulations do not disturb the integrity of the skin lipid bilayers and are not washed out while cleaning the skin. In the sense of modern strategies of cosmetics, these formulations get by with a minimum of auxiliary compounds, which put only a strain on the skin. Moreover, compatibility means embedding lipids and hydrophilic agents in the horny layer and being in accordance with the natural situation.

Remarkably, phosphatidylcholine need not be applied in high concentrations because the experience shows that formulations are stable at lower amounts. Also, there is a cumulative effect in the horny layer with repeated application of phosphatidylcholine. In many cases, liposomes, nanoemulsions, and DMS are compatible with each other in a sense that they can be used as a sort of construction kit. So these formulations are believed to still have a great future in cosmetic science. How far new findings about the importance of the choline moiety of phosphatidylcholine [16] will impact skincare research and development cannot be estimated today.

REFERENCES

1. Lasic DD. Liposomes and niosomes. In: Rieger MM, Rhein LD, eds. Surfactants in Cosmetics. 2d ed. New York: Marcel Dekker, 1997:263–283.
2. Wendel A. Lecithins, phospholipids, liposomes in cosmetics, dermatology and in washing and cleansing preparations. Augsburg: Verlag fuer chemische Industrie, 1994.
3. Wendel A. Lecithins, phospholipids, liposomes in cosmetics, dermatology and in washing and cleansing preparations. Part II. Augsburg: Verlag fuer chemische Industrie, 1997.
4. Braun-Falco O, Korting HC, Maibach HI, eds. Liposome Dermatics. Berlin: Springer-Verlag, 1992.
5. Ghyczy M, Nissen H-P, Biltz H. The treatment of acne vulgaris by phosphatidylcholine from soybeans, with a high content of linoleic acid. J Appl Cosmetol 1996; 14:137–145.
6. Lautenschlaeger H. Kuehlschmierstoffe und Hautschutz—neue Perspektiven. Mineraloeltechnik 1998; (5):1–16.
7. Cosmetic Ingredient Review. Lecithin and Hydrogenated Lecithin. Washington: The Cosmetic, Toiletry, and Fragrance Association, 1996.
8. Lautenschlaeger H. Liposomes in dermatological preparations. Part II. Cosmet Toilet 1990; 105(7):63–72.
9. Japanese patent 199104364104. Nippon Surfactant Kogyo KK, 1992.
10. German patent 4021082. Lautenschlaeger, 1990.

11. Kutz G. Galenische Charakterisierung ausgewaehlter Hautpflegeprodukte. Pharmazeutische Zeitung 1997; 142(45):4015–4019.
12. Wallhaeusser KH. Praxis der Sterilisation, Desinfektion—Konservierung. 5th ed. Stuttgart: Georg Thieme Verlag, 1995:43, 394.
13. Roeding J. Properties and Characterisation of Pre-Liposome Systems. In: Braun-Falco O, Korting HC, Maibach HI, eds. Liposome Dermatics. Berlin: Springer-Verlag, 1992:110–117.
14. German patent 4021083. Lautenschlaeger, 1990.
15. Feingold KR. Permeability barrier homeostasis: its biochemical basis and regulation. Cosmet Toilet 1997; 112(7):49–59.
16. Blusztajn JK. Choline, a vital amine. Science 1998; 281:794–795.

18

Topical Delivery by Iontophoresis

Véronique Préat and Rita Vanbever
Université Catholique de Louvain, Brussels, Belgium

INTRODUCTION

Passive permeation of drugs across the skin is limited by the low permeability of the stratum corneum. Transdermal and topical delivery of drugs are presently applicable to only a few drugs with appropriate balance hydro/lipophilicity, small size, no charge, and relatively high potency [1,2].

Strategies have been developed to increase transdermal and topical delivery across or into the skin. They consist of increasing the permeability of the skin or providing a driving force acting on the drug. Chemicals methods (e.g., penetration enhancers) or physical methods (e.g., iontophoresis, sonophoresis, or electroporation) have been shown to significantly enhance transdermal transport [2–4].

Iontophoresis is a noninvasive technique that uses a mild electric current to facilitate transdermal delivery of drugs for both systemic and local effects. Iontophoretic transport of drugs has been extensively studied [5–8]. It has the potential to overcome many of the barriers to topical drug absorption [6–13]. This chapter will focus on local delivery by iontophoresis as an aid to penetration of topically applied drugs. The mechanisms and the parameters affecting iontophoretic transport will be reviewed. The role of iontophoresis in clinical practice and cosmetics will be discussed.

IONTOPHORESIS

Iontophoresis may be defined as the administration of molecules through the skin by the application of an electric current [5–8].

An iontophoretic system has three basic components: 1) the source of electric current, 2) an active reservoir containing the active and an electrode as well as a counter electrode in a return reservoir, and 3) a control unit. The current used for iontophoretic delivery is applied for minutes or hours with current density ranging from 0.1 to 0.5 mA/cm². Miniaturized systems of approximately 10 cm² including a battery have been developed for transdermal drug delivery. For the topical delivery of actives, the current source can be an external power supply and a larger area can be treated by the current.

The principle of iontophoresis is mainly based on electrorepulsion: the electric field drives the molecules into the skin. Positive ions will be repelled from the positive electrode, called the anode, and attracted to the cathode, or the negative electrode. Negatively charged compounds will be repelled from the cathode. Neutral compounds can also be delivered by electro-osmosis [3].

Iontophoresis has been widely studied for transdermal drug delivery. It has been used to achieve systemic concentration sufficient for a desired therapeutic effect. Iontophoresis has also been successfully used in clinical medicine to achieve topical delivery of drugs for several decades. It has found widespread use in physical therapy and dermatology. Large quantities of a medication are targeted to a localized treatment region, minimizing the systemic level of the medication. The literature supports the concept that iontophoresis is a method of choice for drug application in the therapy of surface tissue [9–13].

The rationales for topical drug delivery by iontophoresis are as follows: 1) to deliver a locally high concentration of an active—the delivery of the drug is enhanced by iontophoresis by one to three orders of magnitude as compared with passive diffusion; 2) to control delivery of the active by current application—inter- and intraindividual variations can be reduced; 3) to extend transdermal transport to low and medium (<5000) molecular weight hydrophilic compounds [5–8,14,15].

MECHANISMS OF IONTOPHORETIC TRANSPORT

Theoretical Mechanisms of Iontophoretic Transport

The electrically induced transport of an ion across a membrane results from three mechanisms: (1) diffusion related to a chemical potential gradient, 2) electrical mobility attributable to an electric potential gradient, and 3) solute transfer attributable to a convective solvent flow, i.e., electro-osmosis [5–8,15,16].

$$J_T = J_P + J_E + J_O$$

J_T = total flux
J_P = passive diffusion flux
J_E = electrical flux
J_O = electro-osmotic flux

$$J = -D \, dC/dx - Dzc \, F/RT \cdot d\varepsilon/dx$$

D = diffusion coefficient
c = concentration
z = valence
F = Faraday's constant
R = gaz constant
T = absolute temperature
ε = electrical potential
X = distance

For ionic species, the contribution of passive diffusion is neglible. The major mechanism of active transport by iontophoresis is the electromigration or electrostatic repulsion. However, the contribution of electro-osmotic flow has been reported to be significant for neutral molecules and macromolecules. Because of its negative charges, the skin is permselective to cations, inducing a net convective solvent flow from the anode to the cathode. Hence, neutral molecules can be delivered into or extracted from the skin by cathodal iontophoresis [16–18].

Pathways for Transport

As for conventional transdermal drug delivery, the molecular transport can take place in the stratum corneum by transcellular or paracellular pathways and/or in the appendages (sweat glands and hair follicles). The major route of iontophoretic transport is believed to be the appendageal pathway because of its low electrical resistance [19,20]. However, recent evidence supports the existence of a significant paracellular route [21–23].

PARAMETERS AFFECTING IONTOPHORETIC DELIVERY

Iontophoretic delivery of compounds into or through the skin is affected by the physico-chemical parameters of the active, the formulation of the active, and the electrical parameters of iontophoresis. The parameters affecting iontophoretic transport have been extensively studied and are summarized in Table 1 [5–8,24,25].

The electrical parameters allow control on drug transport. Increasing the current density and/or the duration of current application enhances the delivery of the active into or through the skin. The use of pulsed current rather than constant current can be used to avoid skin polarization, but usually decreases active transport.

The design of the electrodes is also important. Both inert and active electrodes can be used. Inert electrodes, such as platinum or stainless steel, induce electrolysis of water and consequently pH shift of the solutions requiring the presence of a buffer. Active electrodes, such as Ag/AgCl electrodes, require the presence of chloride at the anode. The polarity of the electrodes must be adapted to the charge of the active: anodal delivery for positively charged or neutral molecules and cathodal delivery for negative compounds.

The formulation of the active reservoir as well as counter electrode reservoir also affects iontophoretic transport. Increasing ionization of the active by modifying the pH or decreasing the amount of competitive ions will enhance the transport.

In order to enhance the delivery of an active in the skin, the formulation of the reservoir and counter reservoir and the electrode design have to be optimized. Once the

TABLE 1 Parameters Affecting Iontophoretic Transport

	Parameters increased	Effect on iontophoretic transport
Physicochemical properties of the active	—molecular weight	↘
	—charge	↗
	—partition coefficient	?
Formulation of the active	—pH : ionization	↗
	—competitive ions	↘
	—viscosity	↘
Electrical parameters of iontophoresis	—current density	↗
	—duration of current application	↗
	—current waveform	↘ / ↗
	—electrode design	↘ / ↗
	—area of current application	↗

Source: Ref. 24.

formulation has been optimized and fixed, the control of active delivery can be achieved by modifying the current density and the duration of current application [5]. Hence, the prerequisites for efficient delivery by iontophoresis are 1) a good aqueous solubility, 2) a formulation with a pH allowing the ionization of the active and a low concentration of competitive ions, 3) a polarity of electrodes allowing electrorepulsion (anodal or cathodal iontophoresis for positively or negatively charged compounds, respectively) and/or electro-osmosis (anodal iontophoresis).

EFFECTS OF IONTOPHORESIS ON THE SKIN: SAFETY ISSUES

Evidence for the safety of iontophoresis comes from 1) the long clinical experience with topical iontophoretic delivery, 2) the noninvasive investigations in animals and humans, 3) the biophysical studies of the stratum corneum, and 4) the histological studies.

Effect of Iontophoresis on the Stratum Corneum

The effect of iontophoresis on the stratum corneum structure has been extensively studied by biophysical and histological methods. The effect of iontophoresis on the stratum corneum has recently been reviewed [26]. As shown in Table 2, the major modifications of the stratum corneum induced by iontophoresis include an increased stratum corneum hydration and a disorganization of the lipid lamellae.

Tolerance and Safety Issues Associated with Iontophoresis

The clinical literature on the application of low-intensity current for topical drug delivery supports the fact that iontophoresis is a safe procedure. In general, a minor erythema is observed. The redness disappears progressively within a few hours [31]. The parameters affecting the sensation of current application have been recently reviewed [32].

More recently, noninvasive bioengineering methods have been used in animals as well as in humans to investigate the effect of current application in vivo (Table 3). The barrier function of the skin is hardly modified by iontophoresis as measured by transepidermal water loss. Laser doppler velocimetry and chromametry confirm that a mild and re-

TABLE 2   Influence of Iontophoresis on the Stratum Corneum

Methods	Effect	References
Impedance	Decreased resistance	27
ATR-FTIR	Increased hydration	28, 29
	No change in lipid fluidity	
X-ray scattering		
Small angle	Disorganization of the lipid lamellae, spacing	29
Wide angle	No change in the lipid packing in the lamellae	30
Freeze fracture electron microscopy	Disorganization of the intercellular lipid lamellae	30

Source: Ref. 26.

TABLE 3 Bioengineering Investigations of the Effect of Iontophoresis on the Skin

Methods	Effect	References
Transepidermal water loss	Transient increase (due to an increased hydration)	27, 28, 33–35
Laser Doppler velocimetry	Transient increase	28, 33–35
Chromametry	Transient increase in redness	33, 35

Source: Ref. 26.

versible erythema is induced by current application. The higher the density or the duration of current application, the higher the erythema [28].

In conclusion, the clinical use as well as experimental studies attest to the overall safety of iontophoresis and the absence of long-term side effects. Nevertheless, it should be pointed out that iontophoresis is not without potential injury if not used correctly. The major danger in all iontophoretic treatments is the occurrence of skin irritation and burns. Pain sensation can be relied on as a criterion for the prevention of skin burns as a consequence of excessive densities (>0.5 mA/cm^2). If the electrode metal touches the skin, burns can be caused by excessive current at the site of contact. The solute and the excipients in the solution being delivered can also influence the reaction of the skin [32].

TOPICAL DELIVERY OF DRUGS AND COSMETICS BY IONTOPHORESIS

Topical Iontophoretic Delivery

The main rationale for using iontophoresis for topical delivery is to achieve a higher concentration of the active in the skin. It has been shown that iontophoresis enhances the amount of permeant such as fentanyl, TRH, acyclovir, Ara-AMP, or lidocaine in the stratum corneum, epidermis, and dermis [36–39]. Confocal laser microscopy also shows that iontophoresis enhances the local concentration of fluorescent dye, oligonucleotides, or macromolecules [19,22,23].

Clinical Applications of Topical Iontophoretic Transport

Iontophoresis has been successfully used in medicine to achieve topical delivery of drugs and actives. Most of the clinical applications of iontophoresis were developed in physical therapy and dermatology. The key areas include local anesthesia, hyperhidrosis, and local treatment of inflammation. Efficacy has been shown in clinical studies. In some cases, notably for the delivery of cosmetics, the ability of the medication to penetrate the target tissue in sufficient quantities to produce a clinical effect was not studied in controlled clinical trials.

Tap-water iontophoresis has been widely used for the treatment of hyperhidrosis. It is effective in the management of hyperhidrosis for the axillae, palms, and soles by reducing sweat production with only mild and temporary side effects. The exact mechanism of action remains unknown [40,41]. Current is typically applied in a 10 to 20 min session, which needs to be repeated two or three times per week and followed by a maintenance program [9]. Commercial devices have been marketed. Iontophoresis of actives such as anticholinergic agent and aluminium chloride can increase the average remission.

The successful use of iontophoretic delivery of lidocaine for local anesthesia of the skin has been reported in a variety of situations, including painless venipuncture, painless dermatological procedures such as pulsed-dye ablation of port wine stains, and laceration repairs. The advantages of iontophoresis-induced anesthesia include the painless procedure, the adequate local and low systemic concentration, and the quick onset of action as compared with anesthesia using a eutectic mixture of local anesthetics (10 vs. 60 min) [42–46]. The first drug-iontophoresis device combination approved by the FDA is Iontocaine.

Iontophoresis can also facilitate the penetration of active molecules in the deep tissue underlying the skin. Iontophoresis of dexamethasone sodium phosphate has been reported to be effective for the treatment of patients with musculoskeletal inflammation such as tendinitis, arthritis, or carpal tunnel syndrome [47,48]. Iontophoretic delivery of pilocarpine is extensively used for the diagnosis of cystic fibrosis. It enhances sweat secretion, allowing the measure of chloride concentration in the sweat [49]. Cystic fibrosis indicators are commercially available.

Antiviral drugs such as idoxuridine, acyclovir, or vidarabin can be delivered topically by iontophoresis [10,11,39]. Iontophoresis of Ara-AMP or idoxuridine is efficient in treating HSV1 and HSV2 in mice and orolabial HSV in humans [10,11]. Antiviral-drug iontophoresis could also be useful for the treatment of active zoster lesions and postherpetic neuralgia.

Other applications for topical iontophoresis include the treatment of warts with sodium salicylate [50], calcium deposit with acetic acid [51], improvement of peripheral microcirculation by PGE1 [52,53], treatment of acne scars [54], hypertrophic scars [56,57], or photodynamic therapy with 5 aminolevulinic acid [58].

CONCLUSIONS

Iontophoresis has gained a great deal of attention during the last two decades for both systemic and topical delivery. It offers a convenient and safe means to enhance the topical concentration of drug in the skin and even in deeper underlying tissue as compared with passive diffusion or systemic delivery. Its use to treat local conditions is well known. It is particularly attractive for the delivery of low molecular weight (<1000) hydrophilic solutes at the site of action. Iontophoresis enables precise control of topical delivery by varying electrical current.

The rationales for using iontophoresis to deliver actives in cosmetics and the technology for optimized and controlled iontophoretic transport are well established. However, further double-blind clinical studies are needed to confirm the interest of iontophoresis in specific cosmetic uses.

REFERENCES

1. Hadgraft J, Guy R, eds. Transdermal Drug Delivery. New York: Marcel Dekker, 1989.
2. Guy R. Current status and future prospects for transdermal drug delivery. Pharm Res 1996; 13:1765–1769.
3. Walters K, Hadgraft J, eds. Pharmaceutical Skin Permeation Enhancement. New York: Marcel Dekker, 1993.
4. Barry B, Williams A. Permeation enhancement through skin. In: Swarbick J, Boylan J, eds. Encyclopedia of Pharmaceutical Technology, Vol. 11. 1995:449–493.
5. Sage B. Iontophoresis. In: Swarbick J, Boylan J, eds. Encyclopedia of Pharmaceutical Technology, Vol. 8. 1993:217–247.

6. Singh P, Maibach H. Iontophoresis in drug delivery: basic principles and applications. Crit Rev Therap Drug Carrier Syst 1994; 11:161–213.
7. Singh P, Maibach H. Iontophoresis: an alternative to the use of carriers in cutaneous drug delivery. Adv Drug Del Rev 1996; 18:379–394.
8. Roberts M, Lai M, Cross S, Yoshida N. Solute transport as a determinant of iontophoretic transport. In: Potts R, Guy R, eds. Mechanisms of Transdermal Drug Delivery. New York: Marcel Dekker, 1997:291–349.
9. Banga A. Clinical applications of iontophoresis devices for topical dermatological delivery. In: Banga A, ed. Electrically Enhanced Transdermal Drug Delivery. Francis & Taylor, 1998: 57–74.
10. Gargarosa L, Ozawa A, Ohkido M, Shimomura Y, Hill J. Iontophoresis for enhancing penetration of dermatologic and antiviral drugs. J Dermatol 1995; 22:865–875.
11. Gargarosa L, Hill M. Modern iontophoresis for local drug delivery. Int J Pharm 1995; 123: 159–171.
12. Singh J, Bhatia K. Topical iontophoretic drug delivery: pathways, principles, factors and skin irritation. Med Res Rev 1996; 16:285–296.
13. Costello C, Jeshe A. Iontophoresis: applications in transdermal medication delivery. Phys Ther 1995; 75:554–563.
14. Green P. Iontophoretic delivery of peptides drug. J Control Release 1996; 41:33–48.
15. Phipps JB, Gyory J. Transdermal ion migration. Adv Drug Del Rev 1992; 9:137–176.
16. Pikal M. The role of electroosmotic flow in transdermal iontophoresis. Adv Drug Del Rev 1992; 9:201–237.
17. Hirvonen Y, Guy R. Transdermal iontophoresis: modulation of electroosmosis by polypeptides. J Control Release 1998; 50:283–289.
18. Rao G, Guy R, Glikfeld P, LaCourse W, Leung L, Tamada J, Potts R, Azimi N. Reverse iontophoresis: non invasive glucose monitoring in vivo in humans. Pharm Res 1995; 12:1869–1873.
19. Cullander C. What are the pathways of iontophoretic current flow through mammalian skin? Adv Drug Del Rev 1992; 9:119–135.
20. Scott E, Laplazza A, White H, Phipps B. Transport of ionic species in skin: contribution of pores to the overall skin conductance. Pharm Res 1993; 10:1699–1709.
21. Monteiro-Riviere N. Identification of the pathways of transdermal iontophoretic drug delivery: light and ultrastructural studies using mercuric chloride in pigs. Pharm Res 1994; 11:251–256.
22. Turner N, Ferry L, Price M, Cullander C, Guy R. Iontophoresis of poly-L-lysines: the role of molecular weight? Pharm Res 1997; 14:1322–1331.
23. Regnier V, Préat V. Localization of a FITC-labeled phosphorothioate oligodeoxynucleotide in the skin after topical delivery by iontophoresis and electroporation. Pharm Res 1998; 15: 1596–1602.
24. Préat V, Vanbever R, Jadoul A, Regnier V. Electrically enhanced transdermal drug delivery: iontophoresis vs electroporation. In: Couvreur P, Duchêne D, Green P, Junginger H, eds. Transdermal administration, a case study, Iontophoresis. Paris: Editions de la santé. 1997:58–67.
25. Jadoul A, Mesens J, de Beukelaer F, Crabbé R, Préat V. Transdermal permeation of alnitidan by iontophoresis: in vitro optimization and human pharmacokinetic data. Pharm Res 1996; 13:1347–1352.
26. Jadoul A, Bouwstra J, Préat V. Effects of iontophoresis and electroporation on the stratum corneum. Review of the biophysical studies. Adv Drug Del Rev 1999; 35:89–106.
27. Kalia Y, Nomato LD, Guy R. The effect of iontophoresis on skin barrier integrity: non invasive investigation by impedance spectroscopy and transepidermal water loss. Pharm Res 1996; 13: 957–961.
28. Thysman S, Van Neste D, Préat V. Non invasive investigation of human skin after in vivo iontophoresis. Skin Pharmacol 1995; 8:229–236.

29. Jadoul A, Doucet J, Durand D, Préat V. Modifications induced on stratum corneum by iontophoresis: ATR-FTIR and x-ray scattering studies. J Control Release 1996; 42:165–173.

30. Craane-vanHinsberg W, Verhoef J, Spies F, Bouwstra J, Gooris G, Junginger H, Boddé H. Electroperturbation on the human skin barrier in vitro (II) effects on the stratum corneum lipid ordering and ultrastructure. Micros Res Tech 1997; 37:200–213.

31. Ledger P. Skin biological in electrically enhanced transdermal delivery. Adv Drug Del Rev 1992; 9:289–307.

32. Prausnitz M. The effects of electric current applied to skin: a review for transdermal drug delivery. Adv Drug Del Rev 1996; 18:395–425.

33. Fouchard D, Hueber F, Teillaud E, Marty JP. Effect of iontophoretic current flow on hairless rat skin in vivo. J Control Release 1997; 49:89–99.

34. Vandergeest R, Elshove D, Danhof M, Lavrijsen A, Boddé H. Non-invasive assessment of skin barrier integrity and skin irritation following iontophoretic current application in humans. J Control Release 1996; 41:205–213.

35. Vanbever R, Fouchard D, Jadoul A, De Morre N, Préat V, Marty J-P. In vivo non-invasive evaluation of hairless rat skin after high-voltage pulse exposure. Skin Pharmacol Appl Skin Physiol 1998; 11:23–34.

36. Park N, Gangorasa C, Hill J. Iontophoretic application of Ara-AMP (9b-D-arabinofuranoyl-adenine-5-monophosphate) into adult mouse skin. Proc Soc Exp Biol Med 1977; 156:326–329.

37. Singh P, Roberts M. Iontophoretic transdermal delivery of salicylic acid and lidocaine to local subcutaneous structures. J Pharm Sci 1993; 82:127–131.

38. Jadoul A, Hanchard C, Thysman S, Préat V. Quantification and localization of fentanyl and TRH delivered by iontophoresis in the skin. Int J Pharm 1995; 120:221–228.

39. Volpato N, Nicoli S, Laureri C, Colombo P, Santi P. In vitro acyclovir distribution in human skin layers after transdermal iontophoresis. J Control Release 1998; 50:291–296.

40. Hill A, Baker G, Jansen G. Mechanism of action of iontophoresis in the treatment of palmar hyperhidrosis. Cutis 1981; 28:69–72.

41. Holzle E, Alberti N. Long-term efficacy and side effects of tap water iontophoresis of palmoplantar hyperhidrosis. The usefulness of home therapy. Dermatologica 1987; 175:126.

42. Lener EV, Bucalo B, Kist D, Moy R. Topical anesthetic agents in dermatologic surgery: a review. Dermatologic Surg 1997; 23:673–683.

43. Ashburn M, Gauthier M, Love G, Basta S, Gaylord B, Kessler K. Iontophoretic administration of 2% lidocaine HCl and 1:100,000 epinephrine in humans. Clin J Pain 1997; 13:22–26.

44. Zempsky W, Arand K, Sullivan K, Fraser D, Wana K. Lidocaine iontophoresis for topical anesthesia before intravenous line placement in children. J Pediatr 1998; 132:1061–1063.

45. Greenbaum SS, Bernstein EF. Comparison of iontophoresis of lidocaine with a eutectic mixture of lidocaine and prilocaine (EMLA) for topically administered local-anesthesia. J Dermatolog Surg Oncology 1994; 20:579–583.

46. Irsfeld S, Klement W, Lipfert P. Dermal anaesthesia: comparison of EMLA cream with iontophoretic local anaesthesia. Br J Anaesth 1993; 71:375.

47. Hasson S, Daniels J, Schieb D. Exercise training and dexamethasone iontophoresis in rheumatoid arthritis. Physiotherapy Canada 1991; 43:11–14.

48. Bertolucci L. Introduction of antiinflammatory drugs by iontophoresis: double blind study. J Orthop Sports Phys Ther 1982; 4:103–108.

49. Gibson L, Cooke R. A test for concentration of electrolytes in sweat in cystic fibrosis of the pancreas utilizing pilocarpine by iontophoresis. Pediatrics 1959; 23:545.

50. Gordon A, Weinstein M. Sodium salicylate iontophoresis in the treatment of plantar warts. Phys Ther 1968; 49:869.

51. Kahn J. Acetic acid iontophoresis for calcium deposit. Phys Ther 1977; 57:658.

52. Asai J, Fukuta K, Torii S. Topical administration of prostaglandin E_1 with iontophoresis for skin flap viability. Ann Plast Surg 1997; 38:514–517.

53. Saeki S, Yamamura K, Matsushita M, Niishikimi N, Sakurai T, Nimura Y. Iontophoretic application of prostaglandin E1 for improvement in peripheral microcirculation. Int J Clin Pharmac Ther 1998; 36:525–529.
54. Schmidt JB, Binder M, Macheines UV, Bieglmager C. New treatment of atrophic acne scars by iontophoresis with estriol and tretinoin. Int J Dermatol 1995; 34:53–57.
55. Tannenbaum M. Iodine iontophoresis in reducing scar tissue. Phys Ther 1980; 60:792.
56. Shigeni S, Murakami T, Yata N, Ikuta Y. Treatment of keloid and hypertrophic scars by iontophoretic transdermal delivery of tranilast. Scand J Plast Reconstr Surg Hand Surg 1997; 31:151–158.
57. Zhao L, Hung L, Choy T. Delivery of medication by iontophoresis to treat post-burn hypertrophic scars: investigation of a new electronic technique. Burns 1997; 23(suppl 1):S27–S29.
58. Rhodes L, Tsoukas M, Anderson R, Kollias N. Iontophoretic delivery of ALA provides a quantitative model for ALA pharmacokinetics and PpIX phototoxicity in human skin. J Invest Dermatol 1997; 108:87–91.

19

Mousses

Albert Zorko Abram and Roderick Peter John Tomlinson
Soltec Research Pty Ltd, Rowville, Victoria, Australia

INTRODUCTION

The term "mousse" originated as the French word for foam, and this in fact is a good basic description of an aerosol mousse. A foam is defined as a two-phase system wherein a gas is dispersed in either a liquid or solid phase to form a foam structure. For the purpose of this chapter all aerosol foams will be considered mousses, although the emphasis will be placed on the more recent applications.

Aerosol mousses have wider applications and can suffer greater formulating problems than are generally recognized. One of the first questions to address is: When should consideration be given to formulating a product as a mousse? Possible reasons could include cosmetic attributes, minimization of inhalable particles, ease of dosing, ease of application, and/or ease of spreading. All of these characteristics differentiate a mousse from a lotion, cream, or spray.

MOUSSE ATTRIBUTES

The primary cosmetic attributes of a mousse are its low density and attractive, pure, white appearance. Specific densities of mousses can vary considerably depending on the type and level of propellant(s) and surfactant(s) used. For oil-in-water emulsions this variable gives an ability to produce a wide range of mousse types for any basic emulsion formula. Product characteristics can be fine-tuned from a slowly expanding, dense foam to a rapidly expanding, light, dry foam. By using a low-pressure hydrocarbon such as butane, the former is produced, whereas if propane were used the latter observation would be seen.

A further variable in tuning the cosmetic attributes of a mousse is the nature of the formulation itself. Factors that affect the nature of the emulsion or dispersion will also impact on the visual characteristics of the foam. In shave and moisturizing mousses, which are generally based on alkali or amine neutralized fatty acids, the nature and blend of the fatty acids can markedly vary the appearance of the foam. The use of mixed fatty acids as opposed to single fatty acids can produce denser, creamier foams than would otherwise be the case. Addition of foam boosters such as coconut diethanolamide will also impact on the cosmetic characteristics. Use of humectants such as glycerine and propylene glycol will also tend to produce denser, creamier foams.

In a world that will inevitably become more safety conscious, the minimization of ingestion or inhalation of consumer chemicals is becoming increasingly important. During the late 1960s almost all aerosol hairstyling products were hair sprays. Recognition of ozone depletion led to a reduction in the propellant content of many aerosols. This, in conjunction with a need for marketing innovation, led to the hair mousse. Sales of mousse hair treatments grew over the years to take up 50% of the market in some countries, and it became apparent that many users preferred the mousse variant because it was no longer necessary to hold one's breath while styling the hair.

Quite clearly, many aspects of hairstyling could be achieved with a mousse while eliminating the inhalation of solvents, resins, plasticizers, etc. Recently, we have seen concerns expressed for aerosol spray head-lice products as a result of fears that significant quantities of insecticide could be inhaled. We solved this problem by incorporating the insecticide, synergists, and solvents into an aerosol mousse form, which, in addition to capturing the number-one market position, eliminated the inhalation risk.

Although it is not easy to use metering valves with mousses, the user can achieve reasonable dose control by estimating the volume of mousse dispensed. Consumers quickly learn how to dispense the "right" amount of product for daily tasks such as moisturizing the hands, styling the hair or covering the lower face for shaving. Mousses do, however, present difficulties in terms of metering valves for several reasons. First, metering valves tend to have a small capacity, anywhere between 25 µL to 5 mL. The larger-chamber metering valves are available, particularly in Europe, but are also relatively expensive. When one uses metering valves with a capacity above 1 mL, there is a tendency for residual product in the metering chamber to expand and slowly emerge from the actuator, leading to dripping and mess.

One of the great pleasures of using a mousse product is the ease of application. Even viscous lotions feel lighter and easier to apply as a result of the gas cells producing a "thin film" liquid structure, which collapses with pressure and heat. Variables that contribute to the application characteristics include propellant nature, pressure and quantity, emulsion or vehicle viscosity, and the nature of the formulation excipients and actives. Account must be taken for the required mousse characteristics which will be dependant on the nature of the product. For example, a hairstyling mousse needs to collapse quickly during application because the user wants the resin solution to wet the hair and dry in a controlled but rapid manner. In contrast to this, a shave-mousse user needs a long-lasting foam that will easily spread over the area to be shaved and remain stable during the process of shaving.

A further advantage of mousse systems is the ease with which the mousse can be spread over a large surface area. Again, formulation variables include the propellant type, pressure, and concentration, but, more critically, the viscosity of the product and the nature of the excipients will play an important role. Even with high viscosity, high drag oil phases, the presence of the propellant in the oil phase of oil-in-water emulsions (such as moisturizers and shave foams) tends to reduce the oil phase viscosity during rub-in. In addition to this useful attribute, the thin film nature of the expanded emulsion allows much greater spreadability when compared with an ungassed emulsion.

It is possible to use a portion of low-pressure propellent to keep some waxes and solid fatty acids and alcohols in a liquid state during rub-in. Subsequent loss of propellant leaves these materials free to recrystallize and deliver their cosmetic attributes as waxes. Incorporation of slip agents such as silicones will also help with rub-in and can also be used to allow conventional moisturizing foams to break more rapidly and further aid spreading.

MOUSSE TECHNOLOGY

The mousse product can be defined as a colloidal dispersion of gas in liquid or gas in solid. Mousse products are typically dispensed from pressurized aerosol containers that contain a liquefied propellant (or a suitable compressed gas) that is soluble or miscible with the base formulation. Depending on the propellant concentration, a mousse product can be further classified as either dilute or concentrated. The former exists as spherical bubbles separated by thick, viscous films, whereas the latter is mostly gas phase—consisting of polyhedral gas cells separated by thin liquid films.

Further distinctions of mousse products, with respect to thermodynamic stability, are "unstable" mousses, where solutions of short chain fatty acids or alcohols (which are mildly surface active) drain rapidly from the liquid films surrounding the bubbles, resulting in film rupture and collapse of the foam structure. The other category is "metastable" mousses, where solutions of soaps, synthetic detergents, proteins, and the like form a film that achieves a minimum thickness below which no drainage of the liquid film occurs.

Most cosmetic/therapeutic mousse products contain a significant amount of water (anywhere from 5 to 95% by weight of the overall formulation) that exists in the following forms; (1) a solution with a suitable organic solvent, emulsifier, or solvent/emulsifier combination; or (2) the continuous phase of an oil-in-water emulsion. Mousses can also be prepared without water where a suitably volatile propellant is in solution with a viscous nonvolatile material; as the solution is dispensed from the pressurized container the dissolved propellant has sufficient energy to diffuse from the viscous material. This causes a rapid expansion of the nonvolatile material which then sets because of its inherent viscosity.

Although it is relatively simple to form a foamy product using a combination of water, surfactant, and propellant, there are a number of considerations that must be addressed when formulating a mousse for commercial purposes. One of the most important aspects of formulating such a product is the physical quality of the finished product. It must be consistent throughout the life of the product to ensure consumer satisfaction. That is, the color should not change, the bubble size should not significantly vary, the pH should not change, and there should be no packaging interaction. Although this seems fundamental to the process of product development, there are still large numbers of products that find their way to the market and inevitably disappoint consumers or are recalled because of a lack of thorough testing. The consequences of this can include interruptions to marketing, product launch cancellations, bad press, and even lawsuits.

LIQUID-LIQUID AND LIQUID-GAS INTERFACES

One fundamental necessity of the aerosol mousse is that it must be in the liquid state within the container. This allows the product to flow within the container and be dispensed through the valve. In the case of single-phase products, low viscosity assists with solvation of the propellant within the base formulation. Multiple-phase products, such as emulsions or suspensions, must be formulated to ensure the contents remain homogenous during both manufacture and product application. Reproducible dosing from multiple-phase products is taken into consideration at the commencement of a product development program. A dispersion within a pressurized container is likely to show some signs of sedimentation or creaming during standing so it is important that the contents can be redispersed with gentle agitation. Through the observation of subtle physical changes in the formulation during product development, a homogeneous product that delivers a foam of consistent quality can be prepared.

Surfactants play a very important role in maintaining product uniformity. A simple representation of a surfactant is a molecule that has a hydrophilic head and a hydrophobic tail. The hydrophilic head is typically a hydroxyl group, ethylene oxide chain, or other water-soluble functional group. The hydrophobic tail can be thought of as a saturated hydrocarbon chain that may have additional oil-soluble functional groups attached to the chain. In the case of oil-in-water emulsions, surfactants are dispersed throughout the liquid medium with the hydrophilic heads aligned with the water phase and the hydrophobic tails extending into the surface of the oil droplets. A surfactant layer effectively covers each oil droplet with the hydrophilic heads protruding outward. Sufficient surfactant must be present at the water/oil interface to inhibit coalescence of the oil droplets as they collide.

The surfactant can be a single excipient or a combination of several. The use of more than one surfactant provides a means of establishing the required hydrophile-lipophile balance (HLB) and concentration of the surfactants necessary to form an emulsion with a particular oil phase. Surfactants and oil-phase ingredients have HLB values assigned to them from an empirical scale. Those surfactants that have a HLB value of greater than 10 are generally referred to as hydrophilic whereas those with HLB values below 10 are considered lipophilic. The HLB value for the oil-phase ingredients represents the optimum value a surfactant or combination of surfactants must have to produce an emulsion with the oil and water phases. The HLB for the oil phase can be experimentally determined through monitoring the separation rates of emulsions prepared using different ratios of a set pair of hydrophilic and lipophilic surfactants. The oil-phase HLB value is determined for the surfactant ratio that produces the most stable emulsion. It is calculated by multiplying the fraction of each surfactant present by its respective HLB value and adding the two new values together.

The types of surfactants necessary to produce a spontaneous emulsion are generally selected on a "like dissolves like" principle, where it can be assumed that a match in functional groups between the primary oil-phase ingredient and the hydrophobic tail occurs. Surfactant selection can be simplified somewhat when developing pharmaceutical products through the use of materials conforming to a pharmacopoeial monograph. The range of surfactants for cosmetic products, on the other hand, is quite extensive, so much so that it is possible to select materials from any particular origin (physical or geographical). Industry journals, cosmetic ingredient dictionaries, and literature from raw-material suppliers all represent useful sources of information to assist in narrowing down the task of surfactant selection.

Surfactants are also very important in generating and maintaining the foam structure. As the mousse product is ejected from the aerosol container, it is immediately exposed to a lower-pressure atmosphere. The propellant that has been dissolved or dispersed in the formulation rapidly dissipates and is encapsulated by thin films of the liquid phase. As a result, the foam structure expands away from the surface of the liquid. The presence of surfactant lowers the interfacial tension between the propellant vapor and the liquid phase, enabling thin films to flex and form a matrix of polyhedra. The liquid film comprises the primary liquid phase or continuous phase of an emulsion depending on the characteristics of the base formulation.

Surfactant molecules in the foam structure are aligned with hydrophobic tails pointing away from the surface of the foam and into the center of the individual bubbles that make up the foam structure. By increasing the surfactant concentration of the formulation, a more stable foam structure with finer bubbles can be produced. Lowering the surfactant concentration enables a formulator to prepare a product that liquefies under low shear or a change in temperature. The foam's resistance to flow and subsequent film rupture are directly related to the surfactant concentration, whereas the thickness of the film is related to the cohesive forces that exist within the liquid.

CORROSION AND AEROSOL MOUSSES

Surprisingly, corrosion is not limited to the inside of the aerosol container. There are many instances where the environment in which an aerosol product is stored has led to the packaging's demise. For example, when an exposed tinplate container is stored in a wet or humid area it is not uncommon for the outer surface to rust. Shaving foams are probably the most susceptible mousse product to suffer external corrosion problems because they are often left in the bathroom and are exposed to moisture during handling and storage. Other causes could be from warehousing or transporting products from humid or tropical areas both before and after manufacturing.

Corrosion within the aerosol container can be controlled with an informed selection of packaging and excipients. As a general rule of thumb, if a product is to be formulated between an alkaline and neutral pH, use a lined or unlined tinplate container. If the product is between neutral and acidic pH use a lined aluminium container. Some products do not follow this rule, primarily because they rely entirely on the lining or corrosion passivating ingredients to minimize corrosion. This is typical of hairstyling mousses that use amine-neutralized resins to control hold and high-humidity curl retention and yet are quite alkaline in character.

Water quality is an important issue to address in minimizing the potential for aerosol-can corrosion. Unless you have a foolproof method for controlling corrosion in water containing mousse products, always use deionized or purified water! Trace amounts of chloride ions can wreak havoc on an aqueous aerosol product, ensuring corrosion and leakage of the pressurized containers within months after production. There are many electronegative ions that can have a similar effect, the most common being anionic surfactants. Salt is sometimes added, or formed as a by-product during the preparation and isolation of surfactants and other formulation excipients. If there is an element of doubt as to the existence of chloride ions in a raw material for your mousse formulation, check with the manufacturer; it could save you a lot of time and headaches!

Because of their single-piece construction and simple elegance, aluminium containers with internal coatings are typically used for many mousse products, although there are exceptions. Disinfectant mousses and shave foams have been packaged in lined and unlined tinplate for years. The most common linings for aluminium containers are epoxy phenolic, organosol, and polyamide imide, although other linings including polyethylene are available. Each lining has specific characteristics, and this determines which applications are suitable. Epoxy phenolic and organosol linings are the most common and are approved by most regulatory bodies for food, personal care, and pharmaceutical product contact. Polyamide imide linings are relatively new to aluminium aerosol cans and may not be fully approved for these purposes but, unlike the epoxy phenolic and organosol linings, they are quite resilient to degradation in acidic solutions.

Tinplate aerosol cans are commonly manufactured as three separate components, the base, the dome, and the can wall. A gasket compound seals the base and dome where they join with the can wall. The only negative aspects to this type of can are that a lot of work is done to the individual components before and during the assembly, and some damage can occur in the tinplate and can lining during this process. Also, there are tiny pockets or crevices between the can rims and seam that can inhibit diffusion of product within the container. The consequence of this is that the pockets can act as centers for accelerated corrosion. This issue has been minimized recently, with a new two-piece steel can entering the international market. The potential for liquid phase crevice corrosion has been ameliorated, but it is still quite possible for crevice corrosion to occur in the vapor phase of the can. With the advent of new processing techniques, there is speculation that a single piece or monobloc steel can is not too far away. The two main advantages of tinplate cans are that they are cheaper than aluminium cans and are also magnetic. This latter feature enables tinplate cans to be transported through leak-testing baths on a magnetized conveyor rather than magnetic pucks having to be individually fitted.

TYPES OF MOUSSES

Emulsion Mousses

The use of an oil-in-water emulsion is a convenient starting point for the development of an aqueous aerosol mousse. An important consideration that must be addressed in the development of such a product is the ease with which the product's uniformity can be maintained before dispensing.

During the storage of an aerosol emulsion it is almost inevitable that some separation of the emulsion will occur. In some cases the separated layers will be low in viscosity and hence will be easily redispersed with minimal agitation. However, if the formulation contains excipients that are normally solids at room temperature, there is the possibility that these may crystallize during cold-temperature storage of the finished product. The consequences of this phenomenon are that the oil phase (or possibly water phase) could increase in viscosity to the extent that it is no longer possible to redisperse the separate phases with simple agitation. Crystals may also appear in either phase which, after redispersion is achieved, could potentially block the valve mechanism so that no product can be ejected, or alternatively, product is continually ejected after one actuation (i.e., valve does not cut off).

Shaving foams are a unique example of emulsion mousses in that they contain a very low level of nonvolatile components, yet possess remarkable stability and lubricating properties. A simple shaving foam composition can be prepared with only 5% by weight fatty acid salt, 5% by weight propellant, and the remaining 90% by weight of water. The lubricity of the foam can be enhanced by the addition of emollient oils, polymers, and humectants. In some instances, these can also improve the stability of the foam structure. The density of the foam can also be improved with the incorporation of additional fatty

TABLE 1   Aerosol Shave Foam*

CTFA Name	Function	%w/w
Water	Solvent	to 100%
Potassium hydroxide	pH adjuster	0.44
Triethanolamine	pH adjuster	2.98
Glycerin	Humectant	5.00
Polysorbate-20	Surfactant	1.00
Mineral oil	Emollient	1.50
Coconut acid	Surfactant	0.70
Stearic acid	Surfactant	8.00
Preservative	Preservative	q.s.
Fragrance	Fragrance	q.s.
Propane (and) butane (and) isobutane	Propellant	4.00

* Manufacturing Procedure: Add water, potassium hydroxide, triethanolamine, glycerin, and polysorbate 20 to main mixing vessel. Mix well
and heat to 75°C. In a separate vessel add mineral oil, coconut acid, and
stearic acid, heat to 75°C and mix until uniform. Add hot oil phase to
hot water phase while stirring. Continue stirring and cool to 45°C. Add
preservative and mix until dissolved. Add fragrance, stir until uniformly
dispersed. Correct for water loss, fill product into aerosol can and secure
valve. Add propellant through valve.
Abbreviations: CTFA, The Cosmetic, Toiletry, and Fragrance Association;
q.s., quantum sufficiat, quantum satis.

acid salt, nonionic surfactant, and/or water-soluble polymers. A typical shave foam formulation is given in Table 1.

Quick-Break Mousses

The description ''quick-break'' mousse is a vague term that may be defined by many
different parameters, but typically by physical stability and the inclusion of significant
quantities of an alcohol solvent. When the mousse is dispensed onto a substrate at a temperature below 32°C, it exists as a semisolid mass that can retain its structure for hours.
If the mousse is exposed to heat or shear, the foam structure is disrupted and the product
reverts to a low-viscosity liquid. These characteristics are valuable when developing ther-
mophobic skincare products.

A mousse of this type can exist as either a single- or multiple-phase system with
respect to the formulation packaged in a pressurized container. The single-phase system
typically contains a foaming agent, bodying agent, hydroethanolic solvent, and a hydrocarbon propellant. Without the propellant and below 32°C, the concentrate exists as a pasty
sludge. If the temperature of the concentrate is raised above 32°C the concentrate becomes
a clear, single-phase liquid. This is due to the nature of the solvent system, which has a
certain ethanol to water ratio to dissolve the bodying agent, but only when the temperature
exceeds 32°C. The temperature at which the foam breaks can be controlled by manipulat-
ing the ethanol to water ratio; to increase the melting point of the foam the water level
is increased. Similarly, to reduce the melting temperature of the foam the ethanol level
is increased. This is true if the bodying agent is ethanol-soluble in its own right.

TABLE 2 Quick-Break Mousse*

CTFA Name	Function	%w/w
Emulsifying wax	Surfactant/bodying agent	2.00
Alcohol	Solvent	58.06
Propylene glycol	Humectant	2.00
Water	Solvent	33.94
Propane (and) butane (and) isobutane	Propellant	4.00

* Manufacturing Procedure: Add emulsifying wax, alcohol, and propylene glycol to main mixing vessel. Heat to 35°C while stirring. Heat water in a separate vessel to 35°C. Add water to alcohol phase while stirring. Continue stirring until uniform. Fill product into aerosol can and secure valve. Add propellant through valve and cool to room temperature.
Abbreviation: CTFA, The Cosmetic, Toiletry, and Fragrance Association.

When the propellant is added, a ternary solvent system is established and the formulation reverts to a clear single-phase liquid. The advantage of this system is that, once filled, the product does not need to be shaken before use. We have used this to our advantage when developing skin-disinfectant products. The inverted pressurized container sits in a cradle and is actuated by pressing down on a lever to open the valve.

The single-phase, hydroethanolic quick-break mousse system has a low viscosity inside the pressurized container, which allows for rapid foam development during spraying. When the product is ejected from the can, a rapid change occurs as the propellant boils and diffuses to the surroundings. The pressurized liquid spontaneously foams and the bodying agent precipitates, leaving a crisp, white foam matrix. When the temperature of the foam is increased to 32°C the bodying agent, which has precipitated from the liquid to provide the foam structure, quickly redissolves and the foam begins to melt. Because of the nature of the formulation, the foam is destroyed as heat travels through the structure. A quick-break mousse vehicle is given in Table 2.

This type of formulation can be easily manufactured commercially as either a single phase which is filled warm (above the precipitation temperature of the bodying agent) or by cold-filling the alcohol and water phases separately. In the latter case, the bodying agent is precipitated from the alcohol phase as it mixes with the water. A clear, single-phase liquid forms in the aerosol container with the addition of the propellant.

Multiple-phase systems also require a foaming agent, bodying agent, solvent, and propellant to produce a quick-break foam. This type of formulation shares the characteristics of the emulsion mousse and is only different in the fact that the formulation is fine-tuned to give a foam structure that is more sensitive to heat and shear. Quick-break mousses of this type can be formulated using various approaches. Some of the more popular systems rely on an oil phase that liquefies at skin temperature, using an emulsion system that is inherently unstable, or by incorporating low levels of emulsion destabilizers such as silicone oils.

Hair-Setting Mousses

These are the most common mousse products in the marketplace. They have evolved significantly over the last 30 years and have reached a high level of consumer acceptance.

The formulations were originally based on single-phase, quick-break mousse systems, but because of the residue of bodying agents and surfactants left on the hair, other approaches were also explored. Modern hair-setting mousses rely on aqueous and aqueous ethanol solutions of hair-setting resins and surfactants for their functionality. The propellant usually remains as a separate phase and is readily dispersed in the concentrate with simple agitation of the aerosol container.

Ethanol is used in some hair-setting products at levels up to 20% w/w, and the benefits of this are twofold; first, the need to include a preservative is eliminated if ethanol is present above 10% w/w, and second, the resulting foam dries quicker when the product is applied. Another advantage of including ethanol in a formulation is that it allows fragrances and essential oils to be more effectively solubilized when a surfactant is present. A hair-setting mousse formulation containing tea tree oil is shown in Table 3.

The combination of hair-setting resin and surfactant serve to generate and support the foam structure. Quaternized polymers are included in some products to confer gentle setting properties and conditioning to hair, whereas acrylate or polyvinylpyrrolidone/vinyl acetate (PVP/VA) copolymers are used specifically for setting the hair and maintaining hold in humid conditions. There are numerous additives used in hair-setting mousses to impart sheen, color, and conditioning. Some examples include protein and lanolin derivatives, fragrances, essential oils, and herbal extracts. Many of these can be quite expensive and exotic, and are often present at subfunctional levels to support label claims.

TABLE 3 Hair-Setting Mousse with Tea Tree Oil*

CTFA Name	Function	%w/w
Tea tree (*Melaleuca alternifolia*) oil	Fragrance	1.000
Tocopherol	Antioxidant	0.002
Peg-40 hydrogenated castor oil	Surfactant	2.000
Alcohol	Solvent	20.000
30% Hydroxyethyl cetyldimonium phosphate	Hair conditioner	2.000
20% Polyquaternium-46	Hair conditioner/styling polymer	10.000
Ceteareth-25	Surfactant	0.200
Water	Solvent	54.798
Propane (and) butane (and) isobutane	Propellant	10.000

* Manufacturing Procedure: Add tea tree oil, tocopherol, peg-40 hydrogenated castor oil, and alcohol to main mixing vessel. Mix until a uniform solution is obtained. Add 30% hydroxyethyl cetyldimonium phosphate to main mixing vessel while stirring. Mix until uniform. Add 20% polyquaternium-46 to main mixing vessel while stirring. Mix until uniform. Add ceteareth-25 to main mixing vessel while stirring. Mix until uniform. Add water slowly to main mixing vessel while stirring. Mix until clear and uniform. Fill product into aerosol can and secure valve. Add propellant through valve.
Abbreviation: The Cosmetic, Toiletry, and Fragrance Association.

Postfoaming Mousses

Of the various mousse vehicles available to the formulator, one of the most interesting forms is the hybrid postfoaming mousse. This product is typically dispensed as a gel or cream into which the propellant has been previously emulsified or solubilized. When the gel or cream is rubbed onto warm skin the propellant (postfoaming agent) boils and the product starts foaming. The most notable example of this type of product is the postfoaming shave gel that is dispensed as a translucent, colored gel which expands into a creamy white foam during application.

Postfoaming products are packaged in barrier packages of which there are several variations. The first for mention is what we call a ''bag-in-can'' package. The ''bag'' is supported by the neck-roll of the aerosol container and the product is introduced directly into it. A valve (without diptube) is placed into position and secured to seal the container and hold the bag in place. An additional propellant (of higher pressure) is then injected into the cavity between the bag and the can wall through a bung in the base of the can— this provides the driving force to squeeze the product out of the bag when the valve is opened. The second type of barrier package, the ''pouch-on-valve,'' has a laminated pouch secured to the base of the valve. The pouch/valve combination is placed into an aerosol can and the space between the pouch and can wall is pressurized before securing the valve. Alternatively, propellant can be injected through a bung fitted to the can base or around the valve through a hole and flap arrangement after the product has been filled. The formulation is introduced through the valve into the pouch. The pressure within the aerosol can increases as the pouch is filled and the free volume diminishes. It is important to keep this in mind when prepressurizing this packaging arrangement with nonliquefiable propellants.

The postfoaming agent can be selected from a group of low–boiling point liquids such as butane, isobutane, pentane, isopentane, or hexane. The choice is made with the

TABLE 4   Postfoaming Shave Gel with Tea Tree Oil*

CTFA Name	Function	%w/w
Tea tree (*Melaleuca alternifolia*) oil	Fragrance	1.00
Peg-35 castor oil	Surfactant	10.00
50% Lauryl glucoside	Surfactant	40.00
Water	Solvent	to 100%
1% FD&C Blue No. 1	Colorant	0.10
Citric acid	pH adjuster	0.40
Preservative	Preservative	q.s.
Isopentane	Postfoaming agent	10.00

* Manufacturing Procedure: Add tea tree oil and peg-35 castor oil to main mixing vessel. Heat to 40°C and mix until uniform. Heat 50% lauryl glucoside to 40°C and add to main mixing vessel while stirring. Heat water to 40°C and add slowly to main mixing vessel while stirring. Continue stirring until uniform. Add 1% FD&C Blue No. 1 to main mixing vessel and stir until uniform. Add preservative to main mixing vessel and stir until dissolved. Cool contents of main mixing vessel and isopentane to 4°C. Add isopentane to main mixing vessel slowly while stirring. Continue stirring until uniform. Fill product into ''bag in can'' and secure valve in place. Pressurize container through bung in base with hydrocarbon propellant (pressure 30–40 psig at 21°C).
Abbreviations: CTFA, The Cosmetic, Toiletry, and Fragrance Association; q.s., quantum sufficiat, quantum satis.

product's intended use and its physical characteristics in mind. For a low-viscosity or thixotropic liquid, either the pentane(s) or hexane could be used, whereas for a high-viscosity cream or gel it may be necessary to use the butane(s) to get satisfactory expansion of the foam.

Because of the density difference between the postfoaming agent and the bulk aqueous phase, it is likely that some separation of the two phases will occur. This can be controlled with the use of thixotropic, water-soluble polymers (such as the carbomers or xanthan gum) alone, or in combination with suitable surfactants. Although most of the postfoaming shave products marketed today are based on neutralized fatty acids, it is possible to formulate totally nonionic products. An example of such a product containing Tea tree oil is shown in Table 4.

THE FUTURE OF MOUSSES

Although it is easy to describe the various characteristics and attributes of mousse products, it is difficult to entirely separate this technology from that of other product forms. There are obvious overlaps between mousse technology and the technologies pertinent to solutions, emulsions, and suspensions. The mousse product evolved from a combination of these overlaps as well as an appropriate type of packaging being available. The propellant can be considered simply as a low–boiling point excipient in the formulation. After grasping the ''contents under pressure'' concept, anyone competent in physical chemistry can successfully formulate a mousse product, although there is considerable ''art'' in formulating a product that is commercially successful.

The full potential of aerosol-mousse technology is only beginning to be exploited. Once only a form of presentation novelty, mousse formulations, where direct comparisons with ''conventional'' products have been made, are now showing important, relevant differentiators. Mousse products have in some instances shown to have better efficacy and consumer acceptance than nonaerosol formulations. Clinical studies [5,6] conducted on a scalp psoriasis-treatment mousse have shown greater clinical efficacy and patient acceptability than comparator products. The mousse product is also more likely to be used because it is effective, easy to apply, and well tolerated, thereby further increasing compliance and therapeutic efficacy. Furthermore, it has been shown [7] that an alcohol-based head-lice treatment mousse was able to exert ''a high level of direct ovicidal activity, making it effective with a single application.'' The mousse vehicle was shown to generate synergized pediculicide droplets that were small enough to penetrate the breathing pores of the louse egg shell cap and achieve a greater louse egg mortality than a commercial rinse product.

The various mousse categories previously described are by no means absolute. There are many new product forms in development that are unique in their own right. Microemulsion mousses are one such a vehicle that will offer the advantage of a single-phase system without the need for high levels of volatile organic compounds. Nonaerosol mousses have a presence in the marketplace and can be described simply as aqueous surfactant solutions. Solutions become aerated as liquid passes through a vented pump (or valve) mechanism of the dispenser and a foam with a shampoo-like consistency is formed. Facial cleansing and baby-wash products are suited to this type of mousse technology because of the wet nature of the foam.

Specialized mousse products continue to be developed for cosmetic and pharmaceutical markets, showing a willingness by consumers to try new and effective products. We are currently exploring new ways of using mousse technology to deliver active compounds to the skin for local and systemic use. Therapeutic mousse products for topical and transdermal administration of active compounds are already in the marketplace, and new vehicles are actively being developed. As more approaches to formulating mousse products are explored, greater possibilities are being realized. Products that are cosmetically elegant and efficacious will continue to evolve as more companies explore the possibilities and opportunities of mousse technology.

REFERENCES

1. Johnson Montfort A. The Aerosol Handbook. 2nd ed., Mendham, New Jersey: Wayne Dorland Company, 1982.
2. Balsam MS, Sagarin E, Gershon SD, Rieger MM, Strianse SJ. Cosmetics: Science and Technology. Vol. 1 and 2. 2nd ed., New York: Wiley-Interscience, 1972.
3. DeNavarre Maison G. The Chemistry and Manufacture of Cosmetics. Vol. 3 and 4. 2nd ed. Wheaton, Illinois: Allured Publishing, 1993.
4. Shaw Duncan J. Introduction to Colloid and Surface Chemistry. 4th ed. Oxford: Butterworth-Heinemann Ltd, 1992.
5. Evans Medical Limited, Regent Park, Leatherhead, U.K. Bettamousse Product Monograph, April, 1996.
6. Connetics Corporation. Press Release: Connetics Announces Positive Phase III Data For Novel Formulation of Scalp Psoriasis Treatment. August, 1997.
7. Burgess IF, Brown CM, Burgess NA. Synergised pyrethrin mousse, a new approach to head lice eradication: efficacy in field and laboratory studies. Clin Therapeutics 1994; 16(1):57–64.

20

Cosmetic Patches

Spiros A. Fotinos
Lavipharm, Peania Attica, Greece

GENERAL

The cosmetic patch is a new ''cosmetic form'' that is the result of the natural evolution of this technology in the pharmaceutical field. It appeared in the market just a few years ago, and although its applications are not too many for the time being, they have been already established as the new weapon to fight against the natural imperfections of our skin or to prevent the adverse reaction caused by environmental or other external influences. A broad spectrum of companies, including the major players, distribute at least one cosmetic-patch system. L'Oreal, Estee Lauder, Beiersdorf, Cheseborough-Ponds, Neutrogena, Lavipharm, as well as smaller manufacturers, participate in this special market.

HISTORY AND EVOLUTION

There is a close relation between topical pharmaceutical and cosmetic preparations. This relationship has its origin in the ancient years. Not only the forms (creams, ointments, solutions, liposomes, microemulsions), but also technologies and their production conditions are very close to each other. Under this rationale, the research and development of cosmetic patches started a few years ago. The influence of the pharmaceutical technology is apparent in the case of the cosmetic patches not as simple cosmetic forms but as cosmetic delivery systems. It is not the first time that such a thing has happened. Liposomes and microparticles, for example, had been transferred from other application fields to the pharmaceutical and later to the cosmetic technology fields with successful results. In Figures 1 and 2 we can see the similarities of these two categories regarding the Conventional forms as well as their delivery systems.

Cosmetic patches today, although at the beginning of their evolution and having weaknesses in some cases, represent a convenient, simple, easy, safe, and effective way for cosmetic applications, using one of the most acceptable, modern, and successful delivery technology.

BORDERS BETWEEN PHARMACEUTICAL AND COSMETIC PATCHES

By definition, cosmetic products cannot be used or claimed for the therapy of diseases. Sometimes the companies use claims exceeding the borders between pharmaceutical and

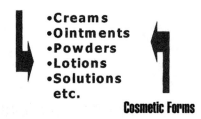

Pharmaceuticals

- **Creams**
- **Ointments**
- **Powders**
- **Lotions**
- **Solutions**
  etc.

Cosmetic Forms

FIGURE 1 Dosage forms "equivalent" for cosmetics and pharmaceuticals.

cosmetic application because the line is very thin between these major classes and/or in the past it was easier to use such terms. The patches could not be the exception to the rule.

Some patches that stand between drug and cosmetic fields, e.g., acne or acneic conditions, are included in this category, and as we will see later, in some countries the actives combining with the claims characterize the classification, although in others products like these are considered to be real cosmetics. We could synopsize some simple rules to draw a bold line between these two classes:

1. Cosmetic patches are not pharmaceutical patches (the same way cosmetic creams are not pharmaceutical creams).
2. Cosmetic patches are designed for cosmetic applications.
3. Cosmetic patches contain cosmetic ingredients only (at concentrations allowed for cosmetic applications).
4. Cosmetic claims have to be confirmed via cosmetic efficacy tests.
5. Additional tests, patch specific, have to be established for cosmetic patches (e.g., peel force, wearing tests, residual solvents).
6. Safety first and efficacy second have to characterize these new forms.

APPLICATIONS OF COSMETIC PATCHES

In theory, cosmetic patches can be applied in most cases for the same use as classical cosmetic products, e.g., wrinkles, aging, dark rings under the eyes, acneic conditions, hydration of specific areas, spider veins, looseness, and slimming. In practice, several of

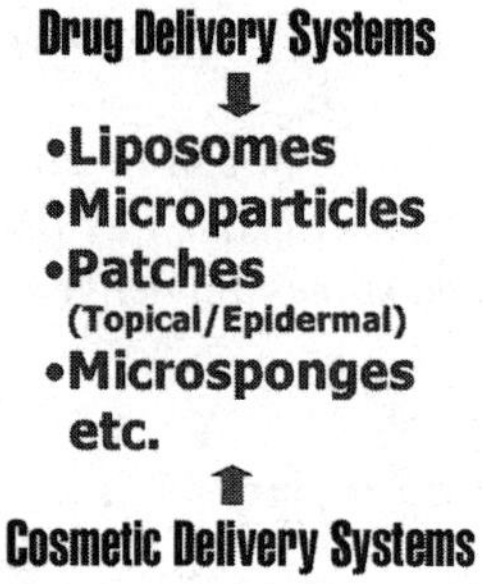

Drug Delivery Systems

- **Liposomes**
- **Microparticles**
- **Patches**
  (Topical/Epidermal)
- **Microsponges**
  etc.

Cosmetic Delivery Systems

FIGURE 2 Delivery systems "equivalent" for cosmetics and pharmaceuticals.

the aforementioned applications have been investigated, with very positive results and a high degree of acceptability from the consumers. The role of the specific form is not to cannibalize or to fully substitute the existing cosmetic forms. The main mission is to provide a breakthrough proposition for the cosmetic category as problem solvers. Someone could compare the cosmetic patches' role with the one of pharmaceutical patches. Where applicable and feasible, the pharmaceutical patches have almost substituted the classical forms because of their superiority over the conventional forms. But they did it because of, e.g., the convenience, better efficacy, less side effects, and the lessened need for use. On the other hand, they never substituted all the existing pharmaceutical forms, each one of which plays its own important role.

We could synopsize by saying that cosmetic patches are destined mainly as problem-solver cosmetic forms, i.e., they are more effective and efficient products with an absolutely and strictly localized action. Applied on the specific site, they limit their action on the specific area (acting topically), protecting at the same time the site and the active(s) itself.

DIFFERENCES BETWEEN CLASSICAL COSMETIC FORMS AND PATCHES

It is known that from the moment classical cosmetics (creams, lotions, etc.) are applied to the skin, they start changing continuously. The air, atmosphere's pollution, humid or dry environment, dust, and anything that can be transferred with it as well as any other factors alter the composition and the form of the product, which results in significant changes to the product's action. Patches, on the other hand, are systems of occlusion even if there is sometimes the need, and we have the possibility, to manufacture breathable or porous patches. Because of this, permeation is getting easier, interactions with the environment are being considerably reduced, and we can expect a more "accurate" and "controlled" overall result.

Using the term "permeation," we mean the possibility that is given to several substances to reach the site of action, without of course confusing this term with the capability of a pharmaceutical patch to introduce the therapeutic substances into the systemic circulation at therapeutic levels. In many cases, this permeation makes the difference between an effective and noneffective form of administration of a cosmetic "active."

DEVELOPMENT OF COSMETIC PATCHES

All of the aforementioned pluses concern "good" cosmetic patches. As always happens with the new trends and the products following them, the low level of knowledge and experience guides several organizations to launch products without proofs of the required quality. As you will find later in the text, cosmetic patches are not pieces of Scotch tape containing one or a combination of cosmetic actives. On the contrary, it has to be an "extremely safe and effective scientific product." As such a product it has to be supported with all the safety and efficacy proofs required.

As a new form or better delivery system, a cosmetic patch requires additional tests not applicable on conventional cosmetic products. Because of the occlusive or semiocclusive character, these patches require a different level of investigation concerning the percentages of the ingredients, the compatibility with the skin, the possible amplified dermal reactions, and so on. Only special people and companies can formulate cosmetic patches. First, what is required is the full and perfect knowledge of the patch technology combined with the same level of knowledge and experience of the cosmetically acceptable ingredients and synergistically acting combinations. Until now, the experience on the patch technology used to be a monopoly of the scientists in the pharmaceutical field. The scientists in the specific pharmaceutical field know very well the correlation between active ingredient and therapy. They used a specific active to treat a specific illness or symptom. Cosmetic technology is "philosophically" different. Although in recent years there have been cosmetically active ingredients with a specific action, conventional cosmetic products use several components, and it is often difficult to make the distinction between "active" and "excipients." At the same time, because there are not real actives as we mean them in the pharmaceutical terminology or the regulations and we cannot use high concentrations of these actives, the cosmetic formulator is obliged to use, in most cases, "its own cocktail" of "cosmetic actives" to achieve the expected result. This is a big conceptual difference between the two types of formulators; the pharmaceutical and the cosmetic. This situation is also going to follow the cosmetic patches formulation. It is expected that several "cocktails of synergistically correct combinations" will play the role of the actives included in the pharmaceutical patches. It is obvious that the case of the cosmetic patch development and the required background cannot be found easily.

TYPES AND CONFIGURATION

There are several ways to describe and categorize a cosmetic patch. It can be characterized from the patch form (e.g., matrix, reservoir), the application purpose and the expected result (e.g., moisturising, anti-wrinkle), the type of its structural materials (synthetic, natural, hybrid), the duration of application (e.g., overnight patch, half-hour patch). Cosmetic marketing is always more inventive in finding attractive terms to characterize a cosmetic product, but even scientifically there is better flexibility regarding the terminology. In practice this category of patches covers the entire field, starting from the small or larger patch-like "facial masques" and finish to the cosmetic patches similar to their pharmaceutical cousins. In between, we can position some patch-like products, or strips for the removal of blackheads from the nose or other problematic areas of the face, or for the stretching of the skin. Another way to classify cosmetic patches is the duration of application, the action, and so on. Table 1 presents a different classification:

Regarding the flexibility of cosmetic patches, Figure 3 shows several and numerous combinations concerning applications as problem solvers, shape, ingredients, and site, among others.

Table 2 presents a "map" of cosmetic patches, covering a big part of their world.

It is obvious from all these examples of cosmetic patches that most are designed

TABLE 1 Examples of Cosmetic Patch Categories

Pore Cleansers
Blackhead removers
Stretching stripes
Short-term patch-like masks
Short-term treatment patches
Overnight treatment patches

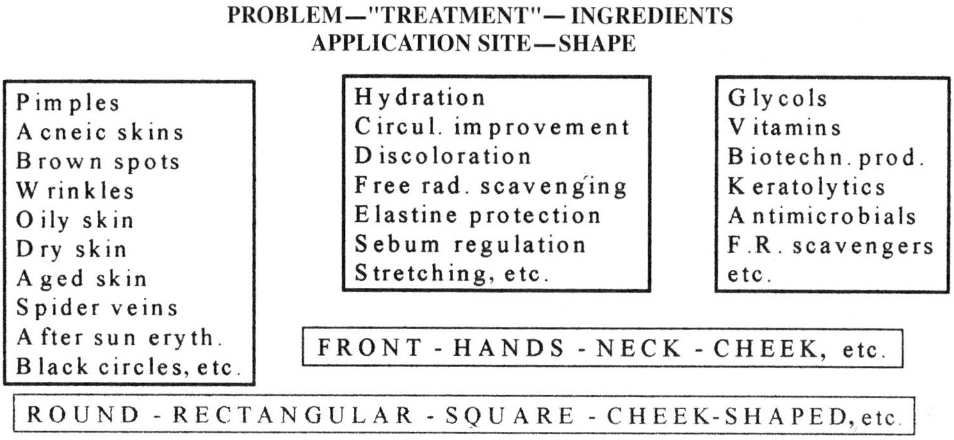

PROBLEM—"TREATMENT"— INGREDIENTS
APPLICATION SITE—SHAPE

Pimples Acneic skins Brown spots Wrinkles Oily skin Dry skin Aged skin Spider veins After sun eryth. Black circles, etc.	Hydration Circul. improvement Discoloration Free rad. scavenging Elastine protection Sebum regulation Stretching, etc.	Glycols Vitamins Biotechn. prod. Keratolytics Antimicrobials F.R. scavengers etc.

FRONT - HANDS - NECK - CHEEK, etc.

ROUND - RECTANGULAR - SQUARE - CHEEK-SHAPED, etc.

FIGURE 3 Versatility of use and applications for cosmetic patches.

TABLE 2 Categories of Functional Cosmetic Patches

Antiblemish Patch
An extremely popular, very small and thin patch for the treatment of pimples and blemishes. Contains a balanced percentage of salicylic acid, anti-irritant, and antimicrobial agents.

Pore Cleansers
Very popular patches applied to the nose; their role is to clean pores and remove sebum plugs.

Pimple Patch
A relatively large and thick patch for the care of pimples and blemishes.

Eye-Contour Patch
Mixture of several beneficial active ingredients for the fast relief of the area under the eyes after a short-term treatment (e.g., half hour).

Antiaging Patch
One of the first cosmetic patches developed and sold. It bases its claims on ascorbic acid contained in the adhesive. Several similar patches have been developed.

Antiwrinkle Patch
Based mainly on the antioxidant action of Vitamin C, as with the antiaging patch, this patch set is suggested for the prevention and treatment of wrinkles.

Lifting Patch
Based on a mixture of glycolic acid, proteins, vitamins, and plant extracts, this large patch is used for the treatment of wrinkles of the neck.

Slimming patch
Thin and transparent, this patch contains a mixture of natural extracts (Fucus vesiculosus, Ginkgo biloba, etc.) and claims a slimming effect.

according to the principle of the matrix patch. This type of patch is thin, has a light weight, has a reasonable production cost, and represents the trend in our days.

STRUCTURAL COMPONENTS OF THE COSMETIC PATCHES

Generally speaking, a matrix patch is composed of three discreet layers:

- The backing film
- The adhesive layer
- The release liner

A matrix patch has the form shown in Figure 4.

Backing Film

The backing film is one of the three layers of a matrix patch. It is the layer that is apparent after the adhesion of the patch on the specific site of the skin. Its main role is to protect the adhesive layer from the influence of external factors; it also provides such characteristics as flexibility, occlusivity, breathability, and printability. Several materials have been used as backing films. The selection of a specific film for use in a cosmetic patch may depend on the following factors:

- Cost
- Stability
- Printability
- Machinability
- Glossy or matte appearance
- Compatibility
- Anchorage to the adhesive
- Transparency
- Opacity
- Occlusivity
- Breathability

Several materials can be used for these purposes depending on the needs already presented.

One of the first and cheapest cosmetic patches used a simple paper layer.

Most of the pore cleansers use nonwoven materials. The reason is obvious: all these systems require wetting the nose before application of the patch. It means that the system has to dry out in order to be able to remove the sebum plugs that stick to the dried layer.

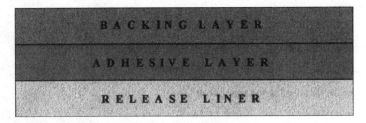

FIGURE 4   Typical structure of a matrix-type patch.

Polyethylene or polyester films are used also in most systems. They do not need to dry out after the application. Sometimes the film used is nontransparent. A white, foamy material is the backing layer of the pimple patch.

In some cases, other more expensive materials have also been tested, such as polyurethane, chlorinated polyethylenes, nylon, and saran. It is very important that the materials used as backing films for cosmetic patches have the same quality specifications with the similar films used for pharmaceutical patches to avoid any adverse reactions of the skin.

Release Liners

The main role of this layer is to protect the product, especially the adhesive layer, before the use of the product. The pharmaceutical patch development has provided a long list of release liners that can be useful for cosmetic patches as well. There are three main classes of release liners according to their composition:

1. Paper based: Glassine paper, densified Kraft super-calendered paper, clay-coated paper, polyolefine coated paper, etc.
2. Plastic based: Polystyrene, polyester (plain, metallicized), polyethylene (low and high density), cast polypropylene, polyvinyl chloride, etc.
3. Composite material based on the combination of several films

All these materials have a common characteristic: one release layer coated on one or both sides depending on the needs of the product and the system itself. This coating is, generally speaking, silicon or polyfluorocarbon. The grade, thickness, coating, and curing methods vary according to the materials and the satisfaction of specific needs.

As mentioned for backing films, this layer has to be compatible with the components of the adhesive layer and should satisfy the specific needs of the product. Sometimes this layer has to be, e.g., printed, scored, perforated, or tinted. The selection of the material and the grade are dictated from similar factors to the ones influencing the selection of the backing layer.

Adhesive Layer

This is the most important layer of a matrix cosmetic patch. The adhesive layer contains not only the adhesive that makes the patch stick to the skin, but in most of cases the cosmetic active ingredients and the additives required for correct formulation of a cosmetic product. Starting with the adhesive itself, the majority of adhesives used in cosmetic patches are taken from the general category of pressure-sensitive adhesives (PSAs). This is a class of adhesives used in several applications, and in all pharmaceutical patches. As its name shows, PSAs are adhesives which, in their solvent free form, remain permanently tacky and stick to the skin with the application of very slight pressure. There are three groups of PSAs: 1) acrylics, 2) silicones, and 3) rubbers. There are numerous members in the three main families of PSAs, but only few can be used for the formulation of cosmetic patches. The reason is that as also happens with pharmaceutical patches, there are so many restrictions on the selection of an adhesive that the useful members are relatively few. The limitations are governed by the mechanical and biomedical properties of the adhesive, as well as the characteristics of compatibility, reactivity, and stability.

The components of the adhesive are also governed by such properties as, solvents, monomers, cross-linkers, and emulsifiers.

There is also another category of cosmetic patches with similar structure, but formulated with a dry-adhesive system other than PSA. In this class we can bring the example of pore cleansers. Here the adhesive layer is created in situ, by wetting the dry adhesive layer with water the same way we stick a stamp on a letter. The components included in the composition of dry adhesives can be found in the classes of synthetic or natural derivatives, e.g., polyvinyl derivatives, starches, celluloses, and sugars.

Pouching Materials

Although this material is not a component of cosmetic patches, its importance for the integrity of the product during its shelf life makes us examine it just after the basic patch components. Almost all cosmetic patches as happens with the pharmaceutical ones, are pouched in pouches. For pharmaceutical patches, the rule is to package one patch in one pouch. With the cosmetic analogues, and in an effort to reduce cost, sometimes patches can be found in the same pouch for more than one application. In this case, it is recommended that the product has stability information for the time interval between the opening of the pouch and the use of the last patch, as well as to foresee some kind of resealable pouch. The materials used for the two categories are similar or the same. One of the differences is the number of packaged patches in one pouch. The protection of the product is the main mission of this packaging material, the role of which is critical for long-term stability of the product.

The pouching material, as has been mentioned, influences a lot of the stability of some sensitive molecules. Sometimes the phenomena of adsorption are noticed because of the affinity of some ingredients with the internal, sealable layer of the pouching laminate. In this case, e.g., AHAs can escape from the adhesive layer and, passing the edge, can be absorbed from the ionomers plastic film of the pouching material. Another protection the pouching material provides is protection from UV radiation by using at least one opaque layer in case of light-sensitive materials, along with protection from oxygen.

Production

The production of cosmetic patches depends on the type of patch, the component characteristics, and the overall configuration of the final product. Because most cosmetic patches are matrix patches, it is useful to follow the general steps of typical production concerning this type of patch. Practically, production starts from the weighing of raw materials and other components, and ends with packaging of the product in the final carton. It is not within the scope of this chapter to go into details in this field, but we can mention the basic steps of the production sequence. Some information is required regarding the critical steps of production, or better the steps that could influence the quality of the product itself. The mixing of cosmetic ingredients and adhesives has to take place under a very slight nitrogen atmosphere (pressure) to avoid oxidation of the ingredients during this phase, but not too high (to avoid inclusion of nitrogen in the mass of the mixture and bubble formation during the drying cycle). Drying is also a critical step because, during this process, the temperature of the coating goes up and the ingredients have to be stable at these conditions. During drying, some of the ingredients are evaporated and/or sublimated. An accurate validated process has to be defined to finally take the patch as it had been designed. The exposure to light has to be limited as well, and the web has to be protected and kept in the predefined conditions before packaging. Of course, all the technology for production of pharmaceutical patches is applicable, but found outside the scope of this chapter.

PRODUCTION STEPS

Production of Casting Solution

This involves the mixing of active ingredient(s), additive(s), and other adjuvants, in the mass of the adhesive in the appropriate size and design production vessel and in the appropriate space.

The bulk could be a solvent or waterborn system, and the basic steps are as follows:

- Weighing
- Mixing
- Deaeration
- Release
- Filtration and transfer to pressure vessel
- Final bulk release

Coating—Drying—Lamination

The casting solution is prepared, released, coated, dried, laminated, and formed to the final rolls according to the specific standard operating procedures (SOPs), and the production records as follows:

- Feeding of the dosing pump, and through this the coating station
- Casting on the release film
- Drying of the coated solution passing through the drying tunnel
- Continuous thickness control and recording
- Lamination with the backing material
- Winding in rolls
- Splitting of the rolls
- Quarantine
- Final control
- Release

Packaging

The process involved in packaging is described as follows:

- Roll feeding
- Punching
- Pouching
- Cartoning
- Boxing

REGULATORY ISSUES

As always happens with new forms, there is some confusion regarding the regulatory status of cosmetic patches. The main reason is that cosmetic patches are not included, for the time being, in the approved forms of cosmetic preparations. Considering the Directive 76/768/EEC, August 1993, which is the official regulation of cosmetic products in the

European Union, a cosmetic product "shall mean any substance or preparation intended to be placed in contact with the various external parts of the human body (epidermis, hair system, nails, lips and external genital organs) or with the teeth and the mucous membranes of the oral cavity with a view exclusively or mainly to cleaning them, perfuming them, changing their appearance and/or correcting body odours or/and protecting them or keeping them in good condition." According to this definition, cosmetic patches, acting similarly to conventional cosmetics, are included with cosmetic products. The confusion starts from paragraph 2 of the same article, stating that; "The products to be considered as cosmetic products within the meaning of this definition are listed in Annex I." In Annex I are included all the conventional forms, but not patches because, at the time of issuing, patches did not exist. So, because cosmetic patches conceptually, according to the cosmetic definition, comply with it, and because cosmetic patches are reality in our days, Annex I has to be revised with the addition of this new category.

Another reason for this confusion is the common origin of patches and transdermal systems. As previously mentioned before, all transdermals are not patches and all patches are not transdermals.

It is true that the first patches were dedicated to transdermal delivery of actives. At the same time, it is true and correct that not all transdermal systems are patches and that not all patches are by definition transdermals. We have the case of Nitro-Bid ointment for the transdermal delivery of nitroglycerin, but at the same time we have "patches" stuck to the skin for diagnostic purposes or for delivering the active to the opposite direction, e.g., to the air to repel mosquitoes or for the topical treatment of pain.

To achieve transdermal delivery and effectiveness, several other factors are required:

- the intrinsic properties of the molecule,
- its concentration in the system,
- the appropriate permeation enhancers,
- the application site,
- the surface area;

and other factors play a very significant role in

- the rate and extent of absorption,
- the ability of the specific active to reach the blood stream, and
- its efficacy and toxicity.

Without forgetting the peculiarity of cosmetic patches as cosmetic delivery systems or forms, we could propose that this new system not be encountered with scepticism and to follow the rules governing other cosmetic preparation. It means that the composition of the formula qualitatively and quantitatively has to follow existing cosmetic regulations, followed by specific tests and controls required especially for patches (e.g., residual solvents, adhesion on the steel, wearability), as well as tests regarding the safety parameters of an occlusive or semiocclusive system.

FUTURE TRENDS

The evolution of cosmetic patches is something expected after the warm acceptance of new cosmetic delivery systems from consumers. There are three axes for their expansion:

1. **The technological field**. It is expected that any new progress on patches, generally speaking, will strongly influence cosmetic patches as well. Even nonpassive cosmetic patches, like the iontophoretic ones, will find in the future several applications for the administration of more sophisticated cosmetic ingredients and actives.

2. **The applications**. For the time being, the applications of cosmetic patches cover a small part of the overall cosmetic applications. It is expected in the future to have a coverage of almost the whole spectrum of cosmetic applications.

3. **The ingredients**. The cosmetic patches, as previously explained, need to present a more potent solution for the cosmetic treatment of skin problems. For this reason, there is the need for the use of very potent ingredients or extracts, that are probably especially designed for the patches in order to achieve a very fast and effective action.

21

Antibacterial Agents and Preservatives

Françoise Siquet
Colgate-Palmolive Technology Center, Milmort, Belgium

Michel J. Devleeschouwer
Free University of Brussels, Brussels, Belgium

INTRODUCTION

The term "antibacterial agent" is largely used to qualify chemical agents that are included in cosmetics or household products to provide them either with a specific bactericidal or bacteriostatic activity during usage. The second function of antibacterial chemicals is to protect the product during its life by providing a preservative efficacy against microbial insults. A particular chemical agent can be used as an active ingredient in antibacterial product or as a preservative to protect the formula from microbial contamination. Taking into account that not only bacteria but also fungi or yeast can be concerned, to cover all germs simultaneously the word "antimicrobial" will be used.

Historically, the first antibacterial products developed were skinwash products such as soap bars, derived from deodorant soap bars. The purpose was not only to clean the skin but also to reduce its microbial flora [1]. During the last 20 years, many different antibacterial or antimicrobial products were marketed. They include toothpastes and mouthwashes, liquid antibacterial soaps, deodorants, and even antibacterial products for dishwashing.

The first part of this chapter will review the different kinds of antibacterial products and the methods to show their efficacy.

The purpose of preservation is to protect all aspects of a product against microbial attack before and during consumer use. Integrity of products in terms of efficacy, fragrance, appearance, and stability must be maintained. The second part of this chapter will review the preservative systems and how to build a well-preserved formula. The test methods for preservative efficacy can be found in Chapter 64 of this book.

ANTIBACTERIAL PRODUCTS

Topical Antimicrobial Products

Most antibacterial soap bars contain triclocarban (TCC) as the active ingredient. In the past, antibacterial soap bars were also formulated with formaldehyde. These were very effective for hospital use, but skin toxicity and irritation were very high. Currently, liquid soaps are formulated with triclosan up to 1% maximum. Safety of the regular use of triclocarban and triclosan in hand-washing products was extensively discussed by the Food and Drug Administration (FDA) [1]. The agency prepared a tentative final monograph in 1994 in which topical antimicrobial products were classified in the following categories: 1) antiseptic handwash or healthcare personnel handwash, 2) patient presurgical skin preparation, and 3) surgical hand scrub. But this meant that products intended to be used in homecare would have to meet the requirements of products for healthcare. In response, two industrial associations, The Cosmetics, Toiletry, and Fragrance Association (CTFA) and the Soap and Detergent Association (SDA), proposed another classification, based on a healthcare continuum model (HCCM) in which the antimicrobial products were related to six categories; two to be used by the general population (antimicrobial handwashes and bodywashes), three for use by healthcare professionals (presurgical preparation, surgical scrubs, and healthcare personnel handwashes), and one category for food handlers. Since then, industry has submitted data to the FDA showing the efficacy of active ingredients used in the six categories; among these ingredients are triclosan, triclocarban, chloroxylenol (PCMX), povidone-iodine, surfactant iodophor, alcohol, and quaternary ammonium compounds [2].

Extensive studies have also been carried out with essential oils as antibacterial agents in soaps. Unfortunately, the data showed that the minimal inhibitory concentration (MIC) for antimicrobial soaps formulated with different essential oils were more than 100 times higher that the MIC obtained on TCC-based soaps when tested against *Staphylococcus aureus* [3].

Deodorants and Antiperspirants

The first antiperspirants appeared on the market at the beginning of the 20th century. They were based on aluminium chloride, which induced skin irritation and fabric damage because of the low pH of the solutions [4]. Several years later, Shelley and colleagues showed that underarm odor was provoked by the growth of the axillae bacterial flora which degraded the apocrine secretions [5]. These bacteria are mainly staphylococci (*S. epidermidis*) and diphteroids from the Corynebacteriaceae family. Antiperspirants can prevent the growth of these degrading bacteria by reducing the available moisture of the axillaries among other mechanisms (see Chap. 56). Some products used the hexaclorophene as an active but its use was discontinued because of its neurotoxic properties [6]. Currently, many contain aluminium salts, or zirconium-aluminium combinations such as Al-Zi-Tri-/ tetra-chlorydrex glycinate as active ingredients. Their low pH (4.0) also helps the antibacterial activity. Antiperspirants are deodorants because they suppress the odor source by reducing perspiration and bacterial growth. Deodorants may or may not have an antimicrobial action; either they are masking products—in this case they contain perfumes or essential oils that hide the odor—or they can contain antibacterial agents which are mainly alcohols and triclosan [6].

Oral Care Products

These are mainly toothpastes and mouthrinses. In general, dental creams serve to clean the teeth, to remove dental stains, and most recently to reduce and/or to prevent gingivitis and to kill the germs responsible for bad mouth odor. Mouthrinses, whether their recommended use is before or after brushing, are also claimed to sanitize the mouth.

Active ingredients used in dental cream are mainly triclosan and chlorexhidine. Other ingredients such as the natural sanguinarine extract also claim a sanitizing effect on the oral flora. The same ingredients can be used in mouthrinses, but most also contain alcohol to ensure a good antiseptic effect of the product. It is interesting to observe that fluorinated dental creams without any specific active ingredient also exhibit antimicrobial activity [7]. This could be related to their fluoride content which, in association with the surfactant system in the formula, release antibacterial active cationic systems.

Dishwashing Products

Among the antibacterial household products that have recently appeared on the market, antibacterial hand dishwashing liquids have become increasingly popular. Even if these products are not true cosmetics, during the dishwashing, they are in direct contact with the skin for a certain time. From a safety point of view, they can be considered as rinse-off cosmetics.

Furthermore, some products on the market have a double claim: "dishwashing liquid and antibacterial liquid soap." They are classical dish liquids based on anionic and non-ionic surfactants, to which one or more antibacterial agents have been introduced. Some of these formula have been optimized to maintain their cleaning/degreasing performance on dishes and to fight bacteria on the hands, in the washing solution, and on washing implements. Ingredients used can be Triclosan, essential oils, or others. The use levels are chosen to ensure a good balance between a maximum efficacy, a low skin toxicity, and keeping good cleaning performances.

Methods to Show Antimicrobial Product Efficacy

In vitro and in vivo tests can be used to show the efficacy of antimicrobial products. Only the in vitro tests will be considered here because they are applicable to all antibacterial products. A detailed review of the in vivo tests, useful for topical antibacterials, can be found in Ref. 1.

—*The minimal inhibitory concentration (MIC) test* principle is to determine the MIC of the test product by performing serial dilutions of the latter in growth medium and inoculating each dilution with the test strain. Products are generally tested at twofold serial dilutions. After suitable incubation, the first tube not exhibiting bacterial growth gives the MIC level, generally expressed in ppm (part per million) of product. The test can be carried out using either 2 mL of broth in tubes or 0.5 to 0.1 mL, in microtiter plates [8] or on agar plates. Control samples without any antimicrobials must be included in the test. This test is very useful to compare activities of different products, products from the same category (e.g., soaps) with different actives, or the active ingredients themselves. However, MIC data obtained on formulated products are very subjective and should be interpreted carefully. Usually, test organisms are *Staphylococcus aureus*, *Staphylococcus epidermidis*, and *Escherichia coli*, for topical antimicrobial. *Pseudomonas aeruginosa* and *Salmonella typhimurium* are added for the dishwashing products; for specific claims in the kitchen, *Aspergillus niger* and *Candida albicans* can be used as test strains. To test oral care products, the chosen organisms are *Actynomyces viscosus*, *Streptococcus mutans*, and *Streptococcus sanguis*, representatives of the oral flora [7].

—*The zone inhibition test* method is largely used to test the resistance of bacteria to antibiotics [9]. Antibacterial agents or products at different concentrations are applied to a substrate, a paper disk, or directly to the surface of an agar plate previously seeded with the test bacteria. During the incubation, the test product will diffuse into the agar layer and produce a zone of growth inhibition of the micro-organism. The larger the inhibition zone, the higher the efficacy of the product. However, the data are influenced by the diffusion capacity of the product or the active into the agar; oily products will not diffuse at the same rate as aqueous-based products. It is thus very important to use negative and positive controls. The data will be expressed in millimeters of inhibition zone around the disk. The strains used for this test are usually the same that those used for the MIC test. These two methods give a good idea of the bacteriostatic concentrations of the tested product or ingredient.

The requirements from the FDA monograph of 1994 [10] are the MIC test on the active ingredient, the vehicle, and the final formula, associated with a time-kill test methodology to be carried out at several time points over a period of 30 minutes.

—*The time-kill test* determines both the killing kinetics and the activity spectrum of antibacterial formulations. This test is generally performed in suspension. The principle is to place in contact a dilution of the product or the antibacterial agent and a specified bacterial inoculum during a defined period of time. At the end of the contact time, the antibacterial in the mixture is inactivated by dilution into neutralizing broth. Serial dilutions in appropriate broth are performed and the number of survival bacteria enumerated on solid culture media. This method can use different concentrations of test agents and bacterial inocula, and different contact times. In general, the concentrations are chosen so that the final organism/test solution concentration is representative of the use concentration of the product.

In the United States, there is no detailed standardized time-kill test, even if the U.S. Food and Drug Administration (FDA) requested a standard procedure [10]. In response, the American Society For Testing and Materials (ASTM) subcommittee of antimicrobial agents has prepared a draft to standardize the organism inocula, media, neutralizers, and contact times [11].

In Europe, the situation is different: to test the antimicrobial efficacy of products and/or agents, standards exist since more than 20 years in France [12], Holland, Germany, and the United Kingdom. Recently, the Council of Europe has installed a Commission for the Normalization of European Norms [13], which is writing and publishing the European Norms (EN) for testing disinfectants and antiseptics. The requirements for disinfection are 99.99% to 99.999% of killing (4 to 5 log reductions) of the initial inoculum, depending on the test.

These norms are also used by the industry to prove the efficacy of their antibacterial products, but the requirements are less strict: 99 to 99.9% killing (2–3 log reduction). Detailed review of the ENs can be found in Ref. 14.

PRESERVATION AND PRESERVATIVE SYSTEMS

Concept of Active Preservation and Self-Preserving Formula

To ensure effective preservation, the method of choice is to add one or more active antimicrobial ingredients to the product. These ingredients must be compatible with the other ingredients of the formula and must retain efficacy for an extended period of time. They also have to be nontoxic for the consumer.

To choose an active antimicrobial molecule as preservative is not so easy; this molecule must have a good oil-water partition coefficient because the contaminating microbes are living in the aqueous phase of the formula. It must not be inactivated by external factors such as the pH and the manufacturing process [15]. Other factors also have to be considered; such as the packaging, which could affect the preservative activity, the adsorption rate on some components of the formula, the solubility of the preservative molecule and its volatility [15].

Furthermore, the inactivation of the micro-organisms by the preservative should be sufficiently fast to prevent any adaptation or resistance to the preservative system [16]. So, the ideal preservative system must be selected for each formula, taking into account the possible inactivating ingredients or the potentiation capacity of other ingredients. Among these, ethylenediaminetetra-acetic acid (EDTA) is well known to act in synergy with many other chemical preservatives. This potentiation is delivered through the permeation of the cell membrane of gram-negative bacteria. EDTA is a chelating agent and disrupts the outer lipid layer where stability is calcium and magnesium ion dependent. As such, it increases the penetration of the other antimicrobial chemical into the bacterial cell [17,18]. In general, liquid- and emulsion-based cosmetic products are the most susceptible to the development of micro-organisms. Powdered products, such as talc, are also susceptible to contamination and need to be preserved [19].

Another way to preserve a product is to build a ''self-preserved'' formula by using raw materials that are not supporting germ growing and optimizing their relative content. The use of humectants such as glycerin or sorbitol at a sufficient level increases the formula resistance. In a dental cream, a mixture of sorbitol and glycerine, at respective levels of 10% and 12%, is often enough to protect the formula. This is linked to the decrease of the water activity in the formula because of the presence of these humectants [20]. Other ingredients, such as alcohols, cationic detergents, fragrance components, and lipophilic acids (lauric and myristic acids) used as emulsifiers, which have intrinsically antibacterial properties, can contribute to the self-preservation of a cosmetic. This is also true for essential oils like tea tree oil or geraniol or eucalyptol, often used as cosmetic ingredients.

Some physical factors, such as the pH and the formula water activity, can also contribute to build a self-preserved product. Micro-organisms are essentially living at pH of around 5 to 8, and any pH outside this range induces difficult life conditions for bacteria. The water activity or availability is an important factor as the water is a necessary ingredient for bacterial growth. The water availability concept is detailed in Chapter 64 of this book.

Most Commonly Used Preservatives

Table 1 lists the most commonly used chemicals to preserve cosmetic products. Attention must be paid to the regulations; in Europe, the Annex VI of the Cosmetic Directive 79/ 768 lists the chemicals, permanently and provisionally allowed to be used as preservatives in the cosmetic products. For each of them, there is an upper concentration use limit, and for several of them, restrictions are mentioned [21]. In the United States, the use of preservative molecules is regulated by the FDA. The chemical preservatives are too numerous to be listed here; details on preservatives can be found in Ref. 22. These molecules can be used in synergistic mixtures to improve the activity spectrum. For example, the parabens can be used with the imidazolydinil urea, the formaldehyde can be used with

TABLE 1 Most Commonly Used Preservatives

Preservative name	Activity spectrum	Compatible with:	Inactivated by:	Optimum pH
Parabens: esters of benzoic acid	fungi, gram+	cationic	anionic, nonionic, proteins	<7
Imidazolydinil urea Diazolydinil urea	broad, weak against fungi	anionic, nonionic cationic, proteins		4–9
Isothiazolones	broad	anionic, nonionic cationic	bleach, high pH	4–8
Formaldehyde DMDM hydantoin	broad	anionic, nonionic cationic	T° > 60°C	4–9
Benzalkonium Cl	gram+, gram−, weak against molds	nonionic, cationic	anionic, proteins, soaps	4–9
2-bromo-2-nitropropanel, 3-diol	broad	anionic, nonionic cationic	heat, high pH, cysteine, aluminum	<6

Abbreviation: DMDM, dimethyloldimethylhydantoin.

the EDTA, and so on. Most of the preservative manufacturers have developed their own synergistic mixtures of chemicals; this allows them to use lower levels of each chemical and thus decrease the toxicity potential with increased preservative efficacy.

REFERENCES

1. Morrison BM, Scala DD, Fischler G. Topical antibacterial wash products. In: Rieger MM, Rhein LD, eds. Surfactants in Cosmetics, 2d ed. New York: Marcel Dekker, 1997:331–356.
2. Poppe CJ. Ensuring a future for antimicrobials. Soap/Cosmetics/Chemical Specialities 1996; 56–58.
3. Morris JA, Khettry A, Seitz EW. Antimicrobial activity of Arome chemicals and essential oils. J Am Oil Chem Soc 1979; 56:595–603.
4. Jass HE. The history of antiperspirant product development. Cosmet Toilet 1980; 95:25–31.
5. Shelley WB, Hurley HJ, Nichols AC. Arch Derm Shyphilol 1953; 68:430.
6. Orth DS. Cosmetic products that prevent, correct or conceal conditions caused by microorganism. In: Orth DS, ed. Handbook of Cosmetic Microbiology. New York: Marcel Dekker, 1993: 221–323.
7. National Committee for Clinical Laboratory Standards. Methods for Dilution Antimicrobial Susceptibility Tests for Bacteria that Grow Aerobically. Approved Standard M7-A2. 2nd ed. Villanova, PA, 1990.
8. Settembrini L, Gultz J, Boylan R, Scherer W. Antimicrobial activity produced by six dentifrices. General Dentistry 1998; 286–288.
9. Balows A, Hausler WJ, Herrmann KL, Isenberg HD, Shadomy HJ. Manual of Clinical Microbiology, 5th ed. Washington, D.C.: American Society of Microbiology, 1991.
10. Food and Drug Administration (FDA). Tentative final monograph for healthcare antiseptic drug products; proposed rules. Federal Register 59, 31402–31451, June 17, 1994.
11. American Society for Testing and Materials (ASTM). E35.15 Subcommittee on Antimicrobial and Antiviral agents Meeting. April 1995, Denver, CO.
12. Association Française de Normalisation. Normes antiseptiques et Désinfectants. 2d ed. Paris: Tour Europe, Cedex 7, 1989.

13. European Committee for Standardization. Brussels, Belgium: CEN 216, 1998.
14. Siquet F. Disinfection and preservation in detergents. In: Stubenrauch J, Broze G, eds. Handbook of Detergents. Vol. 1. New York: Marcel Dekker, 1999.
15. McCarthy TJ. Formulated factors affecting the activity of preservatives. In: Kabara JJ, ed. Cosmetic and Drug Preservation, Principles and Practices. New York: Marcel Dekker, 1984: 359–387.
16. Orth DS, Lutes CM. Adaptation of bacteria to cosmetic preservatives. Cosmet Toilet 1985; 100:57–59.
17. Kabara JJ. Food grade chemicals in a system approach to cosmetic evaluation. In: Kabara JJ, ed. Cosmetic and Drug preservation, Principles and Practices. New York: Marcel Dekker, 1984: 339–356.
18. Denyer SP, Hugo WB, Harding VD. Synergy in preservative combinations. Internat J Pharm 1985; 25:245–253.
19. Selleri R, Caldini O, Orzalesi G, Facchini S. La conservation du produit cosmétique. Biol Chim Farm 1974; 113:617–627.
20. Orth DS, ed. Handbook of Cosmetic Microbiology. New York: Marcel Dekker, 1993:75–99.
21. European cosmetic directive 76/768EEC.
22. Wallhäuser KH. Antimicrobial preservatives used by the cosmetic industry. In: Kabara JJ, ed. Cosmetic and Drug Preservation, Principles and Practices. New York: Marcel Dekker, 1984: 605–745.

22

General Concepts of Skin Irritancy and Anti-irritant Products

André O. Barel
Free University of Brussels, Brussels, Belgium

INTRODUCTION

In the past, some hazardous materials were used in cosmetics such as lead carbonate, bismuth, and mercurials. Serious adverse reactions to cosmetic ingredients and preparations are actually infrequent. However, side effects do occur and are by no means rare. The unwanted effects of cosmetics can be classified in the following categories [1–4]:

1. Irritation and contact urticaria
2. Contact allergy
3. Photosensitive reaction (photoallergy and photoirritation)
4. Acnegenesis and comedogenesis
5. Color changes of the skin and appendages
6. Systemic side effects
7. Other local side effects

When considering skin-irritation symptoms, we are dealing with nonimmunological mediated inflammation of the skin induced by external agents. Chemical irritants are the major cause, but mechanical, thermal, climatic, and UV and IR light are also important factors or cofactors of irritancy [5]. This nonimmunological skin irritancy reaction comprises two forms: the acute irritant reaction with a monofactorial cause (detergent, acid, oxidant, etc.) and the chronic multifactorial form. The symptoms of skin irritation are well known: erythema, dryness, scaling, itching, burning, and tingling. The clinical symptoms are described by some investigators as objective irritation [1–4]. Because these symptoms are clearly perceptible, in vivo testing in humans can easily and reliably detect strong and moderate irritants for cosmetic ingredients and eliminate these potential hazards. However, most cosmetic-use ingredients do not produce acute irritation from a single exposure because they are mild or very mild and consequently difficult to detect. However, they may produce inflammation after repeated application on the same area of the skin, which is referred to as cumulative irritation.

Application of a cosmetic causing symptoms of burning, stinging, or itching without detectable visible or microscopic changes is designated as a subjective irritation or subclinical irritation [2–4]. This reaction is common in certain susceptible individuals, occurring most frequently on the face. These persons are identified as ''stingers.'' Some of the ingredients that cause this reaction are not generally considered as typical irritants, and will not cause abnormal responses in nonsusceptible individuals. Typically about 10 to 20% of the subjects exposed to a 5% aqueous lactic acid develop a stinging response when applied to the face. Generally, all stingers have reported a history of adverse reactions to facial cosmetics, soaps, and similar products. Prior skin damage caused by UV sunburn, pretreatment with surfactants, and tape stripping increase the intensity of the response in ''stingers.'' Attempts to identify reactive subjects by association with other skin problems such as atopy or with phototype or skin dryness have not been very fruitful [6].

Among the potential adverse reactions of cosmetic ingredients and products such as irritant contact dermatitis, immediate contact reaction (urticaria), allergic contact dermatitis, and acnegenesis and comedogenesis, we will consider particularly adverse reactions of irritancy. It is the purpose of this chapter to 1) describe shortly the different symptoms of irritancy and how to evaluate skin irritants by clinical visual and tactile assessments, by noninvasive bioengineering measurements and by self-perception of skin irritation; 2) to give a short overview of the different chemical ingredients, which are potential cosmetic and occupational skin irritants; 3) to give a description of the different in vivo tests for measuring skin irritation and to test the efficiency of specific anti-irritant products and ingredients, and 4) to give an overview of the different possibilities to conceive anti-irritant cosmetics and treatments.

IRRITANCY AND SKIN IRRITANT EVALUATION AND SYMPTOMS

Methods to evaluate skin alterations induced by topical products can be classified in three categories [7]:

1. Clinical visual and tactile assessments
2. Instrumental noninvasive bioengineering measurements
3. Self-perception by the subjects themselves

Clinical Visual and Tactile Assessments

Several skin modifications induced by irritants can be easily evaluated visually and tactilely, e.g., by skin redness (erythema), skin dryness with increased desquamation, scaliness, and flakiness, and skin roughness or edema. Moderate to very intense signs of skin redness/erythema are the visual manifestations of a skin inflammatory process with vasodilatation of the capillary system and increase of the blood flow. After contact with an irritant (particularly with soaps and detergents), symptoms of skin dryness appear after a certain time with a whitish appearance, flakiness, scaliness, and roughness. In the most severe cases of irritation, fissuring, and cracking can also appear. Edema is the result of an accumulation of fluid from the blood vessels in the upper dermis. It appears only in very severe cases of irritancy, which happens very rarely unless in experimental conditions. The visual and tactile assessments of irritancy are made by dermatologists or trained evaluators. These observations always remain subjective in nature even with trained observers, with well-standardized clinical and experimental protocols and with well-established scoring grades. However, the clinical assessments are precise and very reproducible.

Instrumental Noninvasive Bioengineering Measurements

Many changes in skin properties induced by irritant cosmetic ingredients can be evaluated quantitatively in a noninvasive manner by instrumental techniques. In this section the following techniques will be described: 1) skin redness by reflectance skin colorimetry and by Laser Doppler flowmetry; 2) alterations in the integrity of the barrier function by transepidermal water loss; 3) skin hydration measurements using electrical impedance and skin surface alterations using squamometry; and 4) other bioengineering methods such as elasticity and microrelief.

Skin Redness/Erythema by Measuring Skin Color

Most color measurements of the skin surface are based on reflectance colorimetry instruments, such as tristumulus color analysis, Chromameter Minolta, erythema index, Erythemameter Diastron, Mexameter Courage-Khazaka, and Dermaspectrometer Cortex [8–10].

The Minolta chromameter CR-200, considered by many investigators as a sort of reference instrument, quantifies skin surface color using the three-dimensional CIE color representation with the L*a*b* system. Skin redness is readily evaluated by means of the a* values; erythema is always characterized by an increase of the a* skin color parameter. Different, more simple, reflectance meters (Erythemameter Diastron, Mexameter Courage-Khazaka, and Dermaspectrometer Cortex) are also used [9,11]. These instruments are based on the same optical principle, namely, measurements of light absorption and reflection of respectively the melanin and hemoglobin components of the skin. The specific absorption of melanin and hemoglobin in the visible (green and red) and in the near infrared is determined and these instruments quantify redness by a relative erythema index. The erythema index is proportional to the hemoglobin content of the upper layers of the dermis.

Excellent correlations have been shown between visual clinical scoring and erythema and Chromameter measurements of the a* color parameter [12]. Furthermore, reasonably good correlations were noticed between the a* Chromameter parameter and the erythema index of the simple reflectance meters (Mexameter Courage-Khazaka and Dermaspectrometer Cortex) [9,13].

Measurement of Superficial Blood Flux by Laser Doppler Flowmetry

The hemoglobin of the red blood cells of the upper dermis microcirculation system partially absorbs the light of a helium laser beam. The laser Doppler method measures the shift in frequency of the reflected light of this laser beam. This small frequency shift is proportional to the number and the speed of red blood cells present in the superficial blood microcirculation system. An inflammatory reaction with vasodilatation of the capillaries will produce a marked increase in blood flow [14]. There two types of laser Doppler instruments: the first generation flowmeters, which measure the blood flux of a small spot area of the skin (2–3 mm^2) (Servomed, Sweden, Lisca, Sweden and Moor, United Kingdom), and more recently the development of laser Doppler imaging instruments, which has enabled the two dimensional quantitative measurement of blood microcirculation of a much larger skin area (maximum 10 cm^2) [15]. Good correlations were found between clinical assessments of irritancy and noninvasive bioengineering methods, such as skin color and laser Doppler flowmetry, respectively [16].

Alterations in the Integrity of the Barrier Function

When some irritant cosmetic ingredient comes in contact with the skin, the earliest modifications in the skin structure is an alteration of the lipidic barrier structure of the stratum corneum [17]. The physiological function of this barrier is to protect the skin from the penetration of irritants and to ensure low insensible perspiration of the skin [transepidermal water loss (TEWL)]. When the barrier function of the skin is altered by an irritant, the amount of water vapor passing through the stratum corneum is increased, which is characterized by an increase in TEWL. The two most widely used TEWL instruments are the Evaporimeter (ServoMed, Sweden) and the Tewameter (Courage-Khazaka, Germany). Both TEWL instruments are very sensitive, and the slightest alterations of the barrier function can be measured with this technique (''nonvisible'' subclinical irritation). This happens mostly when extremely mild cosmetic ingredients are tested or when normal-use application protocols are considered [18].

Alterations in the Skin Surface Hydration

The assessment of the hydration status of the superficial layers of the epidermis is an important parameter with which to characterize the skin. The hydration level of the stratum corneum remains more or less constant, taking in consideration the following mechanisms: 1) hydration coming from the deeper layers of the fully hydrated viable epidermis and retarded from evaporation in the stratum corneum by the lipids from the hydrolipidic barrier, 2) hydration due to equilibrium with the external ambient humidity, and 3) the presence of entrapped water bound to the natural moisturing factors (NMF) present in the layers of the stratum corneum. When an irritant cosmetic ingredient, such as a surfactant, interacts with the skin surface, it partially or completely removes the lipidic film coating the surface of these and extracts some NMF components altering the equilibrium mechanism of the hydration of the skin surface. Such a dehydration of the horny layer will have many different consequences, such as 1) increase of the desquamation rate of the corneocytes giving the skin a scaly aspect, 2) a modification of the relief of the skin with a rough and wrinkled appearance, and 3) modifications in the viscoelastic properties of the stratum corneum. The modifications in the hydration level of the stratum corneum have been extensively investigated using bioengineering methods based on the electrical impedance to the skin to an alternating current [19]. Many commercial instruments measure the electrical properties of the skin, such as capacitance, impedance, and conductance methods. The measured electrical properties of the superficial layers of the epidermis (impedance units or arbitrary electrical units) are indirectly related to the amount of water present in the horny layer. When used under standard conditions and in thermostatized experimental rooms, all the instruments are able to provide highly accurate and reproducible hydration values. Excellent correlations were obtained between the visual scoring of skin dryness induced by surfactants in a soap chamber test and instrumental readings [20].

Skin-Surface Stripping Tests

The investigation of skin-surface alterations has made great progress by the development and use of skin-surface stripping systems. The superficial layers of the stratum corneum can be easily collected, and without any damage for the viable epidermis, simply by pressing a sticky tape on the skin (D-Squames). When removing the sticky tape after a few seconds, several layers of corneocytes are collected and can be analyzed. The level of desquamation can be quantified by squamometry, which is the staining of the corneocytes and measuring the amount of color [21]. The degree of cohesion between the corneocytes can be measured by visual scoring under the microscope and by image analysis. With some surfactants, no clinical irritation could be observed; however, they induce significant changes at the surface of the stratum corneum as shown by an increase of the amount of corneocytes and a deorganization/loss of the intercorneocyte cohesion [21,22].

Other Noninvasive Bioengineering Methods

Other methods are available to measure some symptoms of skin irritancy, but will not be described in this chapter. Skin dryness and roughness as induced by some irritants can be evaluated by the following techniques: (1) measurement of the viscoelastic properties of the upper layers of the epidermis [23], and (2) skin surface microrelief [24–26].

Self-Perception of Skin Irritations

Generally when a finished cosmetic product comes into contact with the skin of potential consumers, it is very unlikely that observable signs of irritation are noticed in normal use. However, the overall perception of the finished product by the consumer is an important criterion for accepting its cosmetic use. In this global perception many different parameters may play a role, some independant of the potential irritancy of ingredients, such as feeling of aesthetic nature, ease of spreading on the skin, viscosity, perfume, and color. However, the subjective perception of skin feel is closely related to the composition of the cosmetic product. Skin feel attributes, such as self-perception of dryness (feels tight, rough, and dry), or irritation (itching and burning), softness, and smoothness are easily perceived by the subjects. In most cases, the subjects are able to perceive very early on the effects of some cosmetics on the skin well before they become clinically observable or measurable by bioengineering techniques. The assessment of the self-perception of the interaction between some cosmetic ingredients with the stratum corneum is performed by means of questionnaires where several skin attributes are evaluated. Some questionnaires are designed to receive an answer Yes or No to each of the attributes, or the subject will have to rate each of the attributes on a 0 to 10 point scale.

FACTORS THAT INFLUENCE SKIN RESPONSIVENESS TO IRRITANTS

Many factors can influence the responsiveness of a consumer's skin to a potential irritant. Some factors are intrinsic, inherent to the subjects themselves (e.g., sensitive skin, atopic skin), the body site, and previous traumas to the considered skin area. Other factors are external, such as composition of product, conditions of exposure, occupation of the subject, and climatic factors [4,5,7]. The reason why these factors are covered in this chapter are evident. Some cosmetics with anti-irritant ingredients are designed for some specific skin sites, such as the face, or considered as seasonal products, such as cosmetics against winter dryness of the skin.

Factors inherent to the constitution of the skin of the subjects that may influence skin responsiveness are numerous. A marked interindividual variability in response to irritants have been reported and ascribed to host-related factors. Considering the interindividual variability of subjects to skin irritants, one must mention here the concept of ''sensitive skin.'' The term sensitive skin clearly has a different meaning for consumers than for cosmetic scientists and dermatologists [4,6]. Consumers use the term *sensitive skin* to indicate that their skin readily experiences adverse reactions or unwanted changes to external factors, such as the use of personal care products. Subjects with sensitive skin tend to more readily develop skin reactions to cosmetics and other topical drugs than do normal persons. Many attempts have been made by cosmetic scientists and dermatologists to describe and demonstrate in a scientific way what sensitive skin is. Visible effects, such as erythema and skin dryness, are noticed. However, half of adverse reactions are purely sensory perceptions, subjective symptoms of stinging, itching, burning, and feelings of dryness with or without visible effects.

Regional Differences in the Sensitivity of Normal Skin

It has been clearly demonstrated that when measuring the potential irritancy of cosmetic ingredients, great regional differences in the sensitivity of normal skin are observed [27,28]. Several factors must be considered in order to explain the observed regional differences in skin sensitivity, such as differences in total skin thickness, skin permeability, the amount and composition of epidermal and sebaceous lipids, blood microcirculation, hydration level of the horny layer, thickness of the horny layer, and desquamation rate and local daily exposure to irritant products. Most skin-irritation phenomena are noticed in the face.

Influence of Gender, Age, and Ethnic Group

Contradictory data are presented in the scientific literature about the influence of ethnic group on skin sensitivity [29]. It has been demonstrated that the irritant response may be higher in babies and children and decrease with age [30]. Concerning skin sensibility to irritants related to gender, many studies show that women are more reactive than men [31,32]. However, this difference could be attributable to the fact that women are more exposed to household chemicals and more frequently use face care cosmetics, rather than related to real physiological differences. Other factors are external to the subject, such as composition of their usual products, conditions of exposure, occupation of the subject, and climatic factors.

Mode of Exposure of the Product on the Skin

Acute skin exposures of a very irritant chemical cosmetic ingredient are very rare and attributable to accidents, inadequate use, or problems in the manufacturing of the cosmetic product. The list of very irritant products are known and must be totally avoided or used at very low concentrations; we will be dealing mostly with subacute and chronic exposure of the skin. Subacute exposure will provoke an immediate impairment of the skin barrier. Repeated exposures to certain cosmetic products with very limited impairment of the skin barrier can induce, after a certain time, significant cutaneous reactions.

Climatic Factors

There is clearly a seasonal or climatic effect on the amplitude of the skin irritation reaction. Generally, much higher irritation reactions are observed in winter than in summer. This difference is related to a dehydration factor: a situation of dryness of the horny layer provoked by ambient air with very low relative humidity. This situation is particulary present on the lower legs and more frequent in older subjects; typical symptoms include winter xerosis, extreme dryness, scaling, and rough skin surface. Furthermore, in the winter the epidermis is more aggressed by extreme temperature changes between the inside and outside world. In the summer period, the upper layers of the epidermis are well hydrated, and the skin is smooth unless excessively exposed to sun damage. Actinic aging of the skin is characterized by various clinical symptoms, including dryness of the skin.

COSMETIC AND OCCUPATIONAL SKIN IRRITANTS

Occupational Skin Irritants

A broad definition of occupational contact irritant dermatitis is contact dermatitis caused wholly or partially by the occupation of the subject. Occupational irritants may cause an acute response that may take from 1 hour to 1 day to appear, and is usually traceable to a single factor. Chronic irritant contact dermatitis may take months or years to appear and is often multifactorial [33]. Hands are involved in 80 to 90% of all cases of occupational contact dermatitis, and in the minority of cases the wrist, forearm, lower leg, or face is the primary site.

The clinical features are described as follows. Many cases of occupational irritant contact dermatitis start as erythema and scaling on the back of joints and adjacent parts of the back of the fingers, as well as in the web spaces between the fingers. A generalized, rather shiny, superficially fissured, scaly fingertip dermatitis is also characteristic of certain forms of irritancy. Exclusive or more severe involvement of the thumb, index finger, and/ or middle finger of the dominant hand (or of the nails) is generally an indication of possible occupational causation [33]. The principal occupational irritants are listed in Table 1.

Cosmetic Skin Irritants

Cosmetics are complex mixtures of chemical compounds. The abundance of commercially available ingredients has created endless variety in cosmetic formulation. The cosmetic substances used in cosmetic products may be arbitrarily divided in great categories of product and/or function. The principal categories of cosmetic irritants are listed in Table 2.

Intolerance to some ingredients is related to symptoms of contact dermatitis and allergic dermatitis. There is not always a clear distinction between these problems. Some cosmetic ingredients present both an irritant character with the additional possibility of allergic reaction (e.g., cinnamic acid derivates). An overview of cosmetic categories causing irritant side effects in descending importance has been given by A. C. de Groot and coworkers [1–3] and are summarized briefly in Table 3. It has clearly been shown that certain categories of cosmetics, taking into account their composition, frequency of use, mode of application on the skin, and skin area to be treated, are more specific candidates for causing symptoms of skin irritation.

A short overview will be given of the potential irritant character of each category of cosmetic ingredients. Some chemicals are used in industry (occupational irritants) as well as in the cosmetic world (cosmetic irritants). Chapter 37 describes the irritancy of the most frequent emulgators and detergents used primarily in cleansing products.

Preservatives/antimicrobials, antioxidants, fragrances, colors, and UV filters are potentially irritant components. However, these components are often present in cosmetic preparations at low concentrations and are consequently not affecting the overall irritation potential of the final product. These substances are more often incriminated for their allergic reactions.

TABLE 1 Common Irritants in Occupational Dermatitis

Skin cleansers	Soaps, detergents, specific cleansers
Industrial cleaning agents	Detergents, emulsifiers, solubilizers, wetting agents, enzymes
Organic solvents	Alkanes, alkenes, halogenalkanes and alkenes, alcohols, ketones, aldehydes, esthers, ethers, toluene, carbon sulfide, petroleum derivates, silicones
Oils	Cutting oils, metal working fluids, lubrificating oils, braking oils
Acids	Severe irritants are sulfuric, chromic, nitric chlorhydric, hyperchloric, fluorhydric and tri-chloroacetic acids; milder irritants are for-mic, acetic, propionic, oxalic, and salycilic acids
Alkaline substances	Soaps, soda, ammonia, sodium, potassium and calcium hydroxides, various amines
Oxidizing agents	Hydrogen peroxide and peroxides, benzoyl per-oxide, sodium (hypo) chlorate and bromate
Reducing agents	Phenols, aldehydes (formaldehyde), thioglyco-lates, hydrazines
Plants	Various plants are potentially irritant, espe-cially the *Euphorbiaceae, Brassicaceae, Ra-nunculeae* families
Products of animal, food proteins, plant, and bacterial origin	Proteolytic enzymes such as pepsine, papaine, trypsine, subtilisine
Physical factors	

Source: Ref. 5.

TABLE 2 Common Potential Cosmetic Irritant Ingredients

Conservatives/antimicrobials
Antioxidants
Fragrance
Colors
UV filters
Lipids
Organic solvents
Emulgators, surfactants, and rheological agents
Humectants and emollients
Specific cosmetic ingredients such as keratolytic agents, tanning and whitening agents

Source: From Refs. 2 and 4.

TABLE 3 Cosmetic Categories
Causing Irritant Side Effects*

Soap
Deodorant/antiperspirant
Moisturizing/emollient
Aftershave
Shampoo
Lipstick
Hair dye
Perfume

* In descending importance.
Source: Refs. 2 and 3.

Lipids/Emollients

Most oils and fats are relatively mild. However, some oils from plant origin are incriminated for their allergic reactions. Emulgators, surfactants and rheological agents. Some surfactants are known to be rather irritant. These substances are usually classsified as follows, going from the most irritating to the mildest:

> cationics
> anionics
> amphoterics
> nonionics

In shampoos and body and shower gels or creams anionic detergents are rarely used alone but rather in combination with amphoterics and nonionic surfactants. In creams and milks nonionic and amphoteric emulgators are essentially used for their mildness.

Humectants

The classical humectants such as NMF are nonirritant. The other humectants such as proteins, hyaluronic acid, chitosan, proteoglycans, and polysaccharides are very rarely irritant components.

Specific cosmetic ingredients, such as keratolytic agents, tanning and whitening agents, etc., can be more irritant.

In the use of AHAs, irritancy increases with concentration and with a decrease in pH, which is controlled by the proportion of free acid to AHA salts. Classic alkaline soaps were potentially irritant because of the rise in skin pH and induction of skin dryness. Modern soaps are actually very mild because they are buffered to neutral or slightly acidic pH and contain lipids such as emollients and humectants.

Solvents in Aftershave Products

The irritancy of these products is easily related to the very high alcohol content (usually more than 50%) of this category of cosmetics. Alcohol dehydrates the skin and the skin that has been predamaged by the wet or dry shaving process.

TESTS FOR MEASURING SKIN IRRITATION

Tests for evaluating the irritation potential of a cosmetic ingredient or a finished product are considered in a progressive approach to the problem [7].

First, a minimum of toxicological information must be obtained from the general available scientific literature and from information derived from in vitro testing and testing on animals. Starting with the premises that the considered ingredient or product is not toxic or very irritant, testing on humans will be envisaged. A short overview of the different published test method will be given in this chapter. Supplementary information concerning the test methods can be found in Chapter 12 and in a recent review article by Paye [7].

Open Epicutaneous Applications

In a second phase of testing, single and eventual repetitive open application tests are normally used for studying new chemicals with a safety purpose in order to determine if this ingredient is likely to cause serious skin irritation [34].

Occlusive Patch Testing

If the product is not irritant in such open epicutaneous applications, it can be considered to use occlusive patch tests in a further phase. The objective of the clinical study is to compare the mildness or irritation potential of a certain cosmetic ingredient with other similar products. For this purpose some level of cutaneous irritation has to be induced. Generally we are dealing with very mild cosmetic products and it is necessary to include in the comparative testing some more irritating products as a positive reference. By using occlusive conditions one induces a better percutaneous diffusion of the test solution through the horny layer. Occlusion increases the hydration of this layer (increase in percutaneous penetration) and slight increase of skin temperature under the occlusive dressing.

Many variants of occlusive patch tests have been described in the literature [7], some of the most used tests are:

- The single 24-hour occlusive test [35,36]
- Successive occlusive applications, such as the Frosch-Kligman soap chamber test [37], the modified soap chamber test [18]
- The 21-day cumulative irritation test [37]
- The 4-hour occlusive test [38]

Skin irritation is evaluated clinically (visual and tactile) for erythema, dryness, scaling, roughness, and edema, and/or by bioengineering methods.

The Exaggerated Use Tests

The occlusive patch tests were developed as a rapid screening test for evaluating the relative irritation potential of cosmetic products and ingredients. However, these conditions do not simulate the normal usage of the test materials, and other test procedures were developed to be closer to realistic use conditions of the product by the consumer [39]. These exaggerated use tests combine the application of the product to its normal way but still in an exaggerated way: the number of applications per day and the total duration and temperature of application is exaggerated in order to induce more skin irritation reactions than expected in normal use. Several protocols have been published, differing in terms of sort of application, number of applications, skin sites, and so on [7]. Most of these exaggerated in-use tests are concerned with soaps and detergents, but can, with the necessary experimental adaptations, be used for other cosmetic preparations, such as the following:

- The forearm wash test [39]
- The flex wash test [40]
- The hand/forearm immersion test [41]

One advantage of these testing methods is the fact that they are carried out on a relatively small number of subjects [12–25].

Home-Use Testing

Even if the exaggerated in-use tests predict with good confidence the skin tolerance of a certain ingredient or product, it is necessary and safer for the manufacturer to run an extended study with a large number of subjects using the product in normal way and in their usual environment, so it is called a "home-use test" or "in-use test."

The panel will be selected among the population of potential users, e.g., for the target group and for the type of treatment. The duration of the testing is generally for a much longer period (weeks and sometimes months). Any unwanted effects of the product on the skin are recorded, such as visible signs of intolerance (redness, dryness, roughness,) as well as nonvisible perceptions such as itching, burning and tightness. Evaluations of these signs are made very regularly (most cases daily) by the subjects themselves and once a week by an expert evaluator. Usually clinical ratings by visual and tactile assessment are made using numerical grades. They can be completed by instrumental noninvasive bioengineering measurements.

STRATEGY OF MAKING ANTI-IRRITANT COSMETICS

Strictly by definition, an anti-irritant is an agent which, by its presence, minimizes the irritating effect of a cosmetic preparation on the skin. The anti-irritant could reflect all mechanisms that have an opposed effect to an irritant insult. Hence, the term could reflect actions such as skin calming, soothing, and healing, and assisting in the recovery of the skin from an irritation provoked by, e.g., contact with soaps and household cleaning products. As has been demonstrated earlier, very often irritant reactions are associated with inflammation, the so-called anti-irritant effect could eventually also mean alleviation from the inflammatory symptoms that arise shortly after the impairment of the skin barrier. The concept of anti-irritant activity also includes skin protection with barrier creams, which decrease irritant potential of some harmful substances encountered in occupational dermatitis [33]. Despite the numerous claims of skincare products for anti-irritant or protective activity, some lack of scientific data is present to substantiate these claims. There is also a lack of suitable standardized clinical protocols to quantify these anti-irritant properties.

The basic principle of development of general anti-irritant cosmetics or cosmetics for sensitive skin is to avoid as much as possible any risk of irritation [4, 42]. The safest way is to use well-tolerated, chemical compounds for the vehicle and active ingredients without history of "skin problems." Allergic reactions and skin irritancy are generally provoked by known specific ingredients, mostly fragrances, colors, and preservatives. The easy task is to remove fragrances and coloring agents; hypoallergenic cosmetics minimize the use of or do not contain these ingredients. Actually, a modern trend in cosmetics is to develop specific cosmetics without preservatives. This challenge can be partially answered in cosmetic preparations with none or low water content: oils, fats, water/oil emulsions, and lipogels using some synthetic lipids and/or essential oils with bactericidal properties as preservatives. With aqueous solutions, hydrogels, and oil/water emulsions, this goal is very difficult to achieve and presently not realized; consequently, these types of cosmetics still contain preservatives.

In order to elaborate an anti-irritant cosmetic preparation or a cosmetic preparation for sensitive skin, we have a choice from the following possibilities:

1. The vehicle must respect the natural, slightly acidic pH of the skin (pH around 5.3) or be neutral, avoiding alkaline preparations.
2. Strengthen or restore the hydrolipidic barrier function of the skin. As described earlier in this chapter, irritancy reactions are often accompanied by modifications of the structure of the intercellular lipids and water binding capacity resulting in an increase of TEWL and consequently higher penetration rate of irritants. Therefore, anti-irritant preparations should restore the disturbed barrier function by providing the appropriate lipids to the lipidic film. Modern skin care products contain endogeneous components of epidermal lipids such as ceramides and gamma linoleic acid. In a general way, lipids are emollients with soothing capacities.
3. Soothing effect by filmogen compounds. The skin surface is anionic in character. Quaternized derivatives of plant proteins or emollients that are positively charged will smooth the skin surface by a filmogen effect.
4. Irritated skin is very often partially dehydrated skin. In order to alleviate the symptoms of dehydration, water is brought back to the horny layer by humectants (NMF) or by occlusive effect of water/oil emulsions, lipogels, or silicone oils.
5. Use of very mild surfactants and emulgators in cosmetic preparations. General use of amphoteric and nonionic emulgators in creams/milks and cleansing products. In the preparation of shampoos and shower gels, use of anionic emulsifiers with an adequate carbon chain length and sufficient degree of ethoxylation in order to reduce irritancy. Another possibility is to use an adequate mixture of several surfactants. A strong antagonism effect occurs when combining the potential irritant anionic surfactants with amphoterics, nonionic, or even other anionic surfactants with resultant decreased skin irritation [7].
6. Use of specific anti-irritant ingredients. There are a lot of soothing ingredients in dermatological treatments mainly from plant origin, such as hamamelis, algae, chamomile, and aloe vera. Polysaccharides, proteoglycans, and glycoproteins with filmogen and hydrating properties can provide a feel of less or nonirritated skin. Polymers, when used at high concentrations, have also been demonstrated as reducing the irritation potential of anionic surfactants, essentially by entrapping high quantities of surfactants into micelles in solution (see Chap. 23).
7. Sun exposure without UV filters can induce or increase irritant reactions of the skin and accelerate actinic aging. The cosmetic industry has developed suncare products with very high sun protection factors that are waterproof and with reasonably good cosmetic acceptance. There are sun protection products with

active UV filters with the lowest allergenic potential, especially developed for sensitive skin with a minimum amount of emulgators and are fragrance free.

IN VIVO STUDIES OF THE ANTI-IRRITATION PROPERTIES OF SOME COSMETIC INGREDIENTS

In vivo evaluation of the anti-irritant and/or anti-inflammatory effect of dermatocosmetic formulations on human skin is usually based on the quantification of the inhibition presented by these products against an artificially induced contact dermatitis [42]. The model irritant for this purpose can be selected out of a wide range of skin-aggravating factors. Irritation of the skin can be provoked after topical application of Peru balsam [43], solutions of anionic surfactants [44,45], nicotinates [46,47], after exposure to UV-B radiation [48,49], skin abrasion [50], or tape stripping [51,52]. There is clearly a difficulty in identifying the conditions under which these various irritants can be used for inducing a "suitable" irritation. The induced irritation should be great enough to be measurable with good reproducibility and to allow quantification of its inhibition by the tested products. The anionic surfactant sodium lauryl sulphate (SLS) has lately become the model irritant of choice, used widely for inducing experimental contact dermatitis in anti-irritation protocols [45,53–55] or as a reference irritant in safety tests ranking the skin irritation potential of soaps and detergents [56–58]. The irritant character of SLS is attributable to the following factors:

1. Modification of the protein and lipid structure of the stratum corneum. Impairment of the highly ordered bilayers and changes in the fluidity of the lipids [59]. Swelling of the horny layer occurs because of protein denaturation and exposure of new water-binding sites of the keratins [54].
2. Alterations in skin permeability [60]. This surfactant is often used as a pretreatment in order to enhance the penetration of topically applied products [45].
3. SLS causes a vascular inflammatory response [61–62]. SLS is not a sensitizer or carcinogenic agent; it causes no systemic toxicity or permanent cosmetic inconvenience to the skin [45]. The great sensitivity of TEWL parameter in quantifying the impairment of the barrier caused by SLS [63] and the property as a primary irritant have led to the large use of this surfactant in studies of experimental irritant contact dermatitis. However, as for other irritants, the induced cutaneous irritation is not completely reproducible. A marked interindividual variability in response has been reported for this irritant and is ascribed to several host-related factors [42, 45, 64]. Furthermore, intraindividual variability within anatomical regions of skin site have been reported [65]. In the experimental study of the anti-irritant properties of a cosmetic ingredient, three different types of clinical protocol are generally used: postirritation treatment protocols, pretreatment protocols, and treatment with the combined introduction of the anti-irritant into the irritant product.

In the postirritation treatment protocol, the considered skin regions are irritated by treatment with SLS during a certain time and with a certain frequency. After the SLS irritation challenge the skin areas are treated with the anti-irritant ingredient or finished product during a certain time and frequency. One irritated area remains untreated and serves as a control and the irritated areas are respectively treated with the vehicle alone and with the vehicle containing the active anti-irritant ingredient. This last site should heal significantly quicker than the vehicle-treated site. In the pretreatment protocol, the considered skin areas are pretreated during a certain time and frequency with either the vehicle alone or the vehicle with the anti-irritant component. A nonpretreated skin area serves as a control. Following this pretreatment the different skin areas are irritated with a SLS solution.

The typical clinical signs of skin irritancy (redness and dryness) are visually assessed by trained evaluators. Furthermore, redness is quantified by skin color (reflectance color-imetry) and microcirculation of the bloof flux by Laser Doppler flowmetry. Alterations in the barrier function are measured by TEWL and hydration is measured by electrical impedance of the skin. In order to obtain a significant measurable irritancy, the SLS challenge is carried under occlusive dressing. It can also be treated by repetitive open applications with the SLS solution. Different anti-irritant experimental protocols are described in the scientific literature [42].

As found in the literature, these studies are often concerned with the anti-irritant properties of plant extracts. Here follows a short overview of the anti-inflammatory/anti-irritant studies described in the literature:

- Anti-inflammatory properties of the active ingredients α-bisabolol and azulene of chamomile oil [66–69]
- Anti-inflammatory and healing effect of a cream containing glycolic extract of six plants (calendula, Roman and German chamomile, linden, cornflower, and millepertuis) [70]
- Anti-inflammatory effect of the active ingredient namely esculoside extracted from horse chestnut [71]
- Anti-inflammatory properties of the active ingredient, namely ursolic acid extracted from rosemary [72]
- Anti-irritant properties of a preparation containing licorice and chamomile against a wide range of daily life skin irritations (aftershave, depilation, solar erythema, and insect stings) [73]

All these studies differ with respect to the irritation challenge and with respect to the anti-irritant treatment. In both type of protocols, namely postirritation treatment and pretreatment with the anti-irritant cosmetic ingredients, significant anti-irritant effects were observed between the treated skin sites and the untreated skin sites used as a reference. With more discriminative protocols (double-blind vehicle-controlled), where the anti-irritancy efficiency of an anti-irritant ingredient solubilized or dispersed in suitable vehicles (water/oil or oil/water) is compared with the efficiency of the vehicle alone, one generally expects that the specific effect of the anti-irritant alone will be very small and not very often significantly different from that of the vehicle alone. To illustrate this statement, we refer to recent work on plant anti-irritants [42]. Manou [42] has studied, in a double-blind vehicle-controlled way, the potential anti-irritant properties of essential oils and glycolic extracts obtained from different plants such as chamomile, sage, clary sage, peppermint, and hyssop. The essential oils were solubilized at a concentration of 3 to 5% in oil/water and water/oil vehicles. The anti-irritant properties were examined according to the postirritation treatment protocols and pretreatment protocols using visual clinical assessments of redness and dryness and bioengineering methods (skin color, laser Doppler flowmetry, TEWL, and hydration). The results do not support the existence of a significant anti-irritant effect of the essential oils tested under these very strict conditions. In general, the treated skin was found to have benefited from the treatment with the vehicle with or without the essential oils, compared with the irritated but untreated skin. These results could be explained taking in account the following points. First, the concentration range of the active anti-irritant ingredients used in these experiments is rather low (3–5%), and are concentrations that can be found in commercial cosmetic preparations. Probably at higher concentrations (5–10%) a significant specific anti-irritant effect will be observed, but because of the problems of high cost of these plant extracts and the possibility of increasing the risk for allergic contact dermatitis, these higher concentrations are rarely used in commercial cosmetic preparations. Secondly, there is always a significant anti-irritant, anti-inflammatory effect on the skin of the lipids and emollients present in the vehicle.

REFERENCES

1. Cosmetics: introduction. In: De Groot AC, Weyland JW, Nater JP, eds. Unwanted Effects of Cosmetics and Drugs Used in Dermatology. Amsterdam: Elsevier, 1994:422.
2. The spectrum of side effects of cosmetics. In: De Groot AC, Weyland JW, Nater JP, eds. Unwanted Effects of Cosmetics and Drugs Used in Dermatology. Amsterdam: Elsevier, 1994:437.
3. The frequency of adverse reactions to cosmetics and the products involved. In: De Groot AC, Weyland JW, Nater JP, eds. Unwanted Effects of Cosmetics and Drugs Used in Dermatology. Amsterdam: Elsevier, 1994:442.
4. Simion FA, Rau AH. Sensitive skin: what it is and how to formulate for it. Cosmet Toilet 1994; 109:43.
5. Frosch PJ. Cutaneous irritation. In: Rycroft RJG, Menné T, Frosch PJ, eds. Textbook of Contact Dermatitis. Berlin:Springer-Verlag, 1995:28.
6. Amin S, Engasser PG, Maibach HI. Adverse cosmetic reactions. In: Textbook of Cosmetic Dermatology, Second Edition. Baran R, Maibach HI, eds. London, United Kingdom: Martin Dunitz, 1998:709.
7. Paye M. Models for studying surfactant interactions with the skin. In: Broze G, ed. Handbook of Detergent Properties. Part A: Properties. Surf Sci Series, vol. 82. New York: Marcel Dekker, 1999:469–509.
8. Bjerring P. Spectrophotometric characterization of skin pigments and skin color. In: Serup J, Jemec CBE, eds. Handbook of Non-Invasive Methods and the Skin. Boca Raton: CRC Press, 1995:373–376.
9. Takiwaki H, Serup, J. Measurement of erythema and melanin indices. In: Serup J, Jemec CBE, eds. Handbook of Non-Invasive Methods and the Skin. Boca Raton: CRC Press, 1995:373.
10. Westerhof W. CIE Colorimeter. In: Serup J, Jemec CBE, eds. Handbook of Non-Invasive Methods and the Skin. Boca Raton: CRC Press, 1995:385.
11. Diffey BL, Oliver RJ, Farr PM. A portable instrument for quantifying erythema induced by ultraviolet radiation. Br J Dermatol 1984; 111:663.
12. Babulak SE, Rhein LD, Scala DD, Simion FA, Grove GG. Quantification of erythema in a soap chamber test using the Minolta Chroma (reflectance) Meter: comparison of instrumental results with visual assessments. J Cosmet Chem 1986; 37:475.
13. Clarys P. Alewaeters K, Barel AO. Comparative study of skin colour using different bioengineering methods. Abstract, 6th Congress of the International Society for Skin Imaging, London, United Kingdom, 1999.
14. Oberg PA, Tenland T, Nilsson GE. Laser Doppler flowmetry: a non invasive and continuous method for blood flow evaluation in microvascular studies. Acta Med Scand Suppl 1984; 687: 17.
15. Wärdell K, Nilsson G. Laser Doppler imaging of skin. In: Serup J, Jemec CBE, eds. Handbook of Non-Invasive Methods and the Skin. Boca Raton: CRC Press, 1995:421.

16. Anderson PH, Abrams K, Bjerring P, Maibach H. A time correlation study of ultraviolet B-induced erythema measured by reflectance spectroscopy and Laser Doppler flowmetry. Photodermatol Photoimmunol Photomed 1991: 8:123.

17. Imokawa G. In vitro and in vivo models. In: Elsner P, Maibach HI, eds. Bioengineering of the Skin: Water and the Stratum Corneum. Boca Raton: CRC Press, 1994:23.

18. Simion FA, Rhein LD, Grove GG, Wojtkowski JM, Cagan RH, Scala DS. Sequential order of skin responses to surfactants during a soap chamber test. Contact Dermatitis 1991; 27:174.

19. Barel AO, Clarys P, Gabard B. In vivo evaluation of the hydration state of the skin. In: Elsner P, Merck HF, Maibach HI, eds. Cosmetics Controlled Efficacy Studies and Regulation. Berlin: Springer, 1999:57.

20. Paye M, Van de Gaer D, Morrison Jr BM. Corneometry measurements to evaluate skin dryness in the modified soap chamber test. Skin Res Technol 1995;1:123.

21. Piérard GE, Piérard-Franchimont C, Saint Leger D, Kligman AM. Squamometry: the assessment of xerosis by colorimetry of D-Squame adhesive discs. J Cosmet Chem 1992; 47:297.

22. Paye M, Goffin V, Cartiaux Y, Morrison Jr BM, Piérard GE. D-Squame strippings in the assessment of intercorneocyte cohesion. Allergologie 1995; 18:462.

23. Barel AO, Lambrecht R, Clarys P. Mechanical function of the skin: state of the art. In: Elsner P, Barel AO, Berardesca E, Gabard B, Serup J, eds. Skin Bioengineering: Techniques and Applications in Dermatology and Cosmetology. Basel: Karger 1998:69.

24. Gasmüller J, Keckes A, Jahn P. Stylus method for skin surface contour measurements. In: Serup J, Jemec CBE, eds. Handbook of Non-Invasive Methods and the Skin. Boca Raton: CRC Press, 1995:83.

25. Corcuff P, Lévêque JL. Skin surface replica image analysis of furrows and wrinkles. In: Serup J, Jemec CBE, eds. Handbook of Non-Invasive Methods and the Skin. Boca Raton: CRC Press, 1995:89.

26. Efsen J, Hansen HN, Christiansen S, Keiding J. Laser profilometry. In: Serup J, Jemec CBE, eds. Handbook of Non-Invasive Methods and the Skin. Boca Raton: CRC Press, 1995:97.

27. Hannuksela M. Sensitivity of various skin sites in the repeated open application test. Am J Contact Derm 1991; 2:102.

28. Van der Valk PGM, Maibach HI. Potential for irritation increases from the wrist to the cubital fossa. Br J Dermatol 1989; 121:709.

29. Berardesca E, Maibach HI. Racial differences in sodium lauryl sulphate induced cutaneous irritation: black and white. Contact Derm 1988; 18:65.

30. Coenraads PJ, Bleumink E. Nater JP. Susceptibility to primary irritants. Contact Derm 1975; 1:377.

31. Rystedt I. Factors influencing the occurrence of hand eczema in adults with a history of atopic dermatitis in childhood. Contact Derm 1985; 12:247.

32. Lantinga H, Nater JP, Coenraads PJ. Prevalence, incidence and course of eczema on the hand and forearm in a sample of the general population. Contact Derm 1984; 10:135.

33. Rycroft RJG. Occupational contact dermatitis. In: Rycroft RJG, Menné T, Frosch PJ, eds. Textbook of Contact Dermatitis. Berlin: Springer-Verlag, 1995; 343.

34. Hannuksela M. Salo H. The repeated open application test (ROAT). Contact Derm 1986: 14: 221.

35. Tronnier H, Heinrich U. Prüfung der hautvertraglichkeit am menschen zur sicherheitsbewertung von kosmetika. Parf Kosmet 1995; 76:314.

36. Tausch I, Bielfeldt S, Hildebrand A, Gasmüller J. Validation of a modified Duhring Chamber Test (DCT) as a repeated patch test for the assessment of the irritant potential of topical preparations. Parf Kosmet 1996; 76:28.

37. Frosch PJ, Kligman AM. The soap chamber test: a new method for assessing the irritancy of soaps. J Am Acad Dermatol 1979; 1:35.

38. York M, Griffiths HA, White E, Basketter DA. Evaluation of human patch test for the identification and classification of skin irritation potential. Contact 1996; 34:204.

39. Lukakovic MF, Dunlap FE, Michaels SE, Visscher MO, Watson DD. Forearm wash test to evaluate the clinical mildness of cleansing products. J Cosmet Chem 1988; 39:355.

40. Strubbe DD, Koontz SE, Murahata RI, Theiler RF. The flex wash test: a method for evaluating the mildness of personal washing products. J Cosmet Chem 1989; 40:297.

41. Clarys P, Van de Straat R, Boon A, Barel AO. The use of the hand/forearm test for evaluating skin irritation by various detergent solutions. Proc Eur Soc Contact Derm, 1992, Brussels, Belgium p. 130.

42. Manou I. Evaluation of the dermatocosmetic properties of essential oils from aromatic plants by means of skin bioengineering methods. Ph.D. thesis, Free University of Brussels (VUB), Brussels, Belgium, 1998.

43. Muizzudin N, Marenus K, Maes D, Smith WS. Use of a chromameter in assessing the efficacy of anti-irritants and tanning accelerators. J Soc Cosmet Chem 1990; 41:369.

44. Mahmoud G, Lachapelle JM, Van Neste D. Histological assessments of skin damage by irritants: its possible use in the evaluation of barrier cream. Contact Derm 1984: 11:179.

45. Lee CH, Maibach HI. The sodium lauryl sulfate model: an overview. Contact Derm 1995; 33:1.

46. Poelman MC, Piot B, Guyon F, Deroni M, Lévêque JL. Assessment of topical non-steroidal anti-inflammatory drugs. J Pharm Pharmacol 1989; 41:720.

47. Smith WP, Maes D, Marenus K, Calvo L. Natural cosmetic ingredients: enhanced function. Cosmet Toilet 1991; 106:65.

48. Bjerring P. Inhibition of UV-B induced inflammation monitored by laser Doppler blood flowmetry. Skin Pharmacol 1993; 6:187.

49. Woodbury RA, Klingman LH, Woodbury MJ, Kligman AM. Rapid assay of the inflammatory activity of topical corticosteroids by inhibition of UV-A induced neutrophil infiltration in hairless mouse skin. I. The assay and its sensitivity. Acta Derm Venereol (Stockholm) 1994; 74: 15.

50. Fleischner AM. Plant extracts: to accelerate healing and reduce inflammation. Cosmet Tioilet 1985, 100:45.

51. Albring M, Albrecht H, Alcorn G, Lücker PW. The measuring of the anti-inflammatory effect of a compound on the skin of volunteers. Meth Find Exp Clin Pharmacol 1983; 5:575.

52. Mao-Quang M, Brown B, Wu-Pong S, Feingold KR, Elias PM. Exogenous nonphysiologic versus physiologic lipids. Divergent mechanism for correction of permeability barrier dysfunction. Arch Dermatol 1995; 131:809.

53. Frosch PJ. Pilz B. Irritant patch test techniques. In: Serup J, Jemec CBE, eds. Handbook of Non-Invasive Methods and the Skin. Boca Raton: CRC Press, 1995:587.

54. Effendy I, Maibach HI. Surfactants and experimental irritant contact dermatitis. Contact Derm 1995; 33:217.

55. Gabard B, Elsner P, Treffel P. Barrier function of the skin in a repetitive irritation model and influence of 2 different treatments. Skin Res Technol 1996; 2:78.

56. Berardesca E, Fideli D, Gabba P, Cespa M, Rabiosi G, Maibach HI. Ranking of surfactant skin irritancy in vivo in man using the plastic occlusion stress test. Contact Derm. 1990; 3:1.

57. DA Basketter, E White, HA Griffith, York M. The identification and classification of skin irritation hazard by human patch test. Second International Symposium on Irritant Contact Dermatitis, Zurich, Switzerland. Allergologie 1994; 17:131.

58. Morrison Jr BM, Paye M. A comparison of three in vitro screening tests with an in vivo clinical test to evaluate the irritation potential of antibacterial soaps. J Soc Cosmet Chem 1995; 46:291.

59. Forslind B. A domain mosaic model of the skin barrier. Acta Derm Venereol (Stockholm) 1994; 74:1.

60. Di Nardo A, Sugino K, Wertz P, Adenola J, Maibach HI. Sodium lauryl sulfate induced irritant contact dermatitis: a correlation study between ceramides and in vivo parameters of irritation. Contact Derm 1996; 35:86.

61. Bruynzeel DP, Van Ketel WG, Scheper RJ, Blomberg Van Der Flier BME. Delayed time course of irritation by sodium lauryl sulfate: observation on threshold reactions. Contact Derm 1982; 8:236.

62. Novak E, Francom SF. Inflammatory response to sodium lauryl sulfate in aqueous solutions applied to the skin of normal human volunteers. Contact Derm 1984; 10:101.

63. Van Der Valk PGM, Kruis-DeVries MH, Nater JP, Bleumink E, De Jong MC. Eczematous (irritant and allergic) reactions of the skin and barrier function as determined by water vapour loss. Clin Exp Dermatol 1985; 10:185.

64. Judge MR, Griffiths HA, Basketter DA, White IR, Rycroft RJG, McFadden JP. Variations in response of human skin to irritant challenge. Contact Dermatitis 1996; 34:115.

65. Van Der Valk PGM, Maibach HI. Potential for irritation increases from the wrist to the cubital fossa. Br J Dermatol 1989; 121:709.

66. Isaac O. Pharmacological investigations with compounds of chamomile: on the pharmacology of alpha-bisabolol and bisabolol oxides. Planta Med 1979; 35:118.

67. Jellinek S. Alpha-bisabolol un agent anti-inflammatoire pour produits cosmétiques. Parfums Cosmétique Arômes 1984; 57:55.

68. Jakovlev V, Isacc O, Flaskamp E. Pharmacological investigations with compounds of chamomile. Investigation of the anti-phlohistic effects of chamazulene and matricine. Planta Med 1983; 48:67.

69. Mann C, Staba EJ. The chemistry, pharmacology and commercial formulations of chamomile. In: Cracker L, Simon JE, eds. Herbs, Spices and Medicinal Plants, Vol 1. Phoenix: Oryx Press, 1986:235.

70. Fleischner AM. Plant extracts: to accelerate healing and reduce inflammation. Cosmet Toilet 1985; 100:45.

71. Esculoside, Veinotonic molecule, treatment of the red blotches of the skin and rosacea. Technical information. Laboratoires Phybiotex, France, 1997.

72. Ursolic acid, a multifunctional anti-inflammatory principle. Technical information. Laboratoires Phybiotex, France, 1997.

73. Cher S. Botanical: Myth and reality. Cosmet Toilet 1991; 106:65.

23

Anti-irritants for Surfactant-Based Products

Marc Paye
Colgate-Palmolive Research and Development, Inc., Milmort, Belgium

In the scientific literature, sodium lauryl sulfate (SLS) is regularly used as the ''gold'' model to induce skin irritation [1]. This is for several reasons:

1. SLS is classified as a skin irritant, Xi-R38 [2],
2. SLS can be obtained in a very pure form, which allows different laboratories to work on the same material,
3. SLS can be easily formulated in various vehicles,
4. Although a few cases were reported [3], allergic reactions to SLS are not frequent, and
5. The level of induced irritation can be more or less controlled by adjusting the concentration [4,5], and any skin damage is rapidly reversible.

However, SLS is not the only surfactant to be an irritant to the skin, and even if some surfactants are not classified as such by the Dangerous Substances Directive [2], in certain conditions and concentrations all surfactants can be regarded as potential irritants to different degrees. This paragraph will, however, mainly focus on anionic surfactants, as they are mostly used in toiletries and require the most attention in order to optimize their skin compatibility in finished products.

Fortunately, nowadays many systems have been developed to minimize the risks of intolerance in hygiene cosmetics or surfactant-based products. This is extremely important because hygiene habits have strongly evolved over the years. Not so long ago, people came into contact with surfactants only once a day maximum with the only objective being to clean themselves; today it is not unusual to see people having several showers a day not only for cleaning themselves but also for pleasure and relaxation. So far, toilet products must be as mild as possible for the skin. Not only are the mildest ingredients used, but finished hygiene products also have to contain one or more of the following anti-irritant systems.

ANTI-IRRITATION BY AN APPROPRIATE COMBINATION OF SURFACTANTS

Although rarely described as an anti-irritation system, this approach, in my view, should be regarded as the most potent one to get a very mild surfactant-based product. The best counterirritants for surfactants are other surfactants. Several investigators have clearly shown such a positive interaction between various surfactants both in vitro [6,7] and in vivo [8–10], as well as with diluted [6–8] and highly concentrated solutions [9,10]. Amphoteric surfactants are probably best known to decrease the irritation potential of anionic ones [11], but nonionic surfactant can have the same effect as well when used at a sufficiently high concentration. More suprisingly, a well-selected anionic surfactant can also reduce the irritation potential of another anionic surfactant, instead of cumulating their effects [9].

The suspected mechanism occurring in this system is linked to the formation of larger and mainly more stable micelles of surfactants when several surfactants are present in the same solution. It has been described in Chapter 36 [12] that surfactants in aqueous solutions tend to assemble by their hydrophobic tail and form micelles. The totality of surfactants is, however, not entrapped into the micelles and the micelles are not static structures. They form and dissociate constantly at a rate depending on the type of surfactants entering into their composition. Importantly, even if micelles are capable of permeabilizing the skin barrier by interacting with the lipids [10], they do not irritate skin by themselves; only the monomers of surfactant can directly interact with the skin proteins and cause irritation. Forming larger and more stable micelles by an appropriate combination of surfactants can thus decrease the relative amount of monomers available to irritate the skin. Such a mechanism is well acccepted, but it would be too simplistic to consider that it is the only one. For instance, the addition of a secondary surfactant milder than the primary one could decrease the binding to skin surface of this latter by occupying and competing for the same binding site. Although such a mechanism has not been clearly shown yet as being a cause for anti-irritation, it looks quite realistic and possible when using two anionic surfactants in view of surfactant binding studies showing that various anionic surfactants saturate the skin surface from a very similar concentration (personal data). Furthermore, a decrease of binding of anionic surfactants to skin surface has been shown by attenuated total reflectance—Fourier transformed infrared spectroscopy (ATR—FTIR) in presence of a secondary surfactant of any type (personal data). However, this could be the consequence of the bulk effect previously described and not a direct cause of anti-irritation.

ANTI-IRRITATION BY POLYMERS OR PROTEINS/PEPTIDES

The counterirritant capability of polymers or proteins on surfactants has been known from literature data for a long time [13–16]. The mechanism by which they function is similar to the one previously described above for surfactant mixtures, being incorporated into the micelles to decrease the relative amount of free monomers into the solutions. Their usual skin substantivity can also involve some hiding of binding site at the surface of the skin for the surfactants.

All polymers are not equally effective to be incorporated into the micelles or to interact with the skin surface; when selecting a polymer/protein, the following parameters should be considered:

1. A better interaction with the micelles is obtained when the hydrophobicity increases [13]
2. A better substantivity with the skin is obtained when the hydrophobicity increases, such as when the polymer is quaternized or cationic or when the net charge or the size of the polymer/protein increases [14–16]

In view of these properties, more hydrophobic and/or larger polymers/proteins are much more effective to depress the skin irritation potential of surfactants. However, in the literature the anti-irritant effect of proteins/polymers onto surfactants has usually been shown in a single surfactant solution, and at a high polymer-surfactant ratio that is often incompatible with a finished product for stickiness, formulation, foaming, or cost reasons. From my experience, many polymers or proteins, described as depressors of irritation, do not bring any additional benefit on the clinical mildness of the product when they are formulated into a finished product that has already been optimized for skin compatibility through an appropriate combination of surfactants. In some cases, however, those polymers have been shown to reduce the penetration of the surfactants into the stratum corneum in conditions where nonexaggerated application tests are run, but not in occlusive patch tests that would enforce such a penetration whether in the presence or absence of a polymer (personal data).

ANTI-IRRITATION BY REFATTENING AGENTS

One of the effects of surfactants on skin is the alteration of its permeability barrier, which can be easily assessed by measuring the transepidermal water loss [17,18]. Using refattening ingredients or skin barrier repairing ingredients in the surfactant-based product can lead to a reduction of irritation if appropriately delivered to the skin surface. Such ingredients are often the basis for barrier cream effect when topically applied before or after contact with an irritant. Some of these ingredients can, however, be formulated into a surfactant system to act directly as anti-irritants in the mixture. The occlusive effect they bring at the surface of the skin delays the water loss and maintains the skin in a less dehydrated state. Furthermore, they can introduce a barrier that can protect the skin against surfactants when running repetitive applications. Several types of refattening ingredients are available and can be formulated in surfactant systems, such as ethoxylated mono-, di-, and triglycerides, fatty alcohols and ethoxylated fatty alcohols, fatty acid esters, lanolin derivatives, or silicone derivatives. A few products containing a high percentage of oil also exist on the market and can possibly play such a role.

ANTI-INFLAMMATORY EFFECT

Ingredients with an anti-inflammatory effect are not specific for surfactants and are described in the other sections of this chapter. Such ingredients act directly at the skin level and it is obvious that they have no anti-inflammatory effect in solution. In order to be effective, they must be delivered to the skin in a bioavailable form and in sufficient amount.

ANTISENSORY IRRITATION

Although much less discussed than the clinical irritation that is characterized by observable or functional alterations, subjective irritation also exists. It does not have great interest for the dermatologists, but for cosmetologists it can be the reason for the success or rejection of their product. Two types of sensory irritation can be observed by the consumer: itching, stinging, or burning sensations, and unpleasant rough, dry tight sensations. Anti-irritant systems for the former sensations are described in Chapter 25 [19]. Regarding the latter sensations, the irritation perception can be addressed in two ways: by reformulating the surfactant system or by introducing ''good'' skin feel additives. Each surfactant provides in itself a specific perception on the skin of the consumer, going from smooth (perception of nonirritated skin) to dry/tight (perception of irritated skin) skin feel. Adapting a combination of surfactants can allow formulators to provide the expected feel. However, if constraints in the choice of surfactants does not allow moving away from an "irritated" feel, it is still possible to add skin feel additives into the product in order for the product to be perceived as smoothing or hydrating the surface of the skin. Skin feel additives have been reviewed in Chapter 35 [20]. In the consumer view, this will often be considered as a milder product.

MAGNESIUM AND DIVALENT CATIONS ARE NOT ANTI-IRRITANTS FOR SURFACTANTS

Magnesium is frequently described as a depressor of skin irritation [21]. Such a false idea is essentially arising from in vitro data based on protein denaturation tests. In those tests, the more a surfactant solution denatures a protein, the more it is predicted to be an irritant for the skin, and magnesium clearly depresses surfactant-induced protein denaturation in vitro [22]. However, when well-controlled in vivo tests are performed to investigate the effect of magnesium directly on human volunteers, it comes out unambiguously that magnesium does not decrease the skin irritation potential of surfactants or surfactant-based products [21]. The in vivo studies included both acute irritation by occlusive patch tests and chronic irritation by repetitive short-term applications of the products. The study compared sodium and magnesium salts of surfactants (e.g., magnesium and sodium lauryl sulfate) in single solutions or incorporated into finished products, and investigated the effect of adding magnesium sulfate to a solution of surfactant. Some preliminary studies with calcium showed a similar behavior as magnesium (personal data) both in vitro and in vivo.

CONCLUSION

This chapter briefly reviews several systems by which it is now possible to control the skin irritation potential of surfactant-based products. This can be done

1. Through a modification of their behavior in solution,
2. Through a modification of their interaction with the surface of the skin,
3. Through a protection of the skin surface via the solution, and
4. Through an action onto the inflammatory process.

This last mechanism is, however, not specific at all to surfactant systems and has been reviewed in other parts of this chapter.

These anti-irritant systems, combined with a selection of mild surfactants, allow the cosmetic formulator to design very mild hygiene products. In the synthesis or chemical transformation of surfactants, it is also possible to modify the surfactant molecule to make it less irritating for the skin. This can be done by modifying the carbon chain length, by grafting fatty chains to the surfactant, or by increasing the ethoxylation level of the surfactant. Such modifications are, however, not directly considered anti-irritant systems, even if their goal and consequence is usually a decrease of the overall irritation potential.

REFERENCES

1. Lee CH, Maibach HI. The sodium lauryl sulfate model: an overview. Contact Dermatitis 1995; 33:1–7.
2. EC Directive 67/548/EEC.
3. Prater E, Goring HD, Schubert H. Sodium lauryl sulfate—a contact allergen. Contact Dermatitis 1978; 4:242–243.
4. Dillarstone A, Paye M. Classification of surfactant-containing products as ''skin irritants.'' Contact Dermatitis 1994; 30:314–315.
5. Agner T, Serup J. Sodium lauryl sulphate for irritant patch testing—a dose-response study using bioengineering methods for determination of skin irritation. J Invest Dermatol 1990; 95:543–547.
6. Rhein LD, Simion FA. Surfactant interactions with skin. Surf Sci Ser 1991; 32:33–49.
7. Rhein LD, Robbins CR, Fernee K, et al. Surfactant structure effects on swelling of isolated human stratum corneum. J Soc Cosmet Chem 1986; 37:125–139.
8. Lee CH, Kawasaki Y, Maibach HI. Effect of surfactant mixtures on irritant contact dermatitis potential in man: sodium lauryl glutamate and sodium lauryl sulphate. Contact Dermatitis 1994; 30:205–209.
9. Dillarstone A, Paye M. Antagonsim in concentrated surfactant systems. Contact Dermatitis 1993; 28:198.
10. Hall-Manning TJ, Holland GH, Rennie G, et al. Skin irritation potential of mixed surfactant systems. Food Chem Toxicol 1998; 36:233–238.
11. Dominguez JG, Balaguer F, Parra JL, Pelejero CM. The inhibitory effect of some amphoteric surfactants on the irritation potential of alkylsulphates. Intl J Cosmet Sci 1981; 3:57–68.
12. Tamura T, Masuda M. Surfactants. In: *Contact Dermatitis*, Chapter 36:417–443.
13. Teglia A, Secchi G. New protein ingredients for skin detergency: native wheat protein-surfactant complexes. Intl J Cosmet Sci 1994; 16:235–246.
14. Teglia A, Mazzola G, Secchi G. Relationships between chemical characteristics and cosmetic properties of protein hydrolysates. Cosmet Toilet 1993; 108:56–65.
15. Goddard ED, Leung PS. Protection of skin by cationic cellulosics: in-vitro testing methods. Cosmet Toilet 1982; 97:55–69.
16. Pugliese P, Hines G, Wielenga W. Skin protective properties of a cationic guar derivative. Cosmet Toilet 1990; 105:105–111.
17. Van der Valk PGM, Nater JP, Bleumink E. Skin irritancy of surfactants as assessed by water vapor loss measurements. J Invest Dermatol 1984; 82:291–293.
18. Kawasaki Y, Quan D, Sakamoto D, et al. Influence of surfactant mixtures on intercellular lipid fluidity and skin barrier function. Skin Res Technol 1999; 5:96–101.
19. Hahn GS. Antisensory anti-irritants. In: *Contact Dermatitis*, Chapter 25:285–288.
20. Zocchi G. Skin-feel agents. In: *Contact Dermatitis*, Chapter 35:388–415.
21. Paye M, Zocchi G, Broze G. Magnesium as skin irritation depressor: fact or artifact? Proceedings of the XXVII Jornadas Anuales del CED, Barcelona, Spain, June 1998, 449–456.
22. Goffin V, Paye M, Piérard GE. Comparison of in vitro predictive tests for irritation induced by anionic surfactants. Contact Dermatitis 1995; 33:38–41.

24

The Case of Alpha-Bisabolol

Klaus Stanzl
DRAGOCO Gerberding & Co. AG, Holzminden, Germany

Jürgen Vollhardt
DRAGOCO Inc., Totowa, New Jersey

INTRODUCTION

In the inflammatory process, monocytes leave the blood and enter the tissue at the site of inflammation as part of the cellular infiltrate. The tissue endothelial cells in inflammation express adhesion molecules to which monocytes adhere, then they penetrate through the endothelium into the tissue along a gradient of inflammation signals. The metabolites of the arachidonic acid cascade (Fig. 1), like leukotriene, prostaglandin, as well as oxygen radicals, play an important role.

Chamomile is one of the most popular plants in medicine as well as in cosmetics. Its active ingredients are essential oils with a blue color coming from chamazulen—yellow flavonoids as well as some coumarins and mucilage among others.

The essential oil has an excellent anti-inflammatory effect according to its chamazulene, ($-$)-α-bisabolol, -oxides, and enindicycloether content [1]. This is the reason why we have chosen chamomile ingredients, and especially Bisabolol, as an example of anti-irritants and how these ingredients actually work.

The major constituents of chamomile are: Matricin, ($-$)-α-bisabolol, bisabololoxides A and B, flavonoids (apigenin, apigenin-7-glucosides), and cis-trans-en-in-dicycloether. Chamazulen is formed from matricin. Matricin will be transferred by steam distillation into chamazulencarbonacid and further to chamazulen during extraction of the essential oil (Fig. 2).

Alpha-bisabolol is a sesquiterpene component (Fig. 3), which was detected by Isaac et al. [2] The antiphlogistic property was demonstrated in several animal tests [3–5]. In an in vitro study, Ammon et al. [6] described the mechanism of the activity of chamomile ingredients. ($-$)-α-Bisabolol works by inhibiting 5-lipoxygenase and cyclooxygenase. There is no inhibition of the 12-lipoxygenase and ($-$)-α-bisabolol does not have any antioxidant properties. The author found that bisabolol is effective at a concentration level of about 30 to 80 micromoles to inhibit 50% of the enzyme activity.

In 1983, Guillot et al. [7] compared the anti-irritant properties of various ingredients used in cosmetic products (Table 1). In this study, he made an emulsion irritating by the

Phospholipid
↓
Phospholipase A₂
↓
Arachidonic Acid
|

↓   ↓   ↓

12-Lipoxygenase
15-Lipoxygenase 5-Lipoxygenase Cyclooxygenase

↓   ↓   ↓

Hydroxyeicosa-tetraenoic acid	Leukotriene	
12-HETE	LTB₄, LTC₄, LTD₄, LTE₄,	Prostaglandin
15-HETE	5-HPETE	Thromboxane
	5-HETE	

FIGURE 1   Arachidonic acid cascade.

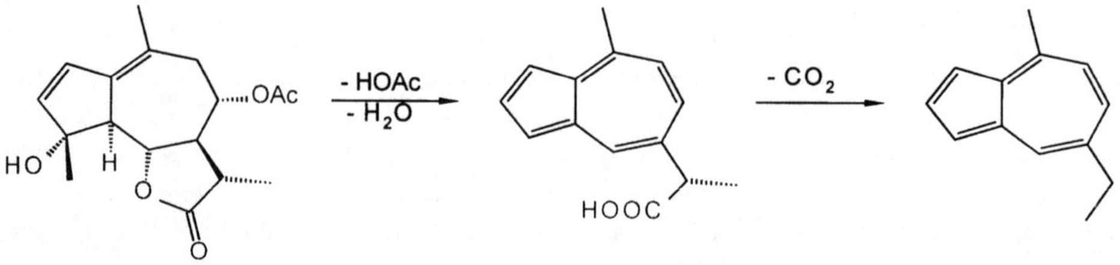

M a t r i c i n   C h a m a z u l e n c a r b o n a c i d   C h a m a z u l e n

FIGURE 2   Transfer of matricin via steam distillation into chamazulen.

► IUPAC-name:
(2S)-6-Methyl-2-((1S)-4-methyl-3-cyclohexenyl)-5-hepten-2-ol

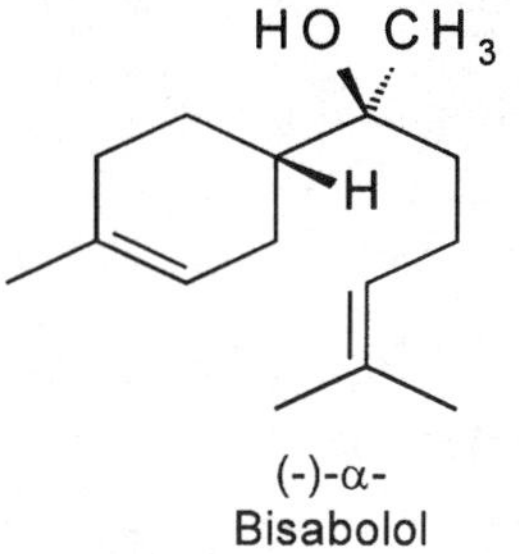

(-)-α-
Bisabolol

FIGURE 3   Chemical structure of (−)-α-bisabolol.

TABLE 1   Anti-irritant Properties of Ingredients Used
in Cosmetic Products

Product	% used	Irritation index
Glycyrrhetinic acid	1.0%	−0.42
Lidocaine	0.5%	−0.79
Phenylsalicylate	0.5%	−0.62
Bisabolol	1.0%	−0.55
Bisabolol	3.0%	−0.25
Azulene	0.2%	−0.21
Guaiazulene	0.1%	−0.13
Panthenol	3.0%	0/−0.13

addition of croton oil in sufficient quantities to provoke a clearly adverse reaction. The primary cutaneous irritation index was close to 2 according to the French method. The smaller the number, the more active the product. Interestingly, he found that bisabolol at 1% was more effective than bisabolol at 3%. Unfortunately, he did not mention what type of bisabolol he tested, because in a study conducted by Jakovlev [8], this investigator demonstrated that the various isomers of bisabolol show different activities. He found that (−) alpha-bisabolol was the most effective isomer. He set the efficacy of (−) alpha-bisabolol as 1,000 and compared the efficacy of the other substances to (−) alpha.

(−) alpha-bisabolol	1,000
(+) alpha-bisabolol	595
(+/−) bisabolol nat.	419
(+/−) bisabolol synth.	493

We conducted a clinical study to demonstrate in vivo the anti-inflammatory effects of natural (−)-α-bisabolol and synthetic bisabolol, which contains four stereoisomeric molecules (Fig. 4). The aim of this study was to find the concentration at which these ingredients are most active. A second test was designed to prove that the synthetic bisabolol also has protective properties against sodium hydroxide–induced irritation.

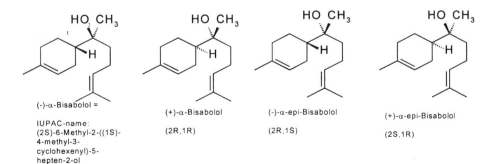

FIGURE 4   Molecular structure of bisabolol isomers.

STUDY OF THE EFFECTIVENESS OF FIVE PRODUCTS CONTAINING BISABOLOL OR SYNTHETIC BISABOLOL ON SLS-INDUCED SKIN IRRITATION: TEST METHOD

Thirty female volunteers at the age of 18 to 63 years with healthy skin were included in the test. The participants were briefed on the study procedures and each gave written informed consent. Measurements were carried out at a temperature of $22 \pm 1°C$ and relative humidity of $60 \pm 10\%$. The test was carried out on the volar forearms. Skin irritation was induced in the test sites by applying sodium lauryl sulphate (SLS) 2% in distilled water under aluminum chamber occlusion. After 24 hours, occlusion was removed, and 2 hours later skin redness and TEWL were recorded. After the initial measurement the five test products were applied, and one area remained untreated. The dose of application was about 2 mg/cm^2. In the following 5 days, the subjects applied the test samples in the morning and in the evening. Measurements were done during the treatment period on days 1, 3, and 5, 2 hours after the last daily application. No use of other cosmetics was allowed on the test sites during the whole test.

EVALUATION OF THE PROTECTIVE EFFICACY OF SYNTHETIC BISABOLOL AGAINST SODIUM HYDROXIDE–INDUCED IRRITATION

Fifteen volunteers between the age of 25 and 44 years with healthy skin were entered into the study. The participants were briefed on the study procedures and gave written informed consent. Measurements were carried out at a temperature of $22 \pm 1°C$ and relative humidity of $60 \pm 10\%$. The test was carried out on the volar forearms. The dose of application was about 2 mg/cm^2. Two products were tested. One contained 0.56% synthetic bisabolol in mineral oil, the other pure mineral oil. Two hours after the application, 50 µL 0.1 M sodium hydroxide (NaOH) was applied to the volar forearms with occlusive aluminum chambers for 12 hours. At the end of exposure, the skin was wiped with a soft paper towel to remove remaining solution, rinsed with distilled water and gently dried with a soft paper towel. Measurements were performed after 15 minutes.

Chromametry

Skin color was assessed with the Minolta Chromameter CR 300 (Minolta, Japan) in compliance with the Commission International de l'Eclairage (CIE) system. A color is expressed in a three-dimensional coordinate system with greed-red (a*), yellow-blue (b*), and L* axes (brightness). In inflamed skin, a positive change on the a* axis is observed. Each value was the average of three recordings.

TEWL

Measurements of TEWL were performed with the Tewameter TM 210 (Courage & Khazaka, Cologne, Germany). Each value was the average of three recordings.

Statistics

Summary statistics procedure was used to determine the center, spread, and shape of the data. Statistical analysis was performed using Wilcoxon matched pairs signed rank test. A *p*-value of less than 0.05 was taken to indicate a significant difference.

717:   mineral oil
498:      0.5%   synthetic Bisabolol in mineral oil
984:      0.1%   synthetic Bisabolol in mineral oil
973:      0.05%   synthetic Bisabolol in mineral oil
251:      0.1125%   (-)-α-Bisabolol in mineral oil

FIGURE 5   Test products to determine the beneficial effect of synthetic bisabolol and (−)-α-bisabolol.

RESULTS OF STUDY 1 (HEALING POWER OF SYNTHETIC BISABOLOL)

Figure 8 shows the result of the TEWL measurements. The application of five test products (Fig. 5) after SLS exposure reduced TEWL in shorter time (after 24 h and 48 h) in comparison with the untreated area ($p < 0.05$). After 120 hours there was no difference between the six test areas. Neither synthetic bisabolol nor natural (−)-α-bisabolol influenced the repair of skin barrier. The measurement of the redness values shows (Fig. 7) that the inflammation was reduced faster (72 h and 120 h) in a dose-dependent manner with the products containing the actives compared with the mineral oil treatment (area 717) and the untreated area. Mineral oil delays the healing process.

RESULTS OF STUDY 2 (PROTECTIVE PROPERTIES OF SYNTHETIC BISABOLOL)

There was an increase of the a*-values in the untreated area after 4 hours indicating that a solution of 0,1 M NaOH−induced strong skin irritation. The redness in the test area with the synthetic bisabolol treatment increased only slightly after NaOH treatment. The Chromameter value a* after NaOH treatment was significantly lower for the test area with

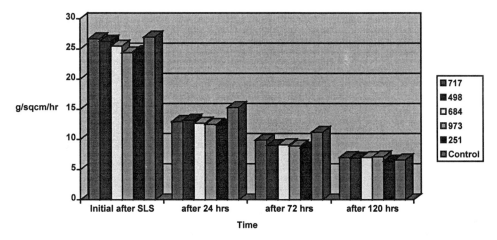

FIGURE 6   TEWL Measurements of five products containing different amounts of synthetic bisabolol/(−)-α-bisabolol.

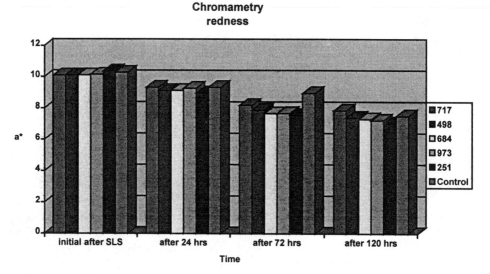

FIGURE 7   Redness assessment of five products containing different amounts of synthetic bisabolol/(−)-α-bisabolol.

Chromametry

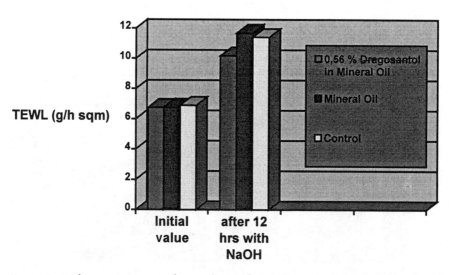

FIGURE 8   Redness assessment of a product with 0.56% synthetic bisabolol in mineral oil in comparison to the untreated area and the mineral oil–treated area.

TEWL

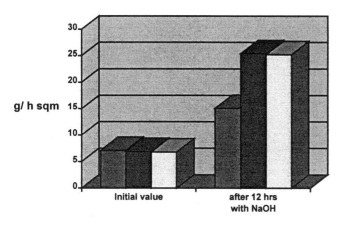
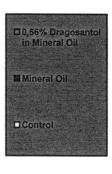

FIGURE 9   TEWL Measurements of a product containing 0.56% synthetic bisabolol in mineral oil compared with mineral oil and the untreated site.

the product, containing synthetic bisabolol, compared with the untreated site. The areas treated with pure mineral oil showed the highest increase in skin redness (Fig. 8). There was an increase in TEWL in all test areas after NaOH treatment. The TEWL values after exposure to NaOH were significantly higher for the untreated area in comparison to the pretreated sites (Fig. 9).

SUMMARY

Synthetic bisabolol and natural $(-)$-α-bisabolol have protective and beneficial effects, which were demonstrated by two new clinical studies. The grade of inflammation was measured with the help of a Minolta Chromameter and the a*-value was used to determine the grade of inflammation. The transepidermal water loss was used to reflect the damage of the skin barrier.

The studies proved that $(-)$-α-bisabolol and synthetic bisabolol reduces the development of an erythema and reduce erythema set by sodium lauryl sulfate. The damage of the skin barrier was also reduced by both products. It is important to mention that the concentration of the synthetic bisabolol and natural $(-)$-α-bisabolol is very essential for the efficacy of the cosmetic product. There is a maximum concentration level for both ingredients. An increase of the concentration beyond this point leads to a reduction in efficacy. For leave-on products, the maximum concentration depending on the base formula is between 0.05% and 0.2%.

Synthetic bisabolol and natural $(-)$-α-bisabolol show a significant substantivity to skin out of a rinse-off product. Therefore, both ingredients can add value to a body wash or shampoo by reducing the well-known irritation effect of certain surfactants. In this case, the maximum concentration level is approximately 0.3%.

REFERENCES

1. Ammon HPT, Kaul R. Pharmakologie der Kamille und ihrer Inhaltsstoffe. Dtsch, Apoth, Ztg, 1992; 132:1–26.
2. Isaac O. Fortschritte der Kamillenforschung. Struktur und Wirkung des (−) Bizabolols. Praeperative Pharmazie 1986; 5:189–199.
3. Wichtl M. Teedrogen, 2. Auflage Wissenschaftliche Verlagsgesellschaft mbH, Stuttgart.
4. Wagner H. Pharmazeutische Biologie, 5. Stuttgart, New York: Auflage Gustav Fischer Verlag.
5. Issac O. Die Kamillentherapie–Erfahrung und Bestätigung Deutsche Apotheker Zeitung, 120 Jahrg., 13. 567.
6. Ammon HPT, Sabieraj J, Kaul R. Kamille–Mechanismus der antiphlogistischen Wirkung von Kamillenextrakten und -inhaltsstoffen. Dtsch. Apoth. Ztg 1996; 136:1821.
7. Guillot et al. Intern J Cosm Sci 1983; 5:255.
8. Jakovlev et al. Planta Medica 1979; 35:125.

25

Anti-irritants for Sensory Irritation

Gary S. Hahn
*University of California at San Diego School of Medicine, San Diego, and
Cosmederm Technologies, LLC, La Jolla, California*

INTRODUCTION

Many chemicals found in cosmetics, personal-care products, pharmaceuticals, and in industrial processes can irritate the skin and mucous membranes of the eye and the respiratory and gastrointestinal tracts. Perhaps the most effective early-warning system that responds to these chemicals is sensory irritation—the rapid-onset stinging, burning, and itching sensations that alert an organism to their exposure to foreign, and potentially injurious, substances. These sensations, even when intense, may occur in the absence of visible signs of irritation or skin damage or, alternatively, may be accompanied by erythema and/or edema [1].

Sensory irritation occurs when thin, unmyelinated, chemically sensitive type-C nociceptors (from the Latin *nocere*, to injure) are activated and transmit a depolarizing signal via the dorsal root ganglia (DRG) in the spinal cord to the brain where stinging, burning, itching, and poorly localized burning pain is appreciated [2]. These sensations are neurologically distinct from the highly localized sharp pain caused by cutting or puncturing the skin that is transmitted by the thinly myelinated A-delta class of nerve fibers [3]. Type-C nociceptors are present throughout the dermis and extend to the outermost layer of the viable epidermis, thus acting as one of the skin's earliest warning systems [4]. When the intensity of the irritant stimulus is sufficiently high, interneurons in the DRG and/or depolarizing signals within the terminal aborization of a single nerve fiber trigger retrograde depolarization down the activated fiber, resulting in the exocytosis of inflammatory mediators at the site of the irritant stimulus [5,6]. The principal mediators in humans include substance P, calcitonin gene-related peptide (CGRP), and neurokinin-A, a member of the substance P family. These mediators, coupled with the neurogenically mediated vasodilatory erythematous "flare" surrounding the irritated site, produce erythema, edema, and activation of immune cells, including mast cells, that contribute to the clinical response of neurogenic inflammation.

THE IDEAL ANTISENSORY ANTI-IRRITANT

The idea antisensory anti-irritant would effectively inhibit stinging, burning, and itching caused by a broad range of acidic, neutral, and basic chemical irritants by reducing the sensitivity of type-C nociceptors. In contrast, it would not inhibit the warning symptom of pain mediated by A-delta nerves, nor would it affect other nerve sensors that mediate tactile, temperature, or vibratory sensations. Since most cosmetic-induced sensory irritation occurs within several minutes after application, the ideal anti-irritant should work within seconds when formulated with the irritant. For broad product use, it should also work when applied as a pretreatment before the irritating formulation and it should work when applied after irritation has occurred. Because cosmetics use a wide range of chemicals, the anti-irritant should be stable in many chemical environments and inexpensive enough to be used in low-cost products. With repeated daily use, the ideal anti-irritant should provide the same effective level of anti-irritant protection (no tachyphylaxis) and, most importantly, it must be safe for broad, unsupervised use.

With the exception of local anesthetics that are regulated as drugs in most countries and may have undesirable side effects and safety concerns, no compounds have been described that are able to broadly inhibit sensory irritation from cosmetics and pharmaceuticals. Because a safe compound capable of blocking sensory irritation and inflammation would provide considerable benefit, I sought to identify compounds that could effectively block sensory irritant reactions. Simple water-soluble strontium salts have proved to be potent and selective inhibitors of chemically induced sensory irritation and neurogenic inflammation in humans and do not produce numbness or loss of other tactile sensations [7–10].

THE FIRST EFFECTIVE ANTISENSORY ANTI-IRRITANTS: STRONTIUM SALTS

Clinical Evaluation of Sensory Irritation

A variety of chemical irritants used in cosmetics were used to induce sensory irritation. All clinical studies were conducted according to double-blind, vehicle-controlled, random treatment assignment protocols in which each subject served as her own control. Test subjects were healthy women, aged 18 to 65, who self-reported a history of sensitive skin and were sensitive to lactic acid facial challenge. Treated skin sites were first washed with Ivory bar soap, followed by sequential application of test materials and sensory irritation evaluation. Statistical analysis of the mean sensory irritation differences between vehicle and strontium-treated groups was conducted using the Wilcoxon Signed Ranks Test for paired comparisons. All subjects provided informed consent and all protocols were reviewed by a safety committee.

Sensory Irritation Scale

Each minute for 10 to 60 minutes, depending on the study, subjects reported the magnitude of sensory irritation (stinging, burning, and itching) according to the following scale:

0 = none		
1 = slight	Transient, barely perceptible irritation	
	Does not bother them	
2 = mild	Definite and continuous irritation	
	Bothers them	
3 = moderate	Distinctly uncomfortable irritation	
	Bothers them and interferes with concentration	
4 = severe	Continuous, intensely uncomfortable irritation	
	Intolerable and would interfere with daily routine	

ACIDIC IRRITANTS

Lactic Acid (7.5%, pH = 1.9) Sensory Irritation on the Face

Alpha-hydroxyacids (AHAs) including lactic and glycolic acids are used in cosmetics and in professionally applied chemical peels to reduce the visible signs of skin aging. To maximize AHA efficacy, the formulation must be acidic, which increases the active "free acid" form of the AHA molecule and, unfortunately, directly contributes to their irritation potential [11,12]. To evaluate the ability of strontium salts to reduce lactic acid sensory irritation, either lactic acid alone (7.5% in 10% ethanol/water vehicle, pH = 1.9), or an identical vehicle at the same pH containing various concentrations of strontium nitrate or strontium chloride was applied (0.1 g) to cheek sites using cotton swabs (6 swipes) extending from the nasolabial fold to the outer cheek. Test materials were applied to the right or left side of subjects' faces sequentially followed by sensory irritation assessment on each side for 10 minutes. A typical time-response curve for lactic acid (7.5%, pH = 1.9) on the face is presented in Figure 1. When the areas under both irritation curves are compared, strontium nitrate inhibited sensory irritation by 68% ($p < 0.01$). Both strontium nitrate and strontium chloride produced dose-dependent inhibition of sensory irritation when mixed with lactic acid (Table 1) [7]. In separate studies, the local anesthetic lidocaine (4%) was used as a positive control. When applied at the same time as the lactic acid, lidocaine did not produce significant inhibition ($<10\%$), presumably because it requires time to be absorbed. When lidocaine (4%) was applied 5 minutes before the lactic acid, lidocaine inhibited by 51% ($p < 0.05$, n = 10).

Strontium Pretreatment on the Face

Many cosmetics such as toners and skin conditioners, are applied immediately before application of potentially irritating products. Incorporation of strontium salts into such a pretreatment product from 1 minute to 15 minutes before the same lactic acid facial challenge produced a substantial level of sensory irritation inhibition (Table 1). In other studies, substantial anti-irritancy was also observed when strontium nitrate was applied several minutes after lactic acid was applied.

When the same lactic acid challenge was used in conjunction with "conventional" anti-irritants used in cosmetics such as green tea (3%), alpha-bisabolol (1%), and glycyrrhizic acid (1%), no significant inhibition was observed ($<10\%$ difference from vehicle control).

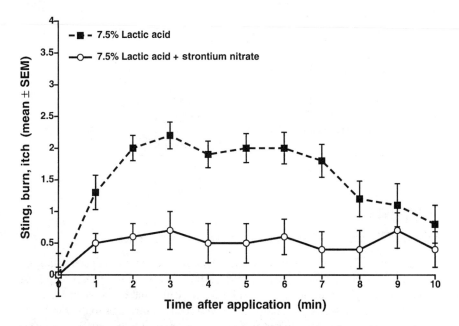

FIGURE 1   Lactic acid alone (closed squares) or with strontium nitrate (250 mM) was applied to the faces of 23 subjects and sensory irritation was assessed every minute for 10 minutes (see text for scale). Each data point represents the mean ±SEM irritation at each minute for all subjects. Total cumulative irritation (area under the curve) was inhibited by 68% ($p < 0.01$).

To determine whether the strontium cation was necessary for the observed antiirritant activity, sodium chloride (250 mM) and sodium nitrate (250 mM) were mixed with the lactic acid and compared with strontium nitrate (250 mM) or strontium chloride (250 mM). In both instances, sodium nitrate or sodium chloride produced insignificant ($<10\%$) inhibition of sensory irritation proving that the nitrate or chloride anions did not produce the observed anti-irritant activity.

Lactic Acid (15%, pH = 3.0) Sensory Irritation on the Face

The anti-irritant activity of strontium salts is also evident for less acidic AHA irritants similar to what could be used in high-potency over-the-counter cosmetic products. When lactic acid (15% in a hydroxyethyl cellulose hydrogel, pH = 3.0) with or without 250 mM (5.3%) strontium nitrate was applied to the faces of 33 subjects, the cumulative irritation inhibition by the strontium-containing solutions was 66% ($p = 0.003$) (Table 2). The incidence of each of the four scores of lactic acid only versus lactic acid plus strontium was: severe: 25 vs. 1 = 96% inhibition; moderate: 59 vs. 2 = 97% inhibition; mild: 48 vs. 5 = 90% inhibition; slight: 22 vs. 48 = 118% increase; and none: 44 vs. 142 = 223% increase.

Glycolic Acid (70%, pH = 0.6) Sensory Irritation on the Arms

High-concentration, low-pH glycolic acid formulations are used by physicians to reduce the visible signs of skin photoaging and to treat moderately severe acne. To maximize

TABLE 1 Inhibition of Sensory Irritation Scores from 7.5% Lactic Acid (pH = 1.9)

| Strontium salt (mM) | Strontium chloride* | | Strontium nitrate* | | 15-Minute pretreatment strontium nitrate* | |
| | Inhibition† | | Inhibition | | Inhibition | |
	% ± SEM	(# subjects, p)	% ± SEM	(# subjects, p)	% ± SEM	(# subjects, p)
500	75 ± 7	(n = 16, $p < 0.005$)	68 ± 6	(n = 24, $p < 0.01$)	58 ± 12	(n = 16, $p < 0.01$)
250	65 ± 12	(n = 17, $p < 0.01$)	74 ± 7	(n = 23, $p < 0.01$)	48 ± 11	(n = 18, $p < 0.01$)
125	64 ± 5	(n = 15, $p < 0.01$)	42 ± 14	(n = 15, $p < 0.01$)	28 ± 16	(n = 15, $p < 0.01$)
63	30 ± 6	(n = 8, $p < 0.01$)	34 ± 8	(n = 16, $p < 0.01$)	17 ± 10	(n = 18, $p < 0.01$)

* Strontium nitrate or strontium chloride hexahydrate was either mixed with the lactic acid vehicle (7.5%, pH = 1.9, 10% ethanol/water) or preapplied to the face in a 10% ethanol/water vehicle 15 minutes before the application of the lactic acid vehicle.

† The total cumulative irritation in each study (scores of 1 + 2 + 3 + 4) for the lactic acid–treated side of the face was compared with the lactic acid + strontium-treated side of the face (areas under the curves) and irritation inhibition was calculated as a percent difference.

TABLE 2 Inhibition of Sensory Irritation Scores by Strontium Nitrate

Irritation score		Lactic acid (15%, pH = 3.0)	Glycolic acid (70%, pH = 0.6)	Capryloyl salicylic acid (1%, pH = 3.5)	Ascorbic acid (30%, pH = 1.7)	Calcium thioglycolate (4%, pH = 12)
				% Inhibition of sensory irritation scores*		
Subjects (#)		33	19	24	20	23
Total scores		363	209	312	110	506
None	(0)	−223†	−381	−74	−260	−65
Slight	(1)	−118	−6	−8	63	40
Mild	(2)	90	43	71	91	76
Moderate	(3)	97	92	31	100	71
Severe	(4)	96	100	58	100	—

* Sensory irritation was induced by lactic acid (15%, pH = 3.0) application to the face, glycolic acid (70%, pH = 0.6) application to arms, capryloyl salicylic acid (1%, pH = 3.5) application to face, ascorbic acid (30%, pH = 1.7) application to the face, and calcium thioglycolate (4%, pH = 12) depilatory application to the legs. For each study, the incidence of each of the four sensory irritation scores (0–4) for the irritant alone and the irritant plus strontium nitrate treatment was compared. Each number represents the percent inhibition of each irritation score incidence induced by strontium nitrate.
† Negative inhibition values represent an increase in the score incidence.

potency, unneutralized glycolic acid solutions are used (e.g., 20%, pH = 1.5 to 70%, pH = 0.6) but all produce potentially severe irritation. For this reason, most patients are exposed to increased concentrations and exposure times over a multimonth period until they reach a "maintenance" exposure (e.g., 70% glycolic acid, pH = 0.6 for 4–6 min) [13]. With strontium nitrate added to such formulations, patients can immediately obtain the benefits of the most potent glycolic acid formulations with very little or no irritation.

To demonstrate the anti-irritant efficacy of strontium in glycolic acid peel solutions, 70% glycolic acid (pH = 0.6) with or without strontium nitrate (20% [945 mM]) was applied to the forearms of 19 subjects on 2 inch by 4 inch rectangular sites and sensory irritation was evaluated every minute for 10 minutes, followed by neutralization with sodium bicarbonate. Within seconds after glycolic acid application (time 0 in Fig. 2), sensory irritation differences were apparent between the two groups (mean ± SEM = 0.53 ± 0.16 for glycolic only vs. 0.16 ± 0.09 for glycolic plus strontium) indicating that strontium had an immediate onset of action. Throughout the remainder of the exposure, strontium strongly inhibited irritation at all time points, and cumulative irritation was inhibited by 75% (p = 0.005). The data in Table 2 presents the percent inhibition of each of the four sensory irritation scores induced by strontium nitrate. During the study, the 19 subjects reported 209 irritation scores. The incidence of each of the four scores of the glycolic acid only versus the glycolic acid plus strontium was: severe: 41 vs. 0 = 100% inhibition; moderate: 50 vs. 4 = 92% inhibition; mild: 44 vs. 25 = 43% inhibition; slight: 47 vs. 50 = 6% increase; none: 27 vs. 130 = 381% increase. In other studies, measurement of skin turnover using the dansyl chloride technique [14] showed that strontium nitrate did not affect the stimulatory effect of glycolic acid on skin turnover.

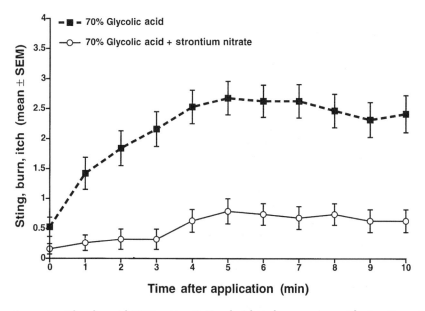

FIGURE 2   Glycolic acid (70%, pH = 0.6) only (closed squares) or with strontium nitrate (20%) (open circles) was applied to the forearms of 19 subjects and sensory irritation was measured every minute for 10 minutes. Each data point represents the mean ±SEM irritation at each minute for 19 subjects. Total cumulative irritation (areas under the curve) was inhibited by 75% (p < 0.005).

Clinical studies of a 70% glycolic acid (pH = 0.6) chemical peel solution with strontium nitrate applied to the whole face in over 150 human subjects demonstrated substantially reduced sensory irritation and erythema without reducing the expected benefits of the peel as judged by clinical response [15,16]. Histological analysis of punch biopsies from skin exposed to AHA formulations containing strontium nitrate (70% glycolic acid, pH = 0.6) every 2 weeks for 8 weeks and 15% lactic acid lotion (pH = 3.2) twice daily at the same facial sites) demonstrated that there was slightly *less* inflammation in the AHA and strontium-treated sites compared with untreated skin in the same individuals [16], thus demonstrating that strontium not only reduced irritation symptoms, but also protected the skin from cryptic damage.

Capryloyl Salicylic Acid–Induced Sensory Irritation

Capryloyl salicylic acid is a covalently modified derivative of salicylic acid with enhanced lipophylicity attributable to the 8 carbon caprylic acid moiety. It is used as a cosmetic exfoliant and is reported to have utility as an acne therapeutic [17]. A cream emulsion base containing capryloyl salicylic acid (1%) with or without strontium nitrate (500 mM) was applied to cheek sites 2 inches by 4 inches extending from the nasolabial fold to the outer cheek of 24 female subjects and sensory irritation was evaluated every 5 minutes for 60 minutes. The data in Table 2 presents the percent inhibition of each of the four sensory irritation scores induced by strontium nitrate. During the entire study, subjects reported 312 sensory irritation scores. The incidence of each of the four scores of the capryloyl salicylic acid versus the capryloyl plus strontium was: severe: 19 vs. 8; moderate: 13 vs. 9; mild: 35 vs. 10; slight: 39 vs. 42; and none: 50 vs. 87. The mean sensory irritation score of the capryloyl salicylic acid reached approximately 0.8 5 minutes after application, peaked at approximately 1.0 from 20 minutes to 35 minutes, and remained at approximately 0.8 until 45 minutes, after which it declined to 0.4 at 60 minutes. Total irritation, calculated as the percent difference of the areas under the 60-minute irritation curves, was inhibited by 46% ($p = 0.002$).

Ascorbic Acid (30%, pH = 1.7) Sensory Irritation on the Face

Ascorbic acid (Vitamin C) is used in many cosmetic products because it is a potent water-soluble antioxidant and can protect the skin against damage from ultraviolet radiation [18]. In vitro studies also show that ascorbic acid can also stimulate collagen synthesis [19]. Because ascorbic acid is most stable and bioavailable in aqueous formulations at a highly acidic pH (e.g., pH < 3) a 30% aqueous solution of ascorbic acid (pH = 1.7) was evaluated for sensory irritation with or without strontium nitrate (250 mM). After application to the face of 20 subjects, the cumulative irritation inhibition by the strontium-containing solutions was 84% ($p < 0.005$) (Table 2). The incidence of each of the four scores of the ascorbic acid only versus the ascorbic acid plus strontium was: severe: 1 vs. 0 = 100% inhibition; moderate: 13 vs. 0 = 100% inhibition; mild: 23 vs. 2 = 91% inhibition; slight: 48 vs. 18 = 63% inhibition; plus none: 25 vs. 90 = 260% increase).

Aluminum Chloride Antiperspirant Application to Axilla

Antiperspirants use aluminum salts alone or in combination with other agents to reduce perspiration. In the moist environment of the axilla, aluminum salts can cause sensory irritation and inflammation [20]. The axilla of 16 subjects was pretreated with 1.0 mL of a strontium nitrate solution (500 mM, pH = 7.3 in 50% ethanol/water vehicle) followed 2 minutes later by a 1 mL application of the aluminum chloride (20%) antiperspirant solution. Sensory irritation was evaluated every 2 minutes for 20 minutes. The incidence of each of the four scores of the aluminum chloride versus the aluminum chloride plus strontium was: severe: 12 vs. 2; moderate: 22 vs. 9; mild: 30 vs. 13; slight: 60 vs. 41; and none: 52 vs. 111. Upon application, sensory irritation reached a mean score of 1 within the first minute and a plateau at approximately 1.5 from minutes 6 to 10, then gradually declined to a score of approximately 1 at 20 minutes. During the study, the 16 subjects reported 352 irritation scores. Total irritation caused by the aluminum chloride calculated as the percent difference of the areas under the 20-minute irritation curves was reduced by 56% when the areas under the irritation curves were compared ($p < 0.005$).

Aluminum/Zirconium Salt Erythema on the Arms

Aluminum salts, with or without zirconium salts, are FDA-approved antiperspirant ingredients and frequently cause both sensory irritation and inflammation [20]. Aluminum/ zirconium salt solution (25%) with or without strontium nitrate (500 mM) or strontium chloride (500 mM) was applied to the arms of 29 subjects using occluded patches for 21 days and the magnitude of visible inflammation was evaluated every day. Inflammation was visually measured according to the following scale:

---

0 =   No evidence of erythema
1 =   Minimal erythema
2 =   Definite erythema
3 =   Erythema and papules

Both strontium nitrate (500 mM) or strontium chloride (500 mM) caused nearly complete inhibition of erythema development during the first week and substantially inhibited erythema during the second and third weeks (Fig. 3). Total erythema caused by the aluminum/ zirconium salts, calculated as the percent difference of the areas under the 21 day irritation curves, was reduced by 64% ($p < 0.0001$) by strontium nitrate and by 66% ($p < 0.0001$) by strontium chloride.

BASIC IRRITANTS
Calcium Thioglycolate Sensory Irritation on the Legs

Chemical depilatories typically use calcium thioglycolate formulated at a basic pH (e.g., 9–12) to dissolve hair keratin [21]. Twenty-three subjects shaved their legs with a safety razor to enhance irritation, then strontium nitrate pretreatment solution (10% w/v, in 10% ethanol/water) or vehicle was applied to 2 inch by 4 inch sites on the lateral portions of the legs. After 2 minutes, 5 grams of depilatory lotion was applied to each leg followed by irritation evaluation every minute for 10 minutes. During the study, the 23 subjects reported 506 irritation scores (Table 2). The incidence of each of the four scores of the depilatory versus the depilatory plus strontium was: severe: 0 vs. 0; moderate: 7 vs. 2 = 71% inhibition; mild: 45 vs. 11 = 76% inhibition; slight: 88 vs. 53 = 40% inhibition; and none: 113 vs. 187 = 65% increase. Total irritation caused by the depilatory, calculated

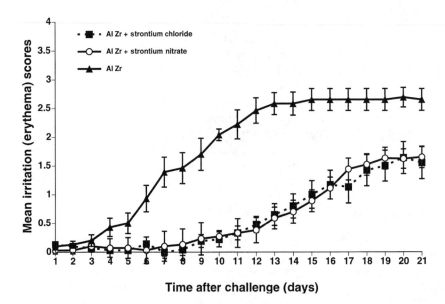

FIGURE 3 Strontium nitrate (500 mM, open circles) or strontium chloride (500 mM, closed squares) was formulated with the aluminum/zirconium salt solution each day when a new patch was applied. Each data point represents the mean ±SEM for 29 subjects. Total cumulative irritation (areas under the curve) was inhibited by 64% ($p < 0.0001$) for strontium nitrate and 66% for strontium chloride ($p < 0.0001$).

as the percent difference of the areas under the 20-minute irritation curves, was reduced by 59% ($p < 0.01$).

NEUTRAL IRRITANTS (HISTAMINE)

Histamine is a potent itch-inducing chemical contained in mast cells and basophils and is released in response to many inflammatory stimuli, including substance P during the neurogenic inflammatory process. It directly activates type-C nociceptors by binding to H1 histamine receptors [22,23]. Strontium nitrate (20%) in water or water alone were used to pretreat 4 by 6 cm sites on the volar forearms of 8 subjects 30 minutes and 5 minutes before intradermal injection of histamine (100 µg in normal saline). Itch was assessed using a visual analog scale for 20 minutes. The mean itch magnitude each minute for all subjects was always less for the strontium-treated sites and reached statistical significance ($p < 0.05$) from minute 12 to the end of the study. The mean difference between the two groups continued to increase until it reached the maximum difference at 20 minutes at which time itch was reduced 52% by strontium ($p < 0.05$) [24].

OCULAR IRRITANTS

The eye is perhaps the most sensitive organ of the body, especially to chemical irritants. When cosmetics, sunscreens, or other topical products are used on the face, they frequently contact the eye and can produce substantial sensory irritation. Preliminary studies of strontium nitrate applied to the human eye indicate that it is a safe and effective anti-irritant. Studies of strontium nitrate in aqueous solution instilled into the eye of humans show that up to 2% strontium nitrate was well tolerated and safe for ocular instillation. Because alpha-hydroxy acids are used in cosmetics around the eye, lactic acid (1%, pH = 4.0) was used as an ocular irritant with or without strontium nitrate (1%) or sodium chloride (1%). In a study of seven subjects, strontium inhibited total cumulative sensory irritation by 63%. In contrast, strontium did not alter the eye's sensitivity to foreign bodies, thus preserving the protective senses of the eye.

STRONTIUM SAFETY

Strontium is the eighth most abundant element in sea water and is found in many foods, especially green leafy vegetables. Average human consumption of strontium in food is estimated to be 0.8 mg to 5 mg a day. Studies in animals and humans show that it is remarkably nontoxic, and in some studies it is estimated to be as safe as calcium. Percutaneous absorption studies of strontium salts indicate that predicted absorption of topically applied strontium salts is far less than would be typically consumed in the diet.

STRONTIUM MECHANISM OF ACTION

Simple salts of the element strontium can effectively suppress sensory irritation caused by chemically and biologically unrelated chemical irritants over a pH range of 0.6 to 12. Because strontium acts within seconds after application, it is likely that it is acting directly on the type-C chemical sensors that transmit stinging, burning, and itching. In animal studies, strontium salts have been reported to directly suppress neuronal depolarization [25,26]. In vivo, strontium is a divalent ion with an ionic radius similar to the divalent calcium ion (1.13 Å vs. 0.99 Å, respectively) [27]. Strontium also resembles calcium's ability to traverse calcium-selective ion channels and trigger neurotransmitter release from nerve endings. In many systems strontium is, however, less potent than calcium and thus can act as an inhibitor of calcium-dependent depolarization [26,28–31]. Strontium may act to block calcium-dependent pathways that lead to neuronal depolarization. Neurons are also known to be sensitive to compounds that alter the electrostatic field surrounding their plasma membrane and ion channels [32]. Because strontium can alter the electrostatic field of ion channels and reduce ion permeation through them [33,34], strontium may suppress irritant-induced depolarization of unmyelinated sensory neurons. Strontium salts may also directly act on non-neuronal cells such as keratinocytes or immunoregulatory inflammatory cells. For example, strontium salts can suppress keratinocyte-derived TNF-α, IL-1α, and IL-6 in in vitro cultures [35].

The fact that strontium can block the rapid intense irritation caused by a 70% (pH = 0.6) glycolic acid chemical peel without causing numbness or other detectable changes in cutaneous sensations suggests that strontium is highly selective in its ability to regulate type-C nociceptors (Fig. 4). In contrast, local anesthetics like lidocaine or procaine not only block irritant sensations, but also block tactile sensations that produce numbness [36]. Recent studies support the concept that strontium is highly selective for only nociceptive subsets of sensory neurons because strontium nitrate (20%) applied to normal skin did not alter sensory thresholds for cold sensations, warmth sensations, or pain caused by cold or heat [24].

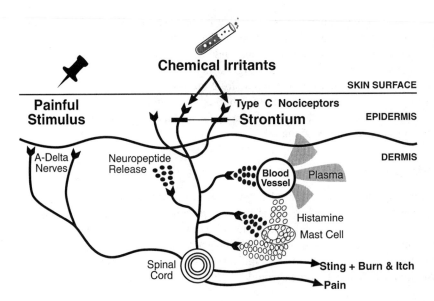

Figure 4 Chemical irritants activate unmyelinated type-C nociceptors and trigger their depolarization. Type-C nociceptors then synapse in the dorsal root ganglia (DRG) of the spinal cord and the signal travels to the brain where it is sensed as sting, burn, or itch. If the stimulation is of sufficient magnitude, interneurons in the DRG send a retrograde signal down the same type-C fibers, which triggers the release of inflammatory substances including substance P, neurokinin A, calcitonin gene-related peptide (CGRP), and other mediators. These substances trigger vasodilation, vascular permeability, and activate inflammatory cells, including mast cells that, in turn, release another set of inflammatory mediators, including histamine, which further activate nociceptive sensory signals and inflammation. Strontium reduces the sensitivity of type-C nociceptors to chemical irritants while not affecting the A-delta nerves that transmit the ability to detect pain.

PRODUCT APPLICATIONS

Burning, stinging, and especially itching sensations are among the most common consumer complaints from cosmetics and topical drugs. The rapid-onset and high-level anti-irritant potency of strontium salts suggest that they will have broad applications in topical products. Throughout the world, cosmetic products are used daily to cleanse and beautify the skin. With the discovery of new, potent, biologically active ingredients, formulators can provide consumers with increased benefit that may resemble that obtained from pharmaceutical products. Unfortunately, irritation frequently accompanies the use of higher concentrations of active ingredients or more potent skin-delivery systems. For people with sensitive skin attributable to inherently dry skin or other causes, the problem is further compounded. In addition to products intentionally applied to the skin, many workers are exposed to chemical irritants in the workplace that can result in considerable occupational disability [37–39].

Strontium salts, particularly strontium nitrate, has proven to be highly effective in reducing irritation, erythema, and inflammation from many irritating ingredients used in topical products and found in the workplace. The first strontium-containing cosmetic products were introduced in the United States, and made available internationally in October

1999. The safety of strontium salts, coupled with their ability to inhibit both sensory irritation and neurogenic inflammation, suggests that they may have therapeutic utility in the treatment of many dermatological conditions. Because the neurogenic inflammation syndrome is believed to be pathogenically important in many other conditions, including allergic contact dermatitis, psoriasis, atopic dermatitis, ocular irritation and inflammation, allergic rhinitis, asthma, rheumatoid arthritis, inflammatory bowel disease and other gastrointestinal disorders [40], strontium salts may have additional therapeutic utility. Strontium salts represent a new class of selective inhibitors of sensory irritation and irritant contact dermatitis without local anesthetic side effects.

REFERENCES

1. Tausk F, Christian E, Johansson O, Milgram S. Neurobiology of the skin. In: Fitzpatrick TB, Eisen AZ, Wolff K, Freedberg IM, Austen KF, ed. Dermatology in General Medicine. Vol. 1. 4th ed. New York: McGraw-Hill, 1993:396–403.
2. Martin JH, Jessell TM. Modality coding in the somatic sensory system. In: Kandel ER, Schwartz JH, Jessell TM, eds. Principles of Neural Science. 3rd ed. New York: Elsevier, 1991: 341.
3. Meyer RA, Campbell JN, Raja SN. Peripheral neural mechanisms of nociception. In: Wall PD, Melzack R, eds. Textbook of Pain. 3rd ed. London: Churchill Livingstone, 1994:13–44.
4. Kennedy WR, Wendelschafer-Crabb G. The innervation of the human epidermis. J Neurol Sci (Netherlands) 1993; 115:184–190.
5. Baluk P. Neurogenic inflammation in skin and airways. J Invest Derm 1997; 2:76–81.
6. Szolcsanyi J. Neurogenic inflammation: reevaluation of axon reflex theory. In: Geppetti P, Holzer P, eds. Neurogenic Inflammation. New York: 1996:33–42.
7. Hahn GS. Strontium is a potent and selective inhibitor of sensory irritation. Derm Surg 1999; 25:1–6.
8. Hahn GS. Modulation of neurogenic inflammation by strontium. In: Kydonieus AF, Willie JJ, eds. Biochemical Modulation of Skin Reactions: Transdermals, Topicals, Cosmetics. New York: CRC Press, 1999:261–272.
9. Hahn GS, Thueson DO. Cosmederm Technologies, Inc., assignee. Formulations and Methods for Reducing Skin Irritation. U.S. patent 5,716,625. Feb. 10, 1998.
10. Hahn GS, Thueson DO, Quick TW. Cosmoderm Technologies, Inc., assignee. Topical Product Formulations Containing Strontium for Reducing Skin Irritation. U.S. patent 5,804,203. Sept. 8, 1998.
11. Thueson DO, Chan EK, Oechsli LM, Hahn GS. The roles of pH and concentration in lactic acid-induced stimulation of epidermal turnover. Dermatol Surg 1998; 24:641–645.
12. Stiller MJ, Bartolone J, Stern R, Kollias N, Gillies R, Drake LA. Topical 8% glycolic acid and 8% L-lactic acid creams for the treatment of photodamaged skin. A double-blind vehicle-controlled clinical trial. Arch Dermatol 1996; 132:631–636.
13. Brody HJ. Chemical Peeling and Resurfacing. 2nd ed. St. Louis, MO: Mosby, 1997:73–108.
14. Jansen LH, Hojyo-Tomoko MT, Kligman AM. Improved fluorescence staining technique for estimating turnover of human stratum corneum. Br J Dermatol 1973; 90:9–12.
15. Rubin MG, Harper RA, Hahn GS. Strontium nitrate in 70% free glycolic acid peels significantly reduces erythema and sensory irritation (Abstr). Poster at American Academy of Dermatology 1999. (Manuscript to be submitted.)
16. Greenway HT, Peterson C, Plis J, Cornell R, Hahn GS, Harper RA. Efficacy of a 70% glycolic acid peel product regimen containing the anti-irritant strontium nitrate (Abst). Poster at American Academy of Dermatology 1999. (Manuscript to be submitted.)
17. Leveque JL, Raincy L, inventors; L'Oreal assignee. Use of salicylic acid derivatives for the treatment of skin aging. US patent 5,262,407. 1993 Nov 16.

18. Gabard DF. Topical melatonin in combination with vitamins E and C protects skin from ultraviolet-induced erythema: a human study in vivo. Br J Derm 1998; 139:332–339.
19. Colven RM, Pinnell SR. Topical vitamin C in aging. Clin Dermatol 1996; 14:227–234.
20. Mueller WH, Quatrale RP. Antiperspirants and deodarants. In: deVavarre MG, ed. The Chemistry and Manufacture of Cosmetics. Vol. 3. 2d ed. Wheaton, IL: Allured Publishing, 1993: 205–228.
21. Rieger MM, Brechner S. Depilatories. In: deVavarre MG, ed. The Chemistry and Manufacture of Cosmetics. Vol. 4. 2d ed. Wheaton, IL: Allured Publishing, 1993:1229–1273.
22. White MV, Kaliner MA. Histamine. In: Gallin JI, Goldstein IM, Snyderman R, eds. Inflammation. New York, 1988:169–193.
23. Schmelz M, Schmidt R, Bickel A, Handwerker HO, Torebjörk HE. J Neuroscience 1997; 17: 8003–8008.
24. Zhai H, Hannon W, Harper RA, Hahn GS, Alessandra P, Maibach HI. Strontium nitrate decreased itch magnitude and duration without effecting thermal pain or sensation in experimentally induced pruritis in man. Contact Dermatitis 2000; 42:98–100.
25. Gutentag H. The effect of strontium chloride on peripheral nerve in comparison to the action of "stabilizer" and "labilizer" compounds. Penn Dent J 1965; 68:37–43.
26. Silinsky EM, Mellow AM. The relationship between strontium and other divalent cations in the process of transmitter release from cholinergic nerve endings. In: Skoryna SC, ed. Handbook of Stable Strontium. New York: Plenum Press, 1981:263–285.
27. Pauling L. Nature of the Chemical Bond and Structure of Molecules and Crystals. 3d ed. Ithica: Cornell University Press, 1960:644.
28. Miledi R. Strontium as a substitute for calcium in the process of transmitter release at the neuromuscular junction. Nature 1966; 212:1233–1234.
29. Meiri U, Rahamimoff R. Activation of transmitter release by strontium and calcium ions at the neuromuscular junction. J Physiol 1971; 215:709–726.
30. Nakazato Y, Onoda Y. Barium and strontium can substitute for calcium in nonadrenaline output induced by excess potassium in the guinea pig. J Physiol 1980; 305:59–71.
31. Mellow AM, Perry BD, Silinsky EM. Effects of calcium and strontium in the process of acetylcholine release from motor nerve endings. J Physiol 1982; 328:547–562.
32. Hille B. Ionic Channels of Excitable Membranes. 2d ed. Sunderland, MA: Sinauer Associates, 1992:445–471.
33. Elinder F, Medeja M, Arhem P. Surface charges of K+: effects of strontium on five cloned channels expressed on Xenopus oocytes. J Gen Physiol 1996; 108:325–332.
34. Reuveny E, Jan YN, Jan YL. Contributions of a negatively charged residue in the hydrophobic domain of the IRK1 inwardly rectifying K+ channel to K+-selective permeation. Biophys J 1996; 70:754–761.
35. Celerier P, Richard A, Litoux P, Dreno B. Modulatory effects of selenium and strontium salts on keratinocyte-derived inflammatory cytokines. Arch Dermatol Res 1995; 287:680–682.
36. Ritchie JM, Greene NM. Local anesthetics. In: Gilman AG, Rall TW, Nies AS, Taylor P, eds. The Pharmacological Basis of Therapeutics, 8th ed. New York: McGraw-Hill, 1993:311–331.
37. Björnberg A. Irritant dermatitis. In: Maibach HI, ed. Occupational and Industrial Dermatology. 2d ed. Chicago: Year Book Medical Publishers, 1987:15–21.
38. Lammintausta K, Maibach HI, Wilson D. Mechanisms of subjective (sensory) irritation: propensity to non-immunologic contact urticaria and objective irritation in stingers. Dermatosen 1988; 36:45–49.
39. Weltfriend SI, Bason M, Lammintausta K, Maibach HI. Irritant dermatitis (irritation). In: Marzulli FN, Maibach HI, eds. Dermatotoxicology. 5th ed. Washington, D.C.: Taylor & Francis 1996:87–118.
40. Geppetti P, Holzer P. Neurogenic Inflammation. Boca Raton: CRC Press, 1996:1–324.

26

Antioxidants

Stefan Udo Weber, Claude Saliou, and Lester Packer
University of California at Berkeley, Berkeley, California

John K. Lodge
University of Surrey, Guildford, Surrey, England

INTRODUCTION

In the field of dermatology, antioxidants are widely used and innovative ingredients in topical applications. This chapter is intended to provide an overview of the current state of research on the use of antioxidants in cosmeceutical applications. The most important antioxidants, vitamin E, vitamin C, thiols, and flavonoids will be introduced and their intriguing cooperation as well as their role in signal transduction events will be discussed.

The body is continuously exposed to oxidants. Endogenous sources arise as a consequence of normal metabolic pathways. For example, mitochondrial respiration produces superoxide and hydrogen peroxide, whilst enzymes such as lipoxygenases, xanthine oxidase, and NADPH oxidase produce hydroperoxides and superoxide respectively. Exogenous oxidants arise from environmental pollutants such as smoke, smog, UV radiation, and the diet. In response to these oxidants, a number of systemic antioxidants are available whose functions are to scavenge reactive oxygen species preventing damage to macromolecules such as lipids, DNA, and proteins. Antioxidant protection arises from molecules synthesized as part of metabolism, e.g., GSH and uric acid; essential vitamins which must be taken in from the diet, e.g., vitamin E and C; and enzymes which decompose reactive oxygen species, e.g., superoxide dismutases, catalase, and the glutathione peroxidases. These systems provide protection in various intra- and intercellular compartments. Usually there is a tight balance between oxidants produced and antioxidant scavenging, however under certain conditions the balance can be tipped in favor of the oxidants, a condition called oxidative stress. Potentially oxidative stress can be caused either by an increase in the number of oxidants, for example as a result of cigarette smoking or UV irradiation, or by a deficiency in antioxidants. This is of major concern since oxidative stress has been implicated in a number of conditions including atherosclerosis, skin cancer, and photoaging.

VITAMIN E

Vitamin is the major lipophilic antioxidant in skin, and it is the most commonly used natural antioxidant in topical formulations. It is found in all parts of the skin, the dermis, and epidermis, as well as in the stratum corneum, and is believed to play an essential role in the protection of biomolecules from oxidative stress.

Vitamin E is a family of 8 naturally occurring isoforms: four tocopherols (α-, β-, γ-, δ-form) and four tocotrienols (α-, β-, γ-, δ-form) (Fig. 1) [1]. All forms consist of a chromanol nucleus that carries the redox-active phenolic hydroxyl group, and a lipophilic tail. While tocopherols contain a phytil side chain, the isoprenoid tail of the tocotrienols is polyunsaturated, making the chain more rigid. The side chain is anchored in lipid membranes while the nucleus is located at the lipid/aqueous interface. Even though the radical scavenging activity of the different isoforms is essentially identical, their biological activity after oral administration differs dramatically [2]. This phenomenon can be explained by the existence of an α-tocopherol transfer protein in the liver that positively selects RRR-α-tocopherol and incorporates it into VLDL which leads to recirculation of the α-tocopherol pool, while this transfer protein does not recognize the other forms, which are therefore excreted more rapidly [3].

In skin, as in the other human organs, α-tocopherol is the predominant form of vitamin E with 5 to 10 higher concentrations than γ-tocopherol. Delivery of vitamin E to the SC occurs in two different modes. On the one hand it stored into differentiating keratinocytes and moves up into the newly formed SC, which leads to a gradient-type distribution of α-tocopherol with decreasing concentrations towards the skin surface [4]. On the other hand, vitamin E is secreted by sebaceous glands and reaches the SC from the outside. In sebaceous gland–rich regions like the face, this delivery mechanism is responsible for the enrichment of the outer SC with vitamin E [5].

Various oxidative stressors have been shown to deplete vitamin E, among other antioxidants. In the epidermis, a dose of at least four minimal erythemal doses (MED) of solar simulated UV radiation (SSUV) is needed to deplete vitamin E [6], while doses as low as 0.75 MED are capable of destroying vitamin E in the human SC [4]. Mouse experiments have shown that a dose of 1 ppm $\times$ 2h of ozone (O_3) depletes SC vitamin E [7]. Since this concentration of O_3 is higher than the naturally occuring levels of tropospheric O_3 the biological relevance of these findings for the skin of humans is not yet clear. A one time application of benzoyl peroxide BPO (10% w/v), a concentration commonly used in the treatment of acne, depleted most of the SC vitamin E in human volunteers [8].

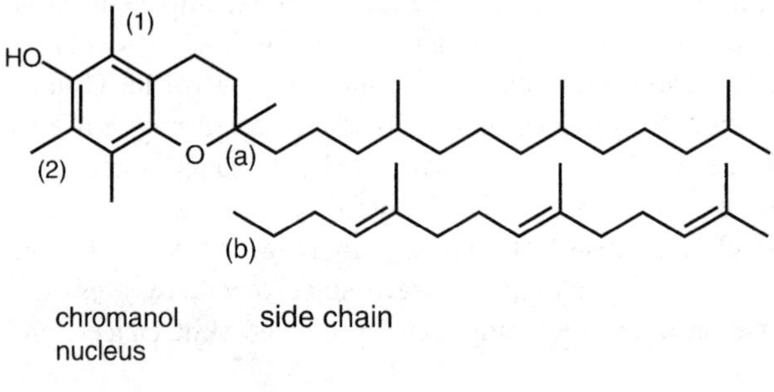

chromanol   side chain
nucleus

Figure 1 Naturally occurring forms of vitamin E. Tocopherols contain a saturated side chain (a), whereas the isoprenoid side chain of tocotrienols is polyunsaturated (b). The α-forms contain both methyl groups on the chromanol nucleus (1,2), whereas the β-forms contain only methyl group (1), the γ-forms only (2), and the δ-forms none.

α-Tocopherol is widely used as an active ingredient in topical formulations. After topical application, it penetrates readily into skin [9]. Since the free form of vitamin E is quite unstable and light-sensitive (it absorbs in the UV-B range), the active hydroxyl group is usually protected by esterification with acetate. This increases the stability but renders the compound redox inactive. When administered orally, vitamin E-acetate is hydrolyzed quantitatively in the intestines [10]. There is some controversy however as to whether α-tocopherol acetate can by hydrolyzed in human skin. Chronic application of α-tocopherol acetate leads to an increase in free vitamin E in both the rat [11] and the mouse [12], where it was recently shown that UV-B increases the hydrolysis of α-tocopherol acetate by induction of nonspecific esterases up to 10 to 30 fold [13]. While one study suggested that bioconversion of α-tocopherol acetate does not occur in human skin [14], significant hydrolysis was demonstrated in recent studies using a human epidermis–tissue culture model [15].

The availability of the free form of vitamin E needs to be considered when analyzing possible health benefits. The majority of studies have been carried out in animal models, while only limited data exists for human studies. Lipid peroxidation is inhibited after topical application of α-tocopherol [16]. Several studies indicate that topically applied α-tocopherol inhibits UVB-induced photodamage of DNA in a mouse model [17] and keratinocyte cultures (trolox) [18]. Protection against Langerhans cell depletion by UV light was observed after topical application of α-tocopherol in a mouse model [19]. α-Tocopherol and its sorbate ester were studied in a mouse model of skin aging. Both antioxidants were found to be effective, sorbate even more so than α-tocopherol [20]. Systemic administration of vitamin E in humans (only in combination with vitamin C) increased the MED and reduced changes in skin blood flow after UV-irradiation [21,22]. Yet several studies indicate that α-tocopherol acetate is not as effective as free vitamin E when applied topically. Inhibition of DNA mutation in mice was 5 to 10 times less effective [18]. Also, in a mouse model, unlike free vitamin E, the acetate form seemed to be ineffective [23]. In summary, even though some health benefits of vitamin E supplementation have been shown, there is still a need for controlled studies in humans under physiological conditions.

Recently, the tocotrienol forms of vitamin E have become a focus of interest, since they have been found to be more efficient antioxidants in some model systems than tocopherols [24]. Even if they are not bioavailable after oral supplementation, topical application circumvents the exclusion by α-TTP in the liver. In fact, free tocotrienols readily penetrate into mouse skin [9], and tocotrienyl acetate is hydrolyzed in skin homogenates and in murine skin in vivo [25]. Topical application of a tocotrienol-rich fraction has been demonstrated to protect mouse skin from UV- and O_3-induced oxidative stress [26,27]. In conclusion, tocotrienols bear a potential that yet remains to be explored.

VITAMIN C

Ascorbic acid or vitamin C is one of the most important water soluble antioxidants and present in high amounts in the skin. While most species are able to produce ascorbic acid, humans lack the enzymes necessary for its synthesis. Deficiency in ascorbic acid causes scurvy, a disease already described in the ancient writings of the Greeks [28]. Apart from the pure antioxidant function ascorbic acid is an essential co-factor for different enzymes. The antioxidant capacity of vitamin C is related to its unique structure (Fig. 2). Due to its pKa1 of 4.25 it is present as a monoanion at physiological pH, which can undergo a

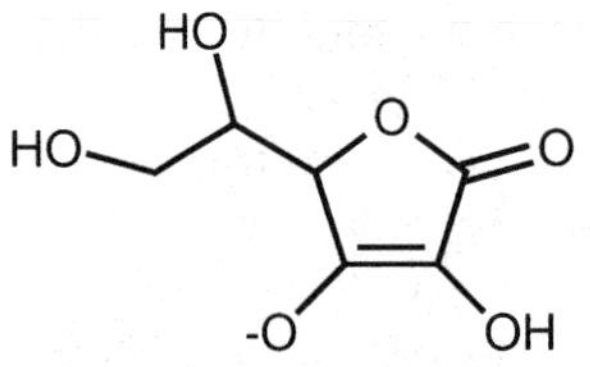

FIGURE 2   Structural formula of vitamin C as the monoanion ascorbate.

one electron donation to form the ascorbyl radical with a delocalized electron and can be further oxidized to result in dehydroascorbic acid. Dehydroascorbic acid is relatively unstable and breaks down if it is not regenerated (see antioxidant network). In vitro ascorbic acid can scavenge many types of radicals including the hydroxyl- (OH$^{\cdot}$), the superoxide- (O$_2^{\cdot-}$) and water soluble peroxyl- (ROO$^{\cdot}$) radicals as well as other reactive oxygen species such as O$_3$, and quenches singlet oxygen. Due to their relative reduction potentials, ascorbate can reduce Fe(III) to Fe(II), which in turn can decompose hydrogen peroxide (H$_2$O$_2$) to the dangerous hydroxyl radical. Therefore, vitamin C can exert pro-oxidant effects in the presence of unbound iron (fenton chemistry).

In the skin, vitamin C is found in all layers. In SC it forms a similar gradient as vitamin E with decreasing concentrations towards the outside. Vitamin C is depleted by O$_3$, UV radiation, and BPO. One of the earliest discoveries of vitamin C benefits in the skin was the observation that it stimulates collagen synthesis in dermal fibroblasts [29]. Recently a pretranscriptional role of vitamin C had been described [30]. Also, vitamin C is essential in the formation of competent barrier lipids in reconstructed human epidermis [31].

Several studies have investigated protective effects of vitamin C against oxidative stress. UVB-induced immunotolerance, as a marker of damage to the immune system, could be abrogated by topical application of vitamin C to murine skin [32]. UVB-induced sunburn cell formation was mitigated by vitamin C in porcine skin [33]. While one study reported a postadministrative protective effect of vitamin C-phosphate against UV-induced damage in mice [34], another study found no such effect in humans [35]. Systemic application of vitamin C in combination with vitamin E protected against UV-induced erythema in humans [21]. In a keratinocyte cell culture system vitamin C reduced UVB-induced DNA damage [18]. In mice, an anticarcinogenic effect of vitamin C was described [36]. However, no data regarding such benefits exists in humans.

Since vitamin C is not very stable, it is difficult to incorporate it into topical formulations. Esterification with phosphate is used to circumvent this limitation. In vitro experiments demonstrated that Mg-ascorbyl-2-phosphate penetrates the murine skin barrier and is bioconverted into free ascorbate [37].

THIOL ANTIOXIDANTS

Thiols share an oxidizable sulphhydryl (SH) group. Glutathione (GSH) is a tripeptide (Fig. 3) whose SH group at the cysteine can be oxidized, forming a disulphide (GSSG) with another GSH molecule. Physiologically, more than 90% of the GSH is in the reduced form. Glutathione peroxidases use GSH oxidation to reduce H$_2$O$_2$ and other water soluble peroxides. The synthesis of GSH by the human cell is stimulated by N-acetyl-cysteine (NAC), which is hydrolyzed to cysteine intracellularly. Moreover NAC acts as an antioxi-

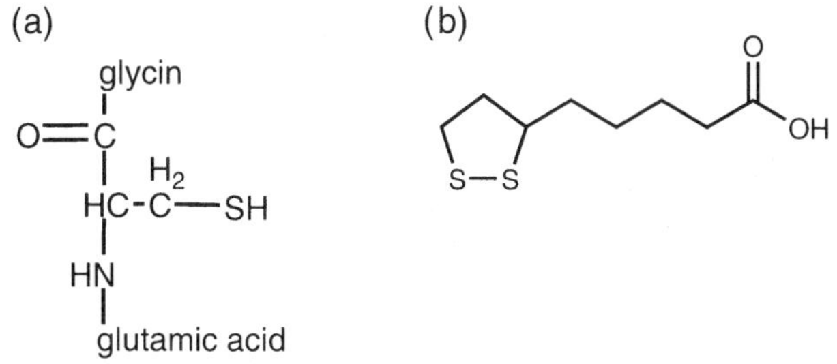

(a)

glycin

```
O=C
    |
    |  H₂
   HC-C—SH
    |
   HN
    |
```
glutamic acid

(b)

FIGURE 3 Chemical structures of thiols: (a) GSH consisting of glycine, cysteine, and glutamic acid; (b) lipoic acid as in its oxidized form as a disulphide.

dant itself. Lipoic acid (1,2-dithiolane-3-pentanonic acid or thioctic acid, LA) is a cofactor of multienzyme complexes in the decarboxylation of α-keto acids. Applied as the oxidized dithiol dehydrolipoic acid (DHLA) it is taken up by cells and is reduced by mitochondrial and cytosolic enzymes (NAD(P)H dependent). It thereby forms an efficient cycle, since it can in turn regenerate GSSG to GSH and stimulate the GSH synthesis by improving cysteine utilization [38].

General provisos in the use of thiols in skin applications are the typical smell and the poor solubility of LA in aqueous solutions below pH 7. Yet, several thiol agents have been tested for protective effects in the skin. For oral as well as topical application in mouse models, GSH-ethylesters and GSH-isopropylesters proved to be more efficient than free GSH. Oral supplementation decreased the formation of UV-induced tumors [39] and the formation of sunburn cells [40]. Topical treatment partially inhibited UV-induced immunosupression [41]. NAC was able to reduce UVA-induced DNA damage in fibroblasts [42] and protected mice against UVB-induced immunosuppression after topical application [43] in a mode that did not involve de novo GSH synthesis [44]. Lipoic acid was demonstrated to penetrate into mouse skin [45], while oral supplementation of lipoic acid has actually been shown to have an anti-inflammatory effect in mice [46], to prevent symptoms of vitamin E deficiency in vitamin E–deficient mice [47], and vitamin C and E deficiency in guinea pigs [48].

POLYPHENOLS

Flavonoids are widely distributed plant pigments and tannins occurring in barks, roots, leaves, flowers, and fruits. Their roles in plants include photoprotection and contributing to the plant color. Consequently, our diet contains flavonoids which can be found in a variety of foods from green vegetables to red wine [49].

Despite the fact that flavonoids have been used in traditional medicine for several centuries, it was not until 1936 that their first biological activity, the vitamin C–sparing action, was described by Rusznyak and Szent-Györgyi [50]. As a result, they received the name of ''vitamin P.'' Flavonoids, also referred to as plant polyphenols, have been recognized as potent antioxidants. Their free radical-scavenging and metal-chelating activities have been extensively studied. Nonetheless, given their polyphenolic structure (Fig. 4), the electron- and hydrogen-donating abilities constitute the major feature of their antioxidant properties [51]. By opposition to the antioxidants previously described, flavonoids

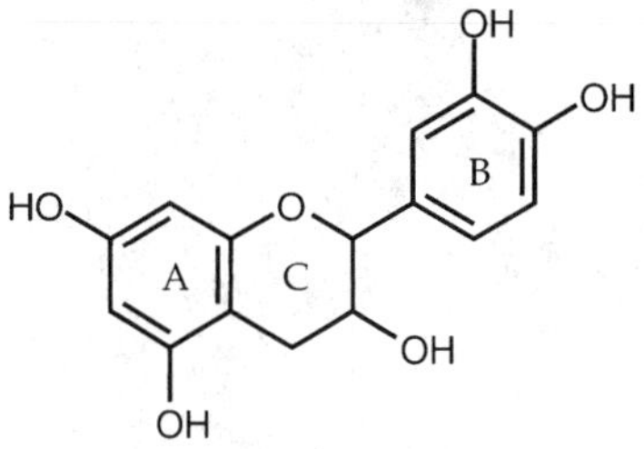

FIGURE 4 Chemical structure of catechin, a flavane, as an example of a flavonoid. Flavanes share a common base structure (rings A, B, C) that is hydroxylated in different patterns.

are not part of the endogenous antioxidant system but still interact with it through the antioxidant network (see the following paragraph).

Among the applications found in traditional medicine, flavonoids account for anti-inflammatory, antiphlogistic, and wound-healing functions [52]. Their effect on skin inflammation has been thought, for a long time, to be limited to the inhibition of the activity of 5-lipoxygenase and cyclo-oxygenase [49]. However, recent studies suggest a more subtle mode of regulation of the inflammatory reaction by flavonoids. In fact, flavonoids such as silymarin, quercetin, genistein, and apigenin are effective inhibitors of NF-κB, a proinflammatory transcription factor, thereby reducing the transcription of proinflammatory genes and preventing inflammation [53–55].

Oral supplementation and topical application of green and black tea polyphenols show beneficial effects against UVR-induced skin carcinogenesis in mice [56–58]. In addition, these flavonoids and silymarin were found to prevent UVR-induced inflammation as well as ornithine decarboxylase expression and activity [59], all of these events being potential contributors to carcinogenesis [60].

Procyanidins, also named condensed tannins, are flavonoids found in, e.g., pine bark (Pycnogenol), grape seeds, and fruits. By direct protein interaction, they were shown to protect collagen and elastin, two dermal matrix proteins, against their degradation [61]. Furthermore, some of these procyanidins exhibit a remarkable effect on follicle hair proliferation [62] thus extending the therapeutic applications of flavonoids to alopecia. Although the flavonoids are not part of our endogenous antioxidant defenses, they display a broad spectrum of properties particularly helpful in preventing UVR-caused deleterious effects in human skin.

THE ANTIOXIDANT NETWORK

When an antioxidant reacts with an oxidant, it is converted to a form that no longer functions as an antioxidant, and is said to be consumed. In order for the oxidized product to function again, it needs to be recycled to its native form. The antioxidant network describes the ability of the antioxidants to recycle and regenerate oxidized forms of each other thereby providing extra levels of protection (Fig. 5). Thus the process is synergistic; the net antioxidant protection is always greater than the sum of the individual effects.

The major systemic antioxidants vitamin E, vitamin C, and glutathione are present in different cellular compartments, and all have the ability to interact with one another. Typically the radicals formed on the antioxidants are more stable and longer lived than the damaging radicals produced in vivo, which is mostly attributable to delocalization of the unpaired electron. Thus they have more chance to interact with each other and be

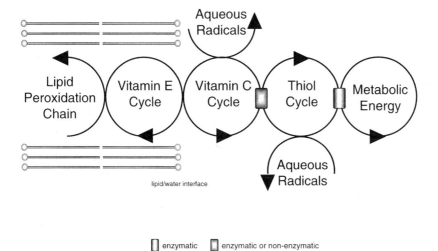

☐ enzymatic ☐ enzymatic or non-enzymatic

FIGURE 5 Schematics of the intertwined action of the antioxidant network. An ascorbate molecule can either recycle the vitamin E radical arising from breaking the lipid peroxidation chain, or scavenge an aqueous radical. Glutathione can either regenerate ascorbate or scavenge a radical enzymatically. Glutathione itself can then be regenerated by the cellular metabolism.

reduced than to react with macromolecules. Vitamin E is the major chain-breaking antioxidant, protecting biological membranes from lipid peroxidation [63], which is a difficult task considering the ratio of phospholipids molecules to vitamin E is about 1500:1. However, vitamin E is never depleted because it is constantly being recycled. When vitamin E becomes oxidized, a radical on vitamin E is formed (chromanoxyl radical). In the absence of networking antioxidants this radical can either become pro-oxidant by abstracting a hydrogen from lipids [64], or react to form nonradical products (consumed). However, a number of antioxidants are known to be able to reduce the chromanoxyl radical and regenerate vitamin E [65]. These include vitamin C [66], ubiquinol, and glutathione (GSH) [67]. Vitamin C, the most abundant plasma antioxidant and first line of defense, can reduce the tocopheroxyl radical, forming the ascorbyl radical. Interactions between vitamins E and C have been shown in various systems both in vivo (reviewed in Ref. 68) and in vitro [69] (reviewed in Ref. 70). The ascorbyl radical is practically inert and oxidizes further to form dehydroascorbic acid. This can be reduced back to native vitamin C by GSH. This process is known to occur both chemically [71] and enzymatically [72] in both erythrocytes [73] and neutrophils induced by bacteria [74]; the latter may relate to a host defense mechanism. Glutathione is the major intracellular antioxidant. Oxidized GSSG is constantly recycled to GSH enzymatically by glutathione reductase, thus providing a constant pool of GSH. Glutathione recycling relies on NAD(P)H as the electron donor. Thus metabolic pathways involved in energy production provide the ultimate electron donors for the antioxidant network. It is also known that GSH can directly recycle vitamin E [65,75], as can ubiquinol [76], another lipophilic antioxidant which itself is recycled in mitochondria as part of the electron transport chain.

Certain supplements are also known to contribute to the network by recycling antioxidants. Lipoic acid is a prime example since this potent antioxidant can recycle ascorbate, GSH, and ubiquinol in vitro (reviewed in Ref. 77). Recently it has been demonstrated that flavonoids may also play a networking role since they are also able to recycle the ascorbyl radical [78]. Thus there exists a very organized defense system against free radical attack, which ultimately serves to protect and recycle antioxidants in various cellular compartments.

REGULATION OF GENE TRANSCRIPTION BY ANTIOXIDANTS

The skin is the largest human organ and permanently exposed to a variety of stresses. Among those, oxidative insults such as ultraviolet radiation and ozone exposure account for the cause of many skin disorders. However, oxidative damage are not responsible for all biological effects engendered by these stressors in the skin. Indeed, ultraviolet radiation (UVR) causes changes in the expression of genes encoding, e.g., proinflammatory cytokines, growth factors, stress response proteins, oncoproteins, and matrix metalloproteinases [79]. Although the immediate target(s) of UVR is/are still unknown, certain kinases and transcription factors can be activated by UVR thereby increasing gene transcription [80]. One transcription factor, NF-κB, appears of particular interest for the skin since the lack of its inhibitory protein, IκBα, is associated with the development of a widespread dermititis in knockout mice [81,82]. Furthermore, reactive oxygen species, such as the ones produced after UVR, are suspected to play an important role in the activation of NF-κB [83]. Consequently, antioxidants have been found to be among the most potent NF-κB inhibitors. However, clinical studies are required in order to assess the effectiveness of these antioxidants, including the flavonoid silymarin, α-lipoic acid and the glutathione precursor *N*-acetyl-*L*-cysteine, on skin inflammatory disorders. Using high-throughput procedures such as the cDNA arrays, for instance [84], the evaluation of the antioxidants on the whole genome is henceforth possible. These studies will only confirm the hypothesis that antioxidants are responsible for a much broader action spectrum than their antioxidant functions per se and extend their role on more subtle regulatory mechanisms of the gene expression.

PERSPECTIVES

The general role of antioxidants in the protection against oxidative stress is well established. In skin applications antioxidants are a promising tool to mitigate oxidative injury. Even though a growing amount of literature deals with skin protection by antioxidants, there is still a need for investigation. In particular, clinical human studies need to be carried out to show the efficacy of antioxidants in topical formulations.

ACKNOWLEDGMENT

We would like to thank Nancy Han for editing the manuscript.

REFERENCES

1. Brigelius-Flohe R, Traber MG. Vitamin E: function and metabolism. FASEB J 1999; 13: 1145–1155.
2. Traber MG, Rader D, Acuff RV, Ramakrishnan R, Brewer HB, Kayden HJ. Vitamin E dose-response studies in humans with use of deuterated RRR-alpha-tocopherol. Am J Clin Nutr 1998; 68:847–853.
3. Traber MG, Ramakrishnan RR, Kayden HJ. Human plasma vitamin E kinetics demonstrate

rapid recycling of plasma RRR-alpha-tocopherol. Proc Natl Acad Sci USA 1994; 91:10005–10008.

4. Thiele JJ, Traber MG, Packer L. Depletion of human stratum corneum vitamin E: an early and sensitive in vivo marker of UV induced photo-oxidation. J Invest Dermatol 1998; 110: 756–761.

5. Thiele JJ, Weber SU, Packer L. Sebaceous gland secretion is a major physiological route of vitamin E delivery to the skin. J Invest Dermatol 1999; 113:1006–1010.

6. Shindo Y, Witt E, Han D, Packer L. Dose-response effects of acute ultraviolet irradiation on antioxidants and molecular markers of oxidation in murine epidermis and dermis. J Invest Dermatol 1994; 102:470–475.

7. Thiele JJ, Traber MG, Polefka TG, Cross CE, Packer L. Ozone-exposure depletes vitamin E and induces lipid peroxidation in murine stratum corneum. J Invest Dermatol 1997; 108:753–757.

8. Thiele JJ, Rallis M, Izquierdo-Pullido M, et al. Benzoyl peroxide depletes human stratum corneum antioxidants. J Invest Dermatol 1998; 110:674.

9. Traber MG, Rallis M, Podda M, Weber C, Maibach HI, Packer L. Penetration and distribution of alpha-tocopherol, alpha- or gamma-tocotrienols applied individually onto murine skin. Lipids 1998; 33:87–91.

10. Traber MG, Serbinova EA, Packer L. Biological activities of tocotrienols and tocopherols. In: Packer L, Hiramatsu M, Yoshikawa T, eds. Antioxidant Food Supplements in Human Health. New York: Academic Press, 1999.

11. Norkus EP, Bryce GF, Bhagavan HN. Uptake and bioconversion of alpha-tocopheryl acetate to alpha-tocopherol in skin of hairless mice. Photochem Photobiol 1993; 57:613–615.

12. Beijersbergen van Henegouwen GM, Junginger HE, de Vries H. Hydrolysis of RRR-alpha-tocopheryl acetate (vitamin E acetate) in the skin and its UV protecting activity (an in vivo study with the rat). J Photochem Photobiol B 1995; 29:45–51.

13. Kramer-Stickland K, Liebler DC. Effect of UVB on hydrolysis of alpha-tocopherol acetate to alpha-tocopherol in mouse skin. J Invest Dermatol 1998; 111:302–307.

14. Alberts DS, Goldman R, Xu MJ, et al. Disposition and metabolism of topically administered alpha-tocopherol acetate: a common ingredient of commercially available sunscreens and cosmetics. Nutr Cancer 1996; 26:193–201.

15. Nabi Z, Tavakkol A, Soliman N, Polefka TG. Bioconversion of tocopheryl acetate to tocopherol in human skin: use of human skin organ culture models. J Dermatol Sci 1998; 16:S207.

16. Lopez-Torres M, Thiele JJ, Shindo Y, Han D, Packer L. Topical application of alpha-tocopherol modulates the antioxidant network and diminishes ultraviolet-induced oxidative damage in murine skin. Br J Dermatol 1998; 138:207–215.

17. McVean M, Liebler DC. Inhibition of UVB induced DNA photodamage in mouse epidermis by topically applied alpha-tocopherol. Carcinogenesis 1997; 18:1617–1622.

18. Stewart MS, Cameron GS, Pence BC. Antioxidant nutrients protect against UVB-induced oxidative damage to DNA of mouse keratinocytes in culture. J Invest Dermatol 1996; 106:1086–1089.

19. Halliday GM, Bestak R, Yuen KS, Cavanagh LL, Barnetson RS. UVA-induced immunosuppression. Mutat Res 1998; 422:139–145.

20. Jurkiewicz BA, Bisset DL, Buettner GR. Effect of topically applied tocopherol on ultraviolet radiation-mediated free radical damage in skin. J Invest Dermatol 1995; 104:484–488.

21. Eberlein-Konig B, Placzek M, Przybilla B. Protective effect against sunburn of combined systemic ascorbic acid (vitamin C) and d-alpha-tocopherol (vitamin E). J Am Acad Dermatol 1998; 38:45–48.

22. Fuchs J, Kern H. Modulation of UV-light-induced skin inflammation by D-alpha-tocopherol and L-ascorbic acid: a clinical study using solar simulated radiation. Free Radic Biol Med 1998; 25:1006–1012.

23. Yuen KS, Halliday GM. Alpha-Tocopherol, an inhibitor of epidermal lipid peroxidation, pre-

vents ultraviolet radiation from suppressing the skin immune system. Photochem Photobiol 1997; 65:587–592.

24. Serbinova EA, Packer L. Antioxidant properties of alpha-tocopherol and alpha-tocotrienol. Methods Enzymol 1994; 234:354–366.

25. Weber SU, Luu C, Traber MG, Packer L. Tocotrienol acetate penetrates into murine skin and is hydrolyzed in vivo. Oxygen Club of California, Book of Abstracts 1999:13.

26. Weber C, Podda M, Rallis M, Thiele JJ, Traber MG, Packer L. Efficacy of topically applied tocopherols and tocotrienols in protection of murine skin from oxidative damage induced by UV-irradiation. Free Radic Biol Med 1997; 22:761–769.

27. Thiele JJ, Traber MG, Podda M, Tsang K, Cross CE, Packer L. Oxone depletes tocopherols and tocotrienols topically applied to murine skin. FEBS Lett 1997; 401:167–170.

28. Sauberlich HE. Pharmacology of vitamin C. Ann Rev Nutr 1994; 14:371–391.

29. Murad S, Grove D, Lindberg KA, Reynolds G, Sivarajah A, Pinnel SR. Regulation of collagen synthesis by ascorbic acid. Proc Natl Acad Sci USA 1981; 78:2879–2882.

30. Davidson JM, LuValle PA, Zoia O, Quaglino D Jr, Giro M. Ascorbate differentially regulates elastin and collagen biosynthesis in vascular smooth muscle cells and skin fibroblasts by pre-translational mechanisms. J Biol Chem 1997; 272:345–352.

31. Ponec M, Weerheim A, Kempenaar J, et al. The formulation of competent barrier lipids in reconstructed human epidermis requires the presence of vitamin C. J Invest Dermatol 1997; 109:348–355.

32. Nakamura T, Pinnel SR, Darr D, et al. Vitamin C abrogates the deleterious effects of UVB radiation on cutaneous immunity by a mechanism that does not depend on TNF-alpha. J Invest Dermatol 1997; 109:20–24.

33. Darr D, Combs S, Dunston S, Manning T, Pinnell S. Topical vitamin C protects porcine skin from ultraviolet radiation-induced damage. Br J Dermatol 1992; 127:247–253.

34. Kobayashi S, Takehana M, Kanke M, Itoh S, Ogata E. Postadministration protective effect of magnesium-L-ascorbyl-phosphate on the development of UVB-induced cutaneous damage in mice. Photochem Photobiol 1998; 67:669–675.

35. Dreher F, Denig N, Gabard B, Schwindt DA, Maibach HI. Effect of topical antioxidants on UV-induced erythema formation when administered after exposure. Dermatology 1999; 198: 52–55.

36. Pauling L. Effect of ascorbic acid on incidence of spontaneous mammary tumors and UV-light–induced skin tumors in mice. Am J Clin Nutr 1991; 54:1252S–1255S.

37. Kobayashi S, Takehana M, Itoh S, Ogata E. Protective effect of magnesium-L-ascorbyl-2 phosphate against skin damage induced by UVB irradiation. Photochem Photobiol 1996; 64: 224–228.

38. Han D, Handelman G, Marcocci L, et al. Lipoic acid increases de novo synthesis of cellular glutathione by improving cytine utilization. Biofactors 1997; 6:321–338.

39. Kobayashi S, Takehana M, Tohyama C. Glutathione isopropyl ester reduces UVB-induced skin damage in hairless mice. Photochem Photobiol 1996; 63:106–110.

40. Hanada K, Sawamura D, Tamai K, Hashimoto I, Kobayashi S. Photoprotective effect of esterified glutathione against ultraviolet B–induced sunburn cell formation in the hairless mice. J Invest Dermatol 1997; 108:727–730.

41. Steenvoorden DP, Beijersbergen van Henegouwen G. Glutathione ethylester protects against local and systemic suppression of contact hypersensitivity induced by ultraviolet B radiation in mice. Radiat Res 1998; 150:292–297.

42. Emonet-Piccardi N, Richard MJ, Ravanat JL, Signorini N, Cadet J, Beani JC. Protective effects of antioxidants against UVA-induced DNA damage in human skin fibroblasts in culture. Free Radic Res 1998; 29:307–313.

43. Steenvoorden DP, Beijersburgen van Henegouwen GM. Glutathione synthesis is not involved in protection by N-acetylcysteine against UVB-induced systemic immunosuppression in mice. Photochem Photobiol 1998; 68:97–100.

44. Steenvoorden DP, Hasselbaink DM, Beijersbergen van Henegouwen GM. Protection against UV-induced reactive intermediates in human cells and mouse skin by glutathione precursors: a comparison of N-acetylcysteine and glutathione ethylester. Photochem Photobiol 1998; 67: 651–656.

45. Podda M, Rallis M, Traber MG, Packer L, Maibach HI. Kinetic study of cutaneous and subcutaneous distribution following topical application of [7,8–14C]rac-alpha-lipoic acid onto hairless mice. Biochem Pharmacol 1996; 52:627–633.

46. Fuchs J, Milbradt R. Antioxidant inhibition of skin inflammation induced by reactive oxidants: evaluation of the redox couple dihydrolipoate/lipoate. Skin Pharmacol 1994; 7:278–284.

47. Podda M, Tritschler HJ, Ulrich H, Packer L. Alpha-lipoic acid supplementation prevents symptoms of vitamin E deficiency. Biochem Biophys Res Commun 1994; 204:98–104.

48. Rosenberg HR, Culik R. Effect of α-lipoic acid on vitamin C and vitamin E deficiencies. Arch Biochem Biophys 1959; 80:86–93.

49. Pietta P. Flavonoids in medicinal plants. In: Packer L, Rice-Evans C, eds. Flavonoids in Health and Disease. New York: Marcel Dekker, 1998:61–110.

50. Rusznyak SP, Szent-Györgyi A. Vitamin P: flavonols as vitamins. Nature 1936; 138:27.

51. Rice-Evans CA, Miller NJ, Paganga G. Structure-antioxidant activity relationships of flavonoids and phenolic acids. Free Radic Biol Med 1996; 20:933–956.

52. Middleton E Jr, Kandaswami C. The impact of plant flavonoids on mammalian biology: implications for immunity, inflammation and cancer. In: Harborne JB, ed. The Flavonoids: Advances in Research Since 1986. London: Chapman & Hall, 1993.

53. Saliou C, Kitazawa M, McLaughlin L, et al. Antioxidants modulate acute solar ultraviolet radiation-induced NF-kappa-B activation in a human keratinocyte cell line. Free Radic Med 1999; 26:174–183.

54. Gerritsen ME, Carley WW, Ranges GE, et al. Flavonoids inhibit cytokine-induced endothelial cell adhesion protein gene expression. Am J Pathol 1995; 147:278–292.

55. Natarajan K, Manna SK, Chaturvedi MM, Aggarwal BB. Protein tyrosine kinase inhibitors block tumor necrosis factor-induced activation of nuclear factor-κB, degradation of IκBα, nuclear translocation of p65, and subsequent gene expression. Arch Biochem Biophys 1998; 352:59–70.

56. Gensler HL, Timmermann BN, Valcic S, et al. Prevention of photocarcinogenesis by topical administration of pure epigallocatechin gallate isolated from green tea. 1996; 26:325–335.

57. Wang ZY, Huang MT, Lou YR, et al. Inhibitory effects of black tea, green tea, decaffeinated black tea, and decaffeinated green tea on ultraviolet B light–induced skin carcinogenesis in 7,12-dimethylbenz[a]anthracene-initiated SKH-1 mice. Cancer Res 1994; 54:3428–3435.

58. Javed S, Mehrotra NK, Sukla Y. Chemopreventive effects of black tea polyphenols in mouse skin model of carcinogenesis. Biomed Environ Sci 1998; 11:307–313.

59. Katiyar SK, Korman NJ, Mukhtar H, Agarwal R. Protective effects of silymarin against photocarcinogenesis in a mouse skin model. J Natl Cancer Inst 1997; 89:556–566.

60. Agarwal R, Mukhtar H. Chemoprevention of photocarcinogenesis. Photochem Photobiol 1996; 63:440–444.

61. Tixier JM, Godeau G, Robert AM, Hornebeck W. Evidence by in vivo and in vitro studies that binding of pycnogenols to elastin affects its rate of degradation by elastases. Biochem Pharmacol 1984; 33:3933–3939.

62. Takahashi T, Kamiya T, Hasegawa A, Yokoo Y. Procyanidin oligomers selectively and intensively promote proliferation of mouse hair epithelial cells in vitro and activate hair follicle growth in vivo. J Invest Dermatol 1999; 112:310–316.

63. Burton GW, Ingold KU. Autoxidation of biological molecules. I. The antioxidant activity of vitamin E and related chain-breaking phenolic antioxidants in vitro. J Am Chem Soc 1981; 103:6472–6477.

64. Bowry VW, Stocker R. Tocopherol-mediated peroxidation—the prooxidant effect of vitamin

E on the radical initiated oxidation of human low density lipoprotein. J Am Chem Soc 1993; 115:6029–6044.

65. Sies H. Strategies of antioxidant defense. Eur J Biochem 1993; 215:213–219.

66. Packer JE, Slater TF, Willson RL. Direct observation of a free radical interaction between vitamin E and vitamin C. Nature 1979; 278:737–738.

67. Wefers H, Sies H. The protection by ascorbate and glutathione against microsomal lipid peroxidation is dependent on vitamin E. Eur J Biochem 1988; 174:353–357.

68. Gey KF. Vitamins E plus C and interacting conutrients required for optimal health. Biofactors 1998; 7:113–174.

69. Kagan VE, Witt E, Goldman R, Scita G, Packer L. Ultraviolet light-induced generation of vitamin E radicals and their recycling. A possible photosensitizing effect of vitamin E in skin. Free Radic Res Commun 1992; 16:51–64.

70. Kamal-Eldin A, Appelqvist L-A. The chemistry and antioxidant properties of tocopherols and tocotrienols. Lipids 1996; 31:671–701.

71. Winkler BS. Unequivocal evidence in support of the nonenzymatic redox coupling between glutathione/glutathione disulfide and ascorbic acid/dehydroascorbic acid. Biochem Biophys Acta 1992; 1117:287–290.

72. Wells WW, Xu DP, Yang YF, Rocque PA. Mammalian thioltransferase (glutaredoxin) and protein disulfide isomerase have dehydroascorbate reductase activity. J Biol Chem 1990; 265: 15361–15364.

73. May JM, Qu ZC, Whitesell RR, Cobb CE. Ascorbate recycling in human erythrocytes: role of GSH in reducing dehydroascorbate. Free Rad Biol Med 1996; 20:543–551.

74. Wang Y, Russo TA, Kwon O, Chanock S, Rumsey SC, Levine M. Ascorbate recycling in human neutrophils: induction by bacteria. Proc Natl Acad Sci USA 1997; 94:13816–13819.

75. Bast A, Haenen GRMM. Regulation of lipid peroxidation of glutathione and lipoic acid: involvement of liver microsomal vitamin E free radical reductase. In: Emerit I, Packer L, Auclair C, eds. Antioxidant in Therapy in Preventive Medicine. New York: Plenum Press, 1990:111–116.

76. Kagan V, Serbinova E, Packer L. Antioxidant effects of ubiquinones in microsomes and mitochondria are mediated by tocopherol recycling. Biochem Biophys Res Commun 1990; 169: 851–857.

77. Packer L, Witt E, Tritschler HJ. α-Lipoic acid as a biological antioxidant. Free Rad Biol Med 1995; 19:227–250.

78. Cossins E, Lee R, Packer L. ESR studies of vitamin C regeneration, order of reactivity of natural source phytochemical preparations. Biochem Mol Biol Int 1998; 45:583–597.

79. Tyrrell RM. UV activation of mammalian stress protein. In: Feige U, Morimoto RI, Yahara I, Polla B, eds. Stress-Inducible Cellular Responses. Basel (Switzerland): Birkhaüser Verlag, 1996:255–271.

80. Herrlich P, Blattner C, Knebel A, Bender K, Rahmsdorf HJ. Nuclear and non-nuclear targets of genotoxic agents in the induction of gene expression: shared principles in yeast, rodents, man and plants. Biol Chem 1997; 378:1217–1229.

81. Beg AA, Sha WC, Bronson RT, Baltimore D. Constitutive NF-kappa-B activation, enhanced granulopoiesis, and neonatal lethality in I-kappa-B-alpha deficient mice. Genes Dev 1995; 9: 2736–2746.

82. Klement JF, Rice NR, Car BD, et al. I-kappa-B-alpha deficiency results in a sustained NF-kappa-B response and severe widespread dermatitis in mice. Mol Cell Biol 1996; 16:2341–2349.

83. Flohé L, Brigelius-Flohé R, Saliou C, Traber M, Packer L. Redox regulation of NF-κB activation. Free Radic Biol Med 1997; 22:1115–1126.

84. Schena M, Heller RA, Theriault TP, Konrad K, Lachenmeier E, Davis RW. Microarrays: biotechnology's discovery platform for functional genomics. Trends Biotechnol 1998; 16: 301–306.

27

Alpha Hydroxy Acids

Enzo Berardesca
University of Pavia, Pavia, Italy

Alpha hydroxy acids (AHAs) constitute a class of compounds that exert specific and unique effects on skin structures. The therapeutic utility of these acids continues to expand; when applied to the skin in higher concentrations they cause detachment of keratinocytes and epidermolysis while application in lower concentration reduces intercorneocyte cohesion and visible stratum corneum desquamation.

The smallest AHA is glycolic acid, which is constituted by two carbons ($H_2C(OH)$-COOH); lactic acid contains three carbons and converts to its keto form, pyruvic acid, and vice versa. Malic acid and tartaric acid consists of four carbon chains, while citric and gluconic acid have six carbon chains [1].

AHAs are found in nature in a variety of species including foods and plants (citric, malic, tartaric, glycolic), animals (cells and body fluids), and microorganisms such as bacteria, fungi, viruses, and algae. AHA are involved in many metabolic processes and participate in essential cellular pathways such as Krebs cycle, glycolysis, and serine biosynthesis. Furthermore, they promote collagen maturation and formation of glucosaminoglycans. Their mechanism of action can be hypothesized via multiple effects [2]:

1. On stratum corneum: low concentration of AHAs diminish corneocyte cohesion. The effect occurs at the lower levels of the stratum corneum and may involve a dynamic process, operative at a particular step of keratinization, like the modification of ionic bonding. The effect is clinically evident as a sheetlike separation of the stratum corneum [3]. Indeed, intercorneocyte bonds are mostly noncovalent. In noncovalent bonds, the bonding force may be ionic or nonionic. AHAs reduce corneocyte cohesion by influencing ionic bonds via three mechanisms: (a) the distance between charges, (b) the number of charges, and (c) the medium between charges. When the stratum corneum becomes hydrated, the distance between corneocytes is increased and therefore cohesion is decreased. Another mechanism involved is the enzymatic inhibition, induced by AHAs, of the reactions of sulphate transferase, phosphototransferase, and kinases which leads to fewer electronegative sulphate and phosphate groups on the outer wall of corneocytes resulting in diminishment of cohesion forces. On the contrary, retinoids reduce intercorneocyte cohesion by breaking down already formed sulphate and phosphate bonds via induction or activation of sulphatase or phosphatase.

2.   On keratinocytes: AHAs stimulate epidermal proliferation possibly by improving energy and redox status of keratinocytes. Changes detected on normal skin after treatment with AHAs [4] are similar to those noted during wound healing [5], in the rebound period after steroid-induced atrophy [6], and in retinoic acid–treated skin [7]. Increase in the overall thickness of viable epidermis as well as in the number of granular layers suggest a stimulation of epidermal turnover. The appearance of Hale's stainable material (GAG-like) in intercellular spaces between spinous and granular cells after treatment with an AHA like ammonium lactate has been reported also in retinoic acid treated skin [7,8].

3.   On fibroblasts: at high concentration and in an appropriate vehicle, AHA induces epidermolysis, epidermal separation, and impact on the papillary dermis and reticular dermis that can lead to dermal changes including the synthesis of new collagen [1]. AHAs might turn on the biosynthesis of dermal glycosaminoglycans and other intercellular substances that could be responsible for eradication of fine wrinkles [9]. It has also been speculated that AHAs might promote collagen synthesis in human skin [9]. Ascorbic acid (an AHA in the lactone form) has been shown to stimulate procollagen synthesis in cultured human fibroblasts [10].

Because of these mechanisms, the cosmetic effects of AHAs on stratum corneum include an increase of plasticization and a decreased formation of dry flaky scales on skin surface. Indeed, a thinner stratum corneum is more flexible and compact; the increased flexibility obtained after topical application of AHAs is not related to an increased water content of the stratum corneum and is maintained even at low relative humidity [11]; this effect is also related to the free acid concentration of the formulation and is not dependent on transcutaneous penetration or sorption of the molecule [12]. The enhanced release of surface corneocytes is not equal for all AHAs and might lead in the long term to a stimulation of epidermal proliferation which increases thickness and metabolic activity of epidermis. The final cosmetic result of this process is an improvement of skin texture associated with increased skin firmness and elasticity.

Optimization of the formulation allows improvement of efficacy: pH is of great importance for achieving good therapeutical results. The suggested range is between 3.0 and 5.0, but lower pH values seem to be also very effective. The lower acid pH level reached in the stratum corneum after application of AHAs helps in dissolving desmosomes

TABLE 1   Mean Values ($\pm$SE) of CBF (Perfusion Units), TEWL (gm^2/h), and Erythema (a* Value)

	CBF		TEWL		Erythema	
	Glycolic	Betameth	Glycolic	Betameth	Glycolic	Betameth
Baseline	109.9 $\pm$ 14.9	101.9 $\pm$ 12.7	19.6 $\pm$ 3.4	18.5 $\pm$ 3.7	17.1 $\pm$ 1.0	17.7 $\pm$ 0.9
Day 5	78.3 $\pm$ 9.9*	52.6 $\pm$ 7.5	11.1 $\pm$ 1.5	10.8 $\pm$ 1.6	15.9 $\pm$ 0.7	16.3 $\pm$ 0.8
Day 10	82.1 $\pm$ 13.9*	38.4 $\pm$ 5.4	12.2 $\pm$ 1.6	8.8 $\pm$ 1.7	16.9 $\pm$ 1.1	15.2 $\pm$ 0.9
Day 15	57.6 $\pm$ 6.5*	35.3 $\pm$ 8.6	9.6 $\pm$ 1.6	8.6 $\pm$ 2.3	14.8 $\pm$ 0.8	14.5 $\pm$ 0.8

* Significant differences in CBF are recorded between glycolic acid–and betamethasone-treated sites during the study [17]. No significant differences appear concerning TEWL and erythema. All treatments induced a significant decrease of the parameters investigated during the study (TEWL, $p < 0.01$ glycolic, $p < 0.005$ betamethasone; CBF, glycolic $p < 0.001$, betamethasone $p < 0.0001$; erythema, glycolic $p < 0.01$, betamethasone $p< 0.009$).

Abbreviations: CBF, cutaneous blood flow; TEWL, transepidermal water loss; SE, standard error.

and/or other linkages between cells increasing therefore cell shedding and AHA activity [13]. Chronic treatment with low pH formula is likely to induce changes in the pH of living epidermis. Several enzymes (e.g., phosphatases, lipases, transforming growth factor beta) have maximum activity at pH 5 or lower and is possible that an acid environment may activate these mechanisms. Other important factors in the development of the product are free acid concentration (the higher the better) [12], the presence of an appropriate delivery system capable to increase penetration of AHA molecule, and the association between AHA and their salts.

Retinoic acid, a well-known and accepted drug for treating photoaging, shows benefits similar to AHAs after long term application. The mechanism of action is different and, even though clinical results may be similar, more complex. Retinoic acid has specific receptors (CRABP) on keratinocytes and fibroblasts; it binds to cell membranes and causes directly or indirectly stimulation of cell metabolism [14]. AHAs are hydrophilic (and diffuse freely throughout the intercellular phase) whereas retinoids are hydrophobic and thus require certain proteins in plasma and skin to act as carriers [14,15]. Retinoids have several side effects including photosensitivity, erythema, irritant dermatitis, and potential teratogenicity. Furthermore, from a cosmetic viewpoint, it takes several months to induce clinically evident cosmetic improvements [16]; AHAs are generally safer, less irritant, nonphotosensitizing, and give cosmetic results after 8 to 10 weeks.

Alpha hydroxy acids have been recently used to treat some skin diseases. Vignoli et al. [17] showed a reduction in psoriasis severity after treatment with glycolic acid as measured by visual scoring and noninvasive instruments (Table 1); in this study, a signifi-

TEWL
Error Bars: ± 1 Standard Error(s)

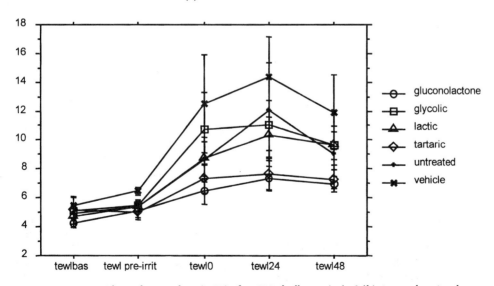

FIGURE 1   Transepidermal water loss (±SE) after SLS challenge ($g/m^2/h$). Lower barrier damage is detected in AHA-treated sites compared to vehicle and untreated areas. ($p < 0.006$). Gluconolactone is significantly lower than glycolic acid at each time point. (hour0 = $p < 0.01$, hour24 = $p < 0.03$, hour48 $p < 0.04$) and than lactic acid at hour 48 ($p < 0.04$). (From Ref. 18.)

cant improvement of transepidermal water loss (TEWL), erythema (a* value), and cutaneous blood flow after treatment with either 15% glycolic acid or betamethasone 0.05%. No significant differences appear in TEWL and erythema between glycolic acid and betamethasone; on the other hand, a significantly decreased CBF is recorded in the sites treated with betamethasone confirming the higher effect of corticosteroid in terms of vasoconstriction and reduction of inflammation.

Prolonged treatment with AHAs can also lead to stratum corneum barrier fortification and increased resistance to chemical irritation; sodium lauryl sulphate (SLS) irritation has been shown to be reduced in AHA-treated sites; a recent study [18] shows that AHAs can modulate stratum corneum barrier function and prevent skin irritation; and the effect is not equal for all AHAs, being more marked for the molecules characterized by antioxidant properties (Fig. 1). This effect has been shown by other keratolytic compounds such as urea [19] and can be related to the increased production of stratum corneum lipids such as ceramides induced by the treatment [20].

Over the years a number of cosmetic or dermatological compounds have gained attention for the capability to treat skin disorders and in particularly skin aging. AHAs are certainly the most intriguing class of compounds that are beginning to be incorporated into the new generation of cosmetic products. Even though many mechanisms are still far from being completely understood and much work remains to be done, the future is promising for these simple molecules.

REFERENCES

1. Van Scott E, Yu RJ. Alpha hydroxyacids: therapeutic potentials. Canadian Dermatol 1989; 1:108–112.
2. Van Scott E, Yu RJ. Hyperkeratinization, corneocyte cohesion and alpha hydroxy acids. J Am Acad Dermatol 1984; 11:867–879.
3. Van Scott E, Yr RJ. Substances that modify the stratum corneum by modulating its formation. In Frost P, Horwitz SN, eds. Principles of Cosmetic for the Dermatologist. St. Louis: Mosby, 1982:70–74.
4. Lavker RM, et al. Effects of topical ammonium lactate on cutaneous atrophy from a potent topical corticosteriod. J Am Acad Dermatol 1992; 26:535–544.
5. Pinkus H. Examination of the epidermis by strip method. J Invest Dermatol 1952; 19:431–447.
6. Zheng P, et al. Morphologic investigations on the rebound phenomenon after corticoid-induced atrophy in human skin. J Invest Dermatol 1984; 82:345–352.
7. Elias PM, Williams ML. Retinoids, cancer and the skin. Arch Dermatol 1981; 117:160–180.
8. Weiss JS, et al. Topical tretinoin improves photoaged skin: a double blind, vehicle controlled study. JAMA 1988; 259:527–532.
9. Van Scott E, Yu RJ. Alpha hydroxy acids: procedures for use in clinical practice. Cutis 1989; 43:222–228.
10. Pinnel SR, et al. Induction of collagen synthesis by ascorbic acid. A possible mechanism. Arch Dermatol 1987; 123:1684–1686.
11. Takahashi M, Machida Y. The influence of hydroxyacids on the rheological properties of the stratum corneum. J Soc Cosmet Chem 1985; 36:177–187.
12. Hall KJ, Hill JC. The skin plasticization effect of 2-hydroxyoctanoic acid. I. The use of potentiators. J Soc Cosmet Chem 1986; 37:397–407.
13. Smith WP. Hydroxy acids and skin aging. Soap/Cosm/Chem Specialties, 54–58, Sept 1993.
14. Puhvel SM, Sakamoto M. Cellular retinoic acid binding proteins in human epidermis and sebaceous follicles. J Invest Dermatol 1984; 82:79–84.

15. Siegenthaler G, Saurat JH. Plasma and skin carriers for natural and synthetic retinoids. Arch Dermatol 1987; 123:1690.

16. Hermitte R. Aged skin, retinoids and alpha hydroxy acids. Cosme Toilet 1992; 107:63–67.

17. Vignoli GP, Distante F, Rona C, Berardesca E. Effects of glycolic acid on psoriasis. Clin Exp Dermatol 1998; 23:190–191.

18. Berardesca E, Distante F, Vignoli GP, Oresajo C, Green B. Alpha hydroxyacids modulate stratum corneum barrier function. Br J Dermatol 1997; 137:934–938.

19. Loden M. Urea-containing moisturizers influence barrier properties of normal skin. Arch Dermatol Res. 1996; 288:103–107.

20. Rawlings AV, Davies A, Carlomusto M, Pillai S, Zhang K, Kosturko R, Verdejo P, Feinberg C, Nguyen L, Chandar P. Effect of lactic acid isomers on keratinocyte ceramide synthesis, stratum corneum lipid levels and stratum corneum barrier function. Arch Dermatol Res 1996; 288:382–390.

28

Colorants

Gisbert Otterstätter
DRAGOCO Gerberding & Co. AG, Holzminden, Germany

The use of coloring agents for decorative purposes is one of the earliest cultural accomplishments of humankind. Even in prehistoric times, colorants could be found not only for art—the famous cave paintings in southern Europe, for example—but also especially for body painting, tattooing, or, to use the modern phrase, for decorative cosmetics. Although there were several historical periods in which those who wore cosmetics were scorned or condemned, its use has nevertheless remained a constant among cultures throughout history. In more recent times, decorative cosmetics have been joined by other cosmetic products whose colors are not intended to conceal or change the appearance of something; instead, these colorants must conform to the statement that a given product makes about itself. While it is true that many first-time purchases are heavily influenced by the way the consumer feels about the color of the product and the attractiveness of its packaging, we nevertheless have some very definite associations between certain products and the colors they should have. Blue would certainly be inappropriate for a soap perfumed with sandalwood; the only color that would do for a pine-scented bubble bath is green; and it is logical to give citrus scents psychological reinforcement by coloring them yellow or yellow-green.

Although the use of colorants* has a long history, a great deal of time passed before their role in cosmetics was legally established. This happened in Germany in 1887 with the enactment of the so-called Color Law, which banned the use of hazardous colorants. The issue of concern that led to this law was primarily pigments containing heavy metals; products of the then-developing color industry were not a genuine consideration. In 1906 a color law was passed in Austria that included various purity specifications and made the use of some coal-tar dyes illegal. In 1907 the use of the first certified food colorants were legalized in the United States, and at the same time purity specifications were also

---

* *Colorants*: general term for all materials that can be used to color. There are three kinds: (1) colorants that are soluble in the medium being colored (in the case of cosmetics, usually water- or oil-soluble), (2) pigments and color lakes that are not soluble in the medium being colored (the latter are usually aluminum hydroxide lakes of water-soluble colorants), and (3) water-dispersible pigments (pigments that yield stable dispersions in water when excipients are added; they can then be processed like soluble colorants).

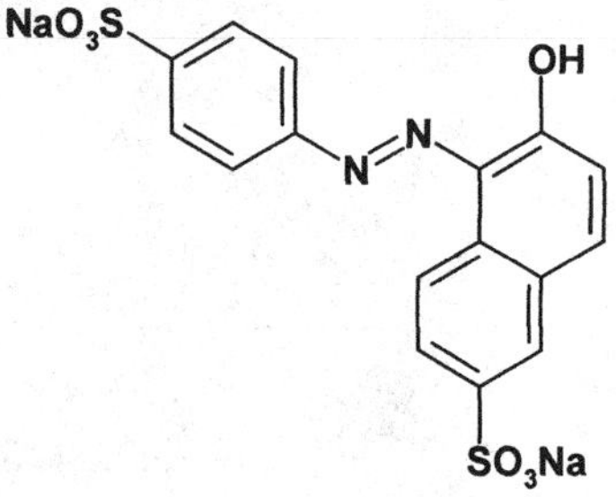

FIGURE 1   Azo colorant yellow-orange S (FD&C Yellow No. 6), C.I. 15985.

determined. The Federal Food, Drug and Cosmetic Act of 1938 first outlined the use of colorants in food, drugs and cosmetics.

The dramatic boom in the development of the color industry led to numerous new colorants and pigments. Because it had become clear that it was not only heavy metals that were dangerous, but the colorants themselves or their initial products could pose a threat as well, after World War II scientific organizations [2] increased their systematic efforts to compile and publish [3] the results of toxicological and dermatological research and encourage further studies. Unfortunately, international cooperation was less intense then than it is today. That means that there are significant differences between the approved colorants for cosmetics in the European Union (EU), the United States, and Japan, for example. An illustration of this is the colorant patent blue V (C.I. 42051), [4] which is approved in the EU for all cosmetic products, [5] but not in the United States or Japan. The same is true of fast yellow (C.I. 13015) and many other European cosmetic colorants. Furthermore, to some extent even approved colorants have different restrictions on their use,* especially for use in the area around the eyes. Table 1 shows the cosmetic colorants in the EU that are also approved for use in the United States and/or Japan. Because they lack fastness, natural colorants (e.g., carotenoids, anthocyans, chlorophylls) play only a minor role in the process of coloring cosmetics. Carmine is an exception (C.I. 75470); the classic red pigment for lipstick is also the only red pigment in the United States that can be used for the eyes.

By comparison, inorganic pigments are used in large quantities. In coloring decorative cosmetics, several products are of vital importance: titanium dioxide (C.I. 77891) in particular—the most important white pigment—the iron oxides and iron hydroxides for the colors yellow (C.I. 77492), and red (C.I. 77491) and black (C.I. 77499), ultramarine (C.I. 77007)—especially in blue and violet—Prussian blue (C.I. 77510), manganese violet (C.I. 77742), coal black (C.I. 77268:1), pearlescent pigments (mica C.I. 77019), and bismuth oxychloride (C.I. 77163). By combining iron oxides, including the addition of titanium dioxide, various brown tones can be created in makeup and toning cremes. The most significant colorant, however, is composed of the organic colorants and pigments which belong to different chemical classes. Mainly these are azo, triarylmethane, anthraquinone, xanthene or phthalocyanine colorants or pigments; occasionally they include indigo derivatives (Figs. 1–6; and Table 1).

---

* In the EU there are four areas of applications: (1) approved for all cosmetic products; (2) not for use around the eyes; (3) not for use near the mucous membranes; and (4) only for brief contact with the skin.

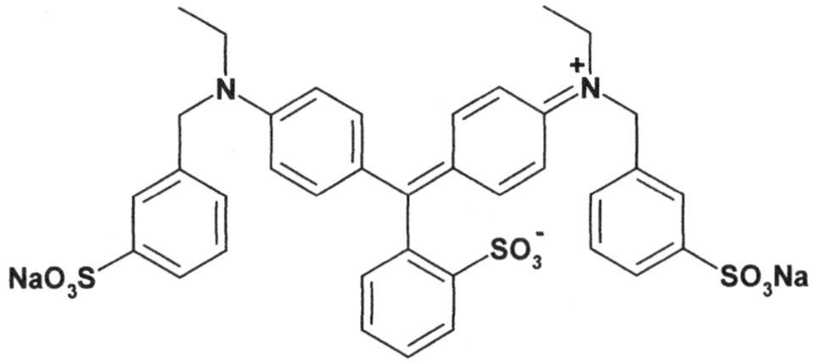

FIGURE 2 Triarylmethane colorant brilliant blue FCF (FD&C Blue No. 1), C.I. 42090.

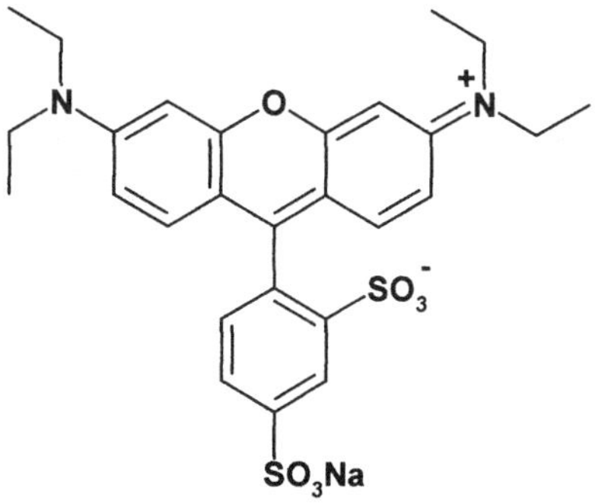

FIGURE 3 Xanthene colorant sulforhodamine B, C.I. 45100.

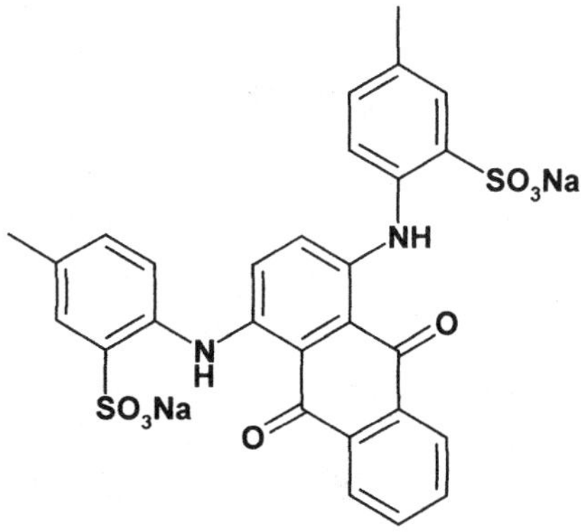

FIGURE 4 Anthraquinone colorant alizarin cyanine green (D&C Green No. 5), C.I. 61570.

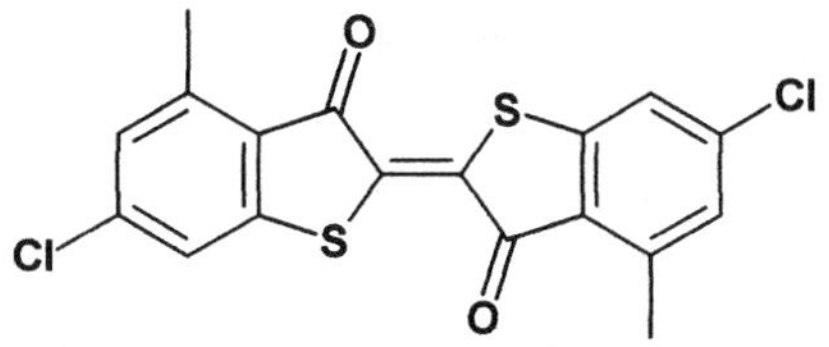

FIGURE 5 Indigo pigment indanthrene brilliant pink R (D&C Red No. 30), C.I. 73360.

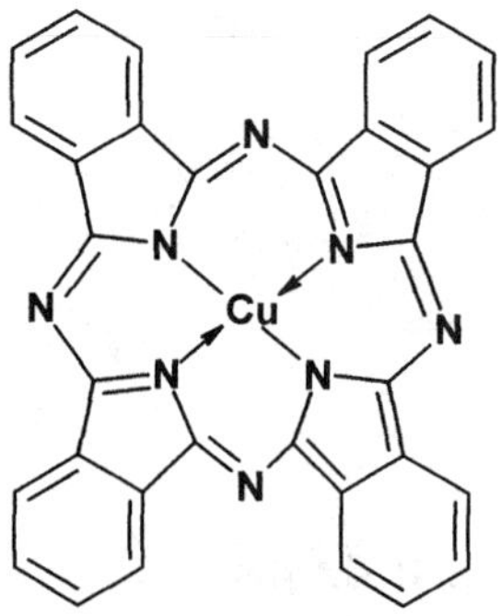

FIGURE 6 Phthalocyanine pigment heliogen blue B (phthalocyanine blue), C.I. 74160.

Regardless of their chemical class, cosmetic colorants are sorted into three groups; this classification is based on their solubility, which determines how they are used: (1) colorants that are soluble in the medium being colored (usually water- or oil-soluble), (2) pigments and color lakes that are not soluble in the medium being colored, and (3) water-dispersible pigments.

Because of the extensive differences in national laws, two major factors must be considered in the development of colored cosmetics: one is technical, and the other is a legal matter. There are three phases to the procedure:

1. After the formulation of the uncolored product has been developed, the decision must be made about the countries in which the product will be marketed.
2. Because not all colorant groups are appropriate for all cosmetics, some are selected (Table 2) and then examined to see which colorant of the respective category is approved in all of the countries where the cosmetic product will be marketed.
3. At this point, the product is colored, and stability tests are then conducted (original packaging, light, heat, etc.). Changing the formulation after successful completion of these tests is strongly discouraged. The testing must be repeated if the risk of unpleasant surprises is to be ruled out.

Although there are approximately 160 approved cosmetic colorants in the EU—many more than in the United States, for example—only a limited number of them is really used. Table 3 shows selected cosmetic product and the colorants that are often and usually added in industry.

Hair-toning and hair-coloring products have a special status among the cosmetics in the EU because the EU guidelines for cosmetics do not apply to these products, especially because common cosmetic colorants have little or no affinity to hair.

Two different kinds of colorants are used to color hair:

1. Oxidation hair colors, which permanently color the hair.
2. Substantive colorants, which only affect the outside of the hair and can be washed out again (semipermanent coloring).

In oxidation hair colors, a colorless initial product penetrates the hair, where a reaction takes place with the aid of hydrogen peroxide (hence the term oxidation hair colors) and

TABLE 1 Cosmetic Colorants in the EU That Are Also Approved in the United States and/or Japan* (as of July 1998)

Color Index Number or name, color, colorant category, solubility	Japan*	U.S.†	Application area in the EU, examples of use
10020 green, water-soluble nitrosonaphthol colorant	Green No. 401 approved (Category III)	Not approved	EU: 3 tenside products
10316 yellow, water-soluble nitro colorant	Yellow No. 403 approved (Category III)	Ext.-D&C Yellow No. 7 not for eyes and lips	EU: 2 soap, tenside products
11680 yellow, azo pigment (also water dispersible)	Yellow No. 401 approved (Category III)	Not approved	EU: 3 soap
11725 orange, azo pigment	Orange No. 401 approved (Category III)	Not approved	EU: 4 soap
12085 red, azo pigment	Red No. 228 approved (Category III)	D&C Red No. 36 not for use near eyes	EU: 1 lipstick (max. 3%)
12120 red, azo pigment	Red No. 221 approved (Category III)	Not approved	EU: 4
14700 red water-soluble azo colorant	Red No. 504 approved (Category III)	FD&C Red No. 4 not for eyes and lips	EU: 1 soap, alcohol-based perfume products
15510 orange, water-soluble azo colorant	Orange No. 205 approved (Category II)	D&C Orange No. 4 not for eyes and lips	EU: 2 tenside products, soap
15620 red, water-soluble azo colorant	Red No. 506 approved (Category III)	Not approved	EU: 4
15630: 1 red (sodium salt), not easily water-soluble azo colorant	Red No. 205 approved (Category II)	Not approved	EU: 1 (max. 3%)
15630: 1 red (barium salt) azo pigment	Red No. 207 approved (Category II)	Not approved	EU: 1 (max. 3%) soap, lipstick, makeup
15630: 2 red (calcium salt) azo pigment	Red No. 206 approved (Category II)	Not approved	EU: 1 (max. 3%) soap, lipstick, makeup
15630: 3 (strontium salt) azo pigment	Red No. 208 approved (Category II)	Not approved	EU: 1 (max. 3%) soap, lipstick, makeup
15800: 1 red (calcium salt) azo pigment	Red No. 219 approved (Category II)	D&C Red No. 31 not for eyes	EU: 3

TABLE 1 Continued

Color Index Number or name, color, colorant category, solubility	Japan*	U.S.†	Application area in the EU, examples of use
15850 red (sodium salt) not easily water-soluble azo colorant	Red No. 201 approved (Category II)	D&C Red No. 6 not for eyes	EU: 1
15850: 1 red (calcium salt) azo pigment	Red No. 202 approved (Category II)	D&C Red No. 7 not for eyes	EU: 1 soap, lipstick, makeup
15865: 2 red (calcium salt) azo pigment	Red No. 405 approved (Category III)	Not approved	EU: 1 soap, lipstick, makeup
15880: 1 red (calcium salt) azo pigment	Red No. 220 approved (Category II)	D&C Red No. 34 not for eyes	EU: 1 soap, lipstick, makeup
15985 orange, water-soluble azo colorant, also as aluminum lake	Yellow No. 5 approved (Category I)	FD&C Yellow No. 6 not for eyes	EU: 1 (food colorant E 110) alcohol-based perfume products
16035 red, water-soluble azo colorant, also as aluminum lake	Not approved	FD&C Red No. 40 also approved for eyes	EU: 1 (food colorant E 129) tenside products, alcohol-based perfume products, mouthwash
16185 red, water-soluble azo colorant, also as aluminum lake	Red No. 2 approved (Category I)	Not approved	EU: 1 (food colorant E 123) tenside products
16255 red, water-soluble azo colorant, also as aluminum lake	Red No. 102 approved (Category I)	Not approved	EU: 1 (food colorant E 124) tenside products, alcohol-based perfume products
17200 blue-red, water-soluble azo colorant, also as aluminum lake	Red No. 227 approved (Category II)	D&C Red No. 33 not for eyes	EU: 1 mouthwash, alcohol-based perfume products, tenside products
18820 yellow, water-soluble azo colorant	Yellow No. 407 approved (Category III)	Not approved	EU: 4
19140 yellow, water-soluble azo colorant, also as aluminum lake	Yellow No. 4 approved (Category I)	FD&C Yellow No. 5 also approved for eyes	EU: 1 (food colorant E 102) tenside products
20170 yellow-brown, water-soluble azo colorant	Brown No. 201 approved, also as aluminum lake (Category II)	D&C Brown No. 1 not for eyes and lips	EU: 3 tenside products
20470 blue-black, water-soluble azo colorant	Black No. 401 approved (Category III)	Not approved	EU: 4 tenside products, soap

26100 red, soil-soluble azo colorant	Red No. 225 approved (Category II)	D&C Red No. 17 not for eyes and lips	EU: 3 oil products
40800 yellow-orange, oil-soluble (also water-dispersible)	Beta-carotene approved (Category I)	Beta-carotene (no FDA certificate) also approved for eyes	EU: 1 (food colorant E 160a) cremes
42053 blue-green, water-soluble triarylmethane colorant, also as aluminum lake	Green No. 3 approved (Category I)	FD&C Green No. 3 not for eyes	EU: 1 mouthwash
42090 blue (sodium salt), water-soluble triarylmethane colorant, also as aluminum lake	Blue No. 1 approved (Category I)	FD&C Blue No. 1 also approved for eyes	EU: 1 (food colorant E 133) tenside products, oral and dental care products
42090 blue (ammonia salt), water-soluble triarylmethane colorant, also as aluminum lake	Blue No. 205 approved (Category II)	D&C Blue No. 4 not for eyes and lips	EU: this ammonia salt is not approved
45100 red, fluorescent water-soluble xanthene colorant, also as aluminum lake	Red No. 106 approved (Category I)	Not approved	EU: 4 tenside products
45190 red-violet, water-soluble xanthene colorant, also as aluminum lake	Red No. 401 approved (Category III)	Not approved	EU: 4 tenside products, soap
45350 yellow, xanthene colorant fluorescent, water-soluble salts, also as aluminum lake; free acid oil-soluble	Yellow No. 201 free acid, Yellow No. 202 (1) sodium salt, Yellow No. 202(2) potassium salt, all approved (Category II)	D&C Yellow No. 7 free acid, D&C Yellow No. 8 sodium salt, both not approved for eyes and lips	EU: 1 (max. 6%) basically only the sodium salt is used: tenside products
45370 orange, xanthene colorant, fluorescent, as sodium salt and free acid (45370:1), water-soluble, also as aluminum lake	Orange No. 201 free acid, approved (Category II)	D&C Orange No. 5 free acid, not for eyes, in lipstick max. 5%	EU: 1 lipstick
45380 red, xanthene colorant, fluorescent, salts and free acid (45380:2) water-soluble, also as aluminum lake	Red No. 223 free acid, Red No. 230(12) sodium salt, Red No. 230(2) potassium salt, all approved (Category II)	D&C Red No. 21 free acid, D&C Red No. 22 sodium salt; sodium salt also approved as color lake; none approved for eyes	EU: 1 lipstick

TABLE 1 Continued

Color Index Number or name, color, colorant category, solubility	Japan*	U.S.†	Application area in the EU, examples of use
45410 red, xanthene colorant, fluorescent, water-soluble salts, also as barium lake and aluminum lake, free acid (45410:1) soluble in ethanol and oils	Red No. 218 free acid, Red No. 231 potassium salt, both approved (Category II); Red. No. 104(1) sodium salt approved (Category I)	D&C Red No. 27 free acid, D&C Red No. 28 sodium salt, both not for eyes	EU: 1 lipstick
45425 red, xanthene colorant, fluorescent, sodium salt water-soluble, free acid (45425:1) soluble in ethanol and oils, also as aluminum lake	Orange No. 206 free acid, Orange No. 207 sodium salt, both approved (Category II), No. 206 not approved as aluminum lake	D&C Orange No. 10 free acid, D&C Orange No. 11 sodium salt, both also approved as color lakes, but not for eyes and lips	EU: 1 lipstick
45430 red, water-soluble xanthene colorant, also as aluminum lake	Red No. 3 approved, also as aluminum lake (Category I)	FD&C Red No. 3 not approved for cosmetics	EU: 1 (food colorant E 127) aluminum lake in lipstick
47000 yellow, oil-soluble quinophthalone colorant	Yellow No. 204 approved (Category I)	D&C Yellow No. 11 not for eyes and lips	EU: 3
47005 yellow, water-soluble quinophthalone colorant, also as aluminum lake	Yellow No. 203 approved also as aluminum lake, barium lake and zirconium lake (Category II)	D&C Yellow No. 10‡ not for eyes	EU: 1 (food colorant E 104) tenside products, soap, permanent and semi-permanent hair products
59040 green, fluorescent, water-soluble pyrene colorant, also as aluminum lake	Green No. 204 approved also as aluminum lake (Category II)	D&C Green No. 8, max. 0.01%, not for eyes and lips	EU: 3 tenside products, soap
60725 blue-violet, oil-soluble anthraquinone colorant	Purple (Violet) No. 201 approved (Category II)	D&C Violet No. 2 not for eyes and lips	EU: 1 oil products
60730 violet, water-soluble anthraquinone colorant	Purple (Violet) No. 401 approved (Category III)	Ext. D&C Violet No. 2 not for eyes and lips	EU: 3 hair, alcohol-based perfume products
61565 green, oil-soluble anthraquinone colorant	Green No. 202 approved (Category II)	D&C Green No. 6 not for eyes and lips	EU: 1 oil products
61570 green, water-soluble anthraquinone colorant, also as aluminum lake	Green No. 201 approved (Category II)	D&C Green No. 5 approved for eyes as well	EU: 1 tenside products, soap

Colorant	US approval	US notes	EU
73000 blue, pigment (indigo, vat-blue colorant)	Blue No. 201 approved (Category II)	Not approved	EU: 1
73015 blue, water-soluble indigo colorant	Blue No. 2 approved, also as aluminum lake (Category I)	FD&C Blue No. 2 not approved for cosmetics	EU: 1 (food colorant E 132) aluminum lake for eye makeup
73360 red, indigo pigment	Red No. 226 approved (Category II)	D&C Red No. 30 not for eyes	EU: 1 toothpaste, lipstick
74160 blue, phthalocyanine pigment (also water dispersible)	Blue No. 404 approved (Category III)	Not approved	EU: 1 eye makeup, toothpaste, soap, tenside products
75120 yellow to orange, oil-soluble carotenoid (also water-dispersible)	Annatto, approved (Category I)	Annatto (no FDA certificate) for eyes as well	EU: 1 (food colorant E 160b) oil products, creams
75130 see 40800			
75170 white, natural organic pigment	Guanine, approved (Category I)	Guanine (no FDA certificate) for eyes also	EU: 1 decorative cosmetics
75470 red, natural anthraquinone pigment, also water-soluble	Carmine, approved (Category I)	Carmine (no FDA certificate) for eyes also	EU: 1 (food colorant E 120) makeup, lipstick
75810 see 75815			
75815 green, water-soluble porphyrine colorant	Sodium copper chlorophylline, approved (Category I)	Potassium sodium copper chlorophylline, (no FDA certificate) max. 0.1%, only approved for oral and dental care products	EU (listed as C.I. 75810) (food colorant E 141): 1, oral and dental care
77000 silver-colored, inorganic pigment	Aluminum powder approved (Category I)	Aluminum powder (no FDA certificate) external application, also for eyes (limitation of the particle size)	EU: 1 (food colorant E 173)
77004 white, pigment	Kaolin approved (Category I)	Kaolin (no FDA certificate), considered cosmetic raw material and not colorant	EU: 1 No known use as a colorant
77007 blue, violet, pink, red and green inorganic pigments	Ultramarine approved (Category I)	Ultramarine (no FDA certificate), also for eyes, but not in products for mouth and lips	EU: 1 makeup, eye cosmetics, lipstick, soap
77019 white to opaque, inorganic pearlescent pigment (mica)	Mica, approved (Category I)	Mica (no FDA certificate), also for eyes	EU (summarized in the EC Guideline with CL 77891): decorative cosmetics

TABLE 1 Continued

Color Index Number or name, color, colorant category, solubility	Japan*	U.S.†	Application area in the EU, examples of use
77120 white, inorganic pigment	Barium sulfate considered cosmetic raw material and not colorant	Barium sulfate considered cosmetic raw material and not colorant	EU: 1 no known use as a colorant
77163 white inorganic pearlescent pigment	Bismuth oxychloride approved (Category I)	Bismuth oxychloride (no FDA certificate) also for eyes	EU: 1 decorative cosmetics
77220 white, pigment	Calcium carbonate considered cosmetic raw material and not colorant	Calcium carbonate considered cosmetic raw material and not colorant	EU: 1 no known use as a colorant
77231 white, inorganic pigment	Calcium sulfate considered cosmetic raw material and not colorant	Calcium sulfate considered cosmetic raw material and not colorant	EU: 1 no known use as a colorant
77266 black, inorganic pigment	Carbon black approved (Category I)	Not approved	EU: 1 decorative cosmetics
77288 green, inorganic pigment	Chromium oxide green, approved for eyes as well, but not around mouth and lips	Chromium oxide greens (no FDA certificate), also for yes, but not around mouth and lips	EU: 1 decorative cosmetics, soap
77289 green, inorganic pigment	Hydrated chromium oxide, approved for eyes as well, but not around mouth and lips	Chromium hydroxide green (no FDA certificate), also approved for eyes, but not around mouth and lips	EU: 1 decorative cosmetics, soap
77400 copper-colored, inorganic pigment	Not approved	Copper powder (no FDA certificate), for external application and also for eyes	EU: 1 decorative cosmetics
77491 red-brown, inorganic pigment	Red oxide of iron approved (Category I)	Synthetic iron oxide (no FDA certificate) also for eyes	EU: 1 (all food colorant E 172) creams, makeup, lipstick, soap
77492 yellow, inorganic pigment	Yellow oxide of iron approved (Category I)		
77499 black, inorganic pigment	Black oxide of iron approved (Category I)		

	Japan	FDA	EU
77510 blue, inorganic pigment	Ferric ferrocyanide approved (Category I)	Ferric ferrocyanide (no FDA certificate), also for eyes, but not around mouth and lips	EU: 1 decorative cosmetics especially eye makeup
77713 white, inorganic pigment	Magnesium carbonate approved (Category I)	Magnesium carbonate considered cosmetic raw material and not colorant	EU: 1 powder
77742 violet, inorganic pigment	Manganese Violet approved for eyes but not around mouth and lips	Manganese Violet (no FDA certificate) also for eyes	EU: 1 decorative cosmetics
77820 silver-colored inorganic pigment	Not approved	Silver (no FDA certificate), max. 1% only for use on nails	EU: 1 (food colorant E 174) no known use as a cosmetic colorant
77891 white, inorganic pigment	Titanium dioxide approved (Category I)	Titanium dioxide (no FDA certificate) also for eyes	EU: 1 (food colorant E 171) creams, makeup, lipstick, powder, soap, toothpaste
77947 white, inorganic pigment	Zinc oxide approved (Category I)	Zinc oxide (no FDA certificate) for external application and also for eyes	EU: 1 no known use as a colorant
Aluminum stearate, calcium stearate, and magnesium stearate white, oil-soluble	Considered cosmetic raw material and not colorant	Considered cosmetic raw material and not colorant	EU: 1 no known use as a cosmetic colorant
Lactoflavin (riboflavin, vitamin B2) yellow, water soluble	Riboflavin approved (Category I)	Not approved	EU: 1 (food colorant E 101) no known use as a cosmetic colorant
Caramel sugar brown, water-soluble	Caramel approved (Category I)	Caramel (no FDA certificate) also used for eyes	EU: 1 (food colorant E 150a–d) rarely also in creams

* Japan: Category I—approved for all cosmetic products, Category II—for external use, Category III—not for use on mucous membranes.
† Unless otherwise indicated and if chemically possible, the corresponding aluminum color lake is also approved.
‡ Because of its perceptual composition of mono-, di-, and trisulfonic acid, D&C Yellow No. 10 does not correspond to the specification of EU-approved food colorant E 104, which is also listed under CI 47005.

TABLE 2

Colorant group	Cosmetic products
Water-soluble colorants	e.g., bath products (shampoo, shower gel, and bubble bath), creams, soap, toothpaste gel, mouthwash
Oil-soluble colorants	e.g., oil products, soap
Pigments	e.g., makeup, powder, lipstick, toothpaste, soap
Color lakes	e.g., eye makeup, lipstick
Water dispersible pigments	soap

TABLE 3

Cosmetic products (selection)	Color	Recommended colorant
	blue	
Bubble bath	yellow	C.I. 42045, 42051, 42090
		C.I. 13015, 19140, 47005, 45350 (fluorescent)
	green	C.I. 61570, 59040 (fluorescent) as well as by mixing blue and yellow colorings
	orange	C.I. 16255, 15985 as well as by mixing yellow and red colorants
	pink/red	C.I. 16255, 16035, 16185
	brown	can be created by mixing red and yellow or orange and blue colorants
	violet	by mixing red and blue, especially C.I. 42090 and 16185.
Recommended dose		0.05–0.3%
Shampoo, shower gel, liquid soap	colors as for bubble bath and also	
	blue	C.I. 61585 and
	pink	C.I. 45100
Recommended dose		0.01–0.05%
Bath salts	blue	C.I. 42090, 42051
	yellow	C.I. 47005, 45350 (fluorescent)
	green	C.I. 61570, also as mixture of blue and yellow colorants
	pink	C.I. 45430
Recommended dose		0.005–0.01%
Oil products	blue	C.I. 60725
	yellow	C.I. 40800
	green	C.I. 75810
	orange	C.I. 75120
	turquoise	C.I. 61565
	red-orange	C.I. 12150
Recommended dose		0.01–0.05%

TABLE 3 Continued

Cosmetic products (selection)	Color	Recommended colorant
Soap	blue	C.I. 61585, 74160, 77007
	yellow	C.I. 10316, 11680, 11710, 21108, 47005, 77492
	green	C.I. 10006, 10020, 59040 (fluorescent), 61570, 74260
	orange	by mixing red and yellow
	red	C.I. 12490, 77491
	black	C.I. 77499, 77268:1
	violet	C.I. 51319 and by mixing blue and red
	white	C.I. 77891
Recommended dose		water-soluble colorants or water dispersible pigments 0.01–0.05% pigments 0.05–0.5%
Toothpaste	blue	C.I. 74160
	green	C.I. 74260
	red	C.I. 73360
	white	C.I. 77891
Recommended dose		0.02–0.05%
Toothpaste gels	blue	C.I. 42051, 42090
Recommended dose		C.I. 0.02–0.05%
Mouthwash	blue	C.I. 42090
	green	C.I. 61570 or a mixture of C.I. 42090 and C.I. 47005
	red	C.I. 16035
Recommended dose		5–20 ppm
Alcoholic perfume products	blue	C.I. 42051, 42090
	yellow	C.I. 47005, 13015, 19140
	orange	C.I. 15985
	red	C.I. 16035, 17200
Recommended dose		5–20 ppm
Lipstick	all pigments (cosmetic application area 1 in the EU)	
Recommended dose		1–10%
Makeup, powder	brown	mixtures of C.I. 77491, 77492, 77499, 77891
Recommended dose		2–10%
Eye makeup	blue	C.I. 77510, 77007
	yellow	C.I. 77492
	red	C.I. 77491, 75470
	violet	C.I. 77742
	black	C.I. 77266, 77268:1, 77499
Recommended dose		5–30%

another colorless initial product. No colorants are used; the color is first created on the inside of the hair.

Substantive colorants are largely cationic and cannot penetrate the hair because their molecules are too large; therefore they only adhere on the outside and can be removed again comparatively easily.

BIBLIOGRAPHY

Colour Index: Third Edition, Vols. 1–4 (1971), Revised Third Edition, Vol. 5–6 (1975); The Society of Dyers and Colourists, P.O. Box 244, Perkin House 82, Grattan Road, Bradford West Yorkshire BD1 2JB/England.

DFG-Farbstoff-Kommission (DFG Dyestuffs Commission), Cosmetic Colorants, 3rd completely revised edition, VCH Weinheim 1991.

Hendry, GAF and Houghton, JD: Natural Food Colorants; Blackie, Glasgow and London 1992.

Lehmann, G, et al.: Identifizierung von Farbstoffen in Hautcremes (Identifying Colorants in Skin Creams); Seifen-Ole-Fette-Wachse, Nr. (Soaps-Oils-Fats-Waxes No.) 16/1986, 565.

Lehmann, G, Binkle, B: Identifizierung von Farbpigmenten in kosmetischen Erzeugnissen (Identifying Color Pigments in Cosmetic Products); Seifen-Ole-Fette-Wachse, Nr. (Soaps-Oils-Fats-Waxes No.) 5/1984, 125.

Loscher, M: Farben—visualisierte Gefühle (Colors—Visualized Feelings); DRAGOCO Report 4/5—1981.

Marmion, DM: Handbook of U.S. Colorants for Foods, Drugs and Cosmetics, Second Edition 1984, ISBN 0–471–09312–2.

Moschl, G, et al.: Perlglanzpigmente für Kosmetika (Pearlescent Pigments for Cosmetics); Seifen-Ole-Fette-Wachse, Nr. (Soaps-Oils-Fats-Waxes No.) 8/1980, 207.

Otterstätter, G: Die Färbung von Lebensmitteln, Arzneimitteln, Kosmetika (Coloring Foods, Drugs, Cosmetics); 2nd revised edition, Behr's Verlag, Hamburg 1995.

Schweppe, H: Handbuch der Naturfarbstoffe—Vorkommen, Verwendung, Nachweis. (Handbook of Natural Colorants—Their Presence, Use and Verification), Landsberg/Lech: Ecomed 1992.

29

Hair Conditioners

Charles Reich and Dean T. Su
Colgate-Palmolive Technology Center, Piscataway, New Jersey

INTRODUCTION

Despite myriad claimed benefits, the primary purpose of a hair conditioner is to reduce the magnitude of the forces associated with combing or brushing hair [1], especially when wet [2,3]. This is generally accomplished by the deposition of conditioning agents that lubricate the hair fiber, diminishing surface friction and, therefore, combing forces [4].

In general, deposition of a conditioning agent also causes the hair to feel softer and more moisturized. Another secondary benefit is the reduction or prevention of flyaway hair [5], especially by cationic conditioners [6]. Increasing ease of combing also makes the hair more manageable, while improving the ability to align the hair fibers in a more parallel configuration can increase hair shine, even if the shine of individual fibers is not increased [7].

A number of other benefits have sometimes been claimed or implied for conditioners including, e.g., repair of damaged hair, strengthening of hair, repair of split ends, and vitamin therapy. Most of these are marketing hype or are based on laboratory conditions or concentrations not found under actual usage conditions. In this chapter, we will confine ourselves to a discussion of only the observable conditioner benefits presented above. The chapter will begin with a discussion of the relationship between hair damage, conditioning and the state of the hair surface. This will be followed by a discussion of the major classes of conditioning agents currently in use. Finally, we will end with a brief discussion of the auxiliary ingredients necessary for the production of a commercial conditioning product.

CONDITIONING AND THE HAIR FIBER SURFACE

Hair Damage

In previous chapters, it has been shown that hair fibers consist of a central cortex that comprises the major portion of the fiber, surrounded by 8 to 10 layers of overlapping cells termed the cuticle. The cortex is responsible for the tensile properties of the hair [8,9], while the state of the cuticle affects a variety of consumer perceivable properties including, e.g., hair feel, shine, and combability.

A major function of conditioners is to protect the hair's structural elements, especially the cuticle, from grooming damage. This type of stress, characterized by chipping, fragmenting, and wearing away of cuticle cells, is probably the single most important source of damage to the hair surface [10–12].

A rather extreme example of combing damage can be seen in Figure 1, which shows the results of an experiment in which a tress of virgin hair was washed with a cleaning shampoo and then combed 700 times while wet. Since hair is more fragile when wet [3] and combing forces are higher [2], combing under these conditions insures maximum damage. It can be seen that damage to the cuticle was extensive with many cuticle cells lifted from the surface, while others were completely torn away by the combing process.

The ability of conditioning agents to protect the hair from this type of damage can be seen in Figure 2, which shows the results of an experiment in which a tress was washed with a high-conditioning "2-in-1" shampoo and then combed 700 times while wet. In this case, because the conditioning agents in the shampoo reduced combing forces, the hair surface is seen to be intact with evidence of only minor chipping and fragmenting of cuticle cells. This demonstrates the important role conditioners can play in maintaining the integrity of the hair fiber.

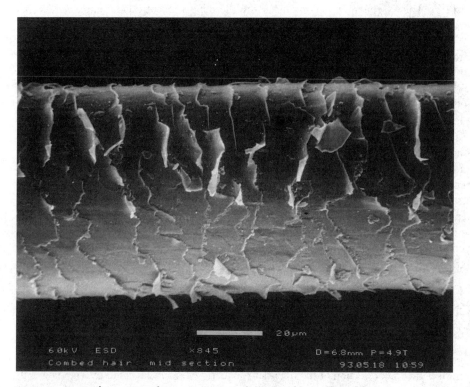

Figure 1 Typical scanning electron micrograph (SEM) of hair taken from a tress washed with a cleaning shampoo and then combed 700 times while wet. Note raised and chipped cuticle cells, and areas where cells have been completely torn away.

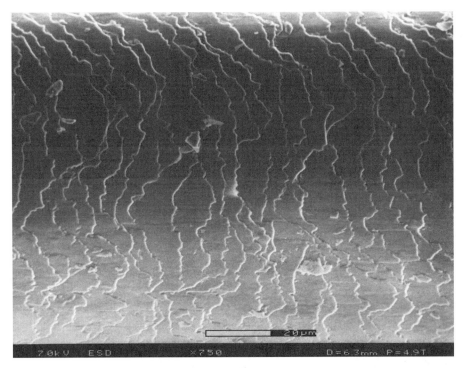

FIGURE 2 Typical SEM photo of hair taken from a tress washed with a high-conditioning 2-in-1 shampoo and then combed 700 times while wet. Note the minimal damage compared with Figure 1.

Hair Damage and the Cuticle Surface

The susceptibility of a hair fiber to grooming damage and the type of conditioner most effective in preventing this damage is affected to a large degree by the nature and state of the hair surface. It is therefore helpful to precede a discussion of conditioning agents with a presentation on the hair surface and how it affects conditioner requirements and deposition.

Virgin Hair Surfaces

Hair that has not been chemically treated is termed virgin hair. The cuticle surface of virgin hair in good condition is hydrophobic [13,14], in large part as a result of a layer of fatty acids covalently bound to the outermost surface of the cuticle (epicuticle) [15,16]. As a result of its protein structure, however, the hair surface has an isoelectric point near 3.67 [17], which insures that the surface will contain negatively charged hydrophilic sites at the ordinary pH levels of haircare products. This mix of hydrophobicity and hydrophilicity affects, of course, the types of conditioning agents that will bind to the virgin hair surface.

The situation is further complicated by the fact that the negative charge density on virgin hair increases from root to tip. This is primarily a result of oxidation of cystine in the hair to cystine S-sulfonate and cysteic acid as a result of exposure to UV radiation in sunlight [18,19]. The tip portions of the hair, being older than the root portions, will have been exposed to damaging [10] UV radiation for a longer period of time and will therefore be more hydrophilic, again affecting the nature of species that can bind to these sites.

In addition to greater UV damage, the tips of hair are also subject to greater combing damage. One reason for this is simply that, being older, the tip portions will have been exposed to more combing. In addition, the surface friction of hair tips is higher (C. Reich, unpublished data) so that combing forces increase as one moves from root to tip. Finally, the ends of hair are subject to unusually high combing stress as a result of entangling during the combing process [2]. This eventually results in destruction of the covalently bound lipid layer and a feeling of dryness at the tips. Because of this, the tip ends of hair require more conditioning than the rest of the fiber. Without sufficient conditioning, the cuticle layer is eventually lost, resulting in a split end. An example is seen in Figure 3, which clearly shows the exposed cortical cells.

Chemically Treated Hair Surfaces

Chemical treatments, perming, bleaching, and permanent dyeing, can all cause significant damage to the hair fiber [3,10,20–22]. In addition to causing tensile damage, all of these treatments, which include oxidative steps, modify the surface of the hair, introducing negative charges as a result of oxidation of cystine to cysteic acid [3,10,20,21,23]. This can result in transformation of the entire fiber surface from a hydrophobic to a hydrophilic character.

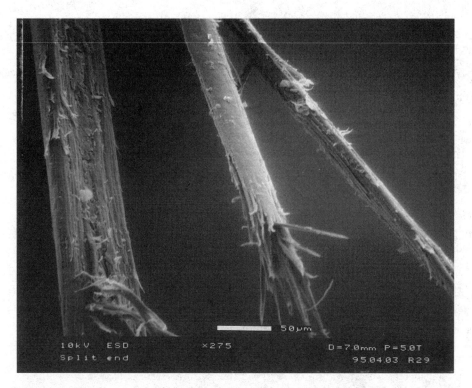

FIGURE 3   SEM photograph of a split end. Note the exposed cortex and the complete loss of cuticle cells on the fiber surface.

All of these treatments also increase surface friction considerably [3,4,24,25] resulting in a significant increase in combing forces. The result is hair that feels rough and dry and is subject to extensive grooming damage. Because of this, treated hair generally requires significantly more conditioning than does virgin hair.

COMMERCIAL CONDITIONERS

The commercial hair conditioners produced to deal with the aforementioned problems have appeared in almost every conceivable form, including thick vaseline pomades; thick, clear, water-soluble gels; spray mists of volatile substances; mousses; lotions; and creams. Conditioners have been marketed as leave-in or rinse-off products. They have also been positioned as pre-shampoo or post-shampoo formulations.

Despite the wide variety of forms available, most commercial conditioners are oil-in-water emulsions in lotion form, having viscosities somewhere between 3000 and 12,000 centipoise. The great majority of these products are of the rinse-off type. In addition, despite different forms and positionings, most commercial conditioners contain the same general classes of conditioning agents with differences mainly in concentrations, numbers of different agents, and the particular members of a conditioning class employed.

The major classes of conditioning agents used in commercial products are surveyed in the following sections.

Cationic Surfactants

Cationic surfactants, in the form of quaternary ammonium compounds, are the most widely used conditioning agents in commercial products [26–28]. Among the reasons for this are their effectiveness, versatility, availability, and low cost.

Important examples of these quats include stearalkonium chloride, cetrimonium chloride, and dicetyldimonium chloride.

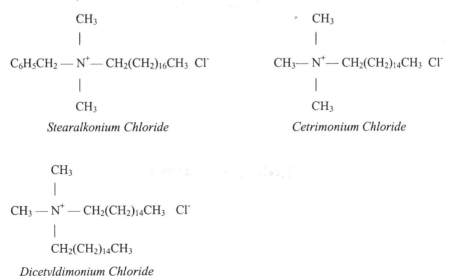

Because of the positive charge on quaternary ammonium compounds such as the above, they are substantive to hair, binding to negative sites on the hair surface. Treatment with these quats, therefore, results in a hydrophobic coating on the fiber that renders the hair softer and easier to comb [29]. Build-up of static charge (flyaway) is also greatly reduced as a result of this surface modification [6].

Another consequence of the positive charge on quats is that deposition increases with increasing negative charge on the hair surface. This is seen in Table 1, which shows the results of an experiment in which hair tresses were treated with 1% stearalkonium chloride and then rinsed. Compared with the roots, 22% more quat was found to bind to the tips of virgin hair, while deposition of stearalkonium chloride on bleached hair was found to be more than twice that on untreated fibers.

This result is important because, as previously discussed, damaged portions of the hair, which generally carry a greater amount of negative charge, require a greater amount of conditioning. The fact that cationic surfactants can supply this increased conditioning, makes them effective on a wide variety of hair surfaces. This is a major factor in the widespread use of these types of conditioning agents.

Conditioner Properties and Hydrophobicity

Many important properties of quaternary ammonium conditioners are related to the degree of hydrophobicity of the lipophilic portion of the surfactant. Thus, increasing the length of the alkyl chain of a monoalkyl quat, and therefore making it more hydrophobic, leads to increased deposition [31–36] on hair. Cetrimonium chloride, as a result, deposits on hair to a greater extent than does laurtrimonium chloride. Increasing the number of alkyl chains also increases deposition, so that tricetylmonium chloride exhibits greater deposition than does dicetyldimonium chloride, which, in turn, is more substantive than the monocetyl quat.

This dependence of deposition on degree of hydrophobicity indicates that van der Waals forces play an important role in deposition of quaternary ammonium conditioners [36]. This conclusion is consistent with the entropy-driven deposition demonstrated by Ohbu et al. [37] and Stapleton [38] for a monoalkyl quat and a protonated long-chain amine.

Increased hydrophobicity also correlates with increased conditioning by quaternary ammonium compounds [31–34,39]. Thus, cetrimonium chloride provides light to medium conditioning, while dicetyldimonium and tricetylmonium chlorides provide heavier conditioning. Detangling and wet combing, in particular, improve significantly from monocetyl to dicetyl to tricetyl quats; differences in dry combing and static charge among these compounds are not as significant.

Increased conditioning with increased hydrophobicity is probably due, in part, simply to increased deposition of quat on hair. Data from Garcia and Diaz [40], however, indicate greater improvements in wet combing from heavier conditioning quats even when present on the hair in much lower amounts than less hydrophobic species. The degree of

TABLE 1   Binding of Stearalkonium Chloride to Human Hair

Type of hair	Quat deposition at roots (mg/g hair)	Quat deposition at tips (mg/g hair)
Virgin hair	0.649	0.789
Bleached hair	1.62	1.83

Source: Ref. 30.

hydrophobicity of a quat must therefore play a direct role in the conditioning efficacy of these compounds [29].

Note that on some types of hair, the greater substantivity of higher conditioning quats can lead to build-up and result in limp, unmanageable hair with repeated use. This is especially true, e.g., for untreated, fine hair. Different quats, or mixtures of conditioning agents, are therefore suitable for different uses or different types of hair. A tricetyl quat might be used, e.g., in an intensive conditioner meant only for occasional use.

The length and number of alkyl chains of quats also determines water solubility of these compounds. Monoalkyl quaternaries up to cetrimonium chloride are water soluble, e.g., distearyldimonium chloride is water dispersible, while tricetylmonium chloride is insoluble in water [34].

Compatibility with Anionics

The quaternium compounds normally used in commercial conditioners are not generally found in shampoos because of incompatibility with common anionic detergents [41]. Introducing hydrophilic groups into the quat can increase compatibility with anionics. An example is the class of ethoxylated quaternaries, termed ethoquats. Typical members of this class are PEG-2 cocomonium chloride, where x + y equals 2 and R is a C12 alkyl chain, and PEG-15 stearmonium chloride where x + y equals 15 and R is a C18 chain.

$$(CH_2\ CH_2O)_xH$$

$$|$$

$$R—N^+—CH_3 \qquad\qquad Cl^-$$

$$|$$

$$(CH_2\ CH_2O)_yH$$

Ethoxylated Quaternary

Both of these quats are compatible with typical anionic detergents. As would be expected from this discussion, however, introducing hydrophilic groups decreases the conditioning efficacy of these materials [31,34]. They are therefore suitable only in light-conditioning formulations. Furthermore, conditioning shampoos based on ethoquats would not be expected to be very effective as a result of low deposition of the detergent-soluble ethoquat complex.

Other detergent-soluble quats have been produced. These include alkylamidopropyl dihydroxypropyl dimonium chlorides [42], lauryl methyl gluceth-10 hydroxypropyl dimonium chloride [43], and even a hydrolyzed ginseng-saponin quaternary derived from Korean ginseng saponin [44]. Although certain advantages have been claimed for these surfactants, particularly low irritation, they all suffer from much the same conditioning limitations as the ethoquats.

Other Cationic Surfactants

In addition to the aforementioned examples, numerous other cationic surfactants are in use or have been proposed for commercial products. One example of a compound that has been receiving increasing use recently is the behentrimonium (C22) quat. This quat exhibits significantly reduced eye and skin irritation compared with the corresponding C18 conditioner. In addition, superior conditioning and thickening properties have been claimed [45].

Another interesting example is hydrogenated tallow octyl dimonium chloride [46]. This material is quite substantive and provides high conditioning as a result of its two hydrophobic chains. Unlike conventional dialkyl quats, however, this particular conditioner is soluble in water as a result of branching (2-ethylhexyl) in the octyl moiety. This makes the compound much easier to formulate into a commercial product.

Stearamidopropyl dimethylamine is another conditioning agent that is found in many commercial conditioners. This material is cationic at the pHs normally used in conditioning products and therefore acts as a cationic emulsifier and, also, as a secondary conditioning agent.

Concern for the environment has led to the synthesis of ester quats that exhibit increased biodegradability and environmental safety. One such example is dipalmitoylethyl hydroxyethylmonium methosulfate, an ester quat based on a partially hydrogenated palm radical [47].

Other cationic surfactants used in conditioners include quats derived from Guerbet alcohols [39] (low to high conditioning depending on length of the main and side alkyl chains), distearyldimonium chloride (high conditioning), and the quaternized ammonium compounds of hydrolyzed milk protein, soy and wheat protein, and hydrolyzed keratin (varying conditioning efficacy depending on alkyl chain length).

Lipophilic Conditioners

Quaternary ammonium surfactants in commercial products are almost never used alone. Instead they are used in combination with long-chain fatty conditioners, especially cetyl and stearyl alcohols [28]. These fatty materials are added to boost the conditioning effects of the quaternary compounds [43]. In one study, e.g., addition of cetyl alcohol to cetrimonium bromide nearly doubled the observed reduction in wet combing forces on hair [48]. In another study, using a novel hydrodynamic technique, Fukuchi et al. [49] found that the addition of cetyl alcohol to a behentrimonium chloride formulation resulted in significantly reduced surface friction.

Several investigators have studied combinations of cationic surfactants and fatty alcohols. Under the right conditions, these mixtures have been found to form liquid crystal mesophases and gel networks [50–54] that can greatly increase viscosity and, at the same time, confer stability upon emulsions. As a result of reduced repulsion between cationic head groups when long chain alcohols are interposed, liquid crystal formation has been observed even at low concentrations [53,54]. The ready formation of these extended structures between quats and cetyl and stearyl alcohols, along with the low cost, stability, and compatibility with cosmetic ingredients of the latter are important reasons why these alcohols are so ubiquitous in conditioning formulations.

Other lipids found in commercial products include, e.g., glycol distearate, triglycerides, fatty esters, waxes of triglycerides, and liquid paraffin.

Cationic Polymers   *Poly quats*

There are numerous cationic polymers that provide conditioning benefits, especially improved wet combing and reduced static charge. Important examples of these polymers are Polyquaternium-10, a quaternized hydroxyethylcellulose polymer; Polyquaternium-7, a copolymer of diallyldimethylammonium chloride and acrylamide; Polyquaternium-11, a copolymer of vinylpyrrolidone and dimethylaminoethyl methacrylate quaternized with dimethyl sulfate; Polyquaternium-16, a copolymer of vinylpyrrolidone and quaternized vinylimidazole; and Polyquaternium-6, a homopolymer of diallyldimethylammonium chloride.

By virtue of their cationic nature, these polymers are substantive to hair. The particular conditioning effectiveness of any of these materials depends on the polymer structure. In one set of studies, deposition on hair was found to be inversely proportional, roughly, to cationic charge density [55,56]. This has been explained by the observation that the higher the charge density, the lower the weight of polymer needed to neutralize all of the negative charge on the hair. Once deposited, however, multiple points of electrostatic attachment makes these polymers harder to remove, especially if charge density is high [30,57]. Care must be taken, therefore, in formulating conditioners containing these materials to avoid overconditioning as a result of build-up with continued use.

As with the preceding monofunctional cationics, deposition of polyquaterniums increases on treated, or damaged, hair [30,57,58]. Unlike common monofunctional quats, however, the first four of these polymers are compatible, to varying degrees, with anionic surfactants [57–61]. As a result, they are used more often in shampoos than in stand-alone conditioners, although they find some use in leave-in conditioners.

Polyquaternium-10 (PQ-10) and Polyquaternium-7 (PQ-7) are two of the most frequently used polymers in commercial shampoos. Both of these polymers form negatively charged complexes [57,59] with excess anionic surfactant, resulting in reduced deposition because of repulsion by the negatively charged hair surface. The magnitude of this effect depends on the particular anionic used, and on the anionic surfactant/polymer ratio. In all cases, however, conditioning from shampoos is significantly less than from stand-alone conditioners.

Despite reduced deposition, Hannah [62] has reported that polyquaternium association complexes formed with SLS resist removal from hair. Build-up and a heavy, coated feel on the hair can therefore result from conditioning shampoos containing polyquats unless they are carefully formulated.

Silicones

The use of silicones in haircare products has increased considerably in the past two decades, although their first incorporation into commercial products dates back to the 1950s. Different types of silicones find use as conditioning agents in a wide variety of products, including conditioners, shampoos, hair sprays, mousses, and gels [63]. One of the most widely used silicones is dimethicone, which is a polydimethylsiloxane. Other important silicones are dimethiconol, which is a dimethylsiloxane terminated with hydroxyl groups, and amodimethicone, which is an amino-substituted silicone.

$$CH_3 - SiO - (SiO)_x - Si - CH_3$$

Dimethicone

$$
\begin{array}{ccccc}
& CH_3 & CH_3 & CH_3 & \\
& | & | & | & \\
HO\!-\!SiO\!-\!&(SiO)_x&\!-\!&(SiO)_y&\!-\!H \\
& | & | & | & \\
& CH_3 & CH_3 & (CH_2)_3 & \\
& & & | & \\
& & & NHCH_2CH_2NH_2 &
\end{array}
$$

Amodimethicone

Most silicones used in haircare products, including those previously mentioned, are insoluble and must therefore be emulsified. To increase ease of product manufacture, many suppliers offer silicones as preformed emulsions, in addition to the pure material. The factors affecting deposition of silicones from such emulsions have been reported by Jachowicz and Berthiaume [64,65].

Conditioning Properties of Silicones

Silicones used in haircare products possess a range of unique properties including lubricity, low intermolecular forces, water insolubility, and low surface tension. These properties permit the silicones to spread easily on the hair surface, forming a hydrophobic film that provides ease of combing, and imparts a smooth, soft feel to the hair without greasiness.

The relative conditioning efficacy of silicones compared to other conditioners was demonstrated by Yahagi [66], who found that dimethicone lowered frictional coefficients and surface energy of virgin hair to a greater extent than did a series of cationic surfactants, including distearyldimonium chloride, a very effective conditioning agent. Dimethicones with molecular weights greater than 20,000 were found to be most effective in reducing surface tension.

Nanavati and Hami [67] measured conditioning on slightly bleached European hair treated with dimethicone fluids and dimethiconol gums. Both types of silicones were found to significantly reduce combing forces on hair. Ease of wet combing was roughly the same for the two silicone treatments, while dimethiconol was found to be more effective in reducing dry combing forces.

Interestingly, under the treatment conditions used (exposure to silicone solutions for 30 sec followed by drying without rinsing), deposition of all silicones studied was found to nearly double if tricetyldimonium chloride was present in the treatment solution. Reduction in combing forces was also doubled, roughly, when silicones were deposited in the presence of quat. This latter effect was found to be synergistic, i.e., it depended on deposition of both silicone and quat, and its magnitude was greater than the sum of the individual conditioner contributions.

Wendel et al. [68] used electron spectroscopy for chemical analysis (ESCA) to demonstrate that the presence of amino groups in silicones considerably increases substantivity of these materials. This is a result of the positive charge developed by these groups at the pHs commonly found in commercial products.

Comparison of conditioning effects of a series of silicone emulsions on bleached and virgin hair was carried out by Hoag et al. [69]. Most of the silicones were dimethicones or amodimethicones, while emulsions were anionic, neutral, or cationic in nature. Diluted emulsions were applied directly to the hair and combing forces measured both before and after rinsing. Prior to rinsing, reduction of combing forces by most emulsions was greater than 80%. This number was decreased after rinsing as a result of partial removal of deposited silicone. Unsurprisingly, the least change in ease of combing was found for cationic emulsions, especially those containing amodimethicone. Combing forces on virgin hair increased less than on bleached hair after rinsing, indicating that the silicones were more substantive to this type of hair. This is also unsurprising considering the hydrophobic nature of these conditioning agents.

Further effects of amodimethicones can be seen in work reported by Berthiaume et al. [70], who studied a series of amodimethicone emulsions in a prototype conditioner formulation. Deposition on hair from the conditioner was found to increase with increasing amine content in the silicone. This increased deposition was found, in half-head tests, to correlate with conditioning efficacy, including wet and dry combing, softness, and detangling. A microemulsion in the test series that provided high conditioning was also shown to significantly reduce the color fading caused by shampooing of temporarily dyed hair.

Other Silicones

Two important silicones not covered in the preceding section are dimethicone copolyol, which is a dimethylsiloxane containing polyoxyethylene and/or propylene side chains, and cyclomethicone, which refers to a class of cyclic dimethyl polysiloxanes ranging from trimer to hexamer. The most commonly used variant is the pentamer.

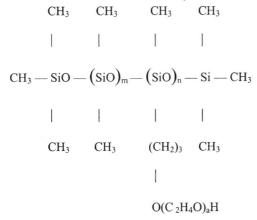

Dimethicone Copolyol

Most commercial dimethicone copolyols are soluble in water and are therefore not very effective in rinse-off products. These silicones find important application, however, in leave-on products, including hair sprays, styling mousses, and gels.

Cyclomethicone is volatile and would not remain on dry hair, especially after blow-drying. It helps other conditioning agents disperse, however, and form films on hair. It also helps improve wet combing and provides transient shine.

2-in-1 Shampoos

Silicones find important application as the primary conditioning agents in 2-in-1 conditioning shampoos. These shampoos, upon their introduction in the latter part of the 1980s, represented a major advance in haircare technology, providing a significantly higher degree of conditioning than was then the norm for conditioning shampoos and, at the same time, leaving a desirable, soft, smooth feel on the hair.

Conditioning from 2-in-1 shampoos is expected to occur primarily at the rinsing stage during which time the shampoo emulsion breaks, releasing the silicone for deposition on hair. This separation of cleaning and conditioning stages permits the shampoo to perform both functions efficiently.

The conditioning agent used most frequently in 2-in-1 shampoos is dimethicone. This silicone can provide good performance in shampoo formulations without building-up excessively on the hair [71]. The level of conditioning from these types of shampoos is lower than that from stand-alone conditioners. This is especially true for treated hair because the greater the degree of negative charge on the hair surface, the lower the substantivity of a hydrophobic material like dimethicone. Many 2-in-1s contain polyquats, which might be expected to increase conditioning on damaged hair. In shampoos with high levels of anionic detergent, however, polyquat performance on treated hair may be no better than dimethicone as a result of formation of the negatively charged polymer complexes discussed in the section on cationic polymers (see p. 338).

Yahagi [66] studied the performance of dimethicone, amodimethicone, and dimethicone copolyols in 2-in-1 shampoos. Ease of combing was found to be similar on hair treated with shampoos containing dimethicone or amodimethicone. Unsurprisingly, soluble dimethicone copolyols did not perform well; insolubility, or at least dispersibility, was required for adequate silicone deposition. In the latter case, dimethicone copolyols were found to provide a somewhat lower level of conditioning than the other two silicones studied, especially once blowdrying was begun. Yahagi also studied silicone effects on foam volume. In these studies dimethicone was found to significantly reduce foam volume in a model shampoo formulation, while amodimethicone and dimethicone copolyol had a minimal effect on foam.

Auxiliary Ingredients

A number of ingredients besides conditioning actives are added to commercial conditioners for functional, aesthetic, and marketing purposes [72]. These include fragrances, dyes, preservatives, thickeners, emulsifying agents, pearlizers, herbal extracts, humectants, and vitamins. Some of these are discussed in the following sections; the literature also contains many examples [28,73–77].

Preservatives

Preservatives are necessary to insure the microbiological integrity of a conditioning product. If the product contains high concentrations of ethyl alcohol (generally 20% or above), additional preservatives are not needed and the product is described as self-preserving.

For other products, a wide variety of preservatives are available; in general, combinations of different preservatives provide the broadest possible protection. Every commercial product that is not self-preserving must be carefully tested over time for adequacy of preservation. Most of the preservatives used in personal-care products are described in the Cosmetic Preservatives Encyclopedia [75].

Thickeners

The section on lipophilic conditioners described thickening as a result of liquid crystal formation in those products containing common quaternary ammonium compounds and fatty alcohols. Cationic conditioning polymers (see p. 338) can also act as thickeners. Many formulations may require additional thickening agents. Hydroxyethylcellulose, a nonionic cellulose ether compatible with cationic surfactants and stable over a wide pH range, is the most common thickening agent added to conditioning products [28]. In addition to providing increased viscosity, this material stabilizes viscosity over time.

Polyamides may also be used to thicken formulations. A commercial product, Sepigel, which contains polyamide, laureth-7, and isoparaffin, can be used to emulsify and thicken lotion or cream conditioners. Other thickeners are described in Ref. 76.

Humectants

Many conditioners contain humectants, which are used to attract moisture. Examples are propylene glycol, glycerine, honey, chitosan, and hyaluronic acid. These materials are not expected to be very effective in rinse-off products.

Emulsifiers

As previously discussed, the fatty alcohol, quat combinations found in common conditioners confer stability on product emulsions. If necessary, other emulsifiers may be added to improve stability. Information on emulsions and emulsifiers may be found in the literature [77,78], as well as from manufacturers' technical bulletins. Most emulsifiers used in conditioners are nonionic, including ethoxylated fatty alcohols, ethoxylated fatty esters, and ethoxylated sorbitan fatty esters.

CONCLUSION

The foregoing sections have surveyed the action and properties of a diverse assortment of commercially available conditioning agents. The availability of a large selection of conditioning materials enables the formulator to tailor products for a wide variety of people having differing conditioning needs and preferences. Thus, a person having short, straight hair in good condition might desire a conditioner primarily to control fly-away. Such a need could be satisfied by one of the ethoquats, which provide light-conditioning benefits together with very good static control. A person having long, heavily bleached hair, on the other hand, would require improved hair feel, ease-of-combing, and manageability. These benefits could best be provided by a trialkyl quat.

Those people sensitive to the feel of their hair might prefer a product containing a silicone as a secondary conditioner. Other people might prefer the convenience of a 2-in-1 shampoo. In many cases, both 2-in-1 shampoos and stand-alone conditioners are used to condition the hair.

There are a number of ways in which one might satisfy the conditioning needs of a target population. It is anticipated that the information in this chapter will help the formulator to quickly choose the best conditioning system for a given purpose. It is also hoped that the material in this chapter will help the formulator to effectively evaluate new conditioning agents and even to work with synthetic chemists as well as suppliers to design new conditioning compounds to solve particular problems.

REFERENCES

1. Robbins CR. Chemical and Physical Behavior of Human Hair. 3d ed. New York: Springer-Verlag, 1994:343.
2. Kamath YK, Weigmann HD. Measurement of combing forces. J Soc Cosmet Chem 1986; 37:111–124.
3. Jachowicz J. Hair damage and attempts to its repair. J Soc Cosmet Chem 1987; 38:263–286.
4. Scott GV, Robbins CR. Effects of surfactant solutions on hair fiber friction. J Soc Cosmet Chem 1980; 31:179–200.
5. Lunn AC, Evans RE. The electrostatic properties of human hair. J Soc Cosmet Chem 1977; 28:549–569.
6. Jachowicz J, Wis-Surel G, Garcia ML. Relationship between triboelectric charging and surface modifications of human hair. J Soc Cosmet Chem 1985; 36:189–212.
7. Reich C, Robbins CR. Interactions of cationic and anionic surfactants on hair surfaces: light-scattering and radiotracer studies. J Soc Cosmet Chem 1993; 44:263–278.
8. Robbins CR, Crawford RJ. Cuticle damage and the tensile properties of human hair. J Soc Cosmet Chem 1991; 42:59.
9. Robbins CR. Chemical and Physical Behavior of Human Hair. 3d ed. New York: Springer-Verlag, 1994:301.
10. Tate ML, Kamath YK, Ruetsch SB, Weigmann HD. Quantification and prevention of hair damage. J Soc Cosmet Chem 1993; 44:347–371.
11. Garcia ML, Epps JA, Yare RS. Normal cuticle-wear pattern in human hair. J Soc Cosmet Chem 1978; 29:155–175.
12. Kelley S, Robinson VNE. The effect of grooming on the hair surface. J Soc Cosmet Chem 1982; 33:203–215.
13. Kamath YK, Danziger CJ, Weigmann HD. Surface wettability of human hair. I. Effect of deposition of polymers and surfactants. J Appl Polym Sci 1984; 29:1011–1026.
14. Wolfram LJ, Lindemann MKO. Some observations on the hair cuticle. J Soc Cosmet Chem 1971; 22:839–850.
15. Negri AP, Cornell HJ, Rivett DE. A model for the surface of keratin fibers. Text Res J 1993; 63:109–115.
16. Shao J, Jones DC, Mitchell R, Vickerman JC, Carr CM. Time-of-flight secondary-ion-mass spectrometric (ToF-SIMS) and x-ray photoelectron spectroscopic (XPS) analyses of the surface lipids of wool. J Text Inst 1997; 88:317–324.
17. Wilkerson VJ. The chemistry of human epidermis. II. The isoelectric points of the stratum corneum, hair, and nails as determined by electrophoresis. J Biol Chem 1935–1936; 112:329–335.
18. Robbins CR, Bahl MK. Analysis of hair by electron spectroscopy for chemical analysis. J Soc Cosmet Chem 1984; 35:379–390.
19. Stranick MA. Determination of negative binding sites on hair surfaces using XPS and Ba^{2+} labeling. Surface Interface Anal 1996; 24:522–528.
20. Horiuchi T. Nature of damaged hair. Cosmet Toilet 1978; 93:65–77.
21. Kaplin IJ, Schwann A, Zahn H. Effects of cosmetic treatments on the ultrastructure of hair. Cosmet Toilet 1982; 97:22–26.
22. Sandhu SS, Ramachandran R, Robbins CR. A simple and sensitive method using protein loss measurements to evaluate damage to human hair during combing. J Soc Cosmet Chem 1995; 46:39–52.
23. Robbins CR. Chemical and Physical Behavior of Human Hair. 3d ed. New York: Springer-Verlag, 1994:120–126, 234–249.
24. Schwartz A, Knowles D. Frictional effects in human hair. J Soc Cosmet Chem 1963; 14:455–463.
25. Robbins CR. Chemical and Physical Behavior of Human Hair. 3rd ed. New York: Springer-Verlag, 1994:341.

26. Quack JM. Quaternary ammonium compounds in cosmetics. Cosmet Toilet 1976; 91(2):35–52.

27. Gerstein T. An introduction to quaternary ammonium compounds. Cosmet Toilet 1979; 94(11):32–41.

28. Hunting ALL. Encyclopedia of Conditioning Rinse Ingredients. Cranford, NJ: Micelle Press, 1987.

29. Foerster T, Schwuger MJ. Correlation between adsorption and the effects of surfactants and polymers on hair. Progr Colloid Polym Sci 1990; 83:104–109.

30. Reich C. Hair cleansers. In: Rieger MM, Rhein LD, eds. Surfactants in Cosmetics. 2d ed. Surfactant Science Series, Vol. 68. New York: Marcel Dekker, 1997:373.

31. Jurczyk MF, Berger DR, Damaso GR. Quaternary ammonium salt. Applications in hair conditioners. Cosmet Toilet 1991; 106:63–68.

32. Finkelstein P, Laden K. The mechanism of conditioning of hair with alkyl quaternary ammonium compounds. Appl Poly Symp 1971; 18:673–680.

33. Jachowicz J. Fingerprinting of cosmetic formulations by dynamic electrokinetic and permeability analysis. II. Hair conditioners. J Soc Cosmet Chem 1995; 46:100–116.

34. Spiess E. The influence of chemical structure on performance in hair care preparations. Parfumerie and Kosmetik 1991; 72(6):370–374.

35. Scott GV, Robbins CR, Barnhurst JD. Sorption of quaternary ammonium surfactants by human hair. J Soc Cosmet Chem 1969; 20:135–152.

36. Robbins CR, Reich C, Patel A. Adsorption to keratin surfaces: a continuum between a charge-driven and a hydrophobically driven process. J Soc Cosmet Chem 1994; 45:85–94.

37. Ohbu K, Tamura T, Mizushima N, Fukuda M. Binding characteristics of ionic surfactants with human hair. Colloid Polym Sci 1986; 264:798–802.

38. Stapleton IW. The adsorption of long chain amines and diamines or keratin fibers. J Soc Cosmet Chem 1983; 34:285–300.

39. Yahagi K, Hoshino N, Hirota H. Solution behavior of new cationic surfactants derived from Guerbet alcohols and their use in hair conditioners. Int J Cosmet Sci 1991; 13:221–234.

40. Garcia ML, Diaz J. Combability measurements on human hair. J Soc Cosmet Chem 1976; 27:379–398.

41. Fox C. An introduction to the formulation of shampoos. Cosmet Toilet 1988; 103(3):25–58.

42. Smith L, Gesslein BW. Multi-functional cationics for hair and skin applications. Cosmet Toilet 1989; 104:41–47.

43. Polovsky SB. An alkoxylated methyl glucoside quaternary. Cosmet Toilet 1991; 106:59–65.

44. Kim YD, Kim CK, Lee CN, Ha BJ. Hydrolysed ginseng-saponin quaternary: a novel conditioning agent for hair care products. Int J Cosmet Chem 1989; 11:203–220.

45. Gallagher KF. Superior conditioning and thickening from long-chain surfactants. Cosmet Toilet 1994; 109:67–74.

46. Jurczyk MF. A new quaternary conditioner for damaged hair. Cosmet Toilet 1991; 106:91–95.

47. Shapiro I, Sajic B, Bezdicek R. Environmentally friendly ester quats. Cosmet Toilet 1994; 109:77–80.

48. Hunting All. Encyclopedia of Conditioning Rinse Ingredients. Cranford, NJ: Micelle Press, 1987:147.

49. Fukuchi Y, Okoshi M, Murotani I. Estimation of shampoo and rinse effects on the resistance to flow over human hair and hair softness using a newly developed hydrodynamic technique. J Soc Cosmet Chem 1989; 40:251–263.

50. Eccleston GM, Florence AT. Application of emulsion theory to complex and real systems. Int J Cosmet Chem 1985; 7:195–212.

51. Eccleston GM. The structure and rheology of pharmaceutical and cosmetic creams. Cetrimide creams: the influence of alcohol chain length and homolog composition. J Colloid Int Sci 1976; 57:66–74.

52. Barry BW, Saunders GM. Kinetics of structure build-up in self-bodied emulsions stabilized by mixed emulsifiers. J Colloid Int Sci 1972; 41:331–342.

53. Barry BW, Saunders GM. The self-bodying action of the mixed emulsifier cetrimide/ceto-stearyl alcohol. J Colloid Int Sci 1970; 34:300–315.

54. Barry BW, Saunders GM. The influence of temperature on the rheology of systems containing alkyltrimethylammonium bromide/cetostearyl alcohol: variation with quaternary chain length. J Colloid Int Sci 1971; 36:130–138.

55. Hossel P, Pfrommer E. Test methods for hair conditioning polymers. In: In-Cosmet. Exhib. Conf. Conf. Proc. Augsburg, Germany: Verlag fuer Chemische Industrie. H. Ziolkowsky, 1994:133–148.

56. Pfau A, Hossel P, Vogt S, Sander R, Schrepp W. The interaction of cationic polymers with human hair. Macromol Symp 1997; 126:241–252.

57. Sykes AR, Hammes PA. The use of Merquat polymers is cosmetics. Drug Cosmet Ind 1980; February: 62–66.

58. Amerchol Corporation Technical Bulletin. Ucare polymers: conditioners for all conditions.

59. Faucher JA, Goddard ED. Influence of surfactants on the sorption of a cationic polymer by keratinous substrates. J Colloid Int Sci 1976; 55(2):313–319.

60. Goddard ED, Faucher JA, Scott RJ, Turney ME. Adsorption of polymer JR on keratinous surfaces—Part II. J Soc Cosmet Chem 1975; 26:539–550.

61. Caelles J, Cornelles F, Leal JS, Parra JL, Anguera S. Anionic and cationic compounds in mixed systems. Cosmet Toilet 1991; 106(4):49–54.

62. Hannah RB, Goddard ED, Faucher JA. Desorption of a cationic polymer from human hair: surfactant and salt effects. Text R J 1978; 48:57.

63. Luoma A, Kara R. Silicones and the perm question. Society of Cosmetic Chemists 1988 Spring Conference on Hair Care, London, UK, April 21–23, 1998.

64. Jachowicz J, Berthiaume MD. Heterocoagulation of silicon emulsions on keratin fibers. J Colloid Int Sci 1989; 133:118–134.

65. Berthiaume MD, Jachowicz J. The effect of emulsifiers on deposition of nonionic silicone oils from oil-in-water emulsions onto keratin fibers. J Colloid Int Sci 1991; 141:299–315.

66. Yahagi K. Silicones as conditioning agents in shampoos. J Soc Cosmet Chem 1992; 43:275–284.

67. Nanavati S, Hami A. A preliminary investigation of the interaction of a quat with silicones and its conditioning benefits on hair. J Soc Cosmet Chem 1994; 43:135–148.

68. Wendel SR, Disapio AJ. Organofunctional silicones for personal care applications. Cosmet Toilet 1983; 98:103–106.

69. Hoag CA, Rizwan BM, Quackenbush KM. Evaluating silicone emulsions for global hair care applications. Global Cosmet Ind 1999; April:44–55.

70. Berthiaume MD, Merrifield JH, Riccio DA. Effects of silicone pretreatment on oxidative hair damage. J Soc Cosmet Chem 1995; 46:231–245.

71. Rushton H, Gummer CL, Flasch H. 2-in-1 shampoo technology: state of the art shampoo and conditioner in one. Skin Pharmacol 1994; 7:78.

72. Hoshowski MA. Conditioning of hair. In: Johnson DH, ed. Hair and Hair Care. Cosmetic Science and Technology Series, Vol. 17. New York: Marcel Dekker, 1997:65–104.

73. Wenninger JA, McEwen GN, eds. CTFA Cosmetic Ingredients Handbook. 3d ed. Washington, DC: Cosmetic, Toiletry and Fragrance Association, 1995.

74. Leung AY. Encyclopedia of Common Natural Ingredients Used in Food, Drugs, and Cosmetics. New York: John Wiley & Sons, 1980.

75. Cosmetic Preservatives Encyclopedia-Antimicrobials. Cosmet Toilet 1990; 105(3):49–63.

76. Lochhead R. Encyclopedia of polymers and thickeners for cosmetics. Cosmet Toilet 1988; 103(12):99–129.

77. McCutcheon's Vol. 1: Emulsifiers and Detergents, North American Edition. Glen Rock, NJ: MC Publishing Co., 1991.

78. Becher P, ed. Encyclopedia of Emulsion Technology. New York: Marcel Dekker, 1985.

30

Hydrating Substances

Marie Lodén
ACO HUD AB, Upplands Väsby, Sweden

INTRODUCTION

Hydrating substances are used in cosmetic products to retard moisture loss from the product during use and to increase the moisture content in material in contact with the product. This function is generally performed by hygroscopic substances, or humectants. In the International Cosmetic Ingredient Dictionary 66 substances are listed as humectants and 76 hygroscopic materials are used to increase the water content of the skin [1]. The resulting effect of the substances depends on their inherent hygroscopicity at different humidity, as well as their volatility and penetration characteristics. Some factors to consider during product development are highlighted in Table 1.

Target body areas for treatment with humectants are dry hair and dry skin. Sometimes mucous membranes also benefit from application of humectants. Dry hair is brittle, rough, has a tendency to tangle, and has hardly any luster. Humidity of the atmosphere is the only source of moisture to hair, except shampooing, and addition of humectants to the hair will therefore facilitate its retention of water. The same is true for the skin, although it is constantly supplied with water from inside of the body. In the stratum corneum a special blend of humectants can be found, which is called natural moisturizing factor (NMF) [2]. NMF can make up about 10% of the dry weight of the stratum corneum cells [2]. Substances belonging to this group are amino acids, pyrrolidone carboxylic acid (PCA), lactates, and urea (Table 2) [2]. NMF is formed from the protein filaggrin and this formation is regulated by the moisture content in the stratum corneum (3). The water held by the hygroscopic substances in the stratum corneum is a controlling factor in maintaining skin flexibility and desquamation (Table 3) [3,4]. This chapter will provide basic information about some commonly used humectants, primarily used for treatment of the skin. Moreover, some safety information will be given.

BUTYLENE GLYCOL

Description

Butylene glycol is a viscous, colorless liquid with a sweet flavor and bitter aftertaste [5,6]. It is soluble in water, acetone, and castor oil, but practically insoluble in aliphatic hydrocarbon [5].

TABLE 1 Parameters to Consider During Product Development

Formulation related	Effect on the target area
Price and purity?	Product claim?
Chemical stability during production and shelf life?	Substantivity in rinse-off products?
Sensitive to heat? UV light? pH?	Penetration characteristics?
Incompatibilities with other ingredients?	Hygroscopicity?
Adsorption to the packaging material?	Adverse effects?
Effects on the preservation system?	

General Use

Butylene glycol is used as humectant for cellophane and tobacco [5]. It is also used in topical products and as solvents for injectable products [6]. Butylene glycol is claimed to be most resistant to high humidity and it is often used in hair sprays and setting lotions [7]. The alcohol also retards loss of aromas and preserves cosmetics against spoilage by micro-organisms [7].

Safety

Human skin patch test on undiluted butylene glycol produced a very low order of primary skin irritation and a repeated patch test produced no evidence of skin sensitization [8]. The substance is reported to be less irritating than propylene glycol [9,10]. Few reports of contact allergy exist, but the substance does not seem to cross-react with propylene glycol [9]. As presently used in cosmetics the alcohol is considered as safe by the Cosmetic Ingredient Review (CIR) Expert Panel [8].

GLYCERIN

Description

In 1779, the Swedish scientist, C. W. Scheele, discovered that glycerin could be made from a hydrolysate of olive oil. The alcohol is a clear, colorless, odorless, syrupy, and hygroscopic liquid [5], that is, about 0.6 times as sweet as cane sugar [5]. It is miscible with water and alcohol, slightly soluble in acetone, and practically insoluble in chloroform and ether.

General Use

Glycerin can be used as a solvent, plasticizer, sweetener, lubricant, and preservative [11]. The substance has also been given intravenously or by mouth in a variety of clinical conditions in order to benefit from its osmotic dehydrating properties [12]. This effect can also be used topically for the short-term reduction of vitreous volume an intraocular pressure of the eye [12]. Concentrated solutions of glycerin is also used to soften ear wax [13]. Suppositories with glycerin (1–3 g) can also promote fecal evacuation [12,13].

TABLE 2 Chemistry of Hygroscopic Substances

Name	CAS No.	MW	Other names	Natural source
Butylene glycol	107-88-0	90.1	1,3-butanediol, 1,3-butylene glycol	
Glycerin	56-81-5	92.1	Glycerol, 1,2,3-propanetriol	Hydrolysis of oils and fats
Lactic acid	50-21-5	90.1	2-hydroxypropanoic acid	Sour milk, tomato juice
Panthenol	81-13-0	205.3	Dexpanthenol, pantothenol	Plants, animals, bacteria
PCA	98-79-3	129.11	L-pyroglutamic acid, DL-pyrrolidonecarboxylic acid, 2-pyrroli-done-5-carboxylic acid	Vegetables, molasses
Propylene glycol	57-55-6	76.1	1,2-propanediol	
Sodium hyaluronate	9067-32-7	5×10^4–8×10^6		Cock's combs, biofermentation
Sorbitol	50-70-4	182.17	D-glucitol	Berries, fruits
Urea	57-13-6	60.08	Carbamide, carbonyl diamide	Urine

Abbreviations: MW, molecular weight; PCA, pyrrolidone carboxylic acid.
Source: Refs. 5, 6, 12.

TABLE 3 Moisture-Binding Ability of Humectants at Various Humidities

Humectant	31%	50%	52%	58–60%	76%	81%
Butylene glycol						38[e]
Dipropylene glycol		12[a]				
Glycerin	13[c]	25[a]	26[b]	35–38[c,f]	67[b]	
	11[b]					
Na-PCA	20[c]	44[a]	45[b]	61–63[c,f]	210[b]	
	17[b]					
Na-lactate	19[b]	56[a]	40[b]	66[f]	104[b]	
Panthenol	3[d]		11[d]		33[d]	
PCA	<1[c]			<1[c]		
Propylene glycol				32[f]		
Sorbitol		1[a]		10[f]		

Abbreviation: PCA, pyrrolidone carboxylic acid.
[a] *Source*: Ref. 28.
[b] *Source*: Ref. 72.
[c] *Source*: Ref. 40.
[d] *Source*: Ref. 35.
[e] *Source*: Ref. 5.
[f] *Source*: Ref. 73.

Effects on the Skin

The importance of glycerin in skincare products is well established. To explain its benefits, early studies have focused on its humectant and the protecting properties. More recently, glycerin has been shown to modulate the phase behavior of stratum corneum lipids and to prevent crystallization of their lamellar structures in vitro at low, relative humidity [14]. Incorporation of glycerin into a stratum corneum model lipid mixture enables the lipids to maintain the liquid crystal state at low humidity [14]. The biochemical consequences of these properties may be to influence the activity of hydrolytic enzymes crucial to the desquamatory process in vivo. Thereby, the rate of corneocyte loss from the superficial surface of human skin increases, probably because of an enhanced desmosome degradation [3].

Repeated tape strippings taken from skin treated with 15% glycerin cream indicates that glycerin diffuses into the stratum corneum to form a reservoir [15]. During some hours after application a decrease in TEWL has been noted [15–18], followed in animal skin by increased values after some hours [18]. Moreover, in human skin its surface profile, electrical impedance, and increase in the coefficient of friction were found to accompany an improvement in the skin condition, as assessed by an expert [16].

Safety

Very large oral or parenteral doses can exert systemic effects, due to the increase in the plasma osmolality resulting in the movement of water by osmosis from the extravascular spaces into the plasma [12]. Glycerin dropped on the human eye causes a strong stinging and burning sensation, with tearing and dilatation on the conjunctival vessels [19]. There is no obvious injury [19], but studies have indicated that glycerin can damage the endothelial cells of the cornea [12]. Before application of glycerin to the cornea, a local anesthetic may be administered to reduce the likelihood of a painful response [12].

HYALURONIC ACID

Description

Hyaluronic acid is a member of the class of amino sugar containing polysaccharides known as the glycosaminoglycans widely distributed in body tissues. Molecular weight is within the range of 50,000 to 8×10^6 depending on source, methods of preparation, and determination [5]. Hyaluronic acid binds water and functions as a lubricant between the collagen and elastic fiber networks in dermis during skin movement. Sodium hyaluronate is a white odorless powder, which forms viscous solutions in water [6]. A 2% aqueous solution of pure hyaluronic acid holds the remaining 98% water so tightly that it can be picked up as though it were a gel [20].

During manufacturing, the large, unbranched, non–cross-linked, water-containing molecule is easily broken by shear forces [20]. The carbohydrate chain is also very sensitive to breakdown by free radicals, UV radiation, and oxidative agents [20]. The manufacturers state that solutions of sodium hyaluronate for injection are stable for 3 years when stored in refrigerator and for 4 weeks when stored at room temperature [12].

General Use

A viscous solution of the sodium salt is used during surgical procedures on the eye and intra-articular injections have been tried in the treatment of osteoarthritis [12]. Topical application of 0.1% solution in patients with dry eye increased tear-film stability and alleviated symptoms of burning and grittiness [12].

Effects on the Skin

High–molecular weight hyaluronic acid solutions form hydrated viscoelastic films on the skin [20]. The larger the molecular size, the greater the aggregation and entanglement of the molecules, and hence, the more substantial and functional the viscoelastic film associated with the skin surface [20]. Because of the high molecular weight, hyaluronic acid will not penetrate deeper than the crevices between the desquamating cells.

Safety

Sodium hyaluronate is essentially nontoxic [6]. When the substance is used as an ophthalmic surgical aid, transient inflammatory ocular response has been described [19].

LACTIC ACID

Description

Lactic acid is colorless to yellowish crystals or syrupy liquid, miscible with water, alcohol, glycerol, but insoluble in chloroform [5,6]. Lactic acid is an α-hydroxy acid (AHA), i.e., an organic carboxylic acid in which there is a hydroxy group at the two, or alpha (α), position of the carbon chain. Lactic acid can exist in a DL, D, or L form. The L and the D forms are enantiomorphic isomers (mirror images). Lactic acid is miscible with water, alcohol, and ether and practically insoluble in chloroform [12]. Lactate is also a component of the natural hygroscopic material of the stratum corneum and constitutes about 12% of this material [2]. Formulations containing lactic acid have an acidic pH in the absence of any inorganic alkali or organic base. pH is increased in several formulations by partial neutralization.

General Use

Lactic acid has been used in topical preparations for several decades because of its buffering properties and water binding capacity [21]. Lactic acid and its salts have been used for douching and to help maintain the normal, acidic atmosphere of the vagina. Lactic acid has also been used for correction of disorders associated with hyperplasia and/or retention of the stratum corneum, such as dandruff, callus, keratosis, and verrucae (viral warts) [12]. It has also been suggested that lactic acid may be effective for adjuvant therapy of mild acne [22]. Also, ethyl lactate has been suggested to be effective in the treatment of acne, because of its penetration into the sebaceous follicle ducts with subsequent lowering of pH and decrease in the formation of fatty acids [23].

Investigators have also reported increases in the thickness of viable epidermis [24,25] as well as improvement in photoaging changes [24,26]. Lactic acid in combination with other peeling agents is used to produce a controlled partial-thickness injury to the skin which is believed to improve the clinical appearance of the skin [27].

Effects on the Skin

In guinea pig footpad corneum, it has been shown that both lactic acid and sodium lactate increase the water holding capacity and skin extensibility [21]. When the pH increases, the adsorption of lactic acid decreases, because of the ionization of the acid [21]. In another study on strips of stratum corneum from human abdominal skin, the uptake of water by sodium lactate was greater than that by lactic acid, but the stratum corneum was plasticized markedly by lactic acid and not by sodium lactate [28].

The concentrations used for treatment of ichthyosis and dry skin have ranged up to 12% [29]. One formulation of 12% ammonium lactate has been approved by the Food and Drug Administration (FDA, 1988) for treatment of ichthyosis vulgaris and dry, scaly skin (xerosis) and for the temporary relief of itching associated with these conditions.

Safety

Lactic acid is caustic to the skin, eyes, and mucous membranes in concentrated form [19]. Compared with other acids, lactic acid has no unusual capacity to penetrate the cornea, so its injurious effect is presumably attributable to its acidity [19].

Immediately after application of an AHA, stinging and smarting may be noticed; this is closely related to the pH of the preparations and the substances in themselves [30–32]. In normal skin, irritation and scaling may be induced when the acids are applied in high concentrations and at low pH [30,33].

PANTHENOL

Description

D-panthenol is a clear, almost colorless, odorless, viscous hygroscopic liquid that may crystallize on prolonged storage [12]. Panthenol is an alcohol that is rapidly converted to

D-pantothenic acid in the body. Panthothenic acid is a water-soluble vitamin, subsequently called vitamin B_5. The substance can be isolated from various living creatures, which gave the reason for its name (panthoten is Greek for "every-where") (Table 2) [34]. Panthenol is very soluble in water; freely soluble in alcohol and glycerol, but insoluble in fats and oils [35]. The substance is fairly stable to air and light if protected from humidity, but it is sensitive to acids and bases and also to heat [35]. The rate of hydrolysis is lowest at pH 4 to 6 [35].

General Use

Panthenol is widely used in the pharmaceutical and cosmetic industry for its moisturizing, soothing, and sedative properties [36]. It is also found in topical treatments for rhinitis, conjunctivitis, sunburn, and for wound healing (ulcers, burns, bed sores, and excoriations) [36]. Usually 2% is used [12]. It can further be used to prevent crystallization at the spray nozzles of aerosols [35].

Effects on the Skin and Hair

Topically applied panthenol is reported to penetrate the skin and hairs and to be transformed into panthothenic acid [35,37]. Pantothenic acid can be found in normal hair [35]. Soaking of hair in 2% aqueous solution of panthenol has been reported to increase the hair diameter up to 10% [38].

Safety

Panthenol has very low toxicity. Panthenol and products containing panthenol (0.5–2%) administered to rabbits caused reactions ranging from no skin irritation to moderate-to-severe erythema and well-defined edema [39]. Low concentrations have also been tested on humans, and those formulations did not induce sensitization or significant skin irritation. Contact sensitization to panthenol present in cosmetics, sunscreens, and hair lotion has been reported, although allergy to panthenol among patients attending for patch testing is uncommon [34,36].

PCA AND SALTS OF PCA

Description

PCA is the cosmetic ingredient term used for the cyclic organic compound known as 2-pyrrolidone-5-carboxylic acid (Table 2). The sodium salt is a naturally occurring humectant in the stratum corneum at levels about 12% of the NMF [2] corresponding to about 2% by weight in the stratum corneum [40]. The sodium salts of PCA are among the most powerful humectants (Table 3). PCA is also combined with a variety of other substances, like arginine, lysine, chitosan, and triethanolamine [1].

Effects on the Skin

The "L" form is a naturally occurring component of mammalian tissue and absorption from cosmetics is in addition to PCA already present in the skin (41). A significant relationship has been found between the moisture-binding ability and the PCA content of samples of stratum corneum [40]. Treatment of solvent-damaged guinea pig footpad corneum with humectant solutions shows that the water held by the corneum decreases in the following order: sodium PCA > sodium lactate > glycerin > sorbitol [21]. Treatment with a cream containing 5% sodium-PCA also increased the water-holding capacity of isolated corneum compared with the cream base [42]. The same cream was also more effective than a control product containing no humectant, and equally effective as a similar established product with urea as humectant, in reducing the skin dryness and flakiness [42].

Safety

In animal studies, no irritation to the eye and skin was noted at concentrations up to 50% and no evidence of phototoxicity, sensitization, or comedogenicity was found [41]. Minimal, transient ocular irritation has been produced by 50% PCA [41]. Immediate visible contact reactions in back skin have also been noted after application of 6.25% to 50% aqueous solutions of sodium PCA [43]. The response appeared within 5 minutes and disappeared within 30 minutes after application. CIR states that the ingredient should not be used in cosmetic products in which N-nitroso compounds could be formed [41].

PROPYLENE GLYCOL
Description

Propylene glycol is a clear, colorless, viscous, and practically odorless liquid having a sweet, slightly acrid taste resembling glycerol [11]. Under ordinary conditions it is stable in well-closed containers and it is also chemically stable when mixed with glycerin, water, or alcohol [5,11].

General Use

Propylene glycol is widely used in cosmetic and pharmaceutical manufacturing as a solvent and vehicle especially for substances unstable or insoluble in water [12,44]. It is also often used in foods as antifreeze and emulsifier [5,12]. Propylene glycol is also used as inhibitor of fermentation and mold growth [5].

Effects on the Skin

Propylene glycol has been tried in the treatment of a number of skin disorders, including ichthyosis [45,46], tinea versicolor [47], and seborrheic dermatitis [48], because of its humectant, keratolytic, antibacterial, and antifungal properties [12,44].

Safety

The estimated acceptable daily intake of propylene glycol is up to 25 mg/kg body weight (WHO) [12]. It is considered a harmless ingredient for pharmaceutical products [11] and safe for use in cosmetic products at concentrations up to 50% [49]. However, clinical data have showed skin irritation and sensitization reactions to propylene glycol in normal subjects at concentrations as low as 10% under occlusive conditions and dermatitis patients as low as 2% [10,49]. The nature of the cutaneous response remains obscure and, therefore, the skin reactions have been classified into four mechanisms: (1) irritant contact dermatitis, (2) allergic contact dermatitis, (3) nonimmunological contact urticaria, and (4) subjective or sensory irritation [50]. This concept allows a partial explanation of effects observed by different investigators [50].

PROTEINS

Description

Proteins and amino acids for cosmetics are based on a variety of natural sources. Collagen is the traditional protein used in cosmetics. Collagen has a complex triple helical structure, which is responsible for its high–moisture-retention properties. Vegetable-based proteins have, in recent years, grown in importance as an alternative to using animal by-products. Suitable sources include wheat, rice, soybean, and oat.

In cosmetics native proteins can be used, but perhaps the most widely used protein types are hydrolyzed proteins of intermediate molecular weight with higher solubility. An increased substantivity is obtained by binding fatty alkyl quarternary groups to the protein. Improved film-forming properties can be obtained by combining the protein and polyvinyl-pyrrolidone into a copolymer. Such modifications may increase the moisture absorption compared with the parent compound. Potential problems with proteins are their odor and change in color with time. Furthermore, as they are nutrients their inclusion in cosmetics may require stronger preservatives.

Efficacy and Safety

Amino acids belong to the NMF and account for 40% of its dry weight [2]. Because of their relatively low molecular weight, they are capable of penetrating the skin and cuticle of the hair more effectively than the higher–molecular-weight protein hydrolysates.

Salts of the condensation product of coconut acid and hydrolyzed animal protein [51] and wheat flour and wheat starch [52] are considered safe as cosmetic ingredients by CIR. The most frequent clinical presentation of protein contact dermatitis is a chronic or recurrent dermatitis [53]. Sometimes an urticarial or vesicular exacerbation has been noted a few minutes after contact with the causative substance [53,54]. Hair conditioners containing quaternary hydrolyzed protein or hydrolyzed bovine collagen have induced contact urticaria and respiratory symptoms [54]. Atopic constitution seems to be a predisposing factor in the development of protein contact dermatitis [53].

SORBITOL

Description

Sorbitol is a hexahydric alcohol appearing as a white crystalline powder, odorless and of fresh and sweet taste [11,12]. Sorbitol is most commonly available as 70% aqueous solution, which is clear, colorless, and viscous. It occurs naturally in fruits and is easily dissolved in water, but not so well in alcohol. It is practically insoluble in organic solvents.

Sorbitol is relatively chemically inert and compatible with most excipients, but it may react with iron oxide and become discolored [11].

General Use

Sorbitol is used in pharmaceutical tablets and in candies when noncariogenic properties are desired. It is also used as sweetener in diabetic foods and in toothpastes. Sorbitol is also used as a laxative intrarectally and believed to produce less troublesome side effects than glycerin [13]. Its hygroscopic properties are reported to be inferior to that of glycerin (Table 3) [21,55].

Safety

When ingested in large amounts (30 g/day) it produces a laxative effect and according to WHO the acceptable daily intake in humans should not exceed 9 grams/day [11].

UREA

Description

Urea is colorless, transparent, slightly hygroscopic, odorless or almost odorless, prismatic crystals, or white crystalline powder or pellets. Urea is freely soluble in water, slightly soluble in alcohol, and practically insoluble in ether [12]. The extraction of pure urea from urine was first accomplished by Proust in 1821 and pure urea was first synthesized by Wöhler in 1828 [56]. Urea in solution hydrolyzes slowly to ammonia and carbon dioxide [12].

General Use

Urea is used as a 10% cream for the treatment of ichthyosis and hyperkeratotic skin disorders [12,56], and in lower concentrations for the treatment of dry skin. In the treatment of onychomycosis, urea is added to a medicinal formulation at 40% as a keratoplastic agent to increase the bioavailability of the drug [57].

Effects on the Skin

An increased water-holding capacity of scales from psoriatic and ichthyotic patients has been observed after treatment with urea-containing creams [58,59].

Concern has been expressed about the use of urea in moisturizers, with reference to the risk of reducing the chemical barrier function of the skin to toxic substances [60]. That urea can increase skin permeability has been shown in several studies, where it has been found to be an efficient accelerant for the penetration of different substances [61–63]. Not all studies, however, support the belief that urea is an effective penetration promoter [64,65], and treatment of normal skin with moisturizers containing 5% to 10% urea has been found to reduce transepidermal water loss (TEWL) and also to diminish the irritative response to the surfactant sodium lauryl sulphate [66,67].

Safety

Urea is a naturally occurring substance in the body, as the main nitrogen containing degradation product of protein metabolism [68]. Urea is an osmotic diuretic and has been used in the past for treatment of acute increase in intracranial pressure due to cerebral edema [12]. No evidence of acute or cumulative irritation has been noted in previous studies on urea-containing moisturizers, but several patients [12–22%] have reported stinging after treatment with 10% urea creams [69,70]. Urea has also shown to give burning reactions on lesioned forearm skin at concentrations used in moisturizers [71].

CONCLUSIONS

A number of interesting humectants are available as cosmetic ingredients. Most of them have a long and safe history of use, and several are also accepted as food additives. A potential drawback of the low–molecular weight substances are their stinging potential, since they may be absorbed into the skin. The high–molecular weight substances usually do not penetrate the skin; instead they are suggested to reduce the irritation potential of surfactants. However, case reports of urticarial reactions have been reported after exposure to modified proteins [54].

The advantage with the larger and chemically modified materials are that they have an increased substantivity to target areas, whereas it is apparent that small amounts of several low–molecular-weight hygroscopic substances have a questionable contribution to the water content of hair and stratum corneum in rinse-off products. Another issue to bear in mind is whether the obtained humectancy is the only mode of action. Some humectants may modify the surface properties and increase the extensibility of stratum corneum without influencing the water content. Furthermore, humectants may also affect specific metabolic process in the skin. One should also keep in mind that humectants can improve the cosmetic properties of the formulation and some of them also facilitate marketing of the product just because of their names.

REFERENCES

1. Wenninger JA, McEwen GN. International Cosmetic Ingredient Dictionary and Handbook. Washington, DC: The Cosmetic, Toiletry, and Fragrance Association, 1997.
2. Jacobi O. Moisture regulation of the skin. Drug Cosmet Ind 1959; 84:732–812.
3. Rawlings AV, Scott IR, Harding CR, Bowser PA. Stratum corneum moisturization at the molecular level. J Invest Dermatol 1995; 103:731–740.
4. Blank IH. Factors which influence the water content of stratum corneum. J Invest Dermatol 1952; 18:433–440.
5. Budavari S. The Merck Index. Rahway: Merck & Co., Inc., 1989.
6. Ash M, Ash I. Handbook of Pharmaceutical Additives. Hampshire: Gower Publishing Limited, 1995.
7. Rietschel RL, Fowler, JF. Fisher's contact dermatitis. Baltimore: Williams & Wilkins, 1995.
8. The Cosmetic Ingredient Review Expert Panel. Final assessment of the safety assessment of butylene glycol, hexylene glycol, ethoxydiglycol, and dipropylene glycol. J Am Coll Toxicol 1985; 2:223–248.
9. Sugiura M, Hayakawa R. Contact dermatitis due to 1,3-butylene glycol. Contact Derm 1997; 37:90.
10. Fan W, Kinnunen T, Niinimäke A, Hannuksela M. Skin reactions to glycols used in dermatological and cosmetic vehicles. Am J Contact Derm 1991; 2:181–183.
11. American Pharmaceutical Association and The Pharmaceutical Society of Great Britain. Handbook of Pharmaceutical Excipients. Baltimore: The Pharmaceutical Press, 1986.
12. Reynolds JEF. Martindale: The Extra Pharmacopoeia. London: The Pharmaceutical Press, 1993.
13. Zimmerman DR. The Essential Guide to Nonprescription Drugs. New York: Harper & Row, 1983.
14. Froebe CL, Simion A, Ohlmeyer H, et al. Prevention of stratum corneum lipid phase transitions in vitro by glycerol—an alternative mechanism for skin moisturization. J Soc Cosmet Chem 1990; 41:51–65.
15. Batt MD, Fairhurst E. Hydration of the stratum corneum. Int J Cosmet Sci 1986; 8:253–264.

16. Batt MD, Davis WB, Fairhurst E, Gerrard WA, Ridge BD. Changes in the physical properties of the stratum corneum following treatment with glycerol. J Soc Cosmet Chem 1988; 39:367–381.

17. Wilson E, Berardesca E, Maibach H. In vivo transepidermal water loss and skin surface hydration in assessment of moisturization and soap effects. Int J Cosmet Sci 1988; 10:201–211.

18. Lieb LM, Nash RA, Matias JR, Orentreich N. A new in vitro method for transepidermal water loss: a possible method for moisturizer evaluation. J Soc Cosmet Chem 1988; 39:107–119.

19. Grant WM. Toxicology of the Eye. Springfield: Charles C. Thomas, 1986.

20. Balazs EA, Band P. Hyaluronic acid: its structure and use. Cosmet Toilet 1984; 99:65–72.

21. Middleton JD. Development of a skin cream designed to reduce dry and flaky skin. J Soc Cosmet Chem 1974; 25:519–534.

22. Berson DS, Shalita AR. The treatment of acne: the role of combination therapies. J Am Acad Dermatol 1995; 32:S31–41.

23. Prottey C, George D, Leech RW, Black JG, Howes D, Vickers CFH. The mode of action of ethyl lactate as a treatment for acne. Br J Dermatol 1984; 110:475–485.

24. Ditre CM, Griffin TD, Murphy GF, et al. Effects of alpha-hydroxy acids on photoaged skin: a pilot clinical, histologic, and ultrastructural study. J Am Acad Dermatol 1996; 34:187–195.

25. Lavker RM, Kaidbey K, Leyden JJ. Effects of topical ammonium lactate on cutaneous atrophy from a potent topical corticosteroid. J Am Acad Dermatol 1992; 26:535–544.

26. Stiller MJ, Bartolone J, Stern R, et al. Topical 8% glycolic acid and 8% L-lactic acid creams for the treatment of photodamaged skin. A double-blind vehicle-controlled clinical trial. Arch Dermatol 1996; 132:631–636.

27. Glogau RG, Matarasso SL. Chemical face peeling: patient and peeling agent selection. Facial Plast Surg 1995; 11:1–8.

28. Takahashi M, Yamada M, Machida Y. A new method to evaluate the softening effect of cosmetic ingredients on the skin. J Soc Cosmet Chem 1984; 35:171–181.

29. Wehr R, Krochmal L, Bagatell F, Ragsdale W. A controlled two-center study of lactate 12% lotion and a petrolatum-based creme in patients with xerosis. Cutis 1986; 37:205–209.

30. Smith WP. Hydroxy acids and skin aging. Cosmet Toilet 1994; 109:41–48.

31. Smith WP. Comparative effectiveness of alpha-hydroxy acids on skin properties. Int J Cosmet Sci 1996; 18:75–83.

32. Frosch PJ, Kligman AM. A method for appraising the stinging capacity of topically applied substances. J Soc Cosmet Chem 1977; 28:197–209.

33. Effendy I, Kwangsukstith C, Lee LY, Maibach HI. Functional changes in human stratum corneum induced by topical glycolic acid: comparison with all-trans retinoic acid. Acta Derm Venereol (Stockh) 1995; 75:455–458.

34. Schmid-Grendelmeier P, Wyss M, Elsner P. Contact allergy to dexpanthenol. A report of seven cases and review of the literature. Dermatosen 1995; 43:175–178.

35. Huni JES. Basel: Roche, 1981.

36. Stables GI, Wilkinson SM. Allergic contact dermatitis due to panthenol. Contact Derm 1998; 38:236–237.

37. Stuttgen G, Krause H. Panthenol. Arch Klin Exp Dermatol 1960; 209:578–582.

38. Driscoll WR. Panthenol in hair products. D&CI 1975; 116:45–49.

39. The Cosmetic Ingredient Review Expert Panel. Final report on the safety assessment of panthenol and pantothenic acid. J Am Coll Toxicol 1987; 6:139–163.

40. Laden K, Spitzer R. Identification of a natural moisturizing agent in skin. J Soc Cosmet Chem 1967; 18:351–360.

41. 1997 CIR Compendium. PCA and Sodium PCA. Washington, D.C.: Cosmetic Ingredient Review, 1997:106–107.

42. Middleton JD, Roberts ME. Effect of a skin cream containing the sodium salt of pyrrolidone carboxylic acid on dry and flaky skin. J Soc Cosmet Chem 1978; 29:201–205.

43. Larmi E, Lahti A, Hannuksela M. Immediate contact reactions to benzoic acid and the sodium salt of pyrrolidone carboxylic acid. Contact Derm 1989; 20:38–40.
44. Cantazaro JM, Smith JG. Propylene glycol dermatitis. J Am Acad Dermatol 1991; 24:90–95.
45. Goldsmith LA, Baden HP. Propylene glycol with occlusion for treatment of ichthyosis. JAMA 1972; 220:579–580.
46. Gånemo A, Vahlquist A. Lamellar ichthyosis is markedly improved by a novel combination of emollients. Br J Dermatol 1997; 137:1011–1031.
47. Faergemann J, Fredriksson T. Propylene glycol in the treatment of tinea versicolor. Acta Derm Venereol (Stockh) 1980; 60:92–93.
48. Faergemann J. Propylene glycol in the treatment of seborrheic dermatitis of the scalp: a double-blind study. Cutis 1988; 42:69–71.
49. Final report of the safety assessment of propylene glycol and polypropylene glycols (PPG-9,-12,-15,-17,-20,-26,-30, and 34). J Am Coll Toxicol 1996; 13:6.
50. Funk JO, Maibach HI. Propylene glycol dermatitis: re-evaluation of an old problem. Contact Derm 1994; 31:236–241.
51. The Cosmetic Ingredient Review Expert Panel. Final report on the safety assessment of potassium-coco-hydrolyzed animal protein and triethanolamine-coco-hydrolyzed animal protein. J Am Coll Toxicol 1983; 2:75–86.
52. The Cosmetic Ingredient Review Expert Panel. Final report on the safety assessment of wheat flour and wheat starch. J Environ Pathol Toxicol 1980; 4:19–32.
53. Janssens V, Morren M, Dooms-Goossens A, Degreef H. Protein contact dermatitis: myth or reality? Br J Dermatol 1995; 132:1–6.
54. Freeman S, Lee M-S. Contact urticaria to hair conditioner. Contact Derm 1996; 35:195–196.
55. Rovesti P, Ricciardi D. New experiments on the use of sorbitol in the field of cosmetics. P & EOR 1959; 771–774.
56. Rosten M. The treatment of ichthyosis and hyperkeratotic conditions with urea. Aust J Dermatol 1970; 11:142–144.
57. Fritsch H, Stettendorf S, Hegemann L. Ultrastructural changes in onchomycosis during the treatment with bifonazole/urea ointment. Dermatology 1992;185:32–36.
58. Swanbeck G. A new treatment of ichthyosis and other hyperkeratotic conditions. Acta Derm Venereol (Stockh) 1968; 48:123–127.
59. Grice K, Sattar H, Baker H. Urea and retinoic acid in ichthyosis and their effect on transepidermal water loss and water holding capacity of stratum corneum. Acta Derm Venereol (Stockh) 1973; 53:114–118.
60. Hellgren L, Larsson K. On the effect of urea on human epidermis. Dermatologica 1974; 149:289–293.
61. Wohlrab W. The influence of urea on the penetration kinetics of vitamin-A acid into human skin. Z Hautkr 1990; 65:803–805.
62. Kim CK, Kim JJ, Chi SC, Shim CK. Effect of fatty acids and urea on the penetration of ketoprofen through rat skin. Int J Pharm 1993; 99:109–118.
63. Beastall J, Guy RH, Hadgraft J, Wilding I. The influence of urea on percutaneous absorption. Pharm Res 1986; 3:294–297.
64. Lippold BC, Hackemuller D. The influence of skin moisturizers on drug penetration in vivo. Int J Pharm 1990; 61:205–211.
65. Wahlberg JE, Swanbeck G. The effect of urea and lactic acid on the percutaneous absorption of hydrocortisone. Acta Derm Venereol (Stockh) 1973; 53:207–210.
66. Lodén M. Urea-containing moisturizers influence barrier properties of normal skin. Arch Dermatol Res 1996; 288:103–107.
67. Lodén M. Barrier recovery and influence of irritant stimuli in skin treated with a moisturizing cream. Contact Derm 1997; 36:256–260.
68. Swanbeck G. Urea in the treatment of dry skin. Acta Derm Venereol (Stockh) 1992; 177 (suppl):7–8.

69. Serup J. A double-blind comparison of two creams containing urea as the active ingredient. Assessment of efficacy and side-effects by non-invasive techniques and a clinical scoring scheme. Acta Derm Venereol (Stockh) 1992; 177(suppl):34–38.

70. Fredriksson T, Gip L. Urea creams in the treatment of dry skin and hand dermatitis. Int J Dermatol 1975; 32:442–444.

71. Gabard B, Nook T, Muller KH. Tolerance of the lesioned skin to dermatological formulations. J Appl Cosmetol 1991; 9:25–30.

72. Rieger MM, Deem DE. Skin moisturizers. II. The effects of cosmetic ingredients on human stratum corneum. J Soc Cosmet Chem 1974; 25:253–262.

73. Huttinger R. Restoring hydrophilic properties to the stratum corneum—a new humectant. Cosmet Toilet 1978; 93:61–62.

31

Ceramides and Lipids

Bozena B. Michniak
University of South Carolina, Columbia, South Carolina

Philip W. Wertz
University of Iowa, Iowa City, Iowa

HISTORICAL PERSPECTIVES

Many published accounts of the composition of lipids from human stratum corneum have been complicated by the almost inevitable presence of sebaceous lipids as well as exogenous contaminants. When stratum corneum samples are obtained from excised skin, there is almost always massive contamination with subcutaneous triglycerides as well as fatty acids derived from the subcutaneous fat. In addition, precautions must be taken to avoid contamination with environmental contaminants such as alkanes and cosmetic components. As a result of these complications, much work has been done with pig skin as a model [1–6].

Young pigs, if properly housed and tended, can be kept clean, and the sebaceous glands are not active. By direct heat separation of epidermis from an intact carcass, it is possible to avoid subcutaneous fat. In terms of general structure, composition, and permeability barrier function, the pig appears to provide a good model for the human. An alternative approach is to use the contents of epidermal cysts [7,8]. This material represents exfoliated stratum corneum lipid that is free of sebaceous and environmental contaminants. If the contents are carefully expressed from the capsule, a contaminant-free sample of stratum corneum lipid can be obtained. Cholesterol sulfate is partially hydrolyzed during the desquamation process; however, this is only a minor stratum corneum component. In either the pig or cyst model, the major lipid components are ceramides, cholesterol, and fatty acids, which represent approximately 45, 27, and 12% of the total lipid, respectively [9]. Other minor components include cholesterol sulfate and cholesterol esters. The fatty acids in either model are predominantly straight-chain saturated species ranging from either 14 (cyst) or 16 (pig) carbons through 28 carbons in length with the 22 and 24 carbon species being the most abundant. The main focus in the rest of this chapter will be on the stratum corneum ceramides.

The first analysis of stratum corneum lipids was performed in 1932 by Kooyman [10], who showed a dramatic reduction in the proportion of phospholipid in stratum corneum compared with the inner portion of the epidermis. Subsequently, Long [11], using the very thick epidermis from cow snout as a model, analyzed lipids from horizontal slices of epithelial tissue. He observed a gradual accumulation of cholesterol and fatty acids in progressing from the basal region toward the surface. Phospholipids initially accumulated, but were degraded as the stratum corneum was approached. In 1965, Nicolaides [12] identified ceramides as a polar lipid component of stratum corneum. This fact was included in a footnote and was largely ignored until the pioneering work of Gray and Yardley in the mid to late 1970s [1,2,13,14]. Among other things, these investigators showed that the ceramides are structurally heterogeneous and contain normal fatty acids, α-hydroxyacids, sphingosines, and phytosphingosines as components. However, individual ceramide types were not well resolved and no definitive structures could be proposed. The first attempt to isolate individual ceramide types and to determine the identities of the individual fatty acid and long-chain base components was conducted in 1979 using neonatal mouse epidermis as a source of lipids [15]. Eight putative ceramide fractions were isolated, and six of these were analyzed. The remaining two were too minor for any analysis. Unfortunately, only normal fatty acids, sphingosines, and dihydrosphingosines were reported for each fraction analyzed. This suggests extensive cross-contamination sufficient to preclude recognition of the actual structural diversity. In 1983, the detailed structures of the ceramides from porcine epidermis were published [3]. Six structurally different types of ceramides were identified, and these included sphingosines, dihydrosphingosines, and phytosphingosines as the base components; normal, α-hydroxyacids, and ω-hydroxyacids as the amide-linked fatty acids; and one ceramide type included an ester-linked fatty acid. Subsequently, it was shown that the same ceramide structural types are present in human stratum corneum, although the proportions are somewhat different [8,15]. More recently it has been shown that in addition to the standard phytosphingosine present in porcine ceramides, the human ceramides also include a variant phytosphingosine, 6-hydroxysphingosine [16].

In 1987 it was discovered that porcine epidermal stratum corneum contains significant levels of covalently bound lipid, the major component of which is an ω-hydroxyceramide [4]. Small amounts of saturated fatty acid and ω-hydroxyacid are also present. A similar situation was shown for human stratum corneum; however, in this case there was a second hydroxyceramide that was shown to contain a variant phytosphingosine [17]. This subsequently proved to be 6-hydroxysphingosine [16]. The free and covalently bound ceramides are discussed in detail in the following section.

CERAMIDES FROM EPIDERMIS

As previously noted, the first comprehensive study of epidermal ceramide structures was directed at the porcine ceramides, which were separated into six chromatographically distinct fractions [3]. Each fraction was analyzed by a combination of chemical, chromatographic and spectroscopic methods, and representative structures are included in Figure 1.

The least polar of the porcine ceramides, ceramide fraction 1, consists of 30- through 34-carbon ω-hydroxyacids amide-linked to a mixture of sphingosines and dihydrosphingosines. The long-chain base component of this ceramide ranges from 16 through 22 carbons in length with 18:1, 20:1, and 22:1 being the most abundant. There is also a fatty acid ester-linked to the ω-hydroxyl group, 75% of which consists of linoleic acid. This species has often been referred to as ceramide 1 or acylceramide, but in the more systematic nomenclature system proposed by Motta et al. [18] this becomes Cer[OSE]. (In this system, the amide-linked fatty acid is designated as N, A, or O to indicate normal, α-hydroxy, or ω-hydroxy, respectively. The base component is designated S or P for sphingosine or

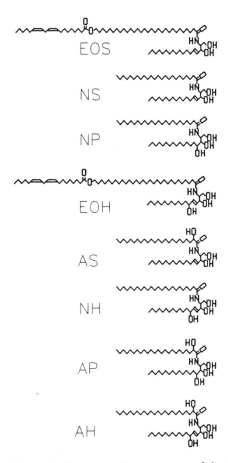

EOS

NS

NP

EOH

AS

NH

AP

AH

FIGURE 1   Representative structures of the free ceramides from human stratum corneum.

phytosphingosine, respectively. It is understood that sphingosines are generally accompanied by dihydrosphingosines in the ceramides.) Cer[OSE] is unusual in two respects: (1) the very long ω-hydroxyacyl portion of the molecule is long enough to completely span a typical bilayer; and (2) a high proportion of the ester-linked fatty acid is linoleic acid. It is thought that this ceramide along with an analogous glucosylated Cer[OSE] in the living layers of the epidermis account for the essential role of linoleic acid in formation and maintenance of the barrier function of the skin [3,19,20]. Specific roles for Cer[OSE] have been proposed in organization of the intercellular lipid lamellae of epidermal stratum corneum [20–22]. In formation of the intercellular lamellae of the stratum corneum, flattened lipid vesicles are initially extruded from the lamellar granules into the intercellular space [23]. These flattened vesicles fuse in an edge-to-edge manner to produce paired bilayers. Cer[OSE] is associated with each of the paired lamellae with both possible orientations.

Approximately half of the Cer[OSE] is oriented with the polar head groups in the outer polar regions of the paired bilayers, whereas the other half of the Cer[OSE] molecules are oriented with the polar head groups in the polar regions in the center of the pair of lamellae. For the Cer[OSE] in the former orientation the ω-hydroxyacyl portion of the molecule will span the bilayer while the linoleate inserts into the other bilayer, thus linking the pair of bilayers together. For Cer[OSE] in the second orientation the linoleate tail is thought to participate in the formation of narrow interdigitated layers that intervene between the paired bilayers. This action of the Cer[OSE] results in the formation of broad-narrow-broad lamellar patterns that are seen in transmission electron micrographs when ruthenium tetroxide is used as a postfixative and which give rise to a 13 nm repeat unit in radiograph diffraction studies [5,6,22].

Porcine ceramide fraction 2 has proven to be Cer[NS]. The fatty acid component is saturated and straight-chained and ranges from 16- through 32-carbons in length. C20:0, C22:0, C24:0, C26:0, and C28:0 are the most abundant, constituting from 9% to 19% of the total fatty acid mass each. The long-chain bases again consist of a mixture of sphingosines and dihydrosphingosines ranging from 16- through 22-carbons in length. The most abundant bases are 18:0, 18:1, 20:0, and 20:1.

Porcine ceramide fraction 3, Cer[NP], contains the same range of fatty acids found in Cer[NS], but the long-chain base component is now a phytosphingosine with no double bond and a third hydroxyl group on carbon 4. The phytosphingosines found here range from 16- through 24-carbons long, and the most abundant are 20:0 and 22:0.

Porcine ceramide fractions 4 and 5 both proved to be Cer[AS], but they differed in terms of the chain length distributions of the α-hydroxyacid component. The chromatographically more mobile fraction 4 contained 24- through 28-carbon α-hydroxyacids amide-linked to sphingosines and dihydrosphingosines, whereas ceramide fraction 5 contains α-hydroxypalmitic acid amide-linked to sphingosines and dihydrosphingosines. Ceramide fraction 4 also contains somewhat longer bases with major amounts of 20:0 and 20:1, whereas ceramide fraction 5 contains mainly 16- through 18-carbon bases. This difference in carbon content results in chromatographic separation into two fractions, even though the basic structural type is the same in each.

Finally, the most polar of the pig ceramide fractions consists of α-hydroxyacids amide-linked to phytosphingosine, Cer[AP]. The α-hydroxyacids present in Cer[AP] range from 16- through 28-carbons in length, but the 24- and 26-carbon entities account for approximately 70% of the total fatty acid mass. The phytosphingosines have a chain-length distribution similar to that already described for Cer[NP].

Subsequently, the human stratum corneum ceramides were investigated and were shown to produce a similar, though not identical, pattern on thin-layer chromatograms [15]. Notably, the human fraction most closely matching porcine ceramide fraction 3 is somewhat broader and less symmetrical. The material most closely matching porcine ceramide fractions 4 and 5 merged into one broad peak, and was designated ceramide 4/5. This was shown to reflect a more continuous chain-length distribution among the α-hydroxyacid component of Cer[AS] as opposed to the bipolar distribution found in the pig. The most polar human fraction similar to porcine ceramide fraction 6 appeared as an incompletely resolved doublet. These two components were designated ceramides 6I and 6II. Subsequently it has been shown the ceramide fraction 6II contains the variant phyto-sphingosine—6-hydroxysphingosine [16]. The Motta system of nomenclature has been extended to include this new long-chain base as H [16]. So ceramide 6I is Cer[AP], and ceramide 6II becomes Cer[AH]. Human ceramide fraction 3 has been shown to contain a minor amount of a 6-hydroxysphingosine-containing acylceramide, Cer[OHE] [16], in addition to Cer[NH]. Likewise, ceramide fraction 4/5 contains Cer[NH] [24] in addition to Cer[AS] [15]. These additional ceramides containing 6-hydroxysphingosine can be resolved on thin-layer chromatography by use of multiple development regimens.

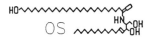

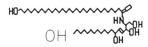

FIGURE 2   Representative structures of the covalently bound ceramides from human stratum corneum.

In addition to the extractable lipids, there are covalently bound lipids coating the outer surface of the cornified envelope in epidermal stratum corneum. This consists mainly of ceramides. In porcine stratum corneum the principal covalently bound lipid is Cer[OS] derived from Cer[OSE] [4]. In human stratum corneum, in addition to covalently bound Cer[OS], a second more polar covalently bound ceramide was found [17]. This was later shown to be Cer[OH] [16]. Representative structures of Cer[OS] and Cer[OH] are presented in Figure 2.

LIPIDS FROM OTHER KERATINIZED TISSUES

The hair and nails contain cholesterol sulfate and ceramides generally similar to those in the stratum corneum as their principal polar lipid components [25]. Unfortunately, the ceramides from these epidermal appendages have not been characterized in detail.

Hair contains 18-methyleicosanoic acid covalently bound to the outer surface of the cuticle cells in human as well as other mammalian hair [21]. The attachment is apparently through thioester linkages. This covalently bound lipid layer provides a hydrophobic outer surface for the hair shaft.

In the oral cavity, the regions of the hard palate and gingiva are covered by a keratinizing epithelium that closely resembles the epidermis in many ways [5]. The stratum corneum in these regions, like epidermal stratum corneum, contains ceramides, cholesterol and fatty acids as major lipid components; however, unlike epidermal stratum corneum, the oral stratum corneum also contains relatively high proportions of phospholipids and glycosylceramides. The ceramides in the oral stratum corneum include the same structural types found in epidermal stratum corneum in similar relative proportions, except that in the oral tissue the proportion of Cer[OSE], the acylceramide, is much lower. It is thought that this lowered proportion of Cer[OSE] accounts for the fact that the broad-narrow-broad lamellar pattern that is characteristic of the intercellular lipids of epidermal stratum corneum is never seen in oral stratum corneum.

COMMERCIALLY AVAILABLE CERAMIDES

There are presently no commercial sources of the ceramides based on 6-hydroxysphingosine.

A variety of ceramides based on phytosphingosine produced by a fermentation technique are commercially available from Cosmoferm, a group company of Gist-brocades based in Delft, the Netherlands. These include an acylceramide, Cer[EOP], which consists of a 27-carbon ω-hydroxyacid amide-linked to phytosphingosine and bearing ester-linked stearic acid on the ω-hydroxyl group. There are also two ceramides of the type Cer[NP]. One of these contains stearic acid and the other oleic acid amide-linked to phytosphingosine. Finally, this supplier also produces N-2-hydroxystearoyl-phytosphingosine, Cer[AP]. These specific ceramides are routinely available; however, it is also possible to customize any of these general structural types to include different fatty acids.

There are several commercial sources of ceramides or ceramide analogues similar to the ceramide type Cer[NS]. For example, SEDERMA of Parsippany, New Jersey produces a synthetic ceramide consisting of N-stearoyl-dihydrosphingosine and sold as ceramide 2. This synthetic ceramide is partially racemic at carbon-3 of the base component; however, the stereochemical configuration at this carbon is at least 70% R, which is the configuration in natural dihydrosphingosine.

FUTURE DIRECTIONS

Presently, ceramides are being used in skin moisturizers and at least one line of hair care products. It has been documented that ceramides are important in the permeability barrier of the skin and the water-holding properties of the stratum corneum [26,27]. It seems likely that the interest in ceramides for incorporation into cosmetic products will result in the introduction of additional, novel ceramide formulations for use in skin and hair care. In addition, it can be anticipated that ceramides will eventually be incorporated into other personal care products, such as stick deodorants, or cosmetic products, such as lipstick. This will likely lead to commercial availability of additional ceramide structural variants that more closely resemble all of the ceramide types that have been identified in human stratum corneum.

REFERENCES

1. Gray GM, Yardley HJ. Different populations of pig epidermal cells: isolation and lipid composition. J Lipid Res 1975; 16:441–447.
2. Yardley HJ, Summerly R. Lipid composition and metabolism in normal and diseased epidermis. Pharmacology & Therapeutics 1981; 13:357–383.
3. Wertz PW, Downing DT. Ceramides of pig epidermis: structure determination. J Lipid Res 1983; 24:759–765.
4. Wertz PW, Downing DT. Covalently bound ω-hydroxyceramide in the stratum corneum. Biochim Biophys Acta 1987; 917:108–111.
5. Law S, Wertz PW, Swartzendruber DC, Squier CA. Regional variation in content, composition and organization of porcine epithelial barrier lipids revealed by thin-layer chromatography and transmission electron microscopy. Arch Oral Biol 1995; 40:1085–1091.
6. Bouwstra JA, Cheng K, Gooris GS, Weerheim A, Ponec M. The role of ceramides 1 and 2 in the stratum corneum lipid organization. Biochim Biophys Acta 1996; 1300:177–186.
7. Nicolaides N, Levan NE, Fu WC. The lipid pattern of the wen (keratinous cyst of the skin). J Invest Dermatol 1968; 50:189–194.
8. Wertz PW, Swartzendruber DC, Madison KC, Downing DT. The composition and morphology of epidermal cyst lipids. J Invest Dermatol 1987; 89:419–425.
9. Wertz PW, Downing DT. Stratum corneum: biological and biochemical considerations. In: Hadgraft J, Guy RH, eds. Transdermal Delivery Systems. New York: Marcel Dekker, 1988: 1–22.
10. Kooyman DJ. Lipids of the skin. Some changes in the lipids of epidermis during the process of keratinization. Arch Dermatol Syphilol 1932; 25:444–450.

11. Long VJW. Variations in lipid composition of different depths of the cow snout epidermis. J Invest Dermatol 1970; 55:269–273.

12. Nicolaides N. Skin lipids. II. Class composition of samples from various species and anatomic sites. J Am Oil Chem Soc 1965; 42:691–702.

13. Gray GM, Yardley HJ. Lipid compositions of cells isolated from pig, human, and rat epidermis. J Lipid Res 1975; 16:434–440.

14. Gray GM, White RJ. Glycosphingolipids and ceramides in human and pig epidermis. J Invest Dermatol 1977; 70:336–341.

15. Wertz PW, Miethke MC, Long SA, Strauss JS, Downing DT. The composition of the ceramides from human stratum corneum and from comedones. J Invest Dermatol 1985; 84:410–412.

16. Robson KJ, Stewart ME, Michelsen S, Lazo ND, Downing DT. 6-Hydroxy-4-sphengenine in human epidermal ceramides. J Lipid Res 1994; 35:2060–2068.

17. Wertz PW, Madison KC, Downing DT. Covalently bound lipids of human stratum corneum. J Invest Dermatol 1989; 91:109–111.

18. Motta SM, Monti M, Sesana S, Caputo R, Carelli S, Ghidoni R. Ceramide composition of the psoriatic scale. Biochim Biophys Acta 1993; 1182:147–151.

19. Wertz PW, Downing DT. Glycolipids in mammalian epidermis: structure and function in the water barrier. Science 1982; 217:1261–1262.

20. Kuempel D, Swartzendruber DC, Squier CA, Wertz PW. In vitro reconstitution of stratum corneum lipid lamellae. Biochim Biophys Acta 1998; 1372:135–140.

21. Wertz PW. Integral lipids of hair and stratum corneum. In: Zahn H, Jolles P, eds. Hair: Biology and Structure. Basel: Birkhauser, 1996:227–237.

22. Bouwstra JA, Gooris GS, Dubbelaar FE, Weerheim AM, Ijzerman AP, Ponec M. Role of ceramide 1 in the molecular organization of the stratum corneum lipids. J Lipid Res 1998; 39:186–196.

23. Landmann L. The epidermal permeability barrier. Anat Embryol 1988; 178:1–13.

24. Stewart ME, Downing DT. A new 6-hydroxy-4-5-sphingemine-containing ceramide in human skin. J Lipid Res 1999; 40:1434–1439.

25. Wix MA, Wertz PW, Downing DT. Polar lipid composition of mammalian hair. Comp Biochem Biophys 1987; 86B:671–673.

26. Lintner K, Mondon P, Girard F, Gibaud C. The effect of a synthetic ceramide-2 on transepidermal water loss after stripping or sodium lauryl sulfate treatment: an in vivo study. Int J Cosmet Sci 1997; 19:15–25.

27. Imokawa G, Akasaki S, Minematsu Y, Kawai M. Importance of intercellular lipids in water-retention properties of the stratum corneum: induction and recovery study of surfactant dry skin. Arch Dermatol Res 1989; 281:45–51.

32

Natural Extracts

Jürgen Vollhardt
DRAGOCO Inc., Totowa, New Jersey

INTRODUCTION

Natural extracts have played an important role since ancient times. Egyptian hieroglyphs over 3000 years old [1] offer formulas showing how treatment products were prepared with extracts from plants. For quite some time natural materials were the only possible raw materials available in cosmetic formulations. The very prosperous development of synthetic chemistry and manufacturing, which started around the beginning of the century, has led to a dramatic increase in materials of synthetic origin and with highly targeted functionality.

Up until the late 1960s, cosmetic formulators and consumers still did not perceive the benefits of traditional, plant-based therapies. This all changed starting in the early 1970s when consumers quickly returned ''back to nature.'' The dramatic changes in consumer perceptions that started some 30 years ago are still strong as ever. This evolutionary change in the society is reflected in a strong interest by the consumer in cosmetic care formulations having a ''natural'' benefit. The trend toward ''nature'' is paralleled by a fast-growing scientific knowledge about plant constituents, human molecular biology, and cell physiology.

Identification and commercialization of new efficacious materials are nowadays stronger than ever, and guided by looking at active principles found in native plant species. Using natural plant extracts in a cosmetic product offers the potential for improved product performance in addition to an appealing marketing story. The success of many mass and prestige products based largely on plant materials is testimony to this fact.

It is important to note however, that not everything that originates from nature can automatically be considered beneficial or safe. Expertise is needed in the selection and application of natural extracts.

DEFINITION

By definition, an extract is the product of a purification procedure that is able to be isolated from a given matrix. One might think of using the entire plant, e.g., dried leaves or ground plant material, for a given cosmetic application. The disadvantages of doing so might be poor application properties attributable to solid particles in the formulation, potential microbiological problems, and/or the requirement of a significantly elevated level of plant material to deliver the same active constituents as an extract would. Using purified extracts for cosmetic formulations is therefore much more convenient and safe.

CATEGORIZING EXTRACTS

There are several ways to categorize plant extracts. Some of the most common methods of differentiation are as follows:

1. Application area (e.g., anti-inflammatory, antimicrobial, moisturizing)
2. Botanical name and family together with origin
3. Extraction method used (e.g., infusion, percolation, maceration, solvents used, steam distillation)

KEY STEPS IN PRODUCTION AND INFLUENCES ON QUALITY

A number of sophisticated approaches exist on how to isolate a specific extract from herbs. However, there are some common steps.

Plant Cultivation, Harvesting, and Collecting

The process begins simply with the growing plant itself. This happens at random out in the fields or by cultivation. Although "wild crafting" is still a method used for some species, cultivated plants can be harvested much more easily. Wild crafting additionally leaves the risk of collecting the wrong species and getting impure plant material for extraction. By using analytical methods, one is able to identify the purity of the herb. To minimize contamination, the collectors should be well educated about their work. One of the major factors that must always be considered is the concern of overharvesting. The major concerns of farmers as well as commercial customers is the continued availability of raw material. Proper cultivation of plants in a controlled environment offers greater security that plant species can be made available. Today many plants are also available that are "organically grown." Because no pesticides, chemical fertilizers, or chemical growing aids are used, there is a greater assurance that a minimum of such residues will be found in the extract. However, because analytical methods have become increasingly sensitive (concentration in the parts per trillion range can now routinely be detected), even some traces might be detected in those qualities as well.

Both of these methods, wild crafting and cultivating, are sensitive to seasonal changes and may produce different levels of active constituents depending on the time of year as well as the quality of the soil conditions. However, one of the most important points is the time of harvest. It should be at the peak of the activity level of the plant. Analytical techniques are available today that offer the farmer accurate information on when the right time for harvesting is.

Drying

In most cases plants are dried before extraction. The drying process results in a loss of between 60% to 80% of its weight as moisture and the plant actives are being concentrated by up to three to four times based on weight. Generally, mild conditions are used, usually between 100 and 140°F (38–60°C). In some cases, fresh plant material might be required for extraction (usually whenever sensitive constituents could be totally damaged by drying). Specific examples are extracts with a special sensory profile for perfumery or flavor compositions, as well as extracts showing enzymatic activity. In those cases, fresh plant material has to be used. This requires a well-organized infrastructure for a ''just in time'' processing in order to avoid breakdown by micro-organisms. Generally, fresh plant extraction takes place during the harvest period of the plant and results in unused extraction capacity during the rest of the year, which might increase production costs.

Drug Preparation for Extraction

Whenever an active is found in only one part of a plant, garbling has to be performed to rid those parts of the plant that should not enter the extraction. For a high-yield extraction, most often the dried drug particles have to be prechopped or minced and then put into a grinding system. Thermal stress during the process should be avoided. Therefore, some mills use liquid nitrogen.

Extraction

Water Extraction

Usually the process is performed with cold (maceration) or hot (infusion) water on dried and broken plant material. This method delivers polar, water-soluble molecules from the source. Hot-water extraction offers the advantage of sterilization, as well as a potential disadvantage of heat-accelerated chemical reactions, which can induce breakdown or transformation of active constituents.

Solvent Extraction

A variety of solvents can be used, e.g., ethanol, isopropanol, acetone, or hexane. Generally, less polar components are extracted than with water. Hexane is particularly well suited to dissolve unpolar components like oils and waxes. The extraction of polar constituents with alcohols or mixtures of alcohol and water is often more selective than the extraction with pure water. However, in some cases a certain degree of oils and waxes are also extracted, which leads to difficult application properties. Solvent residues are a concern to be checked in these types of extracts. A special case to consider is the extraction using supercritical CO_2. Its polarity could be varied via changing temperature and pressure between hexane and ether. Because it is a gas it does not leave solvent residues. Unpolar substrates and smaller molecules, e.g., essential oils, could be extracted very selectively and commonly show only a minimum of color. The high-pressure jacketed extraction vessels and longer process times usually make this technology more expensive.

Steam Distillation

This method easily separates volatile compounds from all others. It has been used since ancient times to gain essential oils from plants. The process is started with the plant being placed into boiling water; steam is feted directly into the flask and the condensate with all the volatiles is collected. The process usually takes several hours and requires heating up to 100°C. This might lead to chemical changes as, e.g., seen for the steam distillation of chamomile by the formation of the blue azulene from a colorless precursor (matricin).

Extract Concentration and Drying of Extracts

If necessary, solvents could be removed from the extract by, e.g., thin-layer distillation or spray drying. Both technologies place only minimal thermal stress on the extract. Thin-layer distillation even allows the removal of traces of organic solvents from a liquid formulation to yield the required level of extract. Liquid extracts with a suitable water activity usually require the addition of a preservative to prevent bacterial growth. Chemical reactions, e.g., polycondensation, may occur in the liquid phase. Solid-spray dried extracts offer good microbiological and chemical stability compared with liquid extracts, but in some cases there are difficulties in incorporating these powders into clear cosmetic systems. If there are no stability concerns, liquid extracts might offer a cost benefit because they spare the process step of concentration.

ANALYTICAL TECHNIQUES

Analytical techniques, such as high-performance liquid chromatography (HPLC) and to some extent gas chromatography (GC), provide a very useful tool to check quality as well as to make certain the presence of a plant constituent in a consumer product. HPLC is usually the preferred method, because it is very sensitive and provides reliable and quantitative data on the content of a certain compound. Thin-layer chromatography (TLC or HPTLC) is sometimes suitable as well if the mixture is not too complex and only a rough semiquantitative identity of the active is needed. A very powerful analytical device is the combination of HPLC with mass spectrometry (HPLC-MS). This approach allows a fast, highly selective detection and quantification. This system is also able to separate complicated molecular structures in complex mixtures.

CONSTITUENTS TO AVOID

Undesired constituents, which might have entered the process chain at some stage, can be pesticides, fungicides (agrochemical treatment), polycondensated aromatic compounds (flame drying), heavy metals, aflatoxins (microbiological, carcinogenic metabolites), and specific plant constituents with known toxic side effects. The manufacturer of an extract should specify the absence of such impurities, respectively, toxic compounds, and guarantee certain legal limits for them.

STANDARDIZATION

If the beneficial constituents of an extract are known, establishing specific quality standards is not difficult. It has to be assured by a suitable analytical technique that the extract contains a certain level of these active constituents. By way of an example, the anti-inflammatory constituents of oat extract (*Avena sativa*) have recently been discovered [2]. This was a difficult task because the chemistry of oat is quite complex. The active in oat belongs to a group of compounds called avenanthramides [3]. Only a few parts per million (ppm) are necessary to achieve a significant redness reduction of a UV-induced erythema [2]. Knowing now the active principle, it is possible to drive the extraction process in a way of receiving the highest quality extract in regard to its activity level as well as giving a minimum guarantee on the amount of active in the extract. Standardization provides the cosmetic formulator a better guarantee of consistent raw material and ultimately product performance.

Sometimes there is more than one active in an extract. Chamomile, e.g., contains several anti-inflammatory constituents [4]. The two major compounds are bisabolol and apigenin-7-glucoside. Standardization of a chamomile product could include either all compounds that have a similar level of activity or only the most active.

Not all discussions regarding standardization are as clear as with the previous examples. In some cases, the cause for activity (as well as the active constituent) has yet to be proven. One example of a substance that continues to cause controversy concerns a common plant: *Aloe barbadensis*. Its efficacy is well documented in various in vivo studies, whereas the active principle has not yet been fully elucidated [5]. Standardization and analysis are therefore less easy to perform [6], and a well-defined production process is important here to always receive the same quality.

In some cases where the active is currently unknown, it might be possible to standardize on another constituent. This substance could be typical for the particular species but not necessarily responsible for the plant extract's activity. The logic behind that is if there are variations regarding the level for the typical standard, the unknown active may vary with the same magnitude. This might not always be correct but is a reasonable working basis. At least this gives a rough tool to check the amount of plant used to produce the extract by comparing the level in the crude drug with that of the extract. It has to be in line with the drug/extract ratio, which should be specified by the manufacturing company. Moreover, it is one very helpful criterion to assure detection of a plant in a consumer product as well. To give an example, willowherb (*Epilobium angustifolium* [7]) is known for its anti-inflammatory efficacy, although the exact reason for its activity is uncertain [8,8a]. However, the plant contains a very typical constituent, called oenothein B [9]. This specific tannin could serve as a monitor for the quality of the extract as well as an identification tool.

There also exists a group of plant extracts for which it is hard to find characteristic constituents suitable for analysis. An example is cucumber extract. It contains mucilaginous polysaccharides, which are difficult to analyze. The minimum requirements for documentation of consistency of extracts with unknown active or lead compound(s) should include the botanical name of the species extracted, location of growth, process used for extraction, drug/extract ratio, stability data, data on impurities, safety data, and legal status.

EFFICACY TESTING

With the large variety of natural extracts it is possible to cover the full spectrum of cosmetic benefits. For details on claim substantiation see Chapter 65 of this book. An insight of possible claims can be offered only by in vivo studies. However, with the help of in vitro test data, prediction of in vivo activities could be made. Therefore, in vitro testing is of particular interest for research on previously undiscovered activities in plant extracts as well as for substantiation of previously described ones. Many physiological processes in human skin could meanwhile be modeled and monitored. Examples include the inflammation cascade by messenger molecules (IL-1α, PGE$_2$, LTB$_4$), collagen/elastin production from fibroblasts (ELISA for procollagen), collagen matrix degradation (MMP activity), antioxidant potential, or melanin formation.

INFORMATION SOURCES

Quite informative sources for cosmetic chemists are the sections in pharmacopoeial or medicinal plant handbooks [10] dealing with plant extracts and preparations. Botanical handbooks might give useful general information about the plant used for the extract. Another useful source is the Internet, either in searching for information on a particular species with the available search engines or by using free databases [11].*

FINAL REMARKS

Considering natural extracts for consumer products requires an inspiring relationship with nature and science. Specific know-how is required to ensure the safe incorporation of a substance in a cosmetic formulation. Natural extract suppliers should be called on to offer guidance of proper concentrations as well as regulatory status of the material they offer. The ultimate goal of the use of a natural extract is to provide the basis for a better cosmetic product that can benefit the consumer.

REFERENCES

1. Ebbell B. trans. rhe Papyrus Ebers. Copenhagen: Levin & Munksgaard, 1937. Bryan, C.P., tr. 1931. rhe Papyrus Ebers. New York: D. Appleton & Co.
2. Vollhardt J, Redmond M, Fielder D. Proceedings of the 21st IFSCC Congress 2000, Verlag für chemische Industrie. Augsburg, Germany: H. Ziolkowsky, GmbH.
3. Collins FW. Oat phenolics: avenanthramides, novel substituted n-cinnamoylanthanilate alkaloids form oat groats and hulls. J Agric Food Chem 1989; 37:60–66.
4. Ammon HPT, Kaul R. Pharmakologie der kamille und ihrer inhaltsstoffe. Deutsche Apoth Ztg 1992; 132:1–26.
5. (a) Reynolds T. The compounds on aloe leaf exudates: a review. Observations on the phytochemistry of the aloe leaf-exudate compounds. Bot J Linnean Soc 1985; 90:157–199. (b) Joshi SP. Chemical constituents and biological activity of *Aloe barbadensis*: a review. J Med Aromatic Plant Sci 1998; 20:768–773. (c) Yagi A. Bioactive components of aloe vera. Aromatopia 1997; 24:50–52. (d) Park MK, Park JH, Shin YG, Lee SK. Chemical constituents of aloe species. Seoul Univ J of Pharma Sci 1996; 21:43–63.
6. Ross SA, Elsohly MA, Wilkins SP. Quantitative analysis of aloe vera mucilaginous polysaccharide in commercial aloe vera products. J AOAC Intl 1997; 80:455–457.
7. Hetherington M, Steck W. Natural Chemicals from Northern Prairie. Saskatoon, Canada: Fytokem Products Inc., 1997.
8. Hetherington M, Dudka G, Steck W. New functional substances form Canadian Willowherb. Pasadena: SCC Meeting, Sept. 28, 1997.
8a. Juan H, Sametz W, Hiermann A. Agents and Actions 1988; 23:106–107.
9. Ducrey B, Marston A, Gohring S, Hartmann RW, Hostettmann K. Inhibition of 5α reductase and aromatase by the ellagitannins oenothein A and oenothein B form Epilobium spec. Planta Medica 1997; 63:111–114.
10. (a) Bradley PR. British Herbal Compendium: A Handbook of Scientific Information on Widely Used Plant Drugs. Dorset, UK: British Herbal Medicine Association, 1992. (b) Wichtl M, Grainger Bisset N, eds. Herbal Drugs and Phytopharmaceuticals. Boca Raton: CRC Press, 1994. (c) Hocking GM. A dictionary of natural products. Terms in the field of pharmacognosy relating to natural medicinal and pharmaceutical materials and the plants, animals and minerals from which they are derived. Medford, NJ: Plexus Publishing, Inc., 1997. (d) Harborne JB, Baxter H. Dictionary of Plant Toxins. Chichester: John Wiley & Sons, 1996. [See also Phyto-

---

* General information about herbs: http://www.herbnet.com, http://www.herb-encyclopedia.com, http://www.herbalgram.org/directory.html, http://www.botanical.com.

chemical Dictionary of Harborne and Baxter. 1993.] (e) Duke JA. Handbook of Phytochemical Constituents of GRAS Herbs and Other Economic Plants. Boca Raton: CRC Press, 1992. (f) McIntyre A. Complete Guide to Medicinal Plants for the Health and Beauty of Today's Woman. Barcelona, Spain: Planeta. (g) Graves G. Medicinal Plants: An Illustrated Guide to More Than 180 Herbal Plants. London: Bracken Books, 1996. (h) Millspaugh CF. Medicinal Plants: An Illustrated and Descriptive Guide to Plants Indigenous to and Naturalized in the United States which are used in medicine, Vol. 2. Philadelphia: J. C. Yorston & Co., 1892. (i) Still CC. Botany and healing. Medicinal plants of New Jersey and the region. New Brunswick: Rutgers University Press, 1998. (j) Karnick CR. Pharmacopoeial standards of herbal plants, Vols. 1 and 2. Delhi, India: Sri Satguru Publications, 1994.

11. (a) Economic and Medicinal Botany. University of Maryland. http://www.inform.umd.edu/ PBIO/FindIT/ecmd.html. (b) Missouri Botanical Garden: Research: Databases (Large literature collection). http://www.mobot.org/MOBOT/database.html. (c) Botanical Dermatology Database: Richard J. Schmidt: 1994–1999. http://bodd.cf.ac.uk/. (d) Poisonous plant databases: Cornell University, Poisonous Plants Home Page. http://www.ansci.cornell.edu/plants/ plants.html. (e) http://www.scs.leeds.ac.uk/pfaf/D_other.html. (f) Botanical Museum, Finnish Museum of Natural History. http://www.helsinki.fi/kmus/botecon.html.

33

Rheological Additives and Stabilizers

Ekong A. Ekong, Mohand Melbouci, Kate Lusvardi,
and Paquita E. Erazo-Majewicz
Hercules Incorporated, Wilmington, Delaware

INTRODUCTION

The use of rheological additives such as clays, plant exudates, and natural polymers, to formulate personal-care products dates back to ancient times. These rheological additives are used to thicken the fluid, suspend dispersions of additives in the fluid, and improve the stability of the ensuing dispersion or emulsion as a function of temperature and shear history. An attempt will be made in this chapter to classify the wide array of rheological additives with respect to the actual function they serve in the final product.

THICKENERS

Water and oils form the base fluids in which most personal-care and cosmetic products are formulated. These base fluids are generally classed as viscous or Newtonian fluids in that they possess a characteristic viscosity that is independent of the imposed rate of deformation. Newtonian fluids are also viewed as ideal fluids, in that they flow readily when subjected to very low deformations.

Non-Newtonian fluids on the other hand possess viscosities that are dependent on the rate of deformation and may exhibit other properties such as elasticity, yield stress, and thixotropy not seen in Newtonian fluids.

Newtonian Fluids

A schematic of the viscosity profiles of Newtonian and non-Newtonian fluids is shown in Figure 1. Fluid (a) represents a typical viscosity of the base fluid, which might be water, oils or other low molecular weight solvents. The viscosity of these fluids can be modified by addition of particulates that may strictly change the viscosity index as illustrated by the higher viscosity for fluid (b). When non-interacting buoyant particles are used in these fluids, the viscosity of the dispersion can be predicted using the Einstein relation [1].

$$\mu = \mu_o(1 + 2.5\phi + \ldots) \tag{1}$$

where μ and μ_o are viscosities of the dispersion and medium respectively and ϕ is the volume fraction of the particles. Examples of such rheology-modifying substances include

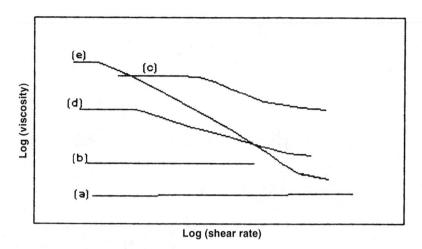

FIGURE 1   Schematic of flow properties of Newtonian and non-Newtonian fluids.

silica gels, fumed silica, carbon black, titanium dioxide and aluminum-magnesium-stearates when used at very small concentrations. Low molecular weight polymers also fit in this category and may be preferred if a smooth or fluid like formulation is desired. Their typical flow curve can also be represented by fluid (b) in Figure 1.

Non-Newtonian Fluids

Unlike Newtonian fluids, non-Newtonian fluids possess shear-rate dependent viscosities. Fluids (c), (d), and (e) in Figure 1 illustrates a range of non-Newtonian profiles observed in personal care formulations. In addition to shear-rate dependent viscosities, non-Newtonian fluids also exhibit elastic stresses when subjected to high shear rates. The usefulness of the elastic response varies with application, as will be illustrated in a later section.

The performance value of rheological additives that impart non-Newtonian characteristics to personal care formulations is demonstrated by the curve in Figure 2. On close

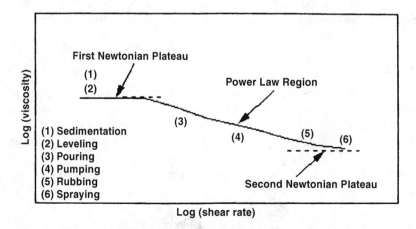

FIGURE 2   Schematic of full flow curve of non-Newtonian fluids.

examination of this figure, it is easy to see why non-Newtonian rheology is more common in personal care formulations than Newtonian (viscous) rheology.

At low shear rates, i.e., near at rest conditions, non-Newtonian fluids exhibit high viscosities that are relatively insensitive to shear rate and characterized by zero shear viscosity. The zero shear viscosity is known to be highly sensitive to the molecular weight and concentration of the rheological additives [2]. The rates of deformation associated with this region include sedimentation and levelling forces, and one can tailor the zero shear viscosity to combat these forces. At moderate shear rates the decrease in viscosity versus shear rate helps when pouring and pumping these fluids. At high shear rates it is found that a second Newtonian plateau in viscosity is reached usually characterised by the so-called infinite viscosity. The shear forces in this area are close in magnitude to forces developed during rubbing and spraying exercises. The low viscosities exhibited by the rheological additives in this region imply low resistance to rubbing and thus a smooth sensation of the substance during its application.

Elasticity

As discussed above, non-Newtonian fluids also exhibit elastic properties, i.e., when subjected to high shear rates, non-Newtonian fluids will exhibit elastic stresses. Figure 3 illustrates the elastic functions of the non-Newtonian fluids (c), (d), and (e) from Figure 1. Note that the elastic response tends to be seen at the higher shear rates.

It is generally observed that fluids that show more shear-thinning properties tend to show more elastic response [3]. This result is well demonstrated on comparison of the viscosity profiles of fluids (c), (d), and (e) in Figure 1 with their normal stress profiles in Figure 3. The rank order of shear-thinning performance for these fluids is fluid (e)>(d) >(c). An identical rank-order of elastic performance is seen for these same fluids in Figure 3.

The desirability of the elastic response will vary with the intended use of the personal care product. In the case of toothpaste, an elastic force is needed to increase extrudate spring back during the tube filling operation in toothpaste production or while dispensing it at home. However, excessive elasticity might not be desirable, as it may make the toothpaste too stringy. High elasticity is needed to stabilize foams, for example in shaving

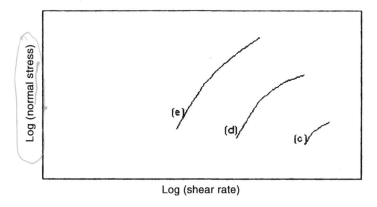

FIGURE 3 Schematic of elastic shear properties of non-Newtonian fluids.

creams, as it provides strength to film at the air/liquid interface in the matrix of bubbles. In the case of creams and lotions, a short texture with less elasticity may be desired.

Examples of substances that impart viscosity as well as elasticity to a fluid are cellulose ethers, xanthan gum, and crosslinked polyacrylic acids. Clays can impart viscosity without elasticity. In the following section, some of the many rheological additives available to personal care formulators will be highlighted. As will be seen, a variety of additives are available in the marketplace that allow formulators to create a range of viscosities and elasticities in the final product.

Interacting particulates such as smectic, hydrophilic and organoclays represent one class of materials used in personal care products that can impart non-Newtonian characteristics to formulations. At a very low concentration, they are known to impart significant viscosity enhancement to the base fluid without any significant elasticity. They typically exhibit a flow curve similar to fluid (C) in Figure 1. It is well-documented [4,5] that these materials cause gelling if used at higher concentrations.

In the case of polymers, their zero shear viscosity, shear-thinning, and elasticity characteristics are a function of their structural characteristics. The rigidity of the polymer, its weight average molecular weight, polydispersity, and degree of branching each play a part in determining these properties.

Water-soluble cellulose ether derivatives such as carboxymethylcellulose (CMC), hydroxyethylcellulose (HEC), hydroxypropyl cellulose, and methylcellulose impart pseudoplastic or shear-thinning rheology to formulations [6a,b]. This characteristic makes these polymers attractive candidates as thickening agents in personal care products.

For instance, this flow characteristic enables a product to pour as a rich, viscous solution from the container, yet be easily applied to a substrate like hair, as its viscosity reduces with shear. These polymers tend to impart high viscosities at low shear. They exhibit moderate shear-thinning behavior, but possess little elasticity at a moderate range of deformation rates, similar to the rheology profile of fluid (d) in Figure 1.

Some of the applications where these polymers are used include shampoos, conditioners, hair spray, and hair-styling gels, toothpastes, and denture adhesives.

This pseudoplastic rheology is particularly beneficial in surfactant-based haircare formulations like shampoos where cellulose ethers can be used to reduce or eliminate inorganic salt added for thickening [7]. Cellulosic thickeners can be used to achieve viscosities higher than possible with salt or even salt combined with alkanolamide. In many cases, even the alkanolamide can be replaced by the cellulose ether [8].

For example, incorporation of 1% hydroxyethylcellulose into a TEA-lauryl sulfate luxury shampoo increased the formulation viscosity from a Brookfield viscosity of 460 cps to a gel with a viscosity of 5300 cps [9].

Additional benefits can also be realised on incorporation of cellulose ethers into formulations. Unlike salt, cellulose ethers do not influence surfactant cloud points, and they can be used to viscosify surfactant systems that are difficult to thicken, such as imidazolidine-derived amphoterics, sulfosuccinates, and highly ethoxylated alkyl ether sulfates [10].

In other haircare applications, such as conditioning hair rinses, addition of a low level of hydroxyethylcellulose polymeric thickener can significantly increase finished product viscosity and improve shelf stability [11].

Cellulose ethers in general have this effect on product viscosity and shelf stability. Methylhydroxypropylcellulose effectively thickens sodium laureth sulfate; a surfactant commonly used in surfactant-based haircare formulations, yielding solutions with excel-

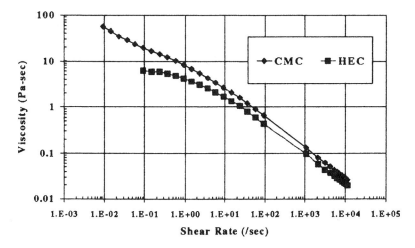

FIGURE 4 Flow properties of 1% cellulosic ether solutions at 25°C.

lent high temperature freeze/thaw stability. Cellulosics achieve this enhanced shelf stability by maintaining the viscosity of the formulation at room temperature, and during freeze/thaw cycling.

A typical rheological profile for two commercially available cellulose ether products, CMC and HEC, are shown in Figure 4. Note that the flow profiles for these materials resemble the profiles for fluids (d) and (e) in Figure 1.

SUSPENDING AGENTS

The storage stability of personal care formulations such as emulsions, suspensions and foams is of prime importance to formulators. Here again, rheological additives have been used widely to prevent sedimentation of solid particulates, prevent coalescence in emulsions, and halt collapse of foams. Rheological substances can impart suspending power to the base fluid. The polymer's yield stress or high viscosity at low shear rates are both used for this purpose. Fluids that possess a yield stress may experience flow only when the imposed stress on the fluid surpasses its yield stress. Below the yield stress the fluid displays solid like properties.

Among the polysaccharides, xanthan gum has been widely used as a suspending aid. Xanthan gum has a double helical structure and undergoes significant hydrogen bonding in solution. At rest or when subjected to very low deformations, a weak three dimensional network structure is the prevailing structure which gives rise to the yield stress [12]. When subjected to higher deformations, this structure can easily be broken down to give rheological behaviour similar to fluid (e) in Figure 1.

Other polysaccharides that exhibit yield stresses are kappa and iota carrageenans. These polysaccharides will also form weak gels and are used in personal care products for stabilization [6].

As discussed in the section on thickeners, cellulose ethers represent another class of polysaccharide-based rheological additives used as suspending aids.

Carboxymethylcellulose imparts a high viscosity at low shear to formulations, enabling it to effectively suspend solids. These characteristics are effectively described by

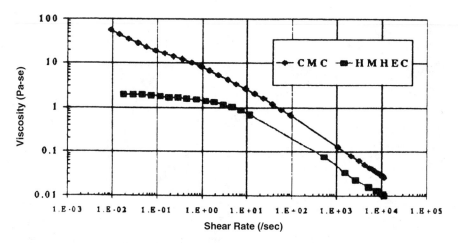

FIGURE 5   Flow properties of 1% cellulosic ether solutions at 25°C.

fluid (e) in Figure 1. CMC has a high capacity for water-binding, and it is generally used to effect rheology and prevent syneresis in high solids formulations [13].

Methylhydroxypropylcellulose has been shown to enhance shampoo lather by way of the water-binding, surface activity, and thermal gelation properties of this cellulose ether. This polymer can stabilize lather by a mechanism known as interfacial gelation [14].

Hydrophobically modified cellulose ethers, such as modified hydroxyethylcellulose, viscosify aqueous phases through both hydrogen-bond network formation and through the formation of three-dimensional networks due to hydrophobic interactions. This dual thickening mechanism makes modified hydroxyethylcellulose particularly effective at suspending solids [15]. The hydrophobic moieties may also associate with surfactant micelles, making modified hydroxyethylcellulose a particularly efficient thickener for surfactant-based systems [16].

Modified hydroxyethylcellulose finds use in many applications, including viscosity and structure development in shampoos, conditioners, and in hand and body lotions [17]. Typical rheological profiles for a modified hydroxethyl cellulose (HMHEC) and CMC are shown in Figure 5.

Salts of cross-linked polyacrylic acids also exhibit considerable yield stresses. However, unlike the other substances, their ensuing structures tend to be much more sensitive to electrolytes [18]. The properties of these materials will be further discussed in the next section.

Colloidal size materials, like fumed silica, are also used for stabilization [5]. Fumed silica can be processed to develop aggregate particles, and thus form weak three-dimensional structures. Stabilization can also be achieved directly by milling the materials to be used in the formulation to colloidal sizes to take advantage of colloidal forces for stabilization.

THIXOTROPIC AGENTS

So far it has been assumed that the non-Newtonian substances discussed are relatively insensitive to the time scale of flow. It is assumed that if the rate of deformation is ramped up and then down, that there will be a superposition of both stress responses. This may not be the case, as will be demonstrated for toothpaste formulations, where the introduction of thixotropes proves quite useful.

As reviewed earlier in this section, viscosity describes the resistance of a liquid to flow and pseudoplasticity relates to the decrease in viscosity observed with increasing shear rates. Thixotropy, however, is a time-dependent phenomenon, defined as:

- The ability of the substance to exhibit lower viscosities as a function of shear rate and duration.
- And its ability to have its structure reformed over a period of time.

For toothpaste, a great effort has been directed towards optimisation of toothpaste physical attributes. These attributes are strongly dependent on rheological characteristics of the toothpaste system, such as viscosity, pseudoplasticity, thixotropy and low shear yield stress.

Various types of rheological additives find their utility in toothpaste formulations. To perform adequately, they must exhibit a strong three-dimensional structure in lean solvent systems while providing the optimum rheological characteristics described above. Toothpaste exhibiting combined properties such as thixotropic behaviour and high yield value are particularly useful.

The main function of thickening and binding agents in toothpaste systems is to impart adequate paste texture and rheology during preparation, storage and utilisation, good stability with no phase separation or syneresis, smooth and shiny aspect, and improved mouthfeel, foamability, and rinsability. These are directly linked with the rheological characteristics of viscosity, pseudoplasticity, thixotropy, and yield stress.

The thixotropy of a toothpaste system can be described by a rheogram representing a plot of shear stress against shear rate. The hysteresis area between the up curve and down curve is defined, as the energy required to break the network structure of the toothpaste. It gives an indication of the degree of thixotropy of the system as given in Figure 6.

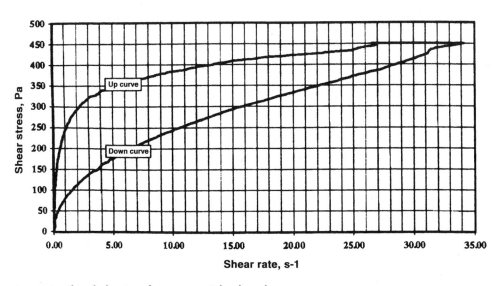

FIGURE 6 Flow behavior of a commercial gel toothpaste.

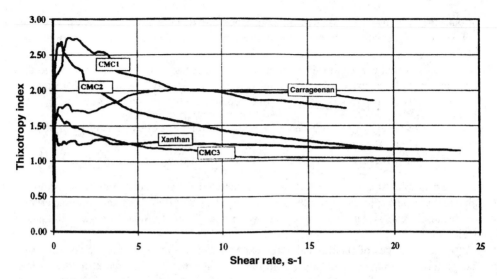

FIGURE 7 Thixotropy of medium water content cream toothpaste.

Five major rheological additive types are currently used in toothpaste systems. They are generally classified into four main categories: 1) natural, 2) modified natural, 3) synthetics, and 4) inorganic. These classes are represented respectively by 1) xanthan gum, carrageenan; 2) cellulose ethers; 3) crosslinked polyacrylic acids; 4) clays and amorphous silicone dioxide.

Figure 7 shows the thixotropic index (TI) of various gums in a cream toothpaste formulation. The thixotropic index is defined as the ratio of the up-curve viscosity to the down curve viscosity measured at the same shear rate. The higher the index, the more thixotropic is the dispersion. For reference a TI of 1.0 means that the dispersion is not thixotropic.

The figure clearly shows CMC 1 gives the most thixotropic structure to this formulation. For cellulose gums, the thixotropic index is shear rate dependent; the extent to which the structure rebuilds is dependent on the shear history to which the gums were subjected.

In comparison with the other gums, xanthan is not thixotropic. The thixotropic index of this formulation is not dependent on the shear rate. The structure is recovered almost instantaneously. Carrageenan has a higher thixotropic index than seen with xanthan gum, but it also recovers its initial structure very quickly.

Interacting fillers such as clay, fumed silica, and aluminum-magnesium hydroxide are also used as thixotropic modifiers in personal care products [19]. These materials tend to form complex networks or gels that show time-dependent rheological properties.

GELLING AGENTS

Hermans [20] suggested that the name gel should be given to systems that display the following features: 1) coherent, two-component systems formed by a solid substance finely dispersed or dissolved in a liquid phase; 2) exhibit solid-like behaviour under the action of mechanical forces; 3) both the dispersed component and the solvent should extend continuously throughout the whole system, each phase being interconnected.

Rheological characterization divides gels into two major classes, strong and weak gels. Strong gels possess the canonical features of true gels. They manifest typical behaviour of viscoelastic solids and rupture beyond a certain deformation value rather than flow. Weak gels resemble strong gels at low deformation rates but their three dimensional networks get progressively broken down at higher deformation rates and they flow as a dispersed system. Physical gels produced by these rheological substances are best described by their viscoelastic properties. Using dynamic oscillatory experiments, the elastic and viscous components of gels can be quantified by G', the elastic modulus which is a measure of energy storage and G", the loss modulus, a measure of energy dissipation at a given deformation. Physical gels will typically show G' to be much higher than G" when measured as a function of frequency. The slope of G' values as a function of frequency best differentiates strong gels from weak gels. Strong gels exhibits a nearly flat G' profile as opposed to weak gels that show a more positive slope [21].

There are several polysaccharides used in personal care formulations that can undergo gelation as a function of ionic strength, pH, and heat treatment. Gelatine, agar, pectins, alginates, and kappa carrageenans will undergo gelation to yield strong gels. Solid air fresheners are a good example of the type of strong gel character achievable with polymers such as carrageenans.

Salts of crosslinked polyacrylic acid, iota-carrageenan, and cellulose ethers, will also form gels and are used in personal care formulations that exploit weak gel properties. They are highly useful in skin creams, shaving gels, hair styling gels, and gel toothpaste formulations.

Literature and formulation ingredients in commercial creams and lotions suggest that a popular approach to providing both emulsification and stabilization is through a three-dimensional surfactant/cosurfactant network. Rheological characterization of commercial creams and lotions, performed using oscillation tests on a controlled stress rheometer, are shown in Figure 8. These results demonstrate the range of rheologies available on combination of different polymeric stabilizers with these surfactant structures [22].

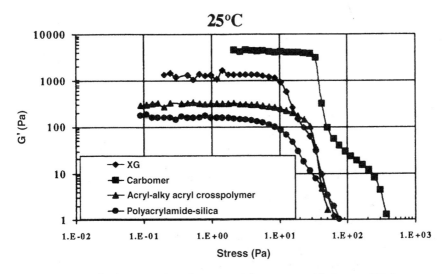

FIGURE 8 **Viscoelastic properties of commercial creams and lotions at 25°C.**

The surfactant-gel network system provides a yield stress, a high degree of elasticity, shear-thinning behavior, and time-dependent structure build-up (thixotropy). These rheological attributes are very important in the consumer's perception of skin feel during lotion application and rub-in.

The primary component of these liquid crystalline gel network systems is a cosurfactant. Cosurfactants are water-insoluble fatty amphiphiles that are too lipophilic to promote o/w emulsions. Cosurfactants combined with a small fraction of a water-soluble surfactant having a high hydrophilic-lipophilic balance (HLB), produce swollen lamellar-gel networks after thermal processing and cooling.

A physical gel forming rheological additive, such as a cellulose ether, cross-linked polyacrylate, clay, or xanthan gum is added to improve temperature stability and modify the rheology of these systems.

A plot of elastic modulus, G' as a function of imposed stress for commercial creams containing xanthan gum (XG), crosslinked sodium polyacrylate (carbomer), Acrylate/ C10-30 alkyl acrylate crosspolymer and polyacrylamide/silica is presented in Figure 8. The elastic modulus, G', at low stresses is a measure of the gel rigidity of the sample. These results serve to distinguish the more solid-like creams, with G' values > 1000 Pa at low shear, from the more liquid-like lotions, with G' values < 1000 Pa at low shear.

Other materials that can form weak gels when given the appropriate mechanical treatment are silica gels and fumed silica. These materials are sometimes used in combination with other polymers to yield weak gels. They are used in toothpaste where it serves a dual role as an abrasive and a rheology modifier. The thickening silicas are the only inorganic products used extensively to structure toothpaste. They provide a good thickening effect and high thixotropic behaviour, but they lack the ability to bind water in the lean solvent slurry. As a result, they are unsuitable for syneresis control. Therefore, a water-soluble organic binder is necessary to modify the toothpaste rheology and to prevent water separation. Carboxymethylcellulose and carrageenans are often combined with silica for this purpose.

Due to the broad performance criteria that personal care products have to meet, most formulators find it necessary to use a mixture of rheological additives to achieve desired properties in final formulations. Mixtures of materials can bring significant synergy in desired properties. In conclusion, rheological additives significantly influence the mechanical, textural, stability, and ultimately the quality of personal care products.

REFERENCES

1. Einstein A. Ann Phys 1906; 19:289–306.
2. Berry GC, Fox TG. Adv Poly Sci 1968; 5:261.
3. Graessley WW. Adv Poly Sci 1974; 16:1.
4. The Benefits of Hectorite Clay, NL Chemical Technical Lit. Hightown, NJ: NL Industries, PB 149. June 1988.
5. Ca-bo-sil Fumed Silica Properties and Functions, Technical Literature. Tuscola, IL: Cabot Corporation, February 1990.
6a. Desmarais AJ, Wint RF. Hydroxyalkyl ethyl ethers of cellulose. In: Industrial Gums. 3d ed. Whistler RL, BeMiller JN, eds. 1992:505.
6b. Feddersen RL, Thorp SN. Sodium carboxymethyl cellulose. In: Industrial Gums. 3d ed. Whistler RL, BeMiller JN, eds. 3d ed. 1992:537.
7. Reng AK, Skryzpak W. Ways to regulate the viscosity of cosmetic preparations. Cosmet Toilet 1979; 94:29–36.

8. Schoenberg T. Formulating without diethanolamides. Household and Personal Products Industry 1998; 35(7):76–79.
9. Performance of Aqualon Water-Soluble Polymers in Shampoos, Aqualon Bulletin VC-526B. September 1989.
10. Hunting ALL. Shampoo thickeners. Cosmet Toilet 1982; 97:53–63.
11. Performance of Natrosol® Hydroxyethylcellulose in Hair-Conditioning Products, Aqualon Bulletin VC-525. October 1987.
12. Davidson RL, ed. Handbook of Water-Soluble Gums and Resins. NY: McGraw-Hill, Inc., 1980:24–27.
13. Aqualon cellulose ethers and their role in toothpaste. Aqualon technical literature 87.507-E2. March 1998.
14. Conklin J, McKnight SM. Cellulose ethers. Household and Personal Products Industry 1988; 25:80–84.
15. Goodwin JW, et al. Polymers in aqueous media: performance through association. Glass JE, ed. Advances in Chemistry Series, 223. Washington, D.C.: American Chemical Society, 1989: 365.
16. AC Sau, Landoll LM. Glass JE, ed. Advances in Chemistry Series, 223. Washington, D.C.: American Chemical Society, 1989:343.
17. Natrosol® *Plus* CS, Grade 330 Modified Hydroxyethylcellulose, Thickener for Hand and Body Lotions, Aqualon Bulletin VC-562A. Wilmington, Delaware: Hercules Inc., October 1992.
18. Laba D, ed. Rheological Properties of Cosmetics and Toiletries. Vol. 13. New York: Marcel Dekker, Inc., 1993.
19. Reference 18, p. 123–145.
20. Hermans PH. Colloid Science. Vol. II. NY: Elsevier Science Publishers, 1949, p. 194.
21. Doublier JL, Choplin L. Carbohydrate Research. A Rheological Description of Amylose Gelation. 1989; 193:215.
22. Barnum PE. Presentation at SCC Mid Atlantic Chapter, Raw Material Symposium "Gums, Polymers & Thickeners for Rheology Modification of Personal Care Products," March 9, 1999.

34

Silicones: A Key Ingredient in Cosmetic and Toiletry Formulations

Janet M. Blakely
Dow Corning S.A., Brussels, Belgium

UNIQUE MATERIALS

Silicone is a generic name for many classes of organo-silicone polymer which consist of an inorganic siloxane (Si—O) backbone with pendant organic groups (usually methyl) (Fig. 1). It is this structure that gives silicones their unique combination of properties and, in particular, their surface properties.

Siloxane Backbone

The prime role of the siloxane backbone is to present the available methyl groups to their best advantage and it does this by virtue of its unique flexibility. In most hydrocarbons, the bond angles are very fixed and steric packing considerations often prevent the available methyls from adopting lowest surface energy orientations. In silicones, the Si—O bond length is significantly longer and the Si—O—Si bond angle flatter than comparable C—C and C—O bonds resulting in a very low barrier to rotation and making the polymer chains very flexible. This flexibility makes many orientations possible and provides "free space" to accommodate different sized substituents or to allow easy diffusion of gaseous molecules; a property useful in the formation of "breathable" films. Coupled with the low intermolecular forces between methyl groups, this flexibility also has a profound effect on the bulk as well as the surface properties of silicones. This is seen in the small variation of physical parameters with temperature and molecular weight, the low freezing and pour points of fluids, the low boiling points, the high compressibility and the retention of liquid nature to unusually high molecular weights. It also makes a number of structural and compositional variations possible, resulting in many families of silicones, including linear and cyclic structures, a wide range of molecular weights and varying degrees of branching or cross linking. Additionally, the siloxane bond is exceptionally strong providing the polymer with a high degree of thermal and oxidative stability and ensuring stability when formulated [1–3].

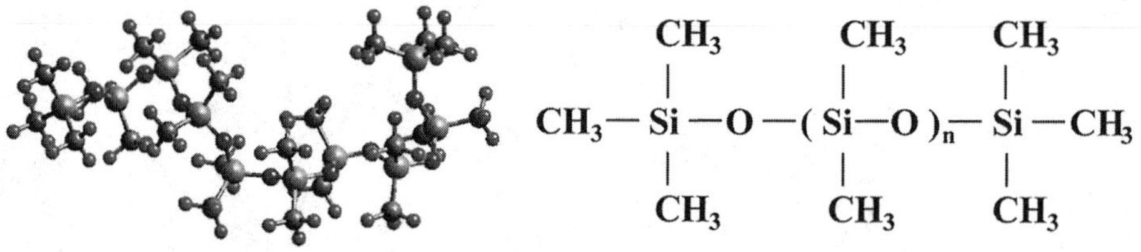

$$CH_3-\underset{\underset{\displaystyle CH_3}{|}}{\overset{\overset{\displaystyle CH_3}{|}}{Si}}-O-(\underset{\underset{\displaystyle CH_3}{|}}{\overset{\overset{\displaystyle CH_3}{|}}{Si}}-O)_n-\underset{\underset{\displaystyle CH_3}{|}}{\overset{\overset{\displaystyle CH_3}{|}}{Si}}-CH_3$$

Dimethicone polydimethylsiloxane (PDMS)

FIGURE 1   Unique chemical structure of silicones.

Pendant Organic Groups

The key function of the organic (methyl) groups is to provide the intrinsic surface activity of the silicones. The order of increasing surface energy for single carbon based groups is $-CF3 > -CF2- > -CH3 > -CH2-$. Liquid surface tension measurements show that, as expected, the order of increasing surface activity is hydrocarbon, followed by silicone, and then by fluorocarbon. Interfacial tension measurements against water, however, show the order of increasing interfacial activity to be fluorocarbon, hydrocarbon, silicone. Silicones do not fit the simple pattern that a reduction in surface energy means an increase in hydrophobicity and interfacial tension because of their backbone flexibility, which allows them to adopt various orientations at different interfaces. The interfacial tension of silicone is also independent of chain length indicating high molecular chain freedom. In addition, critical surface tension of wetting values for silicones have been found to be higher than their liquid surface tension values, meaning that they are able to spread over their own absorbed film. This has an advantage in achieving complete, uniform surface coverage, facilitates the efficient spreading of other materials and results in smooth, lubricating films. In addition, due to the organic groups, the solubility parameters of silicones are significantly lower than those of water and many organic materials making them useful in forming barriers to wash-off or wear and increasing the substantivity of formulations. The introduction of functional groups such as phenyl, alkyl, polyether, amino etc. onto the backbone expands the properties and benefits of silicones further [1–3].

KEY INGREDIENTS IN THE COSMETICS AND TOILETRIES INDUSTRY

Silicones were first used in the cosmetics and toiletries industry in the 1950s, when low levels of medium-viscosity Dimethicone (polydimethylsiloxane) was used to prevent the whitening effect, characteristic of soap-based skin lotions. It was not until the 1970s, when formulators were concerned about the use of CFCs in aerosols, that silicones were considered more seriously as possible ingredients for cosmetic formulations and their unique properties began to be recognized. Since then, the use of silicones has expanded rapidly to virtually all segments and today, 43% of all new products being introduced into the U. S. market contain silicone, with many different types being used [4].

There are five main families of silicones which are used in the cosmetics and toiletries industry today:

1. Cyclomethicones (cyclosiloxanes) are volatile fluids with ring structures. The most commonly used materials are the tetramer, pentamer and hexamer or blends of these. They are good solvents and serve as good carriers for high molecular weight silicones that would otherwise be very difficult to handle. In

addition, they have very low heats of vaporisation compared to water or ethanol giving them a non-cooling feel when drying. Cyclomethicones are classified as non-VOC (volatile organic compounds) in the USA.

2. Dimethicones (polydimethylsiloxanes-PDMS) are linear structures ranging from volatile to non-volatile with increasing molecular weight. Volatile Dimethicones exist as fluids with viscosities of 0.65–2 mm^2/s. Non-volatile Dimethicones exist as fluids with viscosities of 5.0 mm^2/s up to gums. Dimethicone emulsions make handling of the higher molecular weight fluids easier.

3. Silicone blends consist of Dimethiconol or Dimethicone gums or Trimethylsiloxysilicates (highly crosslinked resins) dispersed in lower molecular weight Dimethicones or Cyclomethicones. They have been developed to improve ease of formulation and compatibility of high molecular gums or resins; used for their substantivity.

4. Dimethicone and Vinyldimethicone Crosspolymers or blends are silicone elastomers. They exist in powder form or as elastomeric silicone gels that are swollen with solvent (usually Cyclomethicone). The introduction of different functionalities into such products is also possible. They are used as rheology modifiers in skincare and antiperspirant products, providing a dry, powdery feel to formulations.

5. Functional Silicones:

   (a) Dimethicone Copolyols (silicone polyethers) are fluids or waxes where some of the methyl groups along the siloxane backbone have been replaced with polyoxyethylene or polyoxypropylene groups. The addition of polyoxyethylene substituents increases the hydrophilicity of silicones. Polyoxypropylene substituents are used to balance out this hydrophilicity by increasing the hydrophobic characteristics of the copolymer (16).

   (b) Phenyl Trimethicones are fluids where some of the methyl groups have been replaced by phenyl groups. The phenyl groups increase the refractive index and improve compatibility with organic materials.

   (c) Amodimethicones are fluids where some of the methyl groups have been replaced by secondary and primary amine groups. The polar amine groups have a profound effect on the deposition properties of the silicone, giving it an affinity for negatively charged surfaces, such as the proteinaceous surface of the hair. Emulsions of these fluids are commonly used.

   (d) Alkyl Dimethicones are fluids or waxes where some of the methyl groups have been replaced by alkyl groups. This results in a family of silicone-hydrocarbon hybrids with possibilities for variations in viscosities, softening temperatures and rheological characteristics. They have increased compatibility with organic materials.

   (e) Cyclomethicone (and) Dimethicone Copolyol or Laurylmethicone Copolyol are silicone emulsifiers. They show ampiphilic behaviour and have been designed to emulsify aqueous phases into silicones; usually Cyclomethicone or low-medium polarity organic oils.

SKINCARE, SUNCARE, AND DECORATIVE PRODUCTS

Skin Feel/Emolliency

The main reason that silicones are used in all types of skin care product is because of their sensory properties. Studies on the emollient properties of various materials have shown that silicones deliver greater emolliency values than many commonly used cosmetic ingredients both, during and after application. They are described as smooth, velvety and non-greasy or oily and are able to impart this feel to cosmetic and toiletry formulations, improving the negative feel associated with other ingredients [5].

Cyclomethicones are used for transient effects giving slight lubricity, a light texture, fast spreading and good distribution of the product on application, whilst leaving no residual effects. They are often included in formulations to remove the greasy or oily feel of hydrocarbon-based emollients and are the basis for "oil-free" type claims [6]. They are used in light products for daily use such as facial cleansers, day creams or liquid foundations. Higher molecular weight silicones such as Dimethicone (and) Dimethiconol are used to give a more lubricious, longer lasting effect in richer, more nourishing skin treatment products such as night creams or after-sun products [7]. Silicone elastomers are used to give a dry, powdery feel to skincare formulations [8]. Silicones are also non-comedogenic/non-acnegenic unlike many occlusive, lipophilic fatty emollients which can promote comedone/acne formation on the skin [9].

Substantivity (Long-Lasting/Durability)

High molecular weight Dimethicones or Cyclomethicone (and) Dimethiconols form water-resistant films on the skin which can help prolong the effects of skin care, sun care or decorative products. This substantivity can be improved further by using Alkyl Dimethicones such as Cetyl Dimethicone or C30-45 Alkyl Methicone [7] (see Figure 2). The use of the substantivity of silicones to improve the substantivity of other ingredients in cosmetic and toiletry formulations has been demonstrated in sun care products. The addition of 2.5 wt% Cetyl Dimethicone to an oil-in-water sunscreen formulation shows excellent in vivo resistance to wash-off. The formulation has an in vivo SPF of 21.1 before immersion which reduces to 19.2 only, after immersion for 80 minutes [7] [10].

Cyclomethicones are the basis for long-lasting/non-transfer decorative products, especially lipsticks. They are used to disperse waxes and pigments, improve application and impart a pleasant skin feel, often replacing non-volatile hydrocarbon oils. When they evaporate, a uniform film of waxes and pigments remains which is resistant to transfer and wear [11].

Permeability/Controlled Moisturization/Protection Against Dehydration

Due to the flexibility of the Si—O—Si backbone, the majority of silicones are permeable to water vapour, producing "breathable" films. This is an important parameter for cleansing products or colour cosmetics to avoid clogging pores. The presence of an alkyl group in the chain, however, reduces this permeability, resulting in silicones which can give controlled moisturization, e.g., Stearyl Dimethicone or moisturization (occlusivity) similar to petrolatum e.g. C30-45 Alkyl Methicone [7] [12].

Enhanced Efficacy

Apart from improving the feel and long-lasting benefits of skincare products, silicones can also enhance the efficacy of other ingredients in the formulation. Studies carried out on suncare products have shown that the Alkylmethicones can enhance the in vitro SPF of products containing either organic or inorganic sunscreens. For inorganic sunscreens,

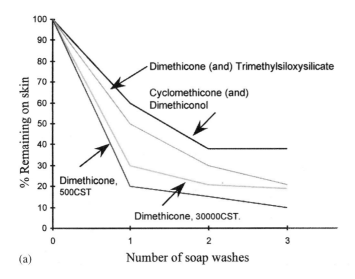

(a)   Number of soap washes

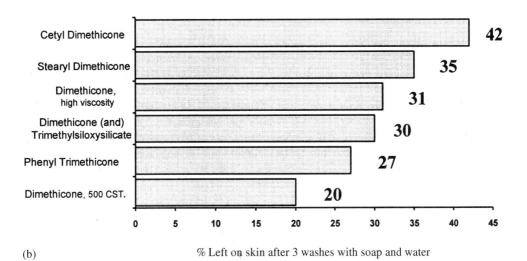

(b)   % Left on skin after 3 washes with soap and water

FIGURE 2   Substantivity of different silicones, FTIR method.

a 100% increase in in vitro SPF was seen with an oil-in-water system containing 2 wt% Cetyl Dimethicone and a 75% increase in the in vitro SPF for a water-in-oil system containing C30-45 Alkyl Methicone [10] [12].

Protection

Dimethicone is listed in the FDA Monograph for Skin Protectant Drug Products for OTC Human Use in the United States [12]. Due to their hydrophobicity, silicones are used in protective hand creams to provide a water-resistant barrier against water-borne contaminants. Recent studies indicate that Cyclomethicone and Dimethicone may also prevent irritation caused by sunscreen agents [13].

Cleansing

The excellent spreading characteristics, dry non-greasy/oily feel, and good solvency of Cyclomethicones make them ideal for use in skin cleansers to help lift and remove dirt without stinging. They can be used alone or in combination with ingredients such as mineral oil. Silicone emulsifiers allow Cyclomethicone to be present in the continuous phase as well as allowing the incorporation of polar ingredients such as water, glycerine etc. This makes the formulation of rinsible foaming facial washes possible [14].

Water-soluble and water-dispersible Dimethicone Copolyols have shown benefits in foaming facial washes. They provide a creamy, more dense foam as well as improving the foam volume. In liquid body cleansing products such as foam baths, shower gels and liquid soaps, they can improve foaming and foam stabilization. They have also been recognized as additives that reduce eye and skin irritation from anionic surfactants [14,15].

Rheology Modification/Structural Integrity (Sticks)

As well as improving the aesthetics of formulations, silicones can also act as rheology modifiers. This is particularly applicable to water-in-oil or water-in silicone-type systems. One such silicone rheology modifier is the C30-45 Alkyl Methicone where 149% and 93% increases in emulsion viscosity have been observed for water-in-silicone and water-in-oil emulsions respectively with 2 wt% of the wax [7]. Rheology modification using 2–4 wt% Stearyl Dimethicone is believed to be part of the reason for the success of this product in enhancing the SPF of sun care products containing organic sunscreens [10]. These waxes are also used to maintain the structural integrity of stick or soft solid products, improving their feel and application. Silicone elastomers can also be used to modify the rheology of skin care and antiperspirant formulations. Such elastomers have the capacity to absorb large amounts of solvents such as Cyclomethicone or low-viscosity Dimethicone without exhibiting any syneresis. It is this property which allows them to successfully thicken formulations. The ability of elastomers to significantly modify the rheology of a formulation combined with their unique powdery feel has led to their use in antiperspirant products.

Formulating Flexibility

Silicones can be used in all types of skin care products ranging from simple oil-in-water gels or emulsions to water-in-silicone and water-in-oil emulsions, from crystal clear to white in colour. Silicone emulsifiers increase this flexibility further. They allow silicones to be present in the continuous phase as well as allowing the incorporation of polar ingredients such as water, glycerine etc. Matching the refractive index of the water phase with the oil phase in such emulsions makes the formulation of clear gels possible and adjusting the phase ratio determines the product form from lotions to gels. This technology is the basis for the clear antiperspirant gels seen on the market today. It is also possible to make non-aqueous emulsions using silicones to deliver hydrophilic ingredients or those that are sensitive to hydrolysis.

HAIRCARE PRODUCTS

Hair Conditioning/Improved Combing

Various types of silicone are used to give different degrees of hair conditioning. Dimethicone Copolyols provide light conditioning due to their solubility in water and low level of substantivity. They can also help reduce eye irritation associated with shampoos and similar products that contain anionic surfactants. Higher molecular weight Dimethicones/ Dimethiconols or Amodimethicones provide a higher level of conditioning due to their insolubility in water and greater substantivity. The latter have an affinity for negatively charged surfaces such as the proteinaceous surface of the hair, which contributes to their substantivity. Evaluation of the average detangling times of Dimethiconol (gum), Amodimethicone and Dimethicone (high viscosity fluid) emulsions at a 4% level in an illustrative two-in-one shampoo formulation indicates that they all show significant improvement over the untreated control tress with the Dimethiconol emulsion providing the best conditioning effect [16,17] (see Figure 3).

Synergistic effects have been observed between quaternary polymers commonly used in shampoos for conditioning and Dimethicone Copolyols. Better detangling results are observed for shampoos containing Dimethicone Copolyol and quaternary polymers than with the quaternary polymers or Dimethicone Copolyols alone [17]. Similar evaluation of silicones in conditioners, indicates that Dimethicone emulsions provides the best conditioning effect in rinse-off products and in permanent waving products, an emulsion of Trimethylsilylamodimethicone significantly reduces the wet and dry combing force.

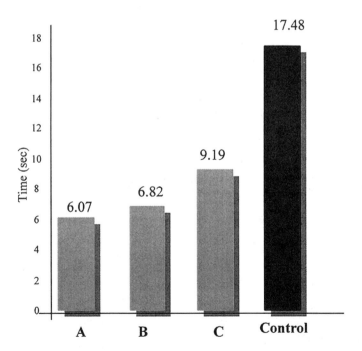

FIGURE 3 Hand detangling results on slightly bleached hair for diluted silicone emulsions. (A) Dimethiconol (and) TEA-Dodecylbenzenesulfonate, (B) Amodimethicone (and) Cetrimonium Chloride (and) Trideceth-12, and (C) Dimethicone (and) Laureth-23 (and) Laureth-4.

Combinations of silicones such as Cyclomethicone, silicone blends and Phenyl Trimethicone are the basis for anhydrous leave-in conditioners, sometimes referred to as "cuticle coat" products [16].

Sensory Enhancement

As in skincare, silicones impart a soft smooth feel to the hair. Sensory evaluations of cuticle coat formulations consisting entirely of blends of silicone showed that, in addition to ease of combing, they improve spreadability, silkiness and softness, gloss and perceived repair of split ends compared to the control [16,18].

Silicones as Drying Aids

Silicones such as Amodimethicone can help hair dry more quickly in comparison to drying aids such as Stearalkonium Chloride, preventing damage due to the use of hair dryers etc. [16].

Foam Boosting

Dimethicone Copolyols can be used to boost the foaming properties of shampoos as well as provide a light conditioning effect [16].

Reduced Flyaway

Tests comparing shampoo formulations containing quaternary polymers to those with quaternary polymers and Dimethicone Copolyols show an improvement in static control with the addition of the silicone. Sensory evaluation has also shown a reduction of flyaway with Dimethicone emulsions [16,18].

Improved Shine

Silicones, in particular Phenyl Trimethicone, are recognized for their ability to enhance hair shine and gloss along with adding softness, manageability, and smoothness to the abraded hair cuticle [16,19].

Natural-Look Fixatives

Because of their low surface tension, silicones spread easily to help fixative products distribute evenly on the surface of hair and improving their effectiveness. They are also used in conjunction with or as a replacement for organic plasticizers. Organic materials tend to be hydrophilic, which diminishes the holding power of a resin. In contrast, the hydrophobic nature of silicones helps repel water so there is less opportunity to reduce the resin's holding properties. The use of Dimethicone Copolyol as a resin plasticizer can also help give hair a more natural look [16].

Longer Lasting Permanent Wave and Coloring Products

Silicones, such as Amodimethicone, can be used to provide a more durable conditioning effect and a longer lasting permanent wave. Pretreatments containing silicone blends help prevent hair damage during the harsh perming process. In hair color products, blends of volatile and non-volatile silicone (Cyclomethicone and Amodimethicone) can be used to seal in the hair cuticle and hold color. The volatile silicone evaporates, leaving behind a smooth, uniform film on the surface of the hair [16,20].

ANTIPERSPIRANT AND DEODORANT PRODUCTS

In addition to the benefits which silicones bring to skin care products such as improved feel, delivery of actives, low residue, formulating flexibility, etc., the following advantages are seen in antiperspirant and deodorant formulations [21].

Anti-whitening

Dimethicones, Phenyl Trimethicone or Alkyl Dimethicones have been shown to reduce/mask the whitening effect caused by antiperspirant salts by matching the refractive index [22].

Improved Spray Characteristics

Low levels of Cyclomethicone (and) Dimethiconol have been demonstrated to reduce the spray width, height, and particle size of antiperspirant pump spray and aerosol formulations, leading to a more directional spray with low mistiness and dustiness [21,23]. The silicone blend may also contribute to the substantivity of the antiperspirant active and lubricate the spray valve to prevent clogging.

Noncooling

The heat of vapourisation of volatile silicones such as Cyclomethicone is much lower than that of water or ethanol meaning that much less energy is required for them to evaporate. This leads to a noncooling effect in formulation [21].

The multifunctional benefits of silicones make them invaluable ingredients in today's cosmetic and toiletry formulations and with the introduction of more and more new silicones, this is a trend which is expected to continue well into the next millenium.

REFERENCES

1. Owen MJ. The surface activity of silicones: a short review. Ind Eng Chem Prod Res Dev 1980; 19:97–103.
2. Owen MJ. Why silicones behave funny. Chemtech May 1981; 11:288–292.
3. DiSapio A. Silicones in Personal Care: An Ingredient Revolution. Brussels: Dow Corning Publication 22-1547.01, 1994.
4. Cosmetic Research, USA News 1997.
5. Goldemberg RL, Pela Rosa CP. Int Soc Cosm Chem 1971; 22:635–654.
6. De Backer G, Ghirardhi D. Goodbye to Grease. Soap, Perfumery and Cosmetic; June 1993.
7. Blakely J, Van Reeth I, Vagts A. The silicone difference in skincare. Inside Cosmetics October/November, 1998; 14–17.
8. Van Reeth I, Dahman F, Lau A, Starch M. Novel Silicone Thickening Technologies: Delivering the Appropriate Rheology Profile to Optimize Formulation Performance. Dow Corning Publication 22-1786-01. Brussels, Belgium, 1999.
9. Lanzet M. Comedogenic effects of cosmetic raw materials. Cosmet Toiletr 1986; 101:63–72.
10. Van Reeth I, Dahman F, Hannington J. Alkymethylsiloxanes as SPF Enhancers. Relationship

Between Effects and Physico-Chemical Properties. International Federation of Societies of Cosmetic Chemists 19th Congress Poster 1996, Sydney.

11. Abrutyn E. Translating Silicone Chemistry to Color Cosmetics. Dow Corning Publication 25-888-97, 1997, Midland, Michigan.

12. Van Reeth I, Marchioretto S, Dahman F, DeSmedt A, Dupont A. Silicones: Enhanced Protection Across Personal Care Applications. IFSCC Poster 1998, Cannes.

13. Nichols K, Desai N, Lebwohl M. Effective sunscreen ingredients and cutaneous irritation in patients with rosacea. Cutis 1998; 61:344–346.

14. Blakely J. The Benefits of Silicones in Facial and Body Cleansing Products. Dow Corning Publication 22-1549-01, Brussels, 1994.

15. Disapio AJ, Fridd P. Dimethicone Copolyols for Cosmetic and Toiletry Applications. IFSCC Paper 1988, London.

16. Marchioretto S. Optimising the Use of Silicones in Haircare Products. Dow Corning Publication 22-1720-01, Brussels, 1998.

17. Marchioretto S, Blakely J. Substantiated synergy between silicone and quats for clear and mild conditioning shampoos. SÖFW October 2, 1997.

18. Thomson B, Vincent J, Halloran D. Anhydrous hair conditioners: silicone-in-silicone delivery systems. Soap Cosmet Chem Specialties 1992; 68:25–28.

19. Reimer BM, Oldinski RL, Glover DA. An Objective Method for Evaluating Hair Shine. Soap Cosmet Chem Specialties (October 1995).

20. Fridd PF, Taylor RM. GB Patents GB2186889 and GB2186890.

21. Abrutyn ES, Bahr BC, Fuson SM. Overview of the Antiperspirant Market: Technology and Trends. Dow Corning Publication 22-1555-01, Brussels, 1994.

22. Abrutyn ES, Bahr BC, Legrow GE, Schulz WJ. US Patent 5, 225, 188; 1993.

23. Spitzer J. US Patent 4, 152, 416; 1979.

35

Skin-Feel Agents

Germaine Zocchi
Colgate-Palmolive Research and Development, Inc., Milmort, Belgium

INTRODUCTION

Skin-feel additives are substances conferring sensorial properties to a skincare product, triggering pleasant perception during application to the skin and after use. Effectiveness of sensory triggers is governed by their substantivity to the skin which occurs either by hydrophobic interaction, charge attraction, or a combination of these two factors. A large variety of cosmetic ingredients function as skin-feel/conditioning additives, comprising lipophilic materials, silicones, water-soluble polymeric substances (including proteins) and their cationic derivatives, and humectants, among others. The Cosmetic, Toiletry and Fragrance Association (CTFA) divides skin conditioning agents into various groups: emollients, occlusive materials, and miscellaneous substances including among others, cationic macromolecules and several surfactants.

This chapter will focus on skin-feel agents for rinse-off products, and more particularly for surfactant-based skin-cleansing products, such as facial cleansers, soap and syndet bars, shower gels and body washes, foam baths (or bubble baths), and bath oils. Shower gels, bars, and facial cleansers first contact the skin, even if only briefly, then are rinsed during the cleaning process; the substantivity of the conditioning agents is crucial to ensure sensory performances, otherwise they will be washed off and the end skin benefit will not be perceived by the user. For bath products intended to be heavily diluted for use, it is difficult to believe that skin-feel agents could function effectively, except perhaps in case of bath oils. Indeed, when bath oils are diluted in water they either float to the surface or lead to a coarse unstable o/w emulsion; when the body emerges from the bath, oils spontaneously stick to the skin because they are incompatible with water and are excluded from the "bathing liquor."

The advent of emollients in body-cleansing liquids occurred with the emergence in the early 1990s of the "body washes" referring to "2 in 1" foaming emulsions; before the development of this new product niche, cationic polymeric materials were the most-used skin-conditioning agents.

Sensorial performance profile of a body-cleansing product comes in a variety of signal attributes:

- Feeling on the skin during use: spreading of a liquid (also related to product rheology), feel of a bar (slipperiness or roughness), foam feel related to foam quality (creaminess, density)
- Skin feel during rinsing, e.g., slipperiness, roughness of the skin, "clean feel" (squeaky feel) left by soaps
- Feel while drying the skin with a towel and feel on damp skin: softness, roughness, stickiness
- After feel and longevity of skin sensations: smoothness, softness, moisturization

All these product attributes are governed at first by e.g., the surfactant nature (amphoterics, nonionics, anionics), their total and relative concentrations, and the clinical mildness for the skin of the surfactant mixture, and can be further influenced or improved by judiciously chosen skin-conditioning agents.

Besides physical, clinical, and organoleptic characteristics of the body-cleansing product, several other imponderable parameters can act on the skin-feel performance and perception, such as usage habits, water hardness, skin condition of the user, and pilosity. Also, consumer expectations in terms of sensorial profile of a product depend on climatic (relative humidity, temperature) and sociodemographic parameters (e.g., sex, occupation, lifestyle, running-water availability), skin type and concerned body part (e.g., face, whole body), and product positioning (e.g., sport, moisturizing, nourishing, others).

Criteria of selection and constraints to be taken into account when choosing skin-feel agents are as follows:

- Solubility and compatibility with the surfactant system
- Sensitivity to electrolytes and pH
- Product physical form: bar, liquid
- Processability (bars) and ease of formulation
- Sensitivity to temperature
- Impact on finished product performance profile:
  on the foam: foam feel, volume and stability, creaminess, bubble structure
  on the product rinsability
  Induction of undesirable and unexpected secondary effects on skin feel when skin is damp (e.g., stickiness)
- Impact on finished product aesthetic:
  on fragrance perception and stability
  on product clarity when relevant
  on viscosity, rheological profile
  on color
- Origin: animal or vegetal, natural or synthetic
- Risk of skin sensitization
- Cost

EMOLLIENTS AND REFATTENERS

Introduction

The CTFA dictionary defines *emollients* as: "cosmetic ingredients which help to maintain the soft, smooth and pliable appearance of the skin; emollients function by their ability to remain on the skin surface or in stratum corneum to act as lubricant, to reduce flaking, and to improve the skin's appearance.'' Emollients are also described as *refatting additives* or *refatteners* in the case of bath products. The word *refattener* refers to substances improving the lipid content of the upper layers of the skin; they prevent defatting and drying out of the skin. Several emollients showing strong lipophilic character are identified as *occlusive* ingredients; they are fatty/oily materials that remain on the skin surface and reduce transepidermal water loss. The CTFA dictionary defines occlusives as: "cosmetic ingredients which retard the evaporation of water from the skin surface; by blocking the evaporative loss of water, occlusive materials increase the water content of the skin.''

Overall, emollients and refatteners are oils and fats derived from natural origins or obtained by chemical synthesis; they are classified in nonpolar (paraffins and isoparaffins) and polar substances (esters and triglycerides); their chemical structure influences the interaction with the skin surface and affects their sensorial properties. As a class, they comprise lipids, oils and their derivatives, fatty acid esters, lanolin derivatives, and silicones and their organofunctional derivatives. Originally, emollients were developed for use in leave-on skin care products; formulation technology can aid the deposition of refatting additives on the skin from wash-off products and avoid that they rinse off with the surfactants; nevertheless, the large dilution factor in both products remains a significant hurdle for skin end benefit perception (except in bath oils).

Emollients and refatteners will provide after feel, but will also influence skin feel during usage, foam feel, and most of the time foam quantity and quality. The more hydrophobic the refattening additive, the more negative its impact on flash foam generation, foam quantity, and stability. In other respects, the more lipidic the material, the better its skin substantivity, and the easier the efficacy documentation; proof and substantiation of claims is of more and more importance in the frame of the Sixth Amendment of European legislation for cosmetics and toiletries.

Lipophilic Emollients and Occlusives

Occlusive materials comprise vegetable oils, triglycerides, mineral oil, natural or synthetic waxes, fatty acid esters, lanolin oil and its derivatives, and polydimethylsiloxanes, among others (Table 1). They form an occlusive layer on the skin, keeping water inside upper stratum corneum layers and consequently acting as moisturizers.

Mineral oil and vegetable oils as well as waxes generally produce heavy and greasy feeling on the skin. Hydrophobic fatty acid esters are an almost unlimited source of synthetic emollients and refatteners; they provide lighter and more pleasant skin feel than oils and waxes. Any fatty acid can be esterified by either ethylene glycol, or propylene glycol, or glycerin polymers, or isopropyl alcohol, or any longer chain alcohol. The feel they impart and their impact on foam is related to the fatty acid chain length; short chains (e.g., isopropyl myristate, octyl octanoate, and cocoate) deliver dryer feel and have lesser impact on foam than longer ones (e.g., stearates and isostearates), which are greasier and detrimental to foam quantity and stability [1].

Hydrophobic emollients are efficacious skin refatteners but not easily formulated in surfactant mixtures commonly used in liquid skin-cleansing product without proceeding to an emulsification step, which most of the time necessitates hot process. Highly hydrophobic refattening additives are not meant for foaming preparations but rather for bath oils. They have a detrimental impact on foam speed, quantity, and stability. Manufacturers circumvent this weakness of lathering capacity by providing a mechanical foaming device with the product: a puff or massage flower [2].

TABLE 1 Emollients and Refatteners

Chemical structures or nature		INCI names
Fats/oils (triglycerides); hydrocarbons; waxes		petrolatum
		ceresin
		mineral oil
		wheat germ oil/wheat germ glycerides
		almond/peach oil
		coconut oil
		jojoba oil
		rape seed/olive/sesame oil
		sunflower/corn/safflower oil
Fatty acid esters: hydrophobic emollient esters	ethylene glycol esters	glycol stearate or palmitate or oleate
	polyethylene glycol esters	PEG-5 octanoate
	propylene glycol esters	propylene glycol myristate or laurate
	polypropylene glycol esters	
	isopropyl esters	PPG-36 oleate
	polyglyceryl esters	isopropyl myristate or laurate or palmitate
	alkyl esters	
		polyglyceryl-10-laurate or myristate
		octyl octanoate
		cetearyl octanoate
		octyl hydroxystearate
Fatty acid mono- and diglycerides		glyceryl oleate
		glyceryl laurate
Ethoxylated triglycerides		PEG-6 caprylic capric triglycerides
		PEG-4 caprylic/capric glycerides
		PEG-45 palm kernel glycerides
		PEG-20 almond glycerides
		PEG-60 corn glycerides
		PEG-18 palm glycerides
		hydroxylated milk glycerides
Ethoxylated mono- and diglycerides: hydrophilic emollient esters	ethoxylated glyceryl esters	PEG-7 glyceryl cocoate
		PEG-8 glyceryl laurate
		PEG-15 glyceryl laurate
		PEG-30 glyceryl cocoate
		PEG-78 glyceryl cocoate
		PEG-20 glyceryl oleate
		PEG-82 glyceryl tallowate
		PEG-200 glyceryl tallowate
Fatty alcohols		lauryl alcohol/oley alcohol
		octyldodecanol
Emollient ethers	ethoxylated/propoxylated fatty alcohols	PPG-5-laureth-5
		PPG-5 ceteth 20
		PPG-8 ceteth 20
	polypropylene glycol ethers	PPG-14 butyl ether
		PEG-4 lauryl ether
		PPG-15 stearyl ether
		PPG-50 cetyl ether
		PPG-3 myristyl ether

Abbreviations: INCI, international nomenclature for cosmetic ingredients; PEG, polyethylene glycol; PPG, polypropylene glycol.

Soaps and syndet bars can easily accommodate waxes and oils without impairing their basic foaming and cleaning functions. Besides beeswax, petrolatum or ceresin, lanolin and jojoba oil, cocoa butter, and mineral oil, are other examples of skin conditioners commonly used in bars. Paraffin wax is often used in soaps and syndets not only for the smooth feel they impart to the finished bar, the mildness they bring to the formulation, but also for the role of plasticizer they play, adding firmness to the bar. Vegetal oils are included as skin-nourishing/refattening agents (e.g., almond, wheat germ, olive oils).

Fatty acid mono- and diglycerides [1,3] are prepared either by transesterification of triglycerides with glycerin or treatment of alkanoate with glycerin. Lipophilic character remains predominant in these esters; depending on chain length, they are soluble in surfactant solutions or they must be emulsified. Besides the improved skin feel they induce, they also reduce defatting of the skin possibly caused by surfactant-based cleansers. Monoglycerides of stearic, lauric, and palmitic acids (glyceryl monostearate, laurate, and palmitate) intervene in the composition of natural lipids of the skin. They adsorb and can be detected on skin after application through a skin-cleaning product [4].

Several mixtures of monoglycerides and mild foaming surfactants are commercially available; they claim improved foam qualities (bubble size, creaminess, and stability) and documentable skin-refattening properties [5,6]. On top of the skin feel improvement they bring, they will also reduce the degreasing effect of cleansers thanks to their lipophilic character and improve the compatibility of the surfactants with the skin [1]. An example of improvement in the skin barrier function and in skin tactile sensations has been shown for glyceryl oleate in a model shower-gel composition [5].

Hydrophilic Lipids

Hydrophilic lipids (Table 1) [1] are preferred for foaming skin-cleansing preparations. Ethoxylation and propoxylation make lipids more compatible with water and more easily soluble in aqueous surfactants solutions. One has to find the right balance between ethoxylation and skin substantivity; the more the lipids are ethoxylated, the more they are soluble, the less the impact on foam and skin substantivity, and the weaker their refattening properties.

Ethoxylated glycerides are obtained either by reaction of natural triglycerides with ethylene oxide (a complex end mixture is then obtained) or by ethoxylation of monoglycerides. They are often referred to as "water-soluble vegetable oils"; their solubility in water will depend on the carbon chain length of starting glycerides and on the degree of ethoxylation.

Low ethoxylated triglycerides are still lipophilic enough to provide good refattening properties, leading to very pleasant skin feel, perceivable at quite high use levels. Ethoxylated mono- and diglycerides generally associate various properties beneficial to the skin. They are more or less refattening the skin, depending on chain length and ethoxylation ratio and act as anti-irritant or mildness additives; they confer slipperiness to the foam. Depending on chain length and ethoxylation degree they are either water dispersible or soluble. Among the low ethoxylates, PEG-7 glyceryl cocoate is one of the mostly used. This emollient depresses irritation of anionic surfactants and shows minimum impact on lathering profile. Higher ethoxylates of longer C chain length (PEG-200 glyceryl tallowate) are still substantive to the skin because of their high molecular weight, as well as provide a smooth feel, but because of their stronger hydrophilic character their refatting properties are less obvious to evidence [7].

Ethoxylated/propoxylated fatty alcohols are useful light emollients: through an appropriate selection of optimum combination between parent alcohol chain length, propoxylation, and ethoxylation degree, these emollients can be formulated up to 2 to 3% in surfactant solutions with minimum impact on foam value.

Lanolin

Lanolin (Table 2) [8,9] is extracted from sheep wool grease; it is a complex mixture of esters of high molecular weight lanolin alcohols (aliphatic alcohols, sterols, and trimethyl sterols) and of lanolin acids; free lanolin alcohols, acids, and lanolin hydrocarbons are minors. Lanolin alcohols and lanolin oil are recommended as superfatting agents in soaps. Ethoxylation of the hydroxyl groups of lanolin or of its derivatives leads to hydrophilic, water-soluble lanolin compounds, offering a broad range of useful emollients to the formulator. Some moderately to highly ethoxylated derivatives, recommended for their good emolliency and moisturization properties, are processable in liquid skin cleansers with limited impact on foam profile; as an example, the 75 mol ethoxylated lanolin does not depress foam and is recommended as skin conditioner in soaps, liquid body-cleansing products, and bubble baths. Medium ethoxylates lanolin alcohols have limited impact on foam performances of body cleansing liquids; lower ethoxylates can be formulated in bars. Propoxylated lanolin alcohols are lipophilic emollients used in soap bars and in other cleansers based on synthetic surfactants.

Alkoxylated lanolin derivatives are obtained by reaction with mixtures of propylene and ethylene oxides in various ratios; they are more soluble than ethoxylated lanolin. They serve as refattening and foam stabilizing agents. Esterification of lanolin fatty acid with isopropyl alcohol provides a range of esters of various molecular weights. Medium molecular weight esters are used as superfatting agents in soaps.

TABLE 2   Emollients and Refatteners

		INCI names
Lecithin		propylene glycol (and) lecithin (and) sodium lauryl sulfate (and) disodium sulfosuccinate (and) cocamidopropyl hydroxysultaine (and) isopropyl alcohol
Lanolin and its derivatives		lanolin oil lanolin alcohol
	ethoxylated lanolin	PEG-75 lanolin
	ethoxylated lanolin alcohols	laneth-16 laneth-25
	propoxylated lanolin alcohols	PPG-30 lanolin alcohol ether
	alkoxylated lanolin	PPG-12 PEG-50 lanolin PPG-40 PEG-60 lanolin oil

Abbreviations: PEG, polyethylene glycol; PPG, polypropylene glycol.

Lecithin

Lecithin (Table 2) is a natural mixture of polar and neutral lipids; the word *lecithin* is also used as the trivial name of a particular phospholipid: phosphatidylcholine. Main vegetable sources of lecithin used in personal-care products are soybean and maize, egg yolk is practically the only animal source of lecithin used in cosmetics and toiletries. The percentage of polar lipids and their fatty acid pattern are characteristic of the lecithin source.

Bare lecithin, a secondary product of Soya oil extraction, typically contains 60 to 70% polar lipids (mainly phospholipids, namely phosphatidylcholine, and glycolipids) and a remaining 25 to 35% Soy oil. This raw lecithin is further fractionated, purified, and chemically modified to allow easier processing and formulation in toiletry products. Emollient, refattening, and moisturizing properties of lecithin are guided by its content in phospholipids.

Lecithin softens, nourishes, and refattens the skin; it provides a nongreasy, long-lasting skin feel and improves foam feel and quality (creaminess, slipperiness, richness). Ready-to-use mixtures of phospholipids in surfactant solutions, free of residual Soya oil, are commercially available for an easy incorporation in liquids or bars; some of these compounds allow formulation of clear products.

Silicone Derivatives

For detailed information about silicones, lecturer will refer to Chapter 34. Only major materials used in body cleansing products will be briefly discussed here [10,11]. Predominant silicones used overall in personal-care products are polydimethyl siloxane, also named *dimethicones*. They are not soluble in water or in surfactant solutions; their incorporation into liquid cleansers requires an emulsification process. The length of dimethylsiloxane polymer chain dictates its molecular weight and hence its viscosity. Most commonly used materials have viscosities ranging from about 100 to several thousands centistokes. High– to medium–molecular weight dimethicones are occlusive, skin-protective emollients; lower molecular weights are dryer emollients, generally preferred for use in skin cleansers. Dimethicones have a detrimental effect on foam profile but are good film-forming agents, lubricants, imparting a nongreasy, nontacky silky feel as compared with ''heavier'' mineral or vegetable oils. They are used in soap bars, where they also aid mold release, and in 2-in-1 shower gels (body washes). Polymethylcyclosiloxanes or cyclomethicones are tetrameric or pentameric oligomers of the same backbone as polydimethylsiloxane, and show the same chemical and physical properties; they are low-viscosity fluids with relatively high volatility because of their low molecular weight and the weak intermolecular attractivity. Because they are not substantive, cyclomethicones are often identified as dry emollients; they deliver light, transient, and dry skin feel during product use.

Formulation of these nonpolar insoluble silicones requests hot emulsification process (nonionic emulsifiers) and proper emulsion stabilization.

Dimethicones are modfied or functionalized with other organic groups to modulate their solubility in water or in surfactant solutions (and consequently make them easier to formulate) and their skin substantivity properties. By adjusting the type and proportion of hydrophilic substituents, the resulting copolymer is soluble or dispersible in aqueous cosmetic products. The combination of the dimethicone structure with polyoxyalkylated substituents (ethylene or propylene oxide) yields dimethicone copolyols, which are copolymers more soluble in water with surface activity. They are foam boosters and stabilizers;

even if they are less film-forming than parent polydimethylsiloxanes, they significantly add to skin sensations during application (use) and provide excellent smooth and silky after feel [12]. They can be used to formulate clear, aqueous products. Blends of polydimethylsiloxanes with volatile and/or water-soluble derivatives are used to design a sensorial profile adapted to the finished product and its end use.

HUMECTANTS

The CTFA dictionary defines humectants as "cosmetic ingredients intended to increase the water content of top layers of the skin" (Table 3). Humectants are hygroscopic substances generally soluble in water. These "moisture attractants" maintain an aqueous film at the skin surface. The primary used humectant in personal-care products is glycerin; it tends to provide heavy and tacky feel which can be overcome by using it in combination with other humectants such as sorbitol.

Less expensive than glycerin, propylene glycol is the second most widely used humectant in cosmetic and toiletry products; it reduces viscosity of surfactant solutions and tends to depress the foam.

Low–molecular weight polyethylene glycol (PEGs from about 10 to 200 PEG units), amino acids and other constituents of skin natural moisturizing factors like sodium PCA and sodium lactate are also applicable for use in surfactant-based skin-cleansing products.

Humectants are not substantive to the skin and are easily rinsed-off after cleaning. Consequently, skin-feel improvement is not obvious to perceive and their efficacy in terms of skin moisturization is difficult to document. Glycerin, propylene glycol, 1,3-butylene glycol, or sorbitol are typically used in body washes, bubble baths, shower gels, or soaps to prevent the dessication of the product itself and the formation of a dry layer at the surface. They also ensure stability and clarity of liquid cleansers at cold temperatures.

Few substantive humectants can be mentioned. They are cationic in nature, which makes them absorbing to the negatively charged skin surface. In the quaternized polyal-

TABLE 3   Humectants

Chemical nature or structure	INCI names
	glycerin
	glycereth-26 and glycereth-7
	propylene glycol
	1,3 butylene glycol
	from PEG-8 to about PEG-200
	sorbitol
	sorbeth-6 to sorbeth-40
	xylitol
Ethoxylated methyl glucose	methyl gluceth-10/methyl gluceth-20
	amino acids
	lactic acid/sodium lactate
	sodium PCA
Substantive conditioning humectants	steardimonium panthenol
	lauryl methyl gluceth-10 hydroxypropyl dimonium chloride
	chitosan-PCA

Abbreviations: PEG, polyethylene glycol; PCA, pyrrolidone carboxylic acid.

koxylated methyl glucose derivative (lauryl methyl gluceth-10 hydroxypropyldimonium chloride), the hydrophilic moiety delivers humectant properties; the hydrophobic chain at the cationic end of the molecule ensures both substantivity and skin conditioning.

Chitosan-PCA is another example. Chitosan is a polycationic (at acidic pH) high–molecular weight polymer produced by deacetylation of chitin, the major constituent of invertebrate exoskeletons. Combining chitosan with pyrrolidone carboxylic acid (PCA) leads to a highly substantive, film-forming humectant material.

POLYMERS

Polymeric materials can interact both with protein of the skin surface and with skin lipids. Parameters influencing the interaction between skin surface and the polymers are as follows:

1. The positive charge density: the more cationic the character of the polymer, the better the polymer interaction with negatively charged skin surface.
2. The hydrophobicity of polymer: grafting of hydrophobic moieties on the polymer backbone favor van der Waals interactions with hydrophobic areas of the keratin.
3. The molecular weight of the polymer: the higher the polymer size, the more its substantivity to the skin (film-forming properties). However, very low–molecular weight polymers can easily penetrate the skin surface chinks and as such adsorb into the superficial stratum disjonctum.
4. The nature of surfactants neighboring the polymer in the finished product: the polymer can interact with surfactants either through their charges or through hydrophobic interactions; also, competition between polymer and surfactants for skin anchoring sites can occur. In both cases, deposition and adsorption of polymer onto the skin surface is weakened.

Natural Polymers and Their Chemically Modified Derivatives

Proteins

Proteins differ by (1) the source; (2) the molecular weight, (3) the amino acid (AA) composition, AA side groups, and electrical charge (more of cationic or of anionic AA); and (4) the chemically attached moieties (quats, fatty chains, silicone, etc.) on the peptide backbone (Table 4) [13–15].

Proteins can be from vegetable or animal origin. The most widely used animal protein is collagen from pork or beef; "marine collagen" (fish) is now an alternative source of collagen to traditional bovine-derived materials. Milk proteins, keratin, and elastin are also considered in cosmetics and toiletries. The shift away from animal-derived ingredients has resulted in an increased interest in plant-derived materials and increasing use of proteins from vegetable sources.

Vegetable/plant proteins are mostly associated with significant amounts of soluble and insoluble carbohydrates because of the extraction process; soluble carbohydrates confer dark color and strong odor to the raw material, and in some commercial grades carbohydrates have been removed. The combination of hydrolyzed vegetable proteins and oligosaccharides produces conditioning additives with synergistic moisturizing action and film-forming properties. Major vegetal starting materials are wheat gluten, almond meal, rice, oat, soya, and maize.

TABLE 4 Natural Polymers and Their Chemically Modified Derivatives

Chemical structure and origin		INCI names
Native proteins	solubilized in anionic surfactants	native wheat protein/lauryl ether sulfate complex
Protein hydrolyzates	animal source	hydrolyzed animal protein hydrolyzed collagen hydrolyzed milk protein
	plant derived	hydrolyzed vegetal protein hydrolyzed wheat protein/oligosaccharide complex hydrolyzed wheat protein and hydrolyzed wheat starch hydrolyzed oats hydrolyzed wheat gluten
Quaternized protein hydrolyzates	animal source	hydroxypropyl trimonium hydrolyzed collagen
	plant derived	hydroxypropyl trimonium hydrolyzed wheat protein
Fatty side chains grafted on protein backbone	native protein	wheat extract (and) stearic (and) sodium chloride
Quaternized fatty chains grafted	protein hydrolyzate	steardimonium hydrolyzed wheat protein or collagen lauryl or cocodimonium hydroxypropyl hydrolyzed collagen alkyl quaternary hydrolyzed soya protein
Copolymers	protein-PVP	hydrolyzed wheat protein/polyvinyl pyrrolidone copolymer
	protein-silicone	hydrolyzed wheat protein hydroxypropyl polysiloxane copolymer
	quaternized copolymer protein-silicone	hydroxypropyl trimonium hydrolyzed wheat protein polysiloxane copolymer

Abbreviation: PVP, polyvinyl pyrrolidone.

Proteins are functional over a wide range of pH. Nevertheless, because they are amphoteric materials, below their isoelectric point they carry a net positive charge which makes them substantive to the negatively charged skin surface. Film-forming properties of proteins and hydrolyzates are related to their molecular weight (the higher, the better). Overall, proteins convey a smoothing and moisturizing effect, and produce a soft and silky feel to the skin. They have a positive effect on foam profile: they increase foam stability, confer creaminess and density, as well as slipperiness to the foam. Proteins and hydrolyzates are also known for their ability to reduce the irritation caused by anionic surfactants and to combat skin dryness induced by detergents [16–19].

Some native proteins, such as elastin, keratin, or vegetable proteins, are insoluble. There exist soluble native collagen species; their use is restricted to some specialized applications. In order to make native proteins suitable for a wide range of applications, they are converted into soluble hydrolyzates by chemical or enzymatic degradation. The sizes of resulting peptides depend on the hydrolysis process used: chemical processes give rise to broader molecular weight distributions and enzymatic digestion to narrower ones. Besides that, native proteins solubilized in various anionic surfactants (by formation of a protein-surfactant complex) are commercially available, allowing easy formulation of these film-forming, moisturizing, mildness additives. A wide range of protein hydrolyzates molecular weights is available, ranging from 500,000 down to 1000 d. Protein hydroly-zates of intermediate molecular weight (average 3000 to 5000 d) are the most widely used; they are less substantive than high–molecular weight proteins but provide smooth skin feel, slippery feel during use, and sensation of skin hydration.

Hydrolyzates are readily soluble and compatible with all classes of surfactants. Most of the commercially available proteins and derivatives have a characteristic odor and color. Furthermore, products formulated with proteins or hydrolyzates should be adequately pre-served.

Chemically Modified Protein Derivatives

In order to increase interaction of proteinic material with skin surface, proteins or hydroly-zates are functionalized or chemically modified. Proteins possess reactive side chain amino and carboxyl groups, which are sites for further modification of their intrinsic properties (Table 4).

Hydrophobic interactions with the skin surface are favored and reinforced by graft-ing fatty carbon chains, and ionic interactions are maximized by grafting cationic moieties onto the protein backbone. Hydrolyzed protein copolymers combine substantivity and film-forming properties of parent proteins with characteristic sensorial properties of com-panion conditioning agents. These macromolecular protein complexes offer greater mois-turizing and conditioning potential as compared with the individual components (20).

Native Proteins Coupled with Fatty Acids.   These lead to macromolecular entity with dual hydrophilic/hydrophobic characteristics and physicochemical properties. Skin substantivity is guided both by the size of the starting protein and by the chain length (the hydrophobicity) of the fatty acid. The macromolecules are surface active and can be formulated in bars or liquids; they produce smooth, long-lasting skin feel. Long-chain fatty acid derivatives tend to decrease foam volume but confer creaminess, richness, and slipperiness to the lather.

Copolymers of Silicone and Proteins.   These are obtained by covalent bonding of low–molecular weight polydimethylsiloxanes on amino groups of (vegetable) protein hydrolyzate. They combine beneficial properties of proteins (anti-irritant effect, substantivity, film-forming, soft afterfeel) with lubricity of silicone [21,22]. Quaternized protein-silicone copolymers are now commercially available.

PVP-Protein Copolymers.   Proteinic component imparts substantivity and polyvinyl pyrrolidone (PVP) modifies the moisture retention and film-forming properties of the resulting copolymer. PVP maximizes film-forming and hydration properties of the protein. The PVP/protein ratio will modulate the profile of performance on the skin and the influence on lathering characteristics of surfactant-based skin cleanser.

Quarternized Protein Hydrolyzates.   Cationic protein hydrolyzates are obtained by reacting the primary amine sites on the protein backbone with a tertiary amine, i.e., hydroxypropyl, propyl trimethyl ammonium, or alkyl trimethyl ammonium [23]. Covalent attachment of quaternary groups strongly increases the cationic character of the protein hydrolyzate, making it further skin substantive and resistant to rinsing step. Covalent attachment of fatty quaternary groups (alkyl dimethyl ammonium) on peptides greatly improves both ionic and hydrophobic interactions with the skin. Alkyl chain can be lauryl myristyl, or stearyl. Alkyl trimonium hydrolyzed proteins are still water-soluble and compatible with all classes of surfactants. These hydrophobically modified cationic protein hydrolyzates are highly adsorbing to skin surface at all pH levels and offer skin substantivity at minimum concentration. They impart pronounced conditioning effect, and the lipophilic moieties provide emollient feel.

Overall, quaternized versions of a protein are many times more substantive than the parent protein hydrolyzate. Quaternization of a protein hydrolyzates raises their isoelectric point (IP) to pH 10 regardless of their initial IP values.

Cationic Guar Gum

Guar gum is a galactomannane polysaccharide derived from the endosperm of Cyamopsis tetragonolobus seeds (Table 5). Depolymerization of the gum by enzymatic or chemical processes allows modulation of its molecular weight, and consequently impacts its solubility, thickening properties, and the clarity of the finished product. Free hydroxyl groups on the polysaccharidic backbone can intervene in esterification and etherification reactions. Hydroxypropyl (HP) side groups improve guar compatibility with electrolytes. Cationic guar derivatives are obtained by reaction of HP guar with epoxypropyltrimethyl ammonium chloride; positive charge density of resulting guar hydroxypropyl trimonium chloride depends on substitution degree. Cationic guar derivatives are film forming, and impart soft, smooth, and silky feel to the skin. Moreover, they act as an anti-irritant for anionic surfactants and soaps, and have a positive effect on foam feel and quality [24,25].

TABLE 5 Natural Polymers and Their Chemically Modified Derivatives

Chemical structure	INCI names	Comments
Cationic cellulose derivatives	Polyquaternium 10	polymeric quaternary ammonium salt of HEC reacted with trimethyl ammonium substituted epoxide
	Polyquaternium 24	polymeric ammonium salt of HEC reacted with lauryl dimethyl ammonium substituted epoxide; average degree of substitution = 1
	PG-hydroxyethyl cellulose lauryl or coco or stearyl dimonium chloride	average degree of substitution > 1
Cationic guar derivatives	guar hydroxypropyl trimonium chloride	
	hydroxypropyl guar hydroxypropyl trimonium chloride	

Abbreviations: INCI, international nomenclature for cosmetic ingredients; HEC, hydroxyethylcellulose.

Cationic Cellulose Derivatives

Polyquaternium 10 is a range of polymeric quaternary ammonium salts of hydroxyethyl cellulose (HEC) reacted with trimethyl ammonium substituted epoxide. Polyquaternium 10 solutions are non-Newtonian and are commercially available 1) in several viscosity grades depending on their molecular weights (they contribute to viscosity of formulations), and 2) with "high" to "moderate" cationic substitution. In vivo tests showed that these cationic cellulosic polymers protect the skin from aggression by anionic surfactants (Table 5) [26,27].

Polyquaternium 24 in a polymeric quaternary ammonium salt of HEC reacted with lauryldimethyl ammonium substituted epoxide. It is a hydrophobically modified polyquaternium 10. The degree of substitution with quaternary fatty chain is average 1 in Polyquaternium 24; a range of alkyl dimonium hydroxypropyl oxyethyl cellulose with higher proportion of substituted fatty quat groups (average degree of substitution is 1.2) is also commercially available.

The presence of fatty side chains on these quaternized cellulose ethers confers on them surface active properties and further participates in their very high skin-substantivity and their film-forming properties. They impart silky, smooth afterfeel. These alkyl quaternary cellulose polymers are soluble in water (longer C chains must be slightly warmed) and compatible with a wide range of surfactants; they have favorable influence on the lathering properties providing creaminess, density, slipperiness, and stability to the foam.

Synthetic Quaternized Polymers

An array of dimethyl diallylammonium chloride (DMDAAC)–based polymers and copolymers is commercially available. Their substantivity, film-forming properties, and resulting skin feel depend on both the molecular weight (ranging from about 400,000 up to 7 million) and the density of positive charges, which also dictates the compatibility of the polymer with anionic surfactants. These polymers generally make foam more dense and stable (Table 6) [28].

Inclusion of acrylamide into DMDAAC homopolymer (Polyquaternium 6 is not compatible with anionics) decreases the positive charge density leading to a skin-conditioning polymer more compatible with anionics (Polyquaternium 7) (29, 30). The same effect is obtained by copolymerizing DMDAAC with either acrylic acid (Polyquaternium 22) or with both acrylamide and acrylic acid (Polyquaternium 39). Polyquaternium 7 is probably one of the most often used synthetic cationic polymer in body-cleansing products; it is highly substantive to the skin, delivering soft, silky, moisturized afterfeel (28).

TABLE 6 Synthetic Quaternized Polymers

INCI names	Chemical structure
Polyquaternium 6	dimethyl diallyl ammonium chloride homopolymer
Polyquaternium 7	acrylamide/dimethyl diallyl ammonium chloride copolymer
Polyquaternium 11	poly(vinylpyrrolidone/dimethylaminoethyl methacrylate)
Polyquaternium 22	acrylic acid/dimethyl diallyl ammonium chloride copolymer
Polyquaternium 39	acrylamide/acrylic acid/dimethyl diallyl ammonium chloride terpolymer

Abbreviation: INCI, international nomenclature for cosmetic ingredients.

Another widely used synthetic cationic polymer in liquids and in bar soaps is a quaternized copolymer of PVP and dimethylaminoethyl methacrylate (DMAEM) (polyquaternium 11). This PVP copolymer is available in molecular weights ranging from 100,000 to 1,000,000.

SURFACTANTS

Amphoteric surfactants are amino acid derivatives; their net charge varies with the pH in solution (Table 7). At pH below the isoelectric point they are positively charged in aqueous

TABLE 7 Surfactants

Chemical class/category	INCI names
Nonionics	
polyhydric alcohol esters	
sucrose esters	sucrose laurate or cocoate
methyl glucose esters	PEG-120 methyl glucose dioleate
	PEG-80 methyl glucose laurate
glucose ethers	alkyl polyglucosides
fatty acid alkanolamides	cocodiethanolamide
Amphoterics	
ampholytes	cocamidopropyl betaine
	olivamidopropyl betaine
	sesamidopropyl betaine
	oleamidopropyl betaine
	isostearamidopropyl betaine
	cocamidopropyl hydroxysultaine
	cocamidopropyldimethyl aminohydroxypropyl hydrolyzed collagen
propionates	alkylamino propionates
	alkyliminodipropionates
imidazoline derivatives	acylamphoacetate
Anionics	
phosphoric acid esters and salts	C9–C15 alkyl phosphate
	PPG-5 ceteth-10 phosphate
	Oleth-3 phosphate
acyl amino acids and salts	
acyl peptides	sodium cocoyl hydrolyzed protein
	sodium lauroyl oat amino acids
	TEA or sodium lauroyl animal collagen amino acids
acyl glutamates	sodium cocoyl glutamate
sarcosinates	sodium cocoyl or lauroyl sarcosinate
taurates	sodium methyl cocoyl taurate
sulfonic acids and salts	
sulfosuccinates	disodium laneth-5 sulfosuccinate
	disodium ricinoleamido MEA-sulfosuccinate
	disodium laureth sulfosuccinate
	disodium PEG-8 palm glycerides sulfosuccinate
isethionates	sodium cocoyl isethionate

Abbreviation: INCI, international nomenclature for cosmetic ingredients.

solution and can consequently adsorb more easily onto the skin. Alkyl chain length can also significantly act on the skin feel; some betaines based on C16/C18 cuts provide more greasy, refattened feel but also have detrimental effect on foam.

Polydimethylsiloxane grafted with a betaine moiety leads to an amphoteric surfactant combining substantivity, refattening properties as well as silicone typical skin feel profile.

Some nonionics are used for their emollient properties and excellent afterfeel; e.g., sucrose and methyl glucose esters as well as sucrose ethers. Fatty acid alkanolamides are often referred to as refatteners; these are not lipids but they confer a greasy slippery feel to the foam and impart a particular afterfeel on the skin that subjectively compares with refatting. Several mild anionic surfactants are known to provide improved skin feel (afterfeel) by themselves, e.g., sarcosinate, taurate, acylglutamate, and isethionate. Fatty acids–protein condensates salts also act as conditioning aids, imparting a pleasant, smooth feel to the skin. The inclusion of fatty acids in soap and syndet bars contributes to enhance skin feel during and after use, and produces creamier lather. Phosphoric acid fatty esters deliver soap-like skin feel: slipperiness during use, and very good rinseability leaving skin feeling "clean" and powdery.

Benefits brought by additional skin conditioning agents are sometimes hidden by a mild or very mild cleaning-surfactant system delivering by itself very good skin feel properties; the sensorial baseline is high to start with and the increment in performance brought by skin feel agent is leveled off, and sometimes not even perceivable. It is, however, important to notice that several mild anionic and most of the nonionic surfactants, if they provide a pleasant afterfeel, are characterized by a "water feel" (feel in solution) that is often unpleasant, with rough and drag feel sensations.

EXFOLIATING AGENTS

Skin scrub agents or body polishers are solid materials from natural origin (fine powder of seeds or shells of different vegetables), or are obtained by chemical synthesis (tiny beads of styrene or polyethylene) (Table 8). When the scrub agent–containing body-cleansing product is rubbed or massaged onto the skin, fine solid particles remove superficial skin horny layer by mechanical abrasion, leaving behind a fresh, smooth skin surface. They are the easiest additives for the consumer to perceive. Scrubbing particles can be suspended in liquid body cleanser thanks to structuring polymers like xanthan gum or carrageenan, which build a viscoelastic network in the surfactant matrix. The scrubbing agent must be carefully selected when formulating facial cleansers. The skin on the face

TABLE 8 Exfoliants/Scrubbing Agents

Apricot/walnut shells powder or flour
Corn cob
Jojoba beads
Polyethylene/styrene beads
Almond meal
Apricot/peach seed powder
Loofah
Maize scape powder

is more sensitive or delicate than that of the rest of the body. For facial application, the formulator should orientate his choices towards, e.g., soft clays or melting jojoba beads.

CONCLUSIONS

The overall skin-feel profile provided by a skin-cleansing product is conditioned by the huge variety of composition constituents. Many have been described in this chapter, but not exhaustively. Other factors can influence the sensations perceived by the consumer, like the presence of electrolytes or of thickening polymers in the product, as well as the water hardness in the user dwelling. It will be the responsibility of the formulator to consider all the potential synergisms or antagonisms in the finished product, in order to deliver the desired skin feel.

REFERENCES

1. Domsch A. Modern bath and shower preparations under dermatological aspects. Seife Öle Fette Wachse 1991; 15:573–576.
2. Gordon G, Schoenberg CO, Winder LC. U.S. patent 5,804,539 (1998). Personal cleansing system comprising a polymeric diamond-mesh sponge and a liquid cleanser with moisturizer. Assigned to the Proctor and Gamble Company.
3. Herbe JF. Produits d'hygiene: les tendances. Parfums Cosmétiques Arômes 1993; 18(113): 37–41.
4. Domsch A. Rückfettung in bade-und-duschpräparaten. Seifen Öle Fette Wache 1986; 112: 163–167.
5. Gassenmeier T, Busch P, Hensen H, Seipel W. Some aspects of refatting the skin; effects oriented to skin lipids for improving skin properties. Cosmet Toilet 1998; 113(9):89–92.
6. Both W, Gassenmeier T, Hensen H, Hörner V, Seipel W, Le Hen Ferrenbach C, Robbe Tomine L. Agents relifidants dans les produits de soin: une nécessité. Parfum Cosmetiques Actualités 1998; 23(142):63–65.
7. Fuller JG. Ethoxylated Mono and Diglycerides in Skin and Hair Care Applications, 15th IFSCC International Congress, London, 1988, Vol. A, paper A5: 43–55.
8. Barnett G. Lanolin and derivatives. Cosmet Toilet 1986; 101(3):23–44.
9. Whalley GR. Take a closer look at lanolin. Household and Personal Products Industry 1998; 36(5):115–118.
10. Wendel SR. Utilisation des silicones dans les cosmétiques et produits de toilette. Parfums, Cosmétiques, Arômes 1984;9(59):67–68.
11. Alexander P. Oils in water. Manufacturing Chemist 1989; 60(3):33–35.
12. Wendel SR, DiSapio AJ. Organofunctional silicones for personal care applications. Cosmet Toilet 1983; 98(5):103–106.
13. Gallagher KF. Hydrolyzed vegetable proteins: a formulator's guide (part 1). Drug Cosmet Ind 1991; 151(8):34–66.
14. Gallagher KF, Jones RT. Hydrolyzed vegetable proteins: a formulator's guide (part 2). Drug Cosmet Ind 1992; 152(12):26–36.
15. Chvapil M, Eckmayer Z. Role of proteins in cosmetics. Int J Cosmet Sci 1985; 7:41–49.
16. Teglia A, Secchi G. New protein ingredient for skin detergency: native wheat protein-surfactant complexes. Int J Cosmet Sci 1994;16:235–246.
17. Tavss EA, Eigen E, Temnikow V, Kligman AM. Effect of protein cationicity on inhibition of in vitro epidermal curling by alkylbenzene sulfonate. J Am Oil Chem Soc 1986; 63(4): 574–579.
18. Eigen E, Weiss S. U.S. Patent 3,548,056 (1970). Skin protecting composition containing a water-soluble partially degraded protein. Assigned to Colgate Palmolive Company.

19. Marsh RA, Mackie GJ, Hale P. U.S. Patent 4,195,077 (1980). Detergent composition comprising modified proteins. Assigned to The Procter and Gamble Company.
20. Gallagher KF, Jones RT. Emerging technology in protein copolymerization. Cosmet Toilet 1993; 108(3):97–104.
21. Jones R. Protein potential. Soap Perfumery Cosmet 1992; 65(4):33–34.
22. Jones R. Dérivés de protéines greffés aux silicones. Parfums Cosmétiques Arômes 1993; 18(109):69–71.
23. Stern ES, Johnsen VL. Cosmetic proteins: a new generation. Cosmet Toilet 1983; 98(5):76–84.
24. Marti ME. Phyto-active cosmetics. Drug Cosmet Ind 1992; 152(2):36–46.
25. Pugliese P, Hines G, Wielinga W. Skin protective properties of a cationic guar derivative. Cosmet Toilet 1990; 105(5):105–111.
26. Faucher JA, Goddard ED, Hannan RB, Kligman AM. Protection of the skin by a cationic cellulose polymer. Cosmet Toilet 1977; 92(6):39–44.
27. Goddard ED. Cationic cellulosic derivatives. Kennedy JF, Phillips GO, Williams PA, eds. Cellulosic Chemical Biochemical and Material Aspects. London: Horwood, 1993:331–336.
28. Alexander P. Cationic polymers for skin & hair conditioning. Manufacturing Chemist 1987; 58(7):24–29.
29. Jack S. The use of Merquat in hair and skin care. Soap Perfumery Cosmet 1985: 58(11):633–636.
30. Sykes R, Hammes PA. The use of Merquat polymers in cosmetics. Drug Cosmet Ind 1980; 126(2):62–136.

36

Surfactants

Takamitsu Tamura and Mitsuteru Masuda

Lion Corporation, Tokyo, Japan

SOLUTION PROPERTIES OF SURFACTANTS

Surfactants for cosmetic use may be grouped into the following six categories: cleaning agents, emulsifying agents, foam boosters, hydrotropes, solubilizing agents, and suspending agents [1]. Most cosmetic products are formulated through the use of these surfactants as main ingredients. This section briefly surveys major surfactants for shampoos and rinses presently on the Japanese market. Basic solution properties of surfactants are then discussed.

Anionic Surfactants

Soaps for detergent have been in use since 3000 BC. Primary detergents in early shampoos before the 1950s were mainly potassium or ammonium salts of fatty acids. These soaps have good foaming performance in pure water, although only slightly so in hard water because of the formation of insoluble metal soaps [2]. Various synthetic surfactants have been developed during the past 50 years. They have come to replace soaps and are soluble even in hard water. The most common synthetic surfactants are alkyl sulfate (AS) and alkyl ether sulfate (AES). These initially appeared on the U.S. market more than 50 years ago, and liquid shampoos subsequently came to be used throughout the country in the 1960s. Ammonium or ethanolamine salts of AS and sodium or ammonium salts of AES were used on a particularly large scale for the preparation of many products. Through the use of ethylene oxide (EO) groups, AS increases solubility and reduces precipitate of Ca salt and foam volume. Increase in solution viscosity is essential for enhancing shampoo appeal to customers. Alkanol amides of fatty acids are effective for viscosity and foam enhancement.

Alpha–olefin sulfonate (AOS) is commonly used as an anionic surfactant in shampoos [3]. A surfactant is a mixture of hydroxyalkane and alkene sulfonates whose structures are shown in Figure 1. AOS exhibits excellent stability at low pH compared with AS or AES and is more soluble in hard water than AS. Increase in solution viscosity has been shown possible through the use of alkanol amides and anionic surfactants in combination.

Various surfactants as supporting ingredients are used in the absence of complete

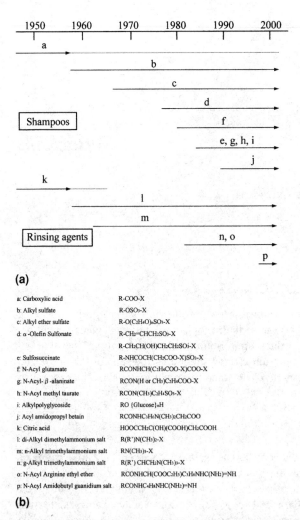

(a)

(b)

a: Carboxylic acid	R-COO-X
b: Alkyl sulfate	R-OSO₃-X
c: Alkyl ether sulfate	R-O(C₂H₄O)ₙSO₃-X
d: α -Olefin Sulfonate	R-CH₂=CHCH₂SO₃-X
	R-CH₂CH(OH)CH₂CH₂SO₃-X
e: Sulfosuccinate	R-NHCOCH(CH₂COO-X)SO₃-X
f: N-Acyl glutamate	RCONHCH(C₂H₄COO-X)COO-X
g: N-Acyl- β -alaninate	RCON(H or CH₃)C₂H₄COO-X
h: N-Acyl methyl taurate	RCON(CH₃)C₂H₄SO₃-X
i: Alkylpolyglycoside	RO {Glucose}ₙH
j: Acyl amidopropyl betain	RCONHC₃H₆N(CH₃)₂CH₂COO
k: Citric acid	HOOCCH₂C(OH)(COOH)CH₂COOH
l: di-Alkyl dimethylammonium salt	R(R')N(CH₃)₂-X
m: n-Alkyl trimethylammonium salt	RN(CH₃)₃-X
n: g-Alkyl trimethylammonium salt	R(R') CHCH₂N(CH₃)₃-X
o: N-Acyl Arginine ethyl ether	RCONHCH(COOC₂H₅)C₃H₆NHC(NH₂)=NH
p: N-Acyl Amidobutyl guanidium salt	RCONHC₄H₈NHC(NH₂)=NH

FIGURE 1 Surfactants for shampoos and rinsing agents on the Japanese market.

functional performances. Alkyl sulfosuccinates exhibit excellent foaming capacity, and their use is attended with low skin irritation provided AS is present [3]. In the 1980s, surfactants with low skin irritation came into popularity. Several amino acids have been developed for surfactant use, such as acyl glutamate [4]. These have excellent foaming, good biodegradability, and low skin irritation. Acyl amino acids such as lauroyl β-ala-ninate [5] and N-methyl β-alaninate [6] are presently in use. N-acyl methyltaurate [7] is also available and has been proven ideal for shampoo use with low skin irritation.

Nonionic and Amphoteric Surfactants

Nonionic surfactants are preferable to those that are anionic, but have found limited use owing to poor foaming capacity for shampoos. Alkanol amides and alkyl amine-oxides are used primarily as foam boosters and stabilizers [3]. Alkyl glucoside may be obtained through reaction of fatty alcohol with glucose; it is mild to the skin and has good foam stability [8].

Amphoteric surfactants are used in combination with anionic and nonionic surfactants to achieve greater shampoo mildness. A typical amphoteric surfactant is N-acyl amidopropyl betaine [3] featured by low skin irritation and foaming enhancement. Alkyl iminodiacetates may be obtained from fatty amines as mild surfactants [9]. The cocoylarginine ethyl ester (CAE) is prepared from arginine and shows high affinity to hair [10,11]. A new mild amphoteric surfactant, Amisafe, is derived from arginine [12] and functions as a cationic surfactant at weakly acidic pH and is readily adsorbed onto hair.

Cationic Surfactants

Because of the negative charge on the surface of hair, cationics strongly bind to hair and are difficult to remove by rinsing. When a shampoo containing soap has been used, acidic rinse containing citric acid may be applied to remove the alkali and metal soaps. Dialkyl ammonium salts are used in rinse formulations for shampoos containing AS and AES as main ingredients [13]. Quaternary ammonium salts containing mono- or dialkyl groups with 16 to 22 carbon atoms are presently in wide use. At the start of the 1980s, a milky lotion-type rinse came into prominent use. It was produced by adding oils to a gel comprising cationic surfactant, fatty alcohol, and water. Novel cationic surfactants are presently being produced. Quaternary ammonium salts made using long-chain Guarbet alcohol form lamellae liquid crystals even in cold water and are readily adsorbed onto hair [14]. Amido guanidine cationic surfactants (AG) with methylene groups as spacers between amide and guanidino groups [15] are available, and there is a hair conditioner containing AG with excellent moisturizing properties even at low humidity.

Micelle Formation and Surfactant Solubility

The high solubility of surfactants in water is very important in the preparation of cosmetic products. Surfactants show characteristic solubility because of the presence of hydrophobic groups, which squeeze out hydrocarbon chains of surfactants to bring about micelle formation [16]. A phase diagram of the two-component system is shown in Figure 2 [17]. At dilute surfactant concentration, micelle formation occurs above a critical temperature and at surfactant concentration above the critical micelle concentration (CMC). In region I, surfactant concentration is too low for micelle aggregation to occur, and consequently the surfactants dissolve into monomers. In region II, surfactant micelles are equilibrated with monomers. In region III, surfactant monomers are present along with precipitated hydrated solid surfactants. That is, the micelles comprise melting hydrated solid surfactants beyond the phase boundary curve between regions II and III. The point where the two phase boundary curves intersect is the Krafft point of a surfactant solution.

Liquid Crystals and Gels

Various intermediate phases may exist between solid and liquid states. At high surfactant concentration in Figure 2, several liquid crystalline phases can be seen to have formed. The liquid crystalline phases of surfactant-water systems are in the liquid state with a long-range repulsive order of one, two, or three [18,19]. With increase in surfactant concentration, the hexagonal (IV), cubic liquid crystalline (V), and lamellae phases (VI) are produced. The hexagonal phase consists of long rod micelles of surfactants hexagonally arranged. The lamellae phase comprises surfactant bilayers separated by water layers. The water layers vary in thickness from 10 Å to several 100 Å. The hexagonal and lamellae

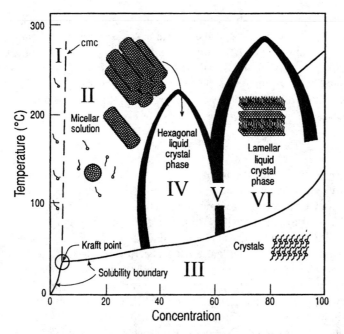

FIGURE 2 Schematic phase diagram of an ionic surfactant. (From Ref. 17.)

phases are optically anisotropic, whereas the cubic liquid crystalline phase is optically isotropic. The cubic phases may take on various structures such as packed spherical micelles in a cubic array, surfactant rods connected in a complex manner to form a continuous network, and bicontinuous networks with positive and negative curvature interfaces [19,20].

In liquid crystalline phases, hydrocarbon chains are in a liquid-like state. When these phases are cooled, a coagel phase consisting of hydrated crystals and a gel phase are formed as shown in Figure 3 [21,22]. The gel phase contains fairly ordered intermediate water, except for hydrated water, between surfactant bilayers. This phase is produced on warming the coagel phase when hydration interactions occur between counter ions. Phase diagrams for octadecyltrimethyl ammonium salts show the stability of the gel phase.

Phase Behavior of Nonionic Surfactants

Increase in nonionic surfactant aqueous solution temperature causes the development of two isotropic phases in solution, above what is called the cloud point. The hydrophilic/hydrophobic balance of a nonionic surfactant may differ considerably at this temperature, and consequently there is characteristic phase behavior in nonionics/hydrocarbon/water ternary systems, as is the case when using a plane of fixed 1:1 weight ratio of oil to water, as shown in Figure 4 [23]. At lower temperature, nonionic surfactants are highly soluble in water and form O/W microemulsions in a water-rich phase with excess oil. At higher temperature, they are highly soluble in oil and form W/O microemulsions in an oil-rich phase with excess water. At the phase inversion temperature, a three-phase system comprises a middle phase microemulsion, a nearly pure water phase, and an oil phase. Phase transition with temperature is indication of potential for cosmetic use.

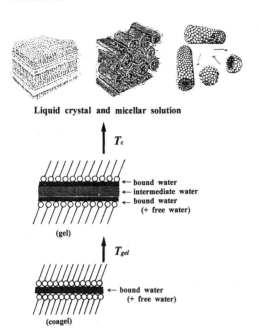

FIGURE 3 Changes in the aggregation of surfactants and water molecules in response to increase in temperature. (From Ref. 21.)

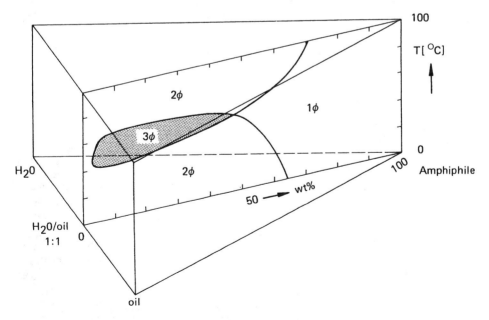

FIGURE 4 Vertical section of the phase prism of a ternary system for $H_2O/Oil = 1/1$. (From Ref. 23.)

FOAMING PROPERTIES OF SURFACTANTS

Foaming is an essential property of shampoos, skin cleansers, aerosols, shaving cream, mouthwash, and toothpaste, and its mechanism and stabilization have been studied [24–26]. This parameter is enhanced by the following [27]: (1) high viscosity in the liquid phase to retard hydrodynamic drainage; (2) high surface viscosity to retard liquid loss between interfaces; (3) surface effects to prevent thinning of liquid film, such as the Gibbs-Marangoni effect; (4) electrostatic and steric repulsion between adjacent interfaces to prevent drainage caused by disjoining pressure; and (5) gas diffusion from smaller to larger bubbles.

Methods for Foaming Assessment

Foam is a dispersion of gas bubbles in a liquid and the liquid film of each bubble is colloidal in size. Surfactant solutions often have the important feature of foaminess. This property may be defined as foam volume produced from a unit foam volume of solution and may be evaluated based on pressure or temperature and the particular method of formation [28,29]. Standard methods of formation are listed in Table 1. The method may be static or dynamic. Foaminess in this study was evaluated based on foam volume and lifetime. These factors are difficult to assess independently by conventional methods. Because of the complexity of the foam system, better methods are being sought.

Dynamic Surface Tension

Surface elasticity is a major factor determining thin liquid film stability [24]. Foam contains many bubbles separated by liquid films that are continuously enforced by dynamic change in the liquid, such as liquid drainage and bubble motion. In the case of surfactant-stabilized aqueous film, stretching causes local decrease in the surface concentration of the adsorbed surfactant. This decrease causes local surface tension increase (the Gibbs elasticity), which acts in opposition to the original stretching force. In time, the original surface concentration of the surfactant is restored. This time-dependent restoration force in thin liquid film is referred to as the Marangoni effect. Dynamic adsorption at the gas/liquid interface must thus be considered in the assessment of foam stability. Although there are various techniques for measuring equilibrium tension [30], the maximum bubble

TABLE 1 Standard Methods for Foaming Assessment

Principle	Classification	Method	Standard
Static methods	Poring	Ross & Miles Test	ASTM standard D 1173-53
		Modified Ross & Miles Test	ISO standard 696-1975(E)
	Shaking	Bottle Test	ASTM standard D 3601-88
	Beating	Perforated Disk Test	DIN standard 53902 part 1
	Stirring	Blemder Test	ASTM standard D 3519-88
Dynamic methods	Air injection	Diffuser Stone Test	ASTM standard D 892-92
			ASTM standard D 1881-86
		Gas Bubble Separation Test	ASTM standard D 3427-86
	Circulation	Recycling and Fall Test	AFNOR draft T73-421

Abbreviations: ASTM, American Society of Testing and Materials; ISO, International Standardization Organization; DIN, Deutsches Institut für Normung; AFNOR, Association Frances Normalization.

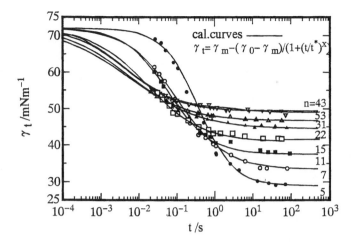

FIGURE 5 Effects of EO units on dynamic surface tension, γ_t, versus bubble surface lifetime, t, for 1 mM aqueous C12En solution at 25°C.

pressure method is used the most for this measurement to monitor dynamic surface tension on a short time scale.

A typical curve of dynamic surface tension shows induction, rapid fall, mesoequilibrium, and equilibrium [31,32]. All these parameters have significant effect on high-speed dynamics. Data for surface tension for aqueous solutions of polyoxyethylene dodecyl ethers (C12En), $C_{12}H_{25}O(C_2H_4O)_nH$, where n = 5 − 53, as a function of time, are presented in Figure 5. Maximum rate of decrease in surface tension $(d\gamma_t/dt)_{max}$, was determined based on the data [33]. Dynamic surface tension (γ_t) at constant surfactant concentration may be obtained as

$$\gamma_t = \gamma_m + (\gamma_0 - \gamma_m)/\{(1 + (t/t^*)^x\} \qquad (1)$$

where γ_t is the surface tension of the solution at time, t; γ_m is the mesoequilibrium surface tension of the solution (where γ_t shows little change—<1mNm^{-1} per 30s—with time), γ_0 is the equilibrium surface tension of the solvent, and t* and n are constants for a given surfactant. The parameter t* is the time for γ_t to reach a value midway between γ_0 and γ_m, and decreases with increase in surfactant concentration. The curves obtained with Eq. (1) are widely fitted for the observed time scale, as shown in Figure 5. The $(d\gamma_t/dt)_{max}$ may be derived from Eq. (2) as

$$(d\gamma_t/dt)_{max} = -x(\gamma_0 - \gamma_m)/4t^* \qquad (2)$$

Foamability and Foam Stability

Methods for foam formation and stability evaluation were established based on various sources of data, such as dynamic surface tension and liquid film movement, respectively, using a laminometer ($L_{lamellae}$). Ross-Miles foam behavior of aqueous C12En solution is shown in Figure 6. Initial foam height increased linearly with EO. Residual foam height decreased sharply with increase in EO. Dynamic surface properties of aqueous C12En solution are shown in Figure 7. The $(d\gamma_t/dt)_{max}$ increased linearly with EO, whereas $L_{lamellae}$ decreased sharply with EO. Dynamic foam behavior by these methods was found

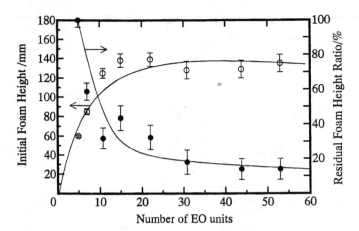

FIGURE 6 Effects of EO units on the Ross-Miles foam behavior for 1 mM aqueous C12En solution at 26°C.

consistent with conventional foam test results. Initial foam height in the Ross-Miles test was in good agreement with $(d\gamma_t/dt)_{max}$, and residual foam height in good agreement with $L_{lamellae}$. Foam formation would thus appear to depend primarily on the rate of adsorption of surfactants onto a gas/liquid interface and foam stability may also be a factor. For nonionic surfactants, initial foam height and stability are less compared with ionic surfactants in aqueous solution because of the large surface area per molecule of surfactant molecule. The effects of area per molecule (A) on foam stability and thinning of vertical films, monitored by FT-IR as a function of time, were examined [34,35]. Data for the Ross and Miles foam stability and aqueous core thickness of vertical foam film at rupture (D_{rup}) as a function of A are shown in Figure 8 [35]. Linear increase in D_{rup} with A was noted, whereas residual foam height sharply decreased with A. Nonionic surfactants that occupy less surface area would thus appear to promote the disruption of foam. Accord-

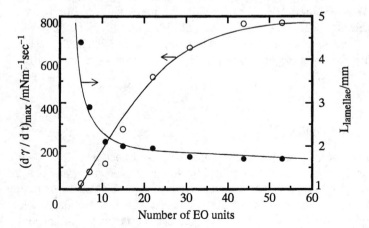

FIGURE 7 Effects of EO units on dynamic parameters for 1 mM aqueous C12En solution at 26°C.

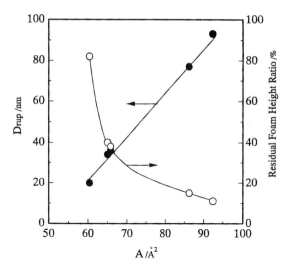

FIGURE 8 Effects of area per molecule (A) on Ross & Miles foam stability (5 min) and aqueous core thickness (D_{rup}) for 1 mM aqueous nonionics solution at ruptured 25°C.

ingly, hydrophobic interactions between surfactant molecules may significantly contribute to foam stabilization.

ADSORPTION OF SURFACTANTS

Adsorption at the solid/liquid interface is an important feature requiring consideration in mechanics, electronics, biological systems, agriculture, foods, and cosmetics. When the adsorption isotherm of a surfactant on a solid surface is measured, several quantitative aspects of surfactant adsorption can be clarified.

Adsorption of Surfactants on Inorganic Solid Surfaces

The surface properties of a solid surface primarily determine the adsorption capacity of a surfactant. There are nonpolar and hydrophobic surfaces, polar and uncharged surfaces, and charged surfaces [36]. Inorganic oxides using cosmetics (e.g., silica, alumina, titania) have charged surfaces. Thus, interactions between a charged surface and ionic surfactant should be understood for controlling the properties on the surface.

The adsorption of SDS onto alumina in aqueous solution has been studied extensively and the mechanisms of adsorption have been made clear [37,38]. The adsorption isotherm of SDS on alumina is presented in Figure 9 and comprises the following four regions [39]: region I with a slope of unity derived from electrostatic interactions between SDS and an oppositely charged solid surface; region II shows steep increase in adsorption attributable to surfactant aggregation at the surface through lateral interactions between hydrocarbon chains—the surface of alumina is not fully covered and there are still positive sites where adsorption may take place; in region III, decrease in the slope of the isotherm attributable to increased electrostatic hindrance of surfactant adsorption is evident—the transition from region II to III corresponds to the isoelectric point of the solid, in which the adsorbent and adsorbate have the same charge; and for region IV, there is maximum

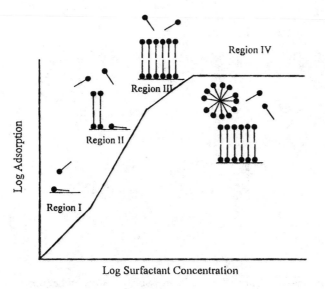

FIGURE 9   Schematic diagram of typical adsorption isotherm. (From Ref. 39.)

surface coverage at cmc and further increase in surfactant concentration has no effect on adsorption density.

Binding of Surfactant to Human Hair

The binding of a surfactant to human hair or wool has been well studied. The thermodynamic aspects of surfactant binding are thus considered in this section. The binding of ionic surfactants to globular proteins has been extensively investigated by thermodynamic analysis of binding interactions [40–44]. In consideration of the fine structure of human hair, surfactants should bind to the cuticle, cortex, and fibrils, all comprising proteins. Thus, continuous binding of a surfactant with human hair would appear the same as that of surfactants with globular proteins.

Binding isotherms of SDS for normal and damaged hair are shown in Figure 10 [45]. SDS bound to cold-waved hair increased remarkably compared with normal and bleached hair. Each isotherm has two regions. Region I shows Langmuir binding attributable to interactions of SDS with ionic sites on the surface of hair. For region II, there was noted sharp increase in adsorption as a result of surfactant aggregation at the surface brought about by lateral interactions between hydrocarbon chains. Damaged hair may possibly be an indication of disruption of disulfide crosslinks. This increase involving the consequent binding of SDS on polypeptides in the hair because of electrostatic repulsion among micelle-like clusters. Rigid disulfide bonds are maintained, and thus such binding was noted to a slight degree for the isotherms of normal hair. The binding isotherms of dodecyltrimethylammonium chloride (DTAC) for normal and damaged hair indicated no increase in binding.

In the Langmuir binding region, the equation of Klotz [Eq. (3)] has quantitative application, as

$$1/\gamma = (1/K \cdot n) \cdot (1/C) + 1/n \tag{3}$$

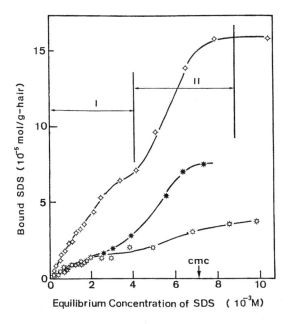

FIGURE 10 Binding of SDS to normal hair (✿), bleached hair (✱), and cold-waved hair (◇) at 25°C.

where γ is total bound surfactants; n, total number of binding sites; K, binding constant; and C, concentrations of surfactants at equilibrium. n and K may be obtained from plot of $1/\gamma$ versus $1/C$. The free energy change, $-\Delta G$, is related to the binding constant as

$$-\Delta G = R \cdot T \cdot \ln K \tag{4}$$

Thermodynamic parameters for binding between surfactants and normal hair are listed in Table 2. n and $-\Delta G$ for anionic surfactants were the same in all cases regardless of alkyl chain length. $-\Delta G$, when SDS was bound to BSA, was twice that in the case of SDS binding to hair. In the case of BSA, electric and hydrophobic interactions contribute to the free energy change of binding. Electrostatic interactions between an anionic surfactant and hair would thus appear quite weak, and no alkyl chains at all would be in a hydrophobic area. n and $-\Delta G$ for cationic surfactants were also the same regardless of alkyl chain length. $-\Delta G$, in the case of DTAC binding to BSA and cationic surfactant binding to keratin powder, were the same as for binding to hair. The force of cationic surfactant

TABLE 2 Thermodynamic Parameters of Binding Between Ionic Surfactants and Normal Hair

Surfactants	n($\times 10^{-5}$ mol/g)	K($\times 10^2$ L/mol)	$-\Delta G$ (KJ/mol)
SDS (C12)	3.1	3.8	14.7
SDeS (C10)	4.0	2.2	13.4
SOS (C8)	3.5	2.9	14.2
DTAC (C12)	2.1	10.0	17.2
DeTAC (C10)	1.7	9.4	16.8

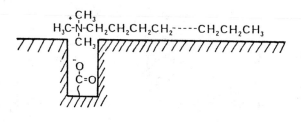

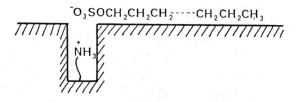

FIGURE 11   Schematic diagrams of the binding of surfactants to human hair.

binding to hair would thus appear to arise mainly from hydrophobic interactions and alkyl chains would not be present in a hydrophobic area on the surface of hair, as also in the case of anionic surfactants. Binding sites for ionic surfactants on hair are shown in Figure 11 [45]. Dissociated carboxyl and amino groups of polypeptides may possibly be present just inside the surface of the hydrophobic layer.

REFERENCES

1. Rieger MM. Cosmetics. In: Kroschwitz JI, Howe-Grant M, eds. Encyclopedia of Chemical Technology. Vol. 7, 4th ed. New York: Wiley, 1992:572–619.
2. Porter MR. Anionics. In: Porter MR, ed. Handbook of Surfactants. London: Blackie, 1994: 99–104.
3. Reich C. Hair cleansers. In: Rieger MM, Rhein LD, eds. Surfactants in Cosmetics: Revised and Expanded. 2d ed. New York: Marcel Dekker, 1997:357–384.
4. Sakamoto K. Application and effect of derivatives of amino acids for hair. Fragrance J 1979; 39:57–62.
5. Yoshimura M, Jokura Y, Hanazawa H, Nozaki T, Okuda M, Imokawa G. Biological characterization of a unique amino acid derivative-surfactant, lauroyl beta-alanine in relation to its cutaneous effect. J Soc Cosmet Chem Jpn 1993; 78:249–254.
6. Ishii M, Takizawa H, Usuba Y, Ishikawa K, Morimoto K, Akiba H. Synthesis and properties of N-acyl-N-alkyl-β-alanine. J Jpn Oil Chem Soc 1968; 17:616–622.
7. Miyazawa K, Tamura U, Katsumura Y, Uchikawa K, Sakamoto T, Tomita K. Anionic surfactants as detergents for scalp and hair. J Jpn Oil Chem Soc 1989; 38:297–305.
8. Kamegai J, Watanabe H, Hanazawa H, Kobayashi H. Properties and applications of nonionic surfactants derived from saccharides to shampoo. J Soc Cosmet Chem Jpn 1993; 27:255–266.
9. Takeuchi K, Shimada M. Solution properties of alkyliminodiacetate. J Jpn Oil Chem Soc 1997; 46:1375–1381.
10. Nakanishi N, Matsuzawa Y, Mikami N. Moisturizing effect of amino acids and their derivatives. Fragrance J 1995; 23:71–80.
11. Infante M^{a}R, Perez L, Pinazo A. Novel cationic surfactants from arginine. In: Krister H, ed. Novel Surfactants: Preparation, Application, and Biodegradability. New York: Marcel Dekker, 1998:87–114.

12. Tabohashi T, Ninomiya R, Imori Y. A novel amino acid derivative for hair care products. Fragrance J 1998; 26:58–63.

13. Scott GV, Robbins CR, Barnhurst JD. Sorption of quaternary ammonium. J Soc Cosmet Chem 1969; 20:135–152.

14. Yahagi K, Hoshino N, Hirota H. Solution behavior of new cationic surfactants synthesized by using long-chain guerbet alcohols in water and their application to hair conditioners. J Soc Cosmet Chem Jpn 1990; 23:301–309.

15. Mitamura J, Suzuki N, Onuma K, Miyake M, Nakamura T, Kiyomiya A. Development of new cationic surfactant "AG" and application for hair conditioners. J Soc Cosmet Chem Jpn 1996; 30:84–93.

16. Degiorgio V. Introduction. In: Degiorgio V, Corn M, eds. Physics of Amphiphiles: Micelles, Vesicles, and Microemulsions. Amsterdam: North-Holland, 1985:1–6.

17. Raney KH. Surfactant requirements for compact powder detergents. In: Showell MS, ed. Powder Detergents. New York: Marcel Dekker, 1998:241–284.

18. Lindman B. Amphiphilic systems. Some basic aspects. In: Degiorgio V, Corn M, eds. Physics of Amphiphiles: Micelles, Vesicles, and Microemulsions. Amsterdam: North-Holland, 1985: 7–23.

19. Laughlin RG. The structures and properties of surfactant phases. In: The Aqueous Phase Behavior of Surfactants. London: Academic Press, 1994:181–237.

20. Fontell K. Cubic phases in surfactant and surfactant-like lipid systems. Colloid Polym Sci 1990; 268:264–285.

21. Kodama M, Seki S. Hyomen Coagel-Ctel-Liquid crystal phase transition and heat properties of amphiphiles. 1990; 22:61–67.

22. Kodama M, Seki S. Thermodynamical investigations on phase transitions of surfactant-water systems: thermodynamic stability of gel and coagel phases and the role of water molecules in their appearance. Adv Colloid Interface Sci 1991; 35:1–30.

23. Kahlweit M, Strey R. The phase behavior of H_2O-Oil-nonionic amphiphile ternary systems. In: Rosano HL, Clausse M, eds. Microemulsion Systems. New York: Marcel Dekker, 1987: 1–13.

24. Malhotra AK, Wasan DT. Interfacial rheological properties of absorbed surfactant films with applications to emulsion and foam stability. In: Ivanov IB, ed. Thin Liquid Films: Fundamentals and Applications. New York: Marcel Dekker, 1988:829–890.

25. Pugh RJ. Foaming, foam films, antifoaming and defoaming. Adv Colloid Interface Sci 1996; 64:67–142.

26. Aveyard R, Clint JH. Foam and thin film breakdown processes. Curr Opin Colloid Interface Sci 1996; 1:764–770.

27. Myers D. Foams. In: Myers D, ed. Surfaces, interfaces, and colloids: principles and applications. New York: VCH, 1991:251–270.

28. Domingo X, Fiquet L, Meijer H. Foam ability/stability of surfactants. Tenside Surf Deter 1992; 29:16–22.

29. Tamura T. The test methods for measuring foaming and antifoaming properties of liquid. J Jpn Oil Chem Soc 1993; 42:737–745.

30. Dukhin SS, Kretzschmar G, Miller R. Experimental technique to study adsorption kinetics. In: Möbius D, Miller R, eds. Dynamics of Adsorption at Liquid Interfaces. Amsterdam: Elsevier, 1995:140–201.

31. Hua H, Rosen M. Dynamic surface tension of aqueous surfactant solutions: I. Basic parameters. J Colloid Interface Sci 1988; 124:652–659.

32. Tamura T, Kaneko Y, Ohyama M. Dynamic surface tension and foaming properties of aqueous polyoxyethylene n-dodecyl ether solutions. J Colloid Interface Sci 1995; 173:493–499.

33. Rosen MJ, Hua XY, Zhu ZH. Dynamic surface tension of aqueous surfactant solutions: IV. Relationship to foaming. In: Mittal KL, Shah DO, eds. Surfactants in Solution. Vol. 11. New York: Plenum, 1991:315–327.

34. Tamura T, Kaneko Y, Nikaido M. Stability factors of foam film in contrast to fluctuation induced by humidity reduction. J Colloid Interface Sci 1997; 190:61–70.

35. Tamura T, Takeuchi Y, Kaneko Y. Influence of surfactant structure on the drainage of nonionic surfactant foam films. J Colloid Interface Sci 1998; 206:112–121.

36. Myers D. Physical properties of surfactants used in cosmetics. In: Rieger MM, Rhein LD, eds. Surfactants in Cosmetics. New York: Marcel Dekker, 1997:29–81.

37. Somasundaram P, Fuerstenau DW. Mechanisms of alkyl sulfonate adsorption at the alumina-water interface. J Phys Chem 1960; 70:90–96.

38. Somasundaram P, Chandar P, Turro NJ. Fluorescence probe studies on the structure of the adsorbed layer of dodecyl sulfate at the alumina-water interface. J Colloid Interface Sci 1987; 117:31–46.

39. O'Haver JH, Harwell H. Adsorption: some expected and unexpected results. In: Sharma R, ed. Surfactant Adsorption and Surface Solubilization. ACS Symposium Ser. 615. Washington, D.C.: ACS, 1995:51–66.

40. Schwuger MJ, Bartnik G. Interaction of anionic surfactants with proteins, enzymes, and membranes. In: Gloxhuber C, ed. Anionic Surfactants: Biochemistry, Toxicology, Dermatology. New York: Marcel Dekker, 1980:1–49.

41. Reynolds JA, Gallagher JP, Steinhardt J. Effect of pH on the binding of N-Alkyl sulfates to bovine serum albumine. Biochemistry 1970; 9:1232–1238.

42. Nozaki Y, Reynolds JA, Tanford C. The interaction of a cationic detergent with bovine serum albumin and other proteins. J Biol Chem 1974; 249:4452–4459.

43. Takagi T, Tsujii K, Shirahama K. Binding isotherms of sodium dodecyl sulfate to protein polypeptides with special performance to SDS-polyacrylamide gel electrophoresis. J Biochem 1975; 77:939–947.

44. Hiramatsu K, Ueda C, Iwata K, Aoki K. The interaction of bovine plasma albumin with cationic detergent. Studies by binding isotherm, optical rotation and difference spectrum. Bull Chem Soc Jpn 1977; 50:368–372.

45. Ohbu K, Tamura T, Mizushima N, Fukuda M. Binding characteristics of ionic surfactant with hair. Colloid Polym Sci 1986; 264:798–802.

37

Classification of Surfactants

Louis Oldenhove de Guertechin
Colgate-Palmolive Research and Development, Inc., Milmort, Belgium

INTRODUCTION

The term ''surfactant'' applies to a group of molecules having both a hydrophilic part and a hydrophobic (or lipophilic) part. Surfactants modify the interfacial properties of the liquids in which they are incorporated; this property stems from their tendency to concentrate at the interfaces separating immiscible phases. Depending on the nature of the hydrophilic moiety ensuring the water-affinity of the molecule, major surfactants can be divided into anionic, cationic, amphoteric, and nonionic classes.

Regarding the hydrophobic moiety of the molecule, it is a hydrocarbon chain in most common surfactants; however, in some more specialized surfactants, this hydrophobic part can be a nonhydrocarbon chain such as a polydimethylsiloxane or a perfluorocarbon. The selection of a surfactant for the development of cosmetic products should be carefully performed, taking into account numerous factors. Among others, one should consider those directly related to functions to be fulfilled (detergency, emulsification, foam quality, rinsability, mildness for skin, skin feel, etc.), and also those related to cost, toxicity, and biodegradability. The aim of this chapter is to provide a classification of various commercially available surfactants. Various textbooks [1–4] or general articles [5,6] may usefully complete this survey.

IONIC SURFACTANTS

Anionic Surfactants

In aqueous solution, anionic surfactants form a negatively charged ion provided the composition pH is neutral to alkaline. The ionized moiety can be a carboxylate, sulfate, sulfonate or phosphate. Among most frequently used surfactants in skin care products, the alkyl sulfates and alkyl ethoxylated sulfates can be mentioned for their high foaming capacity. Anionics are generally used in association with other surfactants (nonionics or amphoterics), which bring improvements in the skin tolerance, in the foam quality, or in the product viscosity.

Other anionics are also used in personal products, as secondary surfactants, often for their milder profile and their low foaming properties (isethionates, sulfosuccinates, taurates, sarcosinates, phosphoric acid esters, acylglutamates, etc.).

Carboxylates

Carboxylate Salts. Surfactants belonging to this class generally derive from oleo-chemistry; carboxylate salts (or soaps) can be directly produced by the alkaline hydrolysis (or saponification) of animal and vegetable glycerides or can result from the neutralization of fatty acids obtained by the acidification of carboxylates.

Saturated sodium soaps are extremely soluble in water up to C_8; they become less soluble up to C_{18} and insoluble above C_{20}. The fatty acids can be either saturated or unsaturated (starting from C_{16} chain lengths). Unsaturated fatty acids are prone to undergo oxidation and form oxides and peroxides, which cause rancidity and yellowing. Potassium soaps and salts of alkanolamines are more fluid and also more soluble than sodium salts. The extremely low solubility of alkaline earth and heavy metals fatty acid salts makes this class of surfactants less appropriate for use in hard water.

$$R-C \overset{\displaystyle O}{\underset{\displaystyle O^{\ominus} \quad M^{\oplus}}{\diagdown}} \qquad \begin{array}{l} M = Na, K, NH_4, etc. \\[2ex] R = CH_3\text{-}(CH_2)_x\text{-} \end{array}$$

Alkyl carboxylate

The main application of fatty carboxylates is found in the soap bars widely used in the world for fabric handwash (generally based on tallow/coconut oil mixtures). Water-soluble soaps are mainly used in skin cleansers (soap bars or liquids), shaving products (sticks, foams, or creams) and deodorant sticks. Mixtures of fatty acids and their salts are used in "acid soaps." Water-insoluble soaps form gels in nonaqueous systems and, because of their hydrophobicity, they can be appropriate surfactants for w/o emulsions.

Ester Carboxylates. This class of surfactants is a subcategory of the previously discussed surfactant group based on carboxylic acids; they are monoesters of di- and tricarboxylic acids. These esters are produced by condensation reactions involving different types of molecules; either an alcohol with a polycarboxylic acid (e.g., tartric or citric acid), or a hydroxyacid (e.g., lactic acid) with a carboxylic acid. The reacting alcohol may have been previously ethoxylated.

$$\begin{array}{l} \qquad\quad \overset{\displaystyle O}{\overset{\displaystyle \|}{CH_2C}}\!-\!O(CH_2CH_2O)_7\!-\!C_{12}H_{25} \\ \qquad\quad | \\ HO\!-\!C\!-\!COONa \\ \qquad\quad | \\ \qquad\quad \underset{\displaystyle \underset{\displaystyle O}{\|}}{CH_2C}\!-\!O(CH_2CH_2O)_7\!-\!C_{12}H_{25} \end{array}$$

Sodium dilaureth-7 citrate

Because of their good foaming properties and substantivity on the hair, ester carboxylates are especially suitable in shampoos; in combination with alcohol ethoxy sulfate (AEOS), they provide reduced skin irritation. Short chain lactylates (i.e., issued from lactyllactic acid) are substantive on the skin and present humectant properties.

Ether Carboxylates. These surfactants are formed by the reaction of sodium chloracetate with ethoxylated alcohols. Because of the addition of ethoxylated groups, ether carboxylates are more soluble in water and less sensitive to water hardness compared with conventional soaps. Also, keeping the best properties of nonionic surfactants, they do not exhibit any cloud point and show good wetting and foam stability. Ether carboxylates do not undergo hydrolysis in the presence of alkali or acids.

$$RO - (CH_2CH_2O)_n\text{-} CH_2\text{- } COONa$$

Alkyl polyglycol ether carboxylate, sodium salt

Ether carboxylates are used as general emulsifier and emulsion stabilizers. In the household, they are used in acidic toilet bowl cleaners. In personal care, they impart mildness, creamy foaming, skin-feel, and hair-conditioning benefits. Therefore, they are especially suitable in shampoos in combination with alcohol ether sulfates and possibly with cationics.

Sulfates

Alkyl Sulfates. Alkyl sulfates are organic esters of sulfuric acid; they vary by the length of the hydrocarbon chain and by the selected counterion. Alkyl sulfates are produced by sulfation of the corresponding fatty alcohols. The properties of alkyl sulfates depend mainly on the chain length and the degree of branching of the hydrocarbon chain, as well as, to a smaller extent, on the nature of the counterions. They are generally good foamers, more especially in hard water; best foam characteristics are obtained in the C_{12}–C_{14} chain length range.

Sodium lauryl sulfate (SLS) has a 12-carbon chain length and is one of the most common surfactants. It is not well tolerated by the skin. When the chain length increases (C_{14}–C_{18} range), surfactant penetrability through the stratum corneum decreases along with the irritation potential of the surfactant, but the foaming capacity is accordingly depressed. Chains with carbon number lower than 12 are better tolerated by the skin than SLS, but are smellier. Combination with other surfactants allows considerable improvement of the skin compatibility of lauryl sulfate while keeping a good foam. It is, however, less frequently used than its ethoxylated counterpart. Lauryl sulfate is available under the form of various salts: sodium lauryl sulfate (SLS), ammonium lauryl sulfate (ALS), magnesium lauryl sulfate [$Mg(LS)_2$], and triethanolamine lauryl sulfate (TEALS). Skin tolerance of lauryl sulfates is as follows: $Mg(LS)_2$ > TEALS > SLS > ALS.

$$
\begin{array}{c}
\text{H} \quad\quad \text{O} \\
| \quad\quad\quad || \\
\text{R--C--O--S--O}^{-} \;\; \text{Na}^{+} \\
| \quad\quad\quad || \\
\text{H} \quad\quad \text{O}
\end{array}
$$

Sodium alkyl sulfate

Alkyl sulfates are used in cosmetics and personal-care areas (e.g., DEA lauryl sulfate in shampoos); they are associated with other surfactants and improve foaming characteristics of detergent systems. Pure SLS (sodium lauryl sulfate) is used in oral care and incorporated in dental creams, essentially as a foaming agent.

Alkyl Ether Sulfates. Alkyl ether sulfates (AES), which are also called alcohol ethoxy sulfates (AEOS), result from the sulfation of an ethoxylated alcohol. Compared with alkyl sulfates, the ether sulfates show higher water solubility, improved foam stability in hard water, and better skin tolerance. The viscosity of surfactant solutions of ether sulfates is much more sensitive to the presence of electrolytes than alkyl sulfates; formulators often take advantage of this opportunity to bring liquid formulations to the desired viscosity by simply adjusting the salt level (e.g., NaCl). The higher the number of ethoxy groups (EO) in the molecule, the lower the surfactant ability to penetrate the stratum corneum and the less irritant for skin it will be. Similar ranking is true for eye irritation. Also, the foaming capacity decreases as ethoxylation degree increases.

$$R\text{-}CH_2\text{-}O\text{-}(CH_2\text{-}CH_2\text{-}O)_n\text{-}SO_3\,Na$$

Sodium alkyl ether sulfate

Alkyl ether sulfates are used in domestic applications such as household cleaners, dishwashing liquids, and fabric care.

Alkyl ether sulfates are also extensively used in personal products such as liquid soaps, shower gels, foam baths, and, more especially, shampoos. Sodium lauryl ether sulfate (SLES) is today the most currently used primary tensioactive, especially under the forms of SLES-2 EO and SLES-3 EO, which combine good foaming and skin compatibility properties.

Amide Ether Sulfates.   The amide ether sulfates are obtained by sulfation of the corresponding ethoxylated amide. The magnesium salts foam well and their skin compatibility is excellent.

$$\left[R-\underset{\underset{O}{\|}}{C}-NH(CH_2CH_2O)_3-SO_3 \right]_2 Mg^{2+}$$

Magnesium PEG-3 cocamide sulfate

Because of their weak lipid removal effect, amide ether sulfates are used in very mild personal cleaners.

Sulfonates

On a chemical standpoint, there is an important difference between the previously discussed alkyl sulfates and the alkyl sulfonates: in the former, the sulfur atom is linked to the carbon chain via an oxygen atom, and in the latter, the sulfur atom is directly linked to the carbon atom.

Alkyl Sulfonates.   Three major types of alkyl sulfonates must be considered: the primary and secondary paraffin sulfonates (PS and SAS) and the α-olefin sulfonates (AOS). The paraffin sulfonates are very water-soluble surfactants, good foamers, and good o/w emulsifiers. Their solutions do not thicken easily upon salt addition. Therefore, they are particularly appropriate to formulate fluid liquids or highly concentrated products. The α-olefin sulfonates (AOS) have general properties fully comparable to LAS (see next section); they are good o/w emulsifiers, wetting, and foaming agents.

$$CH_3 - (CH_2)_m - \underset{\underset{H}{|}}{\overset{\overset{H}{|}}{C}} - SO3\,Na \qquad\qquad CH_3 - (CH_2)_m - \underset{\underset{CH_3(CH_2)_n}{|}}{\overset{\overset{H}{|}}{C}} - SO3\,Na$$

Primary sodium alkyl sulfonate   Secondary sodium alkyl sulfonate

$$\pm 35\% \quad \begin{cases} R-CH_2-CH_2-CH=CH-CH_2-SO_3Na \\ \\ R-CH_2-CH=CH-CH_2-CH_2-SO_3Na \end{cases}$$

$$\pm 65\% \qquad R-CH_2-CH_2-\underset{\underset{OH}{|}}{CH}-CH_2-CH_2-SO_3Na$$

Constituents of α-olefin sulfonate: sodium alkene sulfonates and sodium hydroxy alkane sulfonate

Alkane sulfonates (PS and SAS) are mainly used in Europe in detergent products. Alpha-olefin sulfonates have been mainly used in Asia as surfactants for heavy and light duty laundry detergents, synthetic soap bars, and household products. Because they are less irritating than alkyl-aryl sulfonates, they have also been used in the United States in several personal products (liquid soaps, bubble baths, and shampoos) as alternatives to alcohol ether sulfates. They are also marginally used in oral care formulations.

Alkyl Aryl Sulfonates. Today, the LAS (linear alkylbenzene sulfonate) is the most important surfactant on a volume basis, but its use in personal care is very limited because of a low skin compatibility. It is worth mentioning that some methyl or methyl-ethyl substituted aryl sulfonates, i.e., sodium xylene, toluene, or cumene sulfonates (SXS, STS, or SCS), although not showing typical surfactant properties, are used as hydrotropes (i.e., decreasing hydrophobic effects in aqueous systems).

$$CH_3-(CH_2)_x-CH-(CH_2)_y-CH_3$$

with benzene ring bearing SO_3Na

Sodium linear alkylbenzene sulfonate

Sodium linear alkylbenzene sulfonate (LAS) is a very cost-effective surfactant that is extensively used in a broad variety of detergents for household, fabric care, and institutional and industrial products. Because of its too-high detersive action, LAS has a relatively low compatibility with skin and is only scarcely used in cosmetics except in some antiseborrheic preparations.

Sulfosuccinates. Sulfosuccinates are the sodium salts of alkyl esters of sulfosuccinic acid; they generally result from the condensation of maleic anhydride with a fatty alcohol, followed by a sulfonation with sodium bisulfite $NaHSO_3$. Some variants of sulfosuccinates are derived from other substituted fatty molecules such as fatty alcohol ethoxylates, fatty amines (yielding sulfosuccinamates), or fatty alkanolamides.

$$NaO_3S-\underset{\underset{\underset{\underset{O}{\|}}{C-OR}}{|}}{\overset{\overset{O}{\|}}{CH}-C-OR}$$

Sodium dialkyl sulfosuccinate

Monoesters disodium salts are the most common sulfosuccinates used in cosmetic applications. Monoesters of alkanolamines (sulfosuccinamates) are milder than monoesters of fatty alcohols (sulfosuccinates). Monoesters derived from ethoxylated alcohols or alkanolamides are extensively used in personal products and especially in shampoos; they are known for their mildness and skin-irritation reduction when used in association with other anionic surfactants.

Sulfo Fatty Acid Esters. These surfactants are sometimes known under their abbreviated names: FES for fatty ester sulfonate, MES for methyl ester sulfonate, or ASME for alpha sulfo methyl ester. Most of α-sulfo fatty acid esters derive from fatty acid methyl esters. In general, alkyl esters of α-sulfo fatty acid have excellent detergency (i.e., oil dispersing and emulsifying properties) when the molecule is dissymmetric (as in the case of the α-sulfo methyl esters). On the other hand, the α-sulfo esters, in which the sulfonate group is in the middle of the molecule (as in the case of long-chain alcohol esters), deliver good wetting but poor detergency.

$$R - CH - C \overset{O}{\underset{O-CH_3}{\diagdown}} \qquad R - CH - C \overset{O}{\underset{O-R'}{\diagdown}}$$
$$\qquad | \qquad\qquad\qquad\qquad\qquad | $$
$$\quad SO_3Na \qquad\qquad\qquad\qquad SO_3Na$$

Methyl ester of α-sulfo   Alkyl ester of α-sulfo
fatty acid, sodium salt   fatty acid, sodium salt

Alpha-sulfo methyl ester surfactants deriving from C_{16}–C_{18} fatty acid (e.g., ASMT, the tallowate) are appropriate for use in laundry detergents. ASME is also used in the formulation of syndet bars (laundry bars based on synthetic surfactants).

Fatty Acid Isethionates and Taurides. Fatty acid isethionates are usually prepared by reaction of a fatty acid chloride with sodium isethionate ($HO-CH_2-CH_2-SO_3-Na$), itself resulting from the addition of sodium bisulfite to ethylene oxide. These surfactants are insensitive to water hardness and show good wetting, foaming, and emulsifying properties. In addition, they are very mild and have excellent compatibility with the skin. Taurides (or taurates) are acylamino alkane sulfonates that have chemical structures close to isethionates. They can be used in association with other surfactants to increase the viscosity.

$$\overset{O}{\overset{||}{R-C}}-OCH_2CH_2-SO_3Na \qquad\qquad \overset{O}{\overset{||}{R-C}}-\overset{CH_3}{\overset{|}{N}}-CH_2CH_2-SO_3Na$$

Fatty acid isethionate   Sodium methyl acyl tauride

Acyl isethionates have been used in shampoos and personal cleansers. They are also incorporated in syndet bars together with various soaps. The most currently used is the cocoyl isethionate.

Taurides (or taurates), which have the same expected properties as soaps (except the sensitivity to water hardness), had been extensively used in shampoos but have been replaced by AEOS. Today they are limitedly used in cosmetics mainly in foam baths and toilet bars. Taurides are also used in soap bars especially designed for laundering with seawater, in agriculture, and textile dying.

Phosphate Esters

This class of surfactants includes alkyl phosphates and alkyl ether phosphates.

$$RO-\overset{\overset{\displaystyle O}{\|}}{\underset{\underset{\displaystyle OH}{|}}{P}}-OH \qquad\qquad RO-\overset{\overset{\displaystyle O}{\|}}{\underset{\underset{\displaystyle OR}{|}}{P}}-OH$$

Alkyl phosphoric ester   Dialkyl phosphoric ester

The use of phosphate esters as surfactants is especially useful in applications for which a particular tolerance to pH, heat, or electrolytes is required. They are also used in acidic cleaning products for household as well as industrial applications. Mild for the skin, alkyl phosphates sometimes enter the composition of facial and cleansing products.

Acylamino Acids and Salts

Acyl Glutamates.   These surfactants are formed by acylation of a natural amino acid, the glutamic acid $HOOC\text{-}CH_2\text{-}CH_2\text{-}CH(NH_2)\text{-}COOH$ (or α-aminoglutaric acid). These surfactants are mild for the skin and the eyes, deliver improved skin feel, but are poor foamers.

$$NaOOC-CH_2CH_2\underset{\underset{\underset{\underset{\displaystyle O}{\|}}{C-R}}{\underset{\displaystyle |}{NH}}}{CH}-COONa$$

Sodium acyl glutamate

Acyl glutamates are mainly used in personal products such as shampoos.

Acyl Peptides.   These surfactants are formed from hydrolyzed proteins (e.g., animal collagen). Depending upon the protein hydrolysis process (chemical or enzymatic), the average polypeptide molecular weight can vary from about 350 to 2000 and some free amino acids may be present in the hydrolysate. An acylation reaction occurs on the amine terminal functions and, possibly, on some side groups (e.g., the hydroxyls); it accordingly leaves free carboxyl groups which must be neutralized.

Products containing such surfactants are prone to be contaminated by various germs and have to be properly preserved.

$$R-\overset{\overset{\displaystyle O}{\|}}{C}-[\overset{\overset{\displaystyle X}{|}}{NH}\,CH\,\overset{\overset{\displaystyle O}{\|}}{C}]_x-NH\overset{\overset{\displaystyle X}{|}}{C}H\,\overset{\overset{\displaystyle O}{\|}}{C}-ONa$$

Sodium acyl polypeptide (X= amino acids side groups)

Acyl peptides are mild surfactants designed for the personal-care area; they are especially used in shampoos because of their substantivity on the keratin of hair and, therefore, they effectively deliver the expected benefits of conditioning agents.

Acyl Sarcosides.   Sarcosinates (or salts of acylamino acids) are the condensation products of fatty acids with N-methylglycine $CH_3\text{-}NH\text{-}CH_2\text{-}COOH$ (or sarcosine).

$$R-\overset{\overset{\displaystyle O}{\|}}{C}-\underset{\underset{\displaystyle CH_3}{|}}{N}-CH_2COONa$$

Sodium acyl sarcosinate

Sarcosinates are good surfactants for cosmetic usage because of their mildness to skin, substantivity on skin and hairs when incorporated in formulations around neutral pH, conditioning action, and foaming resistance in the presence of soaps or sebum. Incorporated in shampoos with alkyl sulfates, they boost the lather. Sarcosinates are also used as corrosion inhibitors.

Cationic Surfactants

From a very general standpoint, cationic surfactants differ from anionic and nonionic ones by the fact that they carry a positive charge. Their major interest in cosmetic industry resides in hair care; in this frame, they are use as hair conditioners and antistatic agents. Cationics are also found in the personal-care area as emulsifiers in some cosmetic preparations and as bactericidal agents.

Alkylamines

Primary, secondary, and tertiary alkylamines, and more especially their salts, are included in this surfactant class.

$$R-NH_2 \qquad R-N\overset{\displaystyle CH_3}{\underset{\displaystyle CH_3}{<}} \qquad R-\overset{\overset{\displaystyle O}{\|}}{C}-NH-(CH_2)_3-N\overset{\displaystyle CH_3}{\underset{\displaystyle CH_3}{<}}$$

Alkylamine   Dimethyl alkylamine   Alkylamido dimethyl propylamine

Amines and their salts are mainly used in textile treatment and occasionally in rinse fabric softeners. Salts of amines are used in cosmetics together with other surfactants. Their usage is restricted to specialties; they exhibit conditioning and antistatic properties in haircare applications. Amido-amines are also used in cosmetic products.

Alkylimidazolines

Reaction of a fatty acid with a substituted ethylene diamine forms imidazoline. Heating the resulting, amido-ethylamine yields the imidazoline with a five-member substituted ring. The tertiary nitrogen atom can be quaternized.

$$\begin{array}{ccc} R-C & \!\!\!\!—\!\!\!\! & N-R' \\ \| & & | \\ N & & CH_2 \\ \diagdown & CH_2 & \diagup \end{array}$$

$R' = CH_2CH_2NH_2$ => alkyl aminoethyl imidazoline

$R' = CH_2CH_2OH$ => alkyl hydroxyethyl imidazoline

Imidazolines are cationic o/w emulsifiers. Considered to be irritating they are scarcely used in cosmetics as substantive hair conditioning agents.

Quaternary Ammonium Compounds

Quaternary ammonium compounds form a class of surfactants that contain a positively charged nitrogen atom linked to four alkyl or aryl substituents. The positive charge is permanent, regardless of pH.

Tetra-Alkyl(-aryl) Ammonium Salts. Tetra-alkyl ammonium salts have the structure $[R_1R_2R_3R_4N^+]X^-$ where R_1, R_2, R_3, and R_4 are alkyl or aryl groups and X^- represents an anion. The water solubility of quaternaries mainly depends upon the nature of R substituents. Low solubility quaternaries can adsorb on various substrates and impart various useful conditioning effects (e.g., softening, antistat, corrosion inhibition). With the exception of N-alkyltrimethyl ammonium salts, quaternary surfactants usually show poor detergency, wetting, and emulsifying capacities. Quaternaries are generally not compatible with anionics because of the formation of a water-insoluble complex.

$$\left[R - \overset{\overset{\displaystyle CH_3}{|}}{\underset{\underset{\displaystyle CH_3}{|}}{N^+}} - R' \right] \quad X^-$$

Quaternary compound

The major usage of quaternaries is related to their ability to adsorb on natural or synthetic substrates and fibers. They are widely used as softening agents in rinse fabric softeners. Their softening and antistatic properties are similarly exploited in hair conditioning shampoos or after-shampooing rinses. It is worth noting that, in cosmetic applications, quaternaries may cause ocular and local irritation. Among quaternaries, some are used as germicides and disinfectants (e.g., benzalkonium chloride).

Heterocyclic Ammonium Salts. Heterocyclic quaternaries are derived from heterocyclic aliphatic or aromatic compounds in which a nitrogen atom constitutive of the cycle is quaternized.

$$\left[C_{17}H_{35} - \underset{\underset{\displaystyle N}{|}}{\overset{\overset{\displaystyle CH_2CH_2\,NH\,CO\,C_{17}H_{35}}{|}}{N}} - CH_3 \right]^+ \quad CH_3OSO_3^-$$

Imidazolinium quaternary compound

The quaternaries derived from imidazoline and morpholine are used as hair conditioners and antistatic agents. Those derived from aromatic heterocycles are used as germicides.

Alkyl Betaines. Alkyl betaines, which are N-trialkyl derivatives of amino acids ($[R_1R_2R_3]N^+CH_2COOH$), are classified as cationics because they exhibit a permanent positive charge. Because they also have a functional group able to carry a negative charge in neutral and alkaline pH conditions, they are often regarded—although this position is questionable—as "amphoterics." The positive charge is always carried by a quaternized nitrogen while the anionic site can be a carboxylate (betaine), a sulfate (sulfobetaine or sultaine), or a phosphate (phosphobetaine or phostaine).

Betaines are good foaming, wetting, and emulsifying surfactants, especially in the presence of anionics. Alkylamido betaines deliver more stable foam and are better viscosifiers than alkyl dimethyl betaines. Betaines are compatible with other surfactants and they frequently form mixed micelles; these mixtures often deliver unique properties that are not found in the individual constitutive surfactants.

Betaines have low eye and skin irritation; moreover, the presence of betaines is known to decrease the irritation effect of anionics.

$$R-\overset{\overset{\displaystyle CH_3}{|}}{\underset{\underset{\displaystyle CH_3}{|}}{N^+}}-CH_2COO^-$$

Alkyl dimethyl betaine

$$R-\overset{\overset{\displaystyle O}{\|}}{C}-NH-(CH_2)_3-\overset{\overset{\displaystyle CH_3}{|}}{\underset{\underset{\displaystyle CH_3}{|}}{N^+}}-CH_2\overset{}{\underset{\underset{\displaystyle OH}{|}}{C}}HCH_2SO_3^-$$

Alkylamidopropyl hydroxysultaine

Because of their ability to improve the skin tolerance against irritating anionic surfactants, and also because of their high price, betaines are usually used in association with other surfactants. Betaines are especially suitable in personal-care applications (e.g., shampoos, foam baths, liquid soaps, shower gels), fabric handwash products, and dishwashing products.

Ethoxylated Alkylamines

These surfactants can be considered as cationic or nonionic depending on the degree of ethoxylation and the pH at which they are used. Polyethoxylated amines are formed by ethoxylation of primary or secondary fatty amines.

$$R-\overset{}{\underset{\underset{\displaystyle (CH_2\,CH_2\,O)_x\,H}{|}}{N}}-CH_2\,CH_2\,CH_2\,N\overset{\diagup (CH_2\,CH_2O)_y\,H}{\diagdown (CH_2\,CH_2O)_z\,H}$$

$C_{12}H_{25}N\ [(CH_2CH_2O)_3H]_2$

Laurylamine + 6 EO (or POE 6)   Alkyl propanediamine ethoxylate

The ethoxylated alkylamines have various application fields; they are generally exploited for their capacity of adsorbing on surfaces. In personal care, ethoxylated alkylamines are used as emulsifiers and hair-conditioning agents. Ethoxylated amidoamines find applications in rinse fabric softeners.

Esterified Quaternaries

Esterified quaternaries (or esterquats) are produced by the esterification of the hydroxyl group(s) of secondary or tertiary amino-alcohols with selected fatty acids.

$$\left[\begin{array}{c} H_3C \diagdown \overset{\oplus}{N} \diagup CH_2\text{-}CH_2\text{-}O\overset{O}{\overset{\diagdown}{-}}C\text{-}R \\ HO-H_2C-H_2C \diagup \qquad \diagdown CH_2\text{-}CH_2\text{-}O\underset{O}{\underset{/\!/}{-}}C\text{-}R \end{array} \right] \quad MeSO_4^{\ominus}$$

Esterquat: N-Methyl-N,N-bis[$C_{16/18}$-acyloxy)ethyl]-N-(2-hydroxyethyl)ammonium-methosulfate salt

The esterquats are suitable substitutes for straight quaternaries. They present improved environmental profile and comparable softening properties compared with straight quaternaries.

Amphoteric Surfactants

Amphoteric surfactants are characterized by the fact that these surfactants can carry both a positive charge on a cationic site and a negative charge on an anionic site. The use of amphoteric terminology is still more restrictive: the charge of the molecule must change with pH, showing a zwitterionic form at intermediate pH (i.e., around the isoelectric point). The surfactant properties are accordingly influenced by pH: around the isoelectric point the zwitterionic form takes place, exhibiting the lowest solubility; in alkaline conditions the anionic form is predominant, delivering foam and detergency; and in acidic conditions, the cationic form prevails, providing surfactant substantivity. Although betaines are commonly classified among amphoterics, this classification is improper because these surfactants never exhibit in single anionic form. Amphoteric surfactants are generally used as secondary tensioactives for their foam stabilizing effect, their thickening capacity, and their skin-irritation reduction capacity on alkyl sulfates and alkyl ethoxy sulfates.

Acyl Ethylenediamines and Derivatives

These surfactants are made by the reaction of an alkyl imidazoline with chloroacetic acid (yielding amphoglycinates) or with acrylic acid (yielding amphopropionates).

$$R-\overset{\overset{O}{\|}}{C}-NH-CH_2CH_2-\underset{\underset{|}{\overset{CH_2COONa}{}}}{N}-CH_2CH_2OH$$

Acylamphoacetate

$$R-\overset{\overset{O}{\|}}{C}-NH-CH_2\,CH_2-\underset{\underset{|}{\overset{CH_2\,CH_2\,COO\,Na}{}}}{N}-CH_2\,CH_2\,O\,CH_2\,CH_2\,COO\,Na$$

Acylamphodipropionate

Amphoterics of this class are mainly used in personal products (e.g., coco amphocarboxy glycinate). Incorporated in baby shampoos, they reduce eye irritation. Other applications are fabric softeners, industrial cleaners, and car cleaners.

N-Alkyl Amino Acids or Imino Diacids

These molecules are chemical derivatives of amino acids that can be produced by the reaction of chloroacetic acid or acrylic acid with an alkylamine. Their compatibility with other surfactants is excellent. These surfactants are good emulsifiers and show optimal wetting and detergency under alkaline pH. They are good foamers at neutral and alkaline pH but lose their foaming properties under acidic conditions. They are substantive to surfaces and provide antistatic effects. They provide skin and eye irritancy reduction in combination with anionics.

$$R-NH-CH_2CH_2-COOH \qquad\qquad C_{12}H_{25}-NH-CH_2-COONa$$

Alkyl aminopropionic acid   Sodium coco glycinate

$$R-N\begin{cases} CH_2CH_2CH_2-NH_2 \\ CHCH_2CH_2-C-NH_2 \\ \;\;| \qquad\qquad \| \\ COOH \qquad\;\; O \end{cases} \qquad\qquad R-N\begin{cases} CH_2CH_2-COONa \\ CH_2CH_2-COONa \end{cases}$$

Aminopropyl alkylglutamide   Sodium alkyliminodipropionate

Amphoterics of this class are mainly used in personal products. Polycarboxylates deliver reduced eye irritation and provide hair-conditioning benefits. Their zwitterionic forms are substantive on the hairs.

NONIONIC SURFACTANTS

Nonionic surfactants do not dissociate into ions in aqueous medium. They generally deliver a weak to moderate foam. They are appreciated for their good skin and eye compatibility as well as for their anti-irritant potential when they are combined with anionics in appropriate concentration ratio. Therefore, numerous products for sensitive skin, babies, or the face incorporate nonionics as major surfactants.

Fatty Alcohols

Fatty alcohols are primarily used as a chemical precursor for the production of several other surfactants.

$$R-CH_2-OH$$

Fatty alcohol

Because they are not water soluble, the use of fatty alcohols is very limited in liquid products. They are mainly used as opacifiers, thickening agents, and foam depressors (e.g., lauric alcohol).

Ethers

Alkoxylated Alcohols

This class of surfactants mainly covers ethoxylated or propoxylated alcohols. Ethoxylated alcohols (also called ''polyethyleneglycol ethers'' or ''PEG ethers'') are produced from the reaction of fatty alcohols with ethylene oxide (EO). Similarly, propoxylated alcohols (also called ''polypropyleneglycol ethers'' or ''PPG ethers'') are obtained with propylene oxide (PO). The HLB of ethoxylated alcohols can be adjusted by properly balancing the hydrophilic ethoxylated chain and the hydrophobic fatty chain. Ethoxylate nonionics are compatible with all surfactants. Some beneficial associations with ionic surfactants are often shown.

In the frame of personal-care applications, ethoxylated alcohols often result from the transformation of natural lipids. The nomenclature specific to cosmetic chemicals (i.e., INCI names[1]) is applied to these nonionics: they are denominated by using the root of the fatty acid name terminated by the suffix ''eth'' (contraction of ''ethoxylated''), directly followed by the ethoxylation degree (e.g., laureth-4, oleth-5, myristeth-7). As some raw materials yield on hydrolysis various fatty chain lengths, the names of the derived nonionics are either drawn from the natural source (e.g., laneth-16 for a lanolin-derived nonionic) or from the fusion of the constitutive fatty chains (e.g., ceteareth-20 for a combination of cetyl and stearyl).

$$CH_3 (CH_2)_x - O - (CH_2CH_2O)_n H$$

Alkyl polyethyleneglycol ether or alcohol ethoxylate
(e.g., laureth 20 for x=11 and n=20)

$$CH_3 - \left[CH_2\right]_x \left[O - \underset{\underset{CH_3}{|}}{CH}CH_2\right]_y \left[OCH_2CH_2\right]_z OH$$

EO/PO Alkyl Ether
(e.g., propyleneglycol capreth-4 for x=9, y=1, and z=4)

Applications of ethoxylated alcohols are numerous in industrial as well as in household products. When properly selected, alkoxylated alcohols are also useful for personal products as good emulsifiers and solubilizers. The cosmetic applications remain, however, limited because of their rather weak foaming capacity. Because they are prone to undergo degradation by oxidation, the following precautions can greatly improve the stability of

---

[1] The International Cosmetic Ingredient Dictionary provides a nomenclature of conventional names for cosmetic ingredients that are defined by the CTFA (The Cosmetic, Toiletry, and Fragrance Association).

ethoxylate nonionics: storage in the dark, minimal air contact, low temperature storage, avoiding storage of diluted products, and the addition of an antioxidant.

EO/PO Block Polymers

These polymeric surfactants have some similarity with the previously discussed alkoxylated alcohols. They consist in the combination of the assembly of PPG (hydrophobic part) and PEG chains (hydrophilic part). Such surfactants are known under the denomination "poloxamers" (INCI name) and are called EO/PO block copolymer nonionics. A major property of EO/PO nonionics is their low-foaming profile. As straight EO nonionics, EO/PO copolymers exhibit the cloud point phenomena. EO/PO nonionics are also mild surfactants.

$$HO(CH_2CH_2O)_x \left[\begin{array}{c} CH\ CH_2O \\ | \\ CH_3 \end{array} \right]_y (CH_2CH_2O)_z H$$

Ethoxylated PPG ether

These surfactants are especially useful for applications in which foaming must be significantly depressed, such as automatic dishwashing detergents, laundry detergents, and rinse aids. Because of their mildness, EO/PO block polymers also find applications in cosmetic products. They are generally used as emulsifying, solubilizing, or fluidizing agents.

Alkyl Polyglucosides

Alkyl polyglucosides are most often known by the simple abbreviation APG. APGs are produced by the alkylation of short-chain glucosides resulting from acidic alcoholysis of polysaccharides such as starch. Commercial products consist of mixtures of mono-, di-, and triglucosides. Accordingly the glucosidic chain varies between 1.2 and 3 depending on the production conditions. Surfactants of this class are good emulsifiers and provide good wetting and foaming profiles. Alkyl polyglucosides are compatible with all other surfactants. They show good chemical stability at neutral and alkaline pH, and are impaired under acidic conditions (pH <5).

Alkylpolyglucoside

APGs are used in detergents and personal-care cleansers (e.g., shampoos). They are claimed to be very mild for skin as well as to reduce the skin irritation potential of anionics. Additionally, they impart an excellent skin feel. Their thickening effect in the presence of anionics and their foam stabilization capacity are also exploited in personal-care applications.

Ethoxylated Oils and Fats

This class of surfactants essentially covers ethoxylated derivatives of lanolin (i.e., aliphatic alcohols and sterols, fractionation products of wool fat) and of castor oil (i.e., fatty acids extracted from ricinus seeds). Ethoxylated products of lanolin and castor oil are good and excellent emulsifiers, respectively. These surfactants are mainly used in the cosmetic industry; their major interest is to offer the possibility of claims based on the natural origin of the constitutive surfactant systems.

Alkanolamides

Straight Alkanolamides

Alkanolamides are N-acyl derivatives of monoethanolamine and diethanolamine.

$$R\ CO\ NH\ CH_2CH_2OH \qquad R\ CO\ N {\overset{CH_2CH_2OH}{\underset{CH_2CH_2OH}{}}} \qquad R\ CO\ N{\overset{CH_2CH_2\ OCOR}{\underset{CH_2CH_2OH}{}}}$$

Monoalkanolamide   Dialkanol amide   Ester amide

Alkanolamides have been largely used in household detergent products; their consumption has now significantly declined because of the extensive use of alkyl ethoxylated detergent products. Because of their foam-boosting and viscosity-enhancing capacity in the presence of anionics, alkanolamides are also usefully incorporated in personal care, especially in shampoos.

Ethoxylated Alkanolamides

Reaction of an alkanolamide with ethylene oxide leads to an ethoxylated amide.

$$R\ CO\ NH\ (CH_2CH_2O)_n\ H$$

Polyethoxylated monoalkanolamide

It is more expensive than its corresponding ethoxylated alcohol and has therefore restricted usage. The benefits of thickening, foam stabilization, and dispersibility are exploited in personal-care cleansers.

Esters

In this surfactant class, there are five major subcategories to be considered:

1. Ethoxylated fatty acids
2. Glycol esters, glycerol esters, and ethoxylated derivatives
3. Sorbitan esters and ethoxylated derivatives
4. Alkyl carbohydrates esters
5. Triesters of phosphoric acid

Ethoxylated Fatty Acids

This class of surfactants comprises mono- and diesters that result from the reaction of fatty acids with either ethylene oxide or polyethylene glycol.

$$R-\overset{\overset{\displaystyle O}{\|}}{C}-O-(CH_2CH_2O)_n-H$$

PEG fatty acid ester

$$R-\overset{\overset{\displaystyle O}{\|}}{C}-O-(CH_2CH_2O)_n-\overset{\overset{\displaystyle O}{\|}}{C}-R$$

PEG fatty acid diester

Given their outstanding emulsifying properties, ethoxylated fatty acids are useful in domestic and industrial detergents, more especially in degreasing compositions. If properly balanced, combinations of esters with low and high ethoxylation provide excellent emulsifiers for creams and lotions. They are also used as mild cleaners or viscosifying agents (e.g., PEG-150-distearate). In cosmetics (shampoos), less water-soluble grade (i.e., ethylene glycol monostearate) is used as a pearlescent agent.

Glycol Esters, Glycerol Esters, and Ethoxylated Derivatives

A common point among the surfactants grouped in this class and the following two classes (sorbitan esters and alkyl carbohydrates esters) is that they all derive from the condensation reaction of a polyhydroxyl compound (e.g., glycol, glycerol, sorbitol, sucrose,) with a fatty acid. Some of them can be directly extracted from natural sources. The resulting esters can be additionally ethoxylated to increase their HLB value and, thereby, their solubility in water.

These surfactants show poorer wetting and foaming properties in comparison with alcohol-derived nonionics. Emulsifying properties are excellent. In general, esters and lower ethoxylates are appropriate for w/o dispersions whereas higher ethoxylates are more suitable emulsifiers for o/w dispersions.

$$R-\overset{\overset{\displaystyle O}{\|}}{C}- OCH_2CH_2OH$$

Ethylene glycol ester

$$R-\overset{\overset{\displaystyle O}{\|}}{C}-OCH_2\underset{\underset{\displaystyle CH_3}{|}}{CH}-OH$$

Propylene glycol ester

$$\begin{array}{l} CH_2O-\overset{\overset{\displaystyle O}{\|}}{C}\text{-R} \\ | \\ CHOH \\ | \\ CH_2OH \end{array}$$

Monoglyceride

$$\begin{array}{l} CH_2O-\overset{\overset{\displaystyle O}{\|}}{C}\text{-R} \\ | \\ CHOH \\ | \\ CH_2O-\underset{\underset{\displaystyle O}{\|}}{C}\text{-R} \end{array}$$

1,3-diglyceride

$$\begin{array}{l} CH_2O-\overset{\overset{\displaystyle O}{\|}}{C}\text{-R} \\ | \\ CHO\,(CH_2\,CH_2O)_nH \\ | \\ CH_2O-\underset{\underset{\displaystyle O}{\|}}{C}\text{-R} \end{array}$$

Polyethoxylated 1,3-diglyceride

$$HOCH_2 \underset{\underset{OH}{|}}{CH} CH_2O (CH_2 \underset{\underset{OH}{|}}{CH} CH_2O)_n CH_2 \underset{\underset{OH}{|}}{CH} CH_2O - \overset{\overset{O}{\|}}{C}\text{-}R$$

Polyglyceryl monoester

Because of their high compatibility, these surfactants are widely used in the cosmetic and food industry.

Glycol and glycerol esters are used in the pharmaceutical and cosmetic industries either as emulsifying agents or as oily compounds, refatting agents, emollients, and skin conditioners in various products such as creams, lotions, ointments, and gels. Stearate derivatives also deliver thickening and opacifying properties (e.g., the glyceryl stearate). Some are also used as pearlescent agents (i.e., glycol stearate and distearate). Ethoxylated derivatives are used as solubilizing agents, emulsifiers, and even as emollients. Some show effective thickening effect when combined with other surfactants (e.g., PEG-200 glyceryl stearate).

Sorbitan and Sorbitol Esters and Ethoxylated Derivatives

Sorbitan molecule is generated from the dehydration of the sorbitol molecule, which results in an internal ether bond.

Sorbitol   1, 4 Sorbitan

Sorbitol and sorbitan esters are obtained by acylation of hydroxyl groups, using most frequently natural fatty acids such as lauric, palmitic, stearic, or oleic. These surfactants can be optionally ethoxylated. Acylation (or ethoxylation) can occur on almost all hydroxyl groups present in the original polyol molecule.

1, 4 Sorbitan monoester   1, 4 Sorbitan triester   Polyethoxylated sorbitan

The field of application of sorbitan esters and their ethoxylated derivatives is identical to the one of glycol and glycerol esters (see previous section). The sorbitol esters with a higher degree of ethoxylation (e.g., sorbitol septaoleate 40 EO) are also used as spreading aids in emollient bath oils.

Alkyl Carbohydrates Esters

Surfactants of this class are better known as "sugar esters" or "sucrose esters." The sucrose esters are obtained by transesterification of sucrose with fatty acid methyl esters or triglycerides. Surfactants of this class are good emulsifiers. Of great interest about such surfactants is their natural origin and good biodegradability. It is worth noting that some glucosides surfactants, e.g., the so-called saponins, are already present in nature and directly available from vegetal sources.

Saccharose fatty acid monoester

Sucrose esters are food-grade ingredients and have similar uses as the previously described glycol, glycerol, and sorbitan esters in the food and cosmetic industries. They are very mild surfactants and can be used as emulsifiers or as cleansing agents with emollient properties.

Amine Oxides

Amine oxides are produced by the oxidation of tertiary amines using a 35% hydrogen peroxide solution as the oxidizing agent. Amine oxides remain mainly nonionic in neutral and alkaline conditions (pH >7) but can become weakly cationic under acidic conditions. In current amine oxides, the initial reactives are alkyl dimethyl amines with chain lengths ranging from C_{12} to C_{18}. Amine oxides are compatible with all other surfactants. Amine oxides are also known to increase the skin compatibility of detergent products. A small amount of amine oxide increases the cloud point of nonionics.

Incorporated in shampoos, amine oxides contribute to impart viscosity, reduce eye and skin irritancy, and enhance foam properties (more creamy). They are especially suitable in slightly acidic or neutral formulas.

NONHYDROCARBON SPECIALTY SURFACTANTS

Alkoxylated Polysiloxanes

Surfactants, which can be classified in the chemical group of organosilicones, are structurally derived from polydimethylsiloxanes in which some methyl are replaced by hydrophilic groups that can be of anionic, cationic, or nonionic nature. The nonionic derivatives are mostly represented by the polyether-polydimethylsiloxane-copolymers. The general structure of these surfactants is shown in structure 37. The hydrophilic chain(s) generally contain EO/PO block copolymers.

$$(CH_3)_3\, Si-O-\left[\begin{array}{c} CH_3 \\ | \\ Si-O \\ | \\ CH_3 \end{array}\right]_m \left[\begin{array}{c} CH_3 \\ | \\ Si-O \\ | \end{array}\right]_n Si\,(CH_3)_3$$

$$(CH_2)_p -O- (C_2H_4O)_x - (C_3H_6O)_y - H$$

Polysiloxane-Polyether Copolymer (p generally equals 0 or 3)

These surfactants are specialty ingredients and are used in very different fields (e.g., painting, foam control, phytosanitary products). They are also used in cosmetics and haircare:

1. in cosmetic or personal-care products as emulsifiers in, e.g., protective creams, hydrating body milks, liquid soaps, and shave creams, and
2. in haircare products (e.g., shampoos, conditioners, gels, lotions, foams) to act as combing out auxiliaries, to reduce the irritancy of surfactant system, to provide improved skin feel, or to control the foam. The CTFA-adopted name of these surfactants is *Dimethicone Copolyol.*

Fluorosurfactants

Fluorosurfactants form a distinct group of surfactants besides the conventional surfactants based on hydrocarbon chains. Fluorosurfactants differ from hydrocarbon surfactants by the hydrophobic moiety of the molecule, which is made of perfluoroalkyls chains F—$(CF_2-CF_2)_n-$, in which n ranges from about 3 to about 8. Similarly to conventional surfactants, a rather broad variety of hydrophilic functions (e.g., ethoxylated chains, sulfonates, quaternaries, betaines) can be borne by fluorosurfactants. Depending on their nature, these surfactants show variable emulsifying and foaming characteristics. Although fluorosurfactants have some potential prospects in personal care (e.g., improved hair conditioning), we are not aware of any significant application in this field. We can, however, report their use in barrier creams that require good spreading and stable o/w emulsions.

REFERENCES

1. Ash M, Ash I. Handbook of Industrial Surfactants. An International Guide to More Than 16,000 Products by Trade Name, Application, Composition and Manufacturer. Aldershot: Gower, 1993.
2. Falbe J. Surfactants in Consumer Products. Theory, Technology and Application. Berlin/New York: Springer, 1987.

3. Lange KR. Detergents and Cleaners: A Handbook for Formulators. München: Hanser Publishers, 1994.
4. Porter MR. Handbook of Surfactants. London: Blackie Academic & Professional, 1991.
5. Rieger MM. Surfactant Encyclopedia. 2nd ed. Carol Stream: Allured Publishing, 1996.
6. Anonymous. Surfactant Encyclopedia. 2nd ed. Cosmetic & Toiletries. Carol Stream: Allured Publishing Corp., 1989; 104:67–110.

38

UV Filters

Stanley B. Levy
*University of North Carolina School of Medicine at Chapel Hill, Chapel Hill,
North Carolina, and Revlon Research Center, Edison, New Jersey*

INTRODUCTION

The presence of ultraviolet (UV) filters in skincare and cosmetic products represents a key benefit that cosmetics can provide consumers. The hazards of UV light exposure are well known. It is estimated that the incidence of nonmelanoma skin cancer in the United States exceeds one million cases per year [1]; UV-induced or photoaging accounts for 80% to 90% of visible skin aging [2]. UV radiation damages the skin by both direct effects on DNA and indirectly on the skin's immune system [3].

In animal models, sunscreens prevent the formation of squamous cell carcinomas of the skin [4]. The regular use of sunscreens has been shown to reduce the number of actinic or precancerous keratosis [5] and solar elastosis [6]. Sunscreens also prevent immunosuppression [7]. Double-blind photoaging studies show consistent improvement in the "untreated" control groups partly because of the use of sunscreens by all study subjects [8].

The cosmetic formulator has an expanding menu of active sunscreen ingredients for incorporation into a variety of cosmetic formulations. Selection is restricted by regulatory agencies in the country in which the final product is to be marketed. This chapter will concentrate on reviewing available UV filters.

DEFINITIONS

Ultraviolet radiation (UVR) reaching the Earth's surface can be divided into UVB (290–320 nm) and UVA (320–400 nm). UVA can be further subdivided into UVA I (340–400 nm), or far UVA, and UVA II (320–340 nm), or near UVA.

The sun protection factor (SPF) is defined as the dose of UVR required to produce one minimal erythema dose (MED) on protected skin after application of 2 mg/cm^2 of product divided by the UVR to produce one MED on unprotected skin. A water-resistant product maintains the SPF level after 40 minutes of water immersion. A very water-resistant or waterproof product is tested after 80 minutes of water immersion. If the SPF level is diminished by immersion, a separate SPF level may be listed. A broad-spectrum or full-spectrum sunscreen provides both UVB and UVA protection. Ideally this includes both UVA I and UVA II coverage.

HISTORY

Two UV filters, benzyl salicylate and benzyl cinnamate, were first incorporated into a commercially available sunscreen emulsion in the United States in 1928 [9]. In the early 1930s, phenyl salicylate (Salol) was used in an Australian product [10]. Para-aminobenzoic acid (PABA) was patented in 1943, leading to the development of PABA derivative UV filters. During World War II, red veterinary petrolatum (RVP) was used by the U.S. military, encouraging the development of further UV filters in the postwar period.

In the 1970s, increased interest in commercial sunscreen products led to refinements and consumer acceptance of these products over the next two decades. Facilitated by growing awareness of the hazards of UVR, higher SPF products became the norm. Daily-use consumer products containing UV filters, including moisturizers, color cosmetics, and even haircare products, have become more prevalent in the past decade. Concerns related to the adequacy of sunscreen protection for the prevention of melanoma and photoaging in the last few years has led to greater interest in broad-spectrum sunscreen UV protection throughout the entire UVA range.

REGULATIONS

United States

Sunscreen products in the United States are regulated by the FDA as over-the-counter drugs. The Final Monograph for Sunscreen Drug Products for Over-the-Counter Human Use was recently issued (64 Fed. Reg. 1999: 64: 27,666–27,693), establishing the conditions for safety, efficacy, and labeling of these products. The number of allowable sunscreen ingredients has been reduced (Table 1), reflecting the lack of interest in some of the ingredients in previously issued tentative monographs. Avobenzone and zinc oxide have been added, expanding the available UVA I blockers. Minimum concentration re-

TABLE 1 FDA Sunscreen Final Monograph Ingredients

Drug name	Concentration (%)	Absorbance
Aminobenzoic acid	Up to 15	UVB
Avobenzone	2–3	UVA I
Cinoxate	Up to 3	UVB
Dioxybenzone	Up to 3	UVB, UVA II
Homosalate	Up to 15	UVB
Menthyl anthranilate	Up to 5	UVA II
Octocrylene	Up to 10	UVB
Octinoxate	Up to 7.5	UVB
Octisalate	Up to 5	UVB
Oxybenzone	Up to 6	UVB, UVA II
Padimate O	Up to 8	UVB
Phenylbenzimidazole sulfonic acid	Up to 4	UVB
Sulisobenzone	Up to 10	UVB, UVA II
Titanium dioxide	2 to 25	Physical
Trolamine salicylate	Up to 12	UVB
Zinc oxide	2 to 20	Physical

quirements have been dropped, providing that the concentration of each active ingredient is sufficient to contribute a minimum SPF of not less than 2 to a finished product. A sunscreen product must have a minimum SPF of not less than the number of active sunscreen ingredients used in combination multiplied by 2. Products with SPF values above 30 are allowed, but the SPF declaration for sunscreens with SPF values above 30 are limited to SPF 30 plus. The term ''sunblock'' is now prohibited. It was previously allowed for products that contained titanium dioxide. Consideration of labeling and testing procedures for UVA protection was deferred and will be addressed in the future.

Europe

In Europe, sunscreen products are considered to be cosmetics, their function being to protect the skin from sunburn. The Third Amendment of the European Economic Community (EEC) Directive provides a definition and lists the UV filters that cosmetic products may contain. This list is divided into two parts. Table 2 lists UV filters that are fully permitted updated through the 23rd commission directive of September 3, 1998. Table 3 currently lists the three UV filters that are provisionally permitted through June 30, 1999. The numbers referenced with ''S'' indicate COLIPA numbers (The European Toiletry and Perfumery Association). Unlike the U.S. FDA Monograph, the EEC Directive does not list physical UV filters despite their being used in products to enhance protection.

Australia

In 1992, sunscreens were declared to be drugs in Australia. The latest edition of Australian Standard 2604 was published in 1993 as a joint publication of Australia and New Zealand. Sunscreen products are classified as either primary or secondary, depending on whether the primary function of the designated product is to protect from UVR as opposed to a product with a primary cosmetic purpose. SPF designations greater than 15 are not permitted (SPF 15+ represents the maximum designation). In general, Australian Approved Names (AAN) for allowed active sunscreen ingredients are the same as FDA drug nomenclature with few differences.

Other Countries

Most non-EEC European countries follow the EEC Directive. Many other countries follow U.S. trends with their own provisions. In Japan, sunscreens are classified as cosmetics. Regulations for each individual country need to be consulted for selection of the various UV filters for incorporation into a sunscreen product to be marketed in a given jurisdiction.

MECHANISM OF ACTION

UV filters have been traditionally divided into chemical absorber and physical blockers based on their mechanism of action. Chemical sunscreens are generally aromatic compounds conjugated with a carbonyl group [11]. These chemicals absorb high-intensity UV rays with excitation to a higher energy state. The energy lost results in conversion of the remaining energy into longer lower-energy wavelengths with return to ground state. The evolution of modern sunscreen chemicals represents a prototype study in the use of struc-

TABLE 2   UV Filters That Cosmetic Products May Contain (EEC Directive Annex VII—Part 2)

COLIPA number	Ref. number	Substance	Maximum authorized concentration
S 1	1	4-Aminobenzoic acid	5%
S 57	2	N,N,N-Trimethyl-4-(2-oxoborn-3-ylidenemethyl) anilinium methyl sulphate	6%
S 12	3	Homosalate (INN)	10%
S 38	4	Oxybenzone (INN)	10%
S 45	6	2-Phenylbenzimidazole-5-sulphonic acid and its potassium, sodium, and triethanolamine salts	8% (expressed as acid)
S 71	7	3,3'-(1,4-Phenylenedimethylene)bis[7,7-dimethyl-2-oxo-bicyclo-(2,2,1)hept-1-ylmethanesulphonic acid] and its salts	10% (expressed as acid)
S 66	8	1-(4-Tert-butylphenyl)-3-(4-methoxyphenyl) pro-pane-1,3-dione	5%
S 59	9	Alpha-(2-oxoborn-3-ylidene)toluene-4-sulphonic acid and its salts	10% (expressed as acid)
S 32	10	2-Cyano-3,3-diphenyl acrylic acid, 2-ethylnexyl ester (octocrylene)	10% (expressed as acid)
S 72	11	Polymer of N-(2 and 4)-[(2-oxoborn-3-ylidene)methyl] benzyl acrylamide	6%
S 28	12	Octyl methoxycinnamate	10%
S 3	13	Ethoxylated ethyl-4-aminobenzoate (PEG-25 PABA)	10%
S 27	14	Isopentyl-4-methoxycinnamate (isoamyl p-methoxycinnamate)	10%
S 69	15	2,4,6-Trianilino-(p-carbo-2'-ethylhexyl-1'-oxy)-1,3,5-triazine (octyl triazone)	5%
S 73	16	Phenol,2-(2H-benzotriazol-2-yl)-4-methyl-6-(2-methyl-3-(1,3,3,3-tetramethyl-1-(trimethylsilyl)oxy)-disiloxanyl)propyl (drometrizone trisiloxane)	15%
S 78	17	Benzoic acid, 4,4'-((6-(((1,1-dimethylethyl aminocarbonyl)phenyl)amino)-1,3,5,triazine-2,4-diyl)diimino)bis-bis(2-ethylhexyl)ester	10%
S 60	18	3-(4'-Methylbenzylidene)-d-t camphor (4-methylbenzylidene camphor)	2%
S 61	19	3-Benzylidene camphor (3-benzylidene cam-phor)	2%
S 8	20	2-Ethylhexyl salicylate (octyl-salicylate)	5%

ture-activity relationships to design new active ingredients and has been well reviewed elsewhere [12].

Physical blockers reflect or scatter UVR. Recent research indicates that the newer microsized forms of physical blockers may also function in part by absorption [13]. Some-times referred to as nonchemical sunscreens, they may be more appropriately designated as inorganic particulate sunscreen ingredients.

TABLE 3 UV Filters That Cosmetic Products May Provisionally Contain (Annex VII—Part 2)

COLIPA number	Ref. number	Substance	Maximum authorized concentration
S 8	5	2-Ethylhexyl-4-dimethyl-aminobenzoate	8%
S 40	17	2-Hydroxy-4-methoxybenzo-phenone-5-sulphonic acid and sodium salt (sulisoben-zone and sulisobenzone sodium)	5% (expressed as acid)
S 16	29	4-Isoprypylbenzyl salicylate	4%

NOMENCLATURE

Sunscreen nomenclature can be quite confusing. They may be referred to by their chemical or trade name. In the United States, individual sunscreen ingredients are also assigned a drug name by the OTC Monograph. Annex VII of the European Union (EU) may use either a drug or chemical name. Australia has its own approved list of names (AAN). Table 4 lists the most commonly used names, including their primary listing in the International Cosmetic Ingredient Dictionary (INCI designation) [14].

INDIVIDUAL UV FILTERS

Sunscreen ingredients may be considered by dividing them into larger overall classes by chemical structure. They may also be classified by their absorption spectrum. Although the lists of UV filters approved by the various regulatory agencies may seem quite extensive, fewer are used with any degree of frequency. The discussion that follows will concentrate on those listed in Table 4.

UVB

PABA and Its Derivatives

Para-aminobenzoic acid, or PABA, was one of the first sunscreen chemicals to be widely available. Several problems limited its use. It is very water-soluble, was frequently used in alcohol vehicles, stained clothing, and was associated with a number of adverse reactions. Ester derivatives of PABA, mainly octyl dimethyl PABA or Padimate O, became more popular with greater compatibility in a variety of more substantive vehicles and a lower potential for staining or adverse reactions. Amyl dimethyl PABA or Padimate A is associated with facial stinging [15]. Glyceryl PABA (glyceryl aminobenzoate) is still permitted in the FDA monograph but is no longer available. Octyl dimethyl PABA is a most potent UV absorber in the mid-UVB range. Because of problems with PABA formulations, marketers have emphasized the ''PABA-free'' claim. Although still widely used [16], it is confused with PABA, limiting its use. The decline in the use of this PABA derivative, along with the demand for higher SPF products, has led to the incorporation of multiple active ingredients in a single product to achieve the desired SPF.

Cinnamates

The next most potent UVB absorbers, the cinnamates have largely replaced PABA derivatives. Octinoxate, or octyl methoxycinnamate, is the most frequently used sunscreen ingre-

TABLE 4 Sunscreen Nomenclature

CAS no.	Drug name (FDA)	INCI name	COLIPA no.	EU reference no.	Trade names	Solubility	Spectrum
150-13-0	Para-aminobenzoic acid	PABA	S 1	1	4-Aminobenzoic acid	Hydrophilic	UVB
70356-09-1	Avobenzone	Butyl methoxydibenzyl methane	S 66	8	Parsol 1789	Lipophilic	UVA I
104-28-9	Cinoxate	Cinoxate				lipophilic	UVB
118-56-9	Homosalate	Homosalate	S 12	3	Eusolex HMS	Lipophilic	UVB
134-09-8	Menthyl anthranilate	Menthyl anthranilate			Dermoblock MA, Neo Heliopan, Type MA	Lipophilic	UVA II
6197-30-4	Octocrylene	Octocrylene	S 32	10	Escalol 597, Eusolex OCR, Uvinul N-539-50	Lipophilic	UVB
5466-77-3	Octinoxate	Octyl methoxycinnamate	S 28	12	Neo Heliopan AV, Parsol MCX, Eusolex 2292	Lipophilic	UVB
88122-99-0	Octyl triazone	Octyl triazone	S 69	15	Uvinul T-150	Lipophilic	UVB
118-60-5	Octisalate	Octyl salicylate	S 20	8	Escalol 587, Eusolex BS, Uvinul O-18	Lipophilic	UVB
131-57-7	Oxybenzone	Benzophenone-3	S 38	4	Eusolex 4360, Neo Heliopan, Uvinul M40	Lipophilic	UVB, UVA II
21245-02-03	Padimate O	Octyl dimethyl PABA	S 78	17	Escalol 507, Eusolex 6007	Lipophilic	UVB
27503-81-7	Phenylbenzimidazole sulfonic acid	Phenylbenzimidazole sulfonic acid	S 45	6	Eusolex 232, Neo Heliopan Hydro	Hydrophilic	UVB
4065-45-6	Sulisobenzone	Benzophenone-4	S 78	17	Escalol 577, Uvinul MS 40	Lipophilic	UVB, UVA II

dient [16]. Octyl or ethylhexyl methoxycinnamate is an order of magnitude less potent than Padimate O and requires additional UVB absorbers to achieve higher SPF levels in a final product. Cinoxate (Ethoxy-ethyl-p-methoxycinnamate) is less widely used. When a water-soluble cinnamate is indicated in a formulation, diethanolamine (DEA) methoxycinnamate may be used.

Salicylates

Salicylates are weaker UVB absorbers. They have a long history of use but were supplanted by the more efficient PABA and cinnamate derivatives. They are generally used to augment other UVB absorbers. With the trend to higher SPFs, more octyl salicylate (ethylhexyl salicylate) is being used followed by homomenthyl salicylate. Both materials have the ability to solubilize oxybenzone and avobenzone. Trolamine or triethanolamine (TEA) salicylate has good water solubility.

Camphor Derivatives

Not approved by the FDA for use in the United States, there are six camphor derivatives approved in Europe. 4-methyl-benbenzylidene camphor is the most widely used.

Octocrylene

2-Ethylhexyl-2-cyano-3,3 diphenylacrylate, or octocrylene, is chemically related to cinnamates. It can be used to boost SPF and improve water resistance in a given formulation. Octocrylene is photostabile and can improve the photostability of other sunscreens. It is very expensive and can present difficulties in formulation.

Phenylbenzimidazole Sulfonic Acid

Phenylbenzimadazole sulfonic acid is a water-soluble UVB absorber that can be used in the water phase of emulsion systems, in contrast to most oil-soluble sunscreen ingredients, allowing for a less greasy, more aesthetically pleasing formulation, such as a daily-use moisturizer containing sunscreen. Phenylbenzimidazole sulfonic acid boosts the SPF of organic and inorganic sunscreens. It can also be used in clear gels because of its water solubility.

UVA

Benzophenones

Although oxybenzone or benzophenone-3 absorbs most efficiently in the UVB range, absorption extends well into the UVA II range. It is used primarily as a UVA absorber, but boosts SPF values in combination with other UVB absorbers. Oxybenzone is supplied as a solid material, has poor solubility, and has a relatively low extinction coefficient. Sulisobenzone or benzophenone-4 is water-soluble, somewhat unstable, and used with less frequency.

Menthyl Anthranilate

Anthranilates are weak UVB filters and absorb mainly in the near UVA portion of the spectrum. They are less effective than benzophenones in this range and are less widely used.

Butylmethoxydibenzoylmethane

Avobenzone, or Parsol 1789, has only recently been approved by the FDA for use in OTC sunscreens in the United States, having been used quite extensively in Europe for considerably longer. It provides strong absorption in the UVA I range with peak absorption at 360 nm. Because an agreed-upon standard for measuring UVA protection in the United States does not exist, a minimum-use concentration has been set at 2% with a maximum of 3%.

Avobenzone should not be confused with isopropyl dibenzoylmethane (Eusolex 8020), which had previously been available in Europe. The high incidence of adverse photosensitivity reported with the combination of isopropyldibenzoylmethane and methylbenzylidene camphor by coupled reactions in the late 1980s led to a decrease in its use in commercial [17]. In 1993 its production was discontinued and it is no longer listed in Annex VII. Reported sensitivity to butylmethoxydibenzoylmethane was on the basis of cross-reactivity to isopropyl dibenzoylmethane. Isolated allergy to butylmethoxydibenzoylmethane is rare [17].

Photostability refers to the ability of a molecule to remain intact with irradiation. Photostability is potentially a problem with all UV filters. This issue has been raised specifically with avobenzone [18], with photolysis shown in a specially designed in vitro system [19] that simultaneously irradiates and measures transmittance in situ. This effect may degrade other sunscreens in a formulation. The relevance of this testing to the in vivo situation remains unclear. Overall formulation may be critical in this regard.

Tetraphthalydine Dicamphor Sulfonic Acid

3,3'-(1,4-phenylenedimethylene)bis[7,7-dimethyl-2-oxo-bicyclo-(2,2,1)hept-1-yl]methanesulfonic acid (EU Ref. No. 7) or Mexoryl SX is a UVA blocker more recently available in Europe with comparable efficacy to avobenzone [20].

Physical Blockers

Some of the original sunblocks were opaque formulations reflecting or scattering UVR. Color cosmetics containing a variety of inorganic pigments function in this fashion. Titanium dioxide and zinc oxide are chemically inert and protect through the full spectrum of UVR. They offer significant advantages. Poor cosmetic acceptance limited the widespread use of these two ingredients until recently, when microsized forms have become available. By decreasing particle size of these materials to a microsize or ultrafine grade it is less visible on the skin surface.

Micropigmentary sunblocks function differently than opaque sunblocks of pigmented color cosmetics by absorbing and not simply reflecting or scattering UVR [13]. By varying and mixing particle sizes, differing levels of photoprotection are achieved throughout the UV spectrum. In addition to avobenzone, micropigmentary TiO_2 and ZnO offer the best available protection in the UVA II range.

Photoreactivity has been raised as an issue with these materials. Both TiO_2 and ZnO are semiconductors potentially absorbing light and generating reactive species [21]. These effects have been shown in vitro [22]. Coating these materials reduces their photochemical reactivity. The in vivo relevance of these effects has not been shown and both materials have a long history of safe use.

Titanium Dioxide

TiO$_2$ was the first micropigment extensively used. Advantages include a broad spectrum of protection and inability to cause contact dermatitis. The use of rutile as opposed to anatase crystal forms of titanium dioxide lessens photoactivity. Newer materials are amphiphilic, designed to be dispersed in both water- and oil-emulsion phases. Particle size and uniformity of dispersion is key to achieving SPF. Primary particle size may be 10 to 15 nm with secondary particle assembly to 100 nm. Particle size needs to be less than 200 nm to achieve transparency.

Despite advances in the technology and understanding of these materials, whitening remains a problem secondary to pigment residue. Adding other pigments simulating flesh-tones may partially camouflage this effect. The net effect may be that the user is inclined to make a less heavy application of product, effectively lowering SPF [23]. ''Hybrid'' formulations using a combination of chemical absorbers with inorganic particulates may represent a practical compromise.

Zinc Oxide

Zinc oxide was only recently approved as an active sunscreen agent for the FDA OTC Sunscreen Monograph. Reduced to a particle size of less than 200 nm, light scattering is minimized and the particles appear transparent in thin films [24]. ZnO has a refractive index of 1.9, as opposed to 2.6 for TiO$_2$, and therefore causes less whitening than TiO$_2$. ZnO may attenuate UVR more effectively in the UVA I range [25]. Microfine TiO$_2$ at an equal concentration offers somewhat more protection in the UVB range.

ADVERSE REACTIONS—TOXICITY

In a longitudinal prospective study of 603 subjects applying daily either an SPF 15+ broad-spectrum sunscreen containing octyl methoxycinnamate and avobenzone or a vehicle cream, 19% developed an adverse reaction [26]. Interestingly, the rates of reaction to both the active and vehicle creams were similar, emphasizing the importance of excipient ingredients in the vehicle. The majority of reactions were irritant in nature. Not surprisingly, a disproportionate 50% of the reacting subjects were atopic. Less than 10% of the reactions were allergic, with none of the subjects patch tested actually found to be allergic to an individual sunscreen ingredient.

Subjective irritation associated with burning or stinging without objective erythema from some organic UV filters [27] is the most frequent sensitivity complaint associated with sunscreen use. This is most frequently experienced in the eye area. Longer lasting objective irritant contact dermatitis may be difficult to distinguish from true allergic contact dermatitis. In a postmarket evaluation of sunscreen sensitivity complaints in 57 patients, 20 of the patients had short-lasting symptoms, 26 long-lasting, and 11 mixed or borderline symptoms [28]. Half of the patients were patch and photopatch tested, and only three showed positive reactions to sunscreen ingredients.

Contact and photocontact sensitivity to individual sunscreen ingredients has been extensively reviewed [17]. Considering their widespread use, the number of documented allergic reactions is not high [29]. PABA and PABA esters accounted for many of the early reported reactions, but with a decrease in their use reactions to benzophenones may be increasing [30]. Reactions to dibenzoylmethanes have previously been discussed. Fragrances, preservatives, and other excipients account for a large number of the allergic reactions seen [17].

Virtually all sunscreen ingredients reported to cause contact allergy may be photoallergens [31]. Although still relatively uncommon, sunscreen actives seem to have become the leading cause of photocontact allergic reactions [32,33]. Individuals with pre-existing eczematous conditions have a significant predisposition to sensitization associated with their impaired cutaneous barrier. The majority of individuals who develop photocontact dermatitis to sunscreens are patients with photodermatides [17].

CONCLUSION

A limited menu of UV filters for incorporation into sunscreen products is available to the formulating chemist, depending on regulatory requirements in an individual country or jurisdiction. With the demand for higher SPFs, the trend has been to use more individual and a wider variety of agents in newer products. Recent research in sunscreen efficacy has emphasized the need for products protecting against the full UV spectrum with a limited number of available agents. Regulatory agencies are very slow to approve new ingredients.

Sunscreen efficacy remains very dependent on vehicle formulation. Solvents and emollients can have a profound effect on the strength of UV absorbance by the active ingredients and at which wavelengths they absorb [34]. Film formers and emulsifiers determine the uniformity and thickness of the film formed on the skin surface, which in turn determines SPF level, durability, and water resistance [35]. Lastly, product aesthetics play a large role in product acceptance, particularly with sunscreens being incorporated into daily-use cosmetics. These constraints provide the sunscreen formulator with significant challenges in developing new and improved formulations.

REFERENCES

1. Weinstock MA. Death from skin cancer among the elderly: epidemiological patterns. Arch Dermatol 1997; 133:1207–1209.
2. Yaar M, Gilchrest BA. Aging versus photoaging: postulated mechanisms and effectors. J Invest Dermatol Symp Proc 1998; 3:47–51.
3. Naylor MF, Farmer KC. The case for sunscreens: a review of their use in preventing actinic damage and neoplasia. Arch Dermatol 1997; 133:1146–1154.
4. Gurish MF, Roberts LK, Krueger GG, et al. The effect of various sunscreen agents on skin damage and the induction of tumor susceptibility in mice subjected to ultraviolet irradiation. J Invest Dermatol 1975; 65:543–546.
5. Thompson SC, Jolley D, Marks R. Reduction of solar keratoses by regular sunscreen use. N Engl J Med 1993; 329:1147–1151.
6. Boyd AS, Naylor M, Cameron GS, et al. The effects of chronic sunscreen use on the histologic changes of dermatoheliosis. J Am Acad Dermatol 1995; 33:941–946.
7. Roberts LK, Beasley DG. Commercial sunscreen lotions prevent ultraviolet-radiation–induced immune suppression of contact hypersensitivity. J Invest Dermatol 1995; 105:339–344.
8. Stiller MJ, Bartolone J, Stern R, Smith S, Kollias N, Gillies R, Drake LA. Topical 8% glycolic acid and 8% L-lactic acid creams for the treatment of photodamaged skin: a double-blind vehicle-controlled clinical trial. Arch Dermatol 1996; 132:631–636.
9. Shaath NA. Evolution of modern sunscreen chemicals. In: Lowe NJ, Shaath NA, Pathak MA,

eds. Sunscreens: Development, Evaluation, and Regulatory Aspects. 2d ed. New York: Marcel Dekker, 1997:3–31.

10. Rebut R. The sunscreen industry in Europe: past, present, and future. In: Lowe NJ, Shaath NA, eds. Sunscreens: Development, Evaluation, and Regulatory Aspects. New York: Marcel Dekker, 1990:161–178.

11. Shaath NA. The chemistry of sunscreens. Cosmet Toilet 1986; 101:55–70.

12. Shaath NA. On the theory of ultraviolet absorption by sunscreen chemicals. J Soc Cosmet Chem 1987; 82:193.

13. Sayre RM, Killias N, Roberts RL, et al. Physical sunscreens. J Soc Cosmet Chem 1990; 41: 103–109.

14. Wenninger JA, McEwen GN Jr, eds. International Cosmetic Ingredient Dictionary and Handbook. 7th ed. Washington, DC: The Cosmetic, Toiletry, and Fragrance Association, 1977.

15. Frosch PJ, Kligman AM. A method for appraising the stinging capacity of topically applied substances. J Soc Cosmet Chem 1977; 28:197.

16. Steinberg DC. Sunscreen encyclopedia regulatory update. Cosmet Toilet 1996; 111:77–86.

17. Schauder S, Ippen H. Contact and photocontact sensitivity to sunscreens. Review of a 15-year experience and of the literature. Contact Derm 1997; 37(5):221–232.

18. Deflandre A, Lang G. Photostability assessment of sunscreens. Benzylidene camphor and dibenzoylmethane derivatives. Int J Cosmet Sci 1988; 10:53–62.

19. Sayre RM, Dowdy JC. Avobenzone and the photostability of sunscreen products. Presented at the 7th Annual Meeting of the Photomedicine Society. Orlando, February 26, 1998.

20. Chardoon A, Moyal D, Hourseau C. Persistent pigment-darkening response as a method for evaluation of ultraviolet A protection assays. In: Lowe NJ, Shaath NA, Pathak MA, eds. Sunscreens: Development, Evaluation, and Regulatory Aspects. 2d ed. New York: Marcel Dekker, 1997:559–581.

21. Murphy GM. Sunblocks: mechanisms of action. Photodermatol Photoimmunol Photomed 1999; 15:34–36.

22. Wamer WG, Yin JJ, Wei RR. Oxidative damage to nucleic acids photosensitized by titanium dioxide. Free Radical Biol Med 197; 23:851–858.

23. Diffey BL, Grice J. The influence of sunscreen type on photoprotection. Br J Dermatol 1977; 137:103–105.

24. Fairhurst D, Mitchnik MA. Particulate sun blocks: general principles. In: Lowe NJ, Shaath NA, Pathak MA, eds. Sunscreens: Development, Evaluation, and Regulatory Aspects. 2d ed. New York: Marcel Dekker, 1997:313–352.

25. Mitchnick MA, Fairhurst D, Pinnell SR. Microfine zinc oxide (Z-Cote) as a photostable UVA/ UVB sunblock agent. J Am Acad Dermatol 1999; 40:85–90.

26. Foley P, Nixon R, Marks R, et al. The frequency of reactions to sunscreens: results of a longitudinal population-based study on the regular use of sunscreens in Australia. Br J Dermatol 1993; 128:512–518.

27. Levy SB. Sunscreens for photoprotection. Dermatologic Ther 1997; 4:59–71.

28. Fischer T, Bergstrom K. Evaluation of customers' complaints about sunscreen cosmetics sold by the Swedish pharmaceutical company. Contact Derm 1991; 25:319–322.

29. Dromgoole SH, Maibach HI. Sunscreening agent intolerance: contact and photocontact sensitization and contact urticaria. J Am Acad Dermatol 1990; 22:1068–1078.

30. Lenique P, Machet L, Vaillant L, et al. Contact and photocontact allergy to oxybenzone. Contact Derm 1992; 26:177–181.

31. Fotiades J, Soter NA, Lim HW. Results of evaluation of 203 patients for photosensitivity in a 7.3-year period. J Am Acad Dermatol 1995; 33(4):597–602.

32. Trevisi P, Vincenzi C, Chieregato C, et al. Sunscreen sensitization: a three-year study. Dermatology 1994; 189:55–57.

33. Agrapidis-Paloympis LE, Nash RA, Shaath NA. The effect of solvents on the ultraviolet absorbance of sunscreens. J Soc Cosmet Chem 1987; 38:209–221.

34. Klein K. Formulating sunscreen products. In: Lowe NJ, Shaath NA, ed. Sunscreens: Development, Evaluation, and Regulatory Aspects. New York: Marcel Dekker, 1990:235–266.

35. Klein K. Sunscreen products: formulation and regulatory consideration. In: Lowe NJ, Shoath NA, Pathok MA, eds. Sunscreens: Development, Evaluation, and Regulatory Aspects. 2d ed. New York: Marcel Dekker, 1997:3–31.

39

Vitamins

Alois Kretz and Ulrich Moser
Roche Vitamins Europe Ltd., Basel, Switzerland

INTRODUCTION

Vitamins consist of a mixed group of chemical substances that all occur in nature. Different from most other cosmetic ingredients, they are essential nutrients playing key roles in the metabolism of all human organs, including the largest human organ, the skin. The skin is often the first indicator of a dietary deficiency in one or more vitamins.

Laboratory and clinical studies have shown beneficial effects to the skin for some of the 13 vitamins when topically applied. This scientific evidence is the platform for the incorporation of this substance group in all kinds of cosmetic products.

The most widely used vitamins in cosmetics and toiletries are vitamin A, vitamin E, vitamin C, and panthenol (provitamin B_5). Vitamin E and vitamin C are antioxidants. They neutralize unstable oxygen molecules, the free radicals, thereby preventing the damage these highly reactive substances can cause to the skin. Vitamin A has shown to be effective in preventing, retarding, and restoring changes associated with the aging process, such as dry and scaly skin, photodamage, and the formation of wrinkles. Panthenol is incorporated into skin- hair- lip- and nailcare products mainly for its moisturizing property. In addition, panthenol has wound-healing and anti-inflammatory properties. Although not cosmetic properties, these are welcome side effects, in particular when cosmetics are applied to slightly damaged skin.

VITAMIN E

More than other tissues, the skin is exposed to various aggressive effects of the environment. Chemical and physical agents, such as ultraviolet (UV) light, ozone, heavy metals, and many others, cause permanent stress to the outermost cell layers of the skin. In particular, regular and excessive exposure to UV light induces damage and disease in the tissue. The skin becomes wrinkled, appears older, the immune system is weakened, and, more seriously, skin cancer can develop.

Up to 20% of the solar UVB impinging on the skin reaches the viable cells of the epidermis, and about 10% penetrates to the dermis [1]. An even higher portion of UVA and visible light can reach the dermis. The interaction of UV light with various skin components results in the formation of free radicals.

The skin has enzymatic and nonenzymatic antioxidant systems. These work to prevent the formation of free radicals, which can harm the integrity of the cell structures and with it the normal function of the skin. One nonenzymatic antioxidant is vitamin E.

Chemically, vitamin E (tocopherol) (Fig. 1) is a chromanol derivative. It consists of two functional units, a chromane ring bearing a phenolic OH group and a branched side chain. The hydrocarbon chain is necessary for the proper orientation of tocopherol at its site of activity, whereas the chromanol part provides the antioxidant properties.

Vitamin E has a protector function. It is considered to be essential for the stabilization of biological membranes, particularly those containing large amounts of polyunsaturated fatty acids. Cell membrane lipids in the skin are under constant attack from free radicals formed both in the course of normal biological reactions as well as, in particular, by various external factors. Free radicals can take electrons from membrane lipids, which leads to the impairment of the membranes on one side. On the other side, new free radicals are then formed that continue the destructive work.

Vitamin E is considered the major free-radical chain-breaking antioxidant in membranes. It inactivates peroxyl radicals in the vicinity of the membranes and thus inhibits the propagation of lipid peroxidation. Vitamin E loses thereby its antioxidant power and itself becomes a low-energy radical. This tocopheryl radical is, however, unable to attack other molecules and thus initiate a new free-radical chain reaction. In a next step, the tocopheryl radical gets back its antioxidant properties: it is regenerated by a redox system to the active tocopherol.

Although lost antioxidants are continuously replaced and regenerated, oxidative stress, such as excessive exposure to UV light, can overwhelm the natural cutaneous antioxidant capacity and harm the insufficiently protected tissue. A great number of studies performed during the past 15 to 20 years deal with this problem, and some of them with the role of vitamin E in this process. Investigations include studies on the consequences of low levels of vitamin E in the skin, the influence of external factors on vitamin E concentration, and the possible use of topical vitamin E in the form of tocopherol or its ester vitamin E acetate to reduce or even prevent possible damage to the skin.

In an animal study by Igarashi, low levels of vitamin E increased lipid peroxide levels. Rats deficient in vitamin E showed significantly higher peroxide concentrations than normal animals. UV irradiation of the deficient animals led to a further significant increase [2]. Khettab applied vitamin E to the skin of hairless mice before UV irradiation and observed a reduction in epidermal lipid peroxidation compared with control [3].

Kondo examined the protective effect of vitamin E on UVB damage in human skin fibroblasts in vitro. He found a significant difference in surviving fibroblasts in the presence of 100 and 1000 µg α-tocopherol per mL culture fluid. The results suggest that vitamin E protects human skin fibroblasts against the cytotoxic effects of UVB [4].

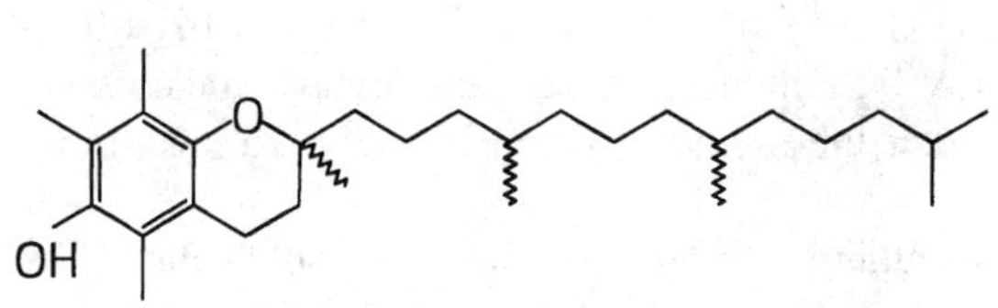

FIGURE 1   Structural formula of dl-α-tocopherol.

Interesting is the result of a study performed by Lopez-Torres et al., in which they investigated the effects of topical tocopherol on epidermal and dermal antioxidants and their ability to prevent UV-induced oxidative damage. Topically applied tocopherol to hairless mice in vivo increased dermal superoxide dismutase activity by 30% and protected epidermal glutathione peroxidase and superoxide dismutase from depletion after UV irradiation. Total and reduced glutathione levels in the epidermis were also increased, as were dermal vitamin C levels. The investigators conclude that topical administration of α-tocopherol protects cutaneous tissues against oxidative damage induced by UV irradiation [5].

Application of pure vitamin E acetate to the skin of hairless mice immediately after UVB irradiation reduced sunburn symptoms such as erythema, skin sensitivity, and skin swelling in a study carried out by Trevithick et al. [6]. Reduced erythema formation after UV irradiation was also reported by Roshchupkin [7] and Pathak [8].

In a human skin model, antioxidant depletion as a result of UV light exposure was shown by Podda [9]. Ubiquinol and ubiquinone in particular, as well as α-tocopherol to a lesser extent, were susceptible and decreased with higher UV light intensities to virtually non detectable levels. Partial impairment of the cutaneous antioxidant defense system, including vitamin E, by UV light was also observed by Fuchs [10].

Clement-Lacroix et al. tested the protector effect of vitamin E on immune suppression in human epidermal cells in vitro. Cultured cells preincubated with or without vitamin E were irradiated with UVA light. The investigators could show that incubation of cell cultures with vitamin E before irradiation partially protected the cells from the immunosuppressive effects of UVA radiation [11]. Finally, Weiser [12] and Miyamoto [13] have shown wound-healing properties of topical vitamin E acetate.

Vitamin E is used in cosmetics for everyday use to strengthen the natural antioxidant potency of the skin and thus to better cope with oxidative stress. Most of the scientific background for the topical use of vitamin E stems from observations in context with UV light. Vitamin E is often used, therefore, in suncare products for improvement of the protection achieved with the sun filters. Even high SPF factors still allow the penetration of some UV light onto and into the skin. Whereas the sun filters absorb or reflect most of the rays on the surface of the skin, vitamin E acts on the inside and reduces the risk of damage that could be caused by rays passing through the sun filter barrier. Vitamin E helps, therefore, in the prevention of symptoms caused by UV-induced skin damage such as wrinkling and irregular pigmentation.

In nature, Vitamin E appears as tocopherols, of which the alpha form has the highest biological potency. The unesterified form is present in wheat germ oil and other vegetable oils that are used in cosmetics as sources of Vitamin E. Most often used is dl-alpha tocopheryl acetate, because this ester is less prone to oxidation than free tocopherol. In the skin, vitamin E acetate is bioconverted into the biologically active antioxidant tocopherol [14,15].

VITAMIN A

Vitamin A (Fig. 2) and its derivatives belong to a large class of structurally related compounds, the retinoids. The term vitamin A is generically used for all derivatives of β-ionone that possess the biological activity of all-trans retinol or are closely related to it. The biological activities of the vitamin A derivatives are expressed in IU (international units.) One IU corresponds to 0.3 μg retinol, 0.34 μg vitamin A acetate, and 0.55 μg vitamin A palmitate.

Vitamin A is best known for its involvement in maintaining normal vision. It exerts, however, a number of other functions in the human organism, of which its activity in the epidermis is of particular interest for cosmetics.

The architecture of the human epidermis is a complex stratified system, its renewal a complex process. Epidermal keratinocytes proliferate and differentiate in a multilayered pattern. These processes are balanced so that new basal cells are formed as the totally cornified cells are shed from the surface of the skin. Proliferation and keratinization of keratinocytes are the two key elements for the build-up of a healthy epidermis. In both processes, vitamin A plays the role of a regulator.

On cell proliferation, vitamin A has a stimulating effect, as has been shown in various studies [16–18]. As little as 10 μg vitamin A acetate suspended in 0.2 mL water applied to normal rat skin led to a clear increase in mitotic activity after only 4 hours. Much more pronounced and longer lasting was the effect with 100 μg vitamin A acetate. However, 24 hours after treatment, the mitotic index had returned to original levels with both concentrations [17]. As can be seen from this study, the effect of vitamin A is dose dependent and disappears after a certain time with decreasing concentration in the tissue. An increase in mitotic activity is the first step in an increase of the number of new keratinocytes formed [19], which results in a thickening of the epidermis [20–23].

In the process of aging, many aspects of the skin structure are altered because of a decreased metabolic activity of the human organism. A thinning of the epidermis is one of the characteristics of aging skin. The skin thereby loses part of its barrier function, and as a consequence of reduced water retention capacity it is often dry, scaly, or even cracks. Vitamin A can counteract this development by stimulating the cell-renewal process.

The effect on the keratinization process was investigated by Fuchs and Green [24]. Removal of vitamin A from the culture fluid of human keratinocyte cell cultures resulted in a reduced cell motility, an increased adhesiveness of the cells, and a prevention of pattern formation. They conclude that the nature of the keratins synthesized by the tissues is regulated by the concentration of vitamin A. Another symptom of skin aging is a decrease in collagen in the connective tissue. Skin collagen decreases linearly by about 1% per year throughout adult life [25]. Topical administration of vitamin A has shown significant dose-related changes in collagen content of the dermis. 0.1% vitamin A palmitate applied to skin of hairless mice for 14 days increased the collagen content by 88%, 0.5% vitamin A palmitate by 101% [20].

Vitamin A not only improves the barrier function of the skin but also its appearance and elasticity. Application of a lotion with vitamin A palmitate to the temples of a group of 40- to 60-year-old volunteers has shown an increase in elasticity by 14% after 2 weeks and by over 22% after 6 weeks [26].

There is evidence that UV light strongly affects vitamin A concentration in epidermis and dermis as was shown in animals and humans [27,28]. Particularly low were the levels when test animals were exposed to UVA near the absorption maximum of vitamin A. The regeneration of normal levels in the depleted tissue is very slow and took more than 1 week in rabbit ear skin [28].

Cluver and Politzer measured the vitamin A concentration in blood serum of humans after 1 hour of exposure to the sun. Depletion was observed immediately after exposure, which lasted at least a further 2½ hours [29]. It can be assumed that, under similar conditions, a depletion also takes place in the skin. The low blood levels could also be an

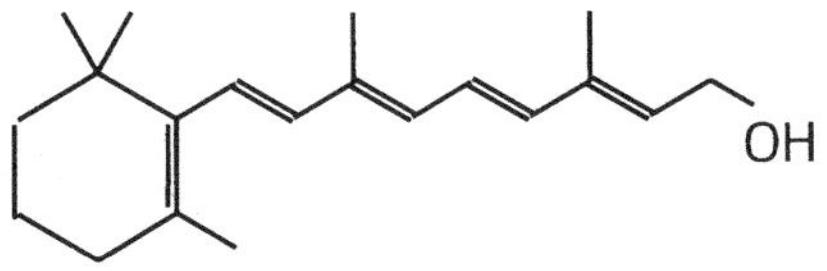

FIGURE 2 Structural formula of vitamin A alcohol.

explanation for the slow restoration of vitamin A in the skin. It cannot be excluded that low vitamin A levels in the skin after regular and excessive sun exposure are implicated in the typical changes seen in photodamaged skin, such as the thickened horny layer and the relatively thin rest of the epidermis. A common practice in treatment of photodamaged skin is the use of vitamin A acid. Although it is not proven, it can be hypothesized that retinoids could be involved in the process of photoaging. In most countries, however, vitamin A acid is classified as a drug and cannot be used in cosmetic products. Whether vitamin A esters have a similar effect to vitamin A acid, and whether they could be used not in the cure but in the prevention of photoaging, is presently under investigation. Some first results are available and show promising results.

Although vitamin A was one of the first vitamins discovered, the molecular mechanism of its activity is still largely unknown. Many attempts have been made to define in biochemical terms the manner in which it induces the differentiation of cells. Uncertainties still exist, but one pathway increasingly seems to explain most of the effects of various retinoids on different cell types. This pathway includes an oxidation of retinol (vitamin A alcohol) to retinal (vitamin A aldehyde), and subsequently a further bioconversion in a controlled mechanism to retinoic acid [30].

In cosmetics, vitamin A is used mainly in the ester forms: vitamin A palmitate and vitamin A acetate, as well as retinol. None of these forms are very stable when exposed to light or warmth. Special attention has to be paid, therefore, to the stabilization of vitamin A–containing cosmetic products and their handling during the manufacturing process. This is particularly true for retinol.

PANTHENOL

Panthenol (Fig. 3) is the biologically active alcohol analogue of pantothenic acid, a vitamin of the B-complex group, which is a normal constituent of skin and hair. Pantothenic acid, also called Vitamin B_5, carries out its function in the body as an element of co-enzyme A, a molecule composed of cysteamine, ATP, and pantothenic acid. This substance is present in all living cells and serves a vital role in the metabolism of a variety of enzyme-catalyzed reactions by which energy is released from carbohydrates, fats, and proteins. Skin manifestations of pantothenic acid deficiency are well known, and include cornification, depigmentation, and desquamation.

Pantothenic acid is an unstable substance. In topical preparations such as skincare, haircare, nailcare, and derma products, pantothenic acid is used in the alcohol form, called panthenol. Its use is based on its dual role as a vitamin precursor and as an ingredient with ideal cosmetic properties. When topically applied, panthenol is absorbed by the skin and can be bioconverted into pantothenic acid [31]. As such it exerts all functions of vitamin B_5.

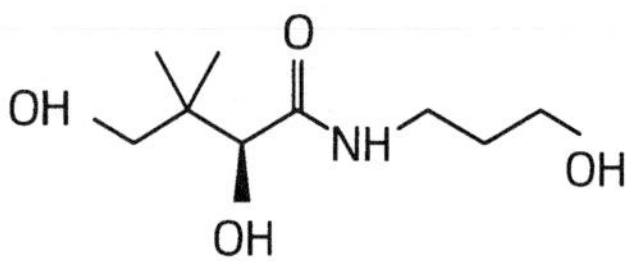

FIGURE 3   Structural formula of D-panthenol.

Because it has a distinct humectant character, panthenol acts as a skin moisturizer [32,33]. This hygroscopic substance not only provides water to the skin surface but it also penetrates deep into the epidermis and brings water to, and retains water in, the inside of the skin. Panthenol imparts a smooth, light feel to the skin without any greasiness or stickiness. Because it is well tolerated by the skin, it is an ideal and widely used ingredient in baby care products as well as in products for sensitive skin.

Topically applied panthenol stimulates epithelization as was shown by Weiser and Erlemann [12]. Superficial wounds treated with creams containing 5% panthenol reduced the healing time by 30% compared with placebo. Favorable effects were also reported in many kinds of skin disorders accompanied by inflammatory reactions such as burns [34], nipple fissures [35], eczemas [36,37], and many others. Another application field of panthenol is, therefore, derma products for wound healing and for soothing of inflammatory disorders where it is usually incorporated in concentrations of 5%. The concentrations in cosmetics vary mainly from 0.3 to 2%.

The use of panthenol in haircare products goes back to the early 1960s, when inflammatory reactions on the scalp were treated with panthenol-containing creams. Panthenol not only showed a soothing effect but also had beneficial effects on the hair.

Pantothenic acid is a natural constituent of human hair [38]. Stuettgen applied tritium-labeled panthenol intracutaneously by injection and could show a transport of radioactive material into the hair [39]. Stangl observed a significant increase of pantothenic acid concentration in the hair after topical application of panthenol over longer periods [38].

Panthenol acts as a humectant for hair. It builds up a thin moisture film on the surface of the hair and gives hair shine without making it greasy. Panthenol also penetrates into the hair cuticle and brings moisture to the cortex. This imparts good pliability and manageability properties to the hair, and improves its resistance to mechanical stress such as combing, brushing, and heat blowdrying.

Panthenol can also contribute to give hair more body. A thickening of the hair after 2 minutes exposure to a 2% water solution of panthenol was shown by means of scanning electron microscopy [39].

The main commercial forms are d-panthenol, dl-panthenol, and ethyl panthenol. All these forms are soluble in e.g., water, ethanol, and propylene glycol, but insoluble in fats and oils. Ethyl panthenol is an ether and available either as d-form or a racemic mixture of d- and l-form. Biological activity has only the d-form, because only d-pantothenic acid is incorporated into coenzyme A.

VITAMIN C

Vitamin C (Fig. 4) is certainly the best-known vitamin. Known also as ascorbic acid, it is a potent antioxidant, a scavenger of superoxide and peroxyl radicals, which are involved in lipid peroxidation in tissues such as the human skin.

Like vitamin E, vitamin C belongs to the natural nonenzymatic antioxidant defense system. Different from the lipophilic properties of tocopherol, ascorbic acid is water-soluble and acts in the more hydrophilic environment of the skin structure.

There is a wealth of literature available on functions of vitamin C in the human organism [41]. Of special interest for the cosmetic industry are those publications dealing with strengthening of the antioxidant system, stimulation of collagen formation, skin lightening, and treatment of hyperpigmentation. Vitamin C has also proven to have good wound-healing properties.

Darr et al. [42] investigated the antioxidant properties of vitamin C in porcine skin. Topical application of ascorbic acid not only resulted in a significant elevation of cutaneous levels of this vitamin but also protected the skin from UVB damage as measured by erythema and sunburn cell formation. In addition, they could show that UVB irradiation reduces the vitamin C levels in the skin. Similar reductions were reported by Podda [9] and to a lesser extent by Fuchs [10].

There are two possibilities of how vitamin C can participate in the inhibition of UV damage when applied to the skin: either it directly reacts with, or quenches, certain free radicals, or it helps to regenerate tocopheryl radicals formed in the course of lipid peroxidation prevention. Vitamin C is, therefore, an attractive molecule for use in skin cosmetics, particularly in combination with vitamin E.

Dermatologists have long observed that skin fibroblasts synthesize less collagen as they age and that too much sun increases the decline. Vitamin C could counteract this decline in two ways. Ascorbic acid is an essential cofactor in the hydroxylation of proline and lysine to form hydroxyproline and hydroxylysine, amino acids of importance to the function of collagen [43]. In addition, vitamin C stimulates the formation of collagen [43]. Thus vitamin C contributes to the formation of a strong matrix of the dermis and can be used in cosmetic products for the maintenance of healthy skin.

Ascorbic acid and its esters are also used as active ingredients in skin bleaching or skin lightening cosmetic products. This use is supported by publications such as that by Takashima et al. [44]. These investigators reported successful skin lightening in patients with chloasma which were treated with an ointment containing 3% magnesium ascorbyl phosphate.

There are mainly two possibilities how ascorbic acid can influence melanin to achieve a lightening of skin color: partial inhibition of formation of new melanin or modification of melanin already present, e.g., by promoting the conversion of formed melanin to the reduced form. Both mechanisms have been investigated and discussed for ascorbic acid [44,45]. Further studies are needed to clarify the exact mode of activity.

The most frequently used forms of vitamin C in cosmetics are ascorbic acid, ascorbyl palmitate, magnesium ascorbyl phosphate, and trisodium ascorbyl phosphate. The cosmetic industry shows great interest in the use of vitamin C, particularly as antioxidant for

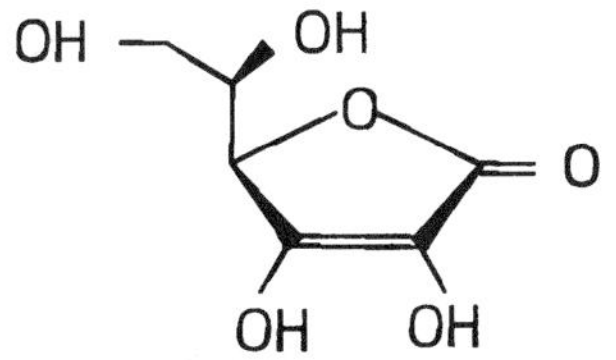

FIGURE 4 Structural formula of L-ascorbic acid.

the skin. Its use, however, has been limited to date due to the insufficient stability of ascorbic acid in aqueous solutions and the prices of some of the more stable derivatives.

OTHERS

Some other vitamins and vitamin precursors used in cosmetic products are biotin, niacinamide, vitamin D, vitamin B_6, beta-carotene, and, in a few products, vitamin K. For all these substances there exists a rationale for their use in cosmetics but there are either no studies or insufficient studies available that prove their efficacy when topically applied.

Systemic use of 2.5 mg biotin per day has shown good effect on brittle nails and has improved hair quality [46–49]. As it has good effect on these keratin structures, it can be assumed that this vitamin could also have interesting effects on the keratinization process in the epidermis.

Beta-carotene is known for its quenching activity on singlet oxygen. It would be an ideal partner for vitamin E and vitamin C to strengthen the antioxidant defense system of the skin. Oral supplementation with beta-carotene over several weeks has shown to reduce the risk of UV-induced skin damage [50].

Unfortunately for cosmetics, beta-carotene is a strong coloring agent and concentrations of more than 0.05% in a cosmetic product can lead to undesirable coloration of the clothes of its users. Low concentrations of beta-carotene are used in some cosmetics as natural coloring agent for creams.

Roccheggiani showed a depression of sebum production with the tripalmitate ester of vitamin B_6 [51]. Vitamin D could be an ideal partner for total sun blockers, as the UV-ray barrier of these products partly prevents the natural formation of vitamin D in the skin. Vitamin D is on the ''list of substances which must not form part of the composition of cosmetic products'' of the European Cosmetic Regulations. It can be used, however, in other countries.

CONCLUSION

Vitamins are a class of naturally occurring active ingredients with well-documented activities when topically applied. They are all essential substances for the well-being and health of the human organism, including the skin.

Thousands of studies have shown the safety and efficacy of systemically and topically used vitamins. In many cases, topical use is the only way to provide sufficient quantities of these highly active protector and care substances to be able to guarantee an optimal functioning of the skin. This is particularly true when the skin is stressed by factors such as UV light or environmental pollutants such as ozone, especially as these factors can often even destroy considerable quantities of the vitamins.

REFERENCES

1. Epstein JH. The pathological effects of light on the skin. In: Free Radicals in Biology III. WA Pryor, ed. New York: Academic Press, 1977; 219–249.
2. Igarashi A, Uzuka M, Nakajima K. The effects of vitamin E deficiency on rat skin. Br J Dermatol 1989; 121:43–49.
3. Khettab N, Amory M-C, Briand G, Bousquet B, Combre A, Forlot P, Barey M. Photoprotective effect of vitamin A and E on polyamine and oxygenated free radical metabolism in hairless mouse epidermis. Biochim 1988; 70:1709–1713.

4. Kondo S, Mamada A, Yamaguchi J, Fukuro S. Protective effect of dl-α-tocopherol on the cytotoxicity of ultraviolet B against human skin fibroblasts in vitro. Photodermatol Photoimmunol Photomed 1990; 7:173–177.

5. Lopez-Torres M, Thiele JJ, Shindo Y, Han D, Packer L. Topical application of α-tocopherol modulates the antioxidant network and diminishes ultraviolet-induced oxidative damage in murine skin. Br J Dermatol 1998; 138:207–215.

6. Trevithick JR, Xiong H, Lee S, Shum DT, Sanford E, Karlik SJ, Norley C, Dilworth GR. Topical tocopherol acetate reduces post-UVB, sunburn associated erythema, edema, and skin sensitivity in hairless mice. Arch Biochem Biophys 1992; 296:575–582.

7. Roschupkin DI, Pistsov MY, Potapenko AY. Inhibition of ultraviolet light-induced erythema by antioxidants. Arch Dermatol Res 1979; 266:91–94.

8. Pathak MA. 1987; unpublished document of Hoffmann-La Roche.

9. Podda M, Traber MG, Weber C, Yan L-J, Packer L. UV irradiation depletes antioxidants and causes oxidative damage in a model of human skin. Free Radical Biol Med 1998; 24:55–65.

10. Fuchs J, Huflejt ME, Rothfuss LM, Wilson DS, Carcamo G, Packer L. Acute effects of near ultraviolet and visible light on the cutaneous antioxidant defense system. Photochem Photobiol 1989; 50:739–744.

11. Clement-Lacroix P, Michel L, Moysan A, Molière P, Dubertret L. UVA-induced immune suppression in human skin: protective effect of vitamin E in human epidermal cells in vitro. Br J Dermatol 1996; 134:77–84.

12. Weiser H, Erlemann G. Acceleration of superficial wound healing by panthenol and zinc oxide. Preprints of the XIVth IFSCC Congress, Barcelona, 1986; 2:879–887.

13. Mijamoto I, Uchida Y, Shinomiya T, Abe T, Nishijima Y. Effects of cosmetics containing bioactive substances on skin. Preprints of the XIVth IFSCC Congress, Barcelona. 1986; 2: 949–959.

14. Norkus EP, Bryce GF, Bhagavan HN. Uptake and bioconversion of α-tocopheryl acetate to α-tocopherol in skin of hairless mice. Photochem Photobiol 1993; 57:613–615.

15. Kramer-Stickland K, Liebler DC. Effect of UVB on hydrolysis of α-tocopherol acetate to α-tocopherol in mouse skin. E J Invest Dermatol 1998; 111:302–307.

16. Lawrence DJ, Bern HA. On the specificity of the response of mouse epidermis to vitamin A. J Invest Derm 1958; 31:313–325.

17. Sherman BS. The effect of vitamin A on epithelial mitosis in vitro and in vivo. J Invest Derm 1961; 37:469–480.

18. Zil JS. Vitamin A acid effects on epidermal mitotic activity, thickness and cellularity in the hairless mouse. J Invest Derm 1972; 59:228–232.

19. Chopra DP, Flaxman BA. The effect of vitamin A on growth and differentiation of human keratinocytes in vitro. J Invest Derm 1975; 64:19–22.

20. Courts DF, Skreko F, McBee J. The effect of retinyl palmitate on skin composition and morphometry. J Soc Cosmet Chem 1988; 39:235–240.

21. Jarrett A, Spearman RIC. Histochemistry of the Skin—Psoriasis. London: English Universities Press, 1964; 41–77.

22. Spearman RIC, Jarrett A. Biological comparison of isomers and chemical forms of vitamin A (retinol). Br J Dermatol 1974; 90:553–560.

23. Kang S, Duell EA, Fisher GJ, Datta SC, Wang Z-Q, Reddy AP, Tavakkol A, Yi JY, Griffiths CEM, Elder JT, Voorhees JJ. Application of retinol to human skin in vivo induces epidermal hyperplasia and cellular retinoid binding proteins characteristic of retinoic acid but without measurable retinoic acid levels or irritation. J Invest Derm 1995; 105:549–556.

24. Fuchs E, Green H. Regulation of terminal differentiation of cultured human keratinocytes by vitamin A. Cell 1981; 25:617–625.

25. Shuster S, Black MM, McVitie E. The influence of age and sex on skin thickness, skin collagen and density. Br J Derm 1975; 93:639–643.

26. Fthenakis CG, Maes DH, Smith WP. In vivo assessment of skin elasticity using ballistometry. J Soc Cosmet Chem 1991; 42:211–222.

27. Berne B, Vahlquist A, Fischer T, Danielson BG, Berne C. UV treatment of uraemic pruritus reduces the vitamin A content of the skin. Eur J Clin Invest 1984; 14:203–206.

28. Berne B, Nilsson M, Vahlquist A. UV irradiation and cutaneous vitamin A: an experimental study in rabbit and human skin. J Invest Derm 1984; 83:401–404.

29. Cluver EH, Politzer WM. Sunburn and vitamin A deficiency. S Afr J Sci 1965; 61:306–309.

30. Olson AJ. Vitamin A. In: Handbook of Vitamins. 2d ed. J Machlin, ed. New York: Marcel Dekker, 1991; 1–57.

31. Burlet E. Die Percutane Resorption von Panthenol (The percutaneous absorption of panthenol). Jubilee Volume Emil Barell 1946; 92–97.

32. Tronnier H. Determination of the hydration effect of a hydrogel with and without d-panthenol. Unpublished document of Hoffmann-La Roche, 1992.

33. Tronnier H. Efficacy of various cream formulations containing panthenol. Unpublished document of Hoffmann-La Roche, 1994.

34. Kline PR. 12 years' experience using pantothenylol topically. Western Med 1963; 4:78–80.

35. Dubecq JP, Detchart M. Etude d'un onguent pantothénique dans la prophylaxie et le traitement des crevasses du sein. La médecine practicienne: special edition 1977; May.

36. Matanić V. Ein Beitrag zur Therapie des Zementekzems. Berufsdermatosen 1963; 11:104–109.

37. Jolibois RP. Etude de l'action d'un onguent à la vitamine B_5 sur les affections cutanées du siège du nouveau-né. Médicine Actuelle 1976; 3:716–721.

38. Stangl E. Ueber den Pantothensaeure-Gehalt menschlicher Kopfhaut (The pantothenic acid content of human hair). Int Z Vitaminforschung 1952; 24:9–12.

39. Stuettgen G, Krause H. Die percutane Absorption von tritium-markiertem Panthenol bei Mensch und Tier (Percutaneous absorption of tritium-labeled panthenol in humans and animals). Archiv fuer klin und exp Dermatologie 1960; 209:578–582.

40. Driscoll WR. Panthenol in hair products. Drug Cosmet Ind 1975; 116:42–45, 149–153.

41. Moser U, Bendich A. Vitamin C. In: Handbook of Vitamins 2d ed. J Machlin, ed. New York: Marcel Dekker, 1991; 195–232.

42. Darr D, Combs S, Dunston S, Manning T, Pinnell S. Topical vitamin C protects porcine skin from ultraviolet radiation-induced damage. Br J Dermatol 1992; 127:247–253.

43. Pinnell SR. Regulation of collagen biosynthesis by ascorbic acid: a review. Yale J Biol Med 1985; 58:553–559.

44. Takashima H, Nomura H, Imai Y, Mima H. Ascorbic acid esters and skin pigmentation. Am Perfum Cosmet 1971; 86:29–36.

45. Takenouchi K, Aso K. The relation between melanin formation and ascorbic acid. J Vitaminol 1964; 10:123–134.

46. Floersheim GL. Treatment of brittle finger nails with biotin. H+G Zeitschrift fuer Hautkrankheiten 1989; 64:41–48.

47. Floersheim GL. An examination of the effect of biotin on alopecia and hair quality. H+G Zeitschrift fuer Hautkrankheiten 1992; 67:246–255.

48. Colombo VE, Gerber F, Bronhofer M, Floersheim GL. Treatment of brittle fingernails and onychoschizia with biotin: scanning electron microscopy. J Am Acad Dermatol 1990; 23:1127–1132.

49. Hochman LG, Scher RK, Meyerson MS. Brittle nails: response to daily biotin supplementation. Cutis 1993; 51:303–305.

50. Gollnick HPM, Hopfenmueller W, Hemmes C, Chun SC, Schmid C, Sundermeier K, Biesalski HK. Systemic beta-carotene plus topical UV-sunscreen are an optimal protection against harmful effects of natural UV-sunlight: results of the Berlin-Eilath study. Eur J Dermatol 1996; 6:200–205.

51. Roccheggiani G. Erfahrungen über die Einwirkung von fettloeslichen Derivaten der Vitamingruppe B auf die Haut (Experiences on the influence of lipid-soluble derivatives of the B group vitamins on the skin). Seifen Oele Fette Wachse 1959; 85:777–779, 819–820.

40

Ellagic Acid: A New Skin-Whitening Active Ingredient

Yoshimasa Tanaka
Lion Corporation, Tokyo, Japan

Melanin is a key factor determining the color of skin. The enzyme tyrosinase plays the most important role in melanin synthesis (melanogenesis) [1,2]. Several tyrosinase inhibitors (chemicals, plant extracts, animal products) have been proposed, based on the view that melanogenesis can be controlled and skin-whitening products developed if tyrosinase activity can be suppressed. However, few have been put to practical use. In practice, it is difficult to develop these candidate materials from in vitro studies to approval for human use, even if inhibitory effects on mushroom-derived tyrosinase or pigment cells can be identified. In addition to showing adequate efficacy and safety, there are many problems to consider, such as stability of the products, production and marketing costs, and perception of the user.

Ellagic acid (EA) (Fig. 1) was approved in 1996 in Japan as the active ingredient of a quasidrug for the prevention of spots and freckles after developing sunburn from exposure to excess sunlight. EA, a naturally occurring polyphenol [3,4] containing four hydroxyl groups, is found in many plants such as strawberry, grape, green tea, eucalyptus, walnut, and tara. Generally, EA is produced by hydrolysis and purification from ellagitannin.

GENERAL PROPERTIES

Ellagic acid is a cream-colored powder slightly soluble in water and ethanol, in alkaline solution and pyridine, and practically insoluble in ether [4]. EA has high antioxidant activity [5], and is listed as a food additive in Japan. The hydroxyl groups of EA can chelate with metal ions [6,7].

IN VITRO STUDIES

Ellagic acid inhibits mushroom-derived tyrosinase competitively and in a dose-dependent manner; the inhibition constant (ki) is 81.6 µM [8]. The decrease in copper concentration and the reduction in tyrosinase activity by EA follow almost parallel patterns. Tyrosinase

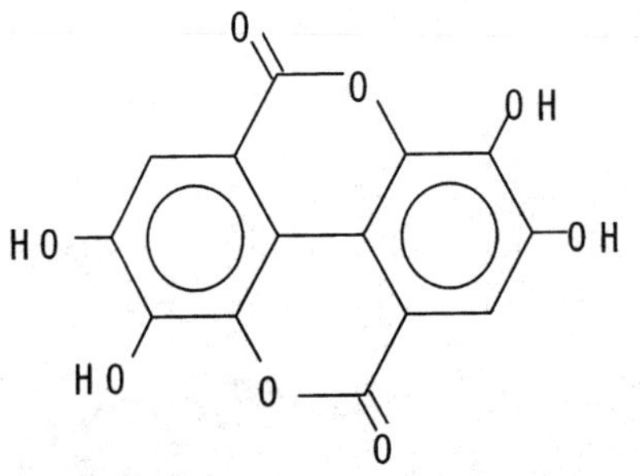

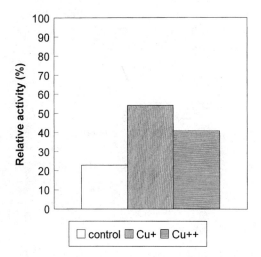

FIGURE 1 Ellagic acid.

activity, after inhibition by EA, partially recovers after addition of cuprous or cupric ion (Fig. 2).

Growth of B16 melanoma cells in culture medium was not suppressed by EA at concentrations of less than 4 μM. At 4 μM, the inhibition of tyrosinase activity was 38.3% and the decrease in melanin concentration 54.4%. Although the color of the cells (reflecting the melanin concentration) became whitened in the presence of EA, cell color reverted to the original shade when EA was removed from the culture medium (Fig. 3). The addition of other metals, in place of the copper compounds, did not lead to recovery of the enzymic activity.

These results show that the inhibitory effect of EA is reversible, effective only in its presence, and specific to copper compounds. It is proposed that EA chelates to copper ion(s) at the active center of tyrosinase, which is a metaloprotein containing copper. Further structural changes then make the tyrosinase inactive. Because the molecular structure of EA is planar, EA may be able to penetrate into the active center of tyrosinase easily. It is clear that EA inhibits tyrosinase because of its molecular structure as well as its ability to chelate with copper.

FIGURE 2 Effects of addition of copper ion on recovery of tyrosinase activity. Cu^+ or Cu^{++} (5 mM) were added to tyrosinase during inhibition by EA.

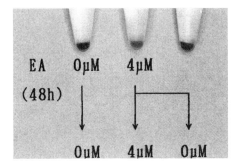

FIGURE 3 Effect of EA on melanoma cells. Cells were incubated with EA (4 μM) for 48 hours. Culture medium was changed to fresh medium in the presence or absence of EA (4 μM) and incubated for an additional 48 hours.

ANIMAL STUDIES

Brownish guinea pigs have melanocytes in their skin and the skin pigmentation is enhanced by ultraviolet (UV) light irradiation, similar to the human situation. The preventative effect of EA on skin pigmentation was investigated by applying EA topically, on the back, for 6 weeks and irradiating by UV for first 2 weeks [8]. The appearance of skin to which EA was applied became similar to normal skin. The melanin content of the skin to which EA had been applied was reduced, not only in the basal layers but also in the stratum spinosum, -granulosum, and -corneum, in comparison with the same structures in control sections to which EA had not been applied. Tyrosinase activity was similar. Furthermore, application of EA to the skin after UV-light irradiation had almost the same affect as applying EA concurrently with the initial irradiation.

According to the results of the studies using the brownish guinea pig, EA is a more efficient skin whitener and suppressor of pigmentation than arbutin or kojic acid, other active skin whiteners, at the same dose level (1%) (Fig. 4).

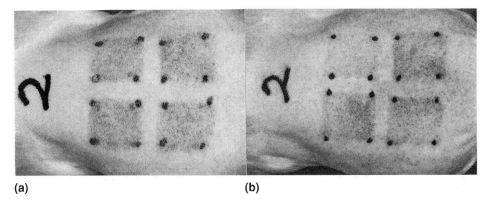

(a) (b)

FIGURE 4 Comparison of effects of some commercially available agents in preventing skin pigmentation induced by UV-light irradiation. Samples were applied for 4 weeks after UV-light irradiation (eight times): (a) before application; (b) after application for 4 weeks; (upper left) ellagic acid, (upper right) vehicle, (lower left) arbutin, (lower right) kojic acid.

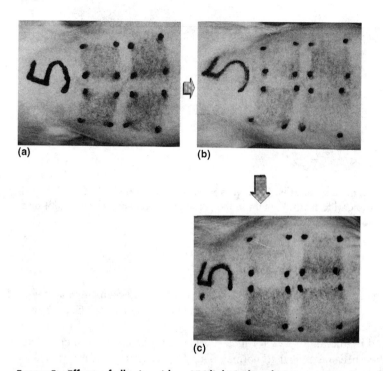

FIGURE 5 Effects of ellagic acid on UV-light induced pigmentation. Samples were applied for 4 weeks (a) after UV-light irradiation (eight times): (upper left) hydroquinone; (upper right) vehicle only; (lower left) control—no EA applied; (lower right) ellagic acid. After application was terminated (b), the same area was irradiated again (c).

Furthermore, the efficacy of EA was almost the same as that of hydroquinone (HQ), a well-known depigmentation agent (Fig. 5). When the same animals were subjected to UV irradiation again after completion of the application phase, normal skin pigmentation was observed in the EA-applied area as well as in the control areas, but only slight pigmentation was seen in the HQ-treated skin. The results of these investigations indicated that EA was not injurious to melanocytes but was a good inhibitor of tyrosinase activity. In comparison, HQ may be toxic to melanocytes.

EFFECT ON HUMAN SKIN

A skin cream containing EA was applied for 6 weeks to the brachium before each irradiation by UV light [9]. The sites were irradiated three times at 1 MED. Skin pigmentation was partially suppressed after only 1 week's application, and completely suppressed after 3 and 6 weeks' application (Fig. 6). Eighty-six percent of the efficacy of EA evaluated by a double-blind controlled test was rated ''moderately preferable'' or better (Fig. 7). Similar efficacy rates were calculated by the image analysis method. Side effects such as depigmentation were not observed throughout the application period.

Thus, EA can prevent the buildup of skin pigmentation after sunburn. It can also be expected to improve the appearance of pigmented skin such as melasma or freckles,

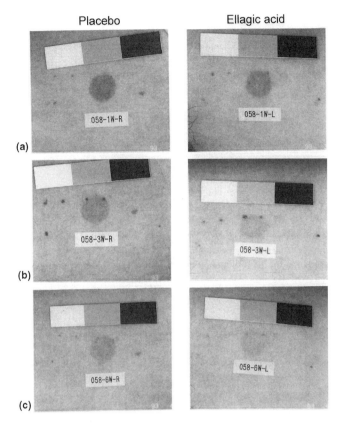

FIGURE 6 **Effect of ellagic acid on UV-light induced skin pigmentation in human.**

for such skin pigmentation is believed to follow similar mechanisms to that of sunburn, at least from the viewpoint of epidermic disorders, even if the mechanism of melasma and so on are not precisely clear. Many impressions that skin pigmentation appears to be lightened have been gathered from users of products containing EA. In practice, the characteristics of melasma, postinflammatory pigmentation, and other conditions appear to be improved by this application. EA is a promising skin-whitening active ingredient.

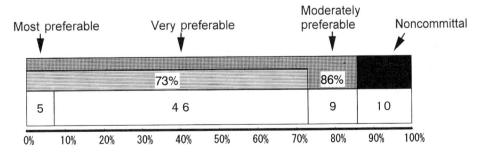

FIGURE 7 **Efficacy for whitening effect on sunburn subjects.**

REFERENCES

1. Nordlund JJ, Boissy RE, Hearing VJ, King RA, Ortonne J-P eds. The Pigmentary System (Physiology and Pathophysiology). New York; Oxford University Press, 1998.
2. Tanaka Y, Masuda M. Trends in skin-whitening agents in Japan. INFORM 1998; 9:306.
3. Bate-Smith EC. Chromatography and systematic distribution of ellagic acid. Chem Ind BIF Rev 1956; April: R32.
4. Zee-Cheng RK-Y, Cheng CC. Ellagic acid. Drugs of the Future 1986; 11:1029.
5. Osawa T, Ide A, Su J-D, Namiki M. Inhibition of lipid peroxidation by ellagic acid. J Agric Food Chem 1987; 35:808.
6. Press RE, Hardcastle D. Some physico-chemical properties of ellagic acid. J Appl Chem 1969; 19:247.
7. Zhang N-Z, Chen Y-Y. Synthesis of macroporous ellagitannic acid resin and its chelating properties for metal ions. J Macromol Sci-Chem 1988; A25(10&11):1455.
8. Shimogaki H, Tanaka Y, Tamai H, Masuda M. In vitro and in vivo evaluation of ellagic acid on melanogenesis inhibition. Int J Cosmet Sci 2000; 22:291.
9. Kamide R, Arase S, Takiwaki H, Watanabe S, Watanabe Y, Kageyama S. Clinical evaluation on the effects of XSC-29 preparation on the pigmentation of the skin by exposure to ultraviolet light. Nishinihon J Dermatol 1995; 57:136.

41

Cosmetics and Interactions with Superficial Epidermis

Jørgen Serup
Leo Pharmaceutical Products, Copenhagen, Denmark

INTRODUCTION

The superficial epidermis is the part of the skin that we see directly. Our appreciation of the condition of the skin, both as consumers and as medical professionals, is primarily dependent on visual inspection. Various examination techniques can be applied additionally [1–3]. Techniques that illustrate the skin condition, such as surface microscopy, assessment of color, scaling, and surface contour, are first-line methods in the evaluation of cosmetic products because of their direct relevance, whereas other methods such as electrical conductance, transepidermal water loss, and pH are second-line or surrogate methods that may only serve as tools in research with a special aim.

From a holistic point of view, consumer appreciation of a cosmetic product is highly complex, and only to a minor degree dependent on true and documented biological effects of the product on skin functions and structures such as the superficial epidermis. Every product has its own aura dependent on culture, society, personal aims, and habits. This is supported by marketing activities of companies in a broad range as well as specifically for a product promoted by the company with a special profile to make profitable business in a market with hundreds or thousands of competitors. The highly complex interaction between psyche, skin, and product is discussed later in this chapter.

EPIDERMIS: THE SUBLIME BARRIER

Barrier functions of various kinds is the sublime function of the epidermis [4]. The barriers of the skin are structurally located in the superficial epidermis. The interface between the superficial epidermis with stratum corneum and the profound epidermis with the stratum Malpighii is the important interface between ambient conditions and environment, including cosmetic product effects, and the internal milieu with many cellular and metabolic functions. The barriers in the superficial epidermis include a temperature moderator and barriers against evaporation of water, uptake of oxygen, expiration of carbon dioxide, penetration of chemicals from the environment (exposures related to occupation and leisure), chemicals contained in products (cosmetics, cosmeceuticals, and drugs), and the penetration of ultraviolet light, which is reflected or scattered in the superficial epidermis. The superficial epidermis also protects against microbes such as bacteria and fungi.

These critically important interfaces in the epidermis are not a simple structure that can be visualized by histology, but by functions and gradients. The epidermis and the skin is also a neurosensory perceptive organ where negative sensations (pain, itching, stinging, burning, hot, cold) and positive sensations (touch, sexual stimulation) are elicited. Cosmetics, cosmeceuticals, and drugs are designed to interact with the different layers of the skin. Cosmetics primarily aim to influence the visible, superficial epidermis, whereas drugs typically aim to influence the inner layers of the skin and heal disease. Some drugs, namely the transdermals, permeate the skin and are absorbed into the blood stream to exert their action at a distant target organ.

It is not clear if cosmetic products and the chemicals ingredient they contain respect epidermal barriers and remain in the superficial epidermis or if they penetrate to deeper layers of the skin. For example, cosmetic products have to penetrate to the dermis in order to smoothen coarse wrinkles. Being present in the dermis, such ingredients or chemicals are expected to be systematically absorbed and reach the blood stream, maybe after metabolism in the skin to some unknow breakdown chemical with unknown action. However, for safety reasons, cosmetic products are normally claimed not to penetrate the dermis to any significant degree.

The interaction between epidermis and the cosmetic product with its various constituents is, as it may be understood, of crucial importance both for the claimed efficacy and the safety of product. Of course, ingredients are selected carefully, and limited to those expected to be harmless.

NATURE OF INTERACTIONS BETWEEN PRODUCTS AND THE SUPERFICIAL EPIDERMIS

Cosmetic products are intended for interaction with the superficial epidermis, and ideally create objective and visible changes. The importance of such changes to be visible to the naked eye and appreciated as improvements was highlighted in the introduction.

The intended, beneficial interactions of cosmetic products with the epidermis are the traditional ones, namely improvement of scaling, improvement of skin color, improvement of wrinkles (fine and coarse), improvement of elasticity, and a range of beneficial effects on the specialized superficial epidermis, namely the hair and nails. These effects are well known. However, interactions of products with the epidermis may also be innocent or irrelevant or directly harmful, with adverse events such as irritant or allergic contact dermatitis or special events such as development of comedoes and acne. Fragrance allergy is now the number two allergy in industrialized countries, with increasing prevalence. Fragrances are, however, contained not only in cosmetic products, but also in a broad range of household products. Harmful effects on the epidermis may be direct or indirect, acute/short term or chronic/long term, predictable and dose dependent (AHA products, urea, and others), or idiosyncratic, occurring unexpectedly in special individuals. Moreover, effects may be objective or subjective, and if subjective, real (stinging, burning, itching, pain) or purely imaginative. The list of effect variables is not complete.

Products of topical pharmaceuticals, in principle, carry the heavy burden of complete preregistrational documentation, whereas cosmetic products reach the market with a small safety dossier only, mirabile dictu non–animal based, but no or very limited formal requirements regarding documentation of efficacy claims.

SELECTED TECHNIQUES FOR THE STUDY OF THE SUPERFICIAL EPIDERMIS

Techniques to study scaling, dryness, transepidermal water loss, skin elasticity, color, and wrinkles, among others, are already well covered in this book and in a number of recent monographs [1–3,5–7]. In each case, techniques need to be adopted and modified relative to the precise purpose of the study protocol. Errors in the use of biophysical methods were more or less the standard some years ago when these techniques were in their infancy, but nowadays the state of the art is to develop, e.g., standard operating procedures, and prestudy validation of the techniques and the design used [8]. Guidelines have been developed and the biophysical methods have today, as a result of this development, acquired acceptance and respect in research and academia.

There are certain study premises to consider:

- A primary claim should be defined, and this should be directly addressed in a study.
- Methods and techniques must be validated before study, and guidelines and proper conduct should be followed.
- The method should be concluded to be valid for the purpose, i.e., accurate, reproducible, linear, and display values within the clinically relevant range.
- The protocols should be orderly and designed with respect to inclusion of, e.g., individuals, blinding, randomization, product application, observation periods, controls, and regression study following active treatment.
- A statistician should be involved and a proper sample size calculation should be conducted.
- Criteria for success relative to the primary study objects should be predefined. Blinding and randomness should be used whenever applicable and despite the use of objective measuring systems.
- It should be clearly understood and defined before study whether a test is used as a first-line method directly to document primary claims or the primary object of clinical relevance, or if the test is used as an indirect or surrogate method, in which case special documentation or arguments are needed to support its relevance for the main claim. The pros and the cons of surrogate parameters should be displayed in an open and balanced discussion.
- In their core design, the conduct and conclusion of studies should not be biased by marketing interests.
- Results should be published irrespective of the outcome.

These modern principles of research are universal, and not only relevant for the study of the superficial epidermis. No good argument has been made for why studies of cosmetic products in humans shall not follow the standards for the study of products on humans as defined by the International Congress of Harmonization (ICH), standards now obligatory in the pharmaceutical industry [9]. In the real world, of course, there is a dilemma between resources and ideal demands, and the good clinical practice (GCP) system is mainly introduced to ensure validity of results and help public control. Studies can easily be high-quality and valid without following GCP, but the GCP remains a master class lesson one can learn from.

THE PSYCHE, SKIN, AND COSMETIC PRODUCT TRIANGLE

It was known for many years that skin well being correlates with physical, social, and mental well functioning. Consumer's use of a cosmetic product on their skin is overall in perspective, and not used by the consumer specifically to improve elastic fibers, electrical conduction, or transepidermal water loss, to maintain a pH of 5.5, or to give her or his kerotinocytes a bigger and rounder shape or whatever the intellectual or pseudointellectual argument for the product might be. Basic biology is a black box for the consumer. Likewise, the consumer does not apply an antiwrinkle cream to improve fine lines of micrometer width, which are only visible under a microscope, but she or he uses an antiwrinkle cream to directly treat visible coarse wrinkles with the overall aim to obtain a young or younger look. The consumer typically has almost no idea about the strong economic forces in the marketplace, where she or he is more or less a gambler in a beauty shop.

There is in cosmetic-product use a triangle with the psyche at the top and the skin and the product at the bottom (Fig. 1). The consumer spontaneously coexists with her or his skin and develops her or his degree of self-esteem relative to the skin depending on her or his intellect and society's coding of her or his psyche. There are many examples of how use of cosmetics vary in different cultures and in different historical periods, and this is, of course, not explained by a different biology of the skin.

Already the application of a cosmetic product is a venue of pleasure and relaxation. The person can for a brief period concentrate on herself or himself and relax, and the massage maneuvre, while spreading an elegant, fragrant scent, is coupled with pleasure and mental satisfaction. Such daily life dreamy meditation is often displayed in announcements for cosmetics where beautiful ladies apply wonderful creams, wordless in their happiness, almost flying in the cosmos. By promoting this way, the producers contribute to daydreams and quality of life, and actually meet with some true needs of the consumers. Cosmetics are used to an enormous degree, much more so than true biological or medical needs of the skin could ever explain or justify on rational grounds.

Thus, it is a difficult dilemma to use objective methods, including biophysical techniques in order to document cosmetics. The role of the methods is bound to be limited, but there remains to exist a distinction between fine and honest products with true claims and documented safety and efficacy, and those products that are just manufactured and sold and which may after all, with an unknown risk, also improve quality of life, despite their limited documentation.

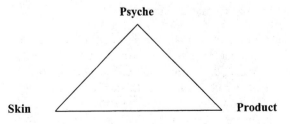

FIGURE 1 The psyche, skin, and cosmetic product triangle.

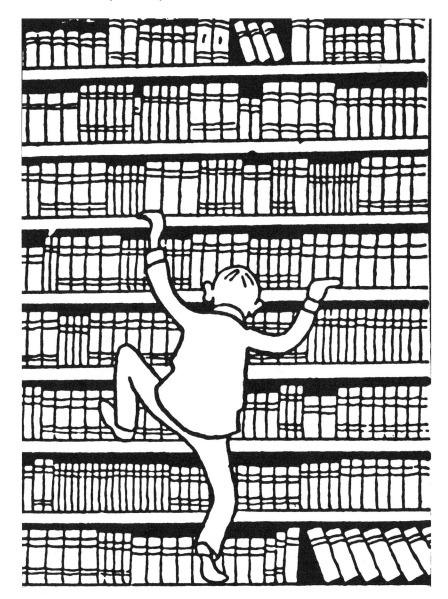

FIGURE 2 The professor's research project on cosmetics.

The dilemma between theory and subjective needs and practice and objective effects has no solution or answer (Fig. 2). There are different angles. This was elegantly expressed by a leading researcher in a French company who said, *"The cosmetic products do less than we say, but more than we think."*

REFERENCES

1. Leveque JL. Cutaneous Investigation in Health and Disease. Noninvasive Methods and Instrumentation. New York: Marcel Dekker, 1989.

2. Serup J, Jemec GBE. Handbook of Non-Invasive Methods and the Skin. Boca Raton: CRC Press, 1995.
3. Elsner P, Barel AO, Berardesca E, Gabard B, Serup J. Skin Bioengineering. Techniques and Applications in Dermatology and Cosmetology. Basel: S. Karger, 1998.
4. Schaefer H, Redelmeier TE. Skin Barrier. Principles of Percutaneous Absorption. Basel: S. Karger, 1996.
5. Berardesca E, Elsner P, Wilhelm KP, Maibach HI. Bioengineering of the Skin: Methods and Instrumentation. Boca Raton: CRC Press, 1995.
6. Elsner P, Berardesca E, Maibach HI. Bioengineering of the Skin: Water and the Stratum Corneum. Boca Raton: CRC Press, 1994.
7. Wilhelm KP, Elsner P, Berardesca E, Maibach HI. Bioengineering of the Skin: Skin Surface Imaging and Analysis. Boca Raton: CRC Press, 1997.
8. Serup J. Bioengineering and the skin: from Standard error to standard operating procedure. Acta Derm Venereol (Stockh) 1994; 185(Suppl):5–8.
9. ICH Harmonised Tripartite Guideline for Good Clinical Practice. Brookwood: Brookwood Medical Publications Ltd, 1996.

42

Skin Cleansing Bars

Joshua B. Ghaim and Elizabeth D. Volz
Colgate-Palmolive Company, Piscataway, New Jersey

INTRODUCTION

Although the origin of soap is not very clear, it is widely accepted that some form of primitive soap-making methods existed several thousand years ago, dating as far back to 2000 BC. For many centuries, soaps were made by heating a mixture of animal fats (tallow) with lye, a basic solution obtained from wood ashes [1]. Until the late eighteenth century, soap was considered a luxury item available only to royalty and the social upper class. Today, soaps are produced using a variety of much more refined processes and different fats and oils, resulting in finished products that deliver consumer-relevant performance benefits with desirable aesthetics [1]. In this section, we will discuss the chemical and physical properties of commercial soap bars with a focus on skin cleansing, the raw materials needed, the manufacturing and process requirements, and the final finished product performance evaluations.

WHAT IS SOAP?

Soap is generally defined as an alkali salt of a long-chain fatty acid. When a fat or oil is saponified, the sodium or potassium salt formed from the long-chain fatty acids is called a soap. The term "soap" refers to a group of neutralized long-chain carboxylic acids, which result from two primary ingredients: an alkali and a triglyceride (fat or oil). The chain length of the aliphatic group is typically between 7 and 21 carbons with one carboxylate carbon, yielding a molecule containing 8 to 22 carbons. The cation associated with the carboxylate head group generally comprises sodium, potassium, or to a lesser extent other cations such as triethanolamine as well as heavy metals and alkali earth metals such as magnesium.

Soap cleans by altering the surface tension of water and emulsifying and suspending soils to be rinsed away. The two ends of soap have different polarities where the long carbon chain end is nonpolar and hydrophobic, whereas the carboxylate salt end is ionic and hydrophilic. When a soap is used to clean grease or dirt, the nonpolar ends of the soap molecules solubilize nonpolar fats and oils that accompany dirt. The water-loving (hydrophilic) salt ends of the soap molecules extend outside where they can be solubilized in water. The soap molecules coat the oil or grease, forming clusters called micelles. The hydrophilic end of the soap molecules provides polarity to the micelles, thus emulsifying them in water. As a result, small globules of oil and fat coated with soap molecules are pulled into the water layer and can be rinsed away.

SOAP RAW MATERIALS

Fats and Oils

The naturally occurring fats and oils used in soap making are glycerides with three fatty acid groups randomly esterified with glycerol (trihydroxy alcohol). The difference between fats and oils is merely one of their physical states: fats are solids and oils are liquids. Fats and oils typically comprise both saturated and unsaturated fatty acid molecules containing between 7 and 21 carbons randomly distributed on the glycerol backbone. Overall, the reaction of caustic (lye) with triglycerides yields glycerin and soap in a reaction known as saponification. This is the most widely used soap making process. The second major soap making process is the neutralization of fatty acids with an alkali. Fats and oils are hydrolyzed (split) with high-pressure steam to yield crude fatty acids and glycerin. The fatty acids are then purified by distillation and neutralized with an alkali to produce soap and water (neat soap) [2–7].

The properties of the resulting soap are determined by the quality and composition of the component fatty acids in the starting fat mixture. In general, chain lengths of less than 12 carbon atoms are more irritating to the skin; conversely, saturated chain lengths greater than 18 carbon atoms form soaps less soluble for ready solution and sudsing. Similarly, a higher proportion of unsaturated fatty acids (e.g., oleic and linolenic) yields soaps susceptible to undesirable atmospheric oxidative changes. For these reasons and the fact that fats and oils are treated as commodities in the open market, the number of fats and oils suitable for commercial soapmaking is limited. The selection of the appropriate starting fats and oils forming the base composition of a soap is key to its quality and performance. Among the fats and oils used throughout the world, beef and sheep tallow are the most common fats, and oils from coconut, palm, soy, and babassu are the most frequently used oils. Soap compositions containing fractions of oils such as palm stearin and other oils with hydrogenation or other upgrading are also in the formulators' arsenal for selection. In the United States, most toilet soaps are made from beef tallow and coconut oil. Some of the common fats and oils used in commercial soapmaking are discussed in the following sections (Table 1).

Tallow

Tallow, which is the principal animal fat in soapmaking, is obtained from the meat processing industry as a result of rendering the body fat from beef and in some cases sheep [8]. In the United States, most toilet soaps are made from beef tallow and coconut oil. The properties of these and other fats are dependent on the constituent fatty acids. Tallow from different sources may vary considerably in color (both initial and after bleaching), titer (solidification point of the fatty acids), free fatty acid content, saponification value (alkali required for saponification), and iodine value (measure of unsaturation). Tallow is composed of mostly long-chain saturated and unsaturated fatty acids—mostly C_{16} (palmitic, 28%), C_{18} (stearic, 18%), and $C_{18:1}$ (oleic, 44%)—providing hardness and thick and creamy long-lasting lather (Table 1).

TABLE 1   Fatty Acid Distribution and Characteristics of Soap Bases

Fatty acid distribution	Tallow	Coconut	Palm oil	Palm stearin	Palm kernel
Caprylic (C-8)		7.4			
Capric (C-10)		6.3			
Lauric (C-12)		47.8			49.7
Myristic (C-14)	2.8	18.3	1.1	1.5	15.7
Palmitic (C-16)	27.8	9.0	43.5	56.5	8.0
Palmitoleic (C-16:1)	3.8			0.2	
Stearic (C-18)	17.9	2.8	4.2	4.8	2.4
Oleic (C-18:1)	43.9	6.3	40.8	29.6	15.2
Linoleic (C-18:2)	2.3	2.0	10.2	7.2	1.5
Linolenic (C-18:3)				0.1	
Characteristics					
Iodine value (IV)	38–48	8–10	50–55	32–40	14–22
Titer, °C	40	26	40	49–51	25
Saponification value (SV)	193–200	251–263	196–209	196–209	240–250
Fatty acid average molecular weight (FA Ave mw)	272	213	270	268	221

Coconut Oil

Coconut oil is one of the most important vegetable oils used in soap making. As previously mentioned, most toilet soaps in the United States are made from tallow and coconut oil. Coconut oil is composed mostly of C_{12} (lauric, 48%) and C_{14} (myristic, 18%) fatty acids, reducing hardness and providing solubility and lather with large bubbles that do not last long (Table 1). Coconut oil is obtained from the dried fruit, copra, of the coconut palm tree.

Palm Oil

Palm oil, which often serves as a substitute for tallow, is obtained from the fruit of the palm tree. It is composed of mostly long chain–length fatty acids—such as C_{16} (palmitic, 44%) and $C_{18:1}$ (oleic, 41%)—providing properties and compositions more similar to tallow than other vegetable oils (Table 1).

Palm Kernel Oil

Palm kernel oil unlike palm oil, is obtained from the center of the nuts of the palm tree and is composed of mostly shorter chain–length fatty acids—such as C_{12} (lauric, 50%) and C_{14} (myristic, 16%)—providing properties and composition similar to coconut oil (Table 1). Palm kernel oil is commonly used as a substitute to coconut oil in the soap-making process.

Palm Stearin

Like palm oil or tallow, palm stearin is composed of mostly long chain–length fatty acids but with lower degree of saturation. Palm stearin is produced by splitting palm oil into palm olein (which is used in foods) and palm stearin. Palm stearin provides properties more similar to tallow than other vegetable oils.

Although the five oils discussed are the most commonly used fats and oils in the soap-making industry, other sources such as lard (hog fat), Babassu oil, rice bran oil, palm kernel olein, and soybean oil are also used throughout the world.

SOAP PHASES

The physicochemical nature of soap has been shown to be critical for the in-use properties. It is generally accepted that four distinct sodium soap crystalline phases exist. These soap phases are referred to as the beta, delta, omega, and liquid crystalline phases. Today, radiographic diffraction (XRD) is considered the simplest and most reliable method for distinguishing the different phases. The phases designate the lattice spacing between the hydrocarbon chains and are predictive of physical properties such as lather, slough, use-up rate, and even the degree of translucency of a soap bar [9]. The large crystals of the omega phase with the liquid phase are formed when neat soap is cooled down (after the drying step). Beta-phase conversion in soap bars depends on several factors, including temperature, type of surfactant, moisture level and number of millings. Delta phase is formed by the recrystallization of saturated higher chain soaps under specific temperature conditions and moisture level. Ferguson et al. first linked XRD measurements to the physical properties and characteristics of soap bars as finished product. For instance, delta phase provides low slough and low wear rate, whereas beta phase has good lather, low wear rate, and high slough [9].

SOAP BASE COMPOSITION AND PERFORMANCE

Product performance profiles are critically dependent on the base composition selection. For example, the relatively less-soluble tallow provides for bar hardness and a dense, stable, small bubbled lather, whereas the more soluble coconut oil provides an easily generated lather consisting of large bubbles. In addition to bar hardness, color, odor, and lather considerations, the formulator must be concerned with the solubility of the soap as it impacts on the use-up and sloughing of the final product. A typical soap bar in the United States uses a tallow/coconut oil base and the ratio of the two components determines lather attributes such as speed, quantity, and richness. An increase of all of these attributes occurs with the increasing proportions of the coconut oil but the higher proportion of coconut oil also results in an increasing degree of irritation to the skin because of the high short-chain–length fatty acid composition. Furthermore, the behavior of the base can be determined not only by the fatty acid chain but also by the cation by which it is neutralized. The cation can also have a significant influence on the solubility and mildness properties of the base. For example, a sodium soap would be harder than a potassium soap of the same carbon chain length [1].

ADDITIVES

Soap manufacturers have developed a variety of formulation approaches to deliver products that better meet the consumer needs of today. Even though the base soap composition has not changed, consumer needs are met by the inclusion of various additives. As with any other product, the stability (physical and chemical state) of the soap-base–additive or even additive-additive mix must be considered during the formulation. There are a variety of additives that are formulated into soap bars to provide additional consumer benefits and/or to modify the performance and aesthetics of the final product. A complete list of functional additives can be found in The Cosmetic, Toiletry and Fragrance Association (CTFA) Cosmetic Ingredient Handbook [10].

Fragrance

Fragrance is by far the most important additive for consumer acceptance of a personal cleansing product. Even though the primary purpose of the selection of a fragrance is to target a specific user group, it is also used to mask the characteristic base odor associated with the fatty acids. Fragrances are compounded from several components including carboxylic acids, esters, aldehydes, ketones, and glycols where the selection of the components could adversely effect the stability and/or the processability of the final product. For instance, fragrances with solvents such as dipropylene glycol (glycol) and diethylpthlate (ester) tend to soften and cloud translucent soap bars [2]. The raw-material manufacturer's ability to provide cleaner base with significantly less base odor has greatly improved in the past two decades, thus allowing soap manufacturers to use less fragrance in the final product or even, in some cases, provide products that are fragrance free. Fragrances are also known to alter the mildness properties of soap bars. For example, a soap bar that targets consumers with sensitive skin has enough fragrance to mask the base odor of the fatty acid while providing some soft perfume that reinforces their mildness properties. The fragrance levels in the soap bar typically range from 0.3% (sensitive skin) to 1.5% (deodorant soaps). Long-term aging studies are always necessary in order to assess the stability of the fragrance in the soap base and its continued ability to mask the base odor.

Free Fatty Acid or Superfatting

Traditional soap bars are alkaline in nature with a pH of around 10. A manufacturing process with excess fatty acid beyond what is needed by the reaction yields a final product with free fatty acid, also known as ''superfatted'' soap. Conversely, a process with caustic in excess of what is needed by the reaction yields a base soap with a slight excess of free caustic. Excess caustic can be neutralized by the addition of excess free fatty acids such as coconut, palm kernel, or stearic acid, or by postaddition of weak acids such as citric or phosphoric acid. Superfatting enhances the lather profile of the soap bar, eliminates free alkali (lowers the pH), and can provide some improvement of skin mildness attributes [1].

Glycerin

Glycerin is a common ingredient formulated into soap bars that dates back to ancient times. As previously discussed, it is the by-product of saponification and thus has always been present in soaps in varying levels [2]. Glycerin is well known for its ability to absorb water (humectancy). This makes it an ideal additive for skincare (moisturization) benefits. Its humectant properties, even at low levels, can alter the rinsability of the soap bar, thus modifying the consumer perception of the product as clean rinsing product.

Colorants and Pigments

The visual appearance of a soap bar is known to influence the consumer acceptance of the product. Because of color differences of some of the base compositions, it is common for most manufacturers to alter the appearance of the final product. This is mostly accomplished by the addition of colorants and opacifying agents. Some of the common additives used to alter the appearance of a soap bar include food and/or cosmetic grade dyes and pigments, as well as lakes and opacifiers such as titanium dioxide and zinc oxide [10].

Preservatives

Soap bases with high proportions of unsaturated fatty acids (e.g., oleic, linoleic, linolenic) [11,12] and the presence of certain soap additives, such as fragrance, tend to be susceptible to undesirable atmospheric oxidative changes. Therefore, preservatives (chelating agents and antioxidants) are necessary to prevent such oxidation from occurring. Some commonly used chelating agents (for trace metals present) in soap bars include ethylenediaminetetraacetate (EDTA); diethylenetriamine pentaacetate (DTPA, also known as pentasodium pentate); sodium etidronate or ethane-1-hydroxy-1,1-diphosphonic acid (EHDP) [13]; citric acid; and magnesium silicate. The most commonly used antioxidants in conjunction with chelating agent in soap bars are butylatedhydroxytoluene (BHT) and, recently, the addition of tetradibutyl pentaerithrityl hydroxyhydrocinnamate [14]. Both of these antioxidants are soluble in fragrances.

Skin Conditioners

As previously mentioned, consumer demand for products that not only cleanse the skin but also provide skin mildness and moisturizing benefits is constantly changing. Therefore, it is common for manufacturers to add ingredients that are known to provide such benefits. We previously discussed two of the most commonly used additives, free fatty acid and glycerin. Other additives that are commonly used in soap bars include the following: vitamin E, aloe, jojoba oil, lanolin, glyceryl stearate, isopropyl esters, sodium cetearyl sulfate, cetyl esters, petrolatum, silicones, beeswax, ceresin, carbomer-934, sodium polyacrylate, cocoa butter, mineral oil, and polyethyleneoxideglycol-12, to name a few [10].

Antimicrobial Agents

Soap bars are very effective in removing microbial flora that are known to cause skin infections, pimples, and malodor during the washing/bathing process. The addition of antimicrobial actives to a soap bar extends this benefit for a longer period of time, mainly between washing/bathing. Because of safety concerns about the different actives used in soap bars, the number of antimicrobial agents used in soap bars has decreased from several in the 1970s to only three today. Trichlorocarbanilide (TCC), trichlorodiphenylhydroxyether (triclosan), and parachloro m-xylenol (PCMX) are commonly used in soap bars today. The selection of which active to use in different products is based on claims or product positioning, efficacy, and cost of the final product. TCC is effective mostly against gram-positive bacteria, whereas triclosan and PCMX have been shown to be effective against both gram-positive and gram-negative bacteria. The use levels of these actives are dependent on the claims associated with the final products and government regulations. For instance, in the United States the maximum use levels allowed for triclosan and TCC are 1.0% and 1.5%, respectively.

Synthetic Surfactants

The formulation of soap bars has become more complex because of the ever-increasing consumer demand of products that not only provide cleansing properties but also skin-conditioning/moisturization benefits. Synthetic surfactants are often used to enhance the performance of soap bars, resulting in improved skin feel, less irritation, and improved quality and quantity of lather. Synthetic surfactants are used at levels ranging from 5% (low-level combar) to 80% (Syndet), which will be discussed in detail in the later sections of this chapter. The selection of a good synthetic surfactant is critical for the performance of the final product. Some examples of commonly used synthetic surfactants in soap bars include sodium cocoyl isethionate, alkyl ether sulfonate and cocomonoglyceride sulfates [15,16].

Other Additives

Several other additives not mentioned in the previous sections are currently being used in soap bars. Some examples include processing aids, binders (gums and resins), fillers (dextrin, salt, talc, etc., for bar hardness), exfoliants, anti-acne actives, and anti-irritants.

SOAP-MAKING/MANUFACTURING PROCESS

The process of making soap begins with the receipt of fats and oils and ends with a soap bar pressed into a desired shape and packaged for sale. There are many unit operations involved in soap making, from distillation (glycerin recovery) to drying to pneumatic conveying. The soap-making process involves the production of neat soap (wet soap) from fats and oils. The soap then goes through drying and finishing steps in order to complete the process. There are two basic routes of commercial soapmaking [17], which are discussed in the following two sections.

Neutral Fat/Oil Route or Saponification

In the saponification process, neutral fats and oils (tallow, palm oil, palm stearin, coconut oil, palm kernel oil) are first upgraded to remove particulate dirt, proteinaceious materials, and other odor and color bodies, and then reacted with caustic (NaOH or KOH) yielding neat soap and free glycerin (Fig. 1a). Saponification can be done in either a batch (kettle) process or a continuous process [1,2].

Fat Splitting/Fatty Acid Route

In this method of soap production, the fats and oils (triglycerides) are hydrolyzed with high-pressure steam (fat splitting) to produce fatty acids and glycerin. The fatty acids are then purified by distillation and neutralized with an alkali to produce soap (neat soap) and water (Fig. 1b). This method of production is most suitable when lower grade fats and oils are used for soap production.

Drying and Finishing

Neat soap produced by one of the processes previously outlined contains over 30% moisture. The soap needs to be dried, typically by vacuum drying to a final moisture level of 8 to 16% for the final finishing steps. Once the neat soap is dried to soap pellets (soap chips), it is transferred into mixers (amalgamators) and the minor additives such as fragrance, color, preservative, antibacterial agents, and other formula additives are added. These additives are mixed with the soap pellets, refined, and extruded into long continuous billet. The billet is cut and pressed into the desired shape and packaged (Fig. 2). Some

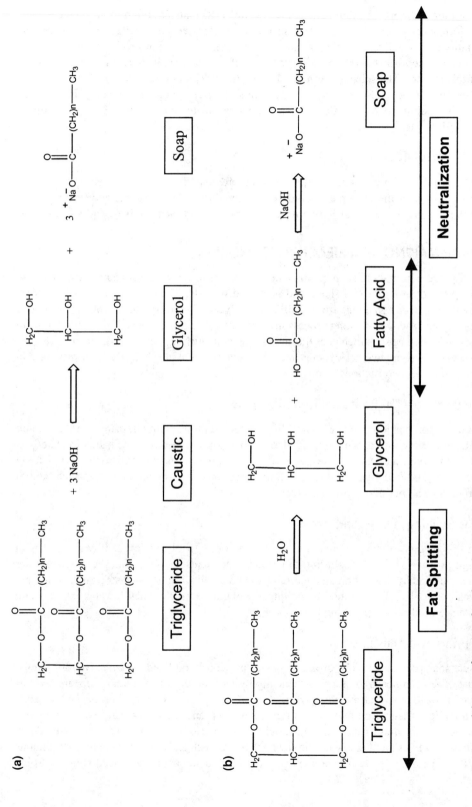

FIGURE 1   (a) Saponification of triglycerides; (b) fat splitting (glycerol as a by-product) and fatty acid neutralization reaction.

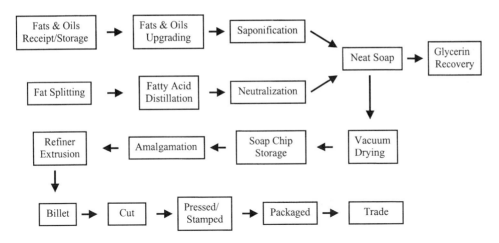

FIGURE 2 Flow chart of the soap manufacturing steps.

soaps are cast instead of cut into shapes. In this case the soap is poured into a mold of desired shape [1,2,18].

FORMULATIONS: REGULAR SOAPS, COMBARS, AND SYNDETS

Soap bars are formulated with a combination of longer carbon chain length fats (tallow, palm oil, palm stearin) and shorter carbon chain length oils (palm kernel oil, coconut oil). Common nomenclature for bar soaps is the ratio of the longer carbon chain length fat to the shorter carbon chain length oil. For example, a bar containing 80% tallow and 20% coconut oil as its soap base would be referred to as an ''80/20'' soap bar. Ratios used typically range from 90/10 to 60/40. The higher coco or palm kernel oil levels in a soap bar not only leads to a higher lathering profile [1] but also to a higher use-up rate due to the high portion of the shorter carbon chain length base. Regular soap bars generally contain approximately 75 to 85% soap. The remainder of the soap bar is made up of water, glycerin, salt, fragrance, and other additives that enhance its aesthetics and performance.

Soap bars are frequently superfatted to ameliorate the harshness of the soap and improve the sensory profiles of the products (see the Free Fatty Acid or Superfatting sections of this chapter). Superfat levels in soaps typically range between 1 and 7%.

Formulation of soap bars has become increasingly complex. As soaps have become more readily available to consumers, the demands on the product performance have increased. Consumer expectations have increased beyond basic cleaning to improved mildness, lathering, deodorant protection, antibacterial protection, and interesting product aesthetics and packaging [2]. Bars produced with synthetic surfactants have improved lathering and rinsing profiles, especially in hard water. At higher levels of synthetic surfactants, the bars exhibit superior mildness versus regular soap. Examples of synthetic bars (syndets) on the market are Dove, Oil of Olay, and Vel. The raw materials and hence the finished product cost of incorporating synthetic surfactants is higher versus soaps. Combination bars, or combars, are designed to incorporate the most desirable properties of plain soap bars and synthetic cleansing bars (Syndets) (Fig. 3). In general, their advantages over conventional soap are superior rinsability and latherability in hard water. Examples of combars on the market include Zest and Lever 2000.

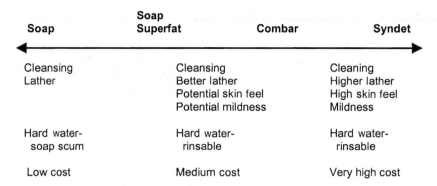

Soap	Soap Superfat	Combar	Syndet
Cleansing Lather	Cleansing Better lather Potential skin feel Potential mildness		Cleaning Higher lather High skin feel Mildness
Hard water- soap scum	Hard water- rinsable		Hard water- rinsable
Low cost	Medium cost		Very high cost

FIGURE 3 Skin cleansing bar formulations and attributes.

The benefits of conventional soap bars are good lathering, thorough cleaning, and low cost compared with bars containing synthetic surfactants (Fig. 3). Some of the shortcomings are: (1) performance dependence on water hardness conditions because of its reactions with calcium and magnesium salts in hard water causing difficulty to rinse "soap scum," and (2) lack of clinical and consumer-perceived mildness benefits. Some people can experience irritation and excessive dryness, especially during periods of low temperature and humidity such as in winter. Synthetic cleansing bars (syndets) generally contain only low levels or no soap. Instead, syndets comprise synthetic surfactants (between 20–80% of the total bar composition), high concentrations of emollients and conditioners, and some fillers and binders [19]. They tend to cleanse and lather well in soft or hard water, and they are unaffected by calcium or magnesium salts which results in better rinsing properties from skin and hard surfaces. Also because of the presence of high levels of skin moisturizers and conditioners, syndets impart more skin after feel, leaving the skin feeling softer and more moisturized.

While all synthetic surfactants overcome the hard-water deficiencies of soap, not all of them are suitable for use in cleansing bars because their effects on skin can be markedly different than soap. Selection criteria that one needs to follow in order to choose a synthetic surfactant for use in soap bars are quite strenuous. In addition to being mild, the surfactant must possess acceptable properties such as surface activity, physical and chemical stability, good odor and color, processability into soap bars, quick lather, and clean skin feel [1]. Some can be too strong and irritating to the skin and can therefore leave the skin feeling dry and damaged. Common anionic synthetic surfactants used in syndets and combars include sodium cocoylisethionate, alkylglycerylether sulfonate, and alkylsulfate. Amphoteric surfactants such as cocamidolpropylbetaine or nonionic surfactants are also sometimes used at low levels. Translucent and transparent soaps incorporate high levels of solubilizers, which tend to control the crystal size and structure, thus allowing the transmittance of light through the product. Examples of solvents added to translucent and transparent soaps include glycerin, sorbitol, triethanolamine, and other sugars [20–22]. These specialty soap products frequently have altered lathering, rinsing and use-up rate characteristics because of the high level of solubilizers in the finished product. Other specialty soaps include the addition of unique aesthetics (marbleized and striated) or the addition of specialty abrasives (e.g., pumice, seaweed) and other botanical or natural ingredients.

BAR SOAP PERFORMANCE EVALUATIONS

Soap bars are evaluated for several characteristics to ensure that they meet consumer needs and expectations.

Lather

The amount of lather, how rapidly a product lathers, and the quality of lather can be judged by a trained panel. This trained panel rates the product on lather quantity, quality, and quickness by rating it on a numerical scale. Typically panelists are trained to rotate a soap bar a fixed number of times and evaluate it for attributes versus benchmark products. This is most useful in the analysis and comparison of formulation similarities and differences as well as competitive products. Variables affecting lather performance of a product include water temperature, water hardness, and method of washing. Trained panelists need to be trained and validated on a regular basis to ensure consistency of their evaluations.

Laboratory methods of lather evaluation include the Ross-Miles foam height test. This requires measuring the foam height of a soap solution that has been inverted in a cylinder for a fixed number of times. Results from this type of test can be misleading because the bar shape and solubility can affect the lather performance in use [1].

Wear Rate/Use-Up

The measurement of how long a bar lasts under normal use conditions is an important attribute to the consumer perceived value. The use-up rate is measured by first weighing the soap bar and then washing the bar for a set number and length of times (for example, 25 washings for 10 sec each). The bar is then dried and weighed again and the use-up or wear rate is reported as the percent weight loss. Soap bar shape and size impact the reported use-up rate. The use-up rate measurement must be controlled for water hardness and temperature. For formulation comparison purposes, it is best to compare soap bars with similar sizes and shapes. Bars can be shaved to the same sizes and shapes in order for the measurement to reflect the true formula influence. To compare how bars will perform in the hands of consumers, actual commercial sizes and shapes should be used.

Slough/Mush

Slough or mush is the undesirable soft part of the bar that results from the hydration of a soap bar as it sits in a wet soap dish. Slough is measured by placing a pre-weighed bar in a high humidity chamber for a fixed period of time, then removing the soft part of the bar and allowing the soap bar to dry. The weight taken before and after determine the slough or mush measured as the percent weight loss. Syndet bars tend to have high slough relative to regular soaps. High humidity conditions exaggerate typical home usage conditions, but help differentiate products and formulations. Slough can also be run at room temperature. Commercial soap bar shapes can be selected by manufacturers to minimize the formation of slough or mush in use conditions.

Cracking

Cracking is the splitting of a bar along the side seams or at any part in the bar during use. Cracking of a soap bar in use conditions is a perceived as a negative by consumers.

Cracking is evaluated by partially submerging bars in water of fixed hardness and temperature for a set period of time. The bars are then dried and evaluated for cracking after one
to two days. Ideally, there should be no cracks present in the soap bars.

Hardness

Bar hardness is a mechanical measure of how resistant the bar is to physical pressure.
Bar hardness can be mechanically measured in finishing trials for machineability as well
as during routine lab evaluations. Bars that are too soft may be difficult to extrude on the
finishing line without significant surface defects.

Bar Feel and Sandiness

Bar soaps are typically evaluated for dry specks and drag. Specks of dry soap (insoluble
soap) can occur during the manufacture of the base soap or syndet or from the additives
in the soap bar. These specks show up as distinct bumps on the surface of the bar. The
bar is washed under controlled water conditions with cooler water bringing out more
obvious dry specks. The bar is both evaluated during wash and after drying for feel and
appearance and rated against standard quality bars.

Sensory Skin Evaluations

Clearly, next to the fragrance preference at the point of purchase, skin feel and lather are
the most important attributes for consumers. Various skin feel attributes from bar soaps
are evaluated by a trained panel of experts. These groups of panelists are trained to evaluate
small (or large) differences in products focusing on a set of defined attributes. Products
are usually compared with a reference product. Examples of attributes evaluated by a
trained panel for skin feel include time to rinse, skin slip, tightness of skin after drying,
and smoothness of skin.

Clinical Evaluations

Clinical Evaluations of soap products are used to determine how effective the products
are on certain attributes, primarily mildness/irritation, skin dryness/tightness, antibacterial
efficacy, and deodorancy. There are several methods of measuring the clinical attributes
of a soap bar ranging from trained panels to biophysical instrumentation [1,2,23].

REFERENCES

1. Spitz L, ed. Soap Technology for the 1990's. Champaign: American Oil Chemists Society,
   1990.
2. Spitz L, ed. Soaps and Detergents: A Theoretical and Practical Review. Champaign: American
   Oil Chemists Society, 1996.
3. Woolatt E. The Manufacture of Soaps, Other Detergents and Glycerin. New York: Halstead,
   1985.
4. Thomsenn EG, Kemp CR. Modern Soap Making. New York: MacNair-Dorland, 1937.
5. Joshi D. U.S. Patent, 4,493,786 (1985).
6. Jungerman E, Hassapis T, Scott R, Wortzman M. U.S. Patent, 4,758,370 (1988).
7. Johnson RW, Fritz E, eds. Fatty Acids in Industry: Process, Properties, Derivatives, Applications. New York: Marcel Dekker, 1989.

8. Patterson HBW. Bleaching and Purifying Fats and Oils: Theory and Practice. Champaign: American Oil Chemists Society, 1993.
9. Ferguson RH, Rosevear FB, Stillman RC. Solid soap phases. Ind & Engineer Chem 1943; 35:1005–1012.
10. Wenninger JA, McEwen GN. CTFA International Cosmetic Ingredient Dictionary and Handbook, 7th ed. Washington, D.C: The Cosmetic, Toiletry and Fragrance Association, 1997.
11. Zaidman B, Kisilev A, Sasson Y, Garti N. Double bond oxidation of unsaturated fatty acids. J Am Oil Chem Soc 1988; 65:611.
12. Rojas-Romero AJ, Morton ID. J Sci Fd Agric 1977; 28:916.
13. U. S. Patent, 3,511,783 (1970).
14. Payne R, Hwang A, Subramanyam R. U. S. Patent, 5,843,876 (1998).
15. Blake-Haskins JC, Scala D, Rhein LD, Robbins CR. J Soc Cosmet Chem 1986; 37:199–210.
16. M Hollstein, Spitz L. J Oil Chemists' Soc October 1982; p. 442.
17. Soap and Detergent Association. Soaps and Detergents Handbook, 2nd ed. 1994.
18. Krawczyk T. Soap Bars Inform May 1996; pp. 478–486.
19. Milwidsky B. Syndet Bars, Happi, May 1985:58–70.
20. U. S. Patent, 2,970,116.
21. Toma K, Hassapis TJ. U. S. Patent, 3,864,272 (1975).
22. Wood-Rethwill JC, Jawarski RJ, Myers EG, Marshal ML. U. S. Patent, 4,879,063 (1989).
23. Kajs TM, Gartsein V. Review of the instrumental assessment of skin: effects of cleansing products. Soc Cosmet Chem 1991; 42(4):249–279.

43

Skin Cleansing Liquids

Daisuke Kaneko and Kazutami Sakamoto
AminoScience Laboratories, Ajinomoto Co., Inc., Kanagawa, Japan

INTRODUCTION

Skin cleansing liquids are products that clean and refresh the skin by removing soil or dirty materials to help keep the skin's physiological condition normal. There are residual metabolites on the skin that are unstable and reactive with oxygen or deposited molecules by sun exposure or skin micro-organisms to form harmful materials to cause skin trouble. Thus cleansing is a necessary daily skincare practice even for normal skin. Furthermore, special care must be taken for sensitive skin or atopic skin because of its vulnerability. In these troubled types of skin, cleanliness must be attained without contributing to their susceptibility [1]. There are different types of cleansing products developed and commonly used depending on the types of materials to be removed from the skin or types of use conditions.

Typical types of commercial skin cleansing products are listed in Table 1 [2]. A most common cleansing product contains a relatively high concentration of surfactants and is applied with water to make foam before washing off thoroughly. Good lathering is the most important feature of these products because sensory feeling of the rich and fine foam is the key factor of repeated use by consumer, although amount and quality of foam are not directly related to the detergency from a physicochemical viewpoint. On the other hand, fine and thick lather serves an important function in shaving foam preparations for smooth razor application. Ease of quick rinse and after-feeling are other factors that rule the quality of skin cleansing products. Refreshed and moist feelings are typical elements that fulfill consumers' desires, and refreshing seems more important for body wash, especially for Japanese consumers.

In terms of formulations for surfactant-type skin cleansers, soap bars have been the most traditional skin cleansers but there are liquid-, paste-, or aerosol-type cleansers getting more popular on the market. Facial cleansing powder—a rather new and niche trend in Japan—contains enzymes to help the cleaning of protein-type deposits because of its anhydrous formula to preserve enzyme activities.

Solvent type is mainly used to remove oily cosmetics applied to the skin. This type is further categorized to cleansing creams, lotions, liquids, or gels. The use of makeup products, such as waterproof or nonstaining and long-lasting lipsticks, require use of spe-

TABLE 1 Types of Commercial Skin Cleansing Products

Product type	Form (formula type)	Features
Surfactant-based type	Solid (soap, transparent soap, neutral soap)	Main type of cleanser: easy to use and feels good, but skin feels tight afterwards.
	Cream · paste (cleansing foam)	Special face cleanser with excellent feeling and lather. It is easy to use. Bases may be selected in the range weakly acidic to alkaline depending on the purpose.
	Liquid or viscous liquid type (cleansing gel)	Weakly acidic to alkaline. The weakly acidic base produces a weak cleanser but the alkaline base produces a strong one. The main type of cleanser for hair and body.
	Granule/powder form (cleansing powder, face cleansing powder)	Easy to use. As they contain no water, papain or other enzyme may be incorporated.
	Aerosol type (shaving foam type, after-foaming type)	There are two types—one that comes out like a shaving foam and the other as a gel which becomes a foam on use (after-foaming type). A double container is used for the after-foaming type.
Solvent-based type	Cream · paste (cleansing cream)	The emulsion type uses mainly O/W emulsion. The type in which oils are made into a gel has high cleansing power. For heavy makeup.
	Milky lotion (cleansing milk); liquid form (cleansing lotion)	O/W emulsion milky lotion. Lighter feeling after use than with cleansing cream. Easy to use. Cleansing lotion. Contains large amounts of nonionic surfactants, alcohol, and humectants. There is also a physical cleansing effect as it is wiped off with cotton. For light makeup.
	Gel (cleansing gel)	The emulsion and liquid crystal types containing a lot of oils have high cleansing power and are rinsed off. They give a light feeling after rinsing off. The water-soluble polymer gel type has low cleansing power.
	Oil (cleansing oil)	Ingredients like surfactants and alcohol are added to the oil in small amounts. Rinsed off. When rinsed off forms O/W emulsion. Soft and moist feeling after use.
Others	Pack (cleansing mask)	Peel-off mask using water-soluble polymers. Skin has strong feeling of being stretched. Removes dirt from skin surface and pores when peeled off.

Source: Ref. 2.

TABLE 2 Main Surfactants Used for Cleansing Products

Type	Ingredients
Anionic Surfactants	Soap
	Polyoxyethylene alkyl ether sulfate
	Acylglutamate
	Acylglycinate
	Acylmethyltaurate
	Acylsurcosinate
	Acylisethionate
Ampoteric surfactants	Alkyl dimethylaminoacetic acid betaine
	Alkyl amidopropyl dimethylaminoacetic acid betaine
Nonionic surfactants	POE alkyl ether
	POE glycerol fatty acid ester
	POE-POP block copolymer

cial cleansers to remove them. Facial packs with cleansing gel that claim gentleness and sufficient cleansing power have been launched in Japan.

SURFACTANT-TYPE SKIN CLEANSERS

Main surfactants used for surfactant-type skin cleansers are listed in Table 2. Soaps are used as a primary surfactant for solid bar cleansers and paste-type cleansers. Sodium soaps are commonly used for solid bars and potassium soaps are mainly for paste-type cleansers or shaving foams. Opaque soft bar is made from triethanolamine soap as gentle facial cleanser. Soaps have excellent lathering properties and superior detergency but some deposit in hard water and cause skin tightness. Additional surfactants are combined with soap in order to improve tightness and give better mildness. Alkylethersulfate, acylisethionate, acylglutamate, acylmethyltaurate, and acylglycinate are commonly combined as a secondary or tertiary surfactant with soap. Acylglutamate has a unique feature as weakly acidic similar to skin pH surfactant and is thus often used as a primary surfactant to give superb mildness for different formulation types.

As of their physicochemical nature, surfactants not only remove soils but also tend to strip useful substances from the skin. Thus excessive solubilization and stripping of skin lipids and natural moisturizing factors (NMF) must be avoided, otherwise destruction of skin-barrier functions would happen. The composition of skin-surface lipids is listed in Table 3 [3] and composition of constitutive lipids in the stratum corneum is shown in Table 4 [4]. Detergency of surfactant should be good enough to remove surface lipid but not to strip minimally constitutive lipids, which are key components of skin-barrier function. Such selective detergency is found for several surfactants and acylaminoacids such as acylglutamate or acylmethyltaurate, which are relatively better in this regard than soap [5,6]. Composition of NMF is shown in Ref. [7]. Acylglutamate showed less stripping of NMF than soap. [8] Changes of skin pH are dependent on the type of surfactant used too. As shown in Figure 1 and 2, water-holding capacity and skin pH by repeated wash with acylglutamate was not affected much while soap changed these two properties seriously.

Formulations are designed to fit for the specific concept to which a product is aimed along with the general requirement as a skin cleanser such as detergency, feeling, viscosity,

TABLE 3 Composition of Human Skin Surface Lipids

Lipid	Average amount (wt%)	Range (wt%)
Triglycerides	41.0	19.5–49.4
Diglycerides	2.2	2.3–4.3
Fatty acids	16.4	7.9–13.9
Squalene	12.0	10.1–13.9
Wax esters	25.0	22.6–29.5
Cholesterol	1.4	1.2–2.3
Cholesterol esters	2.1	1.5–2.6

Source: Ref. 3.

TABLE 4 Composition of Constitutive Lipids in the Stratum Corneum

Lipid	Wt%
Cholesterol esters	1.7
Triglycerides	2.8
Fatty acids	13.1
Cholesterol	26.0
Ceramides	45.8
Glucosylceramides	1.0
Cholesteryl sulfate	3.9
Unidentified	5.7

Source: Ref. 4.

TABLE 5 Analysis of Commercial Paste–Type Facial Cleansers

Sample	Distribution of fatty acid (wt%)				Total fatty acid (wt%)
	C12	C14	C16	C18	
Sample A	5.9	16.8	1.4	6.4	30.5
Sample B	10.9	4.7	9.6	8.5	33.7
Sample C	0.0	15.0	6.9	4.0	25.9
Sample D	5.8	6.4	2.2	3.6	18.0
Sample E	4.9	13.3	3.5	5.8	27.5
Sample F	1.2	23.1	3.9	5.6	33.8

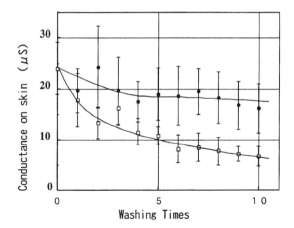

●: Potassium N-Myristoyl-L-Glutamate
☐: Potassium Myristate

FIGURE 1 Effect of surfactant on the moisture content of the skin. Forearms were washed every 20 minutes with 5 mL of surfactant solution (10%) and skin surface conductance was measured by surface hygrometer (Skicon 200; IBS Japan, at 25°C, 40 RH%, n = 6) as indicator of the moisture of the skin.

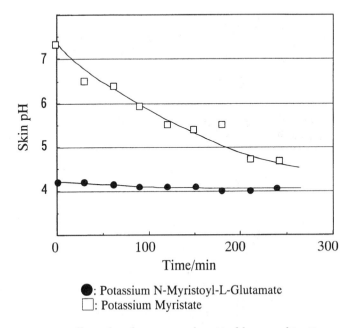

●: Potassium N-Myristoyl-L-Glutamate
☐: Potassium Myristate

FIGURE 2 Effect of surfactants on the pH of human skin. Forearms were washed with 5 mL of surfactant solution (10%) and after that pH of the skin was measured every 20 minutes at 25°C, 40 RH%, n = 6.

stability, safety, and manageability or easiness of use, which are sometimes contradictory to fulfill all at once. Consumers' desire for a natural product requires not only that the ingredients used be natural but also that their appearance be natural-looking or transparent. Such requirements cause further difficulties for the formulation work [9].

Liquid-type skin cleansers have been developed mainly for facial use and diversified further to paste-type or gel-type formulations. Liquid-type body wash was developed first in Japan and spread widely to western markets with rapid growth even to replace significant share of soap bar market. This is among others because of their friendliness of use and added values as natural and mildness concepts.

Following are typical formulas of surfactant-type skin cleansers with their characteristics described:

Formula 1: Soap-Based Liquid Facial Cleanser (Excellent Lathering and Refreshing After-Feel)

Ingredients	%
Lauric acid	2.5
Myristic acid	7.5
Palmitic acid	2.5
Lauric acid diethanolamide	2.0
Propylene glycol	8.0
Potassium hydroxide	3.6
Water	q.s.* to 100
Perfume	q.s.
Preservative	q.s.

Procedure: Add all the ingredients together and heat to dissolve with stirring. Cool down to room temperature.

* q.s., quantum satis (in sufficient amount).

Formula 2: Laurylethersulfate (LES)-Based Liquid Facial Cleanser (Compatible with Hard Water)

Ingredients	%
Sodium polyoxyethylene(3)lauryl ether sulfate (30%)	40.0
Sodium N-lauroylmethyltaurate (30%)	10.0
Coconut acid diethanolamide	3.0
Glycerin	5.0
Sodium chloride	2.0
Water	q.s.* to 100
Perfume	q.s.
Preservative	q.s.

Procedure: Add all the ingredients together and heat to dissolve with stirring. Cool down to room temperature.

* q.s., quantum satis (in sufficient amount).

Formula 3: Acylglutamate-Based Liquid Facial Cleanser Weakly Acidic, Leaves Skin Moist and Supple-Feeling

Ingredients	%
Triethanolamine N-cocoyl-L-glutamate (30%)	30.0
Cocoyl amide propyldimethyl glycine (30%)	30.0
1.3-butylene glycol	5.0
Sodium hydroxide	0.5
Water	q.s.* to 100
Perfume	q.s.
Preservative	q.s.

Procedure: Add all the ingredients together and heat to dissolve with stirring. Cool down to room temperature.

* q.s., quantum satis (in sufficient amount).

Formula 4: Acylglycinate-Based Liquid Facial Cleanser (Excellent Lather and Refreshed After-Feeling Without Tightness)

Ingredients	%
Potassium cocoyl glycinate (30%)	15.0
Potassium laurate	11.0
Potassium myristate	6.0
Glycerin	3.0
Sorbitol (70%)	2.0
Ethylene glycol distearate	2.0
Hydroxypropylcellulose	0.5
Water	q.s.* to 100
Perfume	q.s.
Preservative	q.s.

Procedure: Add all the ingredients together and heat to dissolve with stirring. Cool down to room temperature.

* q.s., quantum satis (in sufficient amount).

Formula 5: Soap-Based Paste-Type Skin Cleanser [10] (Good Foaming and Cleansing Power)

Ingredients	%
Stearic acid	10.0
Palmitic acid	11.0
Myristic acid	12.0
Lauric acid	2.0
Squalane	2.0
Potassium hydroxide	6.0
PEG1500	10.0
Glycerin	20.0
Glycerol monostearate	2.0
POE(30)glycerol monostearate ester	2.0
Water	q.s.* to 100
Perfume	q.s.
Preservative	q.s.

Procedure: Heat fatty acids, emollient, humectants, and preservative together until melted and keep at 70°C (oil phase). Dissolve the alkali in the purified water and add this to the oil phase while stirring. Keep at 70°C until the neutralization reaction is completed. In Table 5, analytical results of the fatty acid compositions for the commercial soap-based paste-type facial cleanser are shown.

* q.s., quantum satis (in sufficient amount).

Formula 6: Acylglutamate-Based Paste-Type Facial Cleanser (Weakly Acidic, Moist and Supple After-Feeling)

Ingredients	%
Sodium N-lauroyl-L-glutamate	35.0
Potassium laurate	5.0
Coconut acid diethanolamide	2.0
1.3-butylene glycol	10.0
Dipropylene glycol	20.0
Polyvinyl pyrolidone	0.5
Water	q.s.* to 100
Perfume	q.s.
Preservative	q.s.

Procedure: Mix polyols and surfactants completely. Add other ingredients and water, then heat to dissolve. Cool to room temperature under reduced pressure with stirring.

* q.s., quantum satis (in sufficient amount).

Formula 7: Acylglycinate-Based Paste-Type Facial Cleanser (Neutral pH, Fresh After-Feeling)

Ingredients	%
Potassium cocoyl glycinate	32.0
Potassium myristate	1.5
Behenyl alcohol	0.5
Citric acid	2.5
1.3-butylene glycol	15.0
Glycerin	17.0
Ethylene glycol distearate	2.5
Water	q.s.* to 100
Perfume	q.s.
Preservative	q.s.

Procedure: Mix polyols and surfactants completely. Add other ingredients and water then heat to dissolve. Cool to room temperature under reduced pressure with stirring.

* q.s., quantum satis (in sufficient amount).

SOLVENT-TYPE SKIN CLEANSERS

Solvent-type cleansers are designed to remove oily residues from cosmetics. Normally these cleansers are applied by hand to remove oily deposits of colors or pigments from the skin, and are then wiped out with tissue or cloth. Water-oil (W/O) emulsions or simple oils work satisfactorily for this purpose but leave skin oily. Thus surfactant-type cleansers are quite often applied after this treatment. The widespread trend of long-lasting cosmetics requires stronger and laborious cleansing with solvent-type cleansers. In order to avoid excess burden to the skin and achieve effective cleansing of oily deposits, (1) solubilization and dispersibility, and (2) washability with water are key properties of solvent-type cleansers, while mildness is mandatory requirement for the product. For the former need, the product should be more lipophilic, and on the contrary for the latter purpose it is better to be rather hydrophilic. To overcome these contradictory tasks, there are several different formulations developed that are W/O emulsions, gels, or liquid crystals with special selections and combinations of oil phase and aqueous phase. The principle of these formulas is to have potent oily phase, which can easily interact and solubilize liquid deposits, when applied to the skin. Thereafter, by the application of an excess amount of water, a mixture will form between the cleanser and the oily deposit, which will easily turn into a hydrophilic mixture (such as a W/O emulsion) [11,12].

Following are typical formulas of solvent-type skin cleansers with their characteristics described:

Formula 8:   Soap-Based Facial Cleansing Lotion (Soap Emulsion)

Ingredients	%
Stearyl alcohol	0.5
Hardened palm oil	3
Liquid paraffin	35
Cholesteryl/behenyl/octyldodecyl Lauroyl glutamate	2
Dipropylene glycol	6
PEG 400	4
Sorption sesquioleate	1.6
POE(20)oleyl alcohol ether	2.5
Carboxyvinyl polymer (1%)	15
Potassium Hydroxide	0.1
Water	q.s.* to 100
Perfume	q.s.
Preservative	q.s.

Procedure: Add the humectants and chelating agent to the purified water and heat to 70°C (water phase). Heat the oil component ingredients together to make solution, add the surfactants, preservative, and perfume, and keep heating to 70°C. Add this mixture to the water phase.

* q.s., quantum satis (in sufficient amount).

Formula 9:   Facial Cleansing Cream (with Arginine to Neutralize Carbomer)

Ingredients	%
Stearic acid	2
Cetyl alcohol	3
Petrolatum	10
Liquid paraffin	38
Isopropyl myristate	10
Propylene glycol	5
Glycerin monostearate	2.5
POE(20)sorbitan monostearate	2.5
Arginine	0.3
Water	q.s.* to 100
Perfume	q.s.
Preservative	q.s.

Procedure: Add the humectant and alkali to the purified water phase. After heating the oil component ingredients together to make a solution, add the surfactants, preservatives, antioxidant, and perfume and keep heating to 70°C. Gradually add this to the water phase.

* q.s., quantum satis (in sufficient amount).

Formula 10: Gel-Type Makeup Remover

Ingredients	%
(A) Glyceryl trictanoate	56.4
Cetyl octanoate	5.0
POE(25)octyldodecyl ether	16.0
Butyl paraben	0.2
(B) POE(10)methyl glucoside	4.0
Glycerin	1.7
Sorbitol (70%)	9.0
Water	7.3
Methyl paraben	0.1
(C) Perfume	0.3

Procedure: Mix (A) components at 80°C to dissolve completely. Mix (B) components separately and dissolve at 80°C completely. Add (A) to (B) with paddle stirring. Gradually cool down while stirring. Add perfume at 55°C; mixture turns to gel at 50 to 45°C.

Formula 11 Body Wash Based on LES

Ingredients	%
Sodium laureth sulfate	40.0
Cocoamidopropylbetain	10.0
Sodium cocoyl glutamate	3.0
Laulamide DEA	3.0
Sodium PCA	2.0
Glycerin	3.0
PEG(150)distearate	0.1
Water	q.s.* to 100
Perfume	q.s.
Preservative	q.s.

Procedure: Add all the ingredients together and heat to dissolve with stirring. Cool down to room temperature.

* q.s., quantum satis (in sufficient amount).

CONCLUSION

A hygiene consumer product must make skin clean and refreshed. There are industrial or heavy-duty cleansers available for skin, often with sufficient mildness but nothing especially elegant. With skin cleansing bars, skin cleansing liquids are the products categorized as cosmetics and personal care. Skin cleansing liquids are more and more chosen by consumers with highly perspective or emotional motives, which is why skin cleansing liquids must carry concepts that appeal to consumers' trendy desires. Cosmetic scientists will continue challenging such difficult tasks to make innovative products, with the encouraging findings that the mental effects of cosmetics use improves quality of life.

REFERENCES

1. Sakamoto K. Surfactant and skin: surfactant suitable for sensitive or atopic skin. J Jpn Cosmet Sci Soc 1997; 21:125.
2. Naito N, Munakata A. Cleansing of sebum and skin treatment. Fragrance J 1988; 92:42.
3. Dawning DT, Strauss JS, Pochi PE. Variability in the chemical composition of human skin surface lipids. J Invest Dermatol 1969; 53:232.
4. Schwartzendruber DC, Wertz PW, Madison KC, Downing DT. Evidence that the corneocyte has a chemically bound lipid envelope. J Invest Dermatol 1978; 88:709.
5. Miyazawa K, Tamura U, Katsumura Y, Uchikawa K, Sakamoto T, Tomita K. Anionic surfactants as detergents for scalp and hair. Yukagaku 1989; 38:297.
6. Miyazawa K, Evaluation of haircare products: shampoo and rinse. J Soc Cosmet Chem Jpn 1995; 29:95.
7. Jacobi OK. About the mechanism of moisture regulation in the horny layer of the skin. Proc Sci Toilet Goods Assoc 1959; 31:22.
8. Nozaki T. Research and development of body cleanser. Fragrance J 1996; 8:24.
9. Fukuda T. Research and development of a face cleanser of liquid type. Fragrance J 1996; 7:24.
10. Mistui T, ed. New Cosmetic Science. Elsevier 1997.
11. Suzuki T, Takai H, Yamazaki S. Formation of fine three-phase emulsions by the liquid crystal emulsification method with arginine-branched monoalkylphosphate. J Colloid Interface Sci 1989; 129:491.
12. Sakai Y, Hashimoto F. Development of a high function make-up remover applying a new polar oil. 40th Ann Sci Conf of Soc Cosmet Chem Jpn, June 17, 1997 Osaka, Japan.

44

Emulsion-Based Skincare Products: Formulating and Measuring Their Moisturizing Benefits

Howard Epstein and F. Anthony Simion
The Andrew Jergens Company, Cincinnati, Ohio

AN OVERVIEW OF EMULSION-BASED SKINCARE PRODUCTS

A variety of skincare products exist in today's marketplace. They fulfill a variety of functions by either acting directly on the skin (e.g., moisturizers) or being a cosmetically elegant vehicle for the delivery of specific active ingredients (e.g., sunscreens or antipuretic or antiacne medicaments). In general, these products may be categorized into three functional groups:

- *Drugs.* To Prevent or ameliorate diseases by altering the structure and/or function of the body.
- *Cosmetics.* To beautify and improve the feeling or sensory aspects of normal and/or nondiseased skin. Dry skin would be included in this category.
- *Cosmeceuticals.* An intermediate classification for cosmetic products that may enhance the function of skin. Currently, this category is not recognized by the United States Food and Drug Administration (FDA) [1].

There is a similar classification in the European Union.

The three product groups can also be classified by their physical properties. Most common forms of skincare products are emulsions. Emulsions are mixtures of two insoluble materials that are stabilized against separation. An example is oil and water, which will not mix unless an intermediate emulsifier is incorporated into the mixture.

Different Types of Emulsions

Emulsifiers can act as solubilizers as well as spreading or dispersing agents. Correct use of emulsifiers permits the formulation of homogeneous mixtures, dispersions or emulsions of oily, waxy substances with water. Solids may be dispersed in liquids or insoluble liquids within other liquids. Greasy anhydrous ointments can be designed to be more washable. These types of properties may be achieved by appropriate selection of emulsifiers, active ingredient, and other compatible ingredients in the vehicle.

Emulsions may be water-in-oil (w/o), oil-in-water (o/w), aqueous gel, and silicone in water. Other products may be formulated as semisolids containing oleaginous ingredi-

TABLE 1 Examples of Vehicle Types

Type of emulsion	Examples
w/o	Cold creams, cleansing, evening, or overnight creams
o/w	Moisturizers, hand and body lotions
Oleaginous	Petrolatum
Water-soluble	Polyethylene glycol-based ointments
Aqueous gels	Lubricating jelly; gelling agents such as carbomers, hydroxyethylcellulose, and magnesium aluminum silicate may be used in the formulation
Absorption bases	Hydrophilic petrolatum; these vehicles may contain raw materials able to function as w/o emulsifiers permitting large quantities of water to be incorporated as emulsified droplets

Source: Ref. 3.

ents, absorption bases, and water-soluble types containing polyethylene glycol. Recently, there has been a growing interest in water-in-oil-in-water (w/o/w), also referred to as multiple emulsions.

Oil-in-water emulsions are the most commonly formulated. These types of emulsions tend to feel less greasy and have a lower cost than other forms because of a higher water content. Water-in-oil (w/o) emulsions have historically been less popular because of a characteristic greasy, oily feel on application to skin. However, the development of newer emulsifiers has enabled a skilled formulator to develop w/o emulsions of a lighter texture. Silicone formulation aids may also be used to form stable water in silicone (w/Si) or w/o emulsions. These silicones are polymeric surface active agents with long bond lengths and wide bond angles. This provides for free rotation of functional groups permitting formulation of w/o and W/Si emulsions with exceptional elegance and good coverage when applied to the skin [2]. This enables formulation of stable emulsions with medium to low viscosity. These different chemical-type emulsions are commonly referred to as vehicles when "cosmetic" active or drug active ingredients are incorporated into them (see Table 1).

Not all emulsifiers behave in the same way. Properties of the emulsifier will determine the emulsion type. Their compatibility with oils having different polarities is also a critical concern. Emulsifiers will impact the desired sensory properties of the product such as color, odor, and desired viscosity (e.g., lotion or cream consistency).

Different Types of Emulsifiers

Emulsifying agents, which are surface active agents (surfactants), are available in a wide range of chemical types. These include nonionic, hydrophilic, lipophilic, ethoxylated, and nonethoxylated. A recent trend is to lower or even eliminate surfactants in an effort to minimize the already low irritation potential of the formulation. It is possible to formulate emulsifier-free emulsions with cross-linked acrylic polymer derivatives. These materials are hydrophilic polymers that are hydrophobically modified by adding an alkylic chain. These molecules, known as polymeric emulsifiers provide additional formulation options for new product development [4].

FORMULATING HYDRATING CREAMS AND LOTIONS

The continuing development of biophysical instrumentation and test techniques has enabled formulation of highly effective skincare formulations. Formulators now have several options with respect to formulating new products. When initiating formulation development, it is important to understand project/product requirements, type of product(s), performance and aesthetic needs, formulation cost constraints, packaging needs, product claims, and formulation safety. To what part of the body will the formulation be applied? What time of day, morning or overnight? Will makeup be applied over the product, and will clothing come into contact with the product? Will the targeted consumer apply a fragrance to the body after application of the product, and if so, will the fragrances conflict? Once these requirements are defined, the formulator can consider active ingredients, emulsion systems, preservative systems, color, and fragrance.

Emulsions allow the formulating chemist to combine otherwise incompatible ingredients into an effective, commercially desirable cosmetic product. Key in product development is the technique used to select appropriate raw materials. Commonly used emulsifying agents are ionic (anionic or cationic) or nonionic. The function of the emulsifying agent is dependent on the unique chemical structure of the emulsifier. Each emulsifier has a hydrophilic (water-loving) and lipophilic (oil-loving) part. Examples of hydrophilic moieties are polyhydric alcohols and polyethylene chains. Lipophilic parts may be a long hydrocarbon chain such as fatty acids, cyclic hydrocarbons, or combination of both. Nonionic agents may have hydrophilic action generated by hydroxyl groups and ether linkages, such as polyoxyethylene chains. Nonionic emulsifying agents can be neutral or acidic, giving formulators greater flexibility regarding pH requirements for cosmetic actives. Nonionics can be used in formulating w/o- or o/w-type emulsions and will help to mitigate the characteristic oily feel of w/o emulsions.

Thousands of emulsifying agents are available on the world market today. Choosing the best agent is the key responsibility of the formulator. Many agents used in the cosmetic and drug industry are classified by a system known as Hydrophilic-Lipophilic Balance (HLB) number. This system, developed in the mid-1950s, is a useful starting point in emulsifier selection. In this system, each surfactant having a specific HLB number is used to emulsify an oil phase having an HLB required for a stable emulsion. Using an emulsifier or combination of emulsifiers matching the required HLB of the oil phase will form a stable emulsion. Limitations to this method include incomplete data for required HLBs of many cosmetic ingredients. Combinations of or single emulsifying agents giving the appropriate theoretical HLB may not be the optimal combination for emulsion stability or product performance. Other emulsifying agents may work better, providing a more elegant formulation with greater efficacy. In addition, theoretical HLB numbers of complex mixtures may not follow a linear additive rule specified in the calculation [2].

In this classification system, emulsifying agents with an HLB of 10 would indicate a more water-soluble agent compared with one having an HLB of 4.

For nonionic detergents of the ester type:

HLB = 20(1-s/a)

s = saponification number of the material

a = acid number of the fatty acid moiety of the product

For ethoxylated esters and ethers when the saponification value is not known:

HLB = E + P/5

E = Percent of ethylene oxide

P = Percent of polyalcohol in the molecule

When the hydrophobic portion contains phenols and monoalcohols without polyalcohols, the equation can be simplified to

$$HLB = E/5$$

Most nonionics fall into this category. Manufacturers who provide HLB values in their product specifications most frequently use the latter formula (see Table 2).

Mixtures of anionic and nonionic agents obtain the best emulsion, whereas mixtures of cationic and nonionic emulsifiers may not be as elegant. Examples of nonionic emulsifiers are alcohol ethoxylates, alkylphenol ethoxylates, block polymers, ethoxylated fatty acids, sorbitan esters, ethoxylated sorbitan esters, and ethoxylated castor oil. The solubility of nonionic surfactants in water can often be used as a guide in approximating the hydrophilic-lipophilic balance and usefulness.

Oil-in-Water Emulsions

Oil-in-water emulsions typically contain 10 to 35% oil phase, and a lower viscosity emulsion may have an oil phase reduced to 5 to 15%. Water in the external phase of the emulsion helps hydrate the stratum corneum of the skin. This is desirable when one desires to incorporate water-soluble active ingredients in the vehicle. Oil droplets in emulsions have a lower density than the phase they are suspended in; to have a stable emulsion it is important to adjust the specific gravity of the oil and water phases as closely as possible. Viscosity of the water phase (external phase) may be increased to impede the upward migration of the oil particles. Addition of waxes to the oil phase will increase specific gravity but have a profound effect on the appearance, texture, and feel on application to skin of the product. Increasing water-phase viscosity is one of the most common approaches. Natural thickeners (alginates, caragenates, xanthan) and cellulosic (carboxymethyl cellulose) gums are used for this purpose.

Carbopol® resin is perhaps the most popular gum thickener for contributing towards emulsion stability, especially at higher temperatures. The addition of a fatty amine to a Carbopol resin will further enhance stability by strengthening the interface of the water

TABLE 2 Relationship Between HLB Range and Water Solubility

Water solubility	HLB Range
No dispensability in water	1–4
Poor dispersion	3–6
Milky dispersion after agitation	6–8
Stable milky dispersion	8–10
Translucent to clear dispersion	10–13
Clear solution	13+

HLB	Application
4–6	w/o emulsifier
7–9	wetting agent
8–18	o/w emulsifier
13–15	detergent
15–18	solublizer

Source: Ref. 5.

and oil phases through partial solubilization into the oil droplets. Electrolytes and cationic materials will have a destabilizing effect on anionic sodium carboxymethyl cellulose and should not be used together. Veegum, an inorganic aluminum silicate material, is also commonly used to thicken emulsions. Carbopol and Veegum may be used together to modify the characteristic draggy feel of Carbopol when used at the higher levels.

Emulsifier blends with HLBs ranging from 7 to 16 are used for forming o/w emulsions. In the blend, the hydrophilic emulsifier should be formulated as the predominate emulsifier to obtain the best emulsion. A popular emulsifier, the glycerol monostearate and polyoxyethylene stearate blend is self-emulsifying and acid-stable. Emulsifiers are called self-emulsifying when an auxiliary anionic or nonionic emulsifier is added for easier emulsification of the formulation. Formulating with self-emulsifying materials containing nonionic emulsifiers permit a wide range of ingredient choice for the formulator, especially with acid systems. In alkaline formulations, polyoxyethylene ether–type emulsifiers are preferred with respect to emulsion stability.

An alternative to glycerol monostearate self-emulsifying emulsifier is Emulsifying Wax, National Formulary (NF). This emulsifier, when used with a fatty alcohol will form viscous liquids to creams depending on the other oil-phase ingredients used. Use levels may vary from 2 to 15%; at lower levels a secondary emulsifier such as the oleths or PEG-glycerides will give good stability. This system is good for stabilizing electrolyte emulsions or when other ionic materials are formulated into the vehicle. Polysorbates are o/w emulsifiers, wetting agents, and solubilizers often used with cetyl or stearyl alcohol at 0.5 to 5.0% to produce o/w emulsions [6].

Water-in-Oil Emulsions

Although less popular than o/w emulsions, these systems may be desirable when greater release of a medicating agent or the perception of greater emolliency is desired. Emulsifiers having an HLB range of 2.5 to 6 are frequently selected. When multiple emulsifiers are used, the predominant one is generally lipophilic with a smaller quantity of a hydrophilic emulsifier. These emulsions typically have a total of 45 to 80% oil phase.

During the last few years, formulators have become interested in more elegant w/o emulsions. This has been achieved by formulating with new emulsifying agents, emollient such as esters, Guerbet alcohols, and silicones. Selection of a suitable emollient depends on ability of the material to spread on skin with low tack, dermal compatibility, and perceived elegance by the user. In achieving this elegance, some researchers suggest a correlation of emollient and molecular weight of the emollients. In these studies, viscosity of w/o creams has correlated with molecular weight of the emollients used in test formulations. High–molecular-weight co-emulsifiers formulated with high–molecular-weight emollients gave more stable w/o emulsions. The polarity of the emollients used was found to be important as well. Emollients or mixtures of emollients with medium polarity gave test lotions the most desirable stability results [7]. Anionic emulsifiers are generally inefficient w/o emulsion stabilizers, because more surface active agents are often needed to stabilize these emulsions. Sorbitan stearates and oleates are effective emulsifiers when used at 0.5 to 5.0% sorbitan isostearates, being branched chain materials, give a very uniform particle size for w/o emulsions.

Multiple Emulsions

Multiple emulsions are of interest to the skincare formulator because of the elegant appearance and less greasy feel of these formulation types. Two types of multiple emulsions are encountered in skincare: (w/o/w), where the internal and external water phases are sepa-rated by oil, and oil-in-water-in-oil (o/w/o) where the water phase separates the two oil phases. The method of preparation for each multiple emulsion type is similar. Benefits of these types of formulations are the claimed sustained release of entrapped materials in the internal phase and separation of various incompatible ingredients in the same formulation.

A suggested technique for forming a w/o/w emulsion is to first create a w/o primary emulsion by combining water as one phase with oil and a lipophilic emulsifier as the second phase in the traditional method. Next, water and a hydrophilic emulsifier are com-bined with the w/o primary emulsion at room or warm (i.e., 40°C) temperature with mixing forming a w/o/w multiple emulsion. These emulsions typically contain about 18 to 23% oils and 3 to 8% lipophilic emulsifier. The continuous oily phase is stabilized with about 0.5 to 0.8% magnesium sulfate. Water-in-oil emulsifiers have an HLB less than 6 and are frequently nonionic or polymeric. Oil-in-water emulsifiers have an HLB greater than 15 and are ionic with high interfacial activity. For o/w/o multiple emulsions, w/o emulsifiers have an HLB less than 6 with similar properties as a w/o/w w/o emulsifier. Oil-in-water emulsifiers have an HLB greater 15 and are nonionic with lower interfacial activity.

Water-in-Silicone Emulsions

Silicone compounds have evolved into a class of specialty materials used for replacements, substitutes, or enhancers for a variety of organic surface-active agents, resulting in the ability to formulate products with unique properties. Previously, silicone compounds were available as water-insoluble oily materials almost exclusively. Newer silicone compounds such as polyethylene-oxide bases grafted to polydimethylsiloxane hydrophobic polymers, known as dimethicone copolyol emulsifiers, have been developed. These types of emulsi-fiers permit formation of water-in-cyclomethicone emulsions. Further work in this field led to adding hydrocarbon chains to silicone polyether polymers. This resulted in improved aesthetics to o/s emulsions. Silicone copolyols exhibit high surface activity and function similarly to traditional emulsifiers. Unlike hydrocarbon emulsifiers with higher molecu-lar weights, high–molecular-weight silicone emulsifiers can remain fluid. This gives very stable viscoelastic films at the w/o interface. The ability to make silicones more formulator-friendly has led to development of several new silicone-based surfactants. Both a water-soluble and an oil-soluble portion are needed to make a surface-active molecule. Silicone surfactants substitute or add silicone-based hydrophobicity, creating a distinctive skin feel and other attributes of typical silicones as well as attributes of fatty surfactants. These emulsions may be prepared in a traditional two-phase method, e.g., 2 to 3% w/w of laurylmethicone copolyol in 23% w/w oil phase can be mixed in a separate water phase with electrolyte to form a hydrating cream. [8]

Water-Soluble Ointment Bases

Polyethylene glycol polymers (PEGs) are available in a variety of molecular weights. These materials are water-soluble and do not hydrolyze or support mold growth. For these reasons, PEGs make good bases for washable ointments and can be formulated to have a soft to hard consistency. Polyethylene glycols dissolve in water to form clear solutions. They are also soluble in organic solvents such as mineral and produce formulations that are more substantive on skin. Polyethylene glycol ointment USP is a mixture of polyethyl-ene glycol 3350 and polyethylene glycol 400 heated to 65°C and cooled and mixed until congealed. To formulate a water-soluble ointment base, water and stearyl alcohol may be incorporated into this base.

Absorption Bases and Petrolatum

Absorption bases can serve as concentrates for w/o emollients, and water may be added to anhydrous absorption bases to form a cream-like consistency. Petrolatum, a component of some absorption bases, has been shown to be absorbed into delipidized skin and to accelerate barrier recovery. Bases can be made washable by addition of a hydrophilic emulsifier. For example, formulation with polysorbate-type emulsifiers with polyoxypropylene fatty ethers will improve washability. These surfactants will form o/w emulsions with rubbing on skin. Water-in-oil petrolatum creams can be formulated by mixing 50 to 55% petrolatum with a sorbitan sesquioleate at 5 to 10%, having an HLB of about 3 to 7 in one phase and water in a second phase. Both phases are blended at 67 to 70°C with mixing.

Other Ingredients

Consumer-perceived benefits of a cream or lotion are often a result of ingredients remaining on the skin after water and other volatile materials have evaporated. Emollients and other skin conditioners are commonly used for this reason. Table 3 lists ingredients frequently used to modify the feel of the emulsion on skin.

Preservative Systems

Most formulations, especially those containing a significant proportion of water, require preservative systems to control microbial growth. Microbial contamination with pathogenic micro-organisms can pose a health risk to the consumer, especially from *Pseudomo-*

TABLE 3 Examples of Moisturizer Ingredients and Their Functions

Ingredient	Use level	Comments
Emollient esters	5–25%	Modify the oily, greasy feel of mineral oil and petrolatum; light to moderate feel on skin
Triglyceride oils	5–30%	Light to heavy feel; often used as spreading agents
Mineral oil/petrolatum	5–70%	Heavy, oily feel; provides occlusion for appropriate vehicles
Silicone oils	0.1–15.0%	Helps to prevent soaping of formulations; improves spread on skin; water-repellent and skin-protective properties
Humectants (glycerin, propylene glycol, sorbitol, polyethylene-glycol)	0.5–15.0%	Moisture-binding properties; helps retard evaporation of water from formulation; viscosity control; impacts body and feel of emulsion
Thickeners (Carbopol, Veegum)	0.1–2.0%	Help obtain viscosity; enhances stability, bodying agents

TABLE 4 Examples of Emulsifiers

Emulsifiers	Properties
Nonionic	
Polyoxyethylene fatty alcohol ethers	Very hydrophobic to slightly hydrophobic
Polyglycol fatty acid esters	Very hydrophobic to slightly hydrophobic
Polyoxyethylene-modified fatty acid esters	Very hydrophilic to slightly hydrophilic
Cholesterol and fatty acid esters	Slightly lipophilic to strongly lipophilic
Glyceryl dilaurate	Secondary emulsifier
Glycol stearate	Secondary emulsifier
Anionic	
Disodium laureth sulfosuccinate	
Sodium dioctyl sulfosuccinate	
Alcohol ether sulfate	
Sodium alkylaryl sulfonate	
Cationic	
PEG-Alkyl amines	
Quaternary ammonium salts	
Self-Emulsifying Bases (Form O/W Emulsions)	
PEG-20 stearate and cetearyl alcohol	
Cetearyl alcohol and polysorbate 20	
Glyceryl stearate SE	
Absorption Bases	
Lanolin alcohol and mineral oil and octyldodecanol	
Petrolatum and ozokerite and mineral oil	

nas infection in the eyes, or from an existing illness. Microbial contamination may cause an emulsion to separate and/or form off-odors. Contaminated products are also subject to recall, which is undesirable from a commercial view point.

Preservatives can be divided into two groups: formaldehyde donors and those that cannot produce formaldehyde. The former group includes DMDM hydantoin, diazolidinyl urea, imidazolidinyl urea, Quaternium 15, and the parabens (esters of p-hydroxybenzoic acid), whereas preservatives such as Kathon GC, phenoxyethanol, and iodopropynyl butylcarbamate work by alternate mechanisms. The formulator is advised to consult appropriate preservative manufacturers to select the optimal preservative system for the emulsion.

ASSESSING MOISTURIZER EFFICACY

Overview of Lotion Function

Hand and body moisturizers have two primary functions. The traditional view of moisturizer function is that they alleviate pre-existing dry skin and prevent its return. Recently, however, reports in the scientific literature have shown that moisturizers can prevent the induction of some signs of irritant contact dermatitis [9,10].

The ability to prevent irritant contact dermatitis has relevance to a significant segment of the population. Epidemiological studies have shown that the prevalence of diagnosable hand and forearm eczema can be as high as 5.4% of the population at any one time, and from 8 to 11% in the preceding year [11,12]. This often has an irritant component especially from repeated exposure to surfactant solutions. Being able to prevent irritation may provide a significant benefit to these individuals, as well as those with dry skin (xerosis), which frequently affects the arms and legs of consumers. Although symptoms are usually less intense than eczema, dry skin probably affects a larger proportion of the population.

Measuring lotions' effects on dryness and primary irritation is key to assessing moisturizer efficacy. Clinical methods have been developed that assess dry skin or its absence via visual scoring by a trained observer and by using biophysical measurements of the skin. Similarly, erythema and stratum corneum barrier damage associated with primary irritation can be measured clinically. Clinical efficacy alone is not sufficient to make a product commercially successful. To appeal to consumers, the lotion must be both efficacious and aesthetically pleasing, i.e., pleasantly scented (or unscented) and have acceptable tactile characteristics during and immediately after application.

Clinical Evaluation of Moisturizer Efficacy

To effectively assess the clinical efficacy of moisturizers, it is important to assess several parameters that relate to skin condition. As lotions can have multiple effects on the skin, using only one modality such as observer scoring may be misleading. For instance, visual observation suggests that Lotion "E" is as effective as Lotion "C" at reducing skin dryness. Skin that was not treated also showed a reduction in visually scored dryness, indicating the effect of prevailing weather conditions. DeSquame® sticky tape (Cuderm Inc, Dallas, TX) and its quantification by image analysis was able to differentiate between the three test sites. DeSquames show that at day 4 (end of treatment phase), Lotion E did not remove corneocytes from the skin's surface as effectively as Lotion C. At day 7, Lotion E was similar to the "No product" site. This suggests that Lotion E may mask the dryness. In contrast, Lotion C caused corneocyte removal at days 4 and 7 (Fig. 1). Visual assessment of skin dryness is useful because it is a direct link to the benefits of moisturization that consumers readily recognize, such as skin flaking, scaling, ashiness, and cracking. These visual assessments should be supplemented with instrumental measures of skin flaking, hydration, surface topography, or elasticity. These instrumental measurements yield a more complete understanding of how moisturizers affect the skin, and can be more easily standardized than observer assessments.

Alleviating Dry Skin

The majority of clinical studies that measure the relief of dry skin after lotion application use either the Kligman regression protocol or a modification [13–17]. Typically these studies start out with dry skin, which is treated for an extended period, followed by a short regression phase during which product usage is discontinued. Kligman originally studied the effect of ingredients and products on the lower legs of 12 to 30 female panelists (Fig. 2). These dry skin sites were treated with an ingredient or lotion (2 mg/cm^2) twice daily for up to 3 weeks. The visual dryness was assessed before treatment (baseline) and at the end of each week. Panelists started with dry skin and the improvement in dryness from baseline was the measure of moisturizing efficacy, or the relief of dryness.

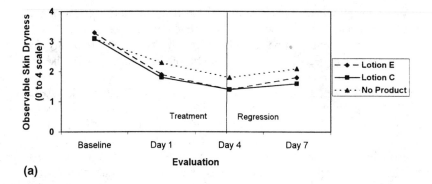

(a)

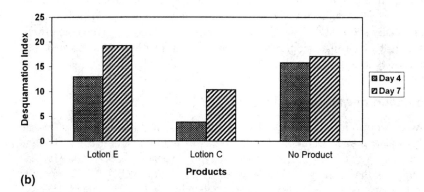

(b)

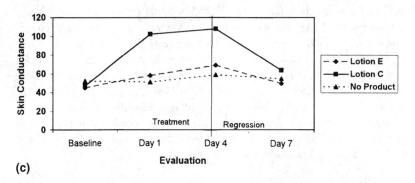

(c)

FIGURE 1 Assessing the ability of two commercially available lotions to alleviate skin dryness using a mini-regression test. (a) Assessment by a trained observer; (b) Assessment of Desquamation Index: harvesting of skin flakes with sticky tape, then quantitation using image analysis; and (c) Evaluation of skin hydration using a Skicon 200 to measure conductance.

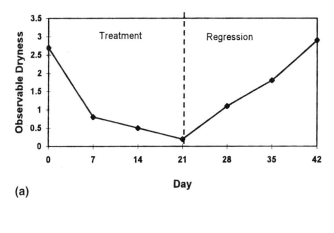

(a)

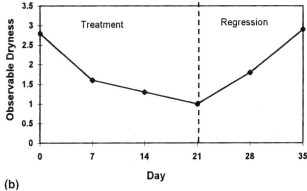

(b)

FIGURE 2 Petrolatum is more effective than lanolin in alleviating dry skin and preventing its return. Methodology: Kligman Regression Test (see Ref. 5). Test material is applied to the lower leg daily for 3 wks. After treatment stops, the legs are followed until the skin's condition regresses to its original level of dryness. Regression takes longer for petrolatum (a) than for lanolin (b).

The prevention of the return of dryness is measured during the regression phase immediately after the treatment period. A slow return to baseline is indicative of an efficacious product with lasting effects. Figure 2 shows the data obtained by Kligman for two cosmetic moisturizing ingredients, petrolatum and lanolin. The data clearly show product efficacy during the treatment and regression phases. During the regression, persistent moisturizing effects are shown 21 days after the last treatment with petrolatum but only 2 weeks for lanolin. Using the regression test, Kligman showed that hydrophobic oils—such as mineral oil or olive oil—alone had little ability to alleviate dry skin. The efficacy of these oils was enhanced when they were formulated with hydrophilic materials into cold creams. Kligman's data suggested that the moisturizer's composition could have a greater influence on its efficacy than the number of applications (dosage). He showed a large range in the ability of ingredients to alleviate dryness, but increasing the dosage had limited effects, especially beyond four applications a day.

The Kligman regression protocol has been modified by several groups to meet different assessment needs. For instance, treatment time can be reduced to 5 days to yield a more rapid assessment of moisturizer efficacy [14,16]. The mini-regression assay is able to show clear differences between two marketed moisturizers and between the treated sites and the untreated site were observed (Fig. 3). Additional assessment methods such as conductance and image analysis of DeSquame sticky tapes should be used to confirm observer scored dryness.

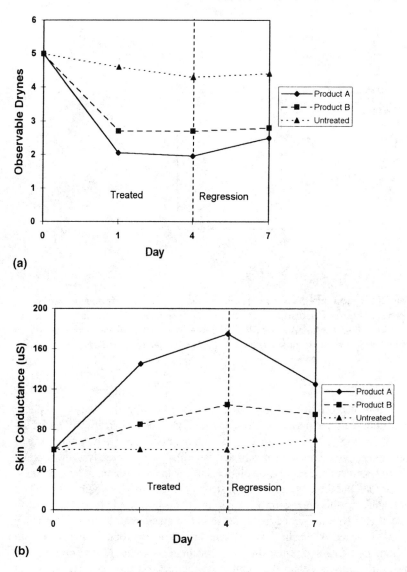

FIGURE 3 Effect of two lotions on: (a) observable skin dryness and (b) skin hydration, as assessed in a mini-regression test. (Data from Ref. 9.)

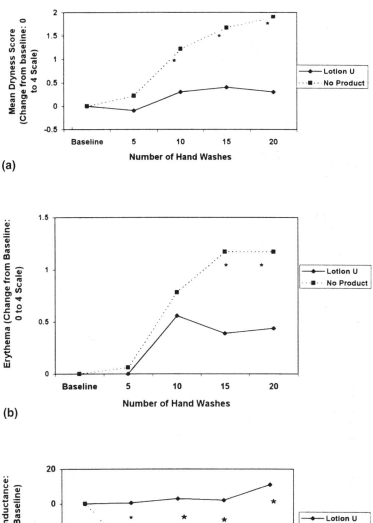

FIGURE 4   Ability of a commercially available lotion to prevent dryness induced by repeated hand washes with an aqueous detergent solution. (a) Lotion U prevents the induction of skin dryness, as assessed by a trained observer; (b) Lotion U prevents the induction of erythema, as assessed by a trained observer; and (c) Lotion U prevents the reduction of skin hydration, as measured by a Skicon 200 conductance meter.

TABLE 5 Bioengineering Methods Currently Used for Assessing Skin Condition

Methodology	Instruments Available*	Parameters Measured	Limitations/Sources of Error	References
Quantification of scaling/flaking	Desquame/sticky tape followed by comparison to a numerical scale or image analysis	Number and thickness of skin flakes	Reproducible application of tape onto skin; materials that interfere with the tape's adhesion to the skin	19
Skin conductance/ capacitance	Skicon 200 Nova Dermal meter Corneometer DermaLab moisture meter	Skin conductance/capacitance, which is a function of water content	Many moisturizer ingredients can affect conductance, either increasing (salt, glycerin) or decreasing it (mineral oil); should be used in environmentally controlled room	20–23
Evaporimetry	Evaporimeter Tewameter DermaLab TEWL probe	Rate of water loss from the skin; measure of stratum corneum barrier function; a critical parameter in anionic surfactant-induced primary irritation	Measures water regardless of source—water evaporating from a lotion immediately after application or subject's sweating, can cause artifacts; should be used in environmentally controlled room	24–28
Skin elasticity	Dermal Torque meter Cutometer Dermaflex Tactile sensor Ballistometer DermaLab elasticity module Gas Bearing Electrodynometer	Viscoelastic properties of the skin; measurements in plane of skin—Dermal Torque meter; the other instruments measure effects perpendicular to skin	Which skin layers are affected, depth of effect; how to relate the parameters measured to skin condition	29–32

Blood flow	Laser Doppler Velocimeter	Measures blood flow near skin's surface	Must be positioned exactly at same place at each measurement; due to use of lasers, cannot be used in eye area	33
Skin color	Minolta Chromameter Erythema meter Mexameter DermaSpectrometer	Measurements of skin color—either of whole color space—Minolta Chromameter, or at specific wavelengths; frequently used to measure primary irritation or tanning/ hyperpigmentation	Best used when observable color changes occur on skin	34–37
Skin surface texture	(1) Silicone replicas followed by analysis by mechanical or optical profilometry; (2) Optical profilometry of the skin—either directly or from photographs		Silicone replicas can damage skin; data is reported as mathematical parameters which can be difficult to interpret	38

* New instruments that may prove useful in the future include:
1. *Magnetic Resonance Imaging*. Specially adapted instrumentation can visualize whole skin and can delineate epidermis. Currently resolution is not sufficient to assess stratum corneum where skin dryness usually manifests itself. Equipment is large and expensive.
2. *Ultrasound*. Measures thickness of skin layers. Use requires hydrating gel on skin's surface to maintain good contact. Currently resolution is not sufficient to assess stratum corneum where skin dryness usually manifests itself.
3. *Confocal Microscopy*. Capable of visualizing cell patterns near skin's surface. Currently pictures are not sufficiently distinct for routine measurements or assessment of stratum corneum effects.

The legs are not the only site that can be used in regression testing. The groups working with both Prall and Grove have used the lower arms to assess moisturizer efficacy. The regression phase of the clinical evaluation may be used to examine the persistence of the moisturization efficacy when skin is stressed by winter weather or washing with soap.

Preventing Skin Dryness and Irritation

There are two main approaches to assessing the ability of a lotion to prevent the induction of skin dryness. First, the rate at which dry skin returns after treatment ceases can be assessed from the regression phase of the Kligman regression test. It is evident that many effective moisturizers and moisturizing ingredients do have a residual effect on the skin and will maintain it in good condition for several days, despite prevailing adverse conditions such as winter weather.

An alternate approach to measure the prevention of dry and irritated skin was developed by Highley et al. [18]. In the Highley Hand Wash protocol, the analysis begins with nondry, healthy skin. The panelists wash their hands with a detergent based cleanser for 1 minute, 5 times a day for several days. Lotions are applied to test sites after the first four washes each day. There are control areas of skin that are washed, but to which no moisturizer is applied. The dryness of the hands are assessed by a trained observer and by instrumental methods, before the first wash of the study (baseline) and approximately 1 hour after the last (fifth) wash each day. Results show that ingredients such as petrolatum and commercial lotions can prevent the induction of dry skin, which can be considerable on the untreated skin (Fig. 4). Products and ingredients can be compared by determining the difference between the sites treated with moisturizers and nonmoisturized skin. Although panels as small as 5 have been used, it is more usual to use panels of 10 or more to enable the data to be statistically analyzed.

Hannuksela and Kinnunen [10] also showed that moisturizers could prevent surfactant induced irritation and speed skin's recovery. Arms were washed with dishwashing liquid for 1 minute, twice a day, for 7 days. The investigators evaluated cleanser-induced irritation using transepidermal water loss (TEWL) as a measure of stratum corneum integrity and Laser-Doppler flowmetry to assess blood flow. They showed that moisturizer application could prevent surfactant induced skin damage and accelerate repair compared with no treatment, but were unable to differentiate between products.

The ability of moisturizers to prevent detergent induced skin dryness has important public health implications. In Denmark, dermatitis is the third leading cause leading occupational disease, and it is reasonable to assume that it has a high incidence in other countries. Such dermatitis which is frequently expressed as hand or forearm eczema, can last for many years as patients are exposed to irritants such as cleansers in both the workplace and at home. Professions that involve frequent hand washings, such as healthcare workers, day-care workers, and cleaners and food preparers, are at particular risk. Frequent, effective moisturization may provide a significant preventative benefit.

Instrumental Evaluations of Moisturizer Efficacy

Instrumental evaluation of skin condition should be used to supplement visual assessments in clinical moisturization studies. They will provide a more complete measure of skin condition that visual scoring alone. Conversely, because each instrumental method measures a physical parameter, care must be taken in using the data to interpret the biological response. For example, conductance is used as a measure of skin hydration, but is reduced when hydrophobic materials such as petrolatum, silicones or mineral oil are applied to the skin. These materials can be effective emmollients and moisturizers, despite the reduction in conductance. Thus multiple bioinstrumental measures should be used simultaneously together with observer scoring, to build a more complete picture of the lotion's effects on the skin.

Table 5 summarizes some of the bioinstrumental methods frequently used in moisturizer studies. This table includes what physical parameters the method assesses, its relationship to skin condition and limitations, and possible artifacts.

Consumer Evaluation of Moisturizer Performance

Consumer testing is a vital tool by which the personal-care industry assesses lotion acceptability. Usage testing provides the most consumer-relevant information available. Not only can moisturization performance be assessed, but information concerning product aesthetics, such as fragrance, appearance, and tactile properties including greasiness and spreadability, is obtained. Such studies yield data on both the intensity of various attributes and whether they are acceptable to the target consumers.

Consumer studies use large panels, frequently hundreds of consumers who use the test moisturizer(s) for a designated period according to their normal routine. Once consumers have tried the product for themselves, they are debriefed with interviews and written questionnaires or in focus groups. Feedback on product attributes such as greasiness, stickiness, and after-feel enables the cosmetic formulator to optimize the products to the needs of the target consumers.

Product Evaluation by a Trained Expert Sensory Panel

Because large-scale consumer testing is time consuming and expensive, product attributes including stickiness, greasiness, and after-feel can be rapidly evaluated by a trained expert sensory panel. One such method is the Skin Feel Spectrum Descriptive Analysis (Skinfeel

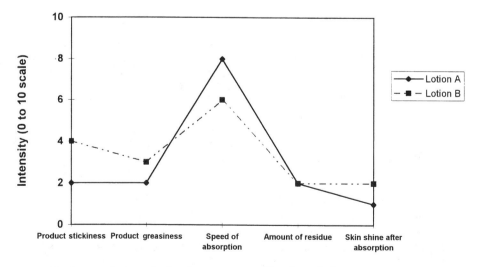

FIGURE 5   Prototypical results for the sensory profile of two lotions.

SDA) used by Meilgaard et al. [19]. This method outlines the product attribute descriptors and scoring scales used to evaluate moisturizers. An expert panel of 8 to 15 persons is required to complete over a 100 hours of training to ensure they can reproducibly quantify moisturizer and skin attributes such as spreadibility, amount of residue, and absorbency, which are scored using a 0-to-10 scale (Fig. 5.) Once the panel is calibrated, they can be used to evaluate competitors' products and optimize new formulas. Validation requires that the sensory panel correctly predict the intensity of attributes from a large-scale consumer test. It should be noted that sensory panels measure attribute intensity only, and do not assess the preference of distinct types of consumer for different products.

REFERENCES

1. Vermeer BJ, Gilchrest B. Arch Dermatol 1996; 132(3):340.
2. Kasprzak R. Drug and Cosmetic Industry (May 1996).
3. Block H. Medicated applications. In: Gennaro AR, ed. Remington's Pharmaceutical Sciences 18th ed. Easton: Mack Publishing Co. PA, 1990, p. 1603.
4. Konish PN, Gruber JV. J Cosmet Sci 1998; 49:335–342.
5. The HLB System. ICI Americas Inc. August 1984.
6. Emulsification of Basic Cosmetic Ingredients. ICI United States Inc., 1975:102–106.
7. Henkel Symposium, October 1991.
8. Silicone Formulation Aids. Dow Corning, 1997.
9. Zhai H, Maibach HI. Moisturizers in preventing irritant contact dermatitis: an overview. Contact Dermatitis 1998; 38:241–244.
10. Hannuksela A, Kinnunen T. Moisturizers prevent irritant dermatitis. Acta Derm Venereol (Stockh.) 1992; 72:42–44.
11. Meding B. Epidemiology of hand eczema in an industrial city. Acta Dermatol Venereol 1990; (suppl) 153:1–43.
12. Lantinga H, Nater JP, Coenraads PJ. Prevalence, incidence and course of eczema on the hands and forearms in a sample of the general population. Contact Dermatitis 1984; 10:135–139.
13. Kligman AM. Regression method for assessing the efficacy of moisturizers. Cosmetics and Toiletries 1978; 93:27–35.
14. Prall JK, Theiler RF, Bowser PA, Walsh M. The effectiveness of cosmetic products in alleviating a range of dryness conditions as determined by clinical and instrumental techniques. Int J Cosmet Sci 1986; 8:159–174.
15. Boisits EK, Nole GE, Cheney MC. The refined regression method. J Cutan Aging & Cosmet Dermatol 1989; 1:155–163.
16. Grove GL. Skin surface hydration changes during a mini regression test as measured in vivo by electrical conductivity. Curr Ther Res 1992; 52:556–561.
17. Grove GL, Jackson R, Czernielewski MD, Tuley M. Poster Presentation at the 53rd Annual Meeting of the American Academy of Dermatology, March 1995.
18. Highley DR, Savoyka VO, O'Neil JJ, Ward JB. A stereomicroscopic method for the determination of moisturizing efficacy in humans. J Soc Cosmet Che 1976; 27:351–363.
19. Schatz H, Altermeyer PJ, Kligman AM. Dry skin and scaling evaluated by D-Squames and image analysis. In: Serup J, Jamec GBE, eds. Handbook of Non-Invasive Methods and the Skin. Boca Raton, CRC Press 1995:153–157.
20. Tagami H. Measurement of electrical conductance and impedance. In: Serup J, Jemec GBE, eds. Handbook of Non-Invasive Methods and the Skin. Boca Raton: CRC Press, 1995:159–164.
21. Barel AO, Clarys P. Meaurement of electrical capacitance. In: Serup J, Jemec GBE, eds. Handbook of Non-Invasive Methods and the Skin. Boca Raton: CRC Press, 1995; 165–170.

22. Morrison BM, Scala DD. Comparison of instrumental methods of skin hydration. J Toxicol Cutan Occular Toxicol 1996; 15:305–314.
23. Loden M, Lindberg M. The influence of a single application of different moisturizers on the skin capacitance. Acta Derm Venereol (Stockh.) 1991; 71:79–82.
24. Pinnagoda J, Tupker RA. Measurement of the transepidermal water loss. (1995) In: Serup J, Jemec GBE, eds. Handbook of Non-invasive Methods and the Skin. Boca Raton: CRC Press, 1995; 173–178.
25. Barel AO, Clarys P. Comparison of methods for measurement of transepidermal water loss. In: Serup J, Jemec GBE, eds. Handbook of Non-Invasive Methods and the Skin. Boca Raton: CRC Press, 1995; 179–184.
26. Grove GL, Grove MJ, Zerwick C, Pierce E. Comparative metrology of evaporimeter and the DermaLab® TEWL probe. Skin Res Tech 1999; 5:1–8.
27. Grove GL, Grove MJ, Zerwick C, Pierce E. Computerized evaporimetry using the DermaLab® TEWL probe. Skin Res Tech 1999; 5:9–13.
28. Simion FA, Rhein LD, Grove GL, Wojtowski J, Cagan RH, Scala DD. Sequential order of skin responses to surfactants in a soap chamber test. Contact Dermatitis 1991; 25:242–245.
29. Agache PG. (1995) Twistometry measurement of skin elasticity. In: Serup J, Jemec GBE, eds. Handbook of Non-Invasive Methods and the Skin. Boca Raton: CRC Press, 1995; 319–328.
30. Barel AO, Courage W, Clarys P. Suction methods for measurement of skin mechanical properties: the cutometer. In: Serup J, Jemec GBE eds. Handbook of Non-Invasive Methods and the Skin. Boca Raton: CRC Press, 1995; 335–340.
31. Elsner P. Skin elasticity. In: Berardesca E, Elsner P. Wilhelm K-P, Maibach HI, eds. Bioengineering and the Skin: Methods and Instrumentation. Boca Raton: CRC Press, 1995:53–64.
32. Omata S, Terunuma Y. New tactile sensor like the human hand and its applications. Sensors and Actuators 1992; 35:9–15.
33. Belcaro G, Nicolaides AN. Laser–doppler flowmetry: principles of technology and clinical applications. In: Serup J, Jemec GBE, eds. Handbook of Non-invasive Methods and the Skin. Boca Raton: CRC Press, 1995:405–410.
34. Takiwaki H, Serup J. Measurement of erythema and melanin indices. In: Serup J, Jemec GBE, eds. Handbook of Non-Invasive Methods and the Skin. Boca Raton: CRC Press, 1995; 377–384.
35. Westerhof W. CIE Colorimetry. In: Eds Serup J, Jemec GBE, eds. Handbook of Non-Invasive Methods and the Skin. Boca Raton: CRC Press, 1995; 385–397.
36. Babulak SW, Rhein LD, Scala DD, Simion FA, Grove GL. Quantitation of erythema in a soap chamber test using a Minolta Chroma (Reflectance) meter: comparison of instrumental results with visual assessments. J Soc Cosmet Chem 1986; 37:475–477.
37. Berardesca E, Maibach HI. Bioengineering and the patch test. Contact Dermatitis 1988; 18:3–9.
38. Corcuff P, Leveque J-L. Skin Surface replica image analysis of furrows and wrinkles. In: Serup J, Jemec GBE, eds. Handbook of Non-invasive Methods and the Skin. Boca Raton: CRC Press, 1995; 89–96.
39. Meilgaard M, Civielle GV, Carr BT. Sensory Evaluation Techniques. Boca Raton: CRC Press, 1987.

45

Anticellulite Products and Treatments

André O. Barel
Free University of Brussels, Brussels, Belgium

INTRODUCTION

Cellulite is a localized condition of subcutaneous fat and connective tissues with the typical visual appearance of the orange-peel look of the skin. Cellulite, or more correctly local lipodystrophy affects mostly women and rarely men, and is considered to be a common aesthetic problem for many women. Cellulite generally appears after puberty and worsens with age. There are preferential places of cellulite: buttocks, thighs, upper part of the arms, knees and more rarely the lower parts of the legs and the back of the neck (Fig. 1). The aims of this chapter are to describe (1) the histological, physiological, and biochemical characteristics of subcutaneous lipodystrophy, (2) the different objective evaluation methods of lipodystrophy, and (3) the different anticellulite treatments available and their efficacy.

CLINICAL VISUAL AND TACTILE SYMPTOMS OF CELLULITE

Upon clinical examination of cellulite, the following symptoms of lipodystrophy can be noticed [1–11].

- Presence of orange-peel skin upon normal visual examination and after pinching of the skin.
- Deep palpation of the skin reveals differences in the mobility of fat tissue: presence of micro- and macronodules and fibrosclerosis.
- Irregularities in skin-surface temperature: touching the skin reveals the presence of cold spots.
- Sometimes presence of painful subcutaneous nodules through deep palpation.

There are different stages in the evolution of cellulite with age. It is difficult to detect cellulite by visual examination and palpation at the first stages: orange-peel skin is not permanently present, and is only visible after pinching the skin.

The clinical symptoms are clearly more visible at later stages of cellulite: permanent orange peel, colder skin areas, diminution in mobility of fat tissue upon palpation and increased skin sensibility.

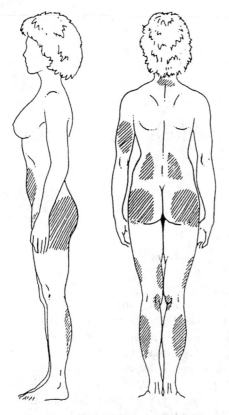

FIGURE 1 Preferential localizations of subcutaneous lipodystrophy in women.

    As a consequence of this, there is a need for sensitive noninvasive bioengineering methods for the detection and evaluation of the degree of cellulite at early stages, and for the objective evaluation of the efficacy of various cosmetic treatments [12,13].

CAUSES OF CELLULITE

Cellulite is probably a multicausal condition and many hypotheses have been proposed regarding the origin of fat lipodystrophy [1–11].

- Sexual differentiation in the histological distribution of subcutaneous fat lobules in women and in men. The differences between the sexes can be found in the structure of the septal connective-fat tissue: the fat lobules in women are larger and more rectangular, whereas men have diagonal septa and smaller lobules. Because cellulite is widely present in women, some investigators consider cellulite to be a secondary sexual characteristic.
- Alterations in the microvascular network (mostly venous blood circulation) in the fat tissue: venous stasis.
- Presence of plasmatic exudate in the subcutaneous connective tissue: noninflammatory edema.

- Alterations in the reticular fibrillar network surrounding the blood vessels and adipocytes: fibrosclerosis. Stiffening and decrease in mobility of fibers.
- Alterations in the interstitial fundamental substance (proteoglycans).
- Modifications and hypertrophy of adipose tissues. Although cellulite is not always synonymous with obesity (skinny persons can sometimes present symptoms of cellulite), there is a relation between cellulite and hypertrophy of fat tissues. Formation of, first, micronodules and, later, of macronodules in adipose tissues.

The combined effect of modifications and hypertrophy of adipose tissues, alterations in the fibrillar connective tissue, and alterations in the microvascular venous network always leads to the presence of cellulite.

HISTOLOGICAL DESCRIPTION OF THE DIFFERENT STAGES OF LIPODYSTROPHY OF FAT TISSUES

Skin-surface contact thermographic pictures using thermographic foils give an indication of the degree of cellulite, because the skin-surface temperature correlates to some extent with the clinical symptoms of cellulite. Based on these thermographic patterns and clinical symptoms, Curri and coworkers proposed a classification of cellulite in four stages [4,5,14,15]. In normal adipose tissues, a fine mesh of blood vessels and lymph vessels supplies this adipose tissue with the necessary nutrients and oxygen, and takes care of the removal of metabolized products. In the early stage of cellulite (stage I), the capillary blood-vessel walls become more permeable, causing leakage of blood plasma from the vessels in between the adipose tissues, which cause an edema in the adipose tissues. In addition, probably, problems with the lymph circulation hampers removal of accumulating fluids. The aggregation of adipose cells and the amplification of the fibrillar network of collagen bundles interconnecting the adipose cells hampers blood circulation leading to some hemostase (stage II).

Adipose cells aggregate into ''micronodules'' surrounded by less-mobile collagen fibers (stage III). The size of these ''micronodules'' is on the order of millimeters. Finally, many of these ''micronodules'' aggregate into ''macronodules'' with larger sizes (2–20 mm) (stage IV). As nerves may be squeezed by this larger nodules, persons with severe cellulite often suffer from sensitive to painful skin.

Stages I, II, and III of lipodystrophy are not considered clinically as pathological symptoms but more as aesthetic–cosmetic problems of the skin. Only in stage IV are clinical symptoms such as an increased skin sensitivity, extensive fibrosclerosis of connective tissue and very advanced edema considered to be light pathology symptoms. Furthermore it is believed that the first stages are more or less reversible, whereas the latter stages are irreversible. However, it must be said that the microscopic description of cellulite and the different stages in the evolution of lipodystrophy, as described by Curri, are not universally accepted [16,17].

OBJECTIVE EVALUATION OF THE SYMPTOMS OF LIPODYSTROPHY OF THE SKIN

In addition to the visual and tactile clinical evaluations of the symptoms of cellulite, various noninvasive bioengineering measurements may be used [11,12].

However, the clinical evaluation of cellulite remains important. The clinical evaluation of cellulite is based on visual examination and palpation of the orange-peel skin with a diminution of the mobility of the hypodermis (appearance of nodules of fat tissues and fibrosclerosis), appearance of differences in skin surface and temperature and patient complaints of hypersensitive skin and pain.

The different noninvasive bioengineering measurements are as follows:

- Contact skin-surface thermographic measurements using liquid crystals
- Non–contact skin-surface thermography of skin surface using infrared video camera
- Microblood circulation using Laser Doppler image analysis
- Ultrasonic skin analysis of skin density
- Measurement of thickness of the hypodermis at 10 to 14 MHz
- Measurement of the surface of the interface between dermis and hypodermis at 20 MHz
- Skin-surface topographical imaging
- Macroscopic normal and digitalized photographic pictures of the skin surface

DESCRIPTION AND VALIDATION OF THE DIFFERENT BIOENGINEERING MEASUREMENTS USED FOR OBJECTIVE EVALUATION OF CELLULITE

Skin-Surface Contact Thermography Using Encapsulated Liquid Crystals in the Evaluation of Cellulite [14,15,18]

The principle of the encapsulated cholesteric liquid-crystal contact thermography consists of different color plates presenting a pattern of different colors corresponding to a temperature range of about 3°C. Application of the color sheet with uniform pressure on the skin surface and photographic recording of the thermographic pattern using a Polaroid camera are carried out. A qualitative global analysis of the thermographic pictures in relation with the different stages of cellulite can be made. A cellulite-free skin-surface thermography shows a uniform color pattern without hypothermic and hyperthermic areas. A cellulite skin-surface thermography shows a nonuniform color pattern with the presence of hypothermic (cold spots) and hyperthermic (warm spots) areas. Quantitative analysis of the thermographic pictures can also be carried out by image analysis. Computerized color-image analysis gives the mean temperature of the thermogram and the number and percent area of the hypo- and hyperthermic areas, respectively, present on a well-defined skin area. As experimentally observed, an anticellulite treatment will induce an increase of the mean temperature of the skin surface and a decrease of the percent hypothermic zones (with a concomitant increase of the percent hyperthermic zones).

This method is rapid, easy to use and inexpensive for screening subjects for cellulite and for confirmation of the clinical diagnosis. However, considering the low accuracy and reproducibility of the photographic pictures, quantitative image analysis of the thermograms is very difficult. One observes large interindividual variations in skin-surface temperature (a large number of subjects is necessary in a study) and long acclimatization time for temperature equilibrium of the skin (influence of external temperature). This method remains a qualitative test of cellulite at different stages.

Validation of Skin-Surface Thermography Using Infrared Thermal Imaging System in the Evaluation of Cellulite

Using an infrared video camera, an infrared thermal image of the skin surface is obtained in a noninvasive manner. The thermographic picture can be quantitatively analyzed [12,13].

In the validation of this infrared video-imaging technique the same problems are encountered as with the contact thermography with liquid crystals such as large interindividual variations in skin-surface temperature, long acclimatization time for temperature equilibrium of the skin, and influence of external temperature.

Validation of Laser Doppler Imaging System in the Evaluation of Cellulite

Using a Laser Doppler Perfusion Imager, an image of the superficial blood circulation can be obtained [12,13]. The He–Ne laser light emitting at 633 nm has a penetration power in the skin of only about 300 μm. This instrument measures the superficial blood flux of the skin (papillary dermis). The blood perfusion of the deeper layers of the skin, such as the hypodermis, cannot be measured with this technique. However, a high correlation is obtained between the skin-surface thermographic pictures and the Laser Doppler imaging system when studying skin with cellulite. However, the measurements are delicate (long measuring times during which the volunteer must remain immobile).

Validation of the Ultrasonic Imaging of the Skin in the Evaluation of Cellulite

A promising method appears to be high-frequency ultrasound C-mode imaging (10–20 MHz). This noninvasive method has been frequently used both clinically and in research for studying the epidermis, dermis and hypodermis [19–21].

Different investigators have used the technique of measuring the thickness of the subcutaneous fatty layer using ultrasound imaging at 10 to 14 MHz [22–26]; however, the determination of the echographic border line between subcutaneous fat and connective tissues/muscles is very delicate. As a consequence, the determination of the mean thickness of the hypodermis is not very accurate. Measurement of the interface between the dermis and the subcutaneous fat using ultrasound imaging at 29 MHz is possible [27,28]. The interface between the echogenic epidermis–dermis and the hypoechoic subcutaneous fat is clearly visible, allowing measurements of skin thickness and of the surface of this border.

Quantification of the surface of the interface between the dermis and the hypodermis (fat tissue) is possible [27,28]. In normal cellulite-free skin, the interface between the dermis and the fat tissue is irregular but rather smooth. In skin with cellulite, this surface is not smooth and very irregular. The surface of this interface is quantified and can be used as a measure of the degree of cellulite.

Measurement of Skin-Surface Topography

Cellulite skin surface presents irregularities (orange-peel skin) and in principle the classic skin-surface roughness measurements, which are used in cosmetic research, can be applied for studying cellulite. It involves stylus profilometry, image analysis by shadow method and optical focus laser profilometry [29–31]. These measurements are carried out on soft or hard skin replicas of general small size (2–3 cm^2 area) and have a limited vertical range of roughness capability (maximum 400–500 μm). These techniques are well suited for the determination of the microrelief of the skin surface (50–200 μm) but not for assessing the skin surface with cellulite. The skin-surface topography of skin with cellulite can be evaluated using photographic pictures, skin-surface contour measurements, and other optical measurements such as Fringe Projection Topography [28,32–34].

The macrorelief of the skin surface can also be evaluated using an optical triangular Laser profilometry. This method involves measurements on large-size soft replicas with an extended vertical range of skin irregularities (up to 8–10 mm). Quantification of the skin surface macrorelief involves a computerized correction for the curvature of the skin surface with cellulite [32].

Normal and Digitalized Macroscopic Photographic Pictures of the Skin Surface

The macrorelief of the skin can be evaluated by taking photographic pictures (classic or digitalized) under standardized experimental conditions. These photographic pictures are then visually graded in a double-blind manner by expert oberservers for the intensity of cellulite (photograding with numerical scales). It has been known for many years that the standardization of classic photographic pictures is not easy, considering the problems of reproducibility of the processing of color film. In addition double-blind visual scoring of these photographic pictures remain subjective. However, some investigators have used photographic pictures in order to evaluate the efficacy of anticellulite treatments [35].

The use of digitalized photographic pictures is aimed to overcome the standardization problems of classic processing of the color film. Macroscopic digitalized photographic pictures (with the use of a CCD camera) of the external part of the thighs were taken after application of a gripping system around the thigh in order to increase the orange-peel look of the skin. The degree of cellulite was photograded by experts using a 0 to 7 scale of intensity of cellulite [24,36].

TREATMENTS OF CELLULITE

Different anticellulite treatments are available [12,13], such as manual and electromechanical deep massage (''pincer-rouler''), manual lymph drainage, sequential pneumatic compression (lymph drainage), electrolipolysis, mesotherapy, and topical applications of dermatocosmetic products with and without massage.

Physiotherapeutic treatments such as deep massage and manual and pneumatic lymph drainage, stimulate the blood and the lymph microcirculation and increase the removal of extra fluid in the adipose tissues. In addition, these massage techniques will retard the further development of fibrosclerosis and the aggregation of fat cells in nodules. These physiotherapeutic treatments are generally combined with the topical use of anticellulite dermatocosmetic products (during massage or pre- or postmassage).

Electrolipolysis and mesotherapy are invasive medical treatments of cellulite; these techniques will not be described in this chapter.

Various topical dermatocosmetic products have been used, generally with massage, in the treatment of cellulite and/or as slimming for many years [37]. A list of the ''active''

TABLE 1   List of Dermatocosmetic Ingredients Most
Frequently Used in Anticellulite Treatments

Caffeine
Barley (*Hordeum vulgare*)
Butcher's broom (*Ruscus aculeatus*)
Centella (*Centella asiatica*)
Cola (*Cola nitida*)
Gingko (*Gingko biloba*)
Green tea (*Thea sinensis*)
Horse chestnut (*Aesculus hippocastanum*)
Horsetail (*Equisetum arvensis*)
Ivy (*Hedera helix*)
Thistle (*Cnicus benedictus*)
Witch hazel (*Hamamelis virginiana*)
Algae
*Fucus vesiculosus, Garcinia combogia, Laminaria flex-
    icaulis*, and *Ascophyllum nodosum*

ingredients mostly used for this purpose [37–38] is given in Table 1. The main purpose of these topical slimming/anticellulite products is to influence the metabolism of the adipocytes. In vitro metabolism studies on fat cells have shown that it is possible to slow down the lipogenesis and to stimulate the lipolysis in different ways [37,39]:

- Diminution of the uptake of glucose by interfering with the membrane-bound glucose transport proteins (e.g., rutin plant flavonoids, Ruta graveolens)
- Stimulation of the hydrolysis of the triglycerides by blocking the enzyme (fosfodiesterase) that hydrolyzes cAMP (e.g., caffeine) and by binding of the membrane-bound beta receptors (Gingko biloba and horse chestnut)
- Inhibition of lipogenesis by binding with the alpha receptors (gingko biloba and horse chestnut).

In addition some of these slimming/anticellulite ingredients present properties of stimulation of the blood and lymph circulation and further inhibit the fibrosclerosis of the fat surrounding collagen matrix. A few examples of typical slimming ingredients are:

- Ivy (*Hedera helix*) stimulation of the lymph circulation
- Butcher's broom (*Ruscus aculeatus*) vasoconstrictive and anti-inflammatory properties
- Horse chestnut (*Aesculus hippocastanum*) and witch hazel (*Hamamelis virginiana*) are also used for their supposed beneficial effects on venous circulation
- Various algae species, such as *Fucus vesiculosus, Laminaria flexicaulis*, and *Ascophyllum nodosum*, are incorporated in anticellulite cosmetic preparations for their hypothetical beneficial effect on the skin surface.

CRITICAL REVIEW OF CLINICAL ANTICELLULITE STUDIES

Very few anticellulite studies that were performed under well-controlled experimental conditions (i.e., double-blind, vehicle-controlled) and under medical and paramedical supervision are published.

A clinical study on 27 female subjects with cellulite at the thighs involving a daily massage with a commercial preparation containing caffeine, *Hedera helix* and Butcher's broom (massage carried out by the subjects themselves) showed after 1 month a significant diminution of the thickness of subcutaneous fat tissues as examined by ultrasonic echography, skinfold and by visual and tactile examination [40].

However, these findings were not confirmed by a similar clinical study carried out on 15 female subjects with cellulite at the thighs using the same cosmetic product in a double-blind vehicle-controlled manner [41]. After 21 days treatment, no significant modifications were observed in skin-surface color (Chromameter), superficial blood flow (Laser Doppler), skin-surface topography (profilometry on skin replicas), and in anthropometric parameters such as thigh perimeter and skinfold.

A double-blind vehicle-controlled clinical study on 15 female volunteers with moderate cellulite at the upper and middle thighs, involving a topical application of a commercial preparation containing mixture of algaes (a 30-min topical application under plastic foil with a thermal electrical blanket) has been published. This typical balneotherapeutic treatment was carried out every 3 days during 3 consecutive weeks under the medical and physiotherapeutic control [42]. A significant decrease in thigh perimeter was observed equally for the vehicle alone and the vehicle with the "active" algaes extract, probably because of the combined effect of plastic foil occlusion and heating with the blanket. No significant modifications were observed in skin-surface color (Chromameter), and superficial blood flow (Laser Doppler) after 3 weeks treatment with the vehicle and the algaes extract.

A double-blind vehicle-controlled clinical study was carried out on 15 female volunteers with cellulite at the upper and middle thighs, involving a manual massage with a cream containing various plant extracts every 3 days during 3 consecutive weeks (massage carried out by a physiotherapist), showed after this period of treatment a significant diminution of the extent of cellulite as examined by skin-surface thermography using liquid crystal sheets [43]. However, no significant differences were obtained between massage treatment with the vehicle containing "active" plant extracts (e.g., ivy, thyme, centella, nettle, horse chesnut, bark, witch hazel) and with the placebo vehicle alone. Recently, a clinical anticellulite study was published consisting of a massage treatment with the help of a hand-held electromechanical apparatus consisting of a low-pressure chamber (200 mBar) and two rollers. The duration of the treatment was 3 months, (three times a week, during 15 minutes on each upper leg (thigh region), on 19 healthy female volunteers with moderate symptoms of cellulite on the thighs. The efficay of this treatment was evaluated using ultrasound measurements at 20 MHz [27].

This electromechanical treatment induces a significant smoothening of the dermis/hypodermis surface after 1, 2, and 3 months treatment. After the treatment was stopped, the dermis/hypodermis surface gradually increased again, which indicates that the effect of this massage on the skin is not permanent.

This modification of the interface structure (smoothening) after this mechanical treatment of the skin can be interpreted as the result of the diminution of the venous stasis (positive effect on the venous microcirculation) and an improvement also of the lymph circulation and prevention of further fibrosclerosis and of aggregation of fat micro- and macronodules. Similar positive improvements as measured by ultrasound echography were obtained after comparable manual-massage treatments and lymph drainage with pressotherapy of cellulite skin located at the thighs [44].

A clinical study was carried out on 55 healthy female volunteers with lipodystrophy on the hips and thighs. The topical anticellulite treatment (massage with a cream containing caffeine, rutin, horse chestnut, and gingko) consisted of a twice daily light massage during 28 days of both legs [40]. The intensity of cellulite was rated by visual skin-surface roughness scoring, skin thickness using a caliper, and the thickness of subcutaneous fat layer. Significant decreases were observed for these 3 experimental parameters after 28 days treatment.

In a double-blind placebo-controlled clinical study, 30 healthy female volunteers with cellulite on the thighs were twice daily treated during 2 months with a massage product containing various plant extracts [24,25]. The intensity of lipodystrophy was rated using photographic digital pictures and thickness of subcutaneous fat tissue by echography. Significant decreases of the mean score of cellulite intensity (photogradation) and the thickness of subcutaneous fat were observed after 2 months treatment only with the active product.

The critical analysis of the efficiency of the different anticellulite treatments generally indicate that similar if not identical improvements of cellulite were observed with the inert massage product and the massage product with the ''active ingredients.'' These findings substantiate the hypothesis that almost all cellulite improvements are attributable to physiotherapeutic treatments such as massage, lymph drainage or thermal occlusion of the skin, and not to the so-called active anticellulite dermatocosmetic ingredients. As a consequence, we must at present time admit that there are very few cosmetic products with a clearly scientifically proven anticellulite activity.

REFERENCES

1. Léonard GJ. La cellulite, Ed; Les éditions de l'homme, Montréal, 1970; 12–222.
2. Bartoletti CA. La cellulite. J Médecine Esthétique 1975; 8:11–16.
3. Merleen JF, Curri SB, Sarteel AM. La cellulite, affection micro-vasculo-conjective. Phlebologie 1979; 32:279–280.
4. Curri SB. Lipödem and zellulitis. In: Foldi M, Tischendorf F, eds. Ein Symposium. Munich; Medizischer Verlag Erdmann-Brenger, 1983:9–77.
5. Curri SB. Ödem, lymphödem und perivaskuläe grundsunstanz. In: Schriftenreihe Manuel Lymphdrainage nach Dr. Vodder, Band 2, Editor. Karl F. Haug Verlag, Heidelberg: 1988:7–101.
6. Gasbarro V, Zamboni P. Varicosités et cellulite: approche thérapeutique combinée. J Médecine Esthétique Chirurgie Dermatologique 1988; 15:49–55.
7. Curri SB, Ryan TJ. Panniculopathy and fibrosclerosis of the femal breast and thigh. In: Ryan TJ, Curry SB, eds. Cutaneous Adipose Tissue. Philadelphia: Lippincott, 1989:107–119.
8. Curri SB, Bombardelli E. Local liposystrophy and districtual microcirculation. Cosmet Toilet 1994; 109:51–65.
9. Parienti IJ, Serres P. La cellulite. Les cahiers de médecine esthétique, Marseille; Solal, 1990: 7–46.
10. Di Salvo RM. Controlling the appearance of cellulite. Cosmet Toilet 1995; 110:50–59.
11. Smith WP. Cellulite treatments. Cosmet Toilet 1995; 110:61–70.
12. Barel AO. Study of subcutaneous fat tissue (normal and lipodystrophy, cellulite) using noninvasive bioengineering methods. Abstract of the 12th International Symposium on Bioengineering and the Skin, Boston, MA, 1998.
13. Barel AO. Etude objective de la lipodystrophie des tissus graisseux au moyen de méthodes de bioenginering non invasives. J Médecine Esthetique 1998; 25:181–189.

14. Ippolito F, Di Carlo A. La thermographie: son utilité comme critère de diagnostic et d'efficacité dans le traitement de la cellulite. J Médecine Esthétique Chirurgie Dermatologique 1984; 11: 81–86.

15. Marzorati V, Curri SB. Contact thermography and cellulitis, technical information IPS, Milan, 1990.

16. Nurnberger F, Muller G. So-called cellulite; an invented disease. J Dermatol Surg Oncol 1978; 4:221–229.

17. Kligman AM. The reality and mythology of cellulite. Abstract of the 12th International Symposium on Bioengineering and the Skin, Boston, MA, 1998.

18. Barel AO, Noël G, Vandermeulen S, Goemare K, Clarys P. The use of contact thermography using liquid crystal in the objective evaluation of a topical anti-cellulitis treatment. Abstract of the 3d Congress International Society for Ultrasound and the Skin, Elsinore, Denmark, 1993.

19. Serup J. Ten years experience with high-frequency ultrasound examination of the skin: development and refinement of technique and equipment. In: Altmeyer P, ed. Ultrasound in Dermatology. Berlin: Springer Verlag, 1992:41–54.

20. Serup J, Keiding J, Fullerton A, Gniadecka M, Gniadecka R, Fornage B. High frequency ultrasound examination of skin: introduction and guide. In: Serup J, Jemec GBE, eds. Non-Invasive Methods and the Skin. Boca Raton: CRC Press, 1995:239–256.

21. Fornage B. Ultrasound examination of the skin and subcutaneous tissues at 7.5 to 10 MHz. In: Serup J, Jemec GBE, eds. Non-Invasive Methods and the Skin. Boca Raton: CRC Press, 1995:279–288.

22. Pittet JC, Perrier C, Schnebert S, Perrier P, Tranquart F, Beau P. Variability of fatty tissue thighness measurements using ultrasonography. Abstract of the 5th meeting of the International Society for Skin Imaging, Vienna, 1997.

23. Perin F, Pittet JC, Perrier P, Schnebert S, Beau P. Ultrasound imaging assessment of adipose tissue thickness variations during the menstrual cycle. Abstract of the 5th Meeting of the International Society for Skin Imaging, Vienna, 1997.

24. Perin F, Perrier C, Pittet JC, Schnebert S, Perrier P, Beau P. Assessment of anti-cellulite treatment efficacy using the photograding of mechanically-accentuated macrorelief of thigh skin. Spincontrol, Tours, France and Parfums Christian Dior, Saint-Jean-de Braye, France. Unpublished results, 1999.

25. Schnebert S, Perin F, Pittet JC, Beau P, Perrier P, Pourcelot L. Evaluation de l'efficacité de produits ou de traitements amincissants par échographie mode B. To be published in Cosmétologie, 1999.

26. Adenola J, Maibach H. Ultrasonography, thermography and the Cutometer in the assessment of cellulite treatments. Abstract of the 12th International Symposium on Bioengineering and the Skin, Boston, MA, 1998.

27. Lucassen G, Van der Sluys W, Van Herk J, Nuijs T, Wierenga P, Barel AO, Lambrecht R. The effectiveness of massage treatment on cellulite as monitored by ultrasound imaging. Skin Res Technol 1997; 3:154–160.

28. Nuijs AM, Van Herk J. Characterizing the texture of cellulite skin. Abstract of the 12th International Symposium on Bioengineering and the Skin, Boston, MA, 1998.

29. Gassmüller J, Kecskes A, Jah P. Stylus method for skin surface contour measurement. In: Handbook of Non-Invasive Methods and the Skin. Serup J, Jemec GBE, eds. Boca Raton: CRC Press, 1995:83–89.

30. Corcuff P. Lévêque JL. Skin surface replica image analysis of furrows and wrinkles. In: Handbook of Non-Invasive Methods and the Skin. Serup J, Jemec GBE, eds. Boca Raton: CRC Press, 1995:89–97.

31. Efsen J, Hansen HN, Christiansen S, Keiding J. Laser profilometry. In: Handbook of Non-Invasive Methods and the Skin. Serup J, Jemec GBE, eds. Boca Raton: CRC Press, 1995:97–107.

32. Mignot J. Three-dimensional evaluation of skin surface: micro- and macrorelief. In: Handbook

of Non-Invasive Methods and the Skin. Serup J, Jemec GBE, eds. Boca Raton: CRC Press, 1995:97–107.

33. Tympanidou P, Tympanidou B. A non contact technique for the objective evaluation of cellulite and local mobilization. Abstract of the 12th International Symposium on Bioengineering and the Skin, Boston, MA, 1998.

34. Lagarde JM, Vié K, Beau P, Zahouani H, Gall Y. Evaluation of a slimming product using multi-scale analysis of 3-D topographical skin imaging with continuous wavelet transformation. Abstract of the 12th International Symposium on Bioengineering and the Skin, Boston, MA, 1998.

35. Endermology and cellulitis. Technical Information LPG Systems, Valence, France.

36. Perrier C, Pittet JV, Schnebert S, Perrier P, Beau P. Photographic assessment of so-called cellulite. Abstract of the 5th Congress of the International Society for Skin Imaging, Vienna, Austria, 1997.

37. Basset F. Amincissants: limites et réalités. Parfums Cosmétiques Actualités 1998; 144:32–37.

38. Tyler VE. The Honest Herbal: A Sensitive Guide to the Use of Herbs and Related Remedies. 3rd ed. New York: Pharmaceutical Product Press, 1993.

39. GlucoBlock, Lipo-Afslankgel met Glucoseremmer. Technical information, Laboratoires Vichy, France, 1999.

40. Clinical study of the efficiency of a cosmetic anti-cellulite treatment (Elancyl MP24). Technical information, Pierre Fabre, France, 1987.

41. Verdaet D. Kritische evaluatie van de ''anti-cellulitische werking'' van een cosmetisch verslankingsprodukt. Licentiate thesis Bachelor in Physiotherapy, Vrije Universiteit Brussel, Brussels, Belgium, 1991.

42. Beelen I, Smeets K. Experimentele studie van het lokaal effect van een cosmetisch algenprodukt op cellulitis door middel van niet invasieve metingen, delen I en II. Licentiate thesis Bachelor in Physiotherapy, Vrije Universiteit Brussel, Brussels, Belgium, 1991.

43. Ghislain N, Vandermeulen S. Objecteve evaluatie van een lokale anti-cellulitis massage behandeling door middel van contact thermografie, delen I en II. Licentiate thesis Bachelor in Physiotherapy, Vrije Universiteit Brussel, Brussels, Belgium, 1996.

44. Debremaeker N. Experimentele studie van een anti-cellulitis lymfedrainage behandeling. Licentiate thesis Bachelor in Physiotherapy, Vrije Universiteit Brussel, Brussels, Belgium, 1996.

46

Antiwrinkle Products

William J. Cunningham

CU-TECH, Mountain Lakes, New Jersey

INTRODUCTION

Skincare products that affect wrinkles are a reality and are well established in consumer, practitioner, and corporate perspectives. In the broadest definition, "products" range from classic and simple cosmetic preparations through vitamins, antioxidants, topical and oral cosmeceutical and pharmaceutical preparations, and even to surgical and laser interventions. Substantiation of product effect ranges from user testimonials through rigorous consumer testing and claim substantiation to classical pharmaceutical trials. Methodologies vary from casual visual and tactile observations to elaborate scoring of specific clinical parameters, and may be enhanced and embellished by use of many sensitive, accurate, reproducible, and validated instrumental techniques. The topic is currently exceptionally rich and expansive.

BACKGROUND

Definition of Wrinkles

Although intuitively obvious, the strict scientific definition of a wrinkle has been somewhat elusive. The consumer easily observes the fine and coarse indented lines of the skin of the face and attributes them to "aging." Although many cultures of the past recognized the damaging effects of sun exposure, only recently, in fact, has science verified the exceptionally strong link between wrinkles and repetitive, chronic, even suberythrogenic ultraviolet irradiation (UVR). Difficult as it is to histologically identify or quantify individual wrinkles, there is much scientific evidence of distinct dermal structural alterations of collagen and elastin that correlate generally with wrinkled skin. Easily conceptualized, the underlying "weaknesses" caused by this damaged infrastructure of the skin allows various length and depth infoldings of the skin to occur as a result of repetitive and chronic contractions of the exceptionally varied superficial musculature of facial expression.

Causes of Wrinkles

All scientific evidence points to UVR as the primary cause of wrinkles and other stigmata of "photoaging," and plausible mechanisms of pathogenesis have been elucidated. The pleotropic effects of UVR on many different cellular and subcellular systems make it difficult however to establish a strictly linear sequence of events, and it is likely that as in most biological systems, interrelated damage and reparative pathways interplay to establish progression, regression, or equilibrium. It is most helpful in rationalizing the potential of various products for prevention or reversal of wrinkles to understand the underlying molecular events. UVR has long been thought to damage skin partly through its generation of reactive oxygen species and subsequent damage to membrane lipids, various cellular proteins, and DNA. It has recently been shown that, within minutes of suberythrogenic UVB exposure, there is induction in human skin of matrix-degrading metaloproteinase messenger RNAs, their translated proteins, and consequent activities, possibly through a complex process involving signal transduction, transcription factors, and cytokine release [1]. Because the metalloproteinases are a large group of zinc-requiring enzymes that includes collagenases, elastases, and several other other proteinases, their induction, required cofactors, and potential inhibitors are logically of considerable interest in wrinkle causation, prevention, and treatment. Repetitive UVR radiation, presumably by chronic production of matrix damage attributable to this mechanism, would then, if inadequately repaired, lead to dermal ''scars'' and thus wrinkle formation [2]. This theory logically leads to many diverse, possible therapeutic interventions to prevent, stabilize, or reverse photoaging, along with its characteristic and prominent stigmatum of wrinkles.

PREVENTION OF WRINKLES OF PHOTOAGING

Quite apart from specific products, elimination of UVR exposure essentially prevents wrinkles. The effect of lifelong UVR avoidance is easily shown by comparison of the never-exposed skin of the buttocks to even suberythrogenic exposed skin of the face in any individual of types I to III skin. Although wrinkles usually appear only after some years of exposure and are noticeable beginning in the second or third decade of life, other seemingly benign yet insidious signs of photoaging, such as freckling, can be shown even in young children, especially those with light skin and high solar exposure as in Australia [3]. Complete avoidance of UVR is impractical, but avoidance during peak solar flux of midday is frequently possible. Protective hats and clothing are practical and highly desirable. Sunscreens of various types have definite utility in reducing UVR damage. Less well established is the potential role of a host of purported preventatives and treatments such as vitamins and antioxidants, many of which would appear to have a theoretical basis for consideration.

SUBSTANTIATION OF ANTIWRINKLE CLAIMS

Clinical Methodologies

Adequate methodologies of many and varied types now exist to accurately, precisely, reproducibly, and validly examine and quantitate the effects of products on wrinkles [4]. Consumers can judge for themselves if a product meets their needs in wrinkle effacement and, even if objective proof of efficacy is lacking, this positive perception is sometimes sufficient. There is a human tendency to estimate the age of other adults primarily by casual estimate of the degree of wrinkling of the skin of the face and, whether applied to others or the self, this quick estimate is fairly accurate [5].

Consumer-panel testing of many types can be quite rigorous and can quantify effect surprisingly effectively. Global grading of overall appearance is performed by using photographically derived scales of severity, with 0 = none, 1 to 3 = mild, 4 to 6 = moderate, and 7 to 9 = severe photodamage [6]. Specific grading of wrinkling and other parameters using visual analogue scales is simple and reproducible when used alone, and can be combined in very elegant clinical-panel testing [7]. The scale may be continuous, rating from 0 to 100 the condition as absent to severe to balanced, with a score of 0 designating no change from baseline, improvement recorded to the right side of 0 (to a maximum of +50 mm), and worsening recorded to the left side of 0 (to a minimum of 50 mm). Pharmaceutically oriented trials have successfully used similar methodologies with good correlation between subject and investigator evaluations.

Instrumentation

The evolving "gold standard" is doubtlessly the area of bioengineering devices. For wrinkling, optical profilometry is the most useful technology and has been widely and successfully used even in large clinical trials [8]. Most commonly, skin replicas of representative areas of wrinkling are evaluated by using image-analysis computer software that reflects wrinkle width and depth [9].

REPRESENTATIVE PRODUCTS FOR WRINKLES

Adequate sun avoidance and sunscreen use are partially prophylactic in the prevention of wrinkle formation. Purely cosmetic and emolliating products may substantially reduce the appearance of wrinkles without change in structure or function of the skin, whereas a number of cosmeceutical and pharmaceutical products fulfill both criteria.

Sunscreens

UVR, even in suberythrogenic doses, is damaging to skin. Prevention of wrinkles, especially in those most genetically predisposed, requires early initiation and lifelong minimization of exposure by sun avoidance and correct use of sunscreens. As multiple wavelengths of UVR are incriminated, it is prudent to use the most complete chemical block that the consumer and physical activity will permit. Substantial block of UVB and UVA is now available in many products, and with the addition of zinc oxide or titanium dioxide, nearly complete block of all damaging wavelengths is achieved.

Cosmetics

Innumerable cosmetic products exist, many of which claim to affect wrinkles and some of which may considerably minimize the appearance of wrinkles. Cosmetics of a simple, occlusive nature may essentially "fill in" the wrinkle valleys; others are of a color or substance that changes reflected light from the wrinkle sufficiently to minimize its appearance. Some products currently regulated as cosmetic contain ingredients such as alpha-hydroxy acids or retinol with potential pharmacological actions, and could more logically be designated cosmeceutical. The effect of removing dead, loosely coherent surface keratinocytes, or of stimulating epidermal or dermal processes, may significantly improve the appearance of wrinkles. It is important to remember that, at least in the United States, if pharmaceutical claims are not stated, the product is legally cosmetic in nature and thus its ingredients and marketing claims may vary considerably and creatively.

Moisturizers

Definite effects on skin appearance, and potentially on structure and function, can be achieved with moisturizers, especially those currently available, many of which are of sophisticated and elegant composition. Improvement in stratum-corneum structure and hydration, and decrease in transepidermal water loss (TEWL) can be quickly achieved and may result in improvement in the appearance of wrinkles.

Alpha- and Beta-Hydroxy Acids

There is substantial evidence that meaningful improvement can be obtained in multiple signs and symptoms of photodamaged skin by the sustained topical application of alpha-hydroxy acids. Specifically, wrinkle effacement has been shown in multiple well-designed and executed clinical trails using clinical and instrumental endpoints [10,11]. Fewer published trials are available that document a similar effect by use of alpha-hydroxy acids, but they nonetheless appear to have utility [12].

Retinoids

Incontrovertible evidence of wrinkle effacement by topical application of retinoids has been extensively shown in numerous large, published clinical trials. Tretinoin (all transretinoic acid) has been the most studied [13,14], but results with topical isotretinoin (13 cis-retinoic acid) appear comparable [15,16]. Retinol, the parent compound, may require metabolism to the purported active transretinoic acid for pharmacological effect and is increasingly incorporated in cosmetic products claiming benefit in wrinkle appearance. Similarly, retinaldehyde has been shown to be active in wrinkle effacement [17]. The most recently marketed retinoids, adapalene and tazorotene, will most likely be studied for similar effect.

Vitamins

Many vitamins, including vitamins A, C, D, and E, are vital in normal metabolic processes, and clinical skin changes resulting from their deficiencies were identified in many cases even in the 1800s. Some of these changes have been shown to be secondary to abnormal keratinization, altered differentiation, or impaired collagen synthesis. Nevertheless, it has been difficult to scientifically confirm cosmeceutical activity or utility of these vitamins under the conditions of normal nutritional status. Retinoids (vitamin A class), which were previously discussed, at pharmaceutical concentrations are the most thoroughly substantiated class in their general effect in photoaging and specific effect on wrinkles.

Vitamin E is an exhaustively studied antioxidant in many systems and could therefore logically be studied in photoaging [18]. Some evidence for pharmaceutical effect in treatment of wrinkles is available. A 4-week study of 5% RRR alpha tocopherol naturally occurring oil-in-water (o/w) cream applied to the crows feet area showed, by optical profilometry, decreased skin roughness, length of facial lines, and depth of wrinkles compared with placebo [19].

An increasing number of vitamin C–containing topical products are being marketed with claims of improvement in skin wrinkling.

Vitamin D analogues have been highly successful in treatment of psoriasis and because of their modulating effect on keratinization, should be studied in photoaging.

Hormones

Estrogens and their diminution at menopause have profound effects, especially on epithelium of the skin and vagina. Wrinkle effacement has been convincingly shown in at least one controlled clinical trail of topical application of 0.01% estradiol or 0.3% estriol-containing preparations [20]. Other studies have shown beneficial changes in skin thickness and texture with topical estrogen application [21,22].

Minerals

That many minerals, such as sodium, potassium, calcium, magnesium, selenium, and zinc, are critical in normal mammalian physiology is well established. A potential cosmeceutical role in improvement of skin appearance has been suggested and requires confirmation [23].

Miscellaneous Agents

Hyaluronic acid is a normal component of epidermis and especially dermis. Stimulation of hyaluronic-acid production in skin by a device that produces a specific pulsed electromagnetic field (electrorydesis) produced improvement in appearance of wrinkles in a small study [24].

Natural cartilage polysaccharides as oral formulations derived from cartilage of marine fish have purported to improve dermal thickness and elasticity [25].

SUMMARY AND CONCLUSIONS

Skincare products now exist that have various degrees of utility for preventing, minimizing the appearance of, or treating wrinkles caused by UVR. Conscientious use of sunscreens can minimize photoaging and wrinkle formation. Rigorous consumer-panel testing can show consistent improvement of the appearance of wrinkles with many products of a purely cosmetic nature. Application of well-established clinical methodologies and increasingly sophisticated instrumental techniques have conclusively shown pharmacologically mediated wrinkle improvement, especially with topical use of retinoids or alphahydroxy acids.

In conclusion, the substantial scientific progress that has driven the development of elegant cosmetic and pharmaceutically active products to ameliorate skin wrinkles warrants optimism for the future. Can the day be far in the future when present cosmetic and cosmeceutical treatments will be eclipsed by specific genetic manipulations to rejuvenate aging skin [26]?

REFERENCES

1. Fisher GJ, Datta SC, Talwar HS, Wang ZQ, Varani J, Kang S, Voorhees JJ. Molecular basis of sun-induced premature skin ageing and retinoid antagonism. Nature 1996; 379:335–339.
2. Fisher GJ, Wang ZQ, Datta SC, Varani J, Kang S, Voorhees JJ. Pathophysiology of premature skin aging induced by ultraviolet light. N Engl J Med 1997; 337(20):1419–1428.

3. Fritschi L, Green A. Sun damage in teenagers' skin. Aust J Public Health 1995; 19(4):383–386.

4. Cunningham WJ. Photoaging. In: Cutaneous Biometrics. New York: Plenum Press. In press.

5. Warren R, Gartstein V, Kligman AM, Montagna W, Allendorf RA, Ridder GM. Age, sunlight, and facial skin: a histologic and quantitative study. [Published erratum appears in J Am Acad Dermatol 1992; 26(4):558.] J Am Acad Dermatol 1991; 25(5 pt 1):751–760.

6. Griffiths CE, Wang TS, Hamilton TA, Voorhees JJ, Ellis CN. A photonumeric scale for the assessment of cutaneous photodamage. Arch Dermatol 1992; 128(3):347–351.

7. Armstrong RB, Lesiewicz J, Harvey G, Lee LF, Spoehr KT, Zultak M. Clinical panel assessment of photodamaged skin treated with isotretinoin using photographs. Arch Dermatol 1992; 128(3):352–356.

8. Grove GL, Grove MJ, Leyden JJ, Lufrano L, Schwab B, Perry BH, Thorne EG. Skin replica analysis of photodamaged skin after therapy with tretinoin emollient cream. J Am Acad Dermatol 1991; 25(2 pt 1):231–237.

9. Grove GL, Grove MJ. Effects of topical retinoids on photoaged skin as measured by optical profilometry. Methods Enzymol 1990; 190:360–371.

10. Ditre CM, Griffin TD, Murphy GF, Sueki H, Telegan B, Johnson WC, Yu RJ, Van Scott EJ. Effect of α-hydroxy acids on photoaged skin: a pilot clinical, histologic, and ultrastructural study. J Am Acad Dermatol 1996; 34(2 pt 1):187–195.

11. Stiller MJ, Bartolone J, Stern R, Smith S, Kollias N, Gillies R, Drake LA. Topical 8% glycolic acid and 8% L-lactic acid creams for the treatment of photoaged skin. Arch Dermatol 1996; 132:631–636.

12. Kligman AM. Salicylic acid: an alternative to alpha hydroxy acids. J Ger Dermatol 1997; 5(3):128–131.

13. Weiss JS, Ellis CN, Headington JT, Tincoff T, Hamilton TA, Voorhees JJ. Topical tretinoin improves photoaged skin: a double-blind vehicle-controlled study. JAMA 1988; 259:527–532.

14. Weinstein GD, Nigra TP, Pochi PE, Savin RC, Allan A, Benik K, Jeffes E, Lufrano L, Thorne EG. Topical tretinoin for treatment of photodamaged skin. Arch Dermatol 1991; 127:659–665.

15. Cunningham WJ, Bryce GF, Armstrong RA, Lesiewicz J, Kim HJ, Sendagorta E. Topical isotretinoin and photodamage. In: Saurat J-H, ed. Retinoids: 10 Years On. Basel: Karger, 1991: 182–190.

16. Sendagorta E, Lesiewicz J, Armstrong RB. Topical isotretinoin for photodamaged skin. J Am Acad Dermatol 1992; 27(6 pt 2):S15–18.

17. Creidi P, Vienne MP, Ochonisky S, Lauze C, Turlier V, Lagarde JM, Dupuy P. Profilometric evaluation of photodamage after topical retinaldehyde and retinoic acid treatment. J Am Acad Dermatol 1998; 39:960–965.

18. Nachbar F, Korting HC. The role of vitamin E in normal and damaged skin. J Mol Med 1995; 73:7–17.

19. Mayer P. The effects of vitamin E on the skin. Cosmet Toilet 1993; 108:99–109.

20. Schmidt JB, Binder M, Demschik G, Bieglmayer C, Reiner A. Treatment of skin aging with topical estrogens. Int J Dermatol 1996; 35(9):669–674.

21. Creidi P, Faivre B, Agache P, Richard E, Haudiquet V, Sauvanet JP. Effect of a conjugated oestrogen (Premarin) cream on aging facial skin. A comparative study with a placebo cream. Maturitas 1994; 19:211–223.

22. Callens A, Vaillant L, Lecomte P, Berson M, Gall Y, Lorette G. Does hormonal skin aging exist? A study of the influence of different hormone therapy regimens on the skin of postmenopausal women using non-invasive measurement techniques. Dermatology 1996; 193(4):289–294.

23. Ma'or Z, Magdassi S, Efron D, Yehuda S. Dead Sea mineral-based cosmetics—facts and illusions. Isr J Med Sci 1996; 32(suppl):S28–35.

24. Ghersetich I, Teofoli P, Benci M, Lotti T. Ultrastructural study of hyaluronic acid before and

after the use of a pulsed electromagnetic field, electrorydesis, in the treatment of wrinkles. Int J Dermatol 1994; 33(9):661–663.

25. Eskelinin A, Santalahti J. Natural cartilage polysaccharides for the treatment of sun-damaged skin in females: a double-blind comparison of Vivida and Imedeen. J Int Med Res 1992; 20(2): 227–233.

26. Zhang L, Li L, Hoffmann GA, Hoffman RM. Depth-targeted efficient gene delivery and expression in the skin by pulsed electric fields: an approach to gene therapy of skin aging and other diseases. Biochem Biophys Res Commun 1996; 220(3):633–636.

47

Artificial Tanning Products

Stanley B. Levy

University of North Carolina School of Medicine at Chapel Hill, Chapel Hill, North Carolina, and Revlon Research Center, Edison, New Jersey

INTRODUCTION

The desire for tanned skin alongside increasing awareness of the hazards of ultraviolet (UV) light exposure has led to renewed interest in artificial tanning products. Better formulations of sunless or self-tanners with improved aesthetics are more widely available. As consumer experience with the newer products has grown this category has become more popular, resulting in an increasing proportion of overall suncare sales. Dihydroxyacetone (DHA) is the active ingredient in sunless or self-tanners, and is responsible for darkening the skin by staining. DHA is classified in the International Cosmetic Ingredient Dictionary and Handbook [1] as a colorant or a colorless dye. Tan accelerators containing tyrosine and other ingredients and tanning promoters containing psoralens require UV exposure and will not be discussed here.

HISTORY

The first mention of DHA as an active ingredient in medicine appeared in the 1920s, when it was proposed as a substitute for glucose in diabetics. In the 1950s the oral administration of DHA was restudied as a diagnostic procedure for glycogen storage disease when it was given in large doses orally [2]. When children in the study spit up this sweet concentrated material, the skin became pigmented in splattered areas on the skin without staining clothing. Aqueous solutions were then applied to the skin directly and the pigmentation reproduced [3]. In the late 1950s, cosmetic tanning preparations first appeared in the marketplace. Cosmetic acceptance of these initial products was limited because of the uneven orange-brown color they imparted to the skin.

CHEMISTRY

Dihydroxyacetone ($C_3H_6O_3$) is a white, crystalline, hygroscopic powder. This 3-carbon sugar forms a dimer in freshly prepared aqueous solution (Fig. 1). With heating to effect a solution in alcohol, ether, or acetone, it reverts to the monomer. The monomeric form is more important in the browning reaction, which leads to the skincolor change [4]. DHA

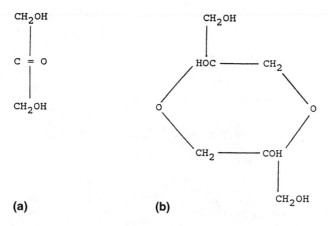

(a)   **(b)**

FIGURE 1   The chemical structure of DHA: (a) monomer, (b) dimer.

is stable between pH 4 to 6, but above pH 7 efficacy is lost with the formation of brown-colored compounds. A buffered mixture at pH 5 is most stable. Heating above 38°C for long periods of time will also effect stability. DHA needs to be stored in a cool, dry place. Glyceraldehyde, the isomer of DHA, is also present in solution [4]. Glyceraldehyde may degrade into formaldehyde and formic acid. In acidic solution (pH 4), this isomerization and consequently these latter undesirable ingredients are minimized.

The Maillard or browning reaction has been defined as the reaction of an amino group of amino acids, peptides, or proteins with the glycosidic hydroxyl group of sugars. DHA in the context of this reaction may be considered a 3-carbon sugar, reacting with free amino groups available as amino acids, peptides, and proteins supplied by the keratin to form products or chromophores referred to as melanoidins [5]. Melanoidins have some physicochemical properties similar to naturally occurring melanin [6].

FORMULATION

The concentration range of DHA in self-tanning products can range from 2.5 to 10%. Lower-concentration products allow the consumer greater latitude with application because they tend to be more "forgiving" of uneven application or rough surfaces. Labeling products as light, medium, or dark can be particularly helpful with the depth of shade a function of DHA concentration.

DHA is predominantly formulated in oil-in-water emulsions. Oils and waxes may reduce the color. Formulating with silicones allows the formulator to obtain the spreadability of oils, which potentially reduces streakiness with application to the skin. Minimizing particle size of the micelles in the chosen emulsion also improves uniformity of spreading on the skin's surface. Based on the chemistry of DHA, formulations should be buffered to an acidic pH (4 to 5) and not heated in manufacturing to temperatures higher than 40°C.

DHA can react with oxygen- and nitrogen-containing compounds, collagen, urea derivatives, amino acids, and proteins. They should be avoided in the formulation of the DHA-containing vehicle. Attempts have been made to take advantage of this effect by using a sulfur-containing amino acid, methionine sulfoxide, in an excipient applied before the application of the DHA-containing cream [7]. Two compartment systems have been patented based on this reaction.

As will all cosmetic products, aesthetics are determined by vehicle formulation. Products may be formulated for dry skin types by the addition of emollients and humectants. Products formulated in gel or alcoholic vehicles may be more suitable for oily skin.

MECHANISM OF ACTION

The site of action of DHA is the stratum corneum. Tape stripping of the skin quickly removes the color [8], as does mechanical rubbing. Deeper staining in areas with thicker stratum corneum and no staining of mucous membranes without a stratum corneum is also consistent with this being the site of action. DHA may be used as a substitute for dansyl chloride as a measure of stratum corneum turnover time [9]. Microscopic studies of stripped stratum corneum and hair reveal irregular pigment masses in the keratin layers [10] known as melanoidins. These melanoidins are formed via the Maillard reaction with DHA as a sugar reacting with the amino groups supplied by the keratin.

APPLICATION

After application of a typical DHA-containing self-tanning lotion, color change may be observed within an hour [11]. This color change may be seen under Wood's light (black light) within 20 minutes. Maximal darkening may take 8 to 24 hours to develop. Individuals can make several successive applications every few hours to achieve their desired color. Color may last as long as 5 to 7 days with a single application. Depending on anatomical application, the same color can be maintained with repeat applications every 1 to 4 days. The face requires fewer applications but more frequent reapplication to maintain color than the extremities. Depth of color varies with the thickness and compactness of the stratum corneum. Palms and soles stain deepest, necessitating washing of hands after application to avoid staining. Hair and nails will color, but not mucous membranes lacking a stratum corneum or keratin layer. Rougher hyperkeratotic skin over the knees, elbows, and ankles will color more unevenly as will older skin with keratoses and mottled pigmentation. Color will also be maintained longer in these areas.

As in the formulation, the pH of the skin before application may have an effect on the tonality of the skin color [4]. Alkaline residues from soaps or detergents may interfere with the reaction between DHA and the amino acids on the skin surface. Wiping the skin surface with a hydroalcoholic, acidic toner just before DHA application may improve results.

Careful directions provided with these products are, therefore, quite important in determining consumer satisfaction. The skin may be prepared with a mild form of exfoliation. Even application is required with lighter application around elbows, knees, and ankles to avoid excessive darkening in these areas. Care also needs to taken around the hairline where lighter hair may darken. Hands need to be washed immediately after use to avoid darkening of the palms, fingers, and nails. Clearly, care, skill, and experience are necessary when using these products.

ADDITIVES

As commonly occurs, growth in this category has compelled both formulators and marketers to seek points of differentiation between their product and that of their competitors. Besides formulating for specific skin types, active treatment ingredients may be incorporated into DHA-containing formulations. Vitamins, botanical extracts, antioxidants, anti-irritants, and even alpha-hydroxy acids may be added to broaden the claims made by a given product. The addition of sunscreen ingredients to self-tanners warrants a more detailed discussion.

SUNSCREEN ACTIVITY

In the United States, the FDA Tentative Final Over-the-Counter Monograph on Sunscreens (Fed Reg. 1993) lists DHA as an approved sunscreen ingredient when used sequentially with lawsone (2-hydroxy-1, 4-napthoquinone). The European Economic Community Directive does not list DHA as a permitted UV filter. DHA itself has at most a modest effect on SPF [12], providing perhaps SPF 3 or 4 protection. The brown color obtained on the skin does absorb in the low end of the visible spectrum with overlap into long UVA and may provide some UVA I protection [13].

Individuals using DHA-containing tanning products need to be cautioned that, despite visible darkening of their skin, these products provide minimal sun protection. Confusion may be compounded by the addition of UV filters to the formulation providing significant sun protection. The stated SPF for the product is applicable for a few hours after application, but not for the days during which the skin color change may remain perceptible.

INDICATIONS

Even with recent improvement in DHA formulations, the color achieved remains dependent on skin type. Individuals of medium complexion with skin phototypes II or III [14], as opposed to those who are lighter or darker, will obtain a more pleasing color. Individuals with underlying golden skin tones will achieve better results than individuals with rosy, sallow, or olive complexions. Older consumers with roughened, hyperkeratotic skin or mottled pigmentation with freckling may be less pleased with their use. Dermatologists regularly recommend these products for tanning as a safe alternative to UV exposure. They may be used to camouflage some skin irregularities such as leg spider veins. Light-to medium-complected patients with vitiligo who show increased contrast with the vitiliginous areas with natural or unavoidable tanning in their normal skin may also benefit. They may even provide some protection for individuals with certain photosensitivity disorders [15].

SAFETY

The visible color change associated with the use of artificial tanning products might suggest to some users that these products are hazardous. Based on the chemistry of DHA and its toxicological profile, it can be considered nontoxic. It reacts quickly in the stratum corneum minimizing systemic absorption. The acute toxicity of DHA was investigated for diabetics in the 1920s with their oral intake well tolerated [6]. The phosphate of DHA is found naturally as one of the intermediates in the Kreb's cycle. Contact dermatitis to DHA has only rarely been reported [16]. As with other topical products with active ingredients, such as sunscreens, much of the reported sensitivity is secondary to other ingredients in the vehicle [17]. Adverse reactions are more likely to occur on the basis of irritation and not true allergy. Ultimately all claims related to product safety are based on testing the final formulation.

ALTERNATIVE TANNING AGENTS

Lawsone found in the henna plant and juglone (5-hydroxy-1,4,-napthoquinone) derived from walnuts also stain hair, skin, and nails. They have been used for centuries for hair coloring. Both substances lack skin substantivity and readily discolor clothing [18]. The skin color they produce does not resemble a natural tan.

Based on the underlying principle of the Maillard reaction, other molecules with a ketone function have been investigated [19]. An alpha-hydroxy group with attaching electron withdrawing groups can also increase reactivity. Substances such as glyceraldehyde and glyoxal [20] have been described but found ineffective. Mucondialdehyde as described by Eichler [21] is an effective agent but is also associated with toxicity, which mitigates against its use [19]. Although several other aldehydes have been shown to have better color properties, stability issues limit their use [19].

CONCLUSION

Increasing consumer awareness as to the hazards of UV light should fuel ongoing interest in self-tanning products. The benign toxicological profile of DHA reinforces the notion that these products represent a safe alternative to a UV-induced tan. The results obtained with these products are dependent on the final formulation, individual application technique, and consumers' complexion type. Greater experience in formulation combined with increasing sophistication on the part of the consumer should lead to continuing growth and satisfaction with the use of these products.

Consumers need to be clearly informed that these products do not offer significant protection against UVB. If formulated with standard sunscreens, consumers should be cautioned that the duration of UV protection is more short-lived than the color change.

REFERENCES

1. Wenninger JA, McEwen GN Jr, eds. International Cosmetic Ingredient Dictionary and Handbook. 7th ed. Washington, D.C.: The Cosmetic, Toiletry, and Fragrance Association, 1997.
2. Guest GM, Cochrane W, Wittgenstein E. Dihydroxyacetone tolerance test for glycogen storage disease. Mod Prob Paediat 1959; 4:169–178.
3. Wittgenstein E, Berry HK. Staining of skin with dihydroxyacetone. Science 1960; 132:894–895.
4. Maes DH, Marenus KD. Self-tanning products. In: Baran R, Maibach HI, eds. Cosmetic Dermatology. London: Martin Dunitz, 1994: 227–230.
5. Wittgenstein E, Berry HK. Reaction of dihydroxyacetone (DHA) with human skin callus and amino compounds. J Invest Dermatol 1961; 36:283–286.
6. Meybeck A. A spectroscopic study of the reaction products of dihydroxyacetone with amino acids. J Soc Cosmet Chem 1977; 28:25–35.
7. Bobin MF, Martini MC, Cotte J. Effects of color adjuvants on the tanning effect of dihydroxyacetone. J Soc Cosmet Chem 1984; 35:265–272.
8. Maibach HI, Kligman AM. Dihydroxyacetone: a suntan-simulating agent. Arch Dermatol 1960; 82:505–507.

9. Pierard GE, Pierard-Franchimont C. Dihydroxyacetone test as a substitute for the dansyl chloride test. Dermatology 1993; 186(2):133–137.
10. Goldman L, Barkoff J, Blaney D, Nakai T, Suskind R. The skin coloring agent dihydroxyacetone. General Practioner 1960; 12:96–98.
11. Levy SB. Dihydroxyacetone-containing sunless or self-tanning lotions. J Am Acad Dermatol 1992; 27:989–993.
12. Muizzuddin N. Marenus KD, Maes DH. UV-A and UV-B protective effect of melanoids formed with dihydroxyacetone and skin. Poster 360 presented at the 55th Annual Meeting of the American Academy of Dermatology, San Francisco, CA, 1997.
13. Johnson JA, Fusaro RM. Protection against long ultraviolet radiation: topical browning agents and a new outlook. Dermatologica 1987; 175:53–57.
14. Fitzpatrick TB. The validity and practicality of sunreactive skin types I through IV. Arch Dermatol 1988; 124:869–871.
15. Fusaro RM, Johnson JA. Photoprotection of patients sensitive to short and/or long ultraviolet light with dihydroxyacetone/naphthoquinone. Dermatologica 1974; 148:224–227.
16. Morren M, Dooms-Goossens A, Heidbuchel M, Sente F. Damas M. Contact allergy to dihydroxyacetone. Contact Dermatitis 1991; 25:326–327.
17. Foley P, Nixon R, Marks R, Frowen K, Thompson S. The frequency of reaction to sunscreens: results of a longitudinal population-based study on the regular use of sunscreens in Australia. Br J Dermatol 1993; 128:512–518.
18. Reiger MM. The chemistry of tanning. Cosmet & Toilet 1983; 98:47–50.
19. Kurz T. Formulating effective self-tanners with DHA. Cosmet & Toilet 1994; 109:11:55–61.
20. Goldman L, Barkoff J. Blaney D, Nakai T, Suskind R. Investigative studies with the skin coloring agents dihydroxyacetone and glyoxal. J Invest Dermatol 1960; 35:161–164.
21. Eichler J. Prinzipien der Haptbraunung. Kontakte (Merck) 1981; 111:24–30.

48

Barrier Creams

Cees Korstanje
Yamanouchi Europe B.V., Leiderdorp, The Netherlands

INTRODUCTION

The expression "barrier cream" is used most often to indicate those creams that are used in the context of prevention of irritant contact dermatitis (ICD) [1]. The use of this type of product, however, is much broader than the medical care circuit (diagnosed patients by dermatologists, general practitioners, or other healthcare professionals), and in fact the major sales of barrier creams is in the segments of skincare and occupational use. In these segments there is quite some mix-up between "barrier creams," "emollients," and "moisturizers," both in use and marketing. However, contemplating on insights gained during the last one and a half decades in both the causes and prevention of ICD [2–6], a more consummated view on treatment options can be given [7,8]. Repeated exposure of the skin to low concentrations of irritants, low temperatures, or friction during daily wear and tear of the skin, may lead to a gradual lowering of treshold for disruption of the skin barrier, and consequently to ICD. This means that it makes sense to distinguish prevention and treatment options for people who are at risk for developing ICD. In this respect persons with a history of (skin) atopy should be considered, along with those whose occupational environments create the aforementioned conditions. It will be evident that prevention of skin barrier problems has two aspects, namely risk avoidance, e.g., by minimizing contact time with irritating conditions and fluids, and protection of the skin, e.g., with gloves or protective products. If despite these measures the skin gets abrogated, it is important to apply products that have the capacity to aid or accelerate skin repair.

Consequently, these principles should be reflected in the definition and choice of topical products used in the management of skin-barrier problems in general and ICD in particular. It is therefore proposed to classify such products as "barrier protective" (BP) and "barrier restorative" (BR) products. In this view, BP products are considered products that guard the skin against the deleterious influences of exogenous stimuli leading to barrier disruption and consequently to the development of ICD. On the other hand, BR products are defined as being intended to restore a disrupted skin barrier. Both types of products can appear as ointments, creams, milks, and foams.

Because of the different functions of BP and BR products in the management of skin-barrier problems, it is noteworthy to consider that this has an impact on the properties that are expected from such products. In this respect it is important to realize that protective

Shielding

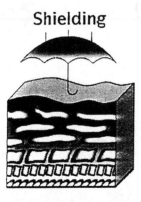

FIGURE 1   The primary function of a protective product.

products have the primary function to shield the skin (Fig. 1), but that this should be accomplished under conditions where people are working in a household or occupational environment. This implies that not only the shielding properties of such preparations, but also whether or not these products can be used under daily working conditions are important. Because occupational conditions may vary tremendously, it is not surprising that this has an impact on what can be called the ''secondary properties'' of BP products, which mean that BP products for e.g., hairdressers, kitchen workers, and slaughterhouse workers should offer the same level of protection but with different wash and wear resistancy as well as cosmetic properties. This requires special products for specific user groups.

In contrast, for BR products there is, in principle, no need for differentiation on the user's occupation, because these products are intended to be used after work. However, because different irritants cause differential structural alterations in e.g., the horny layer of the skin [9], this may require different types of BR formulations. Figure 2 depicts the differences between protective and restorative products. Consequently, product properties can be defined and criteria can be set to comply with.

PROTECTIVE PRODUCTS

Properties

The ideal BP product should be effective, nonsensitizing, nonirritating, easily applied and removed, cosmetically acceptable, and cost efficient. Importantly, BP product characteristics should be designed taking into account both the nature of the irritant and the required

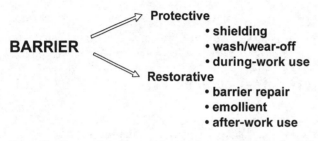

FIGURE 2   Properties of protective and restorative products.

cosmetic properties (e.g., compatible with daily life activities) to guarantee use suitability. This implies that in order to define properties, one should first identify user-group specifications and make an inventory of property—user combinations. An attempt at this is shown in Table 1. Accordingly, product profiles can be defined and assessed as product requirements after testing the product. It is particularly important to realize that the use suitability of BP products is dependent on the fulfillment of all different types of product requirements at the same time. This is not easily accomplished, however. Unfortunately there is an almost inverse relationship between shielding properties and cosmetic acceptability for ointments, creams, and foams, as is depicted in Figure 3.

Formulations

To date, very few preparations have characteristics that make them especially suited for any of the user groups given in Table 1 [10], although some general remarks can be made: current protective products against water-based irritants (soap, alkaline, acids) act in a rather nonspecific way by depositing mineral oils, isopropylmyristate, long-chain alcohols, fats, or waxes on top of the skin or into the outer stratum corneum cell layers in order to create a physical lipids barrier. Water repellants, like silicone oils or perfluoroether, are sometimes included. However, because these are highly inert molecules, high percentages of emulsifier are required to stabilize such formulations. This means that the net increase in protective properties with these supplements is disappointing (water-dragging effect), while high emulsifier concentrations may also cause irritation. More successful attempts have been made by including chemicals that are intended to bind to skin constituents, such as Eucoriol (sodium bischlorophenyl sulfamine), which is included in a water-in-oil (W/O) ointment. A disadvantage is that the product is rather greasy on the skin. The emulsion type of preparations against water-based irritants is usually W/O, although there are some exceptions: a high-fat product in an oil-in-water (O/W) fatty cream*, and a product with petroleum jelly and silicone oil in a gel structure. The latter products have better cosmetic properties. Despite the fair-to-good protective properties offered by W/O products, their poor cosmetic properties make these products less suitable for use by, e.g., hairdressers and hospital nurses.

Recently, O/W emulsions, including CM glucan, a polysaccharide isolated from baker's yeast, was proposed and tested for its protective properties in surfactant-challenged skin [11]. The clinical value of this type of formulation has not been shown, however. In order to increase cosmetic properties for BP products, foam-based products have been developed. An example is a foam containing stearic acid and dimethylpolysiloxane. Unfortunately, comparative tests have shown that the apparent advantage in cosmetic properties for this product does not extend to acceptable protective properties [12].

Cream and gel preparations for the prevention of nickel-induced ICD with ethylene diamine as a chelator have been made and tested in in vitro tests and patch tests [13]. Despite encouraging results in these types of tests, clinical efficacy of this type of preparation has not been shown. For protection against organic solvents, O/W creams are recommended [14], although in efficacy tests using toluene, or poison ivy extracts, this is not well accomplished with currently marketed products [1,10,15], thus casting doubt on this recommendation. Unfortunately, it can be stated that despite the many technological ad-

---

* Product protected by, e.g., Canadian patent 1200504.

TABLE 1 Product Users and Properties Needed to Fulfill Users' Needs for Protective Formulations

| | Product properties* | | | | | | | | |
| | Protective properties against | | | | | | Wash/Wear | | |
Usergroup	Soap solutions	Aggressive chemicals	Diluted acid	Diluted alkali	Dehydrating polar solvents	Apolar solvents	Wash-off	Friction	Cosmetic properties
Cooks, sandwich makers, meat-industry workers	+								
Hairdressers	++	++	+	++			++		++
Packers								++	−/+
Mechanics	+	+	+					+	−
Confectionary workers						++		++	++
Laboratory technicians			+	+	+	+	+		+
Farmers							+	++	−
Graphic-industry workers		++	+	+	+	+		+	−/+
Hospital nurses	+		+	+	+		++		+

* On a scale of −, not important/needed; +, important/needed; ++, very important.

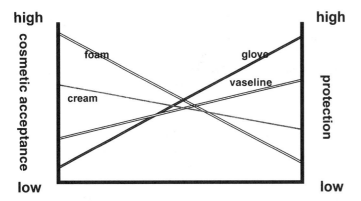

FIGURE 3   Skin-protective properties and suitability in daily-use characteristics for differential topical protective formulations.

vancements that have been made in pharmaceutical and cosmetic topical formulation science, and that have brought a better understanding of composition–properties relationships [16,17,18], this has not yet been translated into efficacious BP products for all user groups.

Test Methods

Sufficiently large field studies proving the efficacy of BP products under real-life conditions are scarce. In fact, the only study that shows the efficacy of a product in this respect is a field study in kitchen workers and cleaners, which showed protective properties of the O/W fatty cream previously mentioned [19]. The availability of reliable laboratory test methods is, therefore, essential, both for classification of products and for the development of new products. Suitable tests should give quantitative read-outs, include appropriate standard preparations and controls, and mimic wear-and-tear conditions when applicable.

Hallmarks for tests with a good predictive clinical value in this respect are the use of low, subtoxic doses of the irritant and repetitive application for 1 to 2 weeks, in absence or presence of pretreatment with test products thus mimicking real-life conditions. If wash-off is important for the target user groups of certain products, modifications can be made, which include washing schemes. After pioneering work by Lachapelle and coworkers [20], Frosch and colleagues have validated a test schedule in human volunteers where pretreatment of the skin with BP products was followed by repetitive treatment with a panel of irritants consisting of diluted solutions of sodium lauryl sulphate, sodium hydroxide, lactic acid, and undiluted toluene [1]. Other groups have used similar approaches on the back or forearm of human volunteers [10,21,22].

In vitro tests for assessing the protective ability of topical products generally have a poor predictive value for the in vivo situation [23]. However, for candidate selection in large-scale industrial development programs, such tests are indispensable to cut time-consuming product-screening procedures. In this respect, a method to test the water-repellent properties of formulations applied on slides dipped into a 1% eosin solution and evaluated for the absorption of color with a chromameter was found valuable as a preselection tool in a development program to identify products against water-based irritants, whereas another test where penetrating dye was assessed after application of the products on a filter paper was of very limited value in this respect (author: unpublished observations). Although some animal tests may be worthwhile because of an obvious good clinical predictability of the results, e.g., the repetitive irritation test in guinea pigs [12], similar information can be obtained in human volunteer studies, avoiding sacrifice of animals.

In an industrial program aimed to develop an O/W cream that should protect against water-based irritants, maintain activity after washing, and with acceptable cosmetic properties, we have used a series of in vitro and human volunteer tests in serial and parallel combination. The test sequence was composed of high-capacity (in vitro) tests as the first selectors, and more laborious tests later on. Firstly, the in vitro eosin dip test was used as mentioned above. Secondly, formulations were tested into an in vivo eosin penetration test (see Fig. 4) and a cosmetic properties test [24]. Formulations that complied with predefined activity and cosmetic standards were taken into a repetitive-irritation test with sodium lauryl sulphate (SLS). The protocol for this test was based on procedures as published by Frosch's group [1], but including a wash-off scheme and with SLS as the only irritant. Typical results for a test run with the eosin penetration test and the repetitive irritation test are given in Figures 4 and 5.

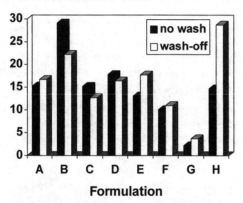

FIGURE 4 Results from a comparison of six experimental protective products (prepared by Yamanouchi Europe B.V., Leiderdorp, The Netherlands). (A, C, D, F, G, H) and two reference products (B, E) in an eosin dye penetration test *with* (first column) and *without* (second column) wash-off schedule. In eight healthy males, 50 μl of the test formulations was applied on 4 areas/arm of 4 × 5 cm. After rubbing in, the left sites of the spots were washed off gently with water. Accordingly, at all sites small paper disks, soaked in 1% eosin solution, were applied. After washing all sites, colorimetry (a* parameter) was performed with a Minolta CR300 colorimeter, and the difference with untreated was noted. (A low value for a* denotes good protective properties.) Preparations used: (A) 45% liquid paraffin/10% carnauba wax/3% glycerin W/O cream; (B) commercial hand cream including among others (a.o.) alcohols, waxes, paraffin, W/O and O/W emulsifiers, glycerin, dimethicone, and water; (C) 25% petroleum jelly in Carbopol 1382 O/W gel; (D) 10% ceresine wax added to an O/W fatty cream; (E) commercial W/O ointment containing mineral oil, petrolatum, Eucoriol, lanolin, Ozokerite; (F) 38% beeswax/34% Miglyol812 O/W oleogel; (G) 100% petroleum jelly; (H) 45% liquid paraffin/3% glycerin W/O cream.

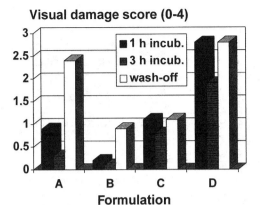

FIGURE 5   Results from a comparison of three experimental protective products (prepared by Yamanouchi Europe B.V., Leiderdorp, The Netherlands) (A, C, D) with a reference product (B) in a repetitive irritation test after five treatment days with SLS and incubation time of 1 h (first bar), 3 h (second bar), and with wash-off treatment (third bar). In this test eight healthy males were treated on 12 spots on the back with rubbing in 50 μl of the four formulations, applied in each column. Each row was allocated to one of the schedules: 1 h incubation, 3 h incubation, or wash-off after 30 min, whereas at 1 h after application 50 μl patches filled with 10% SLS were applied for 30 min. Erythema was scored with a chromameter (Minolta CR300) using the a* scale. Visual damage was scored on a scale from 0–4 (Frosch PJ, Kligman AM. The soap chamber test. J Am Acad Dermatol 1979; 1:35–41). The visual damage scores after five treatment days are given. Preparations used: (A) 4% perfluoroether (FomblinHC) added to an O/W fatty cream; (B) commercial W/O ointment containing a.o. mineral oil, petrolatum, Eucoriol lanolin, Ozokerite; (C) 4% FomblinHC/15% octyl, stearate W/O cream; (D) 4% FomblinHC/18% Miglyol812/15% propyleneglycol O/W cream.

Properties

Based on studies that have been initiated by the group of Elias in San Francisco [25,26], and taken further by others as well [8,27,28], insight has been gathered into mechanisms and components involved in skin repair. Although the body of experiments in this direction was carried out on murine skin, evidence is accumulating that qualitatively similar mechanisms are operative in humans [29,30]. This leads to the view that BR products should have properties directed at re-establishing the broken skin barrier, which is accommodated by restoration of the physical integrity via application of missing basic components of the intracellular lipid matrix in combination with occlusive materials to stimulate repair mechanisms (Fig. 6). The function of the skin barrier is reflected by its ability to prevent excessive water loss. Consequently, transepidermal water loss (TEWL) is the parameter of choice to define the status of the skin barrier in this respect [31]. In this respect, criteria for BR products to comply with are based on the ability to accomplish a significant reduction of TEWL, thus stimulating "early" and "late" recovery [8], e.g., in mouse models [32], and finally in man [30], which go beyond the effect of occlusive products, like petroleum jelly. It should be noted that BR products share some of their purposes with "emollients" [33,34,35], although no strict criteria have been defined for the latter products.

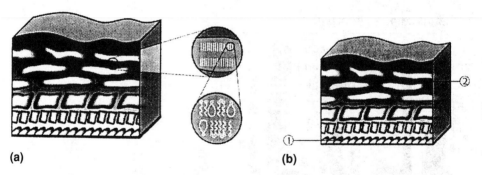

(a)   **(b)**

FIGURE 6   Schematic representation of the structure of the skin and strategies for restoring the barrier.

Formulations

For BR products, formulations containing ceramides, cholesterol, and fatty acids in vehicles that allow the formation of lamellar structures have been proposed [36,37]. Test results for this type of formulation are encouraging [36]. However, clinical results with the first marketed product of this kind* that are underway have to show whether this approach will result in better treatment options for dry skin and damaged skin due to ICD.

Test Methods

Because of the fact that BR products as such are an upcoming category of products, there is not an established view on test methods that should be used to identify and label such products. However, based on the arguments given in this chapter, test methods using mice where recovery of TEWL is studied following breaking of the skin barrier with acetone [26,32] are proposed, whereas human volunteer models using *treatment* instead of *pretreatment* schedules following damaging the skin with irritants [38,29] seem to be appropriate.

REFERENCES

1. Frosch PJ, Kurte A. Efficacy of skin barrier creams (IV). The repetetive irritation test (RIT) with a set of 4 standard irritants. Contact Dermatitis 1994; 31:161–168.
2. Malten KE. Thoughts on irritant contact dermatitis. Contact Dermatitis 1981; 7:238–247.
3. Andersen KE, Benezra C, Burrows D. Contact dermatitis: a review. Contact Dermatitis 1987; 16:55–78.
4. Imokawa G, Akasaki S, Minematsu Y, Kawai M. Importance of intercellular lipids in water-retention properties of the stratum corneum: induction and recovery study of surfactant dry skin. Arch Dermatol Res 1989; 281:45–51.
5. Friedmann PS. Graded continuity or all or none—studies of the human immune response. Clin Exp Dermatol 1991; 16:79–84.
6. Berardesca E, Vignoli GP, Borroni G, Oresajo C, Rabbiosi G. Surfactant damaged skin: which treatment? In: Marks R, Plewig G, eds. The Environmental Threat to the Skin. London: Martin Dunitz, 1992:283–285.

---

* Containing petrolatum, water, paraffin, liquid paraffin, glycerin, sorbitan oleate, carnauba, cholesterol, ceramide-3, oleic acid, palmitic acid, tromethamine, and covered by US patent 5667800.

7. Lachapelle JM. Prevention of allergic contact dermatitis. In: Grob JJ, Stern RS, MacKie RM, Weinstock WA, eds. Epidemiology, Causes and Prevention of Skin Diseases. Oxford: Blackwell Science, 1997:318–323.

8. Halkier-Sorensen L. Occupational skin diseases. Contact Dermatitis 1996; 35(suppl 1):94–97.

9. Fartasch M. Electron microscopic imaging of the skin barrier dysfunction: the structural level. 4th EADV Congress, Satellite symposium: Clinical Management of Skin Barrier Problems, Brussels, Belgium, Oct. 13, 1995.

10. Schlüter-Wigger, Elsner P. Efficacy of 4 commercially available protective creams in the repetitive irritation test (RIT). Contact Dermatitis 1996; 34:278–283.

11. Zülli F, Suter F, Biltz H, Nissen HP. Improving skin function with CM-glucan, a biological response modifier from yeast. Int J Cosmet Sci 1998; 20:79–86.

12. Frosch PJ, Schulze-Dirks A, Hoffmann M, Axthelm I. Efficacy of skin barrier creams (II). Ineffectiveness of a popular ''skin protector'' against various irritants in the repetitive irritation test in the guinea pig. Contact Dermatitis 1993; 29:74–77.

13. Fullerton A, Menné T. In vitro and in vivo evaluation of the effect of barrier gels in nickel contact allergy. Contact Dermatitis 1995; 32:100–106.

14. Forssman T, Gloor M. Hand creams. In: Baran R, Maibach HI, eds. Cosmetic Dermatology. London: Martin Dunitz, 1994:181–187.

15. Smith WB, Baunchalk JM, Grabski WJ. Lack of efficacy of a barrier cream in preventing rhus dermatitis. Arch Dermatol 1993; 129:787–788.

16. Friberg SE. Micelles, microemulsions, liquid crystals, and the structure of stratum corneum lipids. J Soc Cosmet Chem 1990; 41:155–171.

17. Brinon L, Geiger S, Alard V, Tranchant JF, Pouget T, Couarraze G. Influence of lamellar liquid crystal structure on percutaneous diffusion of a hydrophilic tracer from emulsions. J Cosmet Sci 1998; 49:1–11.

18. Junginger HE, Boddé HE, Bouwstra JA. Water in dermatological preparations and its impact on skin. In: Crommelin DJA, Midha KK, Nagai T, eds. Topics in Pharmaceutical Sciences 1993. Stuttgart: Medpharm, 1994:435–458.

19. Halkier-Sorensen L, Thestrup-Pedersen K. The efficacy of a moisturizer (Locobase) among cleaners and kitchen assistants during everyday exposure to water and detergents. Contact Dermatitis 1993; 29:266–271.

20. Mahmoud G, Lachapelle JM, Van Neste D. Histological assessment of skin damage by irritants: its possible use in the evaluation of a ''barrier cream''. Contact Dermatitis 1988; 11:179–178.

21. Allenby CF, Basketter DA, Dickens A, Barnes EG, Brough HC. An arm immersion model of compromised skin (I). Influence on irritation reactions. Contact Dermatitis 1993; 28:84–88.

22. Bettinger J, Gloor M, Gehring W. Influence of a pretreatment with emulsions on the dehydration of the skin by surfactants. Int J Cosmet Sci 1994; 16:53–60.

23. Gehring W, Dördelmann C, Gloor M. Effektivitätsnachweis von Hautschutzpräparaten. [In German]. Allergologie 1994; 17:97–101.

24. Spiertz C, Korstanje C. A method for assessing the tactile properties of dermatological cream bases. J Dermatol Treatment 1995; 6:155–157.

25. Grubauer G, Feingold KR, Elias PM. Relationship of epidermal lipogenesis to cutaneous barrier function. J Lipid Res 1987; 28:746–752.

26. Mao-Qiang M, Feingold KR, Thornfeldt CR, Elias PM. Optimization of physiological lipid mixtures for barrier repair. J Invest Dermatol 1996; 106:1096–1101.

27. EkanayakeMudiyanselage S, Aschauer H, Schmook FP, Jensen JM, Meingassner JG, Proksch E. Expression of epidermal keratins and the cornified envelope protein involucrin is influenced by permeability barrier disruption. J Invest Dermatol 1998; 111:517–523.

28. Fartasch M, Diepgen TL. The barrier function in atopic dry skin. Disturbance of membrane-

coating granule exocytosis and the formation of epidermal lipids? Acta Derm Venereol 1992; 176(suppl):26–31.

29.   Mao-Qiang M, Feingold KR, Wang F, Thornfeldt CR, Elias PM. A natural lipid mixture improves barrier function and hydration in human and murine skin. J Soc Cosmet Chem 1997; 47:157–166.

30.   Di Nardo A, Sugino K, Wertz P, Ademola J, Maibach HI. Sodium lauryl sulphate (SLS) induced irritant contact dermatitis: a correlation study between ceramides and in vivo parameters of irritation. Contact Dermatitis 1996; 35:86–91.

31.   Maibach HI, Bronaugh R, Guy R, Turr E, Wilson D, Jacques S, Chaing D. Noninvasive techniques for determining skin function. In: Drill V, Lazar P eds. Cutaneous Toxicity. New York: Raven Press, 1984; 63–97.

32.   Erlandsen M, Halkier-Sorensen L, De Vringer T. Proc Fourth Congress of the European Soc of Contact Dermatitis, Helsinki, Finland, July 8–11, 1998:49.

33.   Lodén M. Biophysical properties of dry atopic and normal skin with special reference to effects of skin care products. Acta Derm Venereol 1995; 192(suppl):1–48.

34.   Rycroft RJG. Occupational hand eczema: the role of emollients in treatment and prophylaxis. J Dermatol Treatment 1997; 8(suppl 1):S23–S24.

35.   Marks R. How to measure the effects of emollients. J Dermatol Treatment 1997; 8(suppl. 1): S15–S18.

36.   Iwai H, Fukasawa J, Suzuki T. A liquid crystal application in skin care cosmetics. Int J Cosm Sci 1998; 20:87–102.

37.   De Vringer T. A rational design of topical formulations with skin barrier restoration properties. Proc Fourth Congress of the European Soc of Contact Dermatitis, Helsinki, Finland, July 8–11, 1998:152.

38.   Gabard B, Elsner P, Treffel P. Barrier function of the skin in a repetitive irritants model and influence of 2 different treatments. Skin Res Technol 1996; 2:78–82.

49

Skin-Whitening Products

Hongbo Zhai and Howard I. Maibach
University of California at San Francisco School of Medicine,
San Francisco, California

Skin-whitening products have been widely used in the cosmetic field and clinic therapy. They are supposed to either lighten skin (individuals who wish to change or modify their skin color) or depigment skin (treatment for abnormal-hyperpigmentation skin such as melasma, freckles, and senile lentigines). Whitening agents, such as hydroquinone, kojic acid, and ascorbic acid derivatives have shown efficacy in a variety of hyperpigmentary disorders [1–14] but with varying success [1,2,7–9]. Their mechanism of action has been studied in vitro and in vivo [3,10–17]. Recently, their safety of application have been extensively investigated [18–32]. This chapter includes the most popular active ingredients of whitening agents and emphasizes their efficacy and safety.

HYDROQUINONE (1,4-DIHYDROXYBENZENE)

Hydroquinone is a nonvolatile chemical used in the photographic, rubber, chemical, and cosmetic industries. In the late 1930s, it was observed that a chemical used in rubber manufacture, monobenzyl ether of hydroquinone, caused depigmented skin in some workers [1]. The efficacy of hydroquinone (1,4-dihydroxybenzene) as a skin-lightening agent has been established in both human and animal studies. The chemical structure of hydroquinone is shown in Figure 1. Clinically, hydroquinone is applied topically in the treatment of melasma, freckles, and senile lentigines, as well as postinflammatory hyperpigmentation. In the United States, hydroquinone is readily available in concentrations up to 2.0% as an over-the-counter (OTC) drug and by prescription at higher concentrations [1,2]. Thus, hydroquinone is readily applied to the skin for medical and cosmetic reasons [33].

Hydroquinone inhibits the conversion of dopa to melanin by inhibiting the tyrosinase enzyme [1–3]. Other proposed mechanisms are inhibition of DNA and RNA synthesis, degradation of melanosomes, and destruction of melanocytes [2]. Electron microscopic studies of black guinea-pig skin treated with hydroquinone show the anatomic consequences of this action: (1) the melanosome structure is disturbed, resulting in decreased production or increased degradation of these organelles, or both; (2) hydroquinone exposure can ultimately lead to the degradation of the melanocyte; and (3) keratinocytes are spared, showing no apparent injury [1].

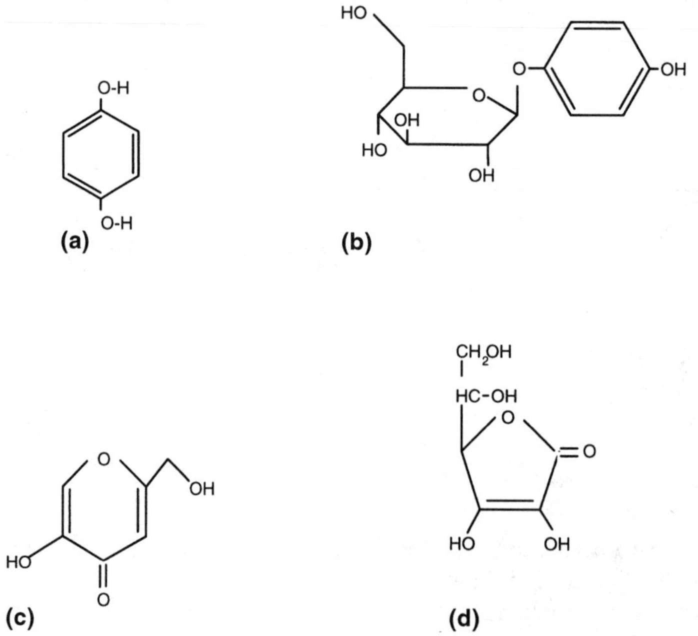

FIGURE 1   Chemical structures of (a) hydroquinone, (b) arbutin, (c) kojic acid, and (d) L-ascorbic acid (vitamin C).

Arndt and Fitzpatrick [4], in a non–placebo-controlled study, compared the efficacy of 2% and 5% hydroquinone cream for treatment of various pigmentary disorders in 56 patients. Results showed that hydroquinone was a moderately effective depigmenting agent in 80% of cases and that there was no difference between the two concentrations in therapeutic efficacy. Two percent hydroquinone was less irritating than 5%. Fitzpatrick et al. [5], in a non–placebo-controlled study, evaluated the efficacy of a 2% cream of stabilized hydroquinone in 93 patients. Sixty-four percent of them showed decreasing hypermelanosis without untoward effects. Sanchez and Vazquez [6] treated 46 patients with melasma using two versions of a 3% hydroalcoholic solution of hydroquinone. In this non–placebo-controlled study, overall improvement was noted in 88% of the patients and moderate-to-marked improvement in 36%. Side effects were minimal. The usage of a sunscreen agent was necessary for therapeutic efficacy. The efficacy of hydroquinone may be improved when it is used in combination with other chemicals as well as tretinoin, salicylic acid, or corticosteroid [1,2]. Kligman and Willis [7] noted an enhanced efficacy with 5% hydroquinone, 0.1% tretinion, and 0.1% dexamethasone in hydrophilic ointment for the treatment of melasma, ephelides, and postinflammatory hyperpigmentation in a non–placebo-controlled study. In contrast, they experienced poor results with each of the aforementioned as monotherapies. However, senile lentigines were resistant to this therapy. Gano and Garcia [8] conducted a 10-week clinical trial in 20 women with melasma. Topical applications of 0.05% tretinoin, 0.1% betamethasone valerate, and 2% hydroquinone were used in a non–placebo-controlled study. There was an objective improvement rate of 65% and a subjective improvement rate of 95%. Side effects were frequent but minimal. Caution is necessary when using potent fluorinated corticosteroids for prolonged periods on the face, because telangiectasia, atrophy, or acne rosacea can develop.

Pathak et al. [9] clinically tested the efficacy of hydroquinone in varying concentrations supplemented with corticosteroids or retinoic acid (tretinoin) in 300 Hispanic women with melasma in a non–placebo-controlled study, and concluded that cream or lotion formulations of 2% hydroquinone and 0.05 to 0.1% retinoic acid provided the most favorable results. In addition, avoidance of sun exposure and constant use of broad-spectrum sunscreens are necessary for the best therapy effects. Recently, Clarys and Barel [34] tested the efficacy of an ascorbate-phytohydroquinone complex in 14 patients with lentigo senile lesions in a non–placebo-controlled study. Objective skin-color changes were evaluated with a chromameter. After 1 month of treatment, a clear depigmentation of the macules was measured. None of the patients reported adverse effects.

Gellin et al. [35] established a reliable in vivo method to predict the depigmenting action of chemicals on mammalian melanocytes. They used black guinea pigs and black mice as animal models to screen the depigmenting capacity of several phenols, catechols, and organic antioxidants. Results showed that complete depigmentation on all test sites was achieved with monomethyl ether of hydroquinone and tertiary butyl catchall in the black guinea pig. Less-pronounced pigment loss was noted with these chemicals in black mice.

To treat some cases, higher concentrations of hydroquinone may be used. The formulations contain concentrations as high as 10% combined with nonfluorinated corticoid creams with or without the additional use of tretinoin or salicylic acid. Extemporaneously compounded preparations are often effective in patients that have failed to respond to lower concentrations of hydroquinone. With controlled use and monitoring, side effects from these preparations have proved minimal [2]. Note, however, that hydroquinone may be quickly oxidized in such formulations.

Hydroquinone occurs in nature as the beta-glucopyranoside conjugate arbutin. Arbutin is a safe and mild agent for treating cutaneous hyperpigmentation disorders, including melasma and UV-induced ephelides [10]. Arbutin is an active ingredient of the crude drug Uvae Ursi Folium-traditionally used in Japan and contained in the leaves of pear tees and certain herbs. The chemical structure of arbutin is shown in Figure 1. Maeda and Fukuda [10] determined the arbutin's inhibitory action on the melanin synthetic enzyme and its effects on melanin intermediates and melanin production in cultured human melanocytes. They indicated that the depigmentation effect of arbutin works through a inhibition of the melanosomal tyrosinase activity, rather than suppression of the expression and synthesis of tyrosinase in human melanocytes. Arbutin was much less cytotoxic than hydroquinone to cultured human melanocytes.

Adverse reactions associated with hydroquinone use include acute and chronic complications. Acute reactions include irritant dermatitis, nail discoloration, and postinflammatory hyperpigmentation [1]. Although commonly assumed to be a common allergen, the documentation of hydroquinone allergic contact dermatitis is weak [1]. Hydroquinone use can also induce hypopigmentation and, rarely, depigmentation of treated surrounding normal skin. However, these changes are temporary and resolve on cessation of hydroquinone treatment, in contrast to monobenzone use, which can cause permanent depigmentation [36]. Hence, the only indication for monobenzone therapy is in the treatment of severe vitiligo.

A more recent concern regarding the use of hydroquinone is the occurrence of hydroquinone-induced ochronosis, a chronic disfiguring condition resulting, in general, from the prolonged use of strong concentrations of hydroquinone [36]. Hydroquinone's acute and chronic toxicity toward higher terrestrial organisms appears to be minimal in humans

[20,21]. An epidemiologic investigation in 478 photographic processors has shown no significant excess mortality, sickness absence, or cancer incidence [20]. The reported nephropathy and cell proliferation, as evidence of carcinogenicity, observed in Fischer 344/N rats [22,23] appear to be strain and sex specific [23]. Hydroquinone was negative in the Ames/Salmonella and Drosophila genotoxicity assays [24]. Others suggest that carcinogenic and teratogenic potentials have been, at present inadequately studied [20,25], and that both hydroquinone and benzoquinone produce cytotoxic effects on human and mouse bone-marrow cells [26]. Hydroquinone readily penetrates human forehead skin in vivo following a single topical exposure in an alcoholic vehicle of 24-hour duration. Elimination was complete within 5 days [19]. Wester et al. [18] determined the topical bioavailability, metabolism, and disposition of hydroquinone on humans in vivo and in vitro; dose recovery in urine was 45.3%, of which the majority was excreted in the first 24 hours.

KOJIC ACID

Kojic acid, a fungal metabolic product, is increasingly being used as a skin-lightening agent in skincare products marketed in Japan since 1988. It was first isolated from Aspergillus in 1907 [31]. The structure is shown in Figure 1. The mode of action of kojic acid is to suppress free tyrosinase, mainly attributable to chelation of its copper [11,16,31], and it has been shown to be responsible for therapy and prevention of pigmentation, both in vitro and in vivo [11,31].

In Japan it is used in nonprescription skincare products up to a concentration of 1%. To increase percutaneous absorption and thus therapeutic activity, it is usually used at the highest concentration allowed [31]. Because it is used intensively in foods (e.g., bean paste, soy, and sake) in some countries, particularly Japan, its oral safety has been studied. Shibuya et al. [28], investigating the mutagenicity of kojic acid by the Ames test, forward mutation test in cultured Chinese hamster cells, and dominant lethal test in mice, concluded that, although kojic acid is a weak mutagen in bacteria, it is nonmutagenic in eukaryotic system either in vivo or in vitro. Abdel-Hafez and Shoreit [30] tested the mycotoxins using the dilution-plate method. Results showed that kojic acid may induce some toxins. Fujimoto et al. [32] examined the tumorigenicity of kojic acid in $B6C3F_1$ mice. Three groups of animals were given 0, 1.5, and 3.0% kojic acid–containing food for 6 weeks; kojic acid groups significantly induced thyroid tumors in $B6C3F_1$ mice. But true adverse effects after human oral ingestion have not been shown. Nakagawa et al. [31] noted that there were no signs of relapse of dermatitis or any other adverse effects on sensitized patients upon ingestion of foods containing kojic acid. However, they reported that topical application of kojic acid may induce allergic contact dermatitis with sensitized patients. They postulated that kojic acid was considered to have a high sensitizing potential, because of the comparatively high frequency of contactsensitivity in patients using 1 or more kojic acid–containing products. Recently, Majmudar et al. [37] used an in vitro model to evaluate the efficacy, stability, and cytotoxicity of whitening agents. They also conducted a non–placebo-controlled clinical study that indicated that kojic acid in an anhydrous base can induce more skin lightening than in the aqueous base.

ASCORBIC ACID (VITAMIN C) AND ITS DERIVATIVES

Ascorbic acid may inhibit melanin production by reducing *o*-quinones [12] so that melanin cannot be formed by the action of tyrosinase until all vitamin C is oxidized. The chemical structure of vitamin C is shown in Figure 1. Although the lightening effect of vitamin C is considered, it is quickly oxidized and decomposes in aqueous solution and is thus not generally useful as a depigmenting agent. Numerous stable derivatives of vitamin C have been synthesized to minimize this problem [12–14,17]. Magnesium-L-ascorby-2-phosphate (VC-PMG) is a vitamin-C derivative that is stable in water, especially in neutral or alkaline solution containing boric acid or its salt [12]. VC-PMG is hydrolyzed by phosphatases of liver or skin to vitamin C and thus exhibits vitamin C-reducing activity [12]. Kameyama et al. [12] investigated the effects of VC-PMG on melanogenesis in vitro and in vivo. Results from this non–placebo-controlled study suggested the topical application of VC-PMG was significantly effective in lightening the skin in 19 of 34 patients with chloasma or senile freckles, and in 3 of 25 subjects with normally pigmented healthy skin.

OTHER AGENTS

Various systemic drugs and natural products may be used as protective agents, such as chloroquine, indomethacin, vitamin C and E, fish oil, and green tea, etc. Topical agents include azelaic acid and melawhite except where previously described [38]. Recently, Kobayashi et al. [39] reported that neoagarobiose could be useful as a novel whitening agent as it has shown moisturizing and whitening effects with low cytotoxicity. Ando et al. [40] evaluated the effects of unsaturated fatty acids on UV-induced hyperpigmentation of the skin in a placebo (vehicle)-controlled study. Skin hyperpigmentation was induced on the backs of guinea pigs by UVB exposure. Oleic acid, linoleic acid, and α-linolenic acid (0.5% in ethanol), or ethanol alone as a control, were then topically applied daily five times per week for 3 successive weeks. Results suggest that the pigment-lightening effects of linoleic acid and α-linolenic acid are, at least in part, attributable to suppression of melanin production by active melanocytes as well as to enhanced desquamation of melanin pigment from the epidermis.

CONCLUSIONS

In general, skin-whitening products are considered modestly effective. High concentrations are not recommended except under a physician's supervision. The application as a combination with certain chemicals (retinoic acid and alpha-hydroxy acids) may enhance lightening. Optimal whitening agents remain a future goal.

REFERENCES

1. Engasser PG, Maibach HI. Cosmetics and dermatology: bleaching creams. J Am Acad Dermatol 1981; 5:143.
2. Grimes PE Melasma. Etiologic and therapeutic considerations. Arch Dermatol 1995; 131:1453.
3. Jimbow K, Obata H, Pathak MA, Fitzpatrick TB. Mechanism of depigmentation by hydroquinone. J Invest Dermatol 1974; 62:436.
4. Arndt KA, Fitzpatrick TB. Topical use of hydroquinone as a depigmenting agent. JAMA 1965; 194:965.
5. Fitzpatrick TB, Arndt KA, el-Mofty AM, Pathak MA. Hydroquinone and psoralens in the therapy of hypermelanosis and vitiligo. Arch Dermatol 1966; 93:589.
6. Sanchez JL, Vazquez MA hydroquinone solution in the treatment of melasma. Int J Dermatol 1982; 21:55.

7. Kligman AM, Willis I. A new formula for depigmenting human skin. Arch Dermatol 1975; 111:40.

8. Gano SE, Garcia RL. Topical tretinoin, hydroquinone, and betamethasone valerate in the therapy of melasma. Cutis 1979; 23:239.

9. Pathak MA, Fitzpatrick TB, Kraus EW. Usefulness of retinoic acid in the treatment of melasma. J Am Acad Dermatol 1986; 15:894.

10. Maeda K, Fukuda M. Arbutin: mechanism of its depigmenting action in human melanocyte culture. J Pharm Exp Ther 1996; 276:765.

11. Cabanes J, Chazarra S, Garcia-Carmona F. Kojic acid, a cosmetic skin whitening agent, is a slow-binding inhibitor of catecholase activity of tyrosinase. J Pharm Pharmacol 1994; 46:982.

12. Kameyama K, Sakai C, Kondoh S, Yonemoto K, Nishiyama S, Tagawa M, Murata T, Ohnuma T, Quigley J, Dorsky A, Bucks D, Blanock K. Inhibitory effect of magnesium L-ascorbyl-2-phosphate (VC-PMG) on melanogenesis in vitro and in vivo. J Am Acad Dermatol 1996; 34:29.

13. Nomura H, Ishiguro T, Morimoto S. Studies on L-ascorbic acid derivatives. II. L-ascorbic acid 3-phosphate and 3-pyrophosphate. Chem Pharm Bull 1969; 17:381.

14. Nomura H, Ishiguro T, Morimoto S. Studies on L-ascorbic acid derivatives. 3. Bis(L-ascorbic acid 3,3′)phosphate and L-ascorbic acid 2-phosphate. Chem Pharm Bull 1969; 17:387.

15. Nakajima M, Shinoda I, Fukuwatari Y, Hayasawa H. Arbutin increases the pigmentation of cultured human melanocytes through mechanisms other than the induction of tyrosinase activity. Pig Cell Res 1998; 11:12.

16. Kahn V. Effect of kojic acid on the oxidation of DL-DOPA, norepinephrine, and dopamine by mushroom tyrosinase. Pig Cell Res 1995; 8:234.

17. Morisaki K, Ozaki S. Design of novel hybrid vitamin C derivatives: thermal stability and biological activity. Chem Pharm Bull 1996; 44:1647.

18. Wester RC, Melendres J, Hui X, Cox R, Serranzana S, Zhai H, Quan D, Maibach HI. Human in vivo and in vitro hydroquinone topical bioavailability, metabolism, and disposition. J Toxicol Environ Health 1998; 54:301.

19. Bucks DAW, McMaster JR, Guy RH, Maibach HI. Percutaneous absorption of hydroquinone in humans: effect of 1-dodecylazacycloheptan-2-one (azone) and the 2-ethylhexyl ester of 4-(dimethylamino)benzoic acid (escalol 507). J Toxicol Environ Health 1988; 24:279.

20. Friedlander BR, Hearne FT, Newman BJ. Mortality, cancer incidence, and sickness-absence in photographic processors: an epidemiologic study. J Occup Med 1982; 24:605.

21. Pifer JW, Hearne FT, Swanson FA, O'Donoghue JL. Mortality study of employees engaged in the manufacture and use of hydroquinone. Int Arch Occup Environ Health 1995; 67:267.

22. English JC, Hill T, O'Donoghue JL, Reddy MV. Measurement of nuclear DNA modification by 32P-postlabeling in the kidneys of male and female Fischer 344 rats after multiple gavage doses of hydroquinone. Fundam Appl Toxicol 1994; 23:391.

23. English JC, Perry LG, Vlaovic M, Moyer C, O'Donoghue JL. Measurement of cell proliferation in the kidneys of Fischer 344 and Sprague-Dawley rats after multiple gavage administration of hydroquinone. Fundam Appl Toxicol 1994; 23:397.

24. Gocke E, King MT, Eckhardt K, Wild D. Mutagenicity of cosmetics ingredients licensed by the European community. Mutat Res 1981; 90:91.

25. Whysner J, Verna L, English JC, William GM. Analysis of studies related to tumorigenicity induced by hydroquinone. Regul Toxicol Pharmacol 1995; 21:158.

26. Colinas RJ, Burkart PT, Lawrence DA. In vitro effects of hydroquinone, benzoquinone, and doxorubicin on mouse and human bone marrow cells at physiological oxygen partial pressure. Toxicol Appl Pharmacol 1994; 129:95.

27. Goffin V, Pierard GE, Henry F, Letawe C, Maibach HI. Sodium hypochlorite, bleaching agents, and the stratum corneum. Ecotoxicol Environ Safety 1997; 37:199.

28. Shibuya T, Murota T, Sakamoto K, Iwahara S, Ikeno M. Mutagenicity and dominant lethal

test of kojic acid: Ames test, forward mutation test in cultured Chinese hamster cells and dominant lethal test in mice. J Toxicol Sci 1982; 7:255.

29. Wei CI, Huang TS, Fernando SY, Chung KT. Mutagenicity studies of kojic acid. Toxicol Letters 1991; 59:213.

30. Abdel-Hafez SI, Shoreit AA. Mycotoxins producing fungi and mycoflora of air-dust from Taif, Saudi Arabia. Mycopathologia 1985; 92:65.

31. Nakagawa M, Kawai K, Kawai K. Contact allergy to kojic acid in skin care products. Contact Dermatitis 1995; 32:9.

32. Fujimoto N, Watanabe H, Nakatani T, Roy G, Ito A. Induction of thyroid tumours in (C57BL/6N × C3H/N)F1 mice by oral administration of kojic acid. Food Chem Toxicol 1998; 36:697.

33. Strauch E, Burke P, Maibach HI. Hydroquinone. J Derm Treatment 2000. Submitted.

34. Clarys P, Barel A. Efficacy of topical treatment of pigmentation skin disorders with plant hydroquinone glucosides as assessed by quantitative color analysis. J Dermatol 1998; 25:412.

35. Gellin GA, Maibach HI, Mislaszek MH, Ring M. Detection of environmental depigmenting substances. Contact Dermatitis 1979; 5:201.

36. Grimes PE. Vitiligo. An overview of therapeutic approaches. Dermatol Clin 1993; 11:325.

37. Majmudar G, Jacob G, Laboy Y, Fisher L. An in vitro method for screening skin-whitening products. J Cosmet Sci 1998; 49:361.

38. Piamphongsant T. Treatment of melasma: a review with personal experience. Int J Dermatol 1998; 37:897.

39. Kobayashi R, Takisada M, Suzuki T, Kirimura K, Usami S. Neoagarobiose as a novel moisturizer with whitening effect. Biosci Biotechnol Biochem 1997; 61:162.

40. Ando H, Ryu A, Hashimoto A, Oka M, Ichihashi M. Linoleic acid and α-linolenic acid lightens ultraviolet-induced hyperpigmentation of the skin. Arch Dermatol Res 1998; 290:375.

50

Interactions with Hair and Scalp

Dominique Van Neste and Ghassan Shaker
Skinterface sprl, Tournai, Belgium

PSYCHOSOCIAL FACTORS INVOLVED IN HAIR COSMETICS

Haircare and psyche reciprocally reflect each other both positively and negatively (bad hair days). Contrary to the bad haircare and negligence of a depressed person or a man in grief, generally people tend to offer themselves the best of haircare when they are feeling happy or when they want to show their internal feelings to others through body language. This is particularly obvious during public appearances and important social gatherings (e.g., parties, marriage ceremonies). Haircare by itself can induce a state of self-confidence and may reflect social status. This may explain significant differences in shampooing regimens, which range from once or twice a week to once a day.

Hair is midway between nature and culture [1]. Haircare attitudes are different from one society to another regardless of economic differences, and from one person to another within societies; e.g., hair loss is not equally perceived by everybody in all societies in the same manner [2–5]. Some people are seriously psychologically affected and ready to spend a fortune in order to cope with the problem, whereas others just do not care at all. In the former group, styling is of high significance as is the selection of cosmetic agents.

The intersocial and interpersonal attitude of adult males towards greying of hair is quite evident, added to the difference in attitude between men and women toward the same problem. However, this is not an exclusivity of mankind; the social significance of hair/pelage/beard/crown is very pronounced in other mammals (e.g., primates, lions). Grooming in humans is specifically a private activity or limited to one professional body (hair stylists).

NATURAL PROPERTIES OF HAIR AND THEIR IMPORTANCE FOR HAIR APPEARANCE

Physical Properties of Hair as a Basis for Appearance and Perception

Optical properties (absorption and reflection of visible light); the role of pigmentation in inducing a contrast between skin and hair; and the role of cuticle, cortex, and medulla are some physical properties playing an important role in hair appearance and perception [6]. Apart from albinos, all normal subjects have melanin. The production of these pigments is genetically determined and results in the production of various proportions of the following: (1) eumelanin, which gives colors from brown to black; and (2) pheomelanin, which gives colors from yellow-red to red. The hair color of each individual depends on the preponderant type of melanin as well as its quantity and distribution in the skin and hair. Melanin is a polymer of high molecular weight, insoluble in water and most solvents. It originates from melanocytes located in the basal cell layer of the hair matrix. Melanogenesis involves a complex sequence of chemical reactions corresponding to an oxidative polymerization catalyzed by certain enzymes; these complex processing phases occur in small vesicles named melanosomes. An intimate relationship must exist between the factors controlling melanocytes and matrix cell activity, because melanosome and pigment transfer from the melanocyte to the hair matrix occur only during the anagen phase of the hair cycle. Hair color also varies with age. There is first an intensification and then a slowdown, or sometimes even a halt, in pigment formation despite the rather constant number of melanocytes. This points to functional and regulatory aspects.

Melanin granules are distributed throughout the hair cortex but in greater concentration towards the periphery [6]. The color of hair is an optical phenomenon attributable to the reflection and refraction of incident light from various interfaces, especially the bulk of melanin contained in the cortex. Newly formed unpigmented hair with no medulla appears yellowish rather than white. This is probably the intrinsic color of dense and well-organized arrangement of keratin fibers [6]. Another important physical factor that helps the ease with which hair can be styled and given a desired shape is the elimination of static electricity, which causes repulsion between individual hairs and is an obstacle to styling and arranging hair [7]. The development of electrical charges on hairs during combing and brushing is a complicated phenomenon that varies according to hair type, surface state, and the humidity of the surrounding environment. A product's antistatic properties can be assessed in vitro by measuring the electrical potential build-up of hair during combing. If opposed electric charges are face to face, matting of hair may occur. There is no way of untangling it and a substantial haircut is the only solution.

Mechanical Properties of Hair Appearance

Hair fibers are generally elliptical, with cross sections having minor and major axis ratio in the range of 0.63 to 0.91, the most elliptical being black hair, the most circular Asian hair. Resistance to longitudinal deformation, bending and torsion stiffness, and hold of set hair are related to fiber diameter. The relationship between the constraint and elongation obtained follows a curve of three regions (preyield, yield, and postyield) according to the stretching force [7]. Fiber breakage occurs mainly in the postyield region. The load values depend on the cohesion of α-keratin. All factors diminishing this cohesion bring the load value down, e.g., wet hair. Examination of load elongation curves helps in studying how hair behaves in the course of various hairdressing procedures including the wide range of temperature, humidity and chemical agents involved.

The hair shaft is a strong enough fiber. It behaves like reinforced wire. Curled black hair is fairly fragile because of the highly twisted configuration and flattening as opposed to Asiatic hair [7]. The disruptive load for hair varies with age, peaking at about 20 years of age.

The length of hair plays a role in perception. A typical example is when the hair is cut short, people usually interpret the perception of stubbles as thickening of the newly produced hair fiber. Instead of the soft feel of a nonchanging full head of hair, one now feels hair growing from day to day. Another misconception among lay people may be so explained: a haircut does not influence hair growth, it is just becoming noticeable.

SPECIFIC ACTIONS OF HAIR COSMETICS ON HAIR SURFACE (CUTICULA), CORTEX, AND MEDULLA

Desirable Actions

The intended desirable effects of cosmetics on hair are very wide and variable. Cleansing, dyeing, perming, bleaching, straightening, dressing, setting, and removing are some of the innumerable aims and claims of hair cosmetics. Some desirable actions are not achievable without inducing some kind of damage to the hair fiber itself, e.g., in permanent or oxidative hair dyeing a degree of damage to the hair cuticle is necessary to introduce the dyes that are targeting the hair cortex. The same is true for bleaching and perming. When the hair cuticle is weakened it cannot be fully restored (Fig. 1), but some cosmetic agents may decrease the abnormal fragility and the rough feel of damaged hair. No better results can be achieved than by cutting away the damaged fibers and letting new hair growth proceed without new harsh procedures (Fig. 2).

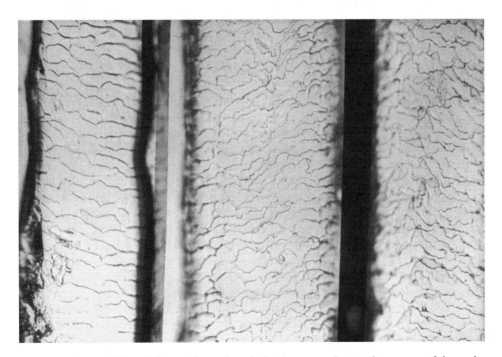

FIGURE 1 The condition of the cuticle on three hair segments taken at the merger of the scalp (left), 1 cm away from it (middle), and 3 cm away (right). Damage of the cuticular scale edges clearly occurs within 3–4 months of exposure to the environment.

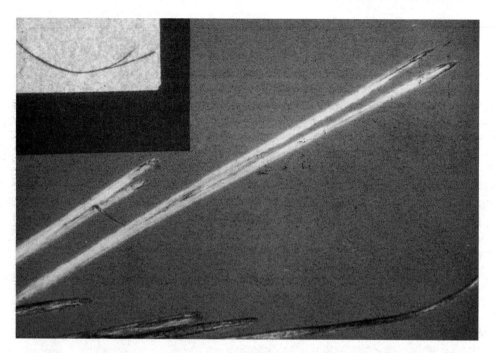

FIGURE 2 Trichoptilosis or split ends. These damaged hair tips frequently occur on long hairs. Lack of cuticle, which normally envelopes the hair fibers, exposes the cortex, a much weaker part of the hair shaft.

Undesirable Action

Hair cosmetics and shampoos in particular are formulated to be nontoxic, nonirritant, and nondamaging to the hair, skin, and eyes. These formulae should not of course, include substances that are systemically toxic following their percutaneous absorption. The integrity of the cuticle is degraded by perming, bleaching, and permanent dyeing, which lead to raising and softening of the cuticle thereby making it vulnerable to mechanical abrasion, e.g., during combing.

Scalp hair may be under excessive physical traction determined by fashion, e.g., tight rollers and tight hairstyles. This can result in temporary hair loss, and if continued over a long period will result in permanent hair loss (thinning). Some examples of this condition have been described by medical literature as chignon alopecia and frontoliminal alopecia.

The hair shaft can be damaged by previous permanent waving or bleaching and thus made more permeable to certain dyes, leading to some unexpected effects, e.g., greencolor from azo dyes, green hair from copper metallic salts, and red hair from chino form. The so-called Bird's Nest hair is a physical phenomenon of felting. This occurs when frictional forces are applied to physically damaged hair especially after the use of a cationic shampoo. A large tangled mass of hair is produced and defies all attempts to unravel it, and the mass has to be cut off. The process can be reproduced experimentally with normal hair. There is no evidence that subjects affected have especially susceptible hair [7].

SPECIFIC ACTIONS OF HAIR COSMETICS ON THE SKIN

Intended Contact with the Skin

Many cosmetic compounds target the skin rather than the hair. Antidandruff and antiseborrehic cosmetic compounds target the scalp skin, not the scalp hair. Many other cosmetics intend to modify the hair/skin system, e.g., preshave and aftershave lotions, along with depilatories, where the effect on hair is always associated with some effect on the skin.

Nonintended Contact with the Skin

Ideally, hair cosmetics should not have contact with the skin, but in practice this is hardly achievable. In some procedures, such as hair dyeing and hair bleaching, skin contact is unnecessary to perform the procedure itself but hardly avoidable during such a procedure.

Many consumers report hair shedding with changes in the shampooing regime. This is not because of a biological process in particular but because of a detachment of telogen hairs, which may modify the usual daily shedding of hair. Another reason for this is that when consumers change products, they tend to be more attentive to the condition of their hair and scalp and attribute any perceived change to the new product, especially if viewed as negative. Properly conducted trials showed that shampooing regimes did not modify hair shedding [8].

The aim of wet and dry shaving is to cut facial hair without harming the skin, which is a frequent adverse side effect of these procedures. These side effects vary in intensity, from a slight irritation—that is going to disappear with time during a process of adaptation—to a very severe and persistent reaction. This will mostly force the consumer to give up using that particular method and select a more "friendly" alternative.

Permanent wave solutions or their neutralizing chemicals can cause chemical burn or necrosis of the scalp epidermis if allowed to contact the scalp skin in certain concentrations for too long. The chemical burn may affect the skin of the scalp, forehead, face, and neck.

Physical burn can result from heated rollers or other apparatus that can cause damage to the superficial layers of the epidermis. The risk of burn also exists during or just after the use of flammable vehicles (e.g., alcoholic lotions) in close proximity to a fire or heat source.

Contact dermatitis to cosmetics in general and to hair cosmetics in particular is not uncommon in clinical dermatology. Following are leading examples from a long list of hair cosmetics reported to be skin sensitizers: hair dyes (p-phenylenediamine, resorcinol), shampoos (surfactants, zinc pyrithione, hydroxyquinolines), hair creams and gels (lanolin, parabens), hair lacquers (benzoin, cyclohexanone-formaldehyde resin), hair lotions (quinine, resorcinol), deodorants (hydroxyquinolines, Irgasan DP 300), bleachers, and shaving lotions (musk ambrette, antimicrobial agents) [9]. Acute and chronic allergic contact dermatitis have been associated with significant though usually transient or reversible hair loss [6]. This is a very often neglected or even unrecognized cause of diffuse hair loss [10].

The irritant effect of cleansing agents is attributable to the removal of surface lipid film and water-holding substances in the stratum corneum. They may denature protein and damage the cell membrane as well. The risk of irritant and allergic contact dermatitis induced by deodorants is greatly enhanced by the natural occlusive properties of body sites such as the armpits.

REFERENCES

1. Dawber R. Shampoos—scientific basis and clinical aspects. Proceedings of the Hair Care Forum Sponsored by Procter and Gamble Ltd, Florence, Italy. London: Royal Society of Medicine Press Limited, 1997.
2. Cash T. The psychological effects of androgenetic alopecia in men. J Am Acad Dermatol 1992; 26:926–931.
3. Cash T, Price V, Savin R. Psychological effects of androgenetic alopecia on women: comparisons with balding men and with female control subjects. J Am Acad Dermatol 1993; 29:568–575.
4. Passchier J. Quality of life issues in male pattern hair loss. Dermatology 1998; 197:217–218.
5. Girman C, Rhodes T, Lilly F, Guo S, Siervogel R, Patrick D, Chumlea W. Effects of self-perceived hair loss in a community sample of men. Dermatology 1998; 197:223–229.
6. Dawber R, Van Neste D, eds. Hair and Scalp Disorders. London: Martin Dunitz Ltd, 1995.
7. Zviak C. The Science of Hair Care. New York: Marcel Dekker, 1986.
8. Kullavanijaya P, Gritiyarangsan P, Bisalbutra P, Kulthanan R, Cardin CW. Absence of effects of dimethicone and non-dimethicone containing shampoos on daily hair loss rates. J Soc Cosmet Chem 1992; 43:195–206.
9. Rycroft RJG. Principle irritants and sensitizers. In: Rook, Wilkinson, Ebling, eds. Textbook of Dermatology. Vol. 1. Oxford: Blackwell Science, 1998:821–860.
10. Tosti A, Piraccini BM, Van Neste D. Telogen effluvium following allergic contact dermatitis of the scalp. Arch Dermatol. In press.

51

Hair Cosmetics

Leszek J. Wolfram
Independent Consultant, Stamford, Connecticut

INTRODUCTION

Throughout recorded history, hair has always been an important element of personal adornment. From the beautifully regular beard curls of the Assyrian kings to the elegant hair cuts of Egyptian pharaohs to the carefully coiffured wigs of the European nobility, hair has been shown, admired, and envied. Over the years, what had been the privilege of the affluent few has become an almost consuming passion of many. The explosive growth of the haircare market since the middle of the twentieth century is the result of deep, socioeconomic changes combined with an increasing focus on personal aesthetics, assisted by affordability of products. The attempt to satisfy the genuine needs of the consumer and the drive for competitive advantage among marketers has led to a variety of grooming aids and products, such as shampoos to cleanse the hair, hair conditioners to make it soft and combable, hair colorants and permanent waves to impart to hair properties it does not have, and hair sprays to keep hair in the desired style. Hair products are in the cosmetic category and, as such, are subject to all laws and regulations that control the labeling and claims of all cosmetic products.

The Structure and Properties of Hair

Hair follicles, which in tens of thousands are deeply invaginated in the scalp tissue, are the essential growth structures of hair. At the base of each follicle, the cells proliferate and, as they stream upwards, the complex and intertwined processes of protein synthesis, structural alignment, and keratinization transform the cytoplasm into the tough fibrous material known as hair. Hair is unique in that its structural and growth characteristics are different between races, sexes, individuals of the same race, areas in the same individuals, and even within the same follicle. The development of hair is a dynamic, cyclical process in which duration of the growth cycle depends not only on the body site, but also on such variables as the individual's age, nutritional habits, and hormonal factors. In the scalp, each hair grows steadily (about 1 cm per month) and continuously for 3 to 5 years (anagen phase); growth then stops and is followed by a brief transient stage (catagen) and a 2- to

4-month resting stage (telogen) during which the old hair is shed. With the onset of the anagen, the new hair starts to grow from the same follicle. The growth process functions independently in each follicle, so hairs are not shed simultaneously as they are in most animals. At any given time, some hairs are growing, some are resting, and some are being shed. Normally, of about 150,000 scalp hairs, 90% are in the anagen phase and the remaining 10% are in the catagen and telogen phases, with 50 to 100 hairs being shed daily. Scalp hair is a fiber of 50-80 µm in diameter and its exterior consists of a layer of flat, imbricated cuticle cells pointing outward from root to tip. This ratched-like structure of the cuticle scales serves as an effective self-cleaning feature and, by interlocking with the scales of the inner root sheath of the follicle, helps to hold the hair firmly in place. The cuticles are thin (0.5 µm), 50 to 60 µm square sheets, attached at their approximal ends to the underlying cortex. Their longitudinal overlap is substantial resulting in an average separation of scale edges of approximately 5 µm. This overlap generates a multilayered shield 3 to 4 µm thick around the hair fiber. The structure of the cuticle fulfills well the role of a protective barrier for hair. A thin film of covalently-bounded lipid on the exterior of the cuticle assures a low friction surface, together with water repellency. Just underneath, the highly cross-linked lamellae of the A-layer and exocuticle augment the mechanical stability of the scales, whereas the soft and water-absorbing endocuticle cushions effects of mechanical impact. The high water swellability of the endocuticle is the likely source of pronounced cuticle lifting on wetting of hair.

Enveloped by this formidable protective sheath of the cuticle layer is hair cortex, which constitutes the bulk of the fiber and is mainly responsible for the mechanical properties of hair. The spindle-shaped cortical cells are arranged parallel to the fiber axis, overlapping each other with frequent interdigitation. They have a unique arrangement of the constituent proteins, comprising intermediate filaments (IF), traditionally termed microfibrills, aligned in the direction of fiber growth and are surrounded by a matrix of IF associated proteins (IFAP). The filaments are composed of high–molecular weight protein chains of low sulfur (cystine) content and possess a high degree of molecular organization (α-helical), whereas the surrounding matrix of IFAP is made up of proteins more extensively cross-linked by cystine lacking definite structural pattern.

During the process of keratinization, the cell plasma membranes are modified to establish a strongly adhesive layer between the adjacent cells known as the cell membrane complex (CMC). This is the only continuous phase in the hair fiber providing adhesion between the cortical cells as well as between and with the cuticle cells.

Dispersed throughout the structure of cortex are melanin pigment particles. Their number, chemical characteristics, and distribution pattern determine the color of hair. In some hairs, coarse hairs in particular, vacuolated medulla cells are present in the central region of the fiber.

Although hair of different racial origin differs in shape, degree of curliness, and color, there is little difference in the underlying chemical properties and fiber structure. The amino-acid composition of the constituent proteins and most physical properties are similar [1,2]. The differences between hair of different ethnic groups are often smaller than the variation in the properties of hair taken from different individuals within one ethnic group.

Compared with Caucasian or Asian hair, African hair is more irregular in the shape of its cross-section. The sharp kinks seen in such hair are often associated with random unevenness of fiber diameter, resulting in weak spots along the fiber length. These are likely to cause problems during combing or chemical treatments.

SHAMPOOS

General Comments

Cleansing is clearly a dominant element of personal hygiene and, when reinforced by the aspect of attractive appearance, translates into a powerful and highly marketable stimulus. Shampooing has become, thus, a factor *sine qua non* in maintaining the aesthetics of hair.

The cleansing task is formidable. A mass of 100,000 to 150,000 flexible fibers has to be cleansed of oily deposits of sebum, sweat, entrapped desquamated scalp cells, along with the residues of mousses, gels, and hair sprays. All this has to be done within the span of a few minutes, leaving the individual hairs clean and free of tangles to which the ratched structure of hair cuticles makes it particularly vulnerable. It should also be kept in mind that although cleansing action is the fundamental assignment of a shampoo formulation, it is by no means the only goal. The promise of hair shine, softness, body, and manageability is inherently tied to product performance. Furthermore, one must not ignore the process of shampooing itself. It is expected to provide a pleasurable experience in working up a rich and lubricous lather that seems almost to caress the hair and leave it, after rinsing, with a touch of refreshing fragrance.

Hair Soiling and Soil Removal

In the course of its residence on the scalp, hair is exposed to a variety of events that contribute to its soiling. Among them are the innate processes of scalp desquamation, sweating, and sebum secretion, which are supplemented by deposition of extraneous substances arising either from environmental pollution (dust and other airborne contaminants) or from hair-grooming preparations, such as oils, waxes, hair spray, and mousse residues. Of all these, sebum, because of to its steady replenishment, greasy characteristics, high adhesiveness to hair, and ability to cement the other soil particulates together and to the hair surface, appears most insidious and thus it is not surprising that its efficacious removal is key in hair cleansing.

The sebaceous glands attached to each of the hair follicles provide a continuous supply [3] of this oily substance to the surface of hair. There are seasonal variations in the amount of sebum secreted [4], but more importantly its output is under hormonal control [3], reaching a maximum at puberty. Oily hair of adolescents is the obvious and often annoying consequence of the high activity of the sebaceous glands, and this at a time in one's life when personal adornment is particularly important. Sebum secreted from the sebaceous ducts spreads within the mass of hair primarily via physical contact between the fibers [5]. Brushing and combing (as well as contact with a pillow) further redistributes the sebum and partly assists in its removal. The quantity of sebum on hair at a particular moment thus reflects the relative efficacy of these two processes (sebum secretion and removal). The term ''oily hair'' often connotes a highly undesirable image of stringy and dull hair with little body and greasy feel. It is, however, worth bearing in mind that such a perception is not universal being strongly influenced by fiber texture and geometry. Thus, a visual appearance of curly African hair can visibly benefit from an increase in oiliness, a fact that is exploited in grooming products for such hair.

Because of the adhesiveness and sticky consistency of sebum-containing soil, its adequate removal by simple mechanical means is virtually impossible, and satisfactory cleansing can only be attained by use of aqueous solutions of detergents. In the broadest sense, all materials used in cleansing that are water and other solvents, soaps and synthetic surfactants, salts, and abrasives may be considered as detergents. However, more specifically, the term ''detergent'' is limited to those surface-active agents that, in addition to the property of lowering surface tension, are effective in deflocculating soil and dirt clumps and keeping them in suspension so that they can be washed away before redepositing on the surface that is being cleaned. This property is exhibited by compounds that contain both a hydrophilic group and a hydrophobic tail that serves as an emulsifying agent. In essence, the removal of soil from hair is governed by the same basic processes that had been previously identified as being involved in laundering of fabrics [6]. Without elaborating on theories underlying the detergency, one should allude to the three fundamental mechanisms that have been proposed to account for the cleansing action of detergents.

1. The ''roll-up'' mechanism [6], particularly relevant to oily deposits in which the progressive wetting of the fiber surface leads to rapid detachment of oil droplets;
2. In the micellar solubilization mechanism [7] the soil is solubilized into micelles that come into contact with the soiled surface. The efficacy of this cleansing mode depends on the availability of sufficient quantity (concentration) of micelles, which does not usually present a problem with conventional shampoo formulations; and
3. The third mechanism [8] invokes the dispersion and emulsification of soil particles penetrated by the diffusing detergent. The amphiphilic components of sebum might enhance cleansing by direct interaction with the molecules of the surfactant.

There is no precise information presently available as to which mechanism is dominant in hair cleansing. Quite possibly all three might be involved, depending on the characteristics of the soil. In any case, the vast majority of shampoo products are formulated to be operative under diverse conditions of detergent action, thus assuring their cleansing efficacy.

Shampoo Ingredients

Almost without exception, shampoos consist of an aqueous solution, emulsion, or dispersion of one or more surfactants together with some additives to enhance performance and aesthetic properties of the product. Additives are used to provide fragrance and color, thicken, opacify, and convey specific tactile attributes. They include stabilizers, foam modifiers, preservatives, conditioning, and antidandruff agents.

Surfactants

Surfactants are long-chain electrolytes and are usually classified according to the nature of their hydrophilic group, which may be anionic, nonionic, amphoteric, or cationic.

Anionic Surfactants

Soaps are salts of fatty acids and, not in the distant past, were the mainstay of shampoo products. In soft water, they lather copiously, cleanse well, and leave the hair in a well-conditioned style. Unfortunately, in hard water the lather is poor, and as the soap combines with calcium or magnesium salts present in hard water it deposits on hair a dulling film. The introduction of synthetic surfactants brought about the end of soap-based shampoos, although some products still contain a small quantity of soap to exploit its conditioning property.

Alkyl sulfates are the most widely used anionic in shampoos, displaying excellent foaming and cleansing properties unaffected by hard water. Lauryl sulfate is the dominate ingredient being present in most shampoo formulations in the form of its ammonium or triethanol ammonium salt at a level of 6 to 18% w/w. Although very effective cleansers, the alkyl sulfates, particularly at high concentrations, have a tendency to irritate the scalp and remove some lipid constituents of hair cuticle. To make the alkyl sulfate-based shampoos milder, they are frequently modified by incorporation of less-irritating alkyl ether sulfates or amphoteric surfactants.

Alkyl ether sulfates are sulfated products of ethoxylated fatty alcohols. They are more water soluble than alkyl sulfates, are excellent solubilizers for fragrances and other oleophilic additives, and are particularly suitable for formulations of clear shampoos. As alluded to earlier, these surfactants are less irritating than the alkyl sulfates and are used, at a higher degree of ethoxylation, in baby shampoos.

Alpha-olefin sulfonates are complex mixtures resulting from sulfonation of alpha-olefins. These detergents exhibit excellent foaming in the presence of sebum, are effective over a wide range of pH, and compare favorably with other surfactants in dermal and eye irritation [9].

Other anionic surfactants worthy of note include alkyl monoglyceride sulfates and alkyl sulfosuccinates. Both are very mild to the skin and, although the former are good foamers and can be used in shampoo formulation in their own right, the latter are primarily used in combination with alkyl sulfates.

Nonionic Surfactants

They are considered to be the mildest of surfactants. Although poor foamers, owing to their good solubilizing and dispersing properties, they have been extensively utilized to supplement the action of the primary cleanser.

Alkanolamides are prepared by condensation of fatty acid (usually lauric) and primary or secondary alkanolamines. Their presence in a shampoo formulation can have a pronounced effect on stabilizing the foam level and improving lather consistency. *Amino oxides* are formed by oxidation of tertiary fatty amines and are used in shampoos primarily as foam modifiers and as antistatic agents to improve the overall manageability of hair.

Polyethoxylated surfactants represent the largest group of nonionics and include the ethoxylated derivatives of alkylphenols, fatty alcohols, fatty esters, and diglycerides. They exhibit excellent detersive power and cleansing properties, but because of poor foaming, their use has been restricted to solubilizing of shampoo fragrances and other oleophilic additives.

Amphoteric Surfactants

Often referred to as ampholytic, these surfactants contain both cationic and anionic groups in one molecule. Because the charge of these surfactants are pH dependent, their properties, such as foaming potential, solubility, and CMC, also vary with the change in pH. Most amphoterics are derivatives of imidazoline or betaine. They are quite compatible with anionic, nonionic, or cationic surfactants, and have been extensively used to formulate mild (baby) shampoos or as mollifying agents in the more irritating anionic compositions.

Shampoo Additives

These are materials incorporated into a shampoo formulation to enhance its aesthetics as well as improve its performance.

Thickeners comprise a broad variety of compounds that are used to increase viscosity of the formulations, modifying their consistency from viscous liquids to thick gels. Among the most frequently used are electrolytes, such as sodium chloride, alkanolamides and water-soluble cellulose derivatives, such as carboxymethylcellulose, hydroxyethylcellulose, carboxy vinyl polymers of the Carbopol type, polyvinyl alcohols, and natural gums, such as tragacanth. Magnesium aluminum silicates have found application as thickeners and suspending agents in antidandruff shampoos.

Opacifiers serve to impart to shampoo a pearlescent or opaque appearance. For this purpose, high-melting, wax-like materials are blended into formulations. Of particular utility in this respect are cetyl and stearyl alcohols and their esters as well as the latex emulsions of vinyl-, styrene-, and acrylic polymers.

The shampoo milieu offers itself as an ideal ground for microbial growth, particularly of the aerobic gram-negative organisms of Pseudomones. This may have a deleterious effect on the shampoo properties, posing at the same time a health hazard to the consumer. The function of preservatives is to inhibit such bacterial development. Although formaldehyde has been one of the most popular and effective preservatives, its use has declined as other compounds have come to the fore. Examples include methyl and propyl parabenes, DMDM hydantoin, quaternium-15, imidazolidynyl urea and others. The selection of a suitable preservative is made through a challenge test in which the product is subjected to the worst possible conditions anticipated during manufacture, shelf storage and actual use.

Other additives. Fragrance is an essential ingredient, often deciding the market appeal and success of the product. Addition of alcohols (ethanol, isopropanol) or glycols may be required to maintain the clarity of clear shampoos, while the presence of sequestering agents like EDTA prevents the formation of insoluble calcium or magnesium soaps when the shampoo is rinsed off the hair. FD&C and D&C dyes are commonly added to enhance the aesthetics of shampoo formulations. "Squeaky" clean feel of shampooed hair is frequently accompanied by difficult combing and substantial "fly away." To overcome this, the shampoos contain "conditioning" additives that are substantive to hair remaining adsorbed on the surface after rinsing. A plethora of materials has been used to this end. To these belong amine oxides, protein hydrolysates, cationic surfactants, cationic polymers, lanolin and its derivatives, as well as natural materials, such as beer, honey, and egg.

Shampoo Formula

It must have become clear from the foregoing that a shampoo product, although straight forward in its purpose, is a complex blend of ingredients carefully chosen and attuned to effectively address the need of individual consumers. Table 1 shows the nature and relative concentration of materials contained in a typical shampoo formulation:

Specialty Shampoos

Baby shampoos place stringent requirements for nonirritancy of the scalp and eye. The majority of products are based on amphoteric detergent systems. Thus, derivatives of

TABLE 1 Typical Shampoo Formulation

Ingredient	Weight %	Function
Ammonium lauryl sulfate	10–20	Primary cleanser
Lauramide DEA	3–5	Foam stabilizer
Methyl paraben	0.08	Preservative
Propyl paraben	0.05	Preservative
Sodium chloride	0.5–1.5	Thickener
Disodium EDTA	0.2	Sequesterant
Fragrance	0.5	Fragrance
FD&C Yellow No. 5	0.001	Colorant
D&C Orange No. 4	0.002	Colorant
Water	to 100.00	Dilutent

imidazoline, betaine, and sulfobetaine are usually combined with nonionic surfactants of the polyoxyethylated alcohol esters class to procure sting-free formulations.

Medicated dandruff shampoos are designed to lessen and alleviate the excessive desquamation of the scalp via inclusion of specific ingredients. These include antimicrobials, such as quaternary ammonium salts; keratolytic agents, e.g., salicylic acid and sulfur, or antiseborrheic compounds like coal tar and resorcinol. Over the past 20 years, the shampoos containing selenium sulfide or zinc pyrithione as anti-dandruff actives have greatly risen in popularity, reflecting both the efficacy of the products and aesthetics of the formulations.

Although so-called conditioning shampoos, or *two-in-one shampoos*, have been on the market for a number of years, offering the feature of hair cleansing and conditioning in a single step, the early versions of such products did not perform to consumers' satisfaction leaving the hair often undercleansed and overconditioned. It was not until the mid-1980s that significant improvements in performance were achieved by emulsifying silicones into an anionic shampoo base. Such products have proved to be efficacious cleansers, and the shampooed hair feels soft and silky and is easy to comb. In some recent renditions of two-in-one products, the silicones have been replaced by quaternized guar gums, cationic polymers, and guaternaries.

Product Forms

In general, the shampoo formulations are relatively simple aqueous systems and, as such, quite amenable to modulation of their physical forms. The latter are often the consequence of market considerations of consumer preferences. Thus, the clarity of clear liquid shampoos conveys the impression of superior cleansing whereas opaque formulations of similar or slightly higher viscosity are suggestive of conditioning qualities. Clear gels are usually sold in compact flexible tubes that are convenient for storage and travel. A class apart are the aerosol dry shampoos that continue to occupy a small niche in the shampoo category. They consist of oil-absorbing powders, such as starch, talc, or clay, which are sprayed on to the hair and after a short while removed by brushing or combing.

Evaluation and Safety

As the work progresses at the formulator's bench, the efficacy of developed shampoo prototypes is being evaluated in the laboratory using established testing procedures. Thus, foamability and lather characteristics are measured in the presence and absence of sebum, gaining some insight into the detersive aspects of the formulas. The properties of shampooed hair, with respect to its luster, combability, body, and fly-away, are instrumentally assessed together with the subjective evaluation of hair appearance. The ultimate proof, however, of the potential success of the formulation is in the practical use. Thus, the consumer evaluation of the product either with outside panelists or in-house testing facility is imperative. The preference of consumers for a particular fragrance is of vital importance and their comments as to the aesthetic characteristics of shampoo and the feel of shampooed hair when combined with the results of laboratory tests provide firm ground for potential product claims.

Shampoo ingredients do not pose a particular hazard with regard to skin or eye safety. The contact time is short and a water rinse follows. The irritation potential of some surfactants has already been alluded to. It is a common practice for most of the manufacturers to make provisions to evaluate their product for skin and eye irritation.

HAIR CONDITIONERS

It is worth noting that the subject of hair ''condition'' appears to be restricted almost entirely to the domain of women's hair. Although, as a woman's ''crowning glory'' the hair evokes in her a particularly profound concern for its beauty, there are at work some more mundane factors. Unlike men's hair, that of a woman's is subject to more frequent and diverse assaults that are injurious to its properties. It is perhaps ironic that except for environmental effects (weathering), most of these are associated with what we call the ''haircare'' practices. Thus, the handling of hair in the course of its daily shampooing, combing and brushing, and blow drying cause, even in the case of intact hair, gradual abrasion of the hair cuticle signaling the onset of hair damage. This process of cuticle loss is particularly evident in longer hair leading often to the generation of split ends. Hair coloring, bleaching, waving, or straightening, although imparting to hair a much sought after different or novel appearance, impair the surface lipid layer of the cuticles, further aggravating the abrasive effects of daily hair regimens. Although gradual, these deleterious effects are additive and further exacerbated by sun exposure.

Clearly, by the use of conditioning shampoos, avoiding practices singularly injurious to the cuticle, such as teasing, and keeping the hair relatively short and shielded from sun, one might, for a considerable length of time, maintain the intact hair in satisfactory condition. Alternatively, one can go a step further and by the use of products designed explicitly for conditioning supplement the benefits obtained from a shampoo and significantly extend their range. A good conditioner eliminates tangling, makes the hair easy to comb and style, eliminates static charge, and, by fostering fiber alignment, enhances the luster and shine of hair. The soft feel of hair and improved manageability are additional important attributes of conditioned hair. It is important to stress that these effects are universal, i.e., irrespective of cosmetic history of hair, whether the hair is intact, waved, colored, or bleached, the conditioner delivers its benefits.

Two general forms of conditioners are currently in use: 1) hair rinses and 2) leave-in products, often referred to as ''deep'' conditioners. Both are applied to freshly shampooed hair. True to their name, the rinse product is rinsed off after a few minutes, whereas the leave-in product is left on the hair for up to 30 minutes, after which it is rinsed off. The purpose of the longer time is to allow the product to penetrate further (thus the name ''deep'') into the hair shaft thereby extending the conditioning effects.

The active ingredients in most conditioners are based on quaternary ammonium salts (cationic surfactants) such as steartrimonium chloride and, cetrimonium chloride, and the like. Because of their great affinity for hair, these compounds bind strongly to the cuticles, providing a low-friction surface, thus making the cuticles slick and less prone to abrasion. Other components present in the conditioning formulations, such as fatty amines, fatty alcohols, and amine oxides, supplement the action of cationic surfactants, adding primarily to the tactile benefits. The leave-in conditioners that are recommended for use on damaged hair frequently contain protein and lanolin derivatives.

Conditioning effects are usually lost in shampooing, and a reapplication is recommended to reinforce the protective effect. Conditioning formulations containing cationic polymers are somewhat longer lasting. The same is true for conditioners based on emulsions of polymeric silicones.

HAIRDRESSINGS

Hairdressing is a broad term describing products applied for final grooming. Including brilliantines, tonics, and gels, this category follows new fashions, hairstyle trends, and is attuned to progress in styling techniques. Hairdressings are applied by spreading the product through the hair with the fingers and then combing through for an even distribution. As they are not rinsed off after application, care must be taken to avoid excessive build-up.

The primary purpose of brilliantines is to add sheen to hair. Thus, the main constituent of these products is oil—usually mineral oil—which is spread on fiber strands increasing their luster and providing grooming effects. Solid brilliantines (pomades) are based on petrolatum to which various waxes are added to attain the desired consistency and texture. Tonics might be viewed as lighter versions of brilliantines and usually consist of alcoholic solutions of various oils. The alcohol wets the hair and after evaporation leaves a thin film of oil. By using synthetic, rather than natural oils, much less greasy formulations can be obtained. Using a high concentration of ethoxylated emulsifiers, grooming oils can also be readily blended into clear gels. On the other hand, setting gels based on hydroalcoholic solutions of carboxyvinyl polymers or methylcellulose ethers are oil free. They range in consistency from liquid to rigid gels and provide a good range of textures, volume, and hold.

Styling Products

Whereas most of the styling needs of short hair are satisfactorily met by a good haircut, those with longer hair require more effort which is, however, well rewarded by the diversity of styles that can be imparted. The underlying principle of all styling processes is hair setting and a few comments on the subject seems appropriate. Hair fibers are flexible and elastic, and when dry bounce back immediately to their original configuration (straight or curly) when bent, extended, or twisted. On wetting, however, they become pliant and malleable and can be readily molded (set) to almost any desired form. On drying, they retain the new shape until exposed to water (moisture) again.

The primary function of all styling products is to assist in the setting process and/or to ensure the stability of the newly imparted configuration. Depending on the type of styling product, different mechanism of action are operative.

Styling Aids

As the name implies, the role of these products are first to facilitate styling the hair and second to keep it in a newly styled shape. Three general product forms represent this category: styling gels, mousses, and styling sprays. Most of the formulations are based on synthetic film-forming polymers and contain a variety of additives to improve film properties and performance. Thus, phtalates and glycols are used as plasticizers. Lanolin derivatives and silicones are added to improve feel and impart some resistance to moisture. The products are applied to wet hair which is styled with fingers or a comb. Usually the more viscous the product, the easier it is to style the hair. As the hair dries and sets in the desired configuration, a polymeric film forms on the surface of hair, cementing adjacent fibers together and thus further stabilizing the newly imparted style.

Table 2 serves as an example of typical styling formulations for a styling gel and a styling mousse.

Hairsprays

Also in this category, polymeric film formers are the backbone of the formulations, although both the intended use and the mode of action are somewhat different from those of styling aids.

These products are applied to dry and already styled (set) hair in the form of fine mist or spray. The spray droplets collide with and become deposited on hair fibers. As they spread on the hair surface, they tend to migrate and accumulate at the points where adjacent fibers are very close or intersect with each other. This results in the formation of minute joints distributed throughout the hair mass. As the solvent evaporates, these joints become rigid bonds welding the fibers together and, thus, preventing the motion of individual hairs relative to each other. This cumulative restraining action of hundreds of

TABLE 2 Typical Formulas of Styling Aids

Ingredient	Weight %	Function
Styling Mousse		
Polyquaternium-11	1.4	Styling ease
Polyquaternium-4	0.6	Film former
Lauramide DEA	0.2	Foam stabilizer
Isosteareth-10	0.2	Foam stabilizer
Dimethicone copolyol	0.15	Styling ease
Fragrance	0.2	Fragrance
DMDH hydantoin	0.2	Preservative
Methyl paraben	0.1	Preservative
Isobutane/propane blend	7.0	Propellant
Water	to 100.00	Solvent
Styling Spray		
Ethylester of PVM/MA copolymer	2.5	Film former
Dimethicone copolyol	0.3	Styling ease
Isopropyl alcohol	5.0	Solvent
Fragrance	0.3	Fragrance
Ethanol	45.0	Solvent
Water	to 100.00	Solvent

such microscopic welds throughout the hair assembly accounts for the style-stabilizing performance of hair sprays, protecting the hair from mechanical deformation,wind, and humidity.

The strength of these hairspray bonds depends on a number of factors, of which the nature of the polymeric resin is of paramount importance. Most of the polymers used form adequately strong bonds at low relative humidity (RH). As the RH increases beyond 80%, however, most resins begin to absorb moisture from the environment, softening the welds. At the same time, water absorption by hair causes rapid relaxation of the set configuration of the fibers and it is the tenacity of the hairspray welds alone that stabilizes the imparted style. Clearly, the polymers that are least sensitive to the plastizing effect of water are likely to be the better performers and are thus preferred for a hairspray product.

It should be stressed that in addition to the intrinsic strength of the resin, other factors may affect bond formation and/or bond toughness. For example, the characteristics of the solvent system used to deliver the resin to hair plays an important role. Efficient weld formation depends on the wetting and spreading properties of the resin droplets on the hair surface. As mentioned earlier, the welds are formed by the accumulation of liquid spray at contact points between fibers. Thus, an aerosol formulation with 30% alcohol and 70% highly volatile propellant will dry much faster than a solvent vehicle with 50% or more alcohol. As the solvent evaporates, the viscosity of droplets increases and mobility decreases. This reduced mobility results in relatively small bonds between adjacent or intersecting fiber which might negatively affect the product performance. One might be led to a conclusion that the spray that stays ''wetter'' longer generates better performing welds. This may hold true for nonaqueous systems as the organic solvents used in hair formulation do not have any adverse effect on the set of the styled hair. With the hydro-alcoholic systems, however, and the water content of over 20% the long ''residence'' time of hairspray droplets on hair may lead to a significant loss of set caused by the selective water absorption by hair fibers.

Although a number of hairspray resins have been developed over the years and many of them have been in use, the combination of regulatory restrictions and increased demands on the aesthetics of product performance has narrowed the field somewhat. Thus the butyl and ethyl esters of poly (vinyl methyl ether/maleic anhydride) copolymers, which for years have been the most widely used polymers in hair sprays, have suffered a rapid decline, being surpassed by octylacrylamide/acrylates/butylaminoethyl methacrylate copolymer. The latter provides excellent holding properties at relatively low resin concentration. For the aerosol hairsprays, the resin of choice is vinyl acetate/crotonates/neodecanoate, which, by modulation of the extent of its neutralization, can substantially modify the film properties.

Essential as it is, the set holding is not the only attribute that has to be considered in formulating hair sprays. Clearly, the aesthetic aspect of sprayed hair cannot be neglected. Thus, the resin film should add shine (gloss) and not dull the hair, nor should the hair become tacky in humid weather. It should resist flaking, but be readily removed by shampoo. By selection of appropriate additives and solvents, both the holding and aesthetic goals can be readily attained. Table 3 provides ingredient listings for typical aerosol and pump sprays.

Safety and Regulatory Issues

All aerosol hairsprays, whether containing hydrocarbon or carbon dioxide propellant, are classified as flammable by virtue of their flame propagative properties. The same is true

TABLE 3   Typical Hair Spray Formulas

Ingredient	Weight %	Function
Aerosol Hairspray		
Poly(vinyl methyl ether)-maleic anhydride ethyl ester	5.0	Film former
Amino methyl propanol	0.2	Neutralizing agent
Dimethyl phthalate	0.4	Plasticizer
Fragrance	0.2	Fragrance
Ethanol	70.0	Solvent
Isobutane/propane	24.2	Propellant
Pump Hairspray		
Octylacrylamine/acrylates/butyl amino ethyl methacrylate copolymer	3.5	Film former
Amino ethyl propanol	0.5	Neutralizing agent
Cetearyl octanoate	0.1	Plasticizer
Fragrance	0.15	Fragrance
Ethanol	80.00	Solvent
Deionized water	15.75	Solvent

of pump sprays on account of their high alcohol content. Appropriate warnings should be displayed on the package informing of potential eye irritancy of the product.

Federal regulation in 1978 that banned the use of chlorofluorocarbons in hairsprays brought about a drastic change in the technology of aerosol hairsprays. New propellants had to be evaluated and formulations developed to accommodate their different properties. The hydrocarbon gases, such as propane, butane, and isobutane have been found to generate the most consistent hairspray pattern, being at the same time compatible with alcohol and current hairspray resins. However, in 1990, both California and New York introduced the concept of volatile organic component (VOC) placing strict limits on allowable VOC content in hair sprays. As the VOC is defined as any organic compound having between 1 and 12 carbon atoms, the VOC restrictions also affect the nonaerosol hairsprays where the ethanol is both the resin solvent and propellant. The decrease in VOC levels is primarily compensated for by the increase in water content of the hairspray, making it wetter, less efficacious, and sticky leaving aside the less aesthetic delivery characteristics. A search is underway to develop new resins that accommodate the high–water content formulas with performance standards equal or approaching those of current sprays.

Permanent Waving

It was perceived a long time ago that wavy hair not only surpasses straight hair in opportunities for more diverse styling, but because of its geometry, it appears more luxurious and, thus, highly desirable. Early records show that the ancient Assyrians wore a mass of curls falling over their shoulders and the beards of men displayed exquisite and highly uniform wave patterns. The earliest recorded methodology of hair waving can be traced to Egyptians who curled their hair with mud and then dried it in the hot sun. The elaborate coiffures of Roman women relied on prototypes of the curling iron. Then, with the advances of the Middle Ages, hair virtually disappeared from view and did not make its reemergence until the time of the Renaissance. But then shortly it hid again—this time under wigs. The latter, made of human hair, were processed to desired configurations by techniques not greatly different from those developed by Egyptians and Romans. It was not until the early 20th century and the pioneering work of Nessler on hot waving that generated stimuli for affordable and simple waving procedures. Basic precepts of modern permanent waving were developed in the 1930s. Over the years, these principles have been further explored and creatively utilized to yield safe and efficacious products.

Hair-Waving Process

The immediate objective of waving is to impart to hair a durable configuration that is different from what the hair exhibits in its native form. Each hair has a geometry that is the result of processes of keratinization and follicular extrusion that transforms a viscous mixture of proteins into strong, resilient, and rigid keratin fiber. In principle, waving can be viewed as a combination of reversal and a stepwise restaging of these processes, as it entails softening of keratin, molding it to a desired shape, and annealing the newly imparted geometry. The underlying mechanism of waving is, thus, essentially molecular and involves manipulation of physicochemical interactions that stabilize the keratin structure.

It might be useful at his point to emphasize the essential difference between waving and setting of hair. Although both cases involve the impartation of new geometry to hair, only water-labile bonds are manipulated in setting, and thus the imparted geometry is moisture sensitive and lost on shampooing. In waving, both the covalent and secondary bonds are involved and the new geometry is stable to repeated washing cycles. The cleavage of covalent bonds (disulphide cross-links of cystine) is conveniently attained by reducing agents that convert them to cysteine residues that can be relinked in the last phase (neutralization step) of the waving process.

In a typical waving procedure, freshly shampooed, damp (but not wet) hair is separated into 30 to 60 tresses. Each tress is wetted with the waving lotion and wound onto plastic rods or curlers with the help of a porous end paper or sponge. The size of the curler determines the character of the resulting wave; the smaller the curler, the tighter the wave. After 10 to 20 minutes, the hair is rinsed thoroughly and, while still on rods, wetted with the neutralizing lotion. The hair is then unwound, rinsed again, and either freely dried or set in the desired style. The waving procedure depends on the type of the waving product used and the desired end result. Thus, instead of wrapping with lotion, the hair can be wound wet and the lotion applied to curled hair. Sometimes a suggestion for a "creep" step is made to obtain a tighter and longer lasting curl. This involves an approximate 30-minute wait between rinsing off the lotion and application of the neutralizer.

The tight curl produced by permanent waving is frequently not the configuration desired for the final hairstyle. Often a water set of a larger curl configuration is superimposed on the wave. Then, as the temporary set begins to relax under the influence of moisture, the change of the hair form towards the tighter, waved configuration counterbalances the forces to straighten the hair with the net result of a greater set stability and more body than if the hair had not been waved.

Waving with Mercaptans as the Active Ingredients

European, American, and large segments of the Asian markets are dominated today by the formulations based on thioglycolic acid (TGA) and its derivatives. The popularity of TGA stems from a number of factors. The long history of use has built an impressive evidence of adequate medical safety. The incidence of injury has been extremely low and so has been the frequency of sensitization. High adaptability of TGA to various formulation types that provided markedly different end benefits coupled with performance reliability and a low price all contributed to its success. The unpleasant odor of TGA has remained it most perceptible drawback. Although some progress has been made in the fragrancing of TGA-based lotions, the results so far are at best mediocre.

Conventional waving lotions contain 0.5 to 0.8M TGA adjusted to pH 9.1 to 9.5. The neutralizing base can be ammonia, alkanol amines, sodium carbonate, or a mixture thereof. Ammonia appears to be more effective than the other bases in facilitating diffusion of TGA through hair. It is also preferred over nonvolatile amines because it escapes during processing and the resultant drop in pH reduces the activity of the lotion with time and thus minimizes the danger of overprocessing.

Over the years, several TGA derivatives (primarily amides and esters) have been tried, but as of now, only one—glyceryl monothioglycollate (GMTG)—is of practical importance and used in so-called acid waves. In terms of waving performance, GMTG works better than TGA at *low pH* under such conditions, however, the resulting wave lacks the crispness and durability of the conventional alkaline TGA wave. This is somewhat compensated for by less hair damage. To increase the efficacy of GMTG, the waving process is often carried out with the aid of heat.

Apart from the weaker waving performance of GMTG, when compared with TGA there are several other disadvantages associated with the use of this mercaptan. Its low water solubility and propensity for hydrolysis necessitates a separate package (container), which represents inconvenience for the consumer and additional cost. Occasional reports of skin sensitization has limited the use of GMTGA to salon applications. Finally, its rather pungent odor has a tendency to stay on the hair even after the neutralization step. Perhaps because of its hydrophobic character, GMTGA may be tightly bound to the apolar domains of the keratin structure, and therefore be more resistant to rinsing.

There are on the market several types of TGA-based formulations that claim point of difference from the conventional lotions. One is called a ''self-timing'' wave, the other a ''self-heating'' or ''exothermic'' wave. Both use TGA under alkaline conditions. The self-timing wave contains, however, dithiodiglycollic acid (DTDGA), which is the oxidation product of TGA. The function of DTDGA is to prevent hair overprocessing without negatively affecting the waving performance. In the United States self-timing formulations command approximately 20% of the market share.

The exothermic wave product contains a small vial of aqueous H_2O_2 (separate from the neutralizer), which is to be added to the waving lotion just before its use. Oxidation of TGA (which in this case is in excess of concentration required for waving), generates some heat as well as small quantities of DTDGA. Although the warmth can be readily perceived on mixing, the heat dissipates quickly as the lotion is applied to hair and equilibriates itself with that of the environment.

The acid wave based on TGA is a conventional TGA formulation adjusted to a lower pH (6.8-8). Unlike the acid wave with its esters (GMTGA), these formulations perform poorly and often require heat to improve the result.

In the Far East, particularly in Japan, the use of cysteine as a waving agent is widespread. This amino acid is claimed to provide a 'natural' and nonodorous alternative to TGA and to wave the hair without damage. Although some of these assertions are doubtlessly true, the waving efficacy of cysteine is mediocre. One can significantly increase its efficacy by the incorporation of a high concentration of urea (2-3M). Most of the Japanese formulations contain, apart from cysteine, hefty amounts of TGA as the effective ingredient.

Waving Formulations with Sulfite as the Active Ingredient

Sulfite, as a permanent setting agent, has found wide application in the wool industry (pleating, lustering, flat setting) well ahead of TGA on account of its effectiveness and lack of odor. Sporadic attempts to use it as a waving agent had not been very successful until the late 1970s when it was successfully introduced. The rapid rise of sulfite products appeared initially to spell demise for conventional TGA formulations. Readily consumer-perceptible attributes, such as lack of odor and low hair damage, combined with the then preference for softer hairstyles greatly favored sulfite systems. A number of companies rushed to the market with offerings of formulations for tight curls, body waves, and hair straighteners. However, attractive as these formulations appeared to be, they could not match the waving efficacy or durability aspects of TGA systems. The TGA-based products regained their ubiquity, although the sulfite product held on to a stable, though small, market share.

It appears appropriate at this junction to re-emphasize that the current methodology of hair waving (ambient temperature, medically safe reagents, short treatment time) relies heavily on the disulfide bond reactivity as the cornerstone of the process. The reductive cleavage of disulfide cross-links is as essential to fiber softening as is their reformation to the stability of newly imparted configuration. Needless to say, throughout the waving process, secondary interactions (hydrogen bonds, salt links, Van der Waals interaction) participate therein, and their more or less intense contributions reflect themselves in the overall efficacy of the process. Nevertheless, so far it is the disulphide bonds that represent the *sine qua non* condition for waving.

Over the years, there have been numerous attempts to explore the ways of permanently altering the configuration of keratin fibers by exclusive manipulation of secondary bonds. Some success has been shown in fibers modified by inclusion of bulky apolar residues, high-temperature steam setting, or by blocking cysteine side chains with hydrophobic maleimides. Except for high-temperature steam setting of wool (in the crimping process), these approaches found little, if any, practical applications either because of the complexity and severity of treatment conditions or because of less-than-acceptable results.

Neutralizing Compositions

The principal active ingredient in most of the neutralizing formulation is acidic hydrogen peroxide at a concentration of 1 to 3 %. Sodium bromate and sodium chlorite are occasionally used on account of their good stability and absence of bleaching power. H_2O_2-compatible conditioning agents, such as cationic surfactants or silicone emulsions, are often included to ensure easy combing, smooth texture, and control of fly-away of the waved hair.

Evaluation of Waving Efficacy

Although "permanent" is the defining adjective of the imparted wave, there are many other considerations that are important in the assessment of wave quality. Among them are tightness of curl, its springiness, feel of the hair, its luster, and combability. Ultimately, the most reliable way of judging the characteristic of a wave is on the head of the consumer, and thus it is not surprising that this subjective approach has always been used as the final evaluative tool of product prototypes. The importance of using the consumer as the testing probe is of particular importance in assessing the wearing characteristics of the imparted wave. So far, no satisfactory laboratory procedures have been developed to accurately mimic this important aspect.

The objective laboratory measurements on both hair tresses and single fibers are the backbone of the development of new prototypes, screening processes, and further evaluation of competitive products.

Single-fiber technique is particularly useful in differentiating between different chemical systems (e.g., TGA vs. sulfite, alkaline vs. acid wave) providing rapid information as to the efficacy of the process. Some measure of the durability can be gained by submitting these microsprings to the action of hot water, detergents, and stress. Using calibrated fibers, the mechanical measurements can provide the first impression of process aggressiveness.

Clearly, hair tresses are required for evaluation of assembly characteristics—combability, fly-away, luster, and feel—as well as for porosity determination by liquid retention. The curl appearance, both wet and dry, can be assessed and appropriate recordings (photographs) made. The tresses are also required for water-setting evaluations where the imparted wave is used as a background to the consequent hair-setting experiments. In this case, conventional techniques of set impartation and durability evaluation in the humidity chamber are used.

The cosmetic history of hair (before waving, straightening, color, bleaching, weathering) influences not only the degree of damage that the waving lotion can inflict, but also the quality of wave it can impart. Both single-fiber techniques and tresses should be used in the manner previously described.

Prevention and/or Masking of Damage

Hair damage has become a constant companion and by-product of most of our hair care practices (e.g., combing, brushing, heat setting, coloring, bleaching), with hair waving making its own contribution. Because the problem of damage is so widespread, there has been vigorous activity over the years to develop some general specific ways of damage repair. So far, none that are effective and reliable are available. A more promising route is that of damage prevention (the word ''alleviation'' would be more appropriate) or damage masking.

Taking a somewhat detached view, one should add that there is no evidence for the epidemic of hair damage with almost any of the cosmetic treatments of hair, and the damage reflected is usually well tolerated by the consumer for the benefits gained. Nevertheless, even from the discussion presented, some measures can be taken to at least limit the damage inherent in the process. Thus, if a gentle wave is required, an acid type of a thiowave or one based on sulfite might be an alternative. With alkaline waving, the potential of acid-buffered salt solution before water rinsing should be considered, primarily for fine or weathered hair. Recovery of disrupted membrane structures can apparently be attained in the use of sulfite waves by using a cysteine after-treatment (a genuine harbinger of damage repair?). Consumers considering combined treatments (e.g., waving and bleaching or haircoloring) should wave the hair first–as the reduction step, irrespective of whether sulfite or TGA is used, is much more damaging to hair with an oxidative cosmetic history.

To mask and/or limit the damage after waving (and hair combing comes here to the fore), the use of both conditioning shampoos and conditioners is imperative. Clearly, the waving formulations containing effective cationic polymers are at an advantage, as every anionic detergent used in the shampoo (and the shampooing process can be quite abrasive to the wave-sensitized cuticle) forms a lubricating complex with the surface-adsorbed polymer.

Finally, as previously indicated hair undergoes faster weathering and sun lightening after waving than before it. Here, sunscreens would come in handy as long as they are delivered from an effective vehicle, such as a hairspray or mousse. The protection attained from sunscreen-containing shampoos or conditioners has been virtually nil up to now.

Hair Straightening

Although the molecular mechanism underlying hair-straightening parallels that of waving or setting of hair, there are some distinct differences in the composition of formulations and, naturally, in the mode of their application. There are essentially two different categories of straightening preparations; 1) those that aim at temporary straightening and 2) those designed to accomplish permanent effects.

Temporary Hair Straightening

The most frequently used technique in this category is hot combing. An oily material (pressing oil) is applied to hair, which is then combed under slight tension with a heated comb. The straightening effect is produced by the combined action of heat and the moisture present in hair. The function of the pressing oil is threefold: 1) to act as a protective heat-transfer agent between the comb and the hair 2) to serve as a lubricant reducing the drag of the comb, and 3) to function as a barrier slowing diffusion into the hair of moisture from the scalp and environment, and thus delaying reversal of the straightening effect. Pressing oils are mostly based on petrolatum and mineral oil blended with some wax and perfume. Frequent combing dulls and damages the hair, leading ultimately to hair breakage.

Permanent Hair Straightening

The most effective class of permanent straighteners (relaxers) is that based on alkali as an active ingredient. Sodium or potassium hydroxide or sodium carbonate in combination with guanidine are used at concentrations of 1.5 to 3% in a heavy cream base. Even though the recommended treatment time is only 5 to 20 minutes, the straightening effects in general, surpass those obtained with either thioglycollates or bisulfites because of the different chemistry of the process and the greater aggressiveness of alkaline relaxers. A 15-minute treatment irreversibly decreases the cystine content of hair to two thirds of its initial value.

The damaging action of strong alkali on hair is not restricted to disulfide bonds alone. Apart from the potential of mainchain scission (peptide bond hydrolysis), the very nature of the base (high pH) leads to a build-up of negative charges in hair that results in increased swelling, which is intensified by concurrent breakdown of the disulfide bonds. Great care must be exercised in the use of alkaline relaxers because even brief contact with skin can cause blistering. It should be pointed out that the chemistry underlying the hair-straightening process with alkaline relaxers is fundamentally different from the systems based on thioglycollates or sulfites. The alkalis (irrespective of their nature, i.e., sodium hydroxide [lye], calcium hydroxide, or guanidine) cleave the disulfide bonds, and this cleavage is almost instantly followed by formation of new (monosulfide) cross-links. The efficacy of this secondary process varies between 50 and 70%, and this, to a great extent, accounts for the observed alkali damage. If the cross-linking step is not accomplished at that time, there is no known way of cross-link reformation at a later stage of the process. The so-called neutralization step in alkaline relaxing should never be confused with that used in thio or sulfite processes, where its main function is bond rebuilding. In the case of alkaline relaxing, the neutralization aims at removing the excess alkali from hair, which is accomplished by acid-containing (or acid-buffered) shampoo.

Alkaline thioglycollate has also been used as the active ingredient in relaxers, although in somewhat different form from that encountered in conventional waving lotions. The latter are always thin, promoting a fast lotion penetration into the tightly wrapped hair on the curler. Relaxers, on the other hand, are formulated into thick (viscous) oil-and-water (o/w) emulsions or creams using a high concentration of cetyl and stearyl alcohols and high–molecular weight polyethylene glycols together with fatty alcohol sulfate as an emulsifier. The cream is worked into the hair while it is combed straight. The high viscosity of the formulation helps to maintain the extended configuration of the hair during processing, which may take from 30 minutes to 2 hours depending on the initial curliness of the hair. In the course of the treatment, the hair is often recombed to assure its straight configuration. Upon thorough rinsing, conventional oxidizing neutralizers (hydrogen peroxide, bromates, or perborates) are used as a final step of the process.

In recent years, hair-straightening compositions based on mixtures of ammonium bisulfite and urea have been introduced and found to be of some use, primarily in the Caucasian hair-straightening market. The recross linking of bisulfite-treated hair is more effectively accomplished with an alkaline rinse (pH 8–10) than with oxidizing agents, although the latter can also be used to destroy the residual sulfite reductant.

Hair Coloring

Not belittling the importance of hair texture and its geometry, it is perhaps not surprising that the quintessence of hair beauty manifests itself in its color. This has been well recognized as much in the distant past as it is now. It is truly remarkable how nature, using the melanin pigment (a substance without an identifiable chromophore) as its primary colorant, has been able, via clever manipulation of physics and chemistry, to generate hundreds of shades ranging from the Scandinavian blondes through Scottish redheads to the intense black hair of Africans and Asians. Still, the need for color enhancement, or indeed its change, continues to exist and is clearly the driving force of the hair-coloring market as reflected by the variety of products available to the consumer.

Setting aside the diversity of claims and application techniques, hair-coloring products fall into two general categories: 1) those that are based on materials that are inherently colored, and 2) those that use colorless precursors and develop their hair coloring characteristics only on interaction with an oxidant. Dyes of the first category are used in temporary (or shampoo-removable) products and semipermanent color formulations (color stable to several shampooings). The second category forms the mainstay of so-called permanent or oxidative hair colors. Their importance lies not only in the durability of the effect, but also in that the natural color of hair can be modified, almost at will, to any desirable hue or shade, whether darker or lighter than the original. This is accomplished in one step through a combination of bleaching of the natural pigment present in the hair and simultaneous color development. Such shade manipulation is clearly not available in the temporary or semipermanent products, the function of which is primarily restricted to the build-up of color intensity. Although semipermanent colorants lack the versatility of oxidative dyes, they are recognized as being gentler to hair because no peroxide is required. In each hair-coloring category, a sizeable number of dyes (or precursors) is required to attain a viable palette of shades. These dyes differ not only in their chromophoric characteristics, but also in their affinity to hair, water solubility, and overall photostability. In color impartation, a delicate balance of constituent dyes is essential to obtain uniform and desirable results. However, subsequent exposure of dyed hair to shampooing, sunlight, perspiration, and simple wear and tear often highlights the differences in properties of dyes that can result in unpredictable color changes.

Temporary Hair Colorants

As the name itself implies, the dyes of this class are scheduled for only a fleeting residence on hair being removed at the first shampoo opportunity. Although the postulate of fast removing precludes the use of low–molecular weight colorants that could penetrate the hair shaft, it nevertheless extends the palette to almost any toxicologically acceptable dye that can be aesthetically formulated into a cosmetic vehicle. In general, food colors, cosmetic colors, pigments, or even textile dyes can be considered. To be avoided are strongly basic dyes that have a tendency toward intensive skin staining and a high affinity for chemically damaged and weathered hair. Table 4 lists some of the dyes currently used in temporary hair products.

Temporary color formulations are of the "leave-on" type, which means that they are applied to hair usually after shampooing and left there to dry. They can be simple solutions of dyes incorporated into a styling mousse, or can be complexed with surfactants whereby more color can be deposited on hair. By the very nature of the application, the intensity of the coloring effect is low, but sufficient, to produce aesthetically pleasing effects. Exposing the colored hair to heat (whether from a blow dryer or bonnet) may bring about some increase in durability of the imparted color to shampooing.

Semipermanent Hair Colorants

This class of dyes, initially designed exclusively for gray-hair coverage, has progressively grown in importance as the formulation changes extended the color palette and improved the durability of the imparted color.

The majority of products features a blend of low–and medium–molecular weight dyes that are capable of penetrating into the hair shaft, thus assuring a moderate degree of fastness. A blend is necessary to achieve the desired color and obtain a match between the roots and the more permeable ends. The dyes that are used are generally nitrophenyldiamines, nitroaminophenols, and, to a lesser extent, aminoantraquinones. Table 5 lists some of the dyes in use.

TABLE 4 Temporary Hair Colorants

Name	Type
FD&C Blue No. 1	Triphenyl methane
D&C Red No. 22	Xanthene
Ext. D&C Yellow No. 7	Nitro
D&C Brown No. 1	Disazo
D&C Green No. 5	Antraquinone
D&C Red No. 33	Azo

Table 5 Semipermanent Hair Colorants

Name	Color
4-nitro-o-phenylenediamine	Yellow
1,4,5,8-tetra amino anthraquinone	Blue
1,4-diamino anthraquinone	Violet
N'-(2-hydroxy ethyl)-2-nitro-p-phenylene diamine	Red

Several product forms are available: lotions, shampoo-in formulations, or mousses. In all cases, the dyes are dissolved or dispersed in a detergent base that contains a thickener so the product stays on the hair without running or dripping. Application time of 20 to 40 minutes is common, after which time the product is rinsed off and frequently followed by a conventional shampoo.

Recently, formulations providing more durable (color stability up to 20 shampoos) effects have become available. They consist of the conventional semipermanent dyes blended with oxidative dye precursors, which in conjunction with dilute hydrogen peroxide produces longer-lasting color moieties. Such products are occasionally referred to as ''demipermanents.'' Unlike the conventional semipermanent products that are sold in single containers, they, in addition to the dye mixture, contain a separate package of the oxidant.

Often included in the semipermanent category is also the only vegetable dye that is permitted to be used in the United States: henna. Henna consists of the dried leaves of the plant *Lawsonia alba*, which grows in North Africa, the Middle East, and India. The active ingredient, lawsone (2-hydroxy-1-4-naphtoquinone), constitutes about 1% of the dried leaves [10]. Using henna, only limited reddish shades can be achieved. In some products, henna is mixed with other dyes to obtain more variety in color. Such products are then subject to the label warnings used for coal-tar dyes.

A mention should also be made of metallic dyes, which are still popular with men. These products usually contain dissolved lead acetate and elemental sulfur. After application to hair and subsequent air exposure, the lead salt reacts to form a mixture of insoluble sulfides and oxides imparting to the hair a darker color, thus providing a gradual gray coverage.

Permanent Hair Colorants

Unmatched by other colorants in the shade palette, durability to shampooing, resistance to fading, and absence of skin staining, the permanent (oxidative) hair colorants have justifiably carved off the largest market share in hair dyes worldwide. Available in a variety of forms (e.g., lotions, gels, shampoos, creams.), these products deliver reliable results that last until the new hair grows out. Most often, the colorant is supplied as a two-component kit consisting of a mixture of colorless dye precursor and of a stabilized solution of hydrogen peroxide. Occasionally, the peroxide is provided in the form of a powder, such as urea peroxide or sodium perborate. The two components are mixed immediately before use, applied to hair, and left for 20 to 40 minutes before being rinsed out with water.

The color formation commences upon mixing and involves complex reactions between precursors and the oxidant. The precursors consist of two classes of reactants: 1) primary intermediates, comprising o- and p-aminophenols and phenylenediamines, which upon oxidation by peroxide form colored quinone imines; and 2) secondary intermediates (couplers). The latter condense with the imines to yield the final dye molecules. While the color-forming reactions take place in the dye mixture, a significant fraction of the dye precursors diffuse rapidly into the hair together with the hydrogen peroxide forming the colorant moieties throughout the hair fiber. The process is carried out at alkaline pH which also favors the bleaching of the melanin pigment by H_2O_2. Table 6 lists some of the primary and secondary intermediates and colors they produce.

Depending on product form, the formulation of the dye base varies. Ammonia and ethanol amines are preferred alkalizing agents, and a mixture of surfactants and solvents are used to solubilize the dyes and assure wetting of hair. A small quantity of reducing agents are added to prevent the auto-oxidation of the dyes during storage. It is important to realize that hydrogen peroxide, which so effectively assists in both the color development and lightening of hair pigment, also displays a less desirable role in causing oxidative hair damage. Although the damage associated with a single application is slight, the cumulative effect of subsequent treatments is quite perceivable.

Hair Repigmenting

The idea of dyeing the hair by melanin has always been alluring. The "natural" aspect of the colorant implied durability of the coloring effect and its insensitivity to haircare regimens, or shade fading—all these have been factors providing continuous incentive to use the potential of such process. Apart from intense patenting in this field, several papers have recently appeared [11,12] that describe such coloring systems as well as the characteristics of repigmented hair. Recently, products based on the principle of melanin repigmentation of hair have appeared on the market, but the information available to date is too scanty to offer a reliable judgment as to the market viability of these products.

Bleaching

The bleaching action of hydrogen peroxide has been already alluded to in the context of permanent hair coloring, and quite satisfactory levels of lightening can be obtained with such products.

To attain a significantly greater level of bleaching, hydrogen peroxide is combined with bleach accelerators or "boosters." The latter are mixtures of ammonium, potassium, or sodium persulfates. The salts are packaged as dry powders and mixed with hydrogen peroxide just before use. Thickeners and alkalizers (usually sodium silicates) are included in the booster package. Processing time depends primarily on the initial hair color and the desired level of lightening. The pH of these formulations is usually much higher than

TABLE 6 Oxidation Dye Colors

| | Colors on hair with | |
Coupler	PPD	p-Aminophenol
Recorcinol	Greenish-brown	Yellow-brown
m-Phenylenediamine	Blue purple	Violet
m-Amino phenol	Red-brown	Light orange
1-Naphtrol	Blue violet	Red-violet
2-Methyl resorcinol	Yellow brown	Yellowish-beige
2-Amino pyridine	Dark grayish-blue	Light grayish-green

that of the permanent hair-color products and so is the concentration of H_2O_2. All of these factors—high concentration of peroxide, presence of oxidizing salts, and high pH of the process—connote significant oxidative damage of hair. After thoroughly rinsing off the bleaching mixture, the hair should be given an acidic "bath" (lemon juice or solution of citric acid or diluted vinegar) followed by a 5 to 10 minute treatment with a "deep" conditioner.

Hair-Color Safety and Regulatory Issues

Because of the allergenic potential of some of the materials used in hair dyes (primarily p-phenylenediamine, or PPD), hair colorants in the United States display on the label as a legal requirement a warning, plus instructions for a 24-hour patch test with the precursors and hydrogen peroxide mixed in the same manner as in use. As required by Section 601(a) of the Federal Food, Drug and Cosmetic Act, the warnings reads as follows:

> This product contains ingredients which may cause skin irritation on certain individuals and a preliminary test according to accompanying directions should be made. This product must not be used for dyeing the eyebrows or eyelashes; to do so may cause blindness.

It should be noted that allergic contact dermatitis to hair dyes appears to be far less common today than decades ago. It has been suggested that PPD, although a strong sensitizer, is not likely to produce skin sensitization because of the short contact time with skin and rapid reaction of PPD with the oxidizing agent and couplers [13].

Concerns as to the possible carcinogenicity of some hair ingredients arose in 1975 when these were reported to be mutagenic for bacteria in bioassays [14]. Presently, it is not clear how significant a risk this poses to users of hair dyes. Because hair dyes have been in common use for over 50 years, epidemiological studies on cancer rates in occupationally exposed groups or the users of hair dyes are of particular value. So far, the results of most of these suggest that hair dyes do not pose a carcinogenic risk [13].

CONCLUDING REMARKS

Available space limits this chapter on hair cosmetics to only a brief overview of what is used and practiced in this broad and important segment of personal-care products. Many aspects of hair chemistry and physics have only been fleetingly discussed, including properties of single hair fibers and their assemblies. The whole area of claim substantiation has been left out, together with the description of physicochemical techniques that are relevant to this subject. For a fuller account on these topics, the reader is referred to an excellent book by Zviak [15] and recent publications on haircare [16] and cosmetic-claim substantiation [17].

REFERENCES

1. Menkart J, Wolfram LJ, Mao I. J Soc Cosmet Chem 1966; *17*:769.
2. Wolfram LJ. (1981) In: Orfanos, Montagna, Stütgen, eds. Hair Research. Berlin: Springer Verlag, 1981:479.
3. Kligman AM, Shelley WD. J Inv Dermatol 1958; *30*:99.
4. Cunliffe WJ, Perera WD, Thackeray P, Williams M, Foster RA, Williams SM. Br J Dermatol 1975; *95*:153.
5. Breuer MM. J Soc Cosmet Chem 1981; *32*:437.

6. Schwartz AM, Perry JW, Belch J. Surface Active Agents and Detergents. Vol. 2. Robert E. Krieger: Huntington, NY; 1977.
7. Preston WC. J Phys Chem 1948; *52*:84.
8. Stevenson DG. J Text Inst 1959; *50*:T548.
9. Zviak C, Vanlerberghe G. In: Zviak C, ed. The Science of Hair Care. New York: Dekker, 1986:57.
10. Stamberg J, Werczberger R, Koltin Y. Mutat Res 1979; *62*:383.
11. Brown K, Mayer A, Murphy B, Schultz T, Wolfram LJ. J Soc Cosmet Chem 1989; *40*:65.
12. Brown K, Marlowe E, Prota G, Wenke G. J Soc Cosmet Chem 1997; *48*:133.
13. Corbett JF. Rev Prog Coloration 1985; *15*:53.
14. Ames BN, Kammen DH, Yannesaki E. Proc Nat Acad Sci USA 1975; *72*:2423.
15. Zviak C, ed. The Science of Hair Care. New York: Marcel Dekker, 1986.
16. Johnson DH, ed. Hair and Hair Care. New York: Marcel Dekker, 1997.
17. Aust LB, ed. Cosmetic Claims Substantiations. New York: Marcel Dekker, 1998.

52

Ethnic Differences in Haircare Products

Joerg Kahre
Henkel KGaA, Düsseldorf, Germany

INTRODUCTION

Hair is undoubtedly one of the most important personal features of people in all cultures. For the past several centuries hair has played an important role. Style, length, and color changes are influenced by fashion trends. Hair often allows for feelings of health and beauty, and thus its influence is of great importance. Therefore hair has been studied greatly as cited in numerous publications. Three major types of hair are known: African, Asian, and Caucasian. The differences between these hair types are related to diameter, geometry, and other physical parameters [1,2]. Closely related to these parameters are biophysical factors, tensile strength, and combing forces, which might be influenced by cosmetic formulations that are applied to hair. Caucasian hair is also called European hair and African hair is also called Negroid hair. The names only summarize the complexity of hair types, e.g., Asian hair is the sum term for Japanese, Chinese, and other Asian ethnic groups. And furthermore, even in such ethnic subgroups we do not really see a single hair quality. Therefore, taking Asian, Caucasian, or African hair is an overall example for the corresponding hair types of these regions. Table 1 shows an overview about the most important hair fiber characteristics [3,4].

The demand for hair care is closely related to the condition and length of the hair and fashion trends. Hair is exposed daily to a wide variety of influences that can damage it to a greater or lesser degree. Especially the surface of hair that has been exposed to environmental influences (e.g., sunlight, combing, blow drying, etc.) or chemical treatments (e.g., cold waving, dyeing, bleaching) carries a stronger negative charge than the surface of untreated hair.

The resulting change in the hair's structure may reduce its natural gloss or cause a mild build-up of static charge, and in extreme cases the hair may break, especially in the region of the tip.

Such changes in the hair's appearance can be avoided by, in the first place, using mild hair-cleansing products or conditioning shampoos. The second protection step, however, is provided by hair aftertreatment products such as hair conditioners or rinses.

The effect of conditioning preparations is restricted to the part of the hair shaft that projects out of the epidermis. Both the cortex and the cuticle of the hair shaft can be negatively affected by the aforementioned influences.

TABLE 1 Hair Fiber Characteristics

	Caucasian	Asian	African
Thickness	fine	coarse	coarse
Curvature	straight to curly	straight to wavy	wavy to wooly
Cross sectional shape	nearly round to slightly oval	nearly round to slightly oval	slightly oval to elliptical
Color	blond to dark brown	dark brown to brown-black	brown-black to black
Cross section area (μm^2)	~70	~90	~70

Chemical hair treatments such as cold waving, bleaching, or the use of straighteners and relaxers have a particularly unfavorable effect on the cortex, because they influence or change, e.g., the disulfide bonds between and in proteins. This generally results in a loss of mechanical strength, a more marked tendency to absorb moisture and therefore to swell, a greater susceptibility to alkalines, and an increase in electrostatic charge [5].

Mechanical stresses such as frequent combing and brushing, blow drying, and intensive exposure to sunlight cause damage to the cuticle; scales either break off completely or along their edges. This makes the hair rougher and reduces its natural gloss [6,7]. An overview of the properties of damaged hair is shown in Figure 1. The requirements to be satisfied by an optimally formulated hair-treatment preparation derive from the listed hair-damaging processes.

Objective test methods are developed to investigate all the effects. Some of the most important methods to understand the actions of hair-treatment preparations are listed in Table 2 [8]. In addition to these tests, cosmetic assessment is usually obtained from the half-head test, the panel test, and the home-use test.

AFRICAN HAIR

The biophysical properties of African hair are more closely related to wool fibers than to the other hair types. African hair shows some special properties as a result of its very curly structure [9–11]. These properties are listed in Figure 2. African hair is treated with hair relaxers, perms, or straighteners in order to get a straight to light curled style. This

- Rough hair surface
- Increased amount of negative charges
- Reduced mechanical solidity

→ Increased combing forces
→ Unfavorable feel
→ Reduced gloss
→ Increased electrostatical loading
→ Higher breaking behavior, split ends

FIGURE 1 Properties of damaged hair.

TABLE 2 Objective Measuring Methods

Term	Objective measuring methods	Measurement parameter
Combability, detangling	Resistance to combing	Wet combing work
		Dry combing work
Strength	Resonance frequency	Modulus of elasticity
	Tensile strength measurement	Elastic range (range of Hooke's law)
	Breaking strength of single hair	Breaking force
	Breaking strength of hair tress	Breaking force
Charging capacity	Faraday cage	Charge difference
Splitting	Electron-scanning microscope	
Gloss	Goniophotometer	Reflection

has an influence on the hair structure. We measured the wet tensile strength of hair tresses after the application of typical hair relaxers. As expected, straighteners and relaxers have a strong influence in decreasing the tensile strength. Relative to untreated hair we found a residual tensile strength of only 60% depending upon the relaxing agent. Thioglycolate (7.5% active at pH 9.3) is milder than sodium hydroxide (2.0% at pH 13.5) and this is better than calcium hydroxide (0.6% active at pH 13.5). A more detailed description of the physical properties and differences of African hair relative to Caucasian hair is reported in the literature [9–11].

Influence of Surfactants and Protein Hydrolysates on African Hair

The use of mild surfactants in shampoos is necessary and avoids additional damage. Applying 2% sodium hydroxide (pH 13.5) to kinky hair resulted in a residual strength of about 73%. Shampooing this hair with a 12% active solution of sodium laureth sulfate (SLES) gave a further decrease of the tensile strength to 64%. If we choose decyl glucoside as surfactant, there is no further damage and a significantly higher wet tensile strength relative to the SLES result.

Adding protein hydrolysates to relaxers or straighteners strongly increases tensile strength. Using 2% active hydrolysed collagen in a 0.6%-containing calcium hydroxide straightener at pH 13.5 resulted in an increase of the wet tensile strength up to 142% relative to the same straightener without hydrolyzed collagen. This is important for the formulation not only for these products, but for shampoos and conditioners in general. The addition of protein hydrolysates to restructure the hair is strongly recommended.

● **Curly structure**

  ➡ **spontaneous knotting**

  ➡ **difficult combing**

  ➡ **less natural luster**

  ➡ **dry hair** (less sebum along hair shaft)

● **High dry combing forces**

FIGURE 2 Characteristics of African hair.

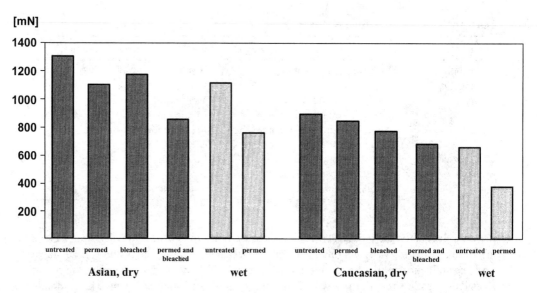

FIGURE 3   Dry and wet tensile strength of single fibers.

DIFFERENCES OF UNTREATED ASIAN AND CAUCASIAN HAIR

Because of the differences in cross-section, we found different wet and dry tensile strengths of single hair fibers. Asian hair shows higher values than Caucasian hair. The application of a perm, bleach, or both results in decreasing tensile forces for both hair types (Fig. 3). The higher values for dry combing forces are found again for Asian hair (Fig. 4). The wet combing work shows comparable results for the untreated hair types.

In addition to these results we measured the bounce of curls. For a natural appearance of hair the physical parameters attenuation, maximum zero amplitude and force of elonga-

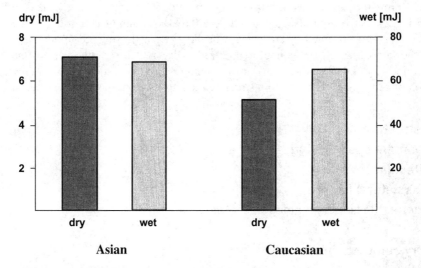

FIGURE 4   Combing work of Asian and Caucasian hair.

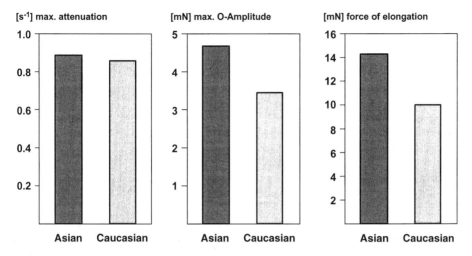

FIGURE 5 Bouncing of Asian and Caucasian hair.

tion are important. If these values are too low, the single hair fibers are not connected to each other. A natural swinging behavior of hair tresses needs entanglements of hair fibers. Therefore, styling products as well as products for fine hair are formulated with polymers. Figure 5 shows the bouncing behavior of untreated hair tresses. Water is used as standard. Differences between Asian and Caucasian hair are detected for the 0-amplitude and the force of elongation. This may be considered a result of the difference in the cross-section of these hair types.

A further difference is split-end generation. As a simulation for the building of split ends 10 washing cycles followed by 3000 combing cycles with a rough comb has been used. Asian hair has a higher tendency for generating split ends by applying this method.

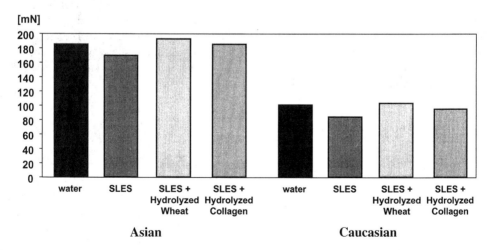

FIGURE 6 Influence of protein hydrolysates and surfactants on the wet tensile strength of permed hair tresses.

TABLE 3   Types of Shampoos and Their Use

Shampoo type	Hair type
Baby shampoo	All baby hair
Shampoo for dry hair	Caucasian, African
Shampoo for fine hair	Caucasian, African
Shampoo for greasy hair	Caucasian, Asian
2-in-1 shampoo	All
Antidandruff shampoo	All
Detangling shampoo	African
Neutralizing shampoo	African
Protective shampoo (after perms, colors, etc.)	All

INFLUENCE OF SURFACTANTS AND PROTEIN HYDROLYSATES

The influence of single surfactants to the tensile strength of Asian and Caucasian hair is tested (Fig. 6). We chose sodium laureth sulfate (2 mol EO—type) as one example for surfactants. First, the hair was permed and then washed with the surfactant. Finally, the tensile strength of the hair tresses was determined. The differences in the absolute values are related to the differences in the cross-section of the hair types. Relative to water, SLES decreases the tensile strength of the hair tresses. This is observed for both hair types.

In a further experiment we added protein hydrolysates to the SLES. The addition of hydrolysates increased the tensile strength of the hair tresses relative to the SLES values. The source of the hydrolysate, animal-based or vegetable-derived, shows no difference in this effect (see Fig. 6). Therefore protein hydrolysates are useful to strengthen hair fibers [12].

EFFECTS OF SHAMPOO

A surfactant plus a protein hydrolysate is not a complete shampoo formulation. Depending on the type of hair they are formulated according to the needs of the different hair qualities. In addition to the ethnic hair quality, hair can be fine, greasy, pretreated etc. Therefore a complete range of different products exists in the market. Table 3 shows various types of shampoos. The following is only a short overview of some formulations and concepts. A basic formulation is shown in Table 4.

TABLE 4   Basic Structure of a Shampoo

Amount (%)	Ingredient	Use
1–3	Preservative	Microbiol, stability
	Color	Sensorial acceptance
	Perfume oil	Sensorial acceptance
0–10	Thickener/auxiliaries	Appearance/product claims
3–5	Cosurfactant	Cleaning, foam
10–15	Basic surfactant	Cleaning, foam
q.s. 100	Water	Handling

TABLE 5 Frame Formulations for a Daily-Use Shampoo

DE/96/161/15 (wt%)		DE/96/161/23 (wt%)	
Decyl glucoside	20.0	Lauryl glucoside	4.8
Ammonium lauryl sulfate	6.5	Sodium laureth sulfate	20.0
Cocamide DEA	3.0	Ammonium lauryl sulfate	11.5
Panthenol (50%)	1.0	Cocamidopropyl betaine	6.7
Polyquaternium-10	0.3	Laurdimonium hydroxypropyl	
Propylen glycol (and) PEG-55	2.5	Hydrolysed wheat protein	3.0
Propylen glycol oleate		Polyquaternium-10	0.3
		Sodium chloride	0.2
Water	q.s. 100		
pH	5.5	Water	q.s. 100
		pH	5.5
		viscosity (mPa.s)	5000
Residual wet combing work Asian hair:	42%		28%
Residual wet combing work Caucasian hair:	40%		52%
Residual dry combing work Asian hair:	40%		104%
Residual dry combing work Caucasian hair:	40%		95%

Daily-Use Shampoos

A daily-use shampoo has to cleanse and condition the hair. It is used frequently, and therefore must be mild. An example for a formulation is listed in Table 5. The influence of this formulation on both hair qualities with respect to dry and wet combing was the same. The reduction of the wet combing forces was sufficient to have an easy combing. The dry combing forces were comparable to the untreated hair. In addition to the objective test results a half-head test on 10 European volunteers was done and a good performance was achieved.

Special Shampoo Products

Fine and Greasy Hair

The appearance of fine hair is described as poor shining, low volume, poor manageability, as well as low tensile strength and problems in the dry combability. In addition to a mild-surfactant base, additives must be incorporated into the formulation to provide easy conditioning, increase dry combability, and thus improve manageability. Furthermore, formulation ingredients must be used that improve the tensile strength of the hair [13]. Cationic protein hydrolysates, specific cationic surfactants compatible with anionic surfactants or pseudo cationics (amphopolymers) are used as slightly conditioning additives. The texture is improved with glucose, alkyl polyglycosides, protein hydrolysates, cationic protein-hydrolysates, or polymers. This formulation concept is summarized in Figure 7.

European hair is finer than Asian hair. If this fine hair type takes up sebum it sticks together. Often greasy hair is also fine hair. Therefore special formulations for this hair type are developed [14]. The formulation concept has to include active ingredients to avoid either the production or uptake of sebum. Often-used ingredients are sulfur products or plant extracts. In formulation DE/94/145/11 (Table 6), the potassium abietoyl hydrolysed collagen is the product that reduces the sebum uptake. The effects with respect to increase the dry

➡ **mild surfactant basis**

➡ **neutral to slightly acid pH value**

➡ **mild conditioning additive**

➡ **high dry combability / body**

➡ **tensile strength improvement**

FIGURE 7   Formulation concept for fine hair.

combing work as well as the wet combing work is sufficient for Caucasian but not Asian hair. By applying this formulation to Asian hair the amount of quaternary polymer has to be slightly increased. This formulation also reduces the uptake of sebum. The action and mechanism for the reduction of sebum uptake is described in the literature [14].

2-in-1 Shampoos

This type of shampoo is very popular. Washing and conditioning is only one step. Therefore these products are well accepted by the consumer. The formulation concept is not so different from the others (Fig. 8). In this case silicones are mostly formulated to achieve the special conditioning effect. New concepts are using monoglycerides in combination with alkyl glucosides and cationic polymers to get this conditioning effect. With such a concept, the build-up effect can be avoided [15]. Formulation DE/94/005/25 is one example tested on Asian and Caucasian hair and one example formulated without the use of silicones. Important is the reduction of wet-combing forces and the increase of the dry-combing forces in order to get a style and volume. The formulation and the results are shown in Table 7. The performance is best on Caucasian hair. For Asian hair the amount of cationic polymer has to be increased.

AFTER HAIR TREATMENTS

Modern preparations are divided into rinse-off types, which are rinsed off after being left to take effect for a certain time, possibly with the help of a slight increase in temperature,

TABLE 6   Shampoo for Fine and Greasy Hair

	DE/94/145/11 (wt%)
Decyl glucoside	10.0
Sodium laureth sulfate	14.3
Cocamidopropyl betaine	10.0
Potassium abietoyl hydrolyzed collagen (PAHC)	5.1
Polyquaternium-10	0.2
Laureth-3	1.0
Sodium chloride	1.0
Water	q.s. 100
pH	5.5

➡ **shampoo and hair rinse**

➡ **mild surfactant bases**

➡ **pearl shine**

➡ **specific cationic surfactants**

➡ **silicone derivatives / emollients**

➡ **cationic polymers**

FIGURE 8 Formulation concept for 2-in-1 shampoo.

and leave-on types, which remain in the hair. In Figure 9 an overview about the hair aftertreatments is listed. We studied the effects of typical conditioners (Table 8). After treatments are used to restructure and improve the hair quality. Such preparations must be effective not only superficially but also below the surface of the hair. Changing the properties of the hair surface can cause improvements in properties such as combability, feel, and manageability, and can reduce the build-up of static charge. Moreover, a protective action can be achieved with chemical hair treatments, and special additives that penetrate inside the hair can improve its mechanical strength. Therefore a schematic formulation makeup is based on the described general requirements derived from hair-damaging processes described in the introduction [16,17].

Cationic surfactants act by being adsorbed onto the surface of negatively charged hair [19,20]. In contrast, active agents such as cationic protein hydrolysates, protein hydrolsates, panthenol, and glucose penetrate at least partially below the surface of the hair.

In order to evaluate differences between conditioners we applied several formulations containing 1.0% active distearoylethyl hydroxyethylmonium methosulfate and 2.5% cetearyl alcohol to Asian and Caucasian hair. The combing work was measured before and after the application of the conditioner. The absolute values for the combing work of Asian and Caucasian hair are different as shown previously in Figure 4. For testing the efficacy it is not important to see the absolute values of combing work; it is more important to know the degree of reduction. This means a residual combing work of 40% is a relative reduction of 60%. All formulations have the same efficacy on Asian and Caucasian hair. There is no significant difference in the relative change of the combing work.

TABLE 7 Example of a 2-in-1 Shampoo

		DE/94/005/25 (wt%)
Sodium laureth sulfate (and) lauryl glucoside		21.0
Glycol distearate (and) glycerin (and) laureth-4 (and) cocamidopropyl betaine		2.0
PEG-7 glyceryl cocoate		1.0
Guar hydroxypropyl trimonium chloride		0.5
Water		q.s. 100
pH		5.5
residual combing work	dry	wet
Asian hair	87%	87%
Caucasian hair	87%	60%

Pretreatments for waving preparations	Prophylaxis
Intermediate treatments for waving prep.	Prophylaxis
Keratin hardeners	Repair
Hot-oil treatments	Repair
Leave-on conditioners	Repair / Prophylaxis
Thermal conditioners	Repair
Rinse-off conditioners	Repair
Hair tip fluids	Repair
Sunscreens	Prophylaxis
Blow-drying lotions	Hair styling
Hair-setting lotion	Hair styling
Hairspray, lacquer	Hair styling
Hair gels	Hair styling
Hair tonic	Hair styling

FIGURE 9   Overview of hair treatment preparations.

TABLE 8   General Conditioner Formulation

Use	Hair rinses	Amount %
Formulation auxiliary	Emulsifier	0–2
Consistency, conditioning agent	Consistency factors	1–5
Emollient, care component	Oily components, auxiliaries	0–3
Conditioning agent	Cationic components	0.5–1.5
Sensorial acceptance	Perfume oil	0–2
Microbiological stability	Color	
	Preservative	
	Water	
	pH value: 3–5	

DE/92/197/6 (wt.-%)		Emollients:	
Lauryl glucoside	2.0	G:	Octyldodecanol
Cetearyl alcohol	3.0	GTEH:	Octanoic Triglyceride
Cetrimonium chloride	4.0	NPC:	Neopentylglycol Dicaprate
Emollient	2.0	302:	Propylenglycol Dicaprylate/Dicaprate
Water	q.s. 100	SN-1:	Cetyl Isooctanoate
		TPEH3:	Trimethylolpropane Triisooctanoate
		PEEH4:	Pentaerythritol Tetraisooctanoate

FIGURE 10   Formulation with emollients in conditioners.

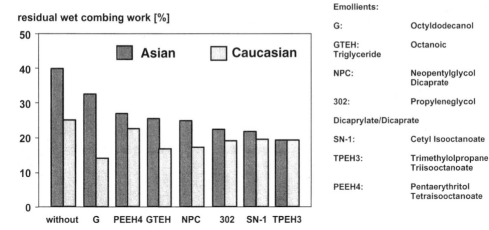

FIGURE 11   Wet combing work/emollients in conditioners.

Further improvements in wet combability properties of hair rinses or hair conditioners can be achieved by adding suitable emollients [18]. The influence of emollients on the conditioning effect of hair aftertreatment preparations was studied with the help of the model formulation DE/92/197/6 shown in Figure 10.

Various emollients were blended into the formulation so that they formed 2% of the total components. The effect of these emollients on wet combability was determined. It can be seen from Figure 11 that the addition of emollients can facilitate a further enhancement of hair-conditioning action.

Relative to emollient-free formulations, a further reduction of 10 to 20% is achieved in the combing work of wet hair. The most marked reduction in wet combing work is

TABLE 9   Conditioners with Active Ingredients

	DE/94/038/43 wt%	DE/94/038/44 wt%	DE/94/038/45 wt%
Distearoylethyl hydroxyethylmonium methosulfate (and) cetearyl alcohol	1.0	1.0	1.0
Cetearyl alcohol	2.1	2.1	2.1
Glyceryl stearate	0.5	—	0.5
Ceteareth-20	0.8	0.8	0.8
Soya sterol	0.7	—	0.7
Hydrolyzed collagen	—	—	2.0
Methyl hydroxypropyl cellulose	0.5	—	0.5
Hydroxypropyl methylcellulose (1% swelling)	—	20.0	—
Laurdimonium hydroxypropyl hydrolyzed wheat protein	—	2.8	—
Water, preservation	q.s. 100	q.s. 100	q.s. 100
Tensile strength of tresses		42.4 (Ncm/g)	51.9 (Ncm/g)
Significance (t-test)		>99.9%	>99.9%

TABLE 10 Leave-On Conditioner

	DE/96/099/4 wt%
Polyacrylamide (and) C13-14 isoparafin (and) laureth-7	3.0
Cocamide DEA	1.0
Glycerin (86%)	5.0
Lauryl glucoside	0.5
Oleyl erucate	0.5
Tocopherol	0.2
Hydrolyzed sweet almond protein	3.0
Laurdimonium hydroxypropyl hydrolyzed wheat protein	0.8
Ethanol (96%)	10.0
Water, preservation	q.s. 100
pH	7.0
Viscosity (Brookfield RVF, 23°C, spindle 4, 10 rpm)	ca. 3000 mPa.s

brought about by high molecular emollients. When the influence of these emollients on the combability of dry hair was studied, it was found that they cause almost no changes.

Not only the hair's characteristics were favorably influenced by the oils in hair rinses, but the physicochemical properties of hair rinses that contain fatty alcohol were also improved. Emollients generally have the effect of stabilizing viscosity during storage.

EXAMPLES OF FORMULATIONS AND EFFECTS

Some further examples of different formulations are listed. If any effects have been measured, these are mentioned. Conditioners for colored, permed, bleached, or straightened hair are given in Tables 9 to 12. These formulations may be used on all ethnic hair types. The listed examples are rinse-off (Tables 9, 10) as well as leave-on (Table 11) conditioners. The so-called liquid hair (Table 12) is a special leave-on product that acts as a restructuring agent for damaged hair. Pretreatments (Table 13) are used to reduce the effects caused by the following application of a perm, bleach, or coloring. They are useful for all ethnic hair types. The last two formulations are shampoos for African hair (Tables 14, 15).

TABLE 11 Hot Oil Treatment

	DE/91/303/11 wt%
Cetrimonium chloride	8.0
Hydroxyethyl cellulose (2% swelling)	20.0
Polysorbate-20	1.5
Hydrolyzed collagen	0.3
D-panthenol (50%)	0.2
Water, preservative, perfume, etc.	q.s. 100

TABLE 12   Liquid Hair (Leave-On)

	DE/94/211/6 wt%
Decyl glucoside	4.0
Laurdimonium hydroxypropyl hydrolyzed collagen	2.0
Hydrolyzed keratin	3.0
Glycerin (86%)	20.0
Ethanol (96%)	5.0
Water, preservative	q.s. 100
pH	5–5.5

TABLE 13   Pretreatment Preparation

	Wt%
Hydrolyzed keratin	2.0
Citric acid	0.1
PEG-hydrogenated castor oil	1.0
Fragrance, preservative, water	q.s. 100

TABLE 14   Detangling Shampoo for African Hair

	Wt%
Ammonium lauryl sulfate	30.0
Cocamidopropyl betaine	10.0
Coco glucoside (and) glyceryl oleate	5.0
Hydrolyzed wheat protein	3.0
Laurdimonium hydroxypropyl hydrolyzed wheat protein	3.0
Water, preservative	q.s. 100
pH	5.5

TABLE 15   Neutralizing Shampoo for African Hair

	Wt%
Ammonium lauryl sulfate	35.0
Cocamidopropyl betaine	10.0
Coco glucoside (and) glyceryl oleate	2.0
Laurdimonium hydroxypropyl hydrolyzed wheat protein	1.0
Hydrolyzed wheat protein	1.0
Polyquaternium-10	0.4
Guar hydroxypropyl trimonium chloride	0.2
Water, preservative	q.s. 100
pH (adjusted with citric acid)	5.5

REFERENCES

1. Taesdale D, Schlüter R, Blankenburg G. Querschnittsparameter von Humanhaaren Teil 1, Ärztl. Kosmetologie 1981; 11:161–170.
2. Taesdale D, Schlüter R, Blankenburg G. Querschnittsparameter von Humanhaaren Teil 2, Ärztl. Kosmetologie 1981; 11:252–259.
3. Hensen H, Kahre J. Haarnachbehandlungsmittel im Überlick, Seifen Öle Fette Wachse 1998; 124, 806–815.
4. Eva Tolgyesi, Coble DW, Fang FS, Kairinen EO. A comparative study of beard and scalp hair. J Soc Cosmet Chem 1983; 34:361–382.
5. Kahre J, Busch P, Salka B, Totani N, Poly W. Asian and caucasian hair—differences of influence for the formulation? Annual Scientific Seminar 1998, preprints, 7.
6. Koester J. Eigenschaften und Anwendung kationischer Haarpflegeadditive. Parfümerie und Kosmetik 1991; 72/4:218–225.
7. Hollenberg D, Müller R. Möglichkeiten zur Beeinflussung der Haarstruktur durch Pflegeprodukte. Seifen Öle Fette Wachse 1995; 121/2:82–89.
8. Busch P, Förster Th, Hensen H, H Th. Müller-Kirschbaum. Tesmann, Subjektiv/objektiv-Bewertung kosmetischer Effekte. Ärztliche Kosmetologie 1990; 20:498–502.
9. Syed AN, Kuhajda A, Ayoub H, Ahmad K. African-American hair. Cosmet Toilet 1995; 110: 39–48.
10. Burmeister F, Bollatti D, Brooks G. Ethnic hair: moisturizing after relaxer use. Cosmet Toilet 1991; 106:49–51.
11. Menkart J, Wolfram LJ, Mao I. Caucasian hair, negro hair, and wool: similarities and differences. J Soc Cosmet Chemists 1966; 17:769–787.
12. Kahre J, Seipel W, Wachter R. Pflanzliche Proteinhydrolysate und Derivate mit universellen Eigenschaften, SEPAWA-Jahrestagung, 35–42, 1995.
13. Hensen H. Surfactant preparations. Eurocosmetics 5/95.
14. Busch P, Hensen H, Fischer D, Ruhnke A, Franklin J. An abietic acid protein condensate for treating greasy hair. Cosmet Toilet 1995; 110:59–63.
15. Both W, Gassenmeier T, Hensen H, Hörner V, Seipel W. Pflegende, lipidhaltige Reinigungspräparate für Haut und Haar, SEPAWA Kongress, 34–38, 1997.
16. Kahre J, Busch P, Totani N, Poly W. Asian and European hair—influence of the difference on the formulation. Poster presentation, IFSCC—Sydney, 1996.
17. Spiess E. The influence of chemical structure on performance in hair care preparations. Parfümerie und Kosmetik 1991; 72:370–376.
18. Busch P, Hensen H, Kahre J, Tesmann H. Alkylpolyglycosides—a new cosmetic concept for mildness and care. Agro-Food-Industry. Sept/Oct 1994; pp. 23–28.

53

Oral-Care Products

Abdul Gaffar
Colgate-Palmolive Company, Piscataway, New Jersey

THE TEETH AND ORAL ENVIRONMENT

Like all mammals, humans generally have two sets of teeth during a lifetime. The first set, known as deciduous, primary, or "milk" teeth, begins to appear in infants between the age of 5 and 9 months. All 20 of these "baby" teeth are generally in place by age $2^1/_2$ years. The second set, or permanent teeth, forms within the gums during the period from infancy to puberty. These teeth, also known as succedaneous teeth, begin to erupt at around age 5, displacing the deciduous set as they appear. There are 32 permanent teeth. An individual will spend 91% of his or her lifetime chewing with these permanent teeth if they are properly cared for. Of the 32 permanent teeth, 16 are located in the upper jaw, or maxillary dental arch, which is part of the cranium, or skull, and is immoveable. The other 16 are located in the mandibular dental arch which is part of the lower jaw and is the moveable part of the skull. Each type of tooth is equally divided between these two dental arches (Figs. 1 and 2).

The Parts of a Tooth

Each tooth consists of three parts: the area above the gum that can be seen, the area below the gum that is not visible, and the constricted portion, or neck, between the other two parts. The crown is the enamel-covered portion of the tooth. The root is the portion of the tooth which, by means of the periodontal ligament, relates to the osseous (bony) structures of the jaw. The root makes up about two thirds of the total length of a tooth (Fig. 3).

The Tissues of a Tooth

A tooth is made up of five different tissues, each with a specific and important function. Serious disease in any of these tissues can affect the entire tooth and result in its decay and/or destruction. These tissues are as follows:

1. Enamel, which is a hard white outer covering surrounds the crown of the tooth and protects it from wearing away as a result of the pressure of chewing. It consists largely (96 to 98 percent) of inorganic substances, mainly calcium and phosphate.

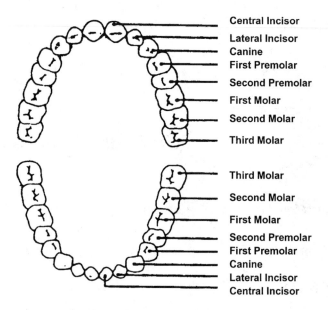

Central Incisor
Lateral Incisor
Canine
First Premolar
Second Premolar
First Molar
Second Molar
Third Molar

Third Molar
Second Molar
First Molar
Second Premolar
First Premolar
Canine
Lateral Incisor
Central Incisor

FIGURE 1   The permanent teeth showing the orderly arrangement of the various types in the upper and lower dental arches.

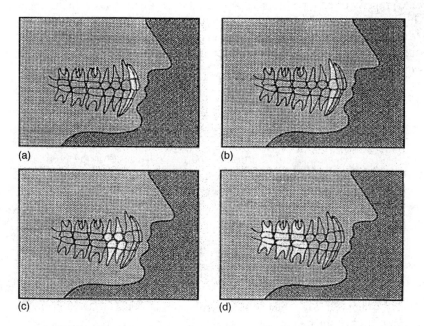

(a)

(b)

(c)

(d)

FIGURE 2   Lateral or side view of the permanent teeth showing the four types of teeth, their arrangement in the dental arch, and differences in size and shape.

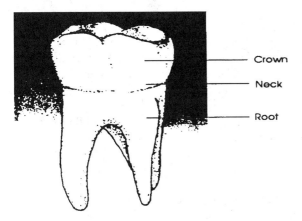

FIGURE 3   **The parts of a tooth.**

2. Dentin, a yellowish bone-like tissue under the enamel, provides support and forms the bulk of the tooth structure, extending almost to its entire length. It is covered by the enamel on the crown and the cementum on the root. Chemically, dentin is composed of 20% organic and 75% inorganic matter, or collagen and calcium phosphate, respectively. The remaining five % is mainly water and other mucosubstances.

3. Pulp, a soft tissue within the center of the crown and root, contains nerves, blood vessels and lymph vessels that produce dentin and provide nourishment for the tooth throughout its life. Because of its rich supply of blood and nerves, the pulp also functions as a defense system against bacterial invasion and as a sensory signal of injury by causing toothache.

4. Cementum, a thin, bone-like tissue that covers the root, serves as a means of attaching the tooth to the surrounding bone.

5. Periodontal ligament, a layer of connective-tissue fibers, stretches between the cementum and the bone connecting the tooth root to the jawbone. It also cushions the tooth from the pressures exerted during chewing (Fig. 4).

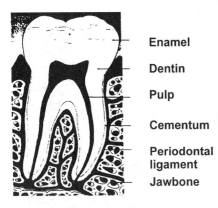

FIGURE 4   **The five tissues of a tooth.**

The Periodontium

The periodontium (from the Greek "peri," meaning "around," and "odous," for "tooth") is a functional system consisting of several different tissues that surround and support the teeth. This system is also called the "attachment apparatus" or the "supporting tissues of the teeth." Anatomically, the term refers only to the connective tissue between the teeth and their bony sockets (Fig. 5).

The tissues that make up the periodontium include the gingiva, the periodontal ligament, the cementum, and the alveolar bone or jawbone. Their good health is of great importance to the overall health of your mouth and the survival of your teeth.

The Gingiva

The gingiva, commonly called the "gums," is the most external part of the periodontium. It is composed of dense fibrous tissue which forms a close ring-like attachment around the necks of the teeth and connects with the epithelial covering (oral mucosa) that lines the mouth. The gingiva is firm in consistency and does not move from its underlying structures. It is covered by a smooth vascular mucous membrane which is tender to the touch and bleeds easily when penetrated or bruised. It also overlays the unerupted teeth, and the pain which occurs during the teething process is the result of the new tooth pushing through this sensitive tissue. Clinically the gingiva is divided into following:

1. Free marginal gingiva which is about 1.5 mm wide and forms the skin-like soft-tissue fold around the teeth. The narrow shallow groove present between the tooth and the free gingiva is known as the gingival sulcus. It is approximately 0.5 mm deep and 0.15 mm wide and surrounds the tooth on all sides. The bottom of the sulcus is made up of cells from the junctional epithelium. The size of this groove or "pocket" is of great importance when determining the health of the periodontium and the stability of the teeth.

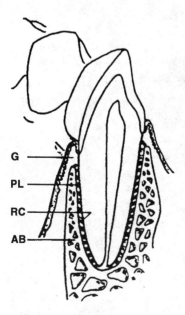

FIGURE 5 A healthy tooth with its periodontium.

2. Attached gingiva which is firmly connected to the hard surface of the tooth by means of a ring of specialized tissue known as the junctional epithelial attachment. The attached gingiva becomes wider with age and may vary considerably among individuals and from tooth to tooth.

3. The cells in the junctional epithelium are continuously being renewed during life and have a turnover rate of every 4 to 6 days. This results in a very permeable tissue which serves as a pathway for the metabolic products produced by the bacteria present in the mouth. This area plays a key role in the maintenance of periodontal health.

4. Interdental gingiva which varies in depth and width and occupies the area between adjacent teeth.

The Periodontal Ligament and the Cementum

The periodontal ligament occupies the space between the root surface of the tooth and the alveolar bone or jawbone. It is composed of connective tissue fibers, blood vessels, nerves and other cells. Its function is to provide the connection between the cementum layer of the tooth and the jawbone, the teeth and the gingiva, and between each tooth and its neighbor. Anatomically the cementum is a part of the tooth, but functionally, it belongs to the tooth-supporting apparatus because the gingival and periodontal ligaments are anchored in it.

The Alveolar Bone

Alveolar bone, also referred to as the jawbone, develops along with the formation of the teeth throughout pregnancy and continues to grow during the eruption of the teeth in childhood. Three types of alveolar bone have been defined: compact bone, trabecular bone, and alveolar bone proper. The trabecular bone provides the major support structure of the teeth and is composed mainly of fatty marrow in adults.

Other Parts of the Mouth

There are several other areas in the mouth which are important. These include the tongue, palate, salivary glands, and the oral mucosa or lining of the mouth or oral cavity itself.

Palate

The palate forms the roof of the mouth and consists of two portions: the hard palate in the front area behind the upper teeth and soft palate at the back at the entrance to the pharynx or throat area. The hard palate separates the mouth from the nasal cavity and serves as the roof of the mouth and the floor of the nose. The soft palate aids in swallowing and sucking functions.

Tongue

The tongue is the main organ of the sense of taste and an important organ of speech. It also assists the teeth in the chewing and swallowing of food. The tongue is situated in the floor of the mouth and is connected to various muscles in the epiglottis and pharynx, or throat. It is covered by mucous membranes, and numerous mucous and serous glands as well as taste-buds. Internally, it consists of fibrous tissue, muscles, blood vessels and nerves (Fig. 6).

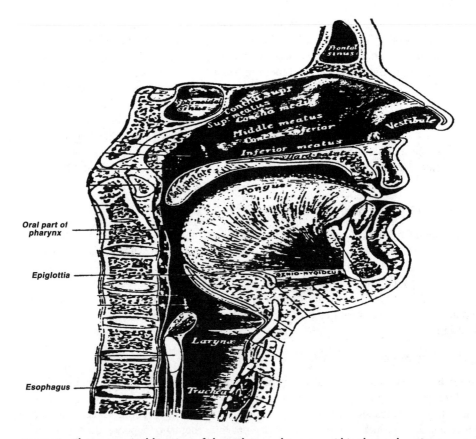

Oral part of
pharynx

Epiglottia

Esophagus

FIGURE 6   The anatomical location of the palate and tongue within the oral cavity.

Saliva and the Salivary Glands

Saliva is a fluid containing water, mucin, protein, salts and enzymes. It is produced and secreted into the oral cavity by three pairs of salivary glands: the submaxillary, sublingual (or submandibular), and parotid glands (Fig. 7).

The submaxillary glands are located beneath the floor of the mouth on the inner side of the jaw. Saliva secreted from these glands enters the mouth through a duct or opening beneath the tongue known as the duct of Wharton. The sublingual glands also are located below the floor of the mouth, but closer to the mid-line and pour their saliva into the mouth through a number of small ducts—the duct of Bartholin and the duct of Rivinus. The parotid glands lie below the ears and along the sides of the jaws. The ducts from these glands enter from the inner cheek opposite the second upper molars.

The salivary glands contain both serous and mucous cells. The secretion from the serous glands is thin and watery while that from the mucous glands contains mucin and is, therefore, thicker and more slimy. These glands are controlled by the autonomic (or involuntary) nervous system and react by reflex to both direct and indirect stimulation. For example, saliva is automatically and directly produced when you take a mouthful of food, but it also can be indirectly produced when you talk about or see some food you particularly like.

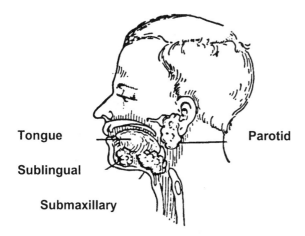

Tongue   **Parotid**

Sublingual

Submaxillary

FIGURE 7   The location of the salivary glands.

Saliva has the following important functions:

- to assist in the digestion of food,
- to prepare food for swallowing by altering its consistency,
- to moisten and lubricate the mouth and lips,
- to cleanse the mouth and teeth from food debris and other foreign materials, and
- to excrete organic and inorganic substances from the body.

The latter function especially can result in serious inflammation of the oral mucosa (the lining of the mouth) and the gums.

Oral Mucosa—The Lining of the Mouth

The oral mucosa, or ''mucous membrane'' lining of the mouth, also has special functions that are important to oral health. This thin, freely movable lining is composed of several layers of epithelial cells. These are the same type of cells found on the outer layers of your skin and which serve as a protective covering. However, within the mouth, this covering lies on a thick layer of ''mucous membranes'' which secrete mucus.

As discussed earlier, mucus contains a protein material known as mucin which is formed within the cytoplasm of these epithelial cells. As the mucin accumulates,the cells become distended until they finally burst, discharging their contents onto the surface of the mouth. The mucus coats the epithelial surface serving as protection against injurious substances in the mouth or as a means to trap small foreign particles.

The production of mucus can be greatly increased by stimulation caused by infection, allergy or temperature. We are all familiar with the increased production of mucus caused by a cold or sore throat. Often, ''cold sores'' or ''canker sores,'' which are small painful ulcerations on the oral mucosa, appear during these illnesses. Therefore, the oral mucosa can also be used as a mirror that reflects the general health of the body.

DENTAL DISEASES WORLDWIDE

Dental diseases including cavities (caries), tartar (calculus), sore gums (gingivitis), and periodontitis (loss of teeth supporting the tissue) are worldwide problems. The annual cost of all dental care in the U.S. exceeds $37 billion, out of which roughly $6 billion is spent to repair the ravages of decay [1]. However, the cost of dental disease cannot simply be measured in monetary terms. Other factors also need to be considered; for example, the loss of teeth leading to impaired chewing ability, speech problems, and changes in facial aesthetics which can cause embarrassment. The well-being of a person may also be compromised due to the associated dental pain, inability to chew properly, and potential of the infection spreading from the mouth to other parts of the body [2].

Currently, a tremendous amount of time is spent by dentists and hygienists to clean the teeth and associated structures to prevent dental disease. Alternative methods to prevent dental diseases which can be used by the general population are being developed to reduce the amount of time spent with the dental professional.

Factors Affecting Delivery of Actives in the Mouth

Before discussing specific product technologies for the prevention and treatment of oral disease, we need to understand the general principles underlying the efficacy and delivery of therapeutic agents in the oral cavity (Fig. 8).

The effective use of active ingredients in oral products is depending upon several factors; some of the major ones are depicted schematically in Figure 8. Normally a therapeutic toothpaste or mouthrinse contains an active ingredient or drug which must be dissolved in the formulation. Mouthrinses currently on the market are aqueous-based formulations but contain numerous other ingredients which must be compatible with the drug. The potential for undesirable interactions between ingredients is a major concern of formulators and manufacturers. Some interactions are specifically designed, such as the increased solubility of poorly water soluble drugs (e.g., triclosan) by adding surfactants and other ingredients to form a microemulsion. However, incompatible ingredients are sometimes unknowingly used, especially in complex formulations where there is an incomplete understanding of the chemistry [3].

The packaging material can also be a source of compatibility problems. Any number of possible interactions can affect, either directly or indirectly, the availability of the drug in the formulation. This can usually be evaluated in the laboratory on new and aged samples of the product. Drugs which are complexed with other materials, although still soluble in the formulation, may exhibit reduced bioavailability in vivo. The term bioavailability is usually used to express a temporal relationship of free drug concentration at the target site. In this case, after mouthrinsing or toothpaste use, the bioavailability is the concentra-

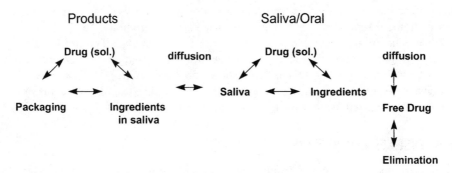

FIGURE 8 Factors affecting delivery of active agents in mouth.

tion of free drug in the environment of the target site and the rapidity at which it disappears. This can be determined providing the site can be sampled and the drug concentration measured in the medium contacting the target site (i.e., saliva, plaque fluid, crevicular fluid).

The duration of exposure may be important. Since most of the dose in the oral product is expectorated, the time in the mouth should be long enough for optimal retention of the drug. This has been determined for some orally used antiseptics such as chlorhexidine and triclosan. In general, 30 to 45 seconds is usually sufficient. Once introduced into the oral environment via a toothpaste/gel/mouthrinse, the residual drug must diffuse in saliva before it can reach its intended site of action. In saliva the drug is then free to interact with salivary components before reaching oral surfaces. In theory, only free available drug can interact optimally with target sites. Such sites include plaque, enamel, the gingival sulcus, gingival tissue, and the mucous membranes.

The amount of drug retained on oral surfaces after use is also thought to be important since subsequent desorption of the drug into the microenvironment of the target site could provide a sustained effect. This will be determined mainly by the substantivity of the particular drug used. Because of the long dosage interval commonly practiced with the product (once or twice a day), highly substantive drugs may have a distinct advantage because of their longer presence in the oral cavity. Superimposed upon this is the normal clearance process by which materials are removed from oral surfaces by salivary flow. The longer a drug can be retained in the environment of the target site in active form, the better chance there is to exert a therapeutic effect.

Evolution of Technologies in Oral Products

Historically, dentifrices or toothpastes were developed to keep the teeth clean and free of stains. The essential ingredients of a toothpaste are: a thickening agent, an abrasive cleaning agent, a surfactant, a humectant, flavor, and active therapeutic agents. One of the first dentifrices contained an abrasive (precipitated calcium carbonate) and a small amount of powdered soap. This toothpaste was irritating to the tissues of the mouth because the pH was relatively high due to its soap content [4]. After the Second World War, many companies undertook scientific research to develop dentifrices which were milder, gentler, and also had therapeutic properties. Instead of soap, a synthetic detergent—sodium lauryl sarcosinate—was introduced in toothpaste. Besides preventing irritation, the synthetic detergent improved the taste and was also shown to control plaque acids which cause cavities. Figure 9 provides an overview of the evolution of technologies in oral products. The category is driven by scientific advances and consumer benefits which have been broadly classified as a good smile (Fig. 9).

Stain Removal and Whitening Toothpastes

There are two types of stains on teeth: (1) stain on teeth (extrinsic stain); and (2) stain in the tooth (intrinsic stain). The extrinsic stain may originate from chromogenic materials from food or drink, while the intrinsic stain could be caused by therapeutic agents, such as tetracycline, or excessive fluoride exposure during teeth development (below age of 5). Several investigators have studied mechanisms of stain formation and developed methods to remove dental stain (Fig. 10) [5].

The evolution of whitening/cleaning technologies in toothpaste and gel is depicted in Figure 10. The most commonly used procedure for removing stains on teeth is the use

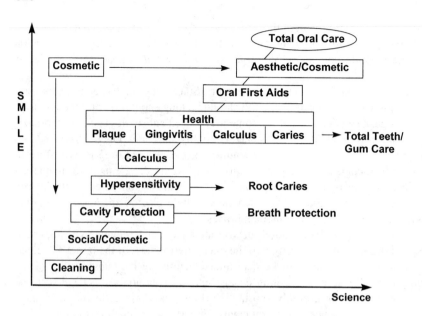

FIGURE 9   Evolution of technologies in oral products.

of abrasives such as silicon dioxide, dicalcium phosphate dihydrate, and aluminum salts such as calcined alumina. All these are used in combination with detergents to remove stains. In the early eighties, calcined alumina or enzymes with or without tartar control ingredient, such as pyrophosphate, were added. Later on, fluoride preparations such as hydrogen peroxide, urea peroxide, or calcium peroxides were added to remove both intrinsic and extrinsic stains. To assess performance, several laboratory tests were developed but none of them correlate with in vivo stain removal on teeth. Therefore, in vivo clinicals are the best way to assess stain removal. Typical results from in vivo studies are depicted in the table below (Table 1).

It can be seen that the addition of calcined alumina with pyrophosphate gave good stain removal in vivo. Another procedure for stain removal in vivo is by reflective spectros-

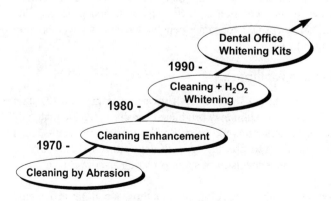

FIGURE 10   Evolution of cleaning/whitening technologies.

TABLE 1   In Vivo Stain Reduction 6 Weeks After Brushing

Dentifrice treatment	% Stain reduction
SiO_2/NaF toothpaste	No change
SiO_2/NaF/tripolyphosphate	14.0
SiO_2/Calcined Alumina/Pyrophosphate	49.0

copy using a Minolta chromameter. The color change is measured by $\triangle E$ (difference in color). The higher the positive value, the whiter the teeth. Using $\triangle E$ in vivo, one would get $\triangle E$ of 2 to 4 with above technologies (in Table 1). If one adds peroxide, the value could reach as high as 6. For the reference, an in-office treatment by a dentist would provide $\triangle E$ of 7 to 8 following two weeks procedure.

Dentifrices to Reduce Offensive Bad Breath

Local mouth odor is caused by oral bacteria reacting with salivary proteins to form volatile sulfur compounds (VSC). Tonzetich has shown that hydrogen sulfide, methyl mercaptan, and dimethyl sulfide [H_2S, CH_3SH and $(CH_3)_2S$, respectively] are the major components of mouth odor. A gas chromatographic method was developed to objectively measure VSC directly from mouth air as an alternative to the organoleptic/sensory method. This instrumental method has, in turn, permitted investigators to carry out studies in a number of areas relevant to human malodor [6]. There are two methods currently available to assess the magnitude of oral malodor. The first is the organoleptic or sensory rating approach, and the second is the GC instrumental method. A study was conducted to determine the correlation between these two methods in a controlled clinical study. An excellent correlation (r = 0.78) has been established between the instrumental method and sensory evaluation. Using the analytical technique, the effect of dentifrices on mouth odor has been evaluated in a variety of clinicals. A baseline reading is taken in the morning. The subjects then brushed with a placebo or an active dentifrice, and then readings are taken three or 12 hours post-treatment to assess the effects. A dentifrice containing the antibacterial triclosan and a copolymer polyvinyl methyl ether maleic acid (PVM/MA) has been developed. This provides sustained reduction in mouth odor. The typical clinical results are summarized in Figure 11 [7].

Therapeutic Dentifrices

Dentifrices to Control Caries (Cavity)

It is well-known that the formation of dental caries is a result of interactions between the tooth enamel, environment (saliva), plaque fluid and ingestion of dietary carbohydrates. These interactions are also important in the formation of dental plaque on teeth. Dental plaque plays an important role in the formation of caries since it is the plaque bacteria which produce acids from sugars. However, the production of acids by plaque bacteria and subsequent dissolution of tooth enamel is not a constant process. Instead, it appears to be cyclical. At a given time, plaque acids attack the enamel surface and deplete it of minerals, creating a small microtrauma at the surface. These areas are actually called incipient caries or white spots and occur long before caries can be detected by dentists or hygienists. If left unchecked, the process eventually results in destruction of the teeth.

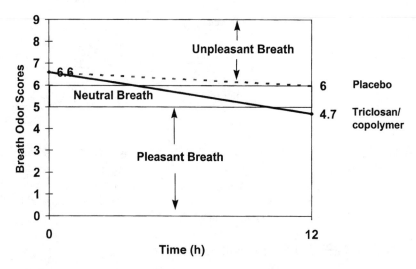

FIGURE 11 Plot of breath odor scores.

Since caries is not a continuous process, early lesions can be repaired through interactions of various elements in the oral environment, that is, supersaturation with respect to calcium phosphate in saliva, fluoride and pH of the plaque fluid [8].

Tooth enamel is not a smooth impervious surface, instead it is porous, and an apparent lack of activity on the surface may mask actual activity below. In order to create a caries lesion, the acids must penetrate the enamel structure, which consists of hydroxyapatite (HA) crystals surrounded by an organic matrix consisting of water, protein and lipid materials and this they do by removing some of the mineral from the crystalline rods below the surface of the teeth. This demineralization weakens the structure and, if unchecked, eventually results in a subsurface lesion often called a white spot which will appear to be chalky and whiter than the normal surrounding tooth surface. Continuation of the demineralization process results in the creation of cavities. This occurs when the surface enamel collapses as the underlying structure of mineral rods can no longer maintain the tooth structure. However, not all white spot lesions progress to cavities, and one of the prime reasons being the process of remineralization which occurs when minerals are redeposited into the enamel that has been weakened by bacterial acids. Remineralization can, therefore, only take place when there has been loss of tooth structure through demineralization. Thus, demineralization and remineralization are continuous processes with loss from, and replacement of, minerals into enamel within the oral environment. The most soluble mineral in the teeth is thereby replaced by the most insoluble calcium phosphate, such as dicalcium phosphate dihydrate (DCPD). If the environment is rich in DCPD, the process of remineralization occurs. This process is greatly enhanced by fluoride ions which convert DCPD into fluorohydroxyapatite which forms onto, and within, the tooth increasing resistance to acid attack [9].

Fluoride increases remineralization by increasing the rate of crystal growth, but to restore tooth structure a supersaturation of calcium phosphate in the environment is also necessary. The process of remineralization has been shown to be controlled by the presence of fluoride and a supersaturation of calcium and phosphate in plaque fluid. Thus, the tooth and environment are in a seesaw battle. Under healthy conditions when supersaturation is high and plaque acids are low, the ambient calcium phosphate (DCPD) in plaque fluid

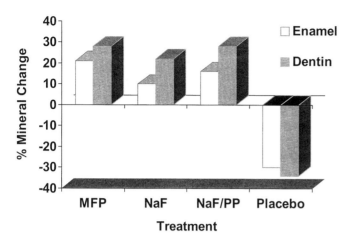

FIGURE 12   Average percent mineral changes for enamel and dentin.

is sufficient to maintain healthy enamel. When the caries challenge is high and plaque is producing more acids, supersaturation with respect to DCPD decreases and demineralization occurs. Fluoride inhibits lesion formation by enhancing the process of remineralization, and this enhancement is greatly influenced by supersaturation of the plaque fluid with respect to HA.

Fluoride dentifrices are capable of adding minerals (remineralization) to early caries lesions. This process can be measured in vivo by using the model of intra-oral remineralization. A dose response effect of fluoride is shown in Figure 12 which shows the percent mineral gains in either enamel or dentine following two weeks use of either 1100 ppm F from MFP (sodium monofluorophosphate) or sodium fluoride, NaF. Both fluoridating systems extend the same degree of mineralization as an equal concentration. Human clinical studies for caries (cavity) prevention require 3 years to document anti-caries effect. In those studies, mean reduction in caries varies from 25 to 40% depending upon the population used in the study and whether or not the study area had water fluoridation. Current efforts are to enhance efficacy of 1000 to 1500 ppm of fluoride in dentifrices with additives such as xylitol, a non-fermentable sugar, or the antibacterial triclosan. These additives have been shown to boost the effectiveness of fluoride in toothpaste (Figs. 12, 13) [10].

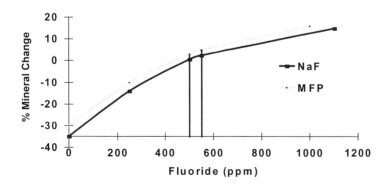

FIGURE 13   Fluoride dose response for MFP and NaF dentifrices.

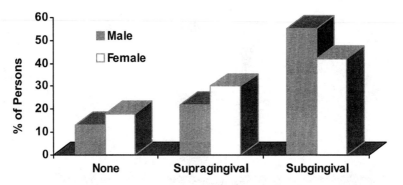

FIGURE 14   Data from "Oral Health of U.S. Adults," NIDR, 1985.

Anticalculus and Anticavity Technologies

Calculus build-up on teeth is a worldwide problem. For nearly 5,000 years since the time of the Sumerians, calculus has been considered an important factor in the etiology of periodontal diseases. Although it is not considered to be a principle cause of periodontal diseases today, calculus is an important contributor to the formation of dental plaque which is implicated in periodontal disease. At a given time, hundreds—even thousands—of hygienists around the world are removing calculus build-up by mechanical cleaning. These procedures are very labor-intensive and may cause a great deal of discomfort to the patient.

The extent and incidence of calculus in the general U.S. population has been shown in a comprehensive oral health survey by the National Institute of Dental Research [11]. The data shown in Figures 14 and 15 indicate the incidence of calculus. Calculus was observed in 34% of school-aged children. In adults, 25 to 30% had calculus build-up above the gingival margin, but 60–65% had deposit below the gingival margin. Older adults showed an even higher incidence. The extent of calculus in the population indicates a need to develop an effective but safe chemical means to prevent calculus build-up on the teeth. This is especially important for the countries where the dentists and hygienists are not readily available (21). Therefore, the development of the technologies to prevent calculus is important around the world from a public health point of view (Figs. 14, 15).

Chemical Composition of Dental Calculi on Teeth and Dental Materials

Dental calculus consists of both organic and inorganic components. The organic portion is a combination of epithelial cells, leukocytes, micro-organisms, and polysaccharides.

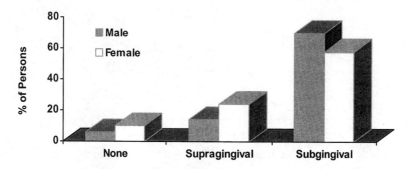

FIGURE 15   Calculus in U.S. population (seniors, "Oral Health of U.S. Adults," NIDR, 1985).

The inorganic part is primarily calcium phosphate salts which include: carbonated hydroxyapatite (CHA), dicalcium phosphate dihydrate (DCPD), and octacalcium phosphate (OCP). The x-ray diffraction patterns and infrared absorption spectra of human dental calculi and the samples obtained from the dentures and tooth surfaces show that the inorganic component of calculus from dentures is principally carbonated hydroxyapatite (CHA), while material from tooth surfaces is a mixed calcium phosphate phase β-TCPC Mg-substituted), CHA, and OCP. The deposits then are primarily basic calcium and phosphate salts [12].

Technologies for the Prevention of Calculus Formation

A general method of removing calculus is by mechanical means. The mechanical means are labor-intensive and painful. Another approach is to develop a chemical way of preventing the formation of the basic phases of calcium phosphates. A large number of agents have been proposed to retard the formation of calculus on to surfaces. These agents are usually compounds which inhibit the formation of calcium phosphate salts to the crystalline phases. Among the most effective inhibitors are pyrophosphate, pyrophosphate plus polymer and zinc salts. In general, agents usually work via a surface effect. The inhibitors adsorb to the growing (calcium phosphate) crystals and they reduce the formation of crystalline phases allowing calcium phosphate to remain in an amorphous phase. In general, two types of tests have been used to evaluate the inhibitors. One test follows the spontaneous formation of HA (Fig. 16) using a supersaturation environment which stimulates the plaque fluid. The second test is a seeded crystal growth for hydroxyapatite which uses the driving force equivalent to saliva environment (Fig. 17). Using these tests, the relative value of efficacy of these inhibitors is summarized, shown in Table 2. It shows that the most active inhibitor is pyrophosphate. Also a combination of pyrophosphate and the copolymer of pyrophosphate and the copolymer (PVM/MA) provides an enhanced efficacy. Zinc salts, on the other hand, require a higher concentration for effectiveness. The relative clinical efficacy of these agents in various dentifrices are summarized in Table 3. Available data from the composite of several clinical studies indicate that calculus inhibition with the pyrophosphate and sodium fluoride combination is roughly in the range of 26%; with the copolymer/pyrophosphate (1.3% soluble pyrophosphate to 3.3%) the

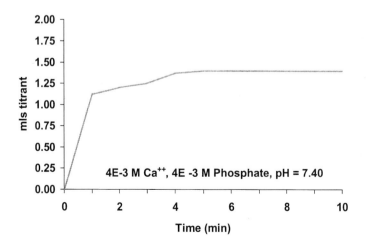

Figure 16 **HAP formation.**

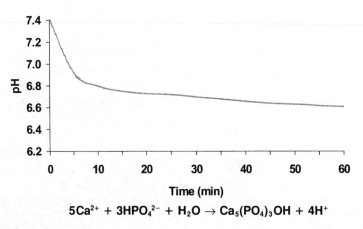

$$5Ca^{2+} + 3HPO_4^{2-} + H_2O \rightarrow Ca_5(PO_4)_3OH + 4H^+$$

FIGURE 17   Crystal growth.

calculus reduction ranged as high as 50%; zinc salts require higher concentration for efficacy (2% or above). With a lower concentration (0.5%), the efficacy against supergingival calculus formation is very poor [13].

Mechanisms of Action of Anticalculus Agents

The mechanism for the inhibition of calculus formation by anticalculus agents are schematically illustrated. The calcium and phosphate from saliva or from plaque fluid precipitate and form a precrystalline phase which matures to crystal phase in the absence of inhibitor. In the presence of inhibitor that amorphous phase is stabilized and the conversion of the crystalline phase is delayed. This is clearly evident from the electronmicrographs of calculus formed in the presence and the absence of inhibitor. In the absence of inhibitor, the crystal size was very large and well-defined; in the presence of an inhibitor, the deposit was very small and has morphology of amorphous calcium phosphate (Fig. 18).

The current technologies used for inhibiting calculus formation also contains fluoride. When the application of a potent inhibitor of calcium and phosphate crystal growth coexists with fluoride, a crystal growth promoter, we need to understand how they work together. The inhibitor prevents the formation of HA. Then how do two agents coexist in the same system and exert the respective effect? Our early data indicated that crystal growth inhibitors work on tooth surfaces while fluoride ion works within teeth. The effect can be explained by the fact that the calculus formation occurs on the teeth (above) where the demineralization occurs in the subsurface region of the enamel (under pellicle). The presence of pellicle on the tooth allows the selective transport of fluoride and the inhibitor. This mechanism has been elucidated by studies of natural inhibitors of crystal growth in

TABLE 2   Calculus-Control Technologies:
Relative Efficacy

Compound	Inhibition (ppm)
Pyrophosphate	4.0
Pyrophosphate + copolymer	3.0
Zinc	60.0

TABLE 3 Clinical Efficacy of Toothpastes in Humans

Toothpaste	Mean reduction in calculus vs. placebo
3.3% pyrophosphate + NaF	26%
3.3% pyrophosphate + 1% PVM/MA/NaF	50%
1.3% pyrophosphate + 1.5% PVM/MA/NaF	47%
0.5% zinc citrate + MFP	14%
2% zinc + sodium fluoride	38–50%

Abbreviation: PVM/MA, copolymer polyvinymethyl maleic acid.
Source: Ref. 13.

saliva. The study indicated that the crystal growth inhibitory effect of the natural inhibitor can be overcome by the addition of fluoride. This effect was neither due to displacement of an adsorbed inhibitor by fluoride nor the activation of secondary growth sides. Rather the effect was explained on the basis of increased driving force of precipitation and incomplete blockage of crystal growth sites on the basis of steric effect. This has now been confirmed via in vivo studies.

Technologies to Reduce Tooth Sensitivity

The next evolution of toothpaste chemistry was developed as a means to prevent pain caused by sensitive teeth; i.e., hypersensitivity. Dentinal hypersensitivity is defined as an acute, localized tooth pain in response to thermal, tactile, or air blast stimulation to exposed dentine surfaces. Normally, the roots of teeth are covered by the gingival or gum tissue but when the gum recedes, the underlying tooth surface is exposed. Once exposed, with time, abrasion and erosion will remove the thin layer of cementum, thus exposing underlying porous dentine. Exposure of the dentine surface to dietary or bacterial acids can expose

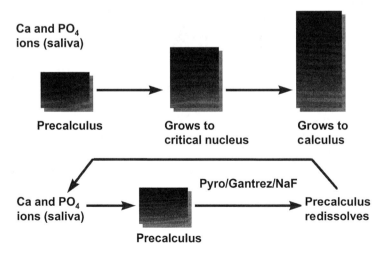

FIGURE 18 Mechanism of pyrophosphate/copolymer/NaF on tartar formation.

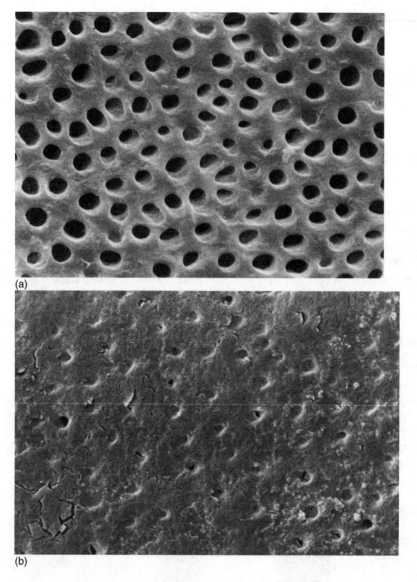

(a)

(b)

FIGURE 19   (a) Open dentinal tubules. (b) Occluded dentinal tubules.

the dentine pores or tubules at the surface. It is well known that exposure and the presence of open tubules (Fig. 19a) on the surface is associated with increased dentinal hypersensitivity. The dentine tubes contain fluid.

Mechanistically, hot or cold stimuli can cause this fluid to expand or shrink, stimulating underlying pulpal nerve resulting in pain. Currently, salts of potassium are available as preventive therapies in OTC toothpaste. Various other agents such as potassium nitrate are believed to cause reduction in nerve activity by altering the threshold of pulpal nerve excitation. These approaches have been combined in a single toothpaste containing potassium nitrate and copolymer which adhere to tooth surfaces. Figure 19b shows occlusion

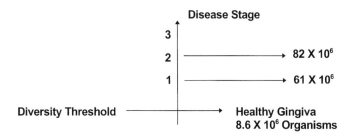

FIGURE 20 Microbiota (health vs. disease).

which can result from in vitro treatment of dentine with such a toothpaste. Unfortunately, this therapy requires two to three weeks treatment before a reduction in sensitivity is observed. Therefore, there is currently a strong need for a fast reactive material in toothpaste which could rapidly reduce dentinal hypersensitivity (Figs. 19a,b) [14].

Multibenefit Technologies in Dentifrices

The next development in dentifrice technology was to incorporate antibacterial agents with fluoride and tartar reducing compounds.

Microbiota of Dental Plaque: Health Versus Disease

The basic research within the past 30 years clearly established the role of dental plaque at the interfaces of tooth/gingiva as the main cause of gingival inflammation, which could lead eventually to periodontitis. The previous studies by Löe et al. [15] and subsequent studies by Syed [16] and Loesche indicated that there was threshold level of bacteria which was compatible with gingival health. When that threshold level of bacteria increased by at least two or three orders of magnitude, then gingival inflammation was initiated. Therefore, the prime purpose of chemical antiplaque agents is to bring the microflora to a healthy level at the gingival interfaces, primarily by reducing the total mass of microbiota at the surface, or by reducing the total number of pathogens at the surface (Figs. 20, 21).

Since dental plaque is principally composed of microorganisms, it is logical to use antibacterials to reduce or prevent plaque formation. The rationale is that the antibacterials will either inactivate bacteria in the existing plaque or prevent colonization. However, early studies clearly showed that 99% of bacteria in the oral cavity must be killed in order to inhibit plaque formation for only 6 hours, provided teeth are brushed twice daily. Since

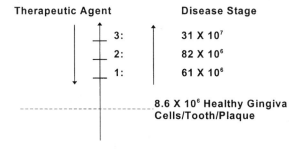

FIGURE 21 Therapeutic strategies.

TABLE 4 Characteristics of
Antibacterials for Plaque Effects

Broad spectrum antibacterial activity
Substantivity to oral surfaces
Good taste
Compatible with toothpaste ingredients
Low toxicity
No disturbance of oral ecology

---

the oral cavity is an open system, the chance of continued reinfection is ever present. Based on recent studies, the general characteristics of antibacterial agents useful for an antiplaque effect can be summarized in Table 4. For an antibacterial antiplaque agent to be effective, a broad-spectrum activity against oral microflora is required, since the microbial composition of the plaque is complex. With cationic antibacterial agents, a minimum inhibitory concentration in the range of 0.1 to 0.5 µg/ml against oral pathogens has been noted. However, the current understanding of the pharmacology of antibacterial antiplaque agents indicates that there are factors other than antibacterial activity in determining sustained antiplaque effect on teeth. These factors include the retention and release of antibacterials on oral surfaces, as well as their efficacy in the presence of the salivary environment. Furthermore, it is important that a given antibacterial does not disturb taste, otherwise the patient's compliance would be very poor. Another consideration for use in oral products is compatibility with polishing agents and surfactants, since both of these ingredients are important for controlling stain on teeth, as well as emulsifying flavor oils, which are incorporated in the oral hygiene products for compliance. Other important considerations are a low toxicity and a minimum potential to disturb the normal microbial oral ecology [17].

Cationic Antibacterial Agents

Among the widely studied agents are cationic antibacterials such as chlorhexidine digluconate (CHDG), benzethonium chloride (BTC), and cetyl pyridium chloride (CPC). CHDG is more effective than BTC or CPC and has higher retention in the oral environment. They also differ with respect to their reaction with salivary protein, which is an important parameter for the retention of cationic antibacterials on oral surfaces; increased retention provides a sustained release of concentrations active against oral pathogens.

Long-term clinical studies have demonstrated the efficacy of cationic antibacterials against plaque, gingivitis and plaque microflora. However, these agents cause unacceptable staining of teeth and an increase in calculus formation. Therefore, their use in oral hygiene products clearly is limited [17].

Noncationic Antibacterial Agents

More recently (during the past 10 years), there has been tremendous interest in non-cationic antibacterials which provide multi-benefits such as plaque, gingivitis, calculus, and caries reduction. This is primarily based on a non-ionic antibacterial agent, triclosan, which has broad-spectrum antibacterial activity against gram-positive and gram-negative bacteria. For triclosan to be effective, a delivery system is required to increase its residence time in the oral cavity. A copolymer of polyvinyl methyl ether (PVM) and maleic acid (MA) has been shown to accomplish that. This copolymer was well-suited for improving the delivery of triclosan, since PVM/MA has been shown to react with hard and soft

TABLE 5 Noncationic Antibacterials: Comparative
Study for In Vivo Plaque Inhibition

Treatment	Mean P on all surfaces $\pm$ SD	SNK group
Placebo	1.46 $\pm$ 0.12	A
0.12% CHDG	0.53 $\pm$ 0.17	B
0.2% SnF$_2$ (rinse)	1.10 $\pm$ 0.16	C
0.06 Triclosan	1.00 $\pm$ 0.14	C
0.06 Triclosan + Gantrez	0.72 $\pm$ 0.17	B
0.06 Triclosan + PVPA	0.67 $\pm$ 0.16	B

Abbreviations: Gantrez, PVM/MA, polyvinyl methyl/maleic acid; PVPA, polyvinylphosphonic acid; SNK, Student Neuman Keuls test; P, plaque index.

surfaces in the oral cavity. In a four-day short-term study of de novo plaque formation, we evaluated a series of different antibacterial agents. We found that triclosan actually needs an improved delivery system, primarily a copolymer, to enhance its retention to both tooth and oral epithelial surfaces [18].

One of the important principles developed is that retention per se is not the only factor in antiplaque activity; the retained concentration has to be active biologically. To demonstrate this principle, we conducted a series of studies to understand how much triclosan was retained post-brushing. In one of the studies, we compared three triclosan formulations, each having a different enhancing system (Table 5). As can be seen in Table 6, even after 14 hours, a significant amount is retained in plaque, a concentration above the MIC's of triclosan for oral bacteria (MIC being 0.3-4 µg/mL). The next important step was to determine whether this retained amount was active biologically. A plaque viability assay was used, in which we exposed the plaque to two fluorescent dyes to discriminate between live and dead bacteria by measuring the ratio of green to red fluorescence. In this study, one could quantitatively measure the ratio and ascertain whether the retained amount was active biologically. In one of the typical studies shown here, brushing with the placebo toothpaste gave some reduction of plaque viability; the triclosan copolymer system gave the highest reduction in viability, and the other systems, such as triclosan/pyrophosphate and triclosan/zinc citrate, were not significantly different from the placebo (Fig. 22). These results have been corroborated by an independent six-month clinical study by Renvert and Birkhed (Table 6) [19].

The mechanism by which the copolymer enhances the delivery of triclosan has been elucidated (Fig. 23). The polymer has two groups: one is the attachment group and the other is the solubilizing group. The solubilizing group retains triclosan in surfactant mi-

TABLE 6 Plaque Triclosan Levels After Brushing (µg/mL)

After brushing	0.3% Triclosan/ copolymer n = 12	0.3% Triclosan/ pyrophosphate n = 12	0.3% Triclosan/ 1% zinc n = 12
2 h	38.83 $\pm$ 18.28*	20.90 $\pm$ 14.14	30.60 $\pm$ 13.6
14 h	4.14 $\pm$ 1.72	2.74 $\pm$ 2.11	3.95 $\pm$ 1.79

* P = 0.05, compared with a placebo toothpaste.

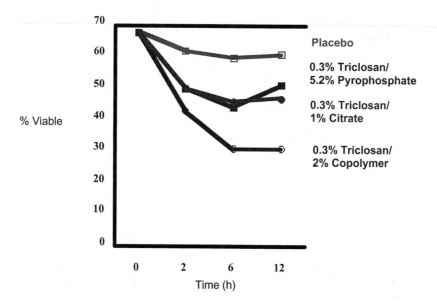

FIGURE 22   Plaque viability study determined via a fluorescent-dye technique.

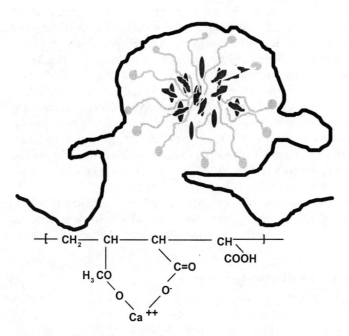

FIGURE 23   Mechanism of retention of triclosan on oral surfaces by the copolymer. The solubilizing group (methoxyether) traps triclosan/surfactant micelle while the attachment group (COOH) binds to calcium in an adherent liquid layer on tooth/enamel interface.

TABLE 7 Therapeutic Mouthrinses

Mouthrinse	Active agents	Typical reduction in the diseases vs. placebo
Fluoride rinses	225 ppm F	50% reduction in caries, children (3 years)
Tartar + calculus	1% pyrophosphate amion; 100 ppm F plus a copolymer of PVM/MA (0.5%)	30–35% reduction in tartar formation after 6 months use
Antiplaque/antigingivitis	0.03 to 0.06 Triclosan + 1% copolymer PVM/MA + fluoride	20–30% reduction in plaque/gingivitis after 3 months of use

celles, and the attachment group reacts with the oral surfaces via calcium in the liquid adherent layer. Triclosan is then slowly released via interactions with salivary environment. In terms of long-term clinical trials, this technology has now been evaluated around the world in 12 six-month plaque/gingivitis studies, three calculus studies, three caries clinical trials, and five long-term studies monitoring the oral microbial population. The results of all these studies indicated that this technology was effective against plaque, gingivitis, calculus, and caries. No side effects of staining or calculus increase were seen. There was also no disturbance of the oral microbial ecology.

One of the most exciting aspects of triclosan is its "double-barrel" effect. This unique antibacterial not only kills bacteria, but also neutralizes the products of bacteria which could provoke inflammation. We have shown that triclosan was a potent inhibitor of both cyclo-oxygenase and lipoxygenase pathways. It not only inhibited these enzymes in vitro but also inhibited the release of their products (prostaglandins and leukotrienes) in gingival fibroblasts which were stimulated by interleukin 1-β. These data were clinically confirmed in a study in which we blocked the antibacterial effect of triclosan but maintained its anti-inflammatory effect. Thus, triclosan has a "double barrel" effect—both antibacterial and anti-inflammatory. This unique feature is not provided so far by other antibacterial, anti-plaque agents [20].

MOUTHWASHING

Mouth rinses currently on the markets are aqueous-based formulation where the therapeutic agents are at lower concentrations than toothpaste. For example, the general population uses toothpaste at 1 g or 1 mL on the brush, but the rinses are used in 10 to 15 mL and some lower concentration of the actives are incorporated. Also, the rinses do not contain polishing agents or thickeners. A typical therapeutic rinse contains surfactants, flavor, active agent, and water. The general principles of active agent delivery which were outlined above also apply for the active agent delivery in the mouthwash. Table 7 summarizes the typical clinical performance vs. a placebo rinse of therapeutic rinse (Table 7).

STRATEGY FOR CLINICAL STUDIES IN ORAL-CARE PRODUCTS

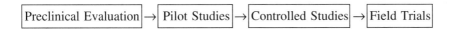

To document the effectiveness of oral products against dental diseases, the strategy for clinical studies is outlined in the above chart. The preclinical studies include laboratory and animal tests. For example, for fluoride efficacy a test would include fluoride uptake in teeth or hydroxyapatite, reduction in enamel solubility following fluoride treatment, followed by an acid challenge. The effectiveness in rats include the effects of topical application of fluoride solution in reducing caries. The pilot studies in humans are done to assess the effectiveness of fluoride to promote mineral deposition or prevent dissolution of artificially created lesions in enamel slabs implanted in partial dentures. Such studies are of 2 to 4 weeks duration and conducted in 20 to 30 subjects per group. If the pilot study significantly enhance remineralization of artificial lesions, control studies in 30 to 60 subjects for 3 to 6 months are conducted with the final formula for efficacy. The parameters could include promotion of mineralization, regression of early cavity lesions, and fluoride uptake in dental plaque and saliva. The field trials are conducted in children (1000 per group) for a period of 3 years to assess the effects on cavity development. For prevention of plaque and gingivitis formation, such trials are conducted for 6 months. The calculus reduction field trials are also conducted for a period of 6 months. Such field trials are of parallel/double-blind design.

FUTURE TRENDS

The global needs for prevention of dental diseases can be met by the development of knowledge in academia and industry and its subsequent applications. With a better understanding of processes occurring in the mouth, we will be able to design better actives and active agent delivery systems for the control of oral diseases. The technological trends are leading toward the goal.

REFERENCES

1. Dental Spending Hits $37 Billion. Am Dent Assoc News, Jan. 6, 1992.
2. Periodontal aspects of systemic health. Symposium proceedings, WD Cohen, ed. Compendium Continuing Education, Fall, 1998.
3. Gaffar A, Afflitto J. General principles for delivery of active agents for mouthrinses. Int Dent J 1996; 42(4):251–256.
4. Fishman SL. Hare's teeth to fluorides, historical aspects of dentifrice use. In: Emery G, Rölla G, eds. Clinical and Biological Aspects of Dentifrice. Oxford: Oxford University Press, 1972: 1–7.
5. Nathoo SA, Gaffar A. Studies on dental stain induced by antibacterial agent and rational approaches for bleaching dental stains. Adv Dent Res 1995; 9(4):462–470.
6. Solis-Gaffar M, Niles HP. Instrumental evaluation of mouth odor in a human clinical study. J Dent Res 1977; 54:851–857.
7. Niles HP, Gaffar A. Relationship between sensory and instrumental evaluation of mouth odor. J Soc Cos Chem 1993; 44:101–107.
8. Gaffar A, Blake-Haskins J, Mellberg J. In vivo studies with dicalcium phosphate dihydrate/ MFP system for caries prevention. Int Dent J 1993; 63(1):81–90.
9. Sullivan RJ, Fletcher R, Barchman R, Legeros RZ. Intra-oral comparison and evaluation of the ability of dentifrices to promote remineralization of caries-like lesions in dentin and enamel. J Clin Dent 1995; 6:135–138.
10. Gaffar A, Blake-Haskins J, Sullivan RJ, Simone A, Saunders F. Cariostatic effects of a xylitol/ NaF dentifrice in vivo. Int Dent J 1998; 48:32–39.

11. Mandel ID. Rinses for the control of supragingival calculus formation. Int Dent J 1992; 42: 270–285.

12. Gaffar A, Legeros RZ, Gambogi RS, Afflitto J. Inhibition of formation of calcium phosphate deposits on teeth and dental materials: recent advances. Adv Dent Res 1995; 9(4):419–426.

13. Volpe AR, Petrone M, Davies RM. A review of calculus clinical efficacy studies. J Clin Dentistry 1993; 4:71–81.

14. Miller S, Gaffar A, Sullivan RJ, Troung T, Stranick M. Evaluation of new dentifrice for treatment of sensitive teeth. J Clin Dent 1994; 5:71–79.

15. Löe H, Theilde E, Jensen SB. Experimental gingivitis in man. J Periodont 1970; 36:177–187.

16. Syed SA, Loesche WJ. Bacteriology of experimental gingivitis: effect of plaque. Info Immun 1978; 21:821–829.

17. Gaffar A, Volpe AR, Lindhe J. Recent advances in plaque/gingivitis control. In: Emery G, Rölla G, eds. Chemical Biological Aspects of Dentifrices. Oxford: Oxford University Press, 1992: 229–247.

18. Gaffar A, Afflitto J, Herles S, Nabi N. Recent advances in plaque, gingivitis, tartar and caries prevention. Int Dent J 1994; 44:63–70.

19. Renvert St, Birkhed D. Comparison of three triclosan dentifrices on plaque, gingivitis and salivary microflora. J Clin Periodont 1995; 23:63–70.

20. Gaffar A, Scherl D, Afflitto J, Coleman EJ. The effects of triclosan on the mediators of gingival inflammation. J Clin Periodont 1995; 22:280–284.

21. Mandel ID. Chemotherapeutic mouthrinses for control of oral disease. Int Dent J 1992; 42(4): 251–285.

54

Decorative Products

Mitchell L. Schlossman
Kobo Products, Inc., South Plainfield, New Jersey

INTRODUCTION

Decorative cosmetics are principally concerned with beautifying and decoration rather than functionality. No discussion of decorative products can be complete without a full understanding of the importance of color, a prime component of every decorative cosmetic. Conventional pigments create color by absorption of certain wavelengths of incident light. The color perceived corresponds to that of the wavelengths reflected. Formulation of decorative cosmetics has been an exciting challenge for cosmetic chemists. Before formulating any color cosmetic product, one must check the current regulations in the country where the proposed product will be sold to make sure all the colors conform to those regulations. The following is a practical guide for the formulator and covers a maximum of technical and regulatory issues in an easy-to-use format.

COLOR

Color-Additive Regulation

In the past, colorants had been used in cosmetics without any consideration being given to their possible toxicity. Today, all countries have regulations that control the type and purity of colors that may be used in cosmetics.

United States: U.S. Food and Drug Administration (FDA)

21 CFR 73, 74; Positive List [1]: Colors listed for general cosmetic use, including eye area only if stated specifically, or external only, meaning no contact with mucous membranes. Hair dyes and true soaps are exempt.

European Union (EU): European Commission (EC)

Directive 76/786, Annex IV [2]; Positive List: Colors listed for ingested use, general, including eye area, external, or rinse-off.
Annex II: Negative List

Japan: Ministry of Health and Welfare (MHW)

MHW Ordinance No. 30 [3]; Positive List, Coal-Tar Colors: Premarket approval by MHW for all other cosmetic ingredients, including inorganic and natural colorants.

Color-Additives Definitions

Primary/Straight Color: A color that is pure, containing no extenders or dilutents.

Dye: A color that is soluble in the medium in which it is dispersed. (e.g., FD&C Blue #1).

Pigment: A color that is insoluble in the medium in which it is dispersed. (e.g., FD&C Blue #1 Al lake, Black iron oxide).

Lake: A water-insoluble pigment composed of a water-soluble straight color strongly absorbed onto an insoluble substratum through the use of a precipitant (e.g., FD&C Blue #1 Al Lake). Generally, 10 to 40% color.*

Toner: A pigment that is produced by precipitating a water-soluble dye as an insoluble metal salt (e.g., D&C Red #6 barium salt, D&C Red #7 calcium salt).

True Pigment: A pigment that, based on its chemistry, precipitates as it is formed (e.g., D&C Red #36).

Extender: A pigment diluted on substrate
1. during manufacture by precipitation, or
2. postmanufacture by intimate milling or mixing.

U.S. Regulations

21 CFR Part 73 [4]: Listing of Color Additives Exempt from Certification

Inorganic pigments, powdered metals, and naturally derived colorants approved for food, drug, and/or cosmetic use. Listed permitted uses are as follows:

- Food
- Ingested/externally applied drugs
- General cosmetic
- Eye area only if mentioned
- External (no mucous membrane), i.e., ultramarines, ferric ammonium ferrocyanide not permitted in lip or bath products

21 CFR Part 74 [5]: Listing of Color Additives Subject to Certification

Synthetic organic dyes and pigments. Each batch must be submitted by the manufacturer to the FDA for certification that specifications are met. Permitted uses as in Part 73.

Four certified organic dyes and their lakes are now permitted for eye-area use:

1. FD&C Blue #1
2. FD&C Red #40
3. FD&C Yellow #5
4. D&C Green #5

21 CFR Part 82 [6]: Listing of Certified Provisionally Listed Colors

Lakes:

FD&C: Aluminum or calcium salt on alumina.

---

* FDA has considered any certified colorant mixed with a diluent to be a lake; e.g., D&C Red 30 Plus talc, and D&C Red #7 CA lake on calcium carbonate.

D&C: Sodium, potassium, barium, calcium, strontium, or zirconium salt on alumina, blanc fixe, gloss white, clay, titanium dioxide, zinc oxide, talc, rosin, aluminum benzoate, calcium carbonate.

A salt prepared from straight color, i.e., D&C Red #6, by combining the color with a basic radical.

Proposed Permanent Listing of Color Additive Lakes (FR Vol. 61 #43), March 4, 1996 [7]

- List substrate, e.g., D&C Red #27 aluminum lake on alumina
- Extenders of insoluble straight colors will no longer be called lakes, e.g., D&C Red #30
- Permit blends of previously certified straight colors in a lake, e.g., FD&C Blue #1 and Yellow #5 aluminum lake
- All lakes to be prepared from previously certified batches of straight color would necessitate process changes for D&C Reds #6, #7, and #34
- Abbreviations permitted for cosmetic ingredient labeling, omitting FD&C, precipitate and substrate designation e.g., Blue 1

European Community

Directive 76/786, as amended [8].

Annex IV

This is a list of coloring agents allowed in cosmetic products.
List by color index number:

Part 1: Permanently listed
Part 2: Provisionally listed

Four fields of application:

1. All cosmetic products
2. All cosmetic products, except those intended to be applied in the vicinity of the eyes, in particular eye makeup and makeup remover
3. Allowed exclusively in cosmetic products intended not to come into contact with mucous membranes (including the eye area)
4. Allowed exclusively in cosmetic products intended to come into contact only briefly with skin (not permitted in nail preparations)

Lakes and Salts

If a color index number is listed in Annex IV, then the pure color plus its salts and lakes are allowed, unless prohibited under Annex II (the list substances that cosmetics may not contain). Exceptions include barium, strontium, and zirconium.

Prohibited under Annex II, but where Footnote 3 appears in Annex IV, "the insoluble barium, strontium, and zirconium lakes, salts, and pigments . . . shall also be permitted." They must pass the test for insolubility which will be determined by the procedure in Article 8. (Insoluble in 0.1 N HCl).

Purity Criteria

Only colors designated by an "E," those also permitted for food use, must meet the general specification for food colors.

<5 ppm	As
<20 ppm	Pb
<100 ppm	Sb, Cu, Cr, Zn, BaSO$_4$ separately
<200 ppm	Of those together
None detectable	Cd, Hg, Se, Te, Th, U Cr^{+6}, or soluble Ba

Sixth Amendment to the directive is currently adopted. Update of purity criteria is being considered, test methods may be stipulated.

Japan

MHW ordinance No. 30 (1966) as amended by MHW ordinance No. 55 (1972) [9].

Positive List

83 Coal-tar colors:

- Must be declared on cosmetic product label
- Fields of application: oral, lip, eye area, external, rinse-off

Inorganic/Natural Colorants

Listing, specifications, test methods:

- Japan standards of cosmetic ingredients (JSCI)
- Comprehensive licensing standards of cosmetics by category (CLS)
- Japan cosmetic ingredient dictionary (CLS)

U.S. Colorants Not Permitted/Restricted in Japan

Pigments

D&C RED #6	Ba Lake
D&C RED #21	Al Lake
D&C RED #27	Al Lake
D&C RED #33	Zr Lake
D&C ORANGE #5	Al Lake

Substrates

Aluminum benzoate	0.5% maximum in lipstick
Rosin	7.0% maximum in lipstick
Calcium carbonate	Not permitted

Inorganic Pigments

In general, inorganic colors are more opaque, more light fast, more solvent resistant, but not as bright as organic colors. They may be affected by alkali and acid. Inorganic colorants are formed from compounds of the transition elements. Color is produced as a result of the ease with which the outer ''d'' electrons can absorb visible light and be promoted to the next higher energy level.

Iron Oxides		
Good stability, opacity	Red	Fe_3O_4
	Brown	
	Burgundy	Fe_2O_3
	Black	Fe_3O_4
	Yellow	FeOOH
Chromium Oxide		
Good stability, opacity	Green	Cr_2O_3
Chromium Hydroxide		
Good stability, lower tinting strength	Aqua	$Cr_2O_{3X}H_2O$
Ultramarines		
Good light stability, lower tinting strength, unstable to acid	Blue	
	Violet	$Na_x(AlSiO_4)_yS_z$
	Pink	
Manganese Violet		
Good light stability, lower tinting strength, unstable to water	Violet	$NH_4MnP_2O_7$
Ferric Ammonium, Ferrocyanide		
Lower light stability, high tinting strength, unstable to alkali and salts, difficult dispersion	Deep Blue	$FeNH_4Fe(CN)_6$
Ferric Ferrocyanide		
Physical/chemical stability as above, precipitated on a substrate (i.e., mica)	Deep Blue	$Fe[Fe(CN)_6]_3$ XH_2O
Titanium Dioxide		
Medium light stability, good chemical stability, high opacity	White	TiO_2 Anatase Rutile

Organic Pigments

Organic pigments are characterized by:

- Transparency
- Variable chemical and physical stability
- ''Clean,'' bright colors

Color is produced by chromophoric groups, generally electron acceptors.

$-N=N-$	$-C=O$
$-NO_2$	$-C=S$
$-NO$	

Shade is modified or intensified by auxochromes, generally electron donors.

—NH$_2$	—OH
—NHR	—OCH$_3$
—NR$_2$	

Categories of Organic Colorants

AZO Colorants: —N=N—

Insoluble (unsulfonated): D&C Red #36; light stable

Soluble (sulfonated): D&C Red #33, FD&C Red #40, FD&C Yellow #5, FD&C Yellow #6; stable to acid, alkali, light, bleed in water

Slightly soluble (sulfonated/insoluble salt): D&C Red #6; D&C Red #7, D&C Red #34; color shift in acid and alkali; light fast; resistant to oil bleed

Oil soluble (unsulfonated): D&C Red #17

Xanthenes

D&C Orange #5; D&C Red; D&C Red #21; D&C Red #27. ''Staining dyes'': structure changes with pH, poor light stability, bleed in solvent

Triarylmethane

FD&C Blue #1, FD&C Green #3 water soluble; poor light stability

Anthraquinone

D&C Green #5; good light stability

Quinoline

D&C Yellow #10, D&C Yellow #11; oil soluble

Indigoid

D&C Red #30; good chemical, light, bleed resistance; exception: acetone soluble

Stability of Organic Pigments

True pigments > Toners > True Lakes
Light: Anthraquinone > Quinone > Indigoid > Azo > Triarylmethane > Xanthene
Heat: True pigments stable to heat.
   Toners: D&C Red #7 Ca lake changes reversibly
   Lakes: D&C Red #27 Al lake changes irreversibly
pH: 4–9
Metal ions: Unstable
Solubility: True lakes tend to bleed in water,
             Fluorescein lakes bleed in solvent

Natural Dyes [10]

Generally used in foods, there is no restriction on their use in cosmetics. For the most part, the resistance of natural dyes to heat, light, and pH instability is much inferior to their synthetic counterparts. A further disadvantage is that they often tend to exhibit strong odors.

Color	Description	Source
Yellow	Curcumim	Turmeric
Yellow	Crocin	Saffron
Orange	Capsanthin	Paprika
Orange	Annatto	Annatto
Orange	Cartenoids	Carrots
Red	Cochineal	Coccus cactii
Red	Betanine	Beetroot
Red	Anthocyanins	Red berries
Green	Chlorophylls	Lucerne grass
Brown	Caramel	Sugars

All of the above are of vegetable origin, with the exception of cochineal which is extracted from the crushed insects *Coccus cactii.*

Color Chemistry and Manufacture

The property of a colorant that makes it absorb more in one part of the visible spectrum than another is its chemical constitution. Molecules, like atoms, exist in different electronic states. Because molecules contain two or more nuclei, they also possess energies of rotation and vibration. This theory applies to both organic and inorganic colorants. With the inorganic colorants, colored compounds are obtained with the ions of the transition elements that have atomic numbers 22 to 29.

Inorganic Pigments

Titanium Dioxide

A brilliant white pigment. Two crystal types occur: anatase and rutile. Two manufacturing processes are used:

1. Sulfate—either crystal may be produced.
2. Chloride—only rutile crystals are formed properties. Crystals of both rutile and anatase are tetragonal, rutile having greater hiding power because of the closer packing of the atoms in the crystal. Refractive indices are 2.55 for anatase and 2.71 for rutile. Opacity is the result of the light-scattering ability of titanium dioxide. Light, heat and chemical stability are excellent. Additionally, in the United States, titanium dioxide is a Category I sunscreen.

Zinc Oxide

Zinc ore is roasted and purified at 1000°C. Two methods of manufacture are used: 1) French (indirect) and 2) American (direct).

Properties. Zinc oxide forms transparent hexagonal crystals; whiteness is attributable to the light scattering of the extremely fine particles. Refractive index is 2.0. Hiding power is less than titanium dioxide. Primary use is for antibacterial and fungicidal properties. Heat and light stability are good. It is soluble in acid and alkali. Zinc oxide in the United States is a Category I skin protectant and a Category III sunscreen.

Iron Oxides

These are used in all types of cosmetic products. By blending black, red, and yellow in certain properties, brown, tans, umbers and sienna may be produced. Yellow iron oxide is hydrated iron II (ferrous) oxide, $Fe_2O_3XH_2O$. It is produced by the controlled oxidation of ferrous sulfate. Red iron oxide is chemically Fe_2O_3 and is obtained by the controlled heating (at about 1000°C) of yellow iron oxide. Black iron oxide is Fe_2O_4 and is a mixture of ferrous and ferric oxide and is prepared by controlled oxidation of ferrous sulfate under alkaline conditions.

Ultramarines

Theoretically they are polysulfide sodium/aluminum sulfosilicates. They range in color from blue to violet, pink, and even green. A mixture is calcined at 800°C to 900°C, for 4 to 5 days. Shades are determined by reaction time, formula variations, and particle size, whereas ultramarine violets and pinks are obtained by treating ultramarine blue with HCl at 275°C, removing some sodium and sulfur from the molecule.

Manganese Violet

Chemically this is $MnNH_4P_2O$. Manufactured by heating manganese dioxide with ammonium dihydrogen phosphate and water. Phosphorus acid is added and the mixture is heated until the violet color develops.

Iron Blue

Chemically ferric ammonium ferrocyanide. $Fe[Fe(Cn)_6]_3$. Sodium ferrocyanide and ferrous sulfate are reacted in the presence of ammonium sulfate. Pigments prepared with sodium or potassium salts are called ferric ferrocyanide.

Chromium Oxide (Cr_2O_3)

A dull yellow green pigment may be prepared by blending an alkali dichromate with sulfur or a carbonaceous material. Reduction to chrome (III) oxide is achieved in a kiln at 1000°C.

Chromium Hydroxide ($Cr_2O(OH)_4$)

A bright bluish green pigment prepared by the calcination of a bichromate with boric acid at 500°C. During cooling, the mass is hydrolyzed with water, yielding a hydrate.

Hydrated Alumina

Chemically Al_2O_3 X H_2O gives little opacity and is almost transparent.

Barium Sulfate

It is relatively translucent and may by used as a pigment extender.

Organic Pigments

These are chiefly conjugated cyclic compounds based on a benzene ring structure, although some heterocyclic ones exist. There are three main types: lakes, toners, and true pigments. Organic pigments are seldom used without a diluent or substrate in order to maintain color consistency from batch to batch. A true pigment is an insoluble compound that contains no metal ions, examples of which are D&C Red #30 and D&C Red #36. They are the most stable. A lake is essentially an insoluble colorant, produced by precipitating a permitted soluble dye to a permitted substrate. In cosmetics, most lakes are based on aluminum, although zinconium lakes are also found. Stability-wise, true aluminum lakes can be affected by extremes of pH, resulting in reforming of the soluble dye or ''bleeding.'' They are fairly transparent and not particularly light-fast. Toners are colorants made with other approved metals besides aluminum, such as barium and calcium. Generally, they are more resistant to heat, light and pH, although extremes of pH can result in shade changes. Generally, many organic colorants are unsuitable for certain cosmetics because of their chemical nature. D&C Red #36 is a typical nonsoluble azo color is not recommended for lipstick because of its very slight solubility in oils and waxes it tends to crystallize upon continual reheating of the lipstick mass. Soluble azo dyes such as FD&C Yellow #5 and #6 Red #33 lakes are often used in lipstick and nail lacquer. Sparingly soluble types such as D&C Red #6 are not highly soluble but the barium lake of Red #6 and the calcium lake of Red #7 are the most popular colors for cosmetics. Colors in this group do not need a substrate to make them insoluble. The D&C Red #6 and #7 lakes are widely used in lipstick and nail lacquer because of high strength, bright hues, good light fasteness, as well as chemical and heat stability. Non–azo-soluble dyes such as D&C Red #21, Orange #5, and Red #27 are all fluoresceins and act as a pH indicator and will change accordingly. They all strain the skin and D&C Red #27 gives the strongest blue stain.

Quality Control of Colorants
Establishment of Standards

- Ensure that product development is performed with material representative of supplier's production
- Before purchase, evaluate at least three lots, establish standard in consultation with the supplier
- Supplier and end user should agree on specifications, standard, and test methods

Test Methods

Shade Evaluation. Methods should predict performance of the colorant under use conditions.

Light Source for Visual Evaluations to Be Specified.

- Dyes: Visual or spectrophotometric evaluation of solutions.
- Pigments: Cannot be evaluated as received due to variable degree of agglomeration. Visual or instrumental evaluation is made of wet and dry dispersions prepared under defined conditions to a defined degree of dispersion.

Vehicles:	Dispersion equipment:
Talc	Osterizer
Nitrocellulose lacquer	Hoover muller,
Acrylic lacquer	Three roll mill, or
Castor oil	Ball mill

Heavy Metals:

Wet chemical
Atomic absorption spectroscopy (AAS)
Inductive coupled plasma (ICP)

Particle Size:

Wet/dry sieve analysis
Optical microscopy
Laser diffraction
Sedimentation

Bulk Density:

Fischer-Scott Volumeter
pH

Pearlescent Pigments and Other Specialty Pigments

Pearlescent Pigments:

The most important requirement for a substance to be pearlescent is that its crystals should be plate-like and have a high refractive index. A thin, transparent, platy configuration allows light to be transmitted. A pearlescent material should have a smooth surface to allow specular reflection and be nontoxic. Generally, when using pearlescent pigments one must use the most transparent formulation, avoiding grinding or milling the pearl pigments and blend pearls complement one another.

1. **Organic Pearls**. These pearls produce a bright silver effect and are obtainable from fish scales as platelets or needles, which are highly reflective. The materials responsible for the pearl effect are crystals of a purine called guanine. Guanine is chiefly used in nail-enamel.

2. **Inorganic Pearls**.

(A) Bismuth oxychloride:
Bismuth oxychloride produces a silvery-grey pearlescent effect and is synthesized as tetragonal crystals. Crystal sizes vary from approximately 8 microns, which give a soft, opaque, smooth luster, and 20 microns, which give a more brilliant sparkling effect. Its major disadvantage in use is poor light stability, which may cause darkening after prolonged exposure. UV absorbs in the finished products are used to overcome this defect. BioCl is chiefly used to pearl nail enamels, lipsticks, blushes, and eye shadows. BioCl may be modified by deposition on mica, titanium dioxide and mica, or talc. Inorganic pigments may be bonded to BioCl then deposited on mica. All these alter the final effect on the finished product.

(B) Titanium dioxide–coated micas:
Titanium dioxide–coated micas are extensively used in decorative cosmetics. They exist in several different forms: (1) silver-titanium dioxide uniformly coats platelets of mica, rutile crystals give a brilliant pearl effect because of a higher refractive index than the anatase grade; and (2)interference pearlescent products can be made by altering the thickness of the film. At a certain thickness, interference of light can take place so that some wavelengths of the incident light are reflected and others transmitted. The colors created are complementary to each other. As the layers become thicker, the reflection goes from silvery white, then yellow-gold, red, blue, and green. Additionally, colorants such as iron oxides can be laminated with this interference film, providing a two-color effect.

3. **Pigment Pearls**. Colored pearls are produced by laminating a layer of iron oxides on titanium dioxide–coated mica, producing a color and luster effect.

4. **Specialty Pigments**. In addition to BioCl and the titanium dioxide–coated mica systems, polyester foil cut into regular shapes, which have been epoxy coated with light fast pigments, have been used for nail enamels and body makeup. Finally, aluminum powder and copper/bronze powder have been used as reflective pigments, especially in eye shadows. For cosmetic-use aluminum powder, 100% of the particles must pass through a 200 mesh screen, and 95% must pass through a 325 mesh (44 millimicron) screen.

Treated Pigments

Surface-treated colors and substrates allowed chemists to enhance the aesthetic and functional qualities of their formulations. The benefits of using these treatments may be divided into two categories: those evident in the finished cosmetic product, and the benefits derived from process improvements. Consumer benefits include hydrophobicity yielding greater wear, improved skin adhesion, smoother product feel, improved optical appearance, moisturization, and ease of application. Processing benefits include ease of dispersion, pressability, less oil absorption, uniformity, and less moisture absorption. The following surface treatments are commercially available:

- Amino Acids (N-Lauroyl lysine, acyl amino acid [11])
   Natural
   Good skin adhesion
   pH balanced
   Heat sensitive
- Fluorochemical (Perfluoropolymethylisopropyl ether perfluoroalkyl phosphate)
   Hydrophobic and lipophobic greatly enhance wear
   Heat and shear resistance
- Lecithin [12]
   Natural
   Exceptionally smooth, silky skin feel, particularly in pressed products
   Heat sensitive, slightly soluble in water
- Metal Soaps (ZnMg Stearate)
   Good skin adhesion
   Enhanced compressibility
- Natural Wax
   Natural
   Moisturizing skin feel
   Good skin adhesion
   Heat sensitive (low m.p.)
- Nylon (pure mechanically coated)
   Smooth skin feel
- Polyacrylate
   Enhanced wetting in aqueous systems
   Feel is not very good
   but is usually used in dispersion
- Polyethylene
   Hydrophobic
   Waxy, smooth skin feel
   Enhanced compressibility
   Heat sensitive
- Silicone (Polymethylhydrogensiloxane; methicone will be chemically bonded and cannot be removed later)
   Hydrophobic
   Achieves full color development
   Main use is to improve wetting
- Other Silicones (No potential for hydrogen evolution)
   Dimethiconol

Absorbed dimethicone
Silicone/lecithin
- Silane
Extremely hydrophobic, lipophilic
No hydrogen potential
- Titanate Ester Isopropyl triisosteryl titanate [13]
Enhances wetting in oil
Smooth skin feel
High pigment loading
Lowers oil absorption of pigments

Microfine/Ultrafine/Nanosized Pigments

These pigments have a primary particle size below 100 nm; larger agglomerates/aggregates can be present. Properties such as surface area, bulk density, vehicle absorption, and UV absorption differ significantly from those of conventional pigment. Microfine titanium dioxide, zinc oxide, and iron oxides can be used in a range of color cosmetics to provide unique visual effects as well as UV protection. In pressed powders and anhydrous and emulsified formulations, significant SPF values can be achieved in formulations having a translucent, natural-looking finish. With microfine pigments, formulations for darker skin tones can be formulated that avoid the ''ashy'' or ''made-up'' appearance caused by conventional opaque pigments.

Light-Diffusing Pigments

Some of the requirements for light-diffusing pigments include a high refractive index, reflection to be diffused, translucency, and its transmission must be primarily diffuse. Skin has a refractive index of 1.60. Examples of light diffusers include $BaSO_4$, silica, silica spheres coated on mica, $TiO_2/BaSO_4$-coated mica, $Al_2OH_3/mica$, ultrafine $TiO_2/mica$, ultrafine $TiO_2/polyethylene$, ethylene acyrates copolymer, polymethyl methacrylate, among others. These products are chiefly used in powders to create illusions and hide wrinkles.

MAKEUP TECHNOLOGY

- Types of Color Cosmetics
Foundation
Blushers
Mascara
Eyeliner
Eye shadow
Lip color
Nail color
- Purpose
Improve appearance
Impart color
Even-out skin tones
Hide imperfections
Protection

- Types of Formulations
    Suspensions
    Aqueous
    Anhydrous
- Emulsions
    Oil-in-water
    Water-in-oil
- Powder
    Pressed
    Loose
- Anhydrous (wax, solvent)
    Stick
    Pan
    Tube

Powder

Powdered cosmetics are generally used to describe face powders, eye shadows, and blushers. When the product is applied to the skin, the shade must not significantly change as it is worn; must feel smooth in use, making it easy to apply; and adhere well for a reasonable time, without reapplication.

Face Powders

Some of the attributes of a satisfactory face powder are the following: (1) gives smoothness to overall texture, (2) gives added skin translucency when excess is buffed, (3) makes the skin appear more refined and finer textured, (4) helps set the makeup base and adds longevity to the makeup overall, and (5) suppresses surface oil and shine. Generally there is a wide range of raw materials used in powdered cosmetics and many of these carry over into the formulation of other decorative cosmetics.

Talc

Talc is the major component of most face powders, eye shadows, and blushers. Chemically it is a hydrated magnesium silicate. Cosmetic talcs are mined in Italy, France, Norway, India, Spain, China, Egypt, Japan, and the United States. Typically, talcs are sterilized by gamma irradiation. Particle size should pass through a 200 mesh sieve. Cosmetic talc should be white, free of asbestos, and have high spreadability or slip with low covering power. Micronized talc is generally lighter and fluffier but less smooth on the skin than regular grades. Although talc is fairly hydrophobic, treated talcs have been used to enhance its texture. In some products, talc is present up to 70% of the formulation.

Kaolin

Kaolin, or china clay, is a naturally occurring, almost white, hydrated aluminum silicate. It does not exhibit a high degree of slip. Kaolin has good absorbency, is dense, and sometimes used to reduce bulk densities in loose-powder products. It provides a matte surface effect that can reduce slight sheen left by some talc products.

Calcium Carbonate

Calcium carbonate, or precipitated chalk, has excellent absorption properties. It provides a matte finish and had moderate covering powder. High levels should be avoided; otherwise an undesirable, dry, powdery feel can result.

Magnesium Carbonate

Magnesium carbonate is available in a very light, fluffy grade that absorbs well and is often used to absorb perfume before mixing into face powders.

Metallic Soap

Zinc and magnesium stearate are important materials for imparting adhesion to face powders. They are usually incorporated at 3 to 10% of the formulation. Stearates add some water repellency to formulas. They are although too-high levels give a blotchy effect on the skin. Zinc stearate, besides imparting adhesions, gives a smoothing quality to face powders. Aluminum stearate and lithium stearates have also been used. High levels can make pressed formulations too hard.

Starch

Starch is used in face powders to give a "peach-like" bloom and to provide a smooth surface on the skin. One problem attributed to rice starch is that, when moistened, it tends to cake. Also, the wet product may provide an environment for bacterial growth.

Mica

Mica is chemically potassium aluminum silicate dihydrate. Cosmetic mica is refined and ground to particles of 150 microns or less. It imparts a natural translucence when used up to 20% in formulations of face-powder blushes. Mica is available as wet ground, which is creamy, or dry ground, which is matte. Sericite is a mineral, similar to white mica in shape and composition. It has a very fine grain size and silky shine. It is soft and smooth and has a slippery feel on the skin. Sericite may be coated with silicone and other treatments for better water repellency and skin adhesion.

Polymers

Polymers are chiefly texture enhancers used at levels of 3 to 40%, depending on whether they are to be included in a loose or pressed powder. Among these polymers, we find Nylon-12 and Nylon-6, lauroyl lysine, boron nitride (makes active ingredients spread more uniformly on inactive bases), polyethylene, polypropylene, ethylene acrylates copolymer (very sheer, will not affect binder in pressed powders, processing temperature less than 85–90°), polymethyl methacrylate (PMMA) and silica beads (can carry oily ingredients into a system, increase wear on oily skin), polyurethane powders, silicone powders, borosilicate, microcrystalline cellulose, acrylate copolymers, Teflon® and Teflon® composites (effective at low concentrations, 1–5%), polyvinylidene copolymers (very light, ultra-low density), and composite powders that are coated on inexpensive beads to reduce costs and increase effectiveness, like nylon/mica, silica/mica, lauryl lysine/mica and boron nitride/

mica. Many of these polymers are treated with silicones, titanates, lecithin, etc. for increased effectiveness.

Colorants

Titanium dioxide and zinc oxide, both pigmentary and ultrafine organics, inorganics, carmine, and pearlescent pigments either predispersed or treated are found in all face powders because the textures of these colorants are not very satisfactory.

Perfumes

The use of perfumes is important for face powder, which requires them because most of the raw materials used are earthy smelling and should be masked. Perfumes should show stability and low volatility.

Preservatives

Preservation of face powders are usually not a problem because they are used dry, but small amounts of antibacterials are recommended. Powdered eye shadows should always contain antibacterials such as parabens, imidazolidinyl urea, and others.

Loose Face Powders

This type has declined in popularity in favor of pressed face-powder products. The smoothness of loose face powder can be enhanced by use of the aforementioned texture enhancers. In the manufacturing process, all ingredients except the pearls, if required, are combined in a stainless steel ribbon blender. Mixing time can be as long as 1 or 2 hours, depending on the size of the batch and evenness of the color. The perfume, if required, is slowly sprayed into the batch, blended until homogenous. The batch is then pulverized through a hammer mill and the color is checked. Color adjustments are made, if necessary, in the ribbon blender, and the batch is repulverized. Any pearl or mica is then added for a final mix. Batch is then stored and made ready for filling into appropriate containers.

Pressed Face Powders

Pressed face powders are more popular than loose powders because of their ease of application and portability. The basic raw materials are the same as loose powder except that one must use a binder to press the cake into a tin-plate godet. If water-based binders are used, aluminum godets should be considered to prevent corrosion. The properties of a binder is as follows: provides creaminess to the powder, aids in compression and adhesion, develops colorants, and enhances water resistance, pick-up, and deposit. If the binder level is too high, it may be difficult to remove the powder with a puff. Also, high levels may lead to glazing of the powder surface, making it waxy looking, with little or no pay-off. Fatty soaps, kaolin, polyethylene, Teflon® synthetic wax, and calcium silicate are some of the binder systems used. Use levels of binder are between 3 to 10%, depending on formulation variables. Silicone-treated pigments have given rise to pressed face powders that may be used wet or dry. When used dry, they are usually smoother than regular pressed powders. When a wet sponge is applied to the cake, no water penetrates the cake; the water is repelled. These "two-way" cakes can be used either as a foundation or face powder. When formulating pressed powders, one must be careful that the raw materials used do not corrode the godets or attack the plastic packaging materials. The manufacture of pressed powders, including the mixing and color-matching process, is similar to loose powders. Sometimes the powder mix is pulverized without binder and then again after its addition. Pearls are usually added during the blending process and preferably without the milling operation which can damage the pearl. If milling a batch containing pearl becomes necessary, it should be done with the mill screen removed. Powder pressing is often times more successful if the powder is kept for a few days to allow the binder system to fully spread, especially when pearls are present. The most common used pressed for face powder are the ALITE-high speed hydraulic press and the KEMWALL, CAVALLA, or VE. TRA. CO. presses. The pressures used and the speed of pressing depends on the characteristics of the individual formulation and the size of the godet.

Powder Blushers

The attributes of blushers are as follows: (1) add color to the face; (2) can give more dimension to the cheekbones; (3) harmonizes the face-balance between eye makeup and lipstick; and (4) creates subtle changes in the foundation look when lightly dusted over the face. Pressed powder blushers are similar to face-powder formulations, except that a greater range of color pigments is used. The three basic iron oxides and one or more of the lakes are used to achieve various blusher shades. Blushers are usually applied with a brush. Manufacture and pressing is similar to face powders. Care should be taken that only nonbleeding pigments be used to avoid skin staining. Total pigment concentration ranges from 2 to 10%, excluding pearls. Pressed-powder rouges were once popular and contained high levels of colorants (10–30%). Usually they are applied from the godet with the finger, so glazing may frequently occur if the rouge is improperly formulated.

Pressed-Powder Eyeshadows

Eye shadows in general have the following functions: (1) adds color and personality to the face; (2) sharpens or softens the eyeball itself; (3) creates the illusion of depth or brings out deep set eyes; (4) creates light and dark illusions for subtle character changes; and (5) can be used wet or dry for different illusions. The technology is similar to other pressed-powder products, but the permitted color range is limited. In the US the only synthetic organic pigments that may be used in eye products are FD&C Red No. 40, FD&C Blue #1, FD&C Yellow #5, and Green #5. Carmine, N.F. is the only natural organic pigment allowed, and all of the inorganic pigments and a wide range of pearls may be used. Preservation is very important in eye-makeup products. Problems of poor adherence to the skin, color matching, and creasing in the eyelid are common when the binder formulation is ineffective with the type and level of pearls used. High binder levels may result in uneven pressing of the godets. In manufacture, formulas with high pearl content should be allowed to settle to remove entrapped air before pressing.

Quality Assurance on Powder Products

Color

Production batch and standard are placed side by side on white paper and pressed flat with a palette-knife. Shades are compared with one another. Shades of eye shadows and blushers are checked on the skin using a brush or wand.

Bulk Density

Carried out on loose powder to ensure that no entrapped air is present so that incorrect filling weights are minimized.

Penetration and Drop Tests

Are carried out on pressed godets. A penetrometer is used to determine the accuracy of the pressure used during filling. A drop test is designed to test the physical strength of the cake. Normally, the godet is dropped on to a wooden floor or rubber matte (1–3 times) at a height of 2 to 3 feet to note damage to the cake.

Glazing and Pay-Off

The pressed cake is rubbed through to the base of the godet with a puff, and any sign of glazing is noted. Pay-off must be sufficient and the powder should spread evenly without losing adhesion to the skin.

Foundation

In general, foundation makeup's chief functions are to hide skin flaws, even-out various color tones in the skin, act as a protectant from the environment, and make the skin surface appear smoother. Requirements for an ideal makeup foundation's application are as follows: (1) should be moderately fast drying to allow for an even application; (2) should be nonsettling, pour easily, be stable in storage; (3) should not feel tacky, greasy, or too dry; (4) it should improve appearance, not artificially; and (5) should have proper "play time" and slip. Depending on the formulations, several contain treated pigments and volatile silicones to add water-resistance properties. There should be shade consistency between the bottle and skin tone. Products should be uniform. Coverage or capacity will vary with skin types; finish on the skin may by matte, shiny, or "dewy." Wear is extremely important—product should not peel-off, go orangy on the skin or rub-off on clothes.

Foundation makeup is available in the following forms:

- **Emulsions**.   O/W, anionic, nonionic, and cationic. W/O; became more popular for water-proofness and contains volatile silicone, hydrocarbones, mineral oil, and light esters.
- **Anhydrous**.   Cream powder and stick.
- **Suspensions**.   Oil and aqueous.

Emulsified Foundations

Composition can vary widely depending on degree of coverage and emolliency desired. Although nonionic (usually not stable), cationic (difficult to make, not on market), and W/O systems have been marketed, most emulsified foundations are anionic O/W emulsions because of the ease of formulation. Anionics possess the following properties:

- emulsion stability
- pigment wetting and dispersion
- easy spreading and blending
- good skin feel
- slippery (soap-like) feeling

Formulation Considerations

1. Prolonged skin contact. Minimize emulsifier levels to avoid irritation.
2. Choose oils based on low *comedogenicity*.
3. Preservation—foundations may be difficult to preserve containing such ingredients as water and gums.

Emulsion Makeup Manufacturing Equipment

- *Pigment Extenders*: hammer mill and jet mill
- *Internal Phase*: propeller mixer/SS steam–jacketed kettle
- *External Phase*: colloid mill, homogenizer/sidesweep, and SS steam–jacketed finishing kettle
- *Emulsification*: sidesweep, homogenizer, and recirculating mill, i.e., colloid mill
- With *high-viscosity systems* planetary mixer is needed

Manufacturing

The coloration of the emulsion base may be handled in different ways: direct pigment, pigment dispersions, mixed pigment blender, and monochromatic color solutions [14]. Each has its advantages and disadvantages. In the direct pigment method, the pigments are weighed directly into the aqueous phase and dispersed or colloid milled; then the emulsion is formed in the usual manner. The major problem is that there are too many color adjustments needed and accurate color matching is difficult. With the pigment dispersion method, the pigment is mixed with talc as a 50:50 dispersion and pulverized to match a standard. This reduces the number of color corrections needed but storage may be a problem as well as the time taken to make these dispersions. During the mixed-pigment blender method, the pigments and extenders are premixed, pulverized, and matched to a standard; it is then dispersed in the aqueous phase of the emulsion and the emulsion is formed in the normal way. The finished shade is color matched at the powder blender stage. Chances of error are reduced. The last method—the monochromatic color solutions—required one to make color concentrates of each pigment in a finished formula. It is easy to color match by blending finished base, but much storage space is needed and the possibility for contamination is increased.

Anhydrous Foundations

Anhydrous foundations are generally powdery, not fluid, and easy to travel with. Ingredients needed include:

1. Emollients. Often texturally light and low viscosity; include oils, esters, and silicones.
2. Waxes.
   (A) Natural: Beeswax, jojoba, orange, carnauba, candelilla, and castor.
   (B) Beeswax derivatives: Dimethicone copolyol beeswax, polyglyceryl-3 beeswax, butyloctanol, and hexanediol beeswax (nice texture, compatibility with silicone material).
   (C) Synthetic: Paraffins, microcrystalline, polyethylene, and "synthetic wax" (highly branched olefin polymers).
   (D) Fatty alcohols and fatty alcohol ethoxylates: Unithox and unilin.

      (E) Fatty esters: Croda (syncrowaxes), koster keunen (kester waxes), Pheonix Chemical, Scher, Flora Tech, and RTD.
3.   Pigments. Often surface treated.
      (A) TiO_2: Pigmentary and ultrafine.
      (B) ZnO: Pigmentary and ultrafine.
      (C) Iron Oxides: Pigmentary and ultrafine (enhances SPF value).
4.   Texturizing Agents. Often surface treated; include nylon, PMMA, sericite, talc, mica, boron nitride, Teflon®, borosilicates copolymer, polyvinylidene copolymer, spherical silica, starches (oats, rice, wheat, corn, dry flo-starch), BiOCl, microcrystalline cellulose, polyurethane powder, and silicone powder.
5.   Wetting Agents. Small amount to be used; include low HLB emulsifiers, polyglyceryl esters, e.g., polyglyceryl-3 diisostearate, hydrogenated lecithin, lanolin alcohols, polyhydroxy stearic acid, and soya sterols.

Basic Formulation	
Emollients (fluids, low melting point waxes, gel-like raws)	30–60%
Waxes	5–10%
Wetting agents	0.50–1.00%
Texturing agents	30–60%

Surface-treated raw materials are frequently used in these types of formulations for the following reasons:

- Improves dispersibility
- Enhances solids loading
    provides drier texture
    creates matte appearance
    improves wear
    overall improved aesthetics

Manufacturing Procedure

1. Emollients, waxes, and wetting agent(s) are introduced into a jacketed kettle and heated until phase is clear and uniform.
2. Pigments and texturizing agents are slowly introduced into the oil phase with higher shear mixing. Continue high shear mixing until dispersion is uniform and colorants are completely "extended."

If surface treatments are temperature-sensitive, care must be taken to prevent the displacement of that treatment from the surface of the powder into the oil phase itself.

EYE MAKEUP

Mascara

1. Brings out the contrast between the iris and the white of the eye, sharpens white of the eye

2. Thickens the appearance of the lashes
3. Lengthens the appearance of the eye
4. Adds depth and character to the overall look
5. Sharpens the color of the eye shadow when worn.

Mascara's performance is usually judged by application, appearance, wear, and ease of removal. It is critical that the proper brush is supplied for the chosen formulation. Generally, mascara and eyeliners consist of one or more film formers, pigment, and the vehicle that mostly evaporates to allow the film to set.

Three Types of Formulations Are Currently in Use

In the past, cake or block mascara was popular. This was basically a wax base with a soap or nonionic emulsifier present so that color could be applied with a wetted brush. Mascara and eyeliners consist of one or more film formers, pigment, and the vehicle that mostly evaporates to allow the film to set.

-   Anhydrous solvent based suspension: waterproof but not smudge-proof and difficult to remove
-   W/O emulsion: also waterproof but not smudge-proof and can be removed with soap and water
-   O/W emulsion: water-based if the film is sufficiently flexible, can be flake-proof and smudge-proof. Water resistance can be achieved with the addition of emulsion polymers, i.e., acrylics, polyvinyl acetates, or polyurethanes.

Oil-in-Water (O/W)

Water Phase
    Water
    Suspending agent: hydroxyethylcellulose
    Film former/dispersing agent: polyvinylpyrrolidone
    Pigment
    Hydrophilic emulsifier: alkali, high HLB nonionic
Wax Phase
    High melting point waxes
    Lipophilic emulsifier: fatty acid, low HLB nonionic, co-emulsifier
    Plasticizer: lanolin or derivatives, liquid fatty alcohol
    Petroleum solvent (optional) as extender for water phase
    Preservative: propyl paraben
Additional Film Former
    Solution polyacrylate (improves flake resistance)
    Emulsion polyacrylate
    Polyurethane
    Polyvinyl acetate
    Rosin derivatives
    Dimethiconol
    Proteins: wheat, soy, corn, keratin, oat, silk
Preservative
    Formaldehyde releaser (not for use in Japan)

Manufacturing

Procedure is generally o/w emulsification procedure except that iron oxides are first wet and milled in the water phase before emulsification and final product goes through a colloid mill, roller mill, or homogenizer.

Solvent-Based

Hard, high melting point waxes
Rosin derivative (optional)
Wetting agent
Pigment
Suspending agent (organoclay)
Volatile solvent (to achieve wax solubility)
  Petroleum distillate
  Cyclomethicone
Preservatives: parabens
Plasticizer: lanolin or derivative, liquid fatty alcohol

Water-in-Oil (W/O)

Wax Phase
  High melting point waxes (carnauba, candellila, polyethylene)
  Rosin derivative (optional)
  Lipophilic emulsifier (lanolin acids, low HLB nonionic)
  Pigment
  Preservative: propyl paraben
  Petroleum solvent, some cyclomethicone
Water Phase
  Hydrophilic emulsifier (alkali, medium HLB nonionic)
  Preservative: methyl paraben
Additives
  Emulsion polymer (optional)
  Preservative: formaldehyde donor (not for use in Japan)

Anhydrous Mascara

Ingredients

- Solvents: Branched chain hydrocarbons and petroleum distillates, isoparaffinic hydrocarbons, and volatile silicones
- Waxes: Beeswax and its derivatives, candelilla, carnauba, paraffin, polyethylene, microcrystalline, castor, synthetic, ceresin, and ozokerite
- Resins: (could be introduced, but do not have to be); Include aromatic/aliphatic, hydrogenated aromatics, polyterpene, synthetic, rosin, acrylics, and silicones
- Gellants: Clays (stearalkonium hectorite, quaternium-18 bentonite, quaternium-18 hectorite), metal soaps (Al, Zn stearates)
- Colorants: Most often use a classic iron oxide without any surface treatment
- Functional Fillers: Spherical particles (PMMA, Silica, Nylon), boron nitride, starches, Teflon®

Purpose

- Provides body to film to enhance thickening properties
- Improves transfer resistance
- Improves deposit on lashes

Basic Formulation:

Solvent(s)	40–60%
Waxes	10–20%
Resin(s)	3–10%
Gellant	3–7%
Colorant(s)	5–15%
Filler(s)	2–10%

Procedure

1. Heat waxes, solvents, and resins in a jacketed kettle until uniform and clear. Slowly add pigments under high shear and mill until dispersion is uniform.
2. Under high shear, add gellant and mill until uniform. Activate gellant with polar additive like propylene carbonate. Under high shear, add fillers and mill until uniform. Cool to desired temperature.

Mascara Componentry

Bottle

PVC-polyvinyl chloride for solvent based and H.D. polyethylene/polypropylene for water-based types.

Brush/Rod/Wiper

Works complementary with each other to deliver required product attributes.

Required for a Thickening Mascara

Larger diameter rod
Larger diameter wiper
Larger brush with significant spacing between the bristles

Suggested for a Defining Mascara

A smaller diameter rod
Smaller diameter wiper
Brush with minimal spacing between the bristles

Brush materials, fiber diameter, brush shape, fiber shape, fiber length, wire diameter, and the number of turns in the wire all affect performance.

Cream Eyeshadows

Generally, cream eye shadows are another form of eye shadow not as popular as the pressed form. Care must be taken in formulation to avoid creasing and other wear problems. In the past, stick eye shadows were popular. They are similar to cream eye shadows but contain high melting point waxes to make them moldable. The ingredients used are as follows.

Ingredients:

- Volatile solvents: Cyclomethicone, hydrocarbons, isoparaffins
- Waxes: Similar to those used in the anhydrous waterproof mascaras, although at lower concentrations
- Emollients: Esters, oils, silicones
- Gellants: Bentonite derivatives, hectorite derivatives
- Colorants and Pearls: Classical
- Fillers: Mica, talc, sericite
- Functional fillers: Boron nitride, PMMA, nylon, starches, Silica, Teflon, Lauroyl lysine

For enhanced textural properties, higher solids loading, and improved application and coverage, use surface-treated raw materials whose coatings are neither temperature nor solvent sensitive. Balance the absorption of fillers to maintain similar textures throughout the shade range.

Basic Formulation

Solvent	35–55%
Gellants	1.50–3.50%
Waxes	7–12%
Emollients	3–8%
Colorants/pearls	5–20%
Fillers	10–20%
Functional fillers	5–15%

The *manufacturing procedure* is identical to that of anhydrous mascaras.

Eyeliners

Eyeliners frame the eye while adding shape to or changing the shape of the eye. They give the illusion of a larger or smaller eye bringing out the color contrast between the iris and white of the eye. Lastly, eyeliners assist in making the lashes appear thicker. Generally, liquid eyeliners are the most popular and will be chiefly outlined. Cake eyeliner was popular in the past and was a wettable pressed cake applied with a wet brush. It contained powder fillers, waxes, resins, and a soap or nonionic. Liquid eyeliners include the following list of ingredients:

- Solvent: Water
- Gellant: Gums (magnesium aluminum silicate and bentonite)
- Wetting agents: Water-soluble esters, and high HLB emulsifiers
- Polyols: Propylene glycol, butylene glycol, and 2-methyl-1, 3 propanediol
- Colorants: Surface treatment is not essential but will enhance ease of dispersibility, maintain fluidity, improve adhesion and may also enhance water resistance. Chiefly, iron oxides and other inorganic are used

- Alcohol: Can solubilize resins and improve dry time
- Film Formers: PVP, PVA, Acrylics, PVP/VA, PVP/Urethanes

Basic Formulations

Water	50–70%
Gellant	0.50–1.50%
Wetting Agent(s)	1–3%
Polyol	4–8%
Colorants	10–20%
Alcohol	5–10%
Film former	3–8%

Manufacturing Procedure

Gellant is premixed with the polyol and added to a heated water phase which also contains the wetting agent. Disperse with high shear until uniform. Add colorants and disperse until uniform. Cool and add alcohol and film former with low shear.

Pencils

Pencils are used in general for coloring the eyebrows and eyelids, although they are now popular as lipsticks, lip liner, and blushers, depending on the hardness of the pencil and the color composition.

Products are nearly always manufactured by a handful of contract manufacturers. The chemists' responsibility is to evaluate the finished product, rather than create one. Evaluation includes shade, texture, sharpenability, wear, application, stability (freeze-thaw and at 40–45°C), and penetration. Generally, extruded pencils are less stable than the molded ones.

Raw Materials

- Oils, esters, silicones
- High–melt point triglycerides
- Stearic acid–helps the extrusion
- Synthetic waxes
- Japan wax
- Bright colorants and pearls in leads increase the variety available in cosmetic pencils
- Fillers, Mica, talc, sericite
- Functional Fillers, boron nitride, Teflon, PMMA, Silicas

Product Types

Product types include eyeliner, lipliner, eyeshadow, lipstick, brow, blush, and concealer
Manufacturing Procedure:

Molded and extruded; significant differences exist in how these products are evaluated initially after manufacturing. Molded pencils set up within a few days. Extruded pencil set up slowly over a few weeks. The molded or extruded lead is placed in a slat of wood grooved lengthwise. A second grooved slat, is glued onto the first slat and pressed together.

LIPSTICKS

Lipsticks add color to the face for a healthier look, shape the lips, and sometimes condition. They Harmonize the face between the eyes, hair, and clothes. Created the illusion of smaller or larger lips depending on the color.

There are two types of lipsticks; classical and volatile based.

The Ingredients in a Classic Lipstick

- Emollients.   Castor oil, esters, lanolin/lanolin oil, oily alcohols (octyl dodecanol), organically modified silicones (Phenyltrimethicone and alkyl dimethicones), Meadowfoam seed oil, jojoba oil and esters and triglycerides
- Waxes.   Candelilla, carnauba, beeswax and derivatives, microcrystalline, ozokerite/ceresein, alkyl silicone, castor, polyethylene, lanolin, paraffin, Synthetic and Ester
- Wax Modifiers.   Work in conjunction with the waxes to improve texture, application and stability include cetyl acetate and acetylated lanolin, oleyl alcohol, synthetic lanolin, acetylated lanolin alcohol, and petroleum (white and yellow)
- Colorants Widely Used.
      D&Cs
         Red #6 and Ba Lake
         Red #7 and Ca Lake
         Red #21 and Al Lake (stains)
         Red #27 and Al Lake (stains)
         Red #33 and Al Lake
         Red #30
         Red #36
         Yellow #10
      FD&Cs
         Yellow #5,6 Al Lake
         Blue #1 Al Lake
      Iron Oxides
      TiO_2
      ZnO
      Pearls
      No Fe Blue, Ultramarines, Mn Violet
- Actives.   Raw materials are added for claims and moisturization; tocopheryl acetate, sodium hyaluronate, aloe extract, ascorbyl palmitate, silanols, ceramides, panthenol, amino acids, and beta carotene
- Fillers (Matting and Texturizing Agents).   Mica, silicas (classic and spherical), nylon, PMMA, teflon, boron nitride, BiOCl, starches, lauroyl lysine, composite powders, and acrylates copolymers

- Antioxidants/Preservatives   BHA, BHT, rosemary extract, citric acid, propyl paraben, methyl paraben, and tocopherol

Classic Lipstick

Formula	Gloss	Matte
Emollients	50–70%	40–55%
Waxes	10–15%	8–13%
Plasticizers	2–5%	2–4%
Colorants	0.5–3.0%	3.0–8.0%
Pearl	1–4%	3–6%
Actives	0–2%	0–2%
Fillers	1–3%	4–15%
Fragrance	0.05–0.10%	0.05–0.10%
Preservatives/Antioxidants	0.50%	0.50%

Procedure

1. Pigments are premilled in either one of the emollients (e.g., castor oil) or the complete emollent phase either by a 3-roller mill, stone mill, or a type of ball mill.
2. Grind phase is added to complete emollient phase and waxes, heated and mixed until uniform (approx. 90–105°C).
3. Pearls and fillers are added to above phases and mixed with shear (if necessary) until homogenous.
4. Add actives, preservatives, fragrance and antioxidants and mix until uniform.
5. Maintain a temperature just above the initial set point of the waxes and fill as appropriate.

Volatile Nontransfer Lipstick

The proper balance of solvents and emollients prevent transfer and prevent lipstick from becoming too dry on the lips [15].

- Solvents.   Isododecane, alkyl silicones, cyclomethicone
- Emollients.   Phenyl trimethicone, esters, alkyl silicones (fluids, pastes), vegetable/plant oils
- Waxes.   Polyethylene, synthetic, ceresin, ozokerite, paraffin (not compatible with some silicones), beeswax, alkyl silicones
- Fixatives.   Silicone resins (MQ type from G.E.), silicone Plus Polymers (SA 70-5, VS 70-5)
- Colorants/Pearls.   Identical to classic lipstick
- Fillers.   Identical to classic lipstick
- Actives.   Identical to classic lipstick
- Preservatives/Antioxidants: Identical to classic lipstick

Solvent Lipstick

Formula

Solvent	25–60%
Emollient	1–30%
Waxes	10–25%
Fixatives	1–10%
Fillers	1–15%
Colorants/Pearls	1–15%
Fragrance	0.05–0.10%

Procedure. Identical to classic lipstick except product should be prepared in a closed vessel to prevent loss of volatile components.

NAIL COLOR

Nail lacquers form the largest group of manicure preparations. They should be waterproof, glossy, adherent, dry quickly, and be resistant to chipping and abrasion. The main constituents include a film former, modifying resin, plasticizer and solvents. Additionally, pigments, suspending agents, and UV absorbers are usually included. Nitrocellulose is the chief film-forming ingredient. Nitrocellulose is derived from cellulose, a polymer made of several anhydroglucose units connected by ether linkages. Nitrocellulose by itself will produce a hard brittle film so it is necessary to modify it with resins and plasticizers to provide flexibility and gloss. The most commonly used modifying resin is para-toluenesulfonamide formaldehyde resin, which is contained at 5 to 10% levels. This resin provides gloss, adhesion, and increases the hardness of the nitrocellulose film. The formaldehyde resin has caused allergies with a small number of consumers so that other modifiers such as sucrose benzoate, polyester resin, and toluene sulfonamide epoxy resin have been used in its place with varying results. Plasticizers used include camphor, glyceryl diesters [16], dibutyl phthalate, citrate esters and castor oil. Other resins such as polyurethanes and acrylics have been used as auxiliary resins. Variations of plasticizers and resins will change the viscosity, dry time, and gloss of the lacquer. Colorants include titanium dioxide, iron oxides, most organics, and pearlescent pigments. Soluble dyes are never used because of their staining effects on skin and nails. In order to reduce settling of the heavier pigments, treatments, such as silicone [17] and oxidized polyethylene [18] have been utilized. Modified clays derived from bentonite and/or hectorite are used to suspend the pigments and make the nail enamel thixotropic and brushable. Solvents, which constitute approximately 70% of nail lacquers, include n-butyl acetate, ethyl acetate, and toluene. Generally, those are cream and pearl nail lacquers. Cream shades may be shear or full coverage with titanium dioxide as the chief pigment. Pearlescent nail polish usually contains bismuth oxychloride and/or titanium dioxide–coated micas and may even contain guanine-natural fish scales. The manufacturing of nail lacquer is usually carried out by specialty manufacturing firms which are familiar with the hazards of working with nitrocellulose and solvents. The manufacture consists of two separate operations: (1) manufacture and compounding of the lacquer base, and (2) the coloring and color matching of shades. Top coats, which are used to enhance gloss, extend wear, and reduce dry time, are usually made with high solids and low boiling point solvents. Cellulose acetate butyrate (CAB) has been used as a substitute for nitrocellulose in nonyellowing top coats but does not adhere as well to the nail [19]. Most top coats are nitrocellulose based. Base coats function to create a nail surface to which nail lacquer will have better adhesion. Different auxiliary resins, such as polyvinyl butyral, have been used in nitrocellulose systems. Fibers, polyamide resins, and other treatment items have been added in order to provide advertising claims, and some may actually alter the effectiveness of the film. In the evaluation of nail enamels the following criteria are used: color, application, wear, dry-time, gloss, and hardness.

FACE PRODUCTS: MAKEUP FORMULARY

Loose Face Powder [20]

Ingredients	W/W%
Zinc stearate	8.00
Magnesium carbonate	1.00
Iron oxides	q.s.
Bismuth oxychloride and mica	25.00
Fragrance	q.s.
Talc to 100.00	
Preservative	q.s.

Procedure

1. Mix ingredient #3 with a portion of ingredient #6; pulverize.
2. Add the other ingredients; mix in a ribbon or double-cone blender until uniform.

Pressed Powder Foundation [21]

Ingredients	W/W%
Part A:	
Talc	6.60
Titanium dioxide	19.20
Mica (and) titanium dioxide	4.80
Iron oxides	11.20
Zinc oxides	6.20
Barium sulfate	13.70
Part B:	
Dimethicone	5.50
Lanolin	8.20
Petrolatum	1.40
Mineral oil	1.40
Isopropyl myristate	1.40
Part C:	
Fragrance	q.s.
Preservative	q.s.

Procedure

1. Mix all of the pigments in Part A together.
2. Add Part B, Part C, Part D with high shear mixing.
3. Press into suitable container.

Two-Way Powder Foundation (Wet and Dry)

Ingredients	W/W%
Sericite	35.0
Talc	24.0
Mica	10.0
Nylon-12	10.0
Titanium dioxide	8.0
Zinc stearate	3.0
Iron oxide pigments, silicone treated	2.0
Cetyl octanoate	q.s.
Squalane	2.0
Octyldodecyl myristate	2.0
Mineral oil	2.0
Dimethicone	2.0
Propyl paraben	0.05
Butyl paraben	0.05
Perfume	q.s.

Procedure

Mix all ingredients except liquid oils and perfume in a blender. Spray or add liquid oils and perfume. Mix and pulverize. Press into pans.

Pressed Face Powder

Ingredients	W/W%
Part A:	
Polymethyl methacrylate	12.00
Talc (and) polyethylene	q.s. to 100.0
Sericite	10.00
Mica (and) polyethylene	5.00
Magnesium stearate	3.00
Mica (and) titanium dioxide	5.00
Kaolin	8.00
Color	q.s.
Part B:	
Dimethicone	6.00
Glyceryl diisostearate	2.00
Tocopherol	0.10
Butyl paraben	0.05
Propyl paraben	0.05

Procedure

Mix A well. Heat B to 80°C. Mix until uniform. Add B to A. Mix well until uniform. Pulverize and sieve. Press into pans.

Liquid Compact Foundation

A hot-pour solid cream foundation that seems to ''liquefy'' when touched. Easy to blend to a sheer finish.

Ingredients	W/W%
Part A:	
Titanium dioxide (and) isopropyl titanium triisostearate	12.99
Yellow iron oxide (and) isopropyl titanium triisostearate	0.33
Red iron oxide (and) isopropyl titanium triisostearate	0.33
Black iron oxide (and) isopropyl titanium triisostearate	0.10
Aluminum starch octenyl succinate (and) isopropyl titanium triisostearate	15.00
Sericite	6.25
Silica	2.00
Part B:	
Squalene	6.50
Dimethicone (5 centistoke)	11.00
Octyl palmitate	18.00
Polyglycerol-3 diisostearate	5.50
Mineral oil	3.00
Hydrogenated coco glycerines	2.00
Microcrystalline wax	4.00
Carnauba	1.00
Part C:	
Nylon-12	12.00
	100.00

Procedure

Micronize Part A until the color is fully developed. Heat Part B with stirring to 195 to 200°F. Continue to stir for 1/2 hour. Add Part A to Part B and mix until homogenous. Cool to 180°F. Add Part C and mix until homogenous. Pour into pans at 165–170°F.

Blusher (Pressed) [22]

Ingredients	W/W%
Talc	65.70
Zinc stearate	8.00
Titanium dioxide	3.50
Iron oxides (russet)	12.00
Iron oxides (black)	0.20
D&C Red No. 6 barium lake	0.30
Titanium dioxide (and) mica	6.00
Methyl paraben	0.10
Imidazolidinyl urea	0.10
Fragrance	0.10
Pentaerythritol tetraisostearate	4.00
	100.00

Procedure

Mix ingredients 1 through 9 well. Pulverize. Place into ribbon blender. Spray into batch number 10 then into number 11. Repulverize. Sieve. Press into pans.

Eye Shadow (Pressed) [23]

Ingredients	W/W%
Mica (and) iron oxides (and) Titanium dioxide	40.5
Talc	32.4
Cyclomethicone (and) dimethicone	13.6
Oleyl Erucate	13.5
	100.00

Procedure

1. Mix and mill all ingredients through a 0.027″ herringbone screen.
2. Press into a suitable container.

Eye Shadow (Pressed) [24]

Ingredients	W/W%
Talc	4.20
Bismuth oxychloride	10.00
Fumed silica	0.50
Zinc stearate	5.00
Titanium dioxide (and) mica	65.00
Methyl paraben	0.10
Propyl paraben	0.10
Imidazolidinyl urea	0.10
Lanolin alcohol	3.75
Mineral oil	9.75
Isostearyl neopentanoate	1.50
	100.00

Procedure

Mix 1 through 8 in a ribbon blender. Mix binders 9 through 11 in a separate container. Spray binders into 1 through 8. Mix until uniform. Pulverize, if necessary, without a screen. Press into pans.

Solvent Mascara [25]

Ingredients	W/W%
(A)	
Petroleum distillate	q.s. to 100.00
Beeswax	18.00
PEG-6 sorbitan beeswax	6.00
Ozokerite 170-D	4.00
Carnauba wax	6.00
Propylparaben	0.10
Glyceryl oleate (and) propylene glycol	1.50
(B)	
Iron oxides	15.00
(C)	
Petroleum distillate (and) quaternum-18 hectorite (and) propylene carbonate	12.50
(D)	
Deionized water	15.00
Methylparaben	0.30
Sodium borate	0.60
Quaternium-15	0.10

Procedure

Mill pigment (B) into (A), which has been heated to 90°C. After (C) has been added slowly and heated with (A), emulsify by adding (D) at 90°C to (A), (B), and (C) mixtures. Continue mixing until cool.

Emulsion-Resistant Mascara [26]

Ingredients	W/W%
(A)	
Deionized water	41.00
Hydroxyethyl cellulose	1.00
Methylparaben	0.30
Aqueous 0.10% phenyl mercuric acetate	4.00
Triethanolamine	1.00
Ammonium hydroxide, 28%	0.50
(B)	
Iron oxides	10.00
Ulltramarine blue	2.00
(C)	
Isostearic acid	2.00
Stearic acid	2.00
Glyceryl monostearate	1.00
Beeswax	9.00
Carnauba wax	6.00
Propylparaben	0.10
(D)	
Quaternium-15	0.10
(E)	
30% Acrylic/acrylate copolymer solution in ammonium hydroxide	20.00
	100.00

Procedure

Mill the pigments of (B) in the water phase (B). Heat to 80°C. Heat the oil phase (C) to 82°C. Emulsify. Cool to 50°C. Add (D), then (E). Cool to 30°C.

Waterproof Eyeliner [27]

Ingredients	W/W%
Beeswax	16.50
PVP/Eicosene copolymer	5.00
Petroleum distillate	35.00
Petroleum distillate (and) quaternium-18 hectorite (and) propylene carbonate	33.50
Preservative	0.20
Titanium dioxide (and) mica (and) ferric ferrocyanide	9.80
	100.00

Procedure

1. Heat ingredients 1 and 2 to 70°C and blend in (3) (n.b. flammable).
2. Blend in (4) with low shear mixing.
3. Cool to 50°C while continuing to mix.
4. Blend in ingredients (2), (5), and (6) and mix until uniform.

Aqueous Eyeliner [28]

Ingredients	W/W%
Part 1	
Ammonium vinyl acetate/actylates copolymer	55.00
Polysorbate 80	1.00
Isopropyl myristate	4.00
Part 2	
Propylene glycol USP	2.50
Methylparaben USP	0.25
Water, deionized	29.50
Hectorite (and) hydroxyethylcellulose	0.25
Iron oxides	7.50
	100.00

Makeup Pencil [29]

Ingredients	W/W%
Part 1	
Cyclomethicone	40.0
Bis phenylhexamethicone	40.0
Diphenyl dimethicone	40.0
Part 2	
Beeswax	15.0
Carnauba	7.0
Ozokerite	7.0
Paraffin	20.0
Mineral oil	q.s. to 100.0
Cetyl alcohol	1.0
Part 3	
Pigments	q.s.
Titanium dioxide	q.s.

Procedure

1. The ingredients of Part 2 are melted and homogenized at 78–82°C, then maintained by a thermostatic bath regulated to 58–62°C.
2. The ingredients of Part 3 are dispersed in Part 1; the mixture is placed in a thermostatic bath at 58–62°C.
3. Part 3 is then added.
4. After homogenization, the whole is cooled in a silicone-treated mold (with dimethicone).

Classic Lipstick [30]

Ingredients	W/W%
Carnauba wax	2.50
Beeswax, white	20.00
Ozokerite	10.00
Lanolin, anhydrous	5.00
Cetyl alcohol	2.00
Liquid paraffin	3.00
Isopropyl myristate	3.00
Propylene glycolricinoleate	4.00
Pigments	10.00
Bromo acids	2.50
Castor oil	q.s. to 100.00

Solvent Lipstick [31]

Ingredients	W/W%
Synthetic wax	6.00
Ceresin	4.00
Isododecane	10.00
Paraffin	3.00
Cetyl acetate/acetylated lanolin alcohol	5.00
Methylparaben	0.30
Propylparaben	0.10
BHA	0.10
D&C Red No. 7 calcium lake	4.00
FD&C Yellow No. 5 aluminum lake	3.00
Titanium dioxide/mica	5.00
Titanium dioxide/mica/iron oxides	3.00
Bismuth oxychloride	10.00
Cyclomethicone	41.50
Isostearyl trimetholpropane siloxy silicate	5.00
	100.00

Procedure

Mix the dry ingredients with the volatiles and silicone ester wax. The waxes and oils are added with heating. The powders are added next. The mixture is then stirred before pouring into molds and allowed to cool.

Cream Nail Enamel [32]

Ingredients	W/W%
n-Butylacetate—solvent	28.23
Toluene—diluent	24.54
Nitrocellulose ½ sec wet—film-former	12.00
Ethyl acetate—solvent	11.00
Toluene sulfonamide/formaldehyde resin—secondary resin	10.00
Acrylates copolymer—resin	0.50
Dibutyl phthalate—plasticizer	5.00
Isopropyl alcohol, 99%—diluent	4.25
Stearalkonium hectorite—suspending agent	1.00
Camphor—plasticizer	1.50
D&C Red No. 6 barium lake—color	0.08
Titanium dioxide	0.75
Iron oxides	0.15
	100.00

Pearlescent Nail Enamel [33]

Ingredients	W/W%
n-Butyl acetate	34.04
Toluene	30.00
Nitrocellulose ½ sec. wet	14.90
Toluene sulfonamide/formaldehyde resin	7.10
Dibutyl phthalate	4.80
Camphor	2.40
Stearalkonium hectorite	1.20
Benzophenone-1	0.20
D&C Red No. 7 calcium lake	0.08
D&C Red No. 34 calcium lake	0.05
FD&C Yellow No. 5 aluminum lake	0.08
Iron oxides	0.15
Bismuth oxychloride (25%)	5.00
	100.00

Acrylic Nail Hardener [34]

Ingredients	W/W%
Ethyl acetate	41.20
Butyl acetate	30.00
Nitocellulose ½ sec. wet	14.00
Toluene sulfonamide/formaldehyde resin	10.00
Dibutyl phthalate	4.00
Camphor	0.50
Acrylates copolymer	0.20
Benzophenone-1	0.10
	100.00

REFERENCES

1. 21 CFR, Parts 1–99. April 1, 1998.
2. EC Cosmetics Directive 76/768/EEC, Annex IV, Part 1. September 3, 1998.
3. MHW Ordinance No. 30. August 31, 1966.
4. 21 CFR Parts 1–99. April 1, 1998.
5. 21 CFR Parts 1–99. April 1, 1998.
6. 21 CFR Parts 1–99. April 1, 1998.
7. 61 *Federal Register* 8372. March 6, 1996.
8. EC Cosmetics Directive 76/768/EEC, Annex IV, Part 1. September 3, 1998.
9. MHW Ordinance No. 30. August 31, 1996.
10. Decorative cosmetics. In: Handbook of Cosmetic Science and Technology. Knowlton JL, Pearce SEM, eds. Oxford: Elsevier Advanced Technology, 1993: 128.
11. Miyoshi R. U.S. Patent No. 4,606,914. 1986.
12. Miyoshi R, Isao Imai. U.S. Patent No. 4,622,074. 1986.
13. Schlossman ML. U.S. Patent No. 4,877,604. 1989.

14. Dweck AC. Foundations—a guide to formulation and manufacture. Cosmetic Toilet 1986; 4: 41–44.
15. Castrogiavanni A, Barone SJ, Krog A, McCulley ML, Callelo JF. U.S. Patent No. 5,505,937. 1996.
16. Castrogiavanni A, Sandewicz RW, Amato SW. U.S. Patent No. 5,066,484. 1991.
17. Socci RL, Ismailer AA, Castrogiavanni A. U.S. Patent No. 4,832,944. 1989.
18. Weber RA, Frankfurt CC, Penicnak AJ. U.S. Patent No. 5,174,996. 1992.
19. Martin FL, Onofrio MV. U.S. Patent No. 5,130,125. 1992.
20. Hunting ALL. Face cosmetics. In: Decorative Cosmetics. Weymouth, Dorset, England: Micelle Press, 1991:3.
21. Personal Care Formulary. GE Silicones Waterford, NY. 1996; p. 151.
22. Knowlton JL, Pearce SEM. Decorative products. In: Handbook of Cosmetic Science and Technology. Oxford: Elsevier Advanced Technology, 1993:143.
23. Personal Care Formulary. GE Silicones, Waterford, NY. 1996; p. 149.
24. Knowlton JL, Pearce SEM. Decorative cosmetics. In: Handbook of Cosmetic Science and Technology. Oxford: Elsevier Advanced Technology, 1993:145.
25. Schlossman ML. Application of color cosmetics. Cosmet Toilet 1985; 100:36–40.
26. Schlossman ML. Application of color cosmetics. Cosmet Toilet 1985; 100:36–40.
27. Hunting ALL. Eye cosmetics. In: Decorative Cosmetics. Weymouth, Dorset, England: Micelle Press, 1991:173.
28. Hunting ALL. Eye cosmetics. In: Decorative Cosmetics. Weymouth, Dorset, England: Micelle Press, 1991:170.
29. Hunting ALL. Eye cosmetics. In: Decorative Cosmetics. Weymouth, Dorset, England: Micelle Press, 1991:174.
30. Bryce DM. Lipstick. In: Poucher's Perfumes, Cosmetics and Soaps. Butler H, ed. London: Chapman & Hall, 1992:234.
31. Castrogiavanni A, Barone SJ, Krog A, McCulley ML, Callelo JF. U.S. Patent No. 5, 505, 937. 1996.
32. Schlossman ML. Manicure preparations. In: Poucher's Perfumes, Cosmetics and Soaps. Butler H, ed. London: Chapman & Hall, 1992:253, 254.
33. Schlossman ML. Manicure preparations. In: Poucher's Perfumes, Cosmetics and Soaps. Butler H, ed. London: Chapman & Hall, 1992:254.
34. Schlossman ML Make-up formulary. Cosmet Toilet 1994; 109:104.

55

Cosmetics for Nails

Douglas Schoon
Creative Nail Design Inc., Vista, California

Robert Baran
Nail Disease Center, Cannes, France

The purpose of this chapter is to present the cosmetics used for the decoration of the nail, of which the nail coating is of prime importance. Fingernail coatings consist of two types [1–3]:

1. Coatings that harden upon evaporation: these products include nail polishes, topcoats and base coats.
2. Coatings that polymerize: nail enhancements are a special type of coating used to create artificial fingernails.

EVAPORATION COATINGS

Base coat, top coat, and nail enamel have similar basic formulas.

They consist of the following:

1. *A film former such as nitrocellulose.* This organic polymer creates a continuous coating over the nail plate. Other nonnitrated cellulosic materials are also used with varying degrees of success, namely cellulose acetate and derivatives. Polyurethanes, polyamides, and polyesters have also been used. However, these cannot match the toughness and surface hardness of nitrocellulose. One of the most commonly used, nitrocellulose has several disadvantages: the surfaces produced by this polymer have low gloss and the films are brittle and adhere poorly to the nail plate. Upon evaporation, nitrocellulose films shrink excessively, which leads to poor adhesion. To overcome these drawbacks, additional film modifiers will offset some deficiencies of the primary film form.

2. *Film modifiers.* They are specifically used to improve adhesion and gloss. The most commonly used modifier is toluene sulfonamide/formaldehyde resin (TSFR), which is considered to be the heart of the product. This thermoplastic resin improves nail-plate adhesion while producing water-resistant, glossy surfaces with improved flexibility. Unfortunately, this resin is the main culprit of users' sensitization. Use of this resin imparts between 0.05 to 0.1% free formaldehyde (as impurity) into the formulation. Therefore, many alternate modifiers have been tried, including toluene/sulfonamide/expoxy resin,

polyester sucrose benzoate, polyesters, acrylic ester oligomers, SAIB, arylsulfonyl methanes, and glyceryl tribenzoate.

3. *Plasticizers.* Plasticizers are chemical flexibilizers for polymer films that improve their durability. They may also improve adhesion and gloss. Dibutyl phthalate and camphor are the most common examples of low–molecular weight, high–boiling point plasticizers. Other examples of plasticizers are castor oil, glyceryl tribenzoate, acetyl tribenzoate citrate PPG-2 dibenzoate, glycerol, citrate esters, triacetin, and a polyether urethane.

4. *Solvents/diluents.* The solid film-forming polymers, upon evaporation, are deposited on the nail plate. The most commonly used solvents are alkyl esters and glycol ethers. Coupling agents (aliphatic alcohols) are useful in varnishes to increase the overall solubility and flow of the system. Diluents are usually nonpolar compounds that will not dissolve nitrocellulose. Toluene was commonly used until the appearance of California Proposition 65. Most companies are now developing toluene-free formulas.

5. *Viscosity modifiers or thixotropic agents.* Ideally, a nail enamel should be gel-like when sitting on the shelf but significantly thin when brushed on. Both consistencies are possible in one bottle by using thixotropic agents such as stearalkonium hectorite.

6. *Color additives.* Colorants should be nonsoluble pigments to prevent staining of the nail plate. Guanine, derived from scales of Atlantic herring, produces pearlescent pigment. Bismuth oxychloride and mica coated with titanium dioxide are used to create iridescent shades.

7. *Base and top coats.* Base coats contain a high percentage of TSFR. They are applied to the nail before application of nail varnish. They are adhesion promoters that improve retention and coating toughness. Top coats use higher levels of film formers, such as nitrocellulose, to maximize surface gloss and hardness. Often the top coat contains UV-absorbing materials.

POLYMERIZING COATINGS

Sculptured Artificial Nails

Liquid-and-powder systems are based on methacrylates. They consist of a liquid monomer (ethyl methacrylate) mixed with a polymer powder (polyethyl and/or polymethyl methacrylate), the latter carrying only the heat-sensitive initiator (usually benzoyl peroxide) to the monomer. UV absorbers are polymer additives that prevent sunlight yellowing. Catalysts speed up polymerization.

Light-Curing Gels

UV or visible light-curing gels are made primarily of urethane acrylate and other acrylated oligomers. Associated with initiator, the catalyst and oligomers are combined into a single product; they come premixed and ready to use. They may be considered a variant of sculptured artificial nails.

Preformed Artificial Nails

These are usually made of ABS plastic, nylon, or acetate, and are adhered to the natural nail with cyanoacrylate monomer. Home-use, retail versions of these tips may be used as temporary natural overlays, not worn for longer than 48 hours on any one occasion. They are more often used as permanent nail-tip extensions. Professional nail technicians usually coat these tips with artificial nail products to create longer lasting nail extensions. Most nail technicians feel it is too time consuming to sculpt nails, and these tips speed the process. The tip can be coated or overlaid with wraps or liquid-and-powder or gel products.

Wraps

Wraps can be used to coat the nail plate or add strength to thin, weak nails. The monomers used to create wraps are cyanoacrylates. In nail wrapping, the free edge of the nail should be long enough to be splinted by the various types of fabrics providing support and added strength to the coating. There are three fabrics in wide use: fiberglass, silk, and linen.

No-Light Gels

These products are wrap monomers that have been thickened to have a gel-like appearance. They should be used and handled as any other wrap product.

Removal of Fingernail Coatings

The most commonly used solvent for removal of nail products is acetone. Warming the solvent with great care can cut product removal time in half. However most gels are difficult to remove because they are highly cross-linked and resistant to many solvents. Therefore, if gel enhancements have to be removed, slowly file (do not drill) the enhancement with a medium-grit file, leaving a very thin layer of product. Soak in warm product remover and, once softened, scrape the remaining product away with a wooden pusher stick [1].

Cuticle Removers

These are lotions or gels containing approximately 0.4% sodium or potassium hydroxide. The lotion is left in place for 1 to 3 minutes and then washed off. Creams containing 1 to 5% lactic acid (pH 3–3.7) are also used.

Nail Whitener

This is a pencil-like device with a white clay (kaolin) core used to deposit color on the undersurface of the free edge of the nail.

REFERENCES

1. Schoon DD. Nail Structure and Product Chemistry. Albany: Milady Publishing, 1996.
2. Baran R, Schoon DD. Cosmetology of normal nails. In: Baran R, Maibach HI. Textbook of Cosmetic Dermatology. London: Martin Dunitz, 1998:213–231.
3. Baran R, Schoon DD. Cosmetics for abnormal and pathological nails. In: Baran R, Maibach HI. Textbook of Cosmetic Dermatology. London: Martin Dunitz, 1998:233–244.

56

Antiperspirants

Jörg Schreiber
Beiersdorf AG, Hamburg, Germany

GENERAL INTRODUCTION

This chapter presents an overview concerning the current knowledge of antiperspirant actives and their interactions with the human axilla. It is my intention to give the interested reader a short introduction about formulation work, drug delivery systems, and application forms developed for antiperspirant actives. The final section lists references that should be useful for anyone who wants to learn more about a specific topic of antiperspirant technology.

BIOLOGY OF SWEAT GLANDS IN THE HUMAN AXILLA

The axilla region of humans contains apocrine, eccrine, and sebaceous glands. Approximately 25,000 sweat glands/axilla can produce up to 12 g sweat/h [1]. The current understanding concerning structure and function of sweat glands is that thermoregulation is only one aspect of the body participating in immmunological, metabolic, and hormonal aspects of human life [2].

Eccrine Glands

This is the organ responsible for the majority of sweat production. It has a sensory and excretory function and can be stimulated by emotional and thermal stimuli [3]. It produces a clear, colorless and odorless liquid containing 98 to 99% water and 1 to 2% inorganic and organic compounds [4]. Inorganic components include NaCl, traces of K^+, Ca^{2+}, Mg^{2+}, Fe^{3+}, and Cu^{2+} ions. Organic components include: lactic acid, citric acid, formic acid, propionic acid, butyric acid, urea, and ammonia. Underarm wetness comes mostly from the secretion of eccrine glands. Antiperspirants reduce the amount of sweat only from eccrine glands.

Apocrine Glands

Apocrine glands are apparently a relict from the phylogenetic development of man. These glands start to produce a milky, viscous fluid during puberty on special locations of the body, especially the underarm pit [5]. In contrast to eccrine glands, the openings of the glands are not at the skin surface but appear at the hair follicle. Decomposition of apocrine sweat by skin bacteria are responsible for the characteristic malodor of human sweat. Apocrine sweat consists among water of proteins, carbohydrates and ammonium salts [6]. Other investigators have reported that these glands secrete lipids, cholesterol, and steroids [7]. Furthermore, it has been shown that androgen-converting enzymes in the apocrine glands are responsible for circulating androgens to dihydrotestosterone [5].

ANTIPERSPIRANTS

Antiperspirants are topically applied products designed to reduce underarm wetness by limiting eccrine sweat production. In the United States these products are regulated by the FDA as over-the-counter (OTC) drugs because they are intended to affect a "function of the body" (in this case, perspiration). Products containing antiperspirant actives have to reduce perspiration to minimum 20% by 50% of the test population under validated test conditions. Test protocols (in vivo clinical trials) to develop a safe and effective product have been designed to substantiate the desired claims [8–14].

Comparative quantitative determination of the activity of sweat glands on the forearm after application of aluminum chlorohydrate solutions is now possible by combining the classic starch iodine visualization technique with digital image analysis [15]. A noninvasive optical technique that allows the analysis of the function of a number of glands simultaneously in vivo was recently reported [16]. A new method for parallel testing of up to eight formulations on the backs of volunteers allows a very fast evaluation of product prototypes [1].

Sweat Reduction by Antiperspirants: Current Model/Theory

The reader should be aware that theories concerning the action of sweat-reducing agents depend strongly on the type of actives (aluminum salts, nonionics, ionic agents). The efficacy of antiperspirants based on aluminum and/or aluminum zirconium salts (see discussion p. 691) can be understood by the formation of an occlusive plug of metal hydroxide in the eccrine duct [17]. Tape-stripping experiments followed by analysis of transmission electron micrographs of an ACH-treated eccrine sweat-gland duct (see discussion p. 691) shows an obstructive amorphous material supporting the theory of a mechanical blockage of sweat glands from diffusion of the soluble ACH solution into the sweat gland and subsequent neutralization to a polymeric aluminum hydroxide gel [18,19]. There seems to be no correlation concerning efficacy of aluminum salts and the location of the plug in the duct because it is known that, compared with ACH, the more effective Al-Zr compounds do not penetrate as deep as the also highly effective $AlCl_3$ solutions [17]. The reader is referred to the literature concerning other theories of sweat reduction by aluminum salts [20].

Active Ingredients for Controlling Underarm Wetness—State of the Art
Buffered Aluminum Salts (ACH)

The first antiperspirant, Ever Dry, based on $AlCl_3$, was introduced to the market in 1903 [21]. The first cream-containing aluminumsulfate was introduced during the 1930s. The acidic pH value (2.5–3.0) was a drawback of these products, leading to skin irritation in the underarm pit. History tells us that the development of actives with a higher pH value, so-called buffered aluminumchlorides (aluminum chlorohydrate, ACH, pH $= 4.0–4.2$) was an appropriate step with the additional benefit of reduced destruction of fabric clothes. The formula of this buffering salt is $\{Al_2(OH)_5\}^+ + \{Cl^-\}$, or more conveniently $Al_2(OH)_5Cl$.

The historical development from $AlCl_3$ to $Al_2(OH)_5Cl$ can be easily understood by the following consideration:

$$AlCl_3 = \tfrac{1}{2}\,Al_2Cl_6 \qquad \text{Substitute 5 } Cl^- - \text{ ions against } OH^- - \text{ ions}$$
$$\Rightarrow Al_2(OH)_5Cl$$

$Al_2(OH)_5Cl$ is a 5/6 basic aluminumtrichloride. The accepted definition of ACH is the ratio of Al to Cl $= 2.1$ to 1.0. Lower levels lead to aluminum dichlorohydrate ($Al_2(OH)_4Cl_2$) or to aluminum sesquichlorohydrate ($Al_2(OH)_{4.5}Cl_{1.5}$—both actives are also generally regarded as safe (GRAS). ACH is supplied as a powder or a 50% solution in water. It can be formulated up to 25% calculated on an anhydrous basis. The 20% aqueous solution reduces perspiration by 35 to 40% on average [22]. Some dyes used in clothing may be acid sensitive and will change color when in contact with an antiperspirant.

The structure of the Lewis acid ACH is very complex because ACH in water forms so-called isopolyoxo-cations with chloride ions as couterions [23–25]. There exists several polymer equilibria of the polycationic aluminum species in water-based systems. Short-chain polycationic species are more effective in reduction of sweat.

Aluminum Zirconium Chlorohydrate-Glycine Complexes (AZG or ZAG)

Aluminum zirconium chlorohydrate is obtained by reaction of ACH with zirconylchloride. Reaction of the former ingredients in the presence of glycine leads ZAG complexes. Glycine is used as a buffering agent. These antiperspirant actives form very complex polymeric structures in water. The actives are defined by the ratio of Al + Zr metal–to–chloride ratio and the Al to Zr atomic ratio. The interested reader is referred to the literature concerning available actives [26,27] and nomenclature of the Al-Zr complexes [21,22]. These antiperspirant actives were developed especially for anhydrous formulations because they show, compared with ACH, enhanced sweat reduction [28–30]. The maximal concentration of ZAG calculated on an anhydrous basis is 20%. They are not allowed to be formulated for use in aerosols.

New Concepts for Controlling Underarm Wetness

Titanium Metal Chelates

The understanding of the complex solution chemistry of aluminum-based antiperspirants gave input to the search for alternative antiperspirant salts. Titanium derivatives like partially neutralized ammonium titanium lactate (ATL) salts were shown to be effective in in-vitro efficacy tests [31]. The titanium metal chelates can be synthesized from the corresponding titanium alkoxides and organic acids followed by neutralization with ammonia. Under acidic to neutral pH conditions the ATL active seems to be relatively stable to hydrolysis and therefore probably a suitable antiperspirant active in water-based or anhydrous drug delivery systems.

Film-Forming Antiperspirant Polymers

So-called polybarrier technology is another approach to reduce perspiration by using a polymer that forms an insoluble occlusive film barrier on the underarm skin [32]. It was mentioned that the occlusive film is a barrier to the passage of moisture. The main advantage of this technology has been described as reduced skin irritation, applicable after underarm shaving, and higher sweat reduction compared with today's classic antiperspirant salts. The preferred polymer is an olefinic acid amide/olefinic acid or ester copolymer–like octylacrylamide/acrylate copolymer (Versacryl™-40). This copolymer can be used alone or in combination with PVP/eicosene-copolymer in sticks, roll-ons, or alcohol-based products [33]. The reduction of sweat depends on the choice of vehicle and exceeds in some formulations 40%.

Lyotropic Liquid Crystals

Certain surfactant/cosurfactant combinations in water form depending on the variables of concentration/temperature instead of micelles lamellar, hexagonal, inverted hexagonal, inverted micellar, or even cubic phases. The cubic phases can be of micellar or bicontinous type [34]. The water domains in lamellar or cubic phases can swell to a certain degree while taking up water. The use of this swelling behavior is the basis of a patent where a surfactant/cosurfactant combination is applied to the underarm pit [35]. Sweat (water) transfers the applied composition to a lyotropic liquid crystal of cubic structure, thus creating a sweat-absorbing system in the axilla. Oleic acid/glycerol monolaurate is one of the surfactant combinations in the patent. Both components are also well known as deodorizers.

DRUG-DELIVERY SYSTEMS AND APPLICATION FORMS FOR ANTIPERSPIRANT ACTIVES

Antiperspirant actives can be formulated in a variety of delivery systems like anhydrous suspensions, water- or hydroalcoholic-based solutions, and emulsions. Typical application forms for antiperspirants are sticks, roll-ons, creams, pump sprays, aerosols, gels, and powders. A new technology for pump sprays is discussed in the chapter 57. On a global basis, the three most important product forms are sticks, roll-ons, and aerosols.

Formulation Work

After the decision for the desired application form has been made the formulator has to decide on the vehicle system for the antiperspirant active. It is the intent of this section to summarize some of the current knowledge concerning influence of actives with the formula, efficacy of different delivery systems, and the function of the ingredients used in antiperspirants.

Antiperspirant actives like ACH or ZAG complexes are soluble in water. Application of a concentrated aqueous solution of an antiperspirant active gives a rather tacky feeling [36]. Reduction of tackiness can be best achieved by silicone oils (cyclomethicones) or ester oils like Di-(2 ethylhexyl) adipate [27]. The acidic pH value (pH 4.0–4.2) has to be taken into account by selecting additional components for the desired drug delivery system. Loss of viscosity and problems of a final formula with color stability are often a hint to change the gellant and/or perfume. Aluminum powders in anhydrous systems (aerosols, suspension sticks) often leave visible white residues on skin or clothing. Liquid emollients, like PPG-14 butylether or the aforementioned adipate ester, minimize these residues. Another approach is to use the solid emollient isosorbide monolaurate (ICI, Arlamol ISML) [37]. In anhydrous aerosol formulations the ACH powder settles down and forms a hard to redisperse cake at the bottom of the aerosol can. Suspending aids like Quaternium-18 Hectorite or Quaternium-18 Bentonite prevents settling of the active and additionly thickens the cyclomethicone oil phase. Usage of fine powders of ACH is another approach to overcome natures law of gravity.

The reader should be aware that hydrophobic ingredients like emollients have an influence on the effectiveness of an antiperspirant active because a cosmetic oil phase or wax can cover the pores of the eccrine duct. The efficacy of an antiperspirant active like ACH is higher in water-containing systems compared with anhydrous formulations. The following rules concerning efficacy might be helpful:

1. Efficacy: Aqueous solution > Anhydrous suspension
2. Since diffusion of an active in the vehicle and from the vehicle to the skin after application has to considered one can further differentiate the expected efficacy trends.
   Efficacy: Aqueous solution > Sprayable O/W emulsion > O/W-emulsion roll-on > O/W-emulsion cream
3. It is accepted that antiperspirant actives in the outer phase of an emulsion have a higher efficacy than in dispersed phase.
   Efficacy: O/W-emulsion > W/O-emulsion
4. In water-free systems the viscosity of the drug delivery system might be of relevance. Suspended ACH in anhydrous vehicles needs to be solubilized after application to the axilla by sweat (water). The effectiveness of suspension sticks depends on the rapidity of active solubilization. The usage of ultrafine powders of ACH is expected to boost efficacy compared with fine powders.
   Efficacy: low viscous suspension > suspension stick

The interested reader is referred to the literature concerning vehicle effects on antiperspirant activity [7,38,39].

Not only lipophilic ingredients might have an influence on the efficacy of a product because it is known that the water-soluble propylene glycol can form complexes or hydrogen bonds with aluminum polycationic species thereby altering the efficacy of the salt [40]. Additionally propylene glycol in high concentrations may result in skin irritations [41]. Successful formulation work aims at finding the right viscosity for the product in the desired application form, a lower viscosity during flow into the underarm pit and a higher viscosity after application so that the product stays where it was applied. Conventional shear shinning flow curves are characteristic for antiperspirant products. The reader is referred to the literature concerning rheology aspects of cosmetic products [42].

Deodorant/Antiperspirant Sticks

It is at present not easy to give the reader an overview about sticks because nowadays there exists many technologies to develop this solid delivery system. In Figure 1 an attempt was made to summarize this area. In the following section only systems of major importance are discussed.

Sticks can be divided into different classes like suspension sticks, gel sticks, and emulsion sticks. Soft sticks have some properties of all three categories (Fig. 1).

Suspension Sticks

Dry deodorants, or antiperspirant solids, are synonyms for an application form where the active in the form of a powder is suspended in a silicone oil phase. Stearyl alcohol is

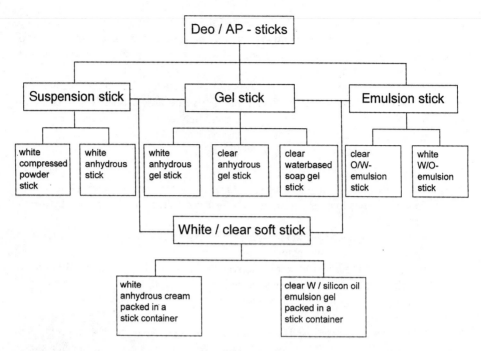

FIGURE 1   Overview of cosmetic Deo/AP-sticks.

usually used as the hardening agent. The molten mass crystallizes into a matrix of stearyl alcohol saturated with the silicone oil and suspended particles [43,44]. Settling of the actives can be reduced by Quaternium-18 Hectorite. Cyclomethicones give the stick a dry, silky feel, and nonvolatile oils like PPG-14 butylether minimize white residues on skin [43]. Low-residue sticks can be obtained by using a combination of high-melting and low-melting waxes and a volatile and nonvolatile silicone-oil combination [45].

Suspension stick	Wt%
Stearyl alcohol	20.0
Cyclomethicone	54.0
PPG-14 butylether	2.0
Hydrog. castor oil	1.0
Talc	2.0
Antiperspirant	20.0
Fragrance	1.0

Gel Sticks

This classes can be subdevided into the groups white anhydrous gel sticks, clear anhydrous gel sticks, clear water-based soapgel sticks. The last mentioned is discussed in the deodorant chapter.

White Anhydrous Gel Sticks.

Shear solids or ultra-clear solids are synonyms for sticks with improved wash-out performance compared with the classic suspension sticks. They contain N-acyl aminoacid amides (N-lauroyl-L-glutamic acid dibutylamide) and 12-hydroxyacid as gelling agents for an oil-phase mixture (e.g., silicone oil/mineral oil). The wash-out agent is an ethoxylated solubilizer like Ceteareth-20. These white sticks turn clear after application to the skin (no-residue stick) [46].

Clear Anhydrous Gel Sticks.

They are quite popular in the United States because clarity is associated by the consumer with a lack of white residue on skin, no dangerous ingredients, and high efficacy. A typical gelling agent is dibenzylidene sorbitol (dibenzyaldehyd monosorbitol acetal, DBMSA). This acetale is not stable in an acidic aqueous environment [47]. The sticks usually contain a high level of alcohol and/or polyols. At high polyol concentration the active is regarded to be solubilized instead of suspended in the gel matrix [48]. An alternative gelling agent is a polyamide [49].

White anhydrous gel sticks	Wt%	Clear anhydrous gel sticks	Wt%
N-Lauroyl-glutamic acid dibutyl amide	5.0	Dibenzylidene sorbitol	2.0
12-Hydroxystearic acid	5.0	Dimethicone copolyol	2.0
Cyclomethicone	40.0	Diisopropyl sebacate	2.0
Hydrog. polyisobutene	15.0	Glycine	1.0
Diisopropyl myristate	15.0	Dipropyleneglycol	10.0
Antiperspirant powder	20.0	Propyleneglycol	33.0
		Antiperspirant powder	50.0

Source: Ref. 58.

Emulsion Sticks:

They can be grouped into clear o/w emulsions, white w/o emulsions, and clear w/s: emulsion gels. The last mentioned is will be discussed shortly.

Clear O/W Emulsions.

They contain a high surfactant combination with the active solubilized in the external water phase. The high concentration of surfactants is a disadvantage; no products based on this technology are known to the author [47].

W/O-Emulsion Sticks.

The water phase containing the active is solubilized by a surfactant like Polyglycerol-4 Isostearate. A typical example for an oil/wax-phase combination is a mixture of silicone oil/stearylalkohol [50].

W/O Emulsion Stick	Wt%
Stearyl alcohol	19.0
Volatile silicone	26.0
Mineral oil	1.0
2-Methyl-2,4 pentandiol	2.0
Polyglyceryl-4 isost.	2.0
ACH solution (50%)	50.0

Source: Ref. 50.

Soft Sticks (Soft Solids, Smooth-Ons)

These sticks can be differentiated into two subgroups: white, anhydrous creams (suspensions) and clear water-in-silicone emulsion gels. Both delivery systems are packed in a container that gives the impression of a stick. The suspension or gel is extruded onto the skin from holes in the top of the stick container to a wide smooth area around the holes.

White, Anhydrous Creams. These creams contain an antiperspirant active, a volatile and nonvolatile silicone oil and a thickener (N-acyl glutamic acid amide).

Clear Water-in-Silicone Emulsion Gels. These formulations can be achieved by adjusting the refractive index of the water and silicone-oil phase. Silicone formulation aids (Dow Corning 3225 C) are mixtures of cyclomethicone and dimethicone copolyol helping to solubilize the active [7,46,48,51]. Low surface tension of cyclomethicones facilitates good spreading of a product on the skin and reduces the tackiness of antiperspirant actives.

Antiperspirant Roll-Ons

Roll-on products can be differentiated into several categories (see Fig. 2). O/W emulsion–based delivery systems are quite popular in Europe, whereas anhydrous suspension roll-ons or transparent water-in-silicone emulsions are preferred in the United States. A new trend concerning the size of the roll-on applicator has been identified. Consumers prefer the big-ball format (3.0–3.5 cm) because of the ease of applying the product to the underarm pit [52]. The popularity of roll-ons in general is due to the nongreasy and nonoily feel in the axilla and the good spreadability of the content on the underarm skin.

Clear Hydroalcoholic Roll-On

This delivery system contains a water/alcohol solution of the antiperspirant active thickened with a water-soluble polymer like hydroxyethylcellulose. The alcohol in the formula gives, compared with the clear aqueous solution–based roll-ons, a fresh sensation in the

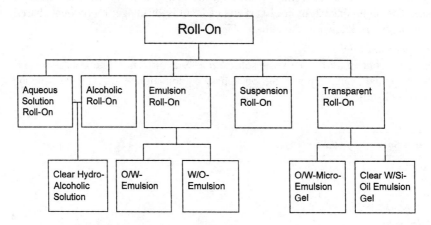

FIGURE 2 Overview of cosmetic Deo/AP-roll-on types.

axilla and faciliates drying of the product. Excellent antiperspirant efficacy is another benefit of hydroalcoholic roll-ons.

O/W Emulsion Roll-On

This delivery system uses ethoxylated surfactants like PEG-40 stearate to solubilize an oil phase like mineral oil. The active is dissolved in the outer phase, allowing the formulation of a highly effective product. In alcohol-free formulated systems microbiological stability has to be checked.

O/W emulsion roll-on	Wt%	Hydroalcoholic roll-on	Wt%
PEG-40 stearate	5.0	Antiperspirant active	20.0
Cetyl alcohol	3.0	PPG-5 ceteth 20	2.0
Mineral oil	2.0	Water	35.4
Polysorbate-80	1.0	Ethanol	42.1
Glycerin	1.5	Hydroxyethylcellulose	.5
Mg-aluminum silicate	.8		
Antiperspirant active	20.0		
Water	66.7		

W/O Emulsion Roll-On

They are weaker in efficacy because the actives are encapsulated and the external oil phase often gives a sticky feeling.

W/Si Emulsion Roll-On

Silicone oils allow to formulate products based on a ''W/O-technology'' because the skin feeling is not comparable to traditional oily components like ester oils or triglycerides. The concentration of the thickener is reduced compared with sticks based on this type. The technology is discussed under soft sticks (see p. 696).

O/W Microemulsion Gel

An alternative approach to transparent products uses the PIT technology. A suitable mixture of surfactants, oils, and water is heated to 60 to 90°C to give a w/o emulsion above the phase inversion temperature (PIT). During cooling the mixture shows phase inversion to give white or transparent o/w emulsions. o/w Microemulsion gels are obtained in the presence of hydrophobically modified water-soluble polymers [53]. The technology is explained in more detail in the deodorant chapter.

Suspension Roll-On

The antiperspirant active in powder form is suspended in cylomethicone. The roll-on can be formulated with or without ethanol. Quaternium-18 Hectorite is used as a thickener to prevent settling of the active. Consumers in the United States prefer this delivery system since it does not give a wet feeling after application and because of the easy drying [39]. Actives like ZAG-complexes give high efficacy underarm products.

Suspension roll-on	Wt%
Volatile silicone	65.0
Quaternium-18 hectorite	13.5
Silica	.5
Antiperspirant powder	20.0
Fragrance	1.0

Antiperspirant Aerosols

Aerosols in Europe and Asia are popular delivery systems for consumers who prefer a hygienic and easy-to-use application form. Typical ingredients for aerosols include isopropylmyristate, isopropylpalmitate, volatile silicone, dimethicone, silica, clays, propylene carbonate, and ethanol. Propellants include propane, butane, and isobutane.

Antiperspirant aerosol	Wt%
Volatile silicone	13.4
Quaternium-18 hectorite	.8
Ethanol	.8
Antiperspirant powder	10.0
Propellant (butane/propane)	75.0

Because acidic aqueous ACH solutions lead to corrosion of the aerosol can, current aerosol antiperspirant products are formulated as water-free suspensions. The active is suspended as a powder in an oil phase like cyclomethicone or in a mixture of ester oils/cyclomethicone. Agglomeration of solid particles and settling of actives can be minimized by usage of suspending agents like fumed silica (amorphous silicon dioxide) or clays (bentonite, hectorite). The clays form a weak gel in the presence of an oil phase that can be destroyed by shaking the aerosol can before usage. The gel structure is reformed on standing, thereby holding the active in suspension. Because the organoclays are agglomerated, shear is needed to deagglomerate the platelets, and a polar activator like propylene carbonate or ethanol is used to disperse them and induce the gelation of the oil phase.

The steps involved to prepare an aerosol product can be summarized in the following sequence [7]:

1. Preparing a bentonite or hectorite clay with the emollient in the presence of the polar activator and shearing the mixture
2. Adding the antiperspirant active until a uniform agglomeration-free suspension is obtained
3. Filling the concentrate into the aerosol can and adding the propellant (pressure filling)

Efficacy studies of aerosols including comparison with other drug delivery systems have been reported in the literature [30]. ZAG-complexes (see discussion p. 691) are not allowed to be used in aerosols.

Environmental Issues

Aerosols contain volatile organic compounds (VOCs) usually in a weight ratio propellant/concentrate of 75/25 [54]. The environmental impact of VOC like the reaction with NO_x in the presence of sunlight causes formation of unwanted ozone in the lower atmosphere. U.S. antiperspirant companies especially were forced to reduce VOC emissions by reformulating and/or exchanging of hydrocarbon propellants to the fluorohydrocarbons 1,1 difluorethane (Propellant 152 a) or 1,1,2,2 tetrafluorethane (Propellant 134 a). The water-soluble dimethoxyethane (DME) is another propellant that is thought to have no impact on the damage of the ozone layer [55].

The current trends in the aerosol market can be summarized as follows:

- Higher ratio of concentrate/hydrocarbon propellant
- Higher amount of silicone oils
- Usage of 1,1 difluorethane (Propellant 152 a)
- Formulations with lower vapor pressure
- Usage of smaller aerosol cans

Aerosols containing 20 to 50% propellants with a concentrate/propellant ratio from 1.0 to 1.0 to 2.3 to 1.0 have been patented [56].

FUTURE TRENDS

Some new trends in the antiperspirant field concerning new actives and delivery systems have been described in this chapter. Improvements of current formulations and innovative concepts will need the ongoing investigation and better understanding of the interaction active/vehicle and vehicle/skin. Improving efficacy and skin compatibility is another major trend in the antiperspirant field. New packaging concepts like the extrudable gels, the big ball applicator for roll-ons, and reduced size aerosol cans with ozone-friendly propellants are probably in a few years state of the art. The influence of perfume components to the skin, the increasing rate of contact allergies attributable to fragrance ingredients have to be closely monitored [57].

REFERENCES

1. Bielfeldt S, Frase T, Gassmüller J. New sensitive method for assessment of antiperspirants with intraindividual comparison of eight formulations. SÖFW 1997; 1237:639–642.
2. Gebhardt W. Do cutaneous coryneform bacteria produce short-chain fatty acids in vitro? Dermatologica 1989; 178:121–122.
3. Sato K, Kang WH, Saga K, Sato KT. Biology of sweat glands and their disorders. I. Normal sweat gland function. J Am Acad Dermatol 1989; 20:537–563.
4. Anonymous. Deodorants and antitranspirants. In: Harry RG, ed. Harry's Cosmeticology. Aylesbury, England: Leonhard Hill Books, 1973:251–275.
5. Barth JH, Kealey T. Androgen metabolism by isolated human axillary apocrine glands in hidradenitis suppurativa. J Dermatol 1991; 125:304–308.
6. Klein RW. pH and perspiration. Cosmet Toilet 1980; 95:19–24.
7. Giovanniello R. Antiperspirants and deodorants. In: Williams DF, Schmitt WH, eds. Chemistry and Technology of the Cosmetics and Toiletries Industry, 2nd edition. London: Blackie Academic Professional, 1996:310–343.

8. Wooding WM, Finkelstein P. A critical comparison of two procedures for antiperspirant evaluation. J Soc Cosmet Chem 1975; 26:255–275.
9. Wooding WM, Finkelstein P. Procedures for evaluation of antiperspirant efficacy. Cosmet Toilet 1976; 91:28–32.
10. Majors PA, Wild JE. The evaluation of antiperspirant efficacy: influence of certain variables. J Soc Cosmet Chem 1974; 25:139–152.
11. Bakiewicz TA. A critical evaluation of the methods available for measurements of antiperspirants. J Soc Cosmet Chem 1973; 24:245–258.
12. Palanker AL. Substantiating the safety of antiperspirants. Cosmet Toilet 1985; 100:43–45.
13. Murphy TD, Levine MJ. Analysis of antiperspirant efficacy test results. J Soc Cosmet Chem 1991; 42:167–197.
14. Wild JE, Bowman JP, Oddo LP, Aust LB. Methods for claim substantiation of antiperspirants and deodorants. Cosmet Sci Technol Ser 1998; 18:131–151.
15. Sauermann G, Hoppe U, Kligman M. The determination of the antiperspirant activity of aluminum chlorohydrate by digital image analysis. Int J Cosmet Sci 1992; 14:32–38.
16. Beck JS, Coulson HF, Hough GL, Mahers EG. Novel technique to investigate individual eccrine sweat gland function in vivo. 19th IFSCC Congress, Sydney, Australia, 1996; 3:95–98.
17. Quatrale RP. The mechanism of antiperspirant action. Cosmet Toilet 1985; 100:23–26.
18. Quatrale RP, Coble DW, Stoner KL, Felger CB. The mechanism of antiperspirant action on aluminum salts II. Historical observations of human eccrine sweat glands inhibited by aluminum chlorohydrate. J Soc Cosmet Chem 1981; 32:107–136.
19. Quatrale RP, Coble DW, Stoner KL, Felger CB. Mechanism of antiperspirant action on aluminum salts III. Historical observations of human sweat glands inhibited by aluminum zirconium chlorohydrate glycine complex. J Soc Cosmet Chem 1981; 32:195–221.
20. Laden K, Felger CB. Antiperspirants and Deodorants. New York: Marcel Dekker, 1988.
21. IFSCC Monograph No 6. Antiperspirants and Deodorants, Principles of Underarm Technology. Weymouth, MA: Micelle Press, 1998.
22. Cuzner B, Klepak P. Antiperspirants and deodorants. In: Butler H. Poucher's Perfumes, Cosmetics and Soaps. Vol. 3, 9th ed. London: Chapman & Hall, 1993:3–26.
23. Teagarden DL, Kozlowski JF, White JL, Hem SL. Aluminum chlorohydrate I: structure studies. J Pharm Sci 1981; 70:758–761.
24. Teagarden DL, Radavich JF, Hem SL. Aluminum chlorohydrate II: physicochemical properties. J Pharm Sci 1981; 70:762–764.
25. Teagarden DL, White JL, Hem SL. Aluminum chlorohydrate III: conversion to aluminum hydroxide. J Pharm Sci 1981; 70:808–810.
26. Woodruff J. On the scent of deodorant trends. Manufacturing Chemists 1994; 65:34–38.
27. Alexander P. Monograph antiperspirants and deodorants. SÖFW 1994; 120:117–121.
28. Klepak P. In vitro killing time studies of antiperspirant salts. SÖFW 1990; 116:478–481.
29. Rosenberg A. Enhanced efficacy antiperspirant actives. Soap Perfume Cosmet 1997; 7:27–30.
30. Fondots DC. Antiperspirants, a look across the Atlantic. Cosmetic Toilet Manuf Worldwide 1993; 108:181–185.
31. Hagan DB, Leng FJ, Smith PM, Snow M, Watson A. Antiperspirant compositions based on titanium salts. Int J Cosmet Sci 1997; 19:271–280.
32. Tranner F. Polybarrier: the future of antiperspirant technology? Soap, Cosmetics, Chemical Specialities. October 1998; 74:56–58.
33. Tranner F. Mineral salt-free topical antiperspirant compositions—comprises water insoluble, occlusive, film-forming polymers. US Patent No. 5508024.
34. Fontell K. Cubic phases in surfactant and surfactant-like lipid systems. Colloid Polym Sci 1990; 268:264–285.
35. Leng FJ, Parrot DT. Antiperspirant materials and compositions. US Patent No. 5593663.

36. Abrutyn ES, Bahr BC. Formulation enhancements for underarm applications. Cosmet Toilet 1993; 108:51–54.
37. ICI Speciality Chemicals. A new emollient for antiperspirant sticks. HAPPI October 1989; 50–51.
38. Osborne GE, Lausier JM, Lawing WD, Smith M. Statistical evaluation of vehicle effect on antiperspirant activity with a limited number of subjects. J Soc Cosmet Chem 1982; 33:179–191.
39. Klepak P. Formulierungsbeispiele bei wasserhaltigen Antitranspirant Kompositionen. SÖFW 1989; 115:415–418.
40. Abrutyn ES, Bahr BC, Fuson SM. Overview of the antiperspirant market. Technology and trends. DCI 1992; 151:40–47.
41. Stephens TJ, Oresago C. Ethnic sensitive skin. Cosmet Toilet 1994; 109:75–80.
42. IFSCC Monograph No 3. An Introduction to Rheology. Weymouth, MA: Micelle Press, 1997.
43. Geria N. Formulation of stick antiperspirants and deodorants. Cosmet Toilet 1984; 99:55–66.
44. Geria N. Antiperspirant sticks. Cosmet Toilet 1996; 111:53–69.
45. Shevade M, Bianchini R, Lee R. Low residue antiperspirant solid stick composition. US Patent No. 5531986.
46. Fox C. OTC products. Cosmet Toilet 1996; 111:53–69.
47. Jungerman E. Clear antiperspirant stick technology. A review. Cosmet Toilet 1995; 110:49–56.
48. Smith J, Madore L, Fuson S. Attacking residue in antiperspirants. DCI 1995; 12:46–51.
49. Fox C. Technically speaking. Cosmet Toilet 1996; 111:23–26.
50. Hourihan JC, Krevald H. Water-in-oil emulsion antiperspirant sticks. US Patent No. 4704271.
51. Fox C. Cosmetic and pharmaceutical vehicles. Cosmet Toilet 1997; 112:31–48.
52. Anonymous. Does size matter? Soap Parf Cosmet 1998; 7:46–51.
53. Schreiber J, Klier M, Wolf F, Diec KH, Gers-Barlag H. Kosmetische oder dermatologische Gele auf der Basis von Mikroemulsionen. DE Patent No. 19509079.
54. Calagero AV. Antiperspirant and deodorant formulation. Cosmet Toilet 1992; 107:63–69.
55. Romanowski R, Schueller R. Aerosols for apprentices. Cosmet Toilet 1996; 111:35–40.
56. Fox C. Technically speaking. Cosmet Toilet 1997; 112:21–25.
57. Johansen JD, Anderson TF, Kjoller M, Veien N, Avnstorp C, Andersen KE, Menne T. Identification of risk products for fragrance contact allergy: a case-referent study based on patient's histories. Am J Contact Derm 1998; 9:80–87.
58. Motley CB. Gel stick compositions comprising optically enriched gellants. US5552136.

57

Deodorants

Jörg Schreiber
Beiersdorf AG, Hamburg, Germany

INTRODUCTION

It is the intention of this chapter to give an overview on the current knowledge about the origin of underarm odor, the biology of the underarm microflora and its interaction with deodorizing agents. The contents of this chapter have been arranged in particular sequence to facilitate the understanding of rational deodorant product development.

BIOLOGY OF THE UNDERARM MICROFLORA

The resident microflora of the human underarm skin consists of up to $10^6/cm^2$ organisms, eg. aerobic cocci, lipophilic diphteroids and varying species of gram-negative bacteria [1]. In the axillae two types of bacterial flora exists—coryneform bacteria and micrococcaceae like *Staphylococus epidermidis*. Coryneform- or *St. epidermidis*-dominated populations are characteristic for human beings. The resident microflora is a quite stable population not varying a lot between both axillaes [2]. The organisms are perfectly adapted to their ecological niche with its higher pH value and higher moisture content compared to other skin areas [3]. Hair in the axilla is according to the literature not a good substrate for bacterial growth, the bacteria prefer to reside on the underarm skin [2]. Moisture is required for bacterial proliferation and is secreted especially from the eccrine sweat glands [4]. The origin of strong compared to low underarm odor is associated with a numerical dominance of Coryneform bacteria [5]. Components of apocrine secretion like e.g. isovaleric acid and androstenone, were proposed to contribute to axillary odor. Hydrolytic exoenzymes of skin bacteria cleave the ester bonds of odorless water soluble precursors of androstenol to the corresponding volatile steroid [6]. Other studies proposed that the key odorants are branched, straight-chain and unsaturated C_6-C_{11} fatty acids [7]. (E)-3-methyl-2-hexenoic acid (E-3M2H) is the most abundant fatty acid compared to the rest of C_6-C_{11} fatty acids that contribute to the axillary odor bouquet. Apocrine sweat extracts have been analyzed and concentrations of 0.5 ng/μl for androstenone and 357 ng/μL for E-3M2H were detected [8]. Volatile odor molecules of E-3M2H found in sweat secretions are transported according to the authors in a nonvolatile fashion to the skin surface. Two apocrine secretion odor binding proteins ($ASOB_1$ and $ASOB_2$) were identified, carrying

3M2H-molecules to the skin surface. Coryneform bacteria liberate the odor molecules from the protein precursor/odorant-complex [8].

The reader should be aware that occurrence of these chemical compounds does not mean that all of us can smell them. Individual differences in odor perception for both isomers of 3M2H [9] and for the steroid androstenone are well known [8]. Approximately 50% of the adult population are not able to smell androstenones, this anosmia to androstenone—or to 3-methyl-2-hexenoic acid—is genetically determined.

DEODORANTS

Deodorants are topically applied products designed to reduce underarm odor. They are considered in the United States as being cosmetics while antiperspirants are treated by the FDA as drugs. Deodorants tend to be less irritating than antiperspirants. In continental Europe the consumer today prefer deodorants compared to antiperspirants. In the United States the trend is approximately reversed.

Concepts for Controlling Underarm Odor: State of the Art

The current knowledge of the biology of the underarm microflora and the origin of underarm odor is the basis for developing strategies against odor formation. Numerous patents and literature articles disclose the incorporation of chemical compounds for their deodorizing properties. It is the intention here to describe and exemplify major strategies, but not all deodorant actives that were developed in the past.

Strategies to reduce underarm odor include the following:

- Antiperspirant active–containing deodorants
- Odor-masking deodorants
- Odor-neutralizing deodorants
- Odor-quenching deodorants
- Esterase inhibitors
- Antimicrobial active-containing deodorants

Antiperspirant Active–Containing Deodorants

Antiperspirant actives like aluminum chlorohydrate or the Al-Zr complexes (see Chapter 56) reduce the secretion of eccrine sweat. Their excellent antimicrobial properties against *St. epidermidis* and coryneform bacteria have been published [10]. The acidity of the aluminum salts may be a major factor in bacterial growth inhibition.

Odor-Masking Deodorants

Fragrance compositions (such as perfumes) have been used to mask odors since ancient times. It is conventional to incooperate 0.2–1.5% of a perfume in body deodorants [11]. They are designed to blend with the underarm odor and thus act as a masking agent. The perception of a perfume may differ significantly between individuals because of different interactions with the skin, washing habits and specific underarm odor. The fragrance materials are blended in order to achieve what is known as "top note," "middle note," and "bottom note" components. The first is the refreshing note upon application while the last are the olfactoric components which stay on after application to the underarm skin.

Perfumes with antimicrobial properties have been described in patents and in the literature [12–14]. An additional benefit, especially for emulsion-based products, is that they might also act as a preservative. The increasing rate of contact allergies against fragrance ingredients should be taken into account using this approach to combat underarm odor [15].

Odor-Neutralizing Deodorants

In Chapter 56 it was mentioned that odorous C_6-C_{11} fatty acids contribute to underarm odor. Chemical neutralization with sodium bicarbonate ($NaHCO_3$) yields the corresponding odorless soaps [16]. This active however is not stable for a long time in aqueous compositions. Patents for deodorant applications and usage of sodium bicarbonate in the presence of antiperspirant actives have been filed [17,18]. Zinc carbonate containing deodorants are also content of a patent [19].

Odor-Quenching Deodorants

Zinc Ricinoleate

Zinc salts of ricinoleic acid have no bacteriostatic or antiperspirant effect [20]. They strongly bind odorous fatty acids, amines and mercaptanes. Ligand-exchange reactions of ricinoleic acid for odor molecules are probably the reason for the quenching properties of zinc ricinoleate [21]. Interactions with perfume components in a deodorant formulation may weaken the desired quenching effect of the odor molecules after topical application to the underarm.

Metal Oxides

The oxides of calcium, magnesium, and zinc form in the presence of fatty acids the corresponding metal soaps [22]. Zinc oxide particles aggregate to form a massive lump. This leads to clogging of aerosol products [23]. Hybrid powders were developed in which the metal oxide covers the surface of a spherical nylon powder [23]. The advantage of this technology is the increased surface area of zinc oxide and thus enhanced odor quenching efficacy and the reduced particle aggregation in aerosols.

Esterase Inhibitors

Zinc Glycinate

The inhibition of exoenzymes from the underarm bacteria (see discussion p. 703) should also result in odor reduction. Zinc glycinate has been described as a suitable active [24]. Antimicrobial tests showed no inhibitory effect against *St. epidermidis* or against the lipophilic diphtheroid bacteria supporting the suggested mechanism against microbial exoenzymes.

Triethylcitrate

The optimal pH value for development of underarm odor caused by coryneform bacteria is approximately about pH 6 in axillary extracts [25]. Shifting the skin surface pH to the acidic side should decrease the activity of skin esterases, proposed to be responsible for degradation of underarm secretions. Triethylcitrate was proposed to form citric acid by an enzymatic process on the underarm skin. In 1991 it was shown that this active has no pH-reducing effect after application to the underarm skin [26]. Nevertheless deodorants containing this active are still in the market.

Antimicrobial Active–Containing Deodorants

This approach is currently the most commonly used strategy to prevent underarm odor. Ethanol is probably one of the best known actives for deodorization [27]. Additional efficacy is normally required for a long term deodorization and this can be achieved by the additional usage of fragrance, an antiperspirant active or other antimicrobial actives (farnesol, phenoxyethanol, etc.).

Triclosan (2,4,4'-Trichloro-2'-Hydroxydiphenylether)

This active has a broad-spectrum antimicrobial activity against most gram-positive and gram-negative bacteria, molds and yeasts. The presence of triclosan in antiperspirant sticks and roll-ons leads to a higher reduction of the bacterial microflora versus the triclosan free antiperspirant composition [28]. Triclosan is also used in skincare products, hand disinfectants and household products [29].

Glyceryl Fatty Acid Ester

Mono- and oligoglyceryl fatty acid ester like glyceryl monocaprylate, -moncaprinate, -monolaurate and diglyceryl monocaprinate are effective deodorizers [30]. Combinations of glyceryl monolaurate with farnesol and phenoxyethanol showed synergistic efficacy effects against coryneform bacteria [31]. The advantage of this ingredient combination over the first generation deodorant actives like triclosan is attributed to their higher biodegradability and their selective bacterial action. These actives are all natural occurring in plants and animal species. In addition, it could be demonstrated that combinations of mono- and oligoglyceryl fatty acid esters with a variety of natural antimicrobials (e.g., wool wax acids) displayed a synergistic antimicrobial efficacy against underarm bacteria and serve as highly effective deodorant actives [32–35]. Products containing such actives have been successfully marketed for a number of years.

Sucrose Fatty Acid Ester

The fatty acid ester of sucrose are well known as emulsifiers in food products [36]. Sucrose can be substituted on eight hydroxyl groups with fatty acids. The antimicrobial potential depends strongly on the substitution degree of the sucrose. Sucrose monostearate and sucrose monolaurate have been described as deodorizers in the literature and in patents [37–39].

Glycerolether

2-Ethylhexyl glycerolether (octoxyglycerol) is a clear liquid with good solubility in cosmetic oils, polyols and alcohol but only moderate solubility in water (0.2%). Synergistic antimicrobial activity with other ingredients has been described [40]. This active has become popular recently in European deodorant formulations.

New Concepts for Controlling Underarm Odor

Ongoing research activities focussing on a better understanding of the interaction between underarm skin/skin microflora and skin microflora/odor formation, in combination with the discovery of highly selective actives allows today more specific designs for deodorant products. In the next sections some of the new trends are discussed in detail.

New concepts for controlling underarm odor include the following:

- Chitosan
- Bacterial enzyme inhibitors
- Odor-inhibiting precursor mimics
- Product- and skin-mediated perfume transformations
- Antiadhesives

Chitosan

Chitin is a natural occurring polysaccharide (e.g., in insects, lobster, crabs, or fungi) containing N-acetylated D-glucosamin units. Deacetylation of the amino group leads to the slightly water soluble chitosan. The deodorizing properties of chitosan and the combination of this active with aluminum salts have been the subject of a patent [41].

Bacterial Enzyme Inhibitors

The enzyme amino acid β-lyase is, according to a patent filed in 1990, a catalyst for the formation of underarm odor [42]. This enzyme is located in odor-releasing bacterial cells and cleaves the apocrine precursors of sweat components, like amino acids with the structure unit $COOH-CH-(NH_2)-CH_2-S-R$, to the corresponding odorous sulfur products. Several classes of enzyme inhibitors like derivatives of hydroxylamines, β-substituted aminoacids, cycloserine and pyridoxal were identified.

Odor-Inhibiting Precursor Mimics

Another approach to the inhibition of the above-mentioned enzyme β-lyase is to provide an alternative substrate for the bacteria that cleave the structure unit $CH(NH_2)CH_2-O-C(O)-R$ instead of the sulfur-containing amino acid sequence [43]. This approach leads to the corresponding non-odorous ingredients, like benzoic acid, or to pleasant odor generating substances, like phenylacetic acid.

Product- and Skin-Mediated Perfume Transformations

The physical and chemical interaction of a perfume with the underarm skin is a very complicated matter. Research activities in this area focused on the question which components of a perfume stay on and above the skin after topical application [44]. Headspace analysis is one of the techniques to gain more informations concerning skin/perfume interactions. It could be demonstrated that the long lastingness of a fragrance can be achieved by using a prodrug (ester, acetale) of a perfume ingredient [45]. The esters or acetales of a fragrance composition hydrolyze on human skin due to the slightly acid pH value. The hydrolysis products (acids, alcohols, aldehydes) impart a pleasant smell to the underarm skin. These product and skin-mediated perfume transformations are especially suitable for alkaline formulations like soap-based deodorant sticks. The advantage of the perfume precursor approach is attributed to a prolonged fragrance impression of a deodorant after topical application to the underarm skin.

Antiadhesives

An alternative concept to reduce the amount of skin bacteria in the underarm skin is the anti-adhesion approach. The understanding of the adhesion mechanisms of the resident underarm microflora to the skin surface is the basis for developing strategies against bacterial adhesion. Numerous skin microorganism adhere preferentially to specific sites on various body surfaces. For example, *S. aureus* and *P. aeruginosa* adhere to collected nasal epithelial cells [46]. *C. xerosis* binds to epidermal cells whereas yeasts species like *Candida albicans* bind to corneocytes. Structures of the skin specifically involved in adherence to the underarm bacteria are thought to be proteins, oligosasccharide structures, lipids and hydrophobic surfaces. Imitation of these adhesion motifs by saccharides, oligosaccharides, polysaccharides and glycoproteins allows to inhibit the bacterial adherence to the skin. Additionally it was discovered recently that among others sucrose ester like sucrose myristate and sucrose laurate have anti-adhesive properties to various microorganism including the typical microflora of the underarm skin [47].

DRUG-DELIVERY SYSTEMS AND APPLICATION FORMS FOR DEODORANT ACTIVES

Products designed to reduce underarm odor can be formulated in a variety of delivery systems such as suspensions, water or hydroalcoholic solutions, and emulsions. Typical application forms are sticks, roll-ons, creams, pump sprays, aerosols, and gels. Sticks, roll-ons, and aerosols are discussed in detail in the antiperspirant chapter. Lowering the amount of an antiperspirant active, like aluminum chlorohydrate, in an antiperspirant is one option to formulate a deodorant. In this case the antiperspirant active has only deodorizing properties and nearly no impact on the eccrine sweat glands. Deodorants can be formulated in acidic, neutral or alcaline environment. Designing a deodorant the formulator should have in mind the following points:

- Long-term deodorization
- No irritation potential
- Good solubility of the active in the delivery system
- Selection of a stable fragrance
- Viscosity control of the product
- Good skin feeling of the product

Protocols for the in vitro and in vivo evaluation of deodorants have been designed. The reader is referred to the literature [48]. A new method for in vivo evaluation of antimicrobial agents was recently developed where the underarm bacteria were translocated to the forearm allowing the simultaneous evaluation of multiple deodorizers in a single individuum [49].

Deodorant Sticks

Deodorant sticks are solidified by 6 to 8% of sodium stearate. The deodorizing agent and a fragrance are dissolved in a hydrophilic carrier. Two stick categories can be differentiated, the ethanol based and the propylene glycol based sticks [50].

Transparency is usually achieved by usage of a high polyol content. Clarifying agents for sticks like PPG-14 butylether, Cocamide DEA, Lauramide DEA, Steareth-100 have been patented [51,52]. Ethanol based sticks are preferred if it is the intent of the formulator to create a cooling sensation for the consumer. Shrinkage of the stick has to be taken into account because of evaporation of the alcohol. Propylene glycol based sticks tend to be more resistant to shrinkage, and solubilization of a fragrance is easier in some instances [53].

Deodorant stick	Wt%	Deodorant stick	Wt%
Water	16.0	Water	3.0
Ethanol	75.5	Propylene glycol	10.0
Deodorizer	1.0	Deodorizer	1.0
Sodium stearate	6.5	Sodium stearate	8.0
Fragrance	1.0	PPG-3 myristyl ether	77.0
		Fragrance	1.0

Deodorant Aerosols

Spray products containing a solution of an antimicrobial active in an ethanol and/or propylene glycol carrier blended with a liquidified propellant are typical for deodorant aerosols. The difference from an antiperspirant active containing aerosol is that the deodorizer is solubilized in an alcohol- or polyol-based formulation and not suspended. Deodorant sprays provide a dry skin feeling to the underarm skin since they are anhydrously formulated.

Typically, 20 to 60% of the sprayable contents of an aerosol reach the skin, since the liquidified hydrocarbon propellant vaporizes as it is sprayed [54]. Propane, butane and isobutane are the most commonly used propellants. They condense to form a clear, colorless and odorless liquid with densities of 0.51 to 0.58 g/mL at 20°C [55]. These propellants are inflammable in the presence of air or oxygen. Labelling of cosmetic aerosols concerning flammability risks of volatile organic compounds (VOCs) and volatile solvent abuse (VSA) is discussed in detail in a recently published review [56]. Aerosol containers can be fabricated from tin-coated steel, tin-free steel (chromium-coated steel) or aluminum. Numerous types of aerosol can corrosion and testing for it was recently discussed in the literature [57]. The environmental issues of aerosols are explained in greater detail in the antiperspirant chapter.

Deodorant aerosol	Wt%
Alcohol	42.0
Laureth-4	0.5
Deodoriser	1.0
Fragrance	0.5
Isobutane	47.6
Propane	8.4

The formulator of an aerosol has to optimize the following parameters to get a dry deodorant product:

- Spray rate
- Spray shape
- Particle size
- Concentrate/propellant ratio
- Fragrance/deodorizer concentration
- Pressure of the aerosol can

Deodorant Pump Sprays

Hydroalcoholic Pump Sprays

An alternative to aerosols are pump sprays. This category is quite popular in Europe whereas it is of lower interest for the consumers in the United States, since they tend to prefer a dry application form, like the anhydrous sticks. Pump sprays allow a good dosage of the formulation to be delivered to the underarm skin in a hygienic way. They consist of low vicosity hydroalcoholic solutions of a deodorizer and a perfume. Usually a solubilizer, like PEG-40 hydrogenated castor oil, is incorporated into the formulation to maintain a clear and homogeneous solution.

Pump spray	Wt%
Water	35.6
Alcohol	60.0
PEG-40 hyd. Castor oil	2.0
Deodorizer	2.0
Fragrance	0.4

PIT-Emulsion Pump Sprays

A disadvantage of hydroalcoholic pump sprays is the alcohol content in the formulation that may contribute to unwanted side reactions especially in the shaved axilla. Beiersdorf AG in Hamburg, Germany introduced into the European market under the brand name "Nivea" a new pump spray based on an emulsion in 1995. The sprayable low viscous deodorant is based on the PIT technology. Suitable mixtures of ethoxylated surfactants, oils and water in the presence of antiperspirant and deodorizing actives are heated to 60–90°C. Cooling the resulting W/O emulsion to room temperature yields via a phase inversion temperature (PIT) process a finely dispersed bluish-white O/W emulsion [58–60]. The droplet size distribution of such PIT emulsions is in the range from 80–250 nm. The above-mentioned pump spray contained a skin-friendly deodorizing combination of glyceryl monocaprinate and wool wax acids (see discussion p. 706) in an alcohol-free delivery system.

PIT-emulsion pump spray	Wt%
Glyceryl stearate, ceteareth-20, ceteareth-10, cetearyl alcohol, cetyl palmitate (Emulgade SE)	4.5
Ceteareth-20	1.0
Dioctyl cyclohexane	5.0
Dicaprylylether	5.0
Deodorizer	2.0
Aluminum chlorohydrate	5.0
Water	77.5

Source: Ref. 60.

Microemulsion Pump Sprays

Hydroalcoholic pump sprays are usually transparent, whereas sprayable PIT-emulsions are white or bluish-white products. Sprayable alcohol-free and additionally transparent pump sprays were recently introduced into the European market (e.g., Basis pH; Beiersdorf AG, Hamburg, Germany). Transparency of an emulsion is achieved when the size of the droplets is below 100 nm. This O/W microemulsion can be obtained with and without the PIT technology but needs careful selection of ingredients and considerable fine-tuning [61]. The main advantage compared to classical microemulsions is the low surfactant concentration (<10%). Furthermore it could be demonstrated that, in the presence of hydrophobically modified water-soluble polymers, the above-mentioned technology allows the formulation of gels, sprayable gels, roll-ons, sticks, and aerosol products [62].

FUTURE TRENDS

The deodorant market has undergone some remarkable changes concerning the principles to reduce underarm odor in the last years. It is expected that the search for effective, skin-friendly actives with a highly selective action against the cutaneous underarm microflora will lead to long-lasting and safe deodorants. Improvements in understanding how microorganism adhere to human skin should facilitate the development of new strategies to reduce underarm odor. Improvements of aerosols with no/low impact to the environment or aerosol alternatives, like sprayable emulsions, are probably in a few years in the portfolio of every deodorant-selling company.

REFERENCES

1. Korting HC, Lukacs A, Braun-Falco O. Mikrobielle Flora und Geruch der gesunden menschlichen Haut. Hautarzt 1988; 39:564–568.
2. Leyden JJ, Mc Ginley KJ, Hölzle E, Labow JN, Kligman AM. The microbiology of human axilla and ist relationship to axillary odor. J Invest Dermatol 1981; 77:413–416.
3. Lukacs A, Korting HC, Lemke O, Ruckdeschel G, Ehret W, Braun-Falco O. The influence of pH value on the growth of *Brevibacterium epidermis* in continous culture. Acta Derm Venerol 1995; 75:280–282.
4. Leyden JJ, Mc Ginley KJ, Nordstrom KM, Webster GF. Skin microflora. J Invest Dermatol 1987; 88:65s–72s.
5. Rennie PJ, Gower DB, Holland KT. In vitro- and in vivo studies of human axillary odor and the cutaneous microflora. Br J Dermatol 1991; 124:596–602.
6. Froebe C, Simone A, Charig A, Eigen E. Axillary malodor production: a new mechanism. J Soc Cosmet Chem 1990; 41:173–185.
7. Zeng XN, Leyden JJ, Lawley HJ, Sawano K, Nohara I, Preti G. Analysis of characteristic odors from human axillae. J Chem Ecology 1991; 17:1469–1491.
8. Spielman AI, Zeng XN, Leyden JJ, Preti G. Proteinaceous precursors of human axillary odor: isolation of two novel odor binding proteins. Experientia 1995; 51:40–47.
9. Wysocki CJ, Zang XN, Preti G. Specifica anosmia and olfactory sensitivity to 3-methyl-2-hexenoic acid: a major component of human axillary odor. Chem Senses 1993; 18:652.
10. Klepak P. In vitro killing time studies of antiperspirant salts. SÖFW 1990; 116:478–481.
11. Geria N. Fragrancing antiperspirants and deodorants. Cosmet Toilet 1990; 105:41–45.
12. Eggensberger H. Duftstoffe und Aromen als multifunktionelle Additive. SÖFW 1996; 122: 789–793.

13. Diehl KH, Oltmanns P, Ramsbotham J. Parfüminhaltsstoffe-eine Alternative für die konservierung von kosmetischen Produkten? SÖFW 1992; 118:546–550.

14. Morris JA, Khettry J, Seitz EW. Antimicrobial activity of aroma chemicals and essential oils. J Am Oil Chem Soc 1979; 96:595–603.

15. Rastogi SC, Johansen JD, Frosch P, Menne T, Bruze M, Lepoitthevin JP, Dreier B, Andersen KE, White IR. Deodorants on the European market: quantitative chemical analysis of 21 fragrances. Contact Dermatol 1998; 38:29–35.

16. Lamp JH. Sodium bicarbonate. An excellent deodorant. J Invest Dermatol 1946; 7:131–133.

17. Berschied JR. Antiperspirant-deodorant cosmetic stick products containing active agent particles in organic matrix, which matched densities for homogeneous products. Patent No. WO 9413256.

18. Winston AE. Microporous alkali metal carbonate powder—comprises particles of average particle size of 0.1–50 microns, surface area of 5–20 sq.m/f, average pore size of 10–500 nm and total pore volume of 0.1–2 cc/g and is useful as lightweight deodorant ingredient. Patent No. WO 9424996.

19. Park AC. Propellant free deodorant composition, for topical application—comprising sparingly water soluble salts or oxide (s) of zinc or magnesium, water absorbing cellulosic polymer and volatile silicone. Patent No. EP 471392 A.

20. Zekorn R. Deowirkstoff auf Basis Zinkricinoleat. Parf Kosmet 1996; 77:682–684.

21. Zekorn R. Zinc ricinoleate. Cosmet Toilet 1997; 112:37–40.

22. Kanda F, Yagi E, Fukuda M, Matsuoka M. Quenching short chain fatty acids responsible for human body odors. Cosmet Toilet 1993; 108:67–72.

23. Kanda F, Nakame T, Matsuoka M, Tomita K. Efficacy of novel hybrid powders to quench body malodors. J Soc Cosmet Chem 1990; 41:197–207.

24. Charig A, Froebe C, Simone A, Eigen E. Inhibitor of odor producing axillary bacterial exoenzymes. J Soc Cosmet Chem 1991; 42:133–145.

25. Rennie PJ, Gower DB, Holland KT, Mallet AI, Watkins WJ. The skin microflora and the formation of human axillary odor. Int J Cosmet Sci 1990; 12:197–207.

26. Lukacs A, Korting HC, Braun-Falco O, Stanzl K. Efficacy of a deodorant and its components. Triethylcitrate and perfume. J Soc Cosmet Chem 1991; 42:159–166.

27. Baxter PM, Reed JV. The evaluation of underarm deodorants. Int J Cosmet Sci 1983; 5:85–95.

28. Cox AR. Efficacy of the antimicrobial agent triclosan in topical deodorant products. J Soc Cosmet Chem 1987; 38:223–231.

29. Nissen HP, Ochs D. Triclosan. Cosmet Toilet 1998; 113:61–64.

30. Dillenburg H, Jakobson G, Klein W, Siemanowski W, Uhlig KH, Wolf F. Cosmetic deodorant preparations containing di- or triglycerin esters. Patent No. EP 666732 A1/B1.

31. Haustein UF, Herrmann J, Hoppe U, Engel W. Growth inhibition of coryneforme bacteria by a mixture of three natural products. Farnesol, glyceryl monolaurate and phenoxyethanol: HGQ. J Soc Cosmet Chem 1993; 44:211–220.

32. Klier M, Schneider G, Traupe B, Voss I, Wolf F. Desodorierende Wirkstoffkombinationen auf der Basis von Wollwachssäuren und Monocarbonsäuren. DE 4305889.2

33. Klier M, Röckl M, Schneider G, Siemanowski W, Traupe B, Uhlig KH, Voss I, Wolf F. Deodorant active substance combinations made from wool grease acids and partial glycerides. EP 689418 A1.

34. Klier M, Röckl M, Traupe B, Wolf W. Deodorizing combinations of agents based on α, ω-alkane dicarboxylic acid and fatty acid partial glycerides. EP 729345 A1.

35. Klier M, Traupe B, Wolf F. Deodorant agent compositions containing α,ω-alcanoic di-acids and mono-carboxylic esters of oligomer glyerols. EP 691125 A1.

36. Friberg SE, Larsson K. Food Emulsions. New York: Marcel Dekker, 1997.

37. Meyer PD, Vianen GM, Baal HCI. Sucrose fatty acid esters in deodorant formulations. Aerosol and Spray Report 1998; 37:18–22.

38. Meyer PD, Vianen GM, Baal HCI. Saccharose-Fettsäureester in deodorants. Parf Kosmet 1997; 78:22–24.
39. Vianen GM, Watraven BW, Meyer PD. Deodorant composition. EP 0750903 A1.
40. Beilfuss W. A multifunctional ingredient for deodorants. SÖFW 1998; 124:360–366.
41. Wachter R, Lehmann R, Panzer C. Desodorierende Zubereitungen. DE 19540296.
42. Lyon S, O'Neal C, van der Lee H, Rogers B. Amino acid β-Lyase enzyme inhibitors as deodorants. WO 9105541.
43. Laney J. O-Acyl Serines as deodorants. WO 9507069.
44. Behan JM, Macmaster AP, Perring KD, Tuck KM. Insight how skin changes perfume. Int J Cosmet Sci 1996; 18:237–246.
45. Suffis R, Barr ML, Ishida K, Sawano K, van Loveren AG, Nakatsu T, Green CB, Reitz GA, Kang RKL, Sato T. Composition containing body activated fragrance for contacting the skin and method of use. US 5626852.
46. Carson RG, Schilling KM, Harichian B, Au V. Biospecific emulsions. US 5416075.
47. Bünger J, Schreiber J, Wolf F. Anti-adhesive active principles. EP 806935 A2.
48. IFSCC Monograph No 6. Antiperspirants and Deodorants. Weymouth, MA: Micelle Press, 1998.
49. Leyden JJ, McGinley K, Foglia AN, Wahrmann JE, Gropper CN, Vowels BR. A new method for in vivo evaluation of antimicrobial agents by translocation of complex dense populations of cutaneous bacteria. Skin Pharmacol 1996; 9:60–68.
50. Calogero AV. Antiperspirant and deodorant formulation. Cosmet Toil 1992; 107:63–69.
51. Dawn R, Morton B. Clear cosmetic stick composition. WO 9427567.
52. Kellner DM. Clear, stable deodorant compositions—containing soap, antimicrobial agent, water, polyhydric alcohol, pentadoxynol 200 and alcanolamide-alkoxylated alcohol mixture. US 5407668.
53. Geria N. Formulation of stick antiperspirants and deodorants. Cosmet Toilet 1984; 99:55–66.
54. Meyer G, Listro JA. Liquid deodorant compositions. WO 9301793.
55. Johnsen MA. The safety assessment of hydrocarbon aerosol propellants. Spray Technology & Marketing. March 1996; pp. 18–24.
56. Redbourn D. Cosmetic aerosol regulations. Living with labelling. Soap Perf Cosmet Sept. 1998; pp. 45–48.
57. Tait WS. Aerosol container corrosion and corrosion testing: what is state of the art? Spray Technology & Marketing Sept. 1997; pp. 47–56.
58. Wadle A, Förster T, von Rybinski W. Influence of the microemulsion phase structure on the phase inversion temperature emulsification of polar oils. Colloids Surf A 1993; 76:51–57.
59. Förster T, von Rybinski W, Tesman H, Wadle A. Calculation of optimum emulsifier mixtures for phase inversion emulsification. Int J Cosmet Sci 1994; 16:84–92.
60. Wadle A, Ansmann A, Jackwerth B, Tesmann H. PIT-Emulgiertechnologie in der Kosmetik Parf Kosmet 1996; 77:250–254.
61. Schreiber J, Eitrich A, Gohla S, Klier M, Wolf F. Cosmetic or pharmaceutical microemulsions. WO 9628131 A2/A3.
62. Schreiber J, Diec KH, Gers-Barlag H, Klier M, Wolf F. Cosmetic and pharmaceutical gels based on microemulsions. WO 9628132 A2/A3.

58

Baby Care

Uwe Schönrock
Beiersdorf AG, Hamburg, Germany

INTRODUCTION

Skin undergoes an extraordinary development. It must grow rapidly and expand dramatically in size to cover the entire developing body. It is exposed to both internal and external environmental influences throughout the entire phase of its existence. However, despite the multitude of regionally specific influences that play a role in the development of skin, there is a remarkable similarity in its developmental pattern and in the ultimate end product of differentiation in every part of the body. The purpose of this chapter is to outline what is known about the development and physiology of baby skin and its implications on our daily care regime of skin at this early stage of life.

THE DEVELOPMENT OF BABY SKIN

The development of skin usually begins 7 to 8 days after fertilization, during which an outer blastodermic layer, the ectoderm, is formed. During the embryonic phase of development, two layers evolve from the ectoderm, the underlying basal layer from which the uppermost skin layer—the epidermis—and the cutaneous appendages develop, along with the periderm, which faces the fetal cavity. When the epidermis is keratinized between week 22 and 24 of pregnancy, the periderm separates itself from most parts of the body. In the third trimenon all cell layers in the epidermis that are typical for mature skin are developed. However, until birth, the stratum corneum has still not developed a significant barrier function. This is made clear when premature babies are observed. One of the biggest problems in preemies is high transepidermal water loss (TEWL), although this decreases exponentially with increasing gestation age. High TEWL in turn may lead to hypothermia and difficulty in fluid balance [1–6].

The mesoderm, a middle layer, develops at day 18 or 19 after fertilization. The mesoderm, with its mesenchymal cells, forms the dermis (corium). Epidermis and dermis are connected by a membrane (basal lamina). Within the third trimenon this contact area (the dermo-epidermal junctional zone) between the dermis and epidermis can now be clearly identified by commencing undulations and by the development of epithelial crests and papillae. The development of the dermis also continues until the birth of the baby. In newborns it is about 60% as thick as in adults [1].

In the embryonic phase the dermis and the underlying subcutis cannot be differentiated from one another. In week 15 of gestation the subcutis can clearly be recognized.
The lobuli network, in which the adipocytes (fat cells) spread, is formed. Within the third
trimenon large fat lobuli develop in the subcutis, which protect the organism from heat
loss in cold conditions. Today it is still not clear what exactly stimulates the adipocytes
to produce fat. The subcutis does not become thicker until after birth, depending on the
baby's nutritional condition [1,2].

The sweat glands begin forming on the palms of the hands and the soles of the feet
between weeks 10 and 12 of gestation. A portion of the excretory glands, however, remains
closed until the end of month 7 of gestation. This is the reason why babies born prematurely have developed, if at all, a limited ability to sweat [2]. They also show a limited
ability to regulate body temperature as well as an increased TEWL, both of which need
to be considered when setting up a daily skincare regime [7]. In contrast, the skin of
preterm and full-term infants usually shows no signs of a physiological deficit.

THE PHYSIOLOGY OF BABY SKIN

Protection Against Water Loss

The following two basic mechanisms account for fluid transport through the skin:

1. Perspiration: active process in which water is excreted through the openings of
   the sweat glands. (Perspiration plays an important role in thermoregulation) [8].
2. TEWL: passive diffusion of water through the skin [9,10].

Gestation age plays an essential role in the birth of a baby [11]. The TEWL decreases
with increasing gestation age. In a fully developed newborn, a TEWL of 6 to 8 g water
per m^2 of skin per hour is low. However, the TEWL is considerably higher in prematurely
born babies, especially those born before week 30 of pregnancy. In the first months of
life, water loss in infants increases slightly. The explanation for this is that the babies
begin to perspire slightly [12].

As the body temperature rises, the permeability of the skin also increases, leading
to higher water loss. As environmental temperatures rise, water evaporates faster. This
fact must be considered especially when caring for newborns. Creams and ointments with
occluding effect can lower TEWL. The application of liquid paraffin on the skin can reduce
TEWL by up to 50%.

Protection Against Percutaneous Absorption of Harmful Substances

In addition to providing protection against water loss, the skin barrier function ensures
that chemical agents, which could harm the organism, cannot penetrate percutaneously
(through the skin). The permeability rate in prematurely born babies is 5 to 50 times higher
than in fully developed newborns. The ratio between body surface and body weight is
almost 2.5 times higher in newborns than in adults. This surface volume ratio is one
of the essential points that must be considered in the application of topically affective
therapeutics. Particularly with treatment of large areas, e.g., of dermatologicals containing
corticoids, there is the danger of increased systemic absorption [13].

With increasing maturation, the epidermal cells develop increased metabolic activity. This means that the activation of enzymes can render potentially harmful substances
harmless. They are modified through oxidation, hydrolysis, reduction, deamination, or

conjugation and thereby inactivated. This enzyme activity is very restricted, especially in prematurely born babies, so that potentially harmful substances can enter the blood stream in an unaltered state if absorbed percutaneously [13].

Protection Against Pathogenic Micro-Organisms

After birth, the body of the baby is exposed to numerous germs. The skin barrier not only protects mechanically against invading micro-organisms, but also through the slightly acidic milieu of the hydrolipidic film on the surface of the skin. The surface of the skin is physiologically populated by specific germs (saprophytes), which are not pathogens but rather a vital microbial defense system on the skin's surface. For optimal living conditions, the saprophytes require an acidic milieu. Directly after birth, however, alkaline values prevail on the surface of the body of the newborn. It can be assumed that these alkaline values result from the vernix caseosa residue. Neither weight at birth nor gestation age seem to have an influence on the pH value. Within the first 24 hours after birth, the pH value drops noticeably. In the first month of life, the pH value then stabilizes at a slightly acidic range (slightly below a pH value of 6) [14].

The natural acid mantle of the skin on the newborn is already developed in the first few days of life, so that pathogenic micro-organisms generally find the conditions unsuitable for their survival. However, the alkaline-neutralizing properties of the skin of newborns and small children is restricted. After contact with alkaline substances (e.g., alkaline soaps), the skin requires a longer time to restore its slightly acidic physiological pH value as compared with adult skin [15].

FREQUENT SKIN PROBLEMS IN NEWBORNS

Diaper Dermatitis

At the beginning of this century, in 1905, a French pediatrician by the name of Jacquet gave the peculiar frequently occurring skin rash in the diaper area the name diaper dermatitis [16]. The skin alterations subcategorized under the diagnosis diaper dermatitis can have a variety of causes. They can be directly related to the contact dermatitis, which is diaper dermatitis in a narrow sense. The occurence can also be unrelated to the use of diapers. Today the factors that enhance this irritating contact dermatitis are known:

1. Diapers that have an occluding effect in an already moist environment, which results in an increased hydration of the stratum corneum.
2. The increased hydration facilitates penetration of xenobiotics.
3. The still very thin epidermis of the newborn reacts sensitively to mechanical stress and friction.
4. The skin barrier function is weakened, and the skin shows an increased irritability.

In addition, an increase of the pH value in the diaper area can also encourage an outbreak of diaper dermatitis. The alkaline urine activates enzymes (lipases and proteases) in the feces, which irritate the skin [17–19].

Boys and girls are equally afflicted with diaper dermatitis. It mainly occurs between 3 and 10 months of age, with a frequency peak between 6 and 9 months. Typically, a skin erythema can be found on the inside of the thighs and on the baby's bottom. The skin is increasingly reddened, has a shiny, glassy appearance, and is wrinkled on the surface.

Corticosteroids are used occasionally in the treatment of diaper dermatitis. In the follow-up treatment, emollients containing zinc oxide are mainly used. Zinc oxide has an astringent, slightly disinfectant effect and offers the skin protection against urine and feces [17–21].

Protective creams containing zinc oxide are usually used to cover the skin of the diaper area with a highly viscous film, which inhibits the penetration of xenobiotics without fully occluding the skin. In order to accomplish this goal, usually water-in-oil (W/O) creams are used, which contain one or more of the following ingredients: petrolatum, lanolin, lanolin alcohol, paraffin oil, natural oils, waxes, zinc oxide, and possibly cod liver oil, vitamins, plant extracts, and titanium dioxide.

Diaper candidiasis is a fungal-infected diaper dermatitis. The most common causative agent is a yeast fungus called *Candida albicans*. It is a known fact that extensive use of antibiotics in newborns and small children increases that incidence of diaper candidiasis. Initially, diaper candidiasis can be treated with a specific antimycotic therapy (nystatin, clotrimazole), then followed up with the healing methods for basic diaper dermatitis as previously described [22].

Neurodermatitis

Neurodermatitis, also called atopic dermatitis, is a skin disease that may occur at a very early age. It can be identified by the so-called milk crust on the reddened, damp skin of the head and cheeks of the newborn. As the first indication of an outbreak of neurodermatitis, the milk crust often provides the starting point for other skin disorders. The skin becomes cracked and transparent, and the permeability increases. Once the skin is damaged, the risk of infection is higher. The skin becomes increasingly dry, transparent, and irritated, with intensified itchiness. The temptation to keep on scratching the skin is usually almost irresistable for small children. Atopic dermatitis is an immunological reaction that affects the skin to an especially large extent. More than 10% of children in industrialized countries are already afflicted, with a rising tendency. The combination of the genetic predisposition and environmental influences as well as psychological and neurovegetative factors can result in an outbreak of this disease [23–25].

Adequate skincare, which reinforces the skin's vital barrier, is a meaningful prophylaxis for avoiding a first outbreak of neurodermatitis in high-risk allergy children. The following measures can help:

- Mild cleansing agents
- Moisturizing emulsions to support the skin's barrier function
- Skincare products with proven skin tolerability
- Skincare products and cleansers with few, carefully selected ingredients, in order to keep the risk of allergies as low as possible [23–25]

THE CARE OF BABY SKIN

The effects of baby-care products can usually be divided into the following categories: cleansing, caring, and protection. Currently, a multitude of product types can be found in the market. Although the shear number of products is overwhelming, there are features they all have in common. The following three sections will deal with product characteristics and general usage advice in the various segments of baby care.

Cleansing

Bath Additives

As soon as the umbilical cord has fallen off, the baby can be bathed [26–29]. However, daily bathing of the baby is not advisable, as this would dry out the skin too much. A bath every 2 to 3 days is sufficient. The bath temperature should lie between 36 and 37°C.

Bath additives usually contain a mixture of various anionic (e.g., fatty alcohol ether sulfates, protein fatty acid condensates), nonionic (e.g., ethoxylated fatty alcohols, fatty acid glycerides), and amphoteric (e.g., betaines) surfactants. Numerous protein hydrolysates, superfatting agents, solubilizing agents, plant extracts, colorants, and perfumes are also found in this product category. In general, bath additives contain mild surfactant mixtures, which neither dry out the skin nor burn in the eyes.

Cleansers for the Diaper Area

Baby oils containing mineral oils as well as oil-impregnated towelets are widely used. (Towelets are usually supplied in dispenser boxes securing product hygiene up to the last towelet used.) Liquid petrolatum is a very desirable ingredient in view of its stability, touch, barrier function, and cost. Liquid petrolatum also has a remarkable occlusivity. Intertrigo areas should therefore be frequently cleansed (1–3 times daily) with oil or oil-containing towelets.

Soft towelets containing mild oil-in-water (o/w) cleansing milks or, alternatively, clear cleansing lotions are also frequently found. They normally contain anionic and/or nonionic surfactants in low concentrations as well as varying amounts of skincare ingredients like plant extracts and protein hydrolysates. These towelets are also offered in dispenser boxes.

Whereas the irritating effect of soaps mainly results from their alkalinity, the use of alkaline-free soaps has shown that all detergents induce a significant delipidizing effect, which can also contribute to skin irritation [26–29].

Liquid cleansers are usually used for cleansing of the face, arm pits, and the genital area. Normally alkaline free, their composition resembles the composition of baby shampoos, whereas the concentration of surfactants is normally higher. The reasoning behind the higher surfactant level lies in the smaller product amount used for cleansing [26–29].

Shampoos

Baby shampoos are usually formulated to be nonirritating to the eyes. This guarantees extraordinary product safety and also ensures that babies do not object to shampooing. Although basically the ingredients used are comparable with the ingredients found in bath additives, the concentration of surfactants is normally lower. Viscosity is adjusted to about 1000 centipoise (cps) to make it hard for the shampoo to migrate into the eyes.

Care

Face and Body Creams/Body Lotions

Face creams are especially important for the protection against environmental influences like sunlight, wind, and cold temperatures, which may dry out baby skin. The composition resembles that of the body-care creams, although the moisturizer content is often higher. The ingredients used are often more compatible with the mucous membranes (especially in the area of the eyes) than in the case of body creams. Body-care creams are frequently used for their excellent superfatting properties. Both o/w and w/o emulsions are found on the market.

Body-care lotions are normally used for large-area body care, e.g., after baby bath. Both o/w and w/o emulsions are found in the market. Classic ingredients used are lanolin, lanolin alcohol, paraffin oil, vaseline, natural and synthetic wax esters, natural oils, fatty alcohols, and emulsifiers (e.g., fatty acid glycerides, ethoxylated fatty alcohols). Many skin-caring, soothing active ingredients are also found.

Protection

Sun Protection

Spending summer vacation at the seashore is a tradition of many families. Unfortunately, the beach is a high-risk environment for future skin cancer because it allows for maximum sunlight exposure. Heat, wind, and humidity are often present. These factors can enhance or intensify UV injury. With or without topical sun-protection measurements, babies and small children should be kept out of direct sunlight. As soon as children begin to explore their environment, it usually becomes impossible to confine them to the shade. In such cases, sunscreens need to be applied.

A wide variety of different o/w and w/o emulsions, hydrogels and oleogels are found in the market using a variety of UV-filter systems. Many products contain broad spectrum (UVA and UVB) sunscreens with a moderate SPF. Products with a water-resistant SPF are favorable at the seashore [30–33].

Cold Protection

Mild facial creams are especially important in the winter for protection against the harsh effects of a dry, cold climate. At freezing temperatures, significant protection against frost bite is obviously helpful. Specific petrolatum-based water-free formulations, which optionally contain zinc oxide and skin-soothing agents like panthenol, can protect the skin at temperatures below freezing.

QUALITY MANAGEMENT IN BABY CARE

Despite careful research with respect to the good skin tolerability of each individual ingredient in baby-care formulations, it should be made certain that this data will also apply to the final product after these ingredients are integrated into the formula. In order to rule out the possibility of contact allergies or sensitizing skin reactions, products are frequently tested using the repeated-insult patch test (RIPT). This test is a validated, recognized method for the testing of skin sensitization. The test preparations are repeatedly applied to the same localization for 3 weeks. After a 2-week break, the test materials are applied once again on another location and the skin is assessed for any allergic reaction that could possibly have been induced [34]. Exposure to sunlight can cause certain ingredients to trigger photoallergic or phototoxic skin reactions. Photopatch or phototoxicity tests enable the detection of UV-induced irritant or allergic skin reactions.

In the elbow-wash test, the skin tolerability of cleansing formulas is tested in the sensitive crease of the elbow under controlled and extreme washing conditions, and compared with a skin-friendly standard product. The evaluation of the skin reaction is performed after repeated washings over a period of 5 days, based on subjective and objective reports [35].

In a clinical application test, skin tolerability as well as the skincare properties of baby products can be tested. At the start, and again after 4 weeks of practical application of baby-care products, dermatological examinations are carried out. Parents are given diaries for the daily evaluation of product properties. Children known to have skin allergies to ingredients in the test products are excluded from the testing.

SUMMARY

Normal baby skin shows no natural inborn deficits that need special treatment. However, the elevated skin permeability in newborns needs to be considered when establishing a routine skincare regime. The sensible use of skin-cleansing and caring products surely needs to be remembered.

However, there is a growing demand for specific dermatological treatments of newborns, as the number of skin disorders (e.g., neurodermatitis) in this age group are on the increase.

REFERENCES

1. Holbrook KA, Sybert VP. Basic science. In: Schachner L, Hansen R, eds. Pediatric Dermatology 2d ed., Vol. 1. New York: Churchill-Livingstone, 1995; 1–70.
2. Holbrook KA. Structure and function of the developing skin. In: Goldsmith LE, ed. Physiology, Biochemistry and Molecular Biology of the Skin. 2d ed., Vol. 1. New York: Oxford University Press, 1991: 63–110.
3. Hammerlund K, Sedin G, Stromberg B. Transepidermal water loss in newborn infants. VII. Relation to postnatal age in very pre-term and full-term appropriate for gestational age infants. Acta Paediatr Scand 1982; 71:369–374.
4. Doty SE, McCormack WB, Seagrave RC. Predicting insensible water loss in premature neonates. Biol Neonate 1994; 66:33–44.
5. Wilson DR, Maibach HI. Transepidermal water loss in vivo. Preterm and term infants. Biol Neonate 1980; 37:180–185.
6. Rutter N, Hull D. Water loss from the skin of term and preterm babies. Arch Dis Child 1979; 54:858–868.
7. Lane AT. Development and care of the premature infant's skin. Pediatr Derm 1987; 4:1–5.
8. Hey EN, Katz G. Optimum thermal environment for naked bodies. Arch Dis Child 1970; 45: 328–334.
9. Hammerlund K, Nilsson GE, Öberg PA, Sedin G. Transepidermal water loss in newborn infants II. Acta Paediatr Scand 1978; 68:371–376.
10. Fanaroff AA, Wald M, Gruber HS, Klaus MH. Insensible water loss in low birth weight infants. Pediatrics 1972; 50:236–245.
11. Dubowitz LMS, Dubowitz V, Golberg C. Clinical assessment of gestational age in the newborn infant. J Pediatr 1970; 77:1–10.
12. Harpin VA, Rutter N. Barrier properties of the newborn infant's skin. J Pediatr 1983; 102: 419–425.
13. Barrett DA, Rutter N. Transdermal delivery and the premature neonate. Crit Rev Therapeutic Drug Carrier Systems 1994; 11(1): 1–30.
14. Tunnessen WW. Practical aspects of bacterial skin infections in children. Pediatr Derm 1985; 2(s):255–265.

15. Braun F, Lachmann D, Zweymüller E. Der Einfluss eines synthetischen Detergens auf den pH der Haut von Säuglingen. Der Hautarzt 1986; 37:329–334.

16. Jacquet L. Traite de Maladie de l'Enfance. Paris: Grauncher & Comby, 1905.

17. Lane AT. Diaper rash: causes and cures. Patient Care 1988:167–173.

18. Honig, PJ. Diaper dermatitis. Postgrad Med 1983; 74(6):79–88.

19. Rasmussen JE. Classification of diaper dermatitis: an overview. Pediatr 1987; 14(Suppl 1): 6–10.

20. Agren MS. Percutaneous absorption of zinc and zinc oxide applied topically to intact skin in man. Dermatol 1990; 180:36–39.

21. Derry JE, McLean WM, Freeman JB. A study of the percutaneous adsorption from topically applied zinc oxide ointment. J Parenteral Enteral Nutri 1983; 7:131–135.

22. Stögmann W. Empfehlungen zur Lokaltherapie banaler Dermatosen im Kindealter. WMW 1984; 1:19–24.

23. Stögmann W. Empfehlungen zur Behandlung und Prophylaxe der Atopischen Dermatitis im Kindesalter. WMW 1989; 18:414–421.

24. Saurat JH. Atopische Dermatitis beim Kind. Annales Nestle 1987; 45:10–28.

25. Queille-Roussel C, Raynaud F, Saurat JH. A prospective computerized study of 500 cases of atopic dermatitis in childhood. Acta Derm Venerol (Stockholm) 1985; 114:87–92.

26. Schneider W. Nutzen und Schaden von Seifen und Syndets. Kosmetologie H 1971; 2:54–56.

27. Debsi S, Jonte G. Skin cleansing and skin care in infants. Ärztl Kosmet 1987; 17(1):65–69.

28. Vergesslich KA, Zweymüller E. Sind die neuen Waschmittel in der Pediatrie von Vorteil? Wiener klinische Wochenzeitschrift 1982; Jg 94, Heft 12; 4:321–359.

29. Cowan ME, Frost MR. A comparison between a detergent baby additive and baby soap on the skin flora of neonates. J Hosp Infect 1986; 7:91–95.

30. Stern RS, Weinstein MC, Baker SG. Risk reduction for nonmelanoma skin cancer with childhood sunscreen use. Arch Dermatol 1986; 122:537–545.

31. Owens DW, Knox JM, Hudson HT, Troll D. Influence of humidity on ultraviolet injury. J Invest Derm 1975; 64:250–252.

32. Freeman RG, Knox JM. The influence of temperature on ultraviolet injury. Arch Derm 1967; 89:858–864.

33. Owens DW, Knox JM, Hudson HT, Troll D. Influence of wind on ultraviolet injury. Arch Derm 1974; 109:200–201.

34. Schelanski H., Schelanski M. A new technique of human patch test. Proc Sci Section 1953; 19:46–49.

35. Lukacovic MF, Dunlpa FE, Michaels SE, Visscher MD,Watson DD. Forearm wash test to evaluate the clinical mildness of cleansing products. J Soc Cosmet Chem 1988; 39:355–366.

59

Cosmetics for the Elderly

Uwe Schönrock
Beiersdorf AG, Hamburg, Germany

INTRODUCTION

Aging is a basic biological process common to all living organisms. Its biochemical mechanisms have yet to be elucidated in detail. Aging is usually understood as an irreversible, progressive loss of homeostatic capacity. By definition, aging affects everyone, but at a variable rate. At present, aging is widely assumed to result partly from a genetically determined program and partly from endogenous and exogenous insults. Both processes occur at the level of individual cells.

At the organ level generally and in the skin specifically, aging is manifested by a loss of maximum metabolic activity and increasing sensitivity or susceptibility to certain diseases and environmental factors. The purpose of this chapter is to outline what is known about morphological and physiological aging of the skin and its implications for a tailored skincare of the elderly.

AGE-ASSOCIATED CHANGES IN HUMAN SKIN
Morphological and Histological Changes

The major aging changes in the morphology of the skin include dryness (roughness and scaliness), wrinkling, and laxity [1]. The most striking and consistent change is a flattening of the dermal-epidermal junction [2]. This results in a considerably smaller surface between the two compartments. This presumably leads to less nutrient transfer and may cause the relatively smaller proliferative compartment in the epidermis. It is also responsible for the lower resistance to shear forces [1]. However, most of the apparent clinical changes associated with advanced age are attributable to chronic sun damage [3,4].

Physiological Changes

An age-associated decrease in the epidermal turnover rate of approximately 30 to 50% between the third and the eighth decade has been determined by a study of desquamation rates at selected body sites [5]. The thymidine labeling index of the epidermis in vivo has been reported to decline nearly 50% during the human life span [6].

Recent studies using highly sensitive techniques for the measurement of sebum secretion rates have documented a decline of approximately 23% per decade [7]. The physiological consequences of decreased sebum production in old age, if any, are unknown [1].

Clinical studies showed that eccrine sweating is markedly impaired with age. Spontaneous sweating in response to dry heat, measured on digital pads, was reduced by more than 70% in healthy old subjects [8], primarily attributable to a decreased output per gland.

The decreased vascular reponsiveness in elderly skin has been documented by clinically assessing vasodilation and transduction after application of standard irritants like histamine [9]. The intensity of erythema after UV exposure also decreases with age [10].

An age-associated decrease in delayed hypersensitivity reactions in human skin is manifested by a relative inability of healthy elderly subjects to develop sensitivity to dinitrochlorobenzene (DNCB), and by their lower rate of patch-test reactions to standard recall antigens. The cutaneous manifestations of immediate hypersensitivity similarly declines with age [1].

Langerhans cells are the epidermal cell population, which is largely responsible for recognition of foreign antigens. An approximately 25 to 50% reduction in the number of epidermal Langerhans cells occurs between early and late adulthood [11] and substantially contributes to the age-associated decrease in cutaneous immune responsiveness. The amount of dermal mast cells likewise decreases with age. The resulting consequences beyond the reduced rate of immediate hypersensitivity reactions, such as a positive ''prick-test'' [12] or acute urticaria, are unknown.

Photoaging

Photoaging is a term used to describe the array of clinical and histological findings in the chronically sun-exposed skin of middle-aged and elderly adults. It has also been called dermatoheliosis [13] and heliodermatitis [14], the latter term reflecting the low-grade inflammatory nature of the process.

Clinical features of actinically damaged skin include coarseness, wrinkling, irregular pigmentation, telangiectasia, and scaliness, as well as a variety of premalignant and malignant neoplasms. The relative severity of these changes varies considerably among individuals. This undoubtedly reflects strong differences in past sun exposure and marked individual differences in vulnerabilities and repair capacities for solar insults. Photoaging usually involves most severely the face, neck, or extensor surface of the upper extremities [15].

THE COSMETIC CARE OF ELDERLY SKIN

Cosmetics for elderly skin can usually be divided into the categories of facecare and bodycare. Currently, a multitude of product types can be found. Although the number of products is overwhelming, there are common features to be mentioned. The following two sections will deal with product characteristics in various segments for the cosmetic care of elderly skin.

Facecare

Skincare

Concepts for cosmetics suited for elderly people are often based on the dry skin conditions typical for elderly skin. Many skincare formulations contain humectants, which enable excellent transient hydrational/moisturizing effects. While lessening the prominence of undesirable surface defects, these formulations have only minor influence on dermal losses. However, evidence is accruing that the following groups of topically applied actives do seem to reverse the degenerative skin changes seen with aging.

By far the most exciting discovery in cutaneous gerontology during the past decade is the effect of tretinoin (all-trans retinoic acid) on the clinical and histological appearance of photoaged skin. Kligman first realized that topical tretinoin improved the appearance of middle-aged women using the drug to control facial acne. Support for the concept was provided by a double-blind vehicle-controlled trial documenting tretinoin's effectiveness on human photoaging. After 4 months of daily application, 0.1% tretinoin cream produced statistically significant improvement in fine and coarse wrinkling, sallowness, and roughness of sun-damaged facial and arm skin [16].

Tretinoin was the first agent shown to reverse age-associated changes in any tissue. This statement must be qualified in that it is unclear whether tretinoin truly reverses aging changes or simply produces new changes that mimic a reversal. It is unclear whether tretinoin affects exclusively sunlight-induced pathologies or a combination of sun damage and intrinsic aging changes [1].

In the past years, estrogen supplementation of the climacteric women has opened new aspects on the wide variability of estrogen effects in various tissues. In skin, estrogens increase vascularization and show effects at various levels of dermal tissue [17,18].

Several attempts have been made to check the skincare efficacy of estriol (0.3%) or estradiol (0.01%) in perimenopausal women. Daily application of a cream over a period of 7 months resulted in a significant increase of skin parameters like skin firmness, wrinkles, and skin moisture content. Hormonal levels showed a slight increase in the prolactin level, whereas the estradiol level was unchanged. Side effects were not found [19,20].

Many further topical actives with excellent antiaging potential are currently used in marketed formulations, the number of which is increasing year after year [21–23].

Skin Cleansing

Active detergent substances contained in cleansing agents for human skin inevitably result in a degreasing of the keratinous layer, so that natural, moisture-retaining substances are also rinsed out in the process. It is, however, possible, by selecting the proper cleansing agents and reducing the frequency and intensity of their application, to reduce the unfavorable influence of various washing procedures on the skin of such elderly persons to a considerable extent.

Facial skin cleansers for elderly skin are usually particularly mild and superfatting. Both surfactant-based and oil-in-water (o/w) emulsion-based formulations are currently found. In the surfactant-based formulations, surfactants like ampholytes, betaines, sulfosuccinates, and various types of alkylpolyglucose are frequently used, whereas o/w emulsion-based formulas frequently contain superfatting agents and various humectants, which secure good cleansing efficacy without drying out the skin.

Bodycare

Skincare

For active care by means of humidity and lipid substitution, mainly o/w and water-in-oil (w/o) emulsions are used, which combine occlusive effects and moisturizing action. In addition to pyrrolidone carboxylic acid salt and urea, other humectant substances such as alpha-hydroxy acid and hyaluronic acid, a highly efficient moisturizer, are frequently found. It is self-evident that such formulation ingredients as glycerine, propylene glycol, and other glycols also contribute to their humectancy.

Polar and unpolar lipids are frequently used in bodycare formulations. They act as emollients, as protective lipids, and as structure formers of the liquid crystalline bilayers between the corneocytes. These three functions are usually performed by fatty alcohols, fatty acids, and short- and long-chain esters, along with triglycerides and waxes. Special effects are frequently delivered by liposomes containing phospholipids, sphingolipids, and ceramides, and lead to the desired long-term effects. This is attributable to special binding mechanisms in the skin, an anchor capacity of transported and/or encapsulated active ingredients, and their slow release.

Skin Cleansing

Bath additives usually contain a mixture of various anionic, nonionic, and amphoteric surfactants. Numerous superfatting agents, solubilizing agents, plant extracts, and perfumes are also found in products within this category. However, only an oil bath for elderly skin may provide skin cleansing and conditioning at the same time. For serious dry-skin conditions, oil baths are indispensable.

A variety of shower products, meanwhile, also contain high amounts of superfatting agents, thus securing their good skin compatibility and low drying-out potential.

SUMMARY

There is an increasing demand for face- and bodycare formulations tailormade for the cosmetic treatment of elderly skin. Modern topical formulations not only deliver excellent moisturizing and superfatting capabilities, but many products, especially facecare products, contain one or more actives counteracting the signs of intrinsic and/or photoaging. However, it is still not clear whether these actives reverse the signs of aging or induce other effects on the skin that mimic a reversal of skin aging.

REFERENCES

1. Gilchrest BA. Physiology and pathophysiology of aging skin. In: Goldsmith LA, ed. Physiology, Biochemistry, and Molecular Biology of the Skin. Vol. 2, 2nd ed. New York, Oxford Press, 1991:1425–1444.
2. Hull MT, Warfel KA. Age- related changes in the cutaneous basal lamina: scanning electron microscopic study. J Invest Derm 1983; 81:378–380.
3. Tindall JP, Smith JG. Skin lesions of the aged and their association with internal changes. J Am Med Assoc 1963; 186:73–76.
4. Beauregard SB, Gilchrest BA. A survey of skin problems and skin care regimes in the elderly. Arch Derm 1987; 123:1638–1643.
5. Tan CY, Statham B, Marks R, Payne PA. Skin thickness measurement by pulsed ultrasound: its reproducability, validation and variability. Br J Derm 1982; 106:657–662.
6. Kligman AM. Perspectives and problems in cutaneous gerontology. J Inv Derm 1979; 73:39–46.
7. Jacobsen E, Billings JK, Frantz RA. Age- related changes in sebum secretion rate in men and women. J Inv Derm 1985; 85:483–485.
8. Silver AF, Motagna W, Karacan I. The effect of age on human eccrine sweating. In: Motagna W, ed. Advances in the Biology of the Skin Aging. Vol. 6. Pergamon Press, 129–137.

9. Grove GL, Lavker RM, Hölzle E, Kligman AM. Use of nonintrusive tests to monitor age-associated changes in human skin. J Soc Cosm Chem 1981; 32:15–19.

10. Gilchrest BA, Stoff JS, Boter NA. Chronologic aging alters the response to UV-induced inflammation in human skin. J Inv Derm 1982; 79:11–15.

11. Thiers BH, Maize JC, Spicer SS, Cantor AB. The effect of aging and chronic sun exposure on human Langerhans cell populations. J Inv Derm 1984; 82:223–226.

12. Barbee RA, Levowitz MD, Thompson HC, Burrows B. Immediate skin-test reactivity in a general population sample. Ann Intern Med 1976; 84:129–133.

13. Gilchrest BA. Skin and Aging Processes. Boca Raton: CRC Press, 1984.

14. Lavker RA, Kligman AM. Chronic heliodermatitis: a morphologic evaluation of chronic actinic dermal damage with emphasis on the role of mast cells. J Inv Derm 1988; 90:325–330.

15. Knox JM, Cockcrall EG, Freeman RB. Etiological factors and premature aging. J Am Med Assoc 1962; 179:630–634.

16. Weiss JS, Ellis CN, Headington JT, Voorhees JJ. Topical tretinoin in the treatment of aging skin. J Am Acad Dermatol 1988; 19:169–175.

17. Schmidt JB. Externe Östrogenapplikation bei Hautalterung im Klimakterium—Ein Therpaieansatz-. H + G. 1993; Band 68; Heft 2:84–87.

18. Artner J, Gitsch E. Über Lokalwirkungen von Östriol. Geburtshilfe und Frauenheilkunde. 1959; 19:812–819.

19. Punnonnen R, Vaajalahti P, Teisala K. Local oestriol treatment improves the structure of elastic fibres in the skin of postmenopausal women. Ann Chir Gynaecol (Suppl.) 1987; 202:39–41.

20. Schmidt JB, Binder M, Demschick G, Biegelmayer C, Reiner A. Treatment of skin aging with topical estrogens. Int J Derm 1996; 35:669–674.

21. Smith WP. Hydroxy acids and skin aging. Cosmet Toilet 1994; 109:41–48.

22. Pierrefriche G, Laborit H. Oxygen free radicals, melatonin, and aging. Exp Gerontol 1995; 30:213–227.

23. Coles LS, Harris SB. Coenzyme Q10 and lifespan extension. In: Klatz RM. ed. Advances in Anti-Aging Medicine. Larchmont, NY, Mary Ann Liebert, Inc., 1996:205–216.

60

EEC Cosmetic Directive and Legislation in Europe

René Van Essche
Free University of Brussels, Brussels, Belgium

THE LAWS OF THE MEMBER STATES RELATING TO COSMETIC PRODUCTS AND THE 6TH AMENDMENT

The Council of the European Communities in regard to the Treaty establishing the European Economic Community (today, the European Union [EU]) and in particular Article 100 thereof has decided to harmonize legislation in the EU [1,2]. The Directive gives a clear definition of cosmetic products: ''Any substance or preparation intended to be placed in contact with the various external parts of the human body or with the teeth and and the mucous membranes of the oral cavity, with a view exclusively or mainly to clean them, perfuming them, changing their appearance and—or correcting body odours and—or protecting them or keeping them in good condition.'' The philosophy of the Directive is that all products should have equal and immediate access to the market throughout the EU provided that they are proven safe for human use. The Directive has been adapted and modified 29 times between 1976 and 1998. The 6th Amendment has made mandatory by January 1, 1997 that cosmetic products may be marketed only if the labeling bears specific information in legible and visible lettering (Article 6) as follows: the name and address or registered office of the manufacturer or the responsible person for marketing in the Union, the nominal content at the time of packaging, the date of minimum durability and the conditions of storage if appropriate, the conditions of use and warnings, the batch number, the function, the list of ingredients in descending order of weight. Article 7a requires that for control purposes the following information be readily accessible to the competent authorities of the Member State: the qualitative and quantitative composition of the product (perfumes may be coded) (good laboratory procedures [GLP], O.J. EU n° L 15, 17—01—87, p. 29), the physicochemical and microbiological specifications of the raw materials and the finished product, the purity and the microbiological control criteria of the cosmetic product, the method of manufacture (good manufacturing procedures, GMP), the person responsible for the manufacturing or first importation into the EU shall possess an appropriate level of qualification, the assessment of the safety (GLP, Council Directive 87—18—EEC of 18 December 1986), the name and address of the responsible person (who must hold a diploma according to Article 1 of Council Directive 89—48— EEC), undesirable effects if existing, and proof of effect by the nature of effect. The competent authority of the Member State shall be notified of the place of manufacture or initial import into the EU of the cosmetic products before the latter are placed on the market, the Poison Information Center shall be informed about the formula, and The European Cosmetic, Toiletry and Perfumery Association (COLIPA) [3] has negotiated that only major deviations from basic formulas shall be indicated (the basic formulas having been given by COLIPA).

The Committee on the Adaptation to Technical Progress of the Directives on the Removal of Technical Barriers to Trade in Cosmetic Products in set up. This Committee is located in Brussels at the European Commission (DG Enterprise, Industry, 200 rue de la Loi, B-1029 Brussels, Belgium, tel; 32 2 299 1111). Article 12 deals with product, that although complying with the Directive, may represent a risk to human health.

The Directive includes seven annexes, and the eighth is pending.

Annex I.   Illustrative list by category of cosmetic products.

Annex II.   List of substances that must not form part of the composition of cosmetic products. 420 substances are listed. On a time-to-time basis, new substances are included in the list. The cosmetics on the market, containing a newly forbidden substance or an authorized substance revised for a lower concentration, are regulated in the sense that they are ''authorized for a short defined period of time, the manufacturing of the cosmetic in question becoming often forbidden.'' Hormones, anesthetics, chloroform, drug type molecules, and, recently, crude and refined coal tar fall in this category.

Annex III.   List of substances that cosmetic products must not contain, except subject to restrictions and conditions. For instance: hydrogen peroxide containing or releasing cosmetics for haircare 12% H_2O_2 is authorized, but for oral hygiene concentration 0.1% only is authorized, and fluorides for oral hygiene products are limited to concentration 0.15% as F.

Annex IV.   List of coloring agents allowed for use in cosmetic products. Four classes are given: (1) all purposes, (2) not for use around the eye, (3) exclusively for products not in contact with mucous membranes, (4) and products briefly in contact with the skin.

Annex V.   List of substances excluded from the scope of the Directive.

Annex VI.   List of preservatives that cosmetic products may contain. For instance, Hexetidine 0.1% as preservative for the product but may be present at higher concentration (justify) as deodorant in soap or antidandruff shampoos.

Annex VII.   List of UV filters that cosmetic products may contain.

Annex VIII.   A proposal for a pictogram calling the attention of the customer to the information for use.

In summary, the Directive covers every cosmetic (see definition) imported or manufactured within the EU. Cosmetics not allowed for children for safety reasons must carry the warning ''not for children'' or ''not below some year of age.'' Samples and testers are handled under the same Directive. National language for the labels is often required, and ingredients may be given in INCI (International Nomenclature for Cosmetic Ingredients). Manufacturing date is not required, expiration date is required for less than 30 months shelflife. In case of damage and in order to deal with emergency situations, a channel of information is built between the Member States through the ''Poison Information Centers'' or some other national medical instances. Cosmetics are controlled regularly on a random basis, by the Competent Authorities either at the manufacturing site in the EU or at the distribution centers, or at the selling points. The methodology for adding new cosmetic ingredients to the existing positive list or modifying the restrictions is as follows: prepare a full dossier from the analytical and safety point of view and submit it to COLIPA [3]. After evaluation, the dossier is sent by the COLIPA ad hoc working party, to the European Commission. At the Commission level the dossier is discussed in the scientific advisory body, the Committee for Cosmetics, and will be published as an amendment in the O.J. EU.

The application may be submitted directly by the applicant to the DG Enterprise, Cosmetic Division in Brussels. The animal testing ban on cosmetic ingredients and combinations is postponed until December 1, 2002. In November 1995, COLIPA [4,5] published two important documents related to the safety information and provision for cosmetics and raw materials in order to prepare the dossiers required by the 6th Amendment. For the provision of safety information for finished products, a process is recommended to be followed by the safety assessor in arriving at the safety assessment. First, a toxicological profile of ingredients must be identified, and second for finished products. For finished products the assessment may take into consideration formulas that can be compared by composition, and a general statement including several products is acceptable.

The information for raw materials is often required at the supplier level. One expects the supplier to consolidate, identity, safety data sheet, toxicology, and human experience (if available). The chairman of the Scientific Committee on Cosmetology of the Commission of the EU, Pr. Loprieno, published in 1992 the views of the Committee [6]. Categories of cosmetic products and exposure levels in use, physicochemical specifications, safety studies in vitro and in vivo, and observation on human subjects are examined in his article, together with toxicokinetics and long-term studies.

The microbiological information on raw materials and finished products is an important part of the dossier [7]. The microbiological quality is identified, by validated methods, for quantitative limits of microorganisms to be 10^3 g or mL and 10^2 g or mL for eye products, baby care, and intimate hygiene, and for qualitative limits the absence of *Pseudomonas aeruginosa*, other gram-negative organisms (enterobacteria), and *Staphylococcus aureus* (*Candida albicans*?).

IMPLEMENTATION OF THE EUROPEAN DIRECTIVE ON COSMETIC PRODUCTS IN THE DIFFERENT MEMBER STATES OF THE EUROPEAN UNION (STATUS JUNE 1998)

The Directive had to be "normally" implemented in the 15 Member States within 18 months after the publication in 1993 (6th Amendment). This was not always the case for nationalistic protection and political reasons. The Council of Europe will call the attention of the "slow" Member States and even the Justice Court of Luxemburg for nonimplementation. A summary of the situation in the 15 Member States and Norway follows—the data hereafter may have been modified recently, but remains a good way to locate Centers and Authorities.

Austria

After the action of the Commission against the Austrian government, the Directive is now fully implemented, excluding the requirement for licensing and the positive list of active substances. Labelling for ingredients still pending. Qualification: broad definition but related to qualification in chemistry, food, and drugs. Competent authority: Bundesministerium fur Gesundheit und Konsumentenschutz, Abteilung II—C—16, Radetzkystrasse 2, A-1030 Wien, tel.: 43 1 71172-4668.

Belgium

Implemented since the publication of the Arrêté Royal of October 15, 1997 published in the Moniteur Belge of January 16, 1998. The Belgian Arrêté Royal is for some points more requiring: labelling of ''tested on animals'' must specify for raw materials and/ or finished product. Import and manufacturing of products not labelled according to the requirements of Article 5 are authorized until July 1, 1999; after that date only products with a manufacturing date anterior to July 1, 1999 will be accepted. Responsible person qualification as the EEC Directive required. Poison Information Center: Centre Antipoison, rue Joseph Stallaert 1, B-1050 Bruxelles Belgium, tel.: 32 2 345 4545. Competent authority: Ministère des Affaires Sociales, de la Santé Publique et de l'Environment, Inspecteur Mr Féroumont, Inspection Générale des Produits Cosmétiques, Cité Administrative de l'État, Quartier Vésale, B-1010 Bruxelles. Belgium, tel.: 32 2 210 4869.

Denmark

Directive implemented in June 1995. Labelling of all ingredients mandatory since January 1, 1998. Product licencing once a year. Qualification requested according to the Cosmetic Directive. Poison information to: Sundhedsstyrelsen, Fredreikssundsvej 378, DK-2700 Bronshoj, Denmark, tel.: 54 44 889111. Competent Authority: Danish Environmental Protection Agency, Strangade 29, DK-1401 Köbenhaven, Denmark.

Finland

Implementation finalized in the Cosmetic Statute 189—96 and the Decision on Cosmetic Products by the Minister of Trade and Industry 191—96. Fee required for notifications (12 categories and 60 sections). After January 1, 1997 notification before marketing. Poisoning information Center: Central University Hospital in Helsinki. Competent Authority: Finnish Consumer Administration Apnasgatan 4, PB 5 FIN-00531 Helsinki (National Agency: 358 9 473341).

France

As of December 12, 1998 no official implementation of the Directive is known in France; however, the Journal Officiel de la République Français has published until recently several ''décrets'' and ''arrêtés'' on manufacturing sites, preparation of the file, dangerous substances, protection agents, and dyes from 1977 until 1995. These publications make the French Laws (Décret n° 77-1558 du 28 décembre 1977) very close to the Directive, which in practice is applied. The arrêté du 27 janvier 1978 (Journal Officiel- N.C. du 7 février 1978) gives the list of the 16 Poison Information Centers. In Paris, the Centre Antipoisons de Paris is located in the Hospital Fernand Vidal, Madame le Professeur Efthymiou, 200 rue du Faubourg-Saint-Denis, F-75010 Paris, France. Competent Authority: Directions Departementales des Affaires Sanitaires et Sociales (DDASS) via Monsieur Luc Lafay, Ministère de l'Emploi et de la Solidarité, Administration Sanitaire et Sociale, Service de l'Information et de la Communication (SICOM), Bureau de la Communication Interne, 1, Place Fontenoy, F-75007 Paris, France, tel.: 33 1 40 567009.

Germany

The Directive 93-35 EEC has been implemented since December 19, 1996. GMP has been mandatory since June 30, 1997. Information file required since June 30, 1998. Last date for products not in accordance on the market is June 30, 1999. Import notification is required since June 30, 1997. Confidentiality for specific ingredients is authorized (perfumes-coded). For colored cosmetics (makeup, etc.) testing on animals is forbidden. Qualification for responsible person includes chemistry, medical, and pharmaceutical sciences, and many others. The Poison Information Center is: IKW, Karistrasse 21, Frankfurt am Main, D-60329, tel.: 49 692556 1323. Competent Authority: BgW, z. Hd Hern Prof. Dr. Heinemeyer, Tielallee 8892, Berlin, D-14195.

Greece

Directive implemented since April 21, 1997. Notification before the marketing of imported products if Greece is the first Member State. Labelling in Greek language is required in case of difficulty to understand foreign language. Poison Information Center address, via the competent authority: National Drug Organisation (EOF), 284 Mesogion avenue, GR-15562 Holargos, Greece, tel.: 301 654 1964.

Ireland

Directive implemented March 1, 1997 for new products and January 1, 1998 for other products. Notification of manufacturing site or first importation. Qualification as requested by the Directive. Competent Authority: Irish Department of Health, The Earlsfort Center, Earlsfort Terrace, IRL-Dublin 2, Ireland, tel.: 353 1676 8490. Poison Information Center not yet identified.

Italy

Implementation of the Directive: May 16, 1997. June 1998 was the latest date for sale of products not in conformation with the Directive. Ethanol must be labelled for Italian products only. Poison Information Center location to be obtained from the competent authority: Ministero di Sanita, Istituto Superiore di Sanita, Via Regina Helena, 299, I-00161 Roma, Italia, tel.: 39 6 493 87114.

Luxemburg

Directive implemented August 3, 1994. Poison Information Center via competent authority: Ministère de la Santé, rue Auguste Lumière 1, L-2546 Luxembourg, tel.: 352 491191.

Netherlands

Directive implemented October 3, 1995. Poison Information Center via competent authority: Inspectie Gezondheidbescherming, Keuringdienst van Waren, Postbus 777, NL-7500 AT Entschede, tel.: 31 53471111.

Portugal

Directive implemented early 1998, Poison Information Center via competent authority: Instituto da Farmacia e do Medicamento, Parque de Saude de Lisboa, av. do Brazil 53, P-1700 Lisboa, Portugal, tel.: 351 1 790 8500.

Spain

The Directive is implemented since the end of 1998 into a Royal Decrete. Notification to be made at the level of the "provinces" who in turn mails a copy to the Dirección General de Farmacia y Productos Sanitarios (DGFPS). Labelling must be understandable to Spanish consumers. Qualification of the responsible person: university degree or equivalent. The information related to poisoning are to be given in urgency to the DGFPS who informs the National Institute for Toxicology (Mahadagonda). Competent Authority: Ministerio de Sanidad y Consumo, Dirección General de Farmacia y Productos Sanitarios, Paseo del Prado 18-20, E-28014 Madrid, Espana, tel.: 34 1 596 4070 (fax preferred for language problems: 34 1 596 1547).

Sweden

Directive implemented since November 4, 1995. Fees 200 Swk per product, maximum 415000 Swk per Company. Poison Information Center: Giftinformationcentrale, Karolinska Sjukuset, Box 60500, S-10401 Stockholm 80, Sweden. Competent Authority: Makamedelsverket (Medical Products Agency) Box 26, Husargatan 8, S-75103, Uppsala, tel.: 46 18174687.

United Kingdom

Directive implemented June 1996, nonconform products accepted until January 1, 1999. Notification for manufacturing site and importation per categories: perfumes, decorative cosmetics, skincare, haircare, and toiletries. Animal testing forbidden from 1998, but the delay will be regulated soon. Qualification: Safety certificates must be signed by pharmacist or a physician holding a United Kingdom diploma. Poison Information Center via competent authorities: Consumer Safety Unit, Department of Trade and Industry, 1, Victoria street London SW1H OET, fax preferred: 44 171 215 0357.

Norway

Not a Member State. Directive implemented in October 1995.

Other European Countries

The Directive 78-768 and the 6th Amendment are applied, sometimes more restrictive in the forbidden molecules. The applicant for importation or local manufacturing is "recommended" to follow the Directive. A hearing with the competent authority, the Ministry of Health, is hardly recommended.

REFERENCES

1. Council Directive of July 27, 1976 on the approximation of the laws of the Member States relating to cosmetic products. (Dir. 76—768—EEC) O.J. EEC September 27, 1976 n° L 262.
2. 6th Amendment to the Directive 76—768, 93—35, June 14, 1993. O.J. EEC June 23, 1993. n° L 151.
3. COLIPA. The European Cosmetic, Toiletry and Perfumery association, rue du Congrès 5-7, B-1000 Brussels, Belgium, tél.: 32 2 227 6610, fax.: 32 2 227 6627, E-mail: colipa@colipa.be.
4. COLIPA. Cosmetic product information requirement in the European Union. Information required for the safety evaluation of cosmetic raw materials 95—242-mc. November 1995.

5. COLIPA. Cosmetic product information requirement in the European Union. The provision of safety information for a cosmetic product 95—200-mc. November 1995.
6. Loprieno N. 1992. Guidelines for safety evaluation of cosmetic ingredients in the EC countries. Food Chem Toxic 1992; 30:809–815.
7. Pr MJ Devleeshouwer. Free University of Brussels, Laboratory of Microbiology and Hygiene. Presentation Colgate, October 4, 1994. Incidence for the cosmetic industry of the 6th Amendment of the European Directive concerning the cosmetics.
8. Poppe K, Van Essche R, Devleeschouwer M, Hanoaq M, De Meerleer M, Feroumont Y-M, Masson PL. Guide Pratique de la mise en oeuvre de la directive européenne sur les produits cosmétiques. Free University of Brussels, Technopol, 1998.

61

Regulatory Requirements for the Marketing of Cosmetics in the United States

Stanley R. Milstein, John E. Bailey, and Allen R. Halper
Office of Cosmetics and Colors, Center for Food Safety and Applied Nutrition (CFSAN), U.S. Food and Drug Administration, Washington, D.C.

SCOPE

This chapter discusses the Federal regulatory requirements for the marketing of cosmetics in the United States, under the laws administered by the U.S. Food and Drug Administration (FDA). Federal control of cosmetics is a complex and shared responsibility, and, although this chapter focuses on the FDA's regulation of cosmetic products and their labeling, it also must take note of the overlapping jurisdictions of its sister agencies, the U.S. Federal Trade Commission (FTC), the U.S. Consumer Product Safety Commission (CPSC), and the U.S. Environmental Protection Agency (EPA). It is clearly beyond the scope of this writing to discuss the role played by the State Legislatures and by the State Attorneys-General, but such discussions are readily available to the interested reader elsewhere (1). The role of ''self-regulation'' in the joint oversight responsibility for cosmetics by the FDA and its stakeholders in the industry is also discussed. Finally, the chapter concludes with a brief mention of international harmonization and its impact on cosmetic regulation in the United States.

BASIC U.S. LEGAL STRUCTURE FOR COSMETICS

The FDA is the principal regulatory agency charged with the enforcement of the *Laws* governing the marketing of cosmetics in the United States. The *Laws* are the basic enabling authority enacted by Congress. For cosmetics, the agency is given the mandate for enforcing the statutory requirements of the 1938 Federal Food and Drug and Cosmetic Act (FD& C Act, also referred to as the ''Act''), the 1960 Color Additive Amendments to the Act, and the 1966 Federal Fair Packaging and Labeling Act (FPLA). Under the authority of these statutes, the FDA has promulgated *Regulations* (or *Rules*) to implement the mandate conferred by the *Laws*. *Guidance Documents*, which include *Policy Statements* (and those documents formerly termed *Advisory Opinions*) have also been issued by the agency. Although not legally binding on the public or on the agency, *Guidance Documents* nonetheless serve to provide the FDA's interpretation of the *Laws* and applicable *Regulations* (see Figure 1).

Federal regulations of cosmetics involves oversight of print, radio, television, and multimedia advertising as well as of product package labeling. The jurisdiction of the FTC to regulate the advertising of cosmetic and "Over-the-Counter" (OTC) Cosmetic-Drug products overlaps that of the FDA, and is largely based upon the portion of Section 5 of the 1914 Federal Trade Commission Act (FTCA) and subsequent amendments and legislation to the FTCA that prohibits "unfair" and "deceptive" acts or practices (2). the FDA and FTC have established a memorandum of understanding (MOU) to clarify the parameters and boundaries of this relationship (3).

FDA also shares its regulatory responsibilities for the regulation of cosmetics and topical personal care products with other Federal agencies. The U.S. Consumer Product Safety Commission (CPSC) exercises regulatory authority over "soap" products not making cosmetic or drug performance claims under the 1960 Federal Hazardous Substances Act (FHSA) and the Consumer Product Safety Act (CPSA) (4e-g); more about the regulation of soap will be discussed later in this chapter. The CPSC also is delegated the authority under the 1970 Poison Prevention Packaging Act (PPPA) for promulgating "child-resistant" packaging (CR Packaging) regulations for cosmetic products and soap products (4a); these regulations are codified at *16 CFR 1700*. In recent years, final rules have been promulgated, requiring CR packaging for nail care products (for example, primers) containing $\geq 5\%$ methacrylic acid (4b), household (artificial nail) glue removers containing acetonitrile (4d), and home cold wave permanent neutralizers containing sodium bromate or potassium bromate (4d). A proposed rule has also been published in the *Federal Register*, which would require CR packaging for fluid cosmetic products (among other categories of household substances) formulated with $\geq 10\%$ of low viscosity hydrocarbons (≤ 100 SUS @ 100 deg. F) (4c). Finally, the Environmental Protection Agency (EPA) has regulatory authority over some multi-functional personal care products, such as cosmetic liquids, lotions, or sprays that are also insect repellants. EPA's authority to

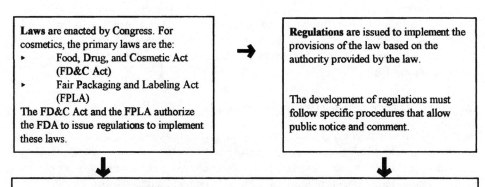

Laws are enacted by Congress. For cosmetics, the primary laws are the:
►   Food, Drug, and Cosmetic Act (FD&C Act)
►   Fair Packaging and Labeling Act (FPLA)
The FD&C Act and the FPLA authorize the FDA to issue regulations to implement these laws.

→

Regulations are issued to implement the provisions of the law based on the authority provided by the law.

The development of regulations must follow specific procedures that allow public notice and comment.

Guidance Documents - Policy Statements
►   These documents serve to provide the agency's interpretation of the law and applicable regulations.
►   Guidance documents and policy statements are not legally binding on the public or the agency.

FIGURE 1 Basic U.S. legal and regulatory structure for cosmetics.

regulate such products is derived from the Federal Insecticide, Fungicide, and Rodenticide Act (FIFRA) (5).

Table 1 summarizes the federal agency interrelationships involved in the regulation of cosmetics in the United States.

BASIC U.S. REGULATORY STRUCTURE FOR COSMETICS

Definitions: Cosmetics, Soaps, and Drugs

The statutory definition of "cosmetic" is given at Section 201 (i) of the FD&C Act as:

> (1) Articles intended to be rubbed, poured, sprinkled, or sprayed on, introduced into, or otherwise applied to the human body or any part thereof for cleansing, beautifying, promoting attractiveness, or altering the appearance, and (2) articles intended for use as a component of any such articles, except that such term shall not include soap.

For reasons discussed earlier in this book (see Chap. 2), the use of the term "cosmetics" refers not only to finished cosmetic products marketed to consumers, but also to constituent ingredients and other components of such finished products (for example, packaging). Under current legal standards, topical products functioning as cosmetics may cleanse, beautify, promote attractiveness, or alter appearance of the human body. The FDA Voluntary Cosmetic Registration Program (VCRP) currently lists 13 subdivided cosmetic product categories, which appear in the codified regulations at *21 CFR 720.4* (see Chap. 2, Table 1).

TABLE 1   U.S. Federal Statutes for Personal Care Products

Cosmetics and OTC drug–cosmetics
    Products, ingredients, packaging, and labeling (FDA, CPSC, BATF[a], EPA[b])
        Federal Food, Drug, and Cosmetic Act (FD&C Act), 1938
        Color Additive Amendments to the FD&C Act, 1960
        Federal Fair Packaging and Labeling Act (FPLA), 1966
        Federal Hazardous Substances Act (FHSA), 1960
        Federal Poisoning Prevention Packaging Act (PPPA), 1970
        Federal Insecticide, Rodenticide, and Fungicide Act (FIFRA)[b], 1947
    Print and media advertising (FTC)
        Federal Trade Commission Act (FTCA), 1914
        Wheeler-Lea Act, 1938
        Magnuson-Moss Warranty-Federal Trade Commission Improvement Act, 1975
Soap Products
    Soap (saponification), FHSA, CPSA
    Soap (detergent, "syndet"[c]), FD&C Act
    Soap (combination saponification + "syndet"), FD&C Act
    Soap (with active drug ingredient), FD&C Act
    Soap (saponification or "syndet" making cosmetic claims), FD&C Act, FPLA

[a] BATF = Bureau of Alcohol, Tobacco, and Firearms (U.S. Dept. of the Treasury), for Specially Denatured Alcohol formulations (see *27 CFR 21*).
[b] Containing pesticide or claiming insect-repellant efficacy.
[c] "Syndet" = synthetic detergent.

"Soap" products are generally exempt from the cosmetic provisions of the FD&C Act, and, indeed, from the definition of "cosmetic" given in the statute. The FDA interprets the term "soap" at *21 CFR 701.20* to apply to products

> Intended for cleansing the human body
> Labeled, sold, and represented solely as soap
> Consisting primarily of alkali metal salts of free fatty acids (i.e., the bulk of its nonvolatile matter that serves as the detergent)
> Detergent properties of which articles are due to the alkali metal salts of free fatty acids

Liquid and solid product formulations consisting of synthetic detergents ("syndets"), combinations of soap and synthetic detergents ("combo" bars) intended not only for cleansing but also claiming other cosmetic product performance attributes (e.g., "beauty bars" or "body bars" claiming to beautify, moisturize, soften, or smooth the skin) must comply with the regulatory requirements applicable to cosmetics (e.g., bear ingredient declarations required at *21 CFR 701.3*). Indeed, even if such detergent or combination soap–detergent products are intended solely for cleansing of the human body, possess the characteristics consumers generally ascribe to "soap," and are identified in labeling as "soap" or some fanciful adaptation of this descriptor (e.g., "sope," "jabon," "liquid soap," etc.), these products are still regulated as cosmetics.

The statutory definition of the term "drug" is given at Section 201 (g)(1) of the FD&C Act, in pertinent part, as:

> (B) articles intended for use in the diagnosis, cure, mitigation, treatment, or prevention in man . . . and (C) articles (other than food) intended to affect the structure or any function of the body of man . . . and (D) articles intended for use as a component of any [such] articles.

Regardless of their respective legal standings as "cosmetics" regulated under the FD&C Act or "soaps" regulated under the CPSA/FHSA, personal-care products that are also intended to treat or prevent disease or otherwise affect the structure or functions of the human body are considered "drugs" and must comply with these provisions of the law as well as any other provisions as cosmetics or soaps, respectively. Most currently marketed cosmetics that are also drugs are OTC drugs (e.g., 'fluoride' anticaries toothpastes, antiperspirant deodorants, antidandruff shampoos, and sunscreen lotions). However, several drug–cosmetics are "new drugs" [6], for which safety and effectiveness had to be proven to the agency before they could be marketed. Analogously, soap products formulated to contain "active ingredients," if intended to cure, treat, or prevent disease, or if intended to affect the structure or any function of the human body, may also be regulated as drugs. This would include, for example "medicated" anti-acne soaps, the "antibacterial" bar and liquid soaps first introduced into the market in the late 1980s [7], and the alcohol-based liquid "hand sanitizers" of the late 1990s [8].

Statutory Controls on Cosmetics

The FD&C Act not only defines the term "cosmetic," but sets forth the basic requirement that cosmetic products introduced into interstate commerce within the United States must be safe for their intended use and properly labeled. The act accomplishes this by explicitly prohibiting the adulteration or misbranding of cosmetics, and the introduction into, or receipt in, interstate commerce of ''adulterated'' or ''misbranded'' cosmetics (see FD& C Act, Sections 601 and 602, respectively).

Adulterated Cosmetics

A cosmetic is ''adulterated'' according to the FD&C Act, Section 601 (a)–(e) if:

It bears or contains any poisonous or deleterious substance, which may render it injurious to users under the conditions of use prescribed in the labeling or under ''customary or usual'' uses

It consists wholly or in part of any filthy, putrid, or decomposed substance

It has been prepared, packed, or held under insanitary conditions whereby it may have become contaminated with filth, or whereby it may have been rendered injurious to health

Its container is composed, wholly or in part, of any poisonous or deleterious substance that may render the contents injurious to health

It is not a hair dye and it is, or bears or contains, a color additive that is unsafe within the meaning of the act

Coal-Tar Hair-Dye Exemption. The FD&C Act exempts so-called ''coal-tar'' hair-dyes from the adulteration provision at Section 601 (a), if they bear the cautionary statement prescribed by law on the label and give ''patch test'' instructions, even if they are irritating to the skin or are otherwise harmful to the human body. The ''coal-tar hair-dye exemption,'' named for the synthetic organic colors originally derived from the coal tar derivative, aniline, to which the exemption was initially applied [9], does not include eyelash and eyebrow dyes since coal-tar derived color additives may cause blindness when used for dyeing the eyelashes or eyebrows (9c). The exemption also does not apply to non-coal tar color additives in hair dyes (9c).

Sources of Adulteration. Cosmetic adulteration may be associated with unintentional trace level contaminants (e.g., N-nitrosamines, or 1,4-Dioxane) of the ingredients (also referred to as 'raw materials') employed in finished cosmetic products [10–12] or to the manner of product formulation. Quality control problems (e.g., pH) or failure to follow good manufacturing practices guidelines [13] can also result in deviations of particular product batches from master formula specifications. In the past four (4) fiscal years (FY96–FY99), the FDA has found that approximately 88% of cosmetic product adulterations subject to voluntary recall actions (see ''Recalls'' in Law Enforcement of FD& C Act Violations, below) were most frequently related to problems of microbiological contamination (see Table 2) [14].

TABLE 2 Cosmetic Product Voluntary Recalls

	FY 1996	FY 1997	FY 1998	FY 1999
Total recalls	26	9	9	9
Microbiology recalls	23	8	8[a]	8
Misbranding recalls	3	1	0	1
Other recalls	0	0	1[b]	0

FY = fiscal year.
[a] 6 Class II Microbiology + 2 Mold.
[b] 1 Class II pH.

Misbranded Cosmetics

A cosmetic is "misbranded" according to the FD&C Act, Sec. 602 (a)–(f) if:

> Its labeling is false or misleading in any particular
>
> Its package label fails to contain the name and place of business of the manufacturer, packer, or distributor, as well as an accurate statement of the quantity of the contents in terms of weight, measure, or numerical count
>
> Any word, statement, or other information required to appear on the label is not prominently and conspicuously placed and in terms likely to be read and understood by the ordinary consumer under customary conditions of purchase and use
>
> Its container is made, formed, or filled in a manner likely to be misleading
>
> It is a color additive, unless its packaging and labeling are in conformity with requirements in the regulations
>
> Its packaging or labeling are in violation of an applicable regulation issued under the 1970 PPPA.

A cosmetic is misbranded as a consumer commodity according to the FPLA, Section 7, if it is introduced or delivered for introduction into commerce in violation of any of the provisions of the law or its implementing regulations, including the requirements contained in Sections 4 and 5 of the FPLA, which provide that the label of a commodity must state:

> The identity of the commodity
>
> The name and place of business of the manufacturer, packer, or distributor
>
> The net quantity of contents (in terms of weight, measure, or numerical count) separately and accurately stated in a uniform location upon the principal display panel (PDP)
>
> The "common or usual name" of the commodity and, if it contains two or more ingredients, the "common or usual name" of each ingredient listed in order of decreasing predominance, with the exception of such ingredients deemed to constitute a "trade secret."

Law Enforcement of FD&C Act Violations

Violations of the adulteration and misbranding provisions of the act may subject the violator to various enforcement tools available to the FDA. These include (but are not limited to) (16c):

> *Warning letters,* subject to public disclosure under the Freedom of Information Act (FOIA), may be posted on the Internet FDA Web site and are regularly publicized in the trade press and industry newsletters such as *The Rose Sheet*
>
> *Targeted establishment inspections* and sampling programs
>
> *Seizure* of cosmetic goods alleged to be in violation of the FD&C Act (civil actions)
>
> *Detention* of imported cosmetics offered for entry into U.S. interstate commerce that appear to be in violation of the law (see, for example, FD&C Act, Section 801(a)
>
> *Injunction* proceedings against firms or individuals, seeking that a company cease present and future manufacture and distribution of cosmetic products until compliance with the law can be assured

Criminal prosecution of responsible persons within violator cosmetic firms

Recalls. Recall and Field Correction are actions taken by a firm to either remove a product from the market or to conduct a field correction. Recalls of cosmetic products, may be conducted on a firm's own initiative or by FDA request. The FDA has no authority under the FD&C Act to order the recall of a defective or possibly harmful cosmetic product, although it can request a firm to recall a product. Resistance to an FDA request for voluntary recall can, however, trigger other enforcement actions by the agency, which have recently been reviewed by Calogero [15]. The FDA has defined policies concerning such voluntary cosmetic (as well as food, drug, and medical device) product recalls; these are codified at *21 CFR 7.45–7.59*, and additional guidance can also be found at the FDA website (*http://www.fda.gov*). The FDA's regulations divide recalls into three categories:

Class I Recall   Products that are clearly dangerous or defective that pose clear or irreversible hazards to the public health; there is reasonable probability that the use of or exposure to a violative product will cause serious adverse health consequences or death *(21 CFR 7.3 (m)(1))*

Class II Recall   Products that are intermediate in their potential for adverse public health consequences, but may cause a temporary or reversible health problem; use of or exposure to a violative product may cause temporary or medically reversible adverse health consequences or where the probability of serious adverse health consequences is remote *(21 CFR 7.3 (m)(2))*

Class III Recall   Products that are unlikely to cause any adverse health reaction but that violate FDA regulations; use of or exposure to a violative product is not likely to cause adverse health consequences *(21 CFR 7.3 (m)(3))*.

Regulatory Controls on Cosmetics

Cosmetics marketed in the United States, whether manufactured domestically or imported from abroad, must be in compliance with the provisions of the FD&C Act, the FPLA, and the regulations published under the authority of these laws. Yet, cosmetics are arguably the least regulated category of articles subject to the jurisdiction of the FD&C Act [16]. There is no premarket approval requirement for cosmetic products or their constituent ingredients under the law. Other than color additives and those few ingredients restricted or prohibited by regulation from use in cosmetics, no mandatory regulatory controls exist on the chemistry and structure substantiation of the ingredients themselves, conditions of manufacture of the finished cosmetic products, or safety testing that the ingredients and products must undergo prior to marketing; no premarket test results need be submitted to the FDA.

The FDA has therefore promulgated regulations and guidance documents to help ensure that only cosmetics that are safe for their intended use and are neither "adulterated" nor "misbranded" enter interstate commerce. These regulatory documents address the following issues.

Cosmetic Safety

Cosmetics are not currently subject to the same FDA safety and effectiveness standards as are drugs, biologics, and medical devices. The FD&C Act does not require that cosmetic manufacturers or marketers test their products for safety, nor does the FDA specify particular test batteries or preclinical (i.e., animal or in vitro alternative tests) and human clinical safety tests by cosmetic product category that marketers must use to substantiate cosmetic product safety. Neither are manufacturers or marketers of cosmetic products required to submit the results of such safety substantiation tests to the agency on a premarket approval basis. Nonetheless, the FDA strongly urges cosmetic manufacturers and/or raw material suppliers to conduct safety substantiation assessments and whatever toxicological or other tests are appropriate to substantiate the safety of their cosmetic products and the ingredients formulated therein prior to marketing them. If the safety of a cosmetic is not *"adequately substantiated,"* the product may be considered misbranded and may be subject to regulatory enforcement action unless the label bears the following statement, using the exclusivity language found at *21 CFR 740.10(a)*:

> *"Warning*—The safety of this product has not been determined."

Cosmetic Ingredients

The FD&C Act provides no statutory authority for the premarket approval of cosmetic ingredients. This is reflected in the FDA's regulations, which are generally silent on the subject of permitted or "positive listed" cosmetic ingredients. With the sole exception of color additives (see *21 CFR 70-82*), which are subject to premarket approval, and a few "negative listed" or prohibited/restricted ingredients at *21 CFR 700* and 21 CFR 250.250 (see Table 3), a cosmetic manufacturer may use virtually any raw material as a cosmetic ingredient (regardless of whether it was specifically designed for use in cosmetic end-use applications) and market the finished cosmetic product without premarket approval [18]. Of course, the marketer of the finished cosmetic product bears legal responsibility for any adverse reactions experienced by consumers or public health consequences that may result from this action. The number of ingredients used in cosmetics has grown exponentially since the early 1970s. For example, the *Eighth (8th) Edition* of the *CTFA*

TABLE 3   Cosmetic Ingredients Prohibited or Restricted in the United States[a]

By regulation (*21 CFR 700, 21 CFR 250.250*)
   Bithionol
   Mercury compounds
   Vinyl chloride
   Halogenated salicylanilides
   Zirconium complexes (aerosol cosmetics)
   Chloroform
   Methylene chloride
   Chlorofluorocarbon propellants
   Hexachlorophene[b]
Miscellaneous ingredients of regulatory concern[a]
   100% Liquid methyl methacrylate monomer (in nail products)[c]
   $\geq 5\%$ Formaldehyde (in nail products)
   Acetylmethyltetramethyltetralin (AETT) (in fragrances)
   Musk ambrette (MA) (in fragrances)
   6-Methylcoumarin (6-MC) (in fragrances)

[a] See *FDA's Cosmetics Handbook*, 1994 Edition, p. 8.
[b] *21 CFR 250.250.*
[c] *Source*: A.R. Halper to J. Nordstrom (President, Nail Manufacturers Council), personal communication, September 20, 1996.

International Cosmetic Ingredient Dictionary (CID) [19], one of the most authoritative tabulations of cosmetic ingredients, contains monographs for approximately 10,500 such raw materials (see Fig. 2).

Color Additives

The term "color additive" is defined in the FD&C Act at Section 201 (t) and by regulation at *21 CFR 70.3 (f)*. Except for "coal tar hair dyes" used to color the hair (of the scalp), the 1960 Color Additive Amendments to the FD&C Act require that color additives used in food, drugs, medical devices, and cosmetics be approved by the FDA for their intended use, a process that requires both chemistry and safety reviews of the color additive by color chemistry and toxicology staff experts at the FDA. A cosmetic containing an "unlisted" color additive (i.e., a color additive that has not been approved by the FDA for its intended use) is considered adulterated and subject to regulatory action. Color additives listed at *21 CFR 73* (predominantly of inorganic (mineral) or botanical origin) are exempt from the FDA's "batch certification" requirements (see *21 CFR 80*). Color additives listed at *21 CFR 74* are largely synthetic organic dyes and pigments (i.e., so-called "coal tar" colors) and are subject to the FDA's "batch certification" requirements at *21 CFR 80*; provisionally listed color additives, including color additive lakes, are listed at *21 CFR 82*. FDA recently published in the *Federal Register* a proposal to permanently list color additive lakes [20]; proposed simplifications in nomenclature for declaring straight colors and their lakes were also included as part of this proposal. It is important to note that all batches of certifiable color additives must actually be tested, certified in the FDA's laboratories for compliance with the identity and specifications established by regulation for that color additive, and issued a certification number before they may be represented and sold as an FDA-certified color additive.

FDA listing regulations for color additives specify permitted end-use applications, which may be general or specific in nature, sometimes with restrictions in permitted uses

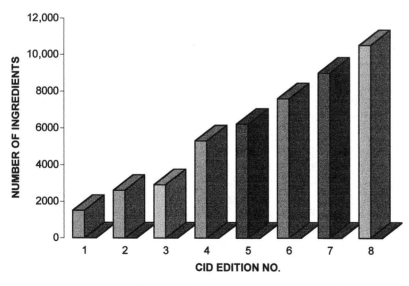

FIGURE 2 Cosmetic ingredient growth. (From J. A. Wenninger and R. C. Canterbery, personal communications.)

or allowed concentrations. Cosmetic color additives, for example, may be listed for general use in imparting color to product formulations, for use in decorative cosmetics intended for external application to the hair and other appendages of the human body (other than the area of the eye), or may be specifically listed, solely or together with other cosmetic product applications, for eye area use [21]. Only color additives specifically authorized by regulation for use in the area of the eye may be legally used for such applications. Only one color additive, dihydroxyacetone (DHA), is specifically listed for an intended use in externally applied cosmetics "to impart a color to the human body"; this finds widespread application in today's "sunless" or "self-tanning" cosmetic products [22]. No color additives are currently approved for use in injectable cosmetic tattoos [23]. Further details about the color additives currently listed (approved) by regulation for use in cosmetics in the United States may be found on the Internet at FDA's website (e.g., http://www.cfsan.fda.gov/cosmetics.html).

Cosmetic Labeling

Cosmetic products distributed in the United States must comply with the labeling regulations published by the FDA under the authority of the FD&C Act and the FPLA [24a]. Section 10(a) of the FPLA gives the FDA authority to require labeling of products considered "consumer commodities"; that is, products regulated under the FD&C Act, which are "customarily produced or distributed for sale through retail sales . . . for consumption by individuals, or use by individuals for purposes of personal care or in the performance of services ordinarily rendered within the household" [24b].

The statute requires that products be honestly and informatively labeled so that consumers can conduct "value comparisons" at the point of purchase; that is, in order to determine what ingredients are in a product and which product among several alternatives being considered for purchase is the best value. This determination includes medical considerations, since the FDA has previously concluded [25] that a cosmetic product or ingredient to which a consumer is allergic (and which the consumer therefore cannot use) has no value to such a consumer.

"Labeling" refers to actual product package labels as well as other written, printed, or graphic material on or accompanying a product (e.g., hangtags, promotional fliers, package inserts). Label statements required under the FD&C Act must appear on both the inside as well as the outside container or wrapper, if any; FPLA requirements need only appear on the label of the outer container or wrapper.

Cosmetic product package labeling regulations enacted under authority of the FD&C Act and/or the FPLA require that cosmetic labels bear certain fields of information that provide the consumer with proper identification and other data that will enhance the consumer's understanding of the product being purchased and facilitate the ability of the consumer to contact the manufacturer or distributor of the product, should there be a need to do so. Although the cosmetic labeling regulations at *21 CFR 701* generally require all labeling information to be written in the English language commonly understood by most American consumers, *21 CFR 701.2 (b)* also provides certain accommodations in the case of articles distributed in Puerto Rico or other territories in which the predominant language is other than English. The required fields of information include the following:

> *Statement of identity* (i.e., common name) rendered in bold type on the cosmetic product principal display panel; note that this is an FPLA requirement for cosmetics, not an FD&C Act requirement per se
> *Name and address of manufacturer* (or packer or distributor)

Net quantity of contents (net weight or count or measure, as customary or as required). English units are mandatory in the United States but a technical amendment to the FPLA under the 1991 American Technology Preeminence Act (ATPA), as revised in 1992 [26a,b], and more recent regulatory proposals to implement the ATPA provisions for FDA-regulated products [26c], now advocate the use of the most appropriate units of the metric international system (SI) of weights or measures, wherever practicable. This proposal includes the dual declaration of net quantity of contents in terms of both English units and the international metric (SI) system of weights or measures

Cosmetic ingredient label declarations (see below)

Warning statements (or cautionary statements) concerning safe use, as required at *21 CFR 740* (see below)

A typical cosmetic product package label exemplifying these features is shown in Figure 3.

Cosmetic Ingredient Label Declarations

Section 5(c)(3) of the FPLA specifically authorizes FDA to promulgate regulations requiring the declaration of all cosmetic ingredients on product package labels of cosmetics considered "consumer commodities" (*loc. cit.*, Ref. 24(b)); these regulations are codified at *21 CFR 701.3*. Exempt from the ingredient declaration requirement are professional cosmetic products, such as hair and skin preparations or makeup products used by cosmetologists, beauticians, or aestheticians on clients at professional establishments such as salons, spas, and theaters, provided that these products are not also sold to consumers through the professional establishments, workplaces, or other miscellaneous beauty supply retail outlets for their consumption at home; such cosmetics are not legally considered "consumer commodities." Similar exemptions apply to "free" (gratis) samples, gifts, cosmetics distributed as free amenities at hotels, and cosmetics and toiletries made available to workers and visitors (but not sold) for on-site use at occupational settings, such as construction sites, hospitals, clinics, etc. However, cosmetic products offered as "gift with purchase" are "consumer commodities" and subject to the ingredient declaration requirement, because the "gift" is only available in conjunction with a retail sale. Professional cosmetic products exempt from the ingredient declaration requirement are frequently labeled "for professional use only."

Ingredient declarations must be "conspicuous" and "prominent" in placement on any appropriate information panel of the outer container, and not less than certain size specifications in relationship to the size and shape of the product package, in order to ensure that the declaration is likely to be read at the time of purchase by the consumer.

FPLA labeling requirements specify that cosmetic ingredients must be declared, in descending order of predominance (see *21 CFR 701.3 [a]*), utilizing ingredient names derived in hierarchical order of precedence from the nomenclature sources specified by regulation (see *21 CFR 701.3 [c]* and *701.30*); alternatively, the ingredients may be grouped and the groups declared according to *21 CFR 701.3 (f)*. The "common or usual" names specified by regulation in the United States are required to be stated in the language understood by American consumers, namely English, except as provided at *21 CFR 701.2 (b)* (see Cosmetic Labeling, p. 746, loc. cit.). Cosmetic ingredients present at one percent or less (≤1%) may be declared after ingredients present at higher levels without regard to order of predominance, and fragrance and flavor, if any, being complex compositions of matter in themselves, may be declared for purposes of product package label-

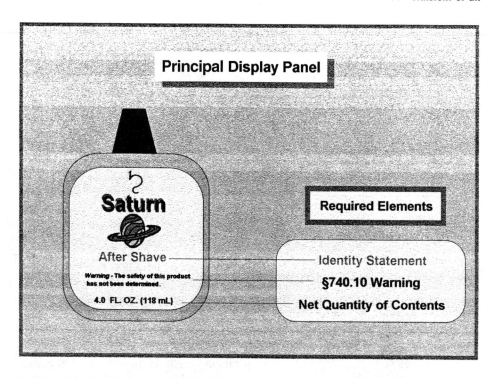

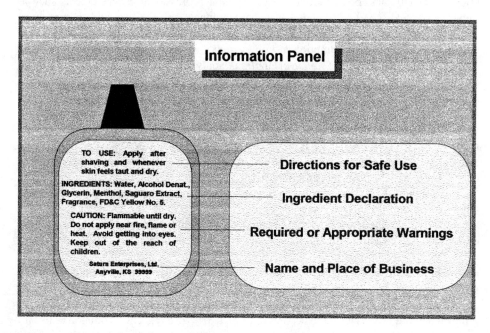

Figure 3   Typical cosmetic label elements. (Note: For illustrative purposes only. See *21 CFR 701* for correct letter heights and proportions.)

ing as "flavor" and "fragrance," respectively. "Incidental ingredients" (see *21 CFR 701.3 [1]*) need not be declared, and those ingredients accepted by the FDA as exempt from public disclosure and granted "confidentiality" or "trade secret" status may be declared as "and other ingredients" (see *21 CFR 720.8*).

"Soap" products meeting the requirements of *21 CFR 701.20(a)(1) and (a)(2)* are exempt from the FPLA requirement for mandatory label ingredient declarations applicable to cosmetics.

The manner of declaration of ingredients in OTC drug–cosmetic products is specified at *21 CFR 701.3(d)*, as recently amended (see 64 FR 13234–13303@13297, March 17, 1999). Drug "active ingredients" present in OTC drug–cosmetic product formulations are declared first, as required at *21 CFR 201.66(c)(2) and (d)* of this chapter, and following the standard-format "Drug Facts" information fields (i.e., "Use(s)," "Warnings," "Directions," and "Other Information"), any "inactive" or cosmetic ingredients are declared in descending order of predominance or grouped, in accordance with the provisions of *21 CFR 701.3(a) and (f)*, respectively. An exception in the manner of declaration of inactive or cosmetic ingredients is provided for, if there is a difference in the labeling provisions in *21 CFR 201.66* and Sections 701.3 or 720.8; under these circumstances, the labeling provisions at *21 CFR 201.66* are controlling (see *21 CFR 201.66(c)(8) and (d)* of this chapter).

Recent efforts to achieve "international harmonization" with cosmetic ingredient nomenclature standards required by the 1976 European Union (EU) Cosmetic Directive [27] and its more recent amendments [28] have resulted in the FDA agreeing to exercise regulatory discretion toward the interim use of parenthetical "dual declarations," employing systematic Linne (Latin) taxonomic genus/species nomenclature for certain categories of ingredients (i.e., botanicals and/or "trivial" ingredients) pending review of a citizen petition submitted by CTFA [29]. Color additives are named using the monograph titles in their respective listing regulations (see *21 CFR 73, 74, 82*), although, here, too, the impact of "international harmonization" efforts has resulted in the FDA agreeing to exercise regulatory discretion towards the interim use of parenthetical "color index (CI) numbers" in a dual declaration [29]. Examples of the new interim "harmonized" ingredient declarations are given in Table 4.

Cosmetic Label Warnings

Cosmetics that may be hazardous to consumers when misused must bear appropriate label warnings and adequate directions for safe use. Manufacturers and marketers of cosmetics have a general responsibility to ensure that the labels of their finished cosmetic products bear a warning statement whenever necessary or appropriate to prevent a health hazard that may be associated with the product (*21 CFR 740.1[a]*). These warning statements must be prominent and conspicuous (*21 CFR 740.2*). Some cosmetics must also bear more specific label warnings or cautions prescribed by regulation. Specific cosmetic product categories requiring such statements currently include:

> Cosmetic products for which adequate substantiation of safety has not been obtained (*21 CFR 740.10*)
> Cosmetics in self-pressurized containers (*21 CFR 740.11*)
> Feminine deodorant sprays (*21 CFR 740.12*)
> Foaming detergent bath products (*21 CFR 740.17*)
> "Coal tar" hair-dyes posing a risk of cancer (*21 CFR 740.18*) [*Effective date stayed at 47 FR 7829, February 23, 1982.*]

TABLE 4 Selected Examples of U.S. Cosmetic Labeling Names, EU Cosmetic Labeling Names, and Proposed Interim Harmonized Cosmetic Labeling Names

U.S. cosmetic ingredient (U.S. INCI labeling name)	EU cosmetic ingredient (EU INCI labeling name)	Proposed interim harmonization (EU/U.S. dual declaration)
Color additives		
FD&C Green No. 3	Cl 42053	Green 3 (Cl 42053)
D&C Orange No. 4	Cl 15510	Orange 4 (Cl 15510)
D&C Blue No. 1 Aluminum Lake	Cl 42090	Blue 1 Lake (Cl 42090)[a]
Ext. D&C Violet No. 2	Cl 60730	Ext. Violet 2 (Cl 60730)
Botanicals		
Peach leaf extract	Prunus persica	Peach (prunus persica) leaf extract
Sambucus nigra extract[b]	Sambucus nigra extract	Sambucus nigra extract
Sweet cherry pit oil	Prunus avium pit oil	Sweet cherry (prunus avium) pit oil
Oat flour	Avena sativa flour	Oat (avena sativa) flour
Denatured alcohols		
SD Alcohol 38B[c]	Alcohol denatured (Alcohol denat.)	Alcohol denatured (Alcohol denat.)
"Trivial" ingredients		
Water	Aqua	Water (aqua)
Fragrance	Parfum	Fragrance (parfum)
Tallow	Adeps bovis	Tallow (adeps bovis)
Yeast extract	Faex	Yeast (paex) extract
Goat milk	Caprae lac	Goat milk (caprae lac)
Beeswax	Cera alba	Beeswax (cera alba)
Honey	Mel	Honey (mel)
Sea salt	Maris sal	Sea salt (maris sal)
Egg oil	Ovum	Egg (ovum) oil
Silk powder	Serica	Silk (serica) powder
Mineral oil	Paraffinum liquidum	Mineral oil (paraffinum liquidum)
Coal tar	Pix ex carbone	Coal tar (pix ex carbone)
Fish extract	Pisces	Fish (pisces) extract
Pigskin extract	Sus	Pigskin (sus) extract
Mink oil	Mustela	Mink (mustela) oil

[a] Annex IV of the EEC Cosmetic Directive 76/768/EEC provides that, for those color additives allowed for use in cosmetic products, the lakes or salts of these coloring agents using substances not prohibited under Annex II or not excluded under Annex V from the scope of the Directive are equally allowed and may also be declared under the same Color Index Number as for the corresponding straight color additive.

[b] Certain botanical (plant) ingredients may have Linne System (Latin genus/species) names that have no English language 'common or usual name' equivalents.

[c] *27 CFR 21.*

Cosmetic suntanning preparations not containing a sunscreen (*21 CFR 740.19*) [*Effective date: May 22, 2000.*]

Tamper-Resistant Packaging

The FDA is given the authority under Sections 601 (a) and (c) and 701 (a) of the FD&C Act to issue package security requirements for cosmetics. Requirements for tamper-resistant packaging for *cosmetic liquid oral hygiene products* (e.g., mouthwashes and breath fresheners) and all *cosmetic vaginal products* (e.g., douches and tablets) were promulgated at *21 CFR 700.25*. Details about such packaging is found in the FDA's *Cosmetics Handbook* [30] and at the FDA website, *http://www.fda.gov.*

Cosmetic Good Manufacturing Practices Guidelines

The FDA has never published current good manufacturing practice (cGMP) regulations for cosmetics, although the agency has actively promoted good manufacturing practices by firms marketing cosmetics in the United States. The agency has published *Cosmetic Good Manufacturing Practice Guidelines*, patterned in pertinent part after the food cGMP regulations [13a] but applicable to the cosmetic manufacturing environment, in the FDA's Cosmetics Handbook [13b]; the latter document references the *FDA Investigation Operations Manual (IOM)* [31]. The *Cosmetic Good Manufacturing Practice Guidelines* is a guidance document reflecting FDA policy, but it is not legally binding, either on the cosmetics industry or on the agency. The FDA has also published drug cGMP regulations [32], which apply to prescription drugs and cosmetic–drugs (i.e., OTC drug products making cosmetic claims).

The Voluntary Cosmetic Registration Program

The FD&C Act does not require cosmetic firms to register manufacturing establishments or formulations with the FDA, nor does it mandate that companies submit product adverse reaction report data. Nevertheless, the FDA has encouraged the voluntary registration of such data as being in the public interest and consistent with the spirit of responsible ''self-regulation'' advocated by the cosmetic industry. In the early 1970s, the FDA developed a three-part system of regulations, under which manufacturers or distributors of cosmetics may submit this information to the agency on a voluntary basis [33]. The three parts of the *Voluntary Cosmetic Registration Program (VCRP)* originally comprised the following:

Part I *Cosmetic Establishment Registration Program (CERP)*, requests that cosmetic manufacturing sites be registered with the FDA (see *21 CFR 710*)

Part II *Cosmetic Product Ingredient Statements (CPIS)*, requests that cosmetic formulations and cosmetic raw material composition statements be registered with the FDA (see *21 CFR 720*). This regulation also set forth the 13 product category codes (PCC) at *21 CFR 720.4* recognized by the FDA as ''cosmetic'' functions. Semi-quantitative raw material disclosures were abandoned and purged from the VCRP database in the early 1990s [34].

Part III *Product Experience Reports (PER),* discontinued in 1996 (35), requested the annual filing of ''reportable'' adverse reactions (see *21 CFR 700.3 [q]*) to the use of cosmetic products by manufacturers which the FDA (euphemistically called 'product experiences' (see *21 CFR 730*). The use of optional 'screening' protocols to be filed with the FDA, designed by individual manufacturers, for use in determining the 'reportability' of experiences, was also provided for in the PER Program (see *21 CFR 700.3 (p), 730.4 (d)(2)*). This data was collected, tabulated, and analyzed for statistical deviations of individual products from industry-wide adverse reaction trends by product category.

Despite its voluntary nature, the VCRP has never enjoyed full industry participation. Table 5 illustrates the VCRP registration statistics for the years 1992–1996, the last five fiscal years during which all parts of the VCRP were in operation. *Part III (PER)* annual filings by firms considered by the FDA to be eligible to participate in the program have

TABLE 5 FDA Voluntary Cosmetic Registration Program (VCRP), FY 1992–FY 1996

	FY 1992	FY 1993	FY 1994	FY 1995	FY 1996
Establishments registered	939	969	954	757	773
Companies filing formulations	800	782	810	806	684
Formulations registered	18,012	18,369	16,929	18,558	15,982
Companies filing product experience reports	114	116	113	97	75

FY, Fiscal Year
Source: J. E. Bailey, Ph.D., personal communication, July 7, 2000.

historically been the lowest of the three parts of the VCRP. *Part III (PER)* was discontinued in 1996 [35] and the VCRP itself was temporarily put into operational abeyance in 1998 due to resource re-allocations within the FDA [36]. With partial funding restoration by the Congress "earmarked" specifically for the FDA's Cosmetics Program, Parts I and II of the VCRP were restarted in 1999 [37], and a new, streamlined electronic World Wide Web-based system to facilitate industry participation is being developed at the time of this writing [38].

Self-Regulation

As the cosmetic industry in the United States has grown and matured, the regulatory paradigm for cosmetics in the United States has evolved from a program based on the *1938 FD&C Act* and lacking Federal pre-market approval authority into a leveraged program of industry "self-regulation," with shared roles played by the FDA's other stakeholders, particularly the cosmetic industry trade associations and consumer advocacy groups. Programs that support industry self-regulation have been initiated by both government and private industry; they include:

> The *FDA Voluntary Cosmetic Registration Program (VCRP) (loc. cit.)*;
> The *Cosmetic Ingredient Review (CIR)*. Originated in the 1970s as a cosmetic industry initiative [39], CIR is a program funded by the CTFA that assesses the safety of cosmetic ingredients, with full albeit *ex-officio* (non-voting) liaison participation by the FDA, industry, and consumer advocate stakeholders. The CIR does not generally assess the safety profiles of ingredients that are reviewed by the FDA as "active ingredients" of drugs (OTC or prescription), nor does it conduct safety assessments of fragrance materials;
> The *Research Institute for Fragrance Materials (RIFM)* evaluates the safety profiles and publishes monographs concerning fragrance materials, while the *International Fragrance Association (IFRA)*, a trade association of national fragrance trade associations, establishes usage guidelines for fragrance materials by industry fragrance houses [40].

The FDA's VCRP and the industry-sponsored *CIR* and *RIFM/IFRA* programs are important components of the government-industry cooperation that characterize current efforts towards the successful implementation of self-regulation of the cosmetic industry in the U.S. Other elements of self-regulation include:

> *Federal Statutes.* The *Lanham Act (1946)* empowers companies to seek judicial redress in the federal district courts for unfair business practices resulting in negative impact on market share [41]. The *Robinson-Patman Act (1936)* enables companies to seek to recoup lost sales and profits ascribed to anticompetitive, predatory pricing tactics [42].
>
> *Advertising Self-Regulation*, NAD/CBBB. Disagreements regarding product performance advertising claims are frequently addressed by competitor/peer-review challenges brought through the self-regulatory protocols of the *National Advertising Division (NAD)*, an arm of the *Council of Better Business Bureaus (CBBB)* [43], and its appeals panel, the *National Advertising Review Board (NARB)*. Failure to resolve advertising controversies through these self-regulatory processes can result in an ultimate referral by the NARB to the FTC. Scrutiny of proposed storyboards prior to being accepted for mass-media air-time is also undertaken by advertising agency legal departments and television/radio network standards and practices boards (e.g., network censors) [44]

The cosmetic industry is characterized by highly competitive marketing strategies and depends on the freedom to rapidly introduce new, innovative cosmetic products to the marketplace without lengthy delays. It is hardly surprising, therefore, that the industry has sought to portray itself as responsible enough to self-police its own manufacturing and marketing practices, or that it has argued [45] that existing laws and FDA regulatory programs concerning cosmetics, together with the industry's commitment to self-regulation and product safety, provide ample consumer protection, given the apparent low risk inherent in cosmetics relative to other categories of products regulated by the FDA. Steinberg [46] advocates compliance within a self-regulatory environment as being in the industry's own self-interest. He observes that regulatory compliance can be a "win-win" end result for the industry, consumers, and regulators alike, and cautions that trying to *"beat the system may succeed in the short term, but it results in significant long-term losses."* Steinberg notes that lost sales, public reputation, and market share are the obvious short-term consequences likely to be suffered by noncompliant firms. Widespread noncompliance can also place the current self-regulatory system itself at risk.

International Harmonization and Future Regulatory Challenges

The U.S. regulatory scheme for cosmetics is based on the axiom that cosmetics marketed in the U.S. are safe for their intended use and unlikely to present a major public health risk [47], which is reflected in the lack of pre-market approval authority for cosmetics included in the original 1938 FD&C Act.

Although many of the regulatory systems of other countries have similar goals to those of the United States, such as protecting public health and safety and promoting trade [48], the means by which these goals are achieved may be quite different from the U.S. system. These differences are often based upon the culture of the particular country and can influence not only specific regulatory requirements, such as labeling, but also the fundamental definition of what constitutes a cosmetic. Several categories of topical prod-

ucts regulated as OTC drugs or OTC drug–cosmetics in the United States, such as sunscreens, skin bleaches, antiperspirants, and antidandruff shampoos [49], are regulated as
cosmetics under the EU Cosmetics Directive of 1976 [27]. Japan, which currently regulates
cosmetics according to a system of premarket approval and licensure rather than the postmarket surveillance system used by the United States or the notification system used by
the EU, allows cosmetics to have some effect on the structure and function of the skin
and hair, provided that the effect is "mild" and provides for a third "quasi-drug" category
of product accommodating "mild," borderline physiological effects, such as hair-growth
promoters [50a]. However, initiatives currently underway in Japan promise to alter the
regulation of cosmetics by shifting to a postmarketing system more nearly aligned with
those in effect in the U.S. and E.U. [50b]. Some regulatory systems currently reflect features of both the U.S. and EU systems; this is true, for example, of the system operative
in Canada [50c]. In some cases, the concept of a regional consortium is being employed
to facilitate international cooperation (such as the Andean Pact and Mercosur groups of
nations in South America) [50d,e]. Still other third-world national regulatory systems are
currently being updated, often using the U.S. or EU regulatory systems as models, to
afford their citizens increased levels of protection.

The unprecedented growth experienced by the cosmetic industry in the 1980s and
1990s has also had its impact on international cosmetic regulation. Corporate consolida-
tions and acquisitions of American companies and domestic product brands by foreign-
based corporations have refashioned the concept of multinational corporations. The economic imperatives of these new "world-class" companies—to expand market penetration
and market share in global overseas markets—have resulted in regulatory challenges in
the international marketplace.

The modification of existing legislation that is viewed as an impediment to international trade, with a goal of alignment and harmonization of national laws and cosmetic
regulations, has emerged as a central tenet of recent and current international negotiations.
Hendrick and Horton [51] observe that:

> Precisely because the regulatory requirements of different countries vary considerably,
> harmonization of regulations among countries is a worthy goal. As we move toward a
> global economy with more countries placing an emphasis on imports and exports, harmo-
> nization would assist in the reduction of barriers to trade.

The United States, a member of the World Trade Organization (WTO) since its formation
in 1995, is a signatory to two principal international trade agreements that are relevant to
the marketing of cosmetics and other FDA-regulated products: the General Agreement
on Tariffs and Trade (GATT) and the North American Free Trade Agreement (NAFTA).
Both the GATT and NAFTA Agreements contain separate agreements on Technical Barriers to Trade (TBT) and Sanitary and Phytosanitary Measures (SBS), whose provisions
seek to eliminate regulations, product standards, and procedures that constitute artificial
technical barriers to trade. Both, however, also reserve to sovereign signatory states the
right to determine whatever level of public health protection they believe necessary for
the benefit of their citizens, agriculture, and environment. In the United States, these initiatives have become important "pillars" of the Vice President's *National Performance
Review (NPR)*, and the FDA, as an agency of the executive branch, has fully supported
these initiatives across all agency programs.

The FDA's policy on the international harmonization of regulatory requirements
and guidelines was published in the *Federal Register* in 1995 [52]; additionally, Section

410(b) of the 1997 FDA Modernization Act (FDAMA) requires that the FDA support the Office of the U.S. Trade Representative (USTR) in meeting with other countries for the purposes of harmonizing regulatory approaches and achieving mutual recognition agreements, to the extent harmonization continues the consumer protections consistent with the FD&C Act [52c]. Agency goals are to simultaneously facilitate international trade and promote mutual understanding, while protecting national interests and establishing a model for resolving issues on the basis of sound scientific evidence in an objective atmosphere. The agency is committed to working toward facilitating the exchange of scientific and regulatory information and knowledge with foreign government officials, and accepting the equivalent standards, compliance activities, and enforcement programs of other countries, provided that the FDA is satisfied such standards, activities, and programs meet the FDA's level of public health protection. However, the FDA is equally committed to the thesis that harmonization activities must not result in a lowering of the gate to furtherance of public health protections afforded by U.S. law (e.g., ''downward harmonization'').

The FDA Office of Cosmetics and Colors (OCAC), which is responsible for administering the cosmetics provisions of the FD&C Act, is committed to seeking implementation of the U.S. Government policies on international harmonization. Outreach conferences with regulatory authorities in Israel, the Andean Pact nations, the EU, Canada, Japan, China, and others have sought to achieve international harmonization through identifying areas of commonality among the regulatory schemes in the various administrations, rather than hoping to arrive at a single global regulatory structure. In particular, two quadrilateral *Cosmetic Harmonization and International Cooperation (C.H.I.C.)* conferences between the United States, the European Union, Canada, and Japan, held in 1999 and 2000, have identified a number of areas of mutual interest, concerning which discussions are continuing at the present time; these areas of mutual interest include:

Memoranda of cooperation (MOC)
Regulatory reform
Animal testing
Cosmetic ingredient nomenclature
Approved color additives
Sunscreens
Drug–cosmetics and quasi-drugs
Safety substantiation
Fragrance allergenicity
International adverse event safety ''alert system''

Further details about the second C.H.I.C. meeting are posted on the FDA's website at the Cosmetics Program Homepage (*http://www.cfsan.fda.gov/cosmetics.html*).

ACKNOWLEDGMENTS

The authors wish to acknowledge the professional assistance in designing the hypothetical product package label for ''Saturn After-Shave Cologne'' by Ms. Donnie K. Lowther, Cosmetic Toxicology Branch, Division of Science and Applied Technology, Office of Cosmetics and Colors. The expert consultations and aid given by Ms. Beth R. Meyers, Technical Editor, Division of Programs and Enforcement Policy, Office of Cosmetics and Colors, FDA-CFSAN in formatting the tables in this chapter and in proofreading this manuscript are also very significant contributions and are deeply appreciated and acknowledged by the authors. Additional guidance by Mr. Richard Jewell, Compliance Officer in the Office of Cosmetics and Colors, and Mr. Charles R. Haynes, Consumer Safety Officer in the Office of Cosmetics and Colors, with respect to field cosmetic inspectional policy and the *Cosmetic Good Manufacturing Practice Guidelines* is also gratefully acknowledged.

DISCLAIMER

The views expressed herein are those of the authors and do not necessarily represent those of the FDA.

REFERENCES AND NOTES

1. a) Jackson EM. Consumer products: cosmetics and topical over-the-counter drug products. In: Chengelis CP, Holson JF, Gad SC, eds. Regulatory Toxicology. New York: Raven Press, 1995:117–119; b) McEwen GN, Murphy EG. The Federal Food, Drug, and Cosmetic Act and the Regulation of Cosmetics. In: Schlossman, ML, ed., The Chemistry and Manufacture of Cosmetics, Volume I, Basic Science, Carol Stream, IL: Allured Publishing Corporation, 2000, p. 82.
2. Hobbs CO. Advertising for foods, veterinary products, and cosmetics. In: Brady RP, Cooper RM, Silverman RS, eds. Fundamentals of Law and Regulation. Vol. 1. Washington, D.C.: Food and Drug Law Institute (FDLI), 1997:347–379.
3. a) Working Agreement Between FTC and FDA, FTC Press Release, Federal Trade Commission, Washington, D.C. June 9, 1954. b) Memorandum of Understanding (MOU) Between the Federal Trade Commission and the Food and Drug Administration Concerning Exchange of Information (FDA-225-71-8003), FDA Compliance Policy Guide 7155m.01, April 27, 1971 (FDA); Approved and Accepted for the FTC May 14, 1971.
4. a) Poison Prevention Packaging Act of 1970 (15 U.S.C. 1471 n, Public Law 91-601, 84 Stat. 1670, December 30, 1970, as amended). b) Household Products Containing Petroleum Distillates and Other Hydrocarbons; Advance Notice of Proposed Rulemaking, 62 FR 8659, February 26, 1997. c) Requirements for Child-Resistant Packaging; Household Products Containing Methacrylic Acid; Proposed Rule, 63 FR 71800, December 30, 1998. d) Requirements for Child-Resistant Packaging; Requirements for Household Glue Removers Containing Acetonitrile and Home Cold Wave Permanent Neutralizers Containing Sodium Bromate or Potassium Bromate, 55 FR 51897, December 18, 1990; e) T.E. Wood, "Regulatory Considerations for Soap Products in the U.S.A.," *Cosmetics and Toiletries,* **104**(12), 75–76, 78–79 (1989); f) Consumer Product Safety Act, 15 U.S.C. Sec. 2051 et. seq. (Pub. L. No. 92-573, October 27, 1972); g) Federal Hazardous Substances Act, 15 U.S.C., Sec. 1261 et. seq. (Pub. L. No. 86-613, July 12, 1960, as amended); codified regulations at 16 CFR 1500.
5. Federal Insecticide, Fungicide, and Rodenticide Act of 1972 (FIFRA, 7 U.S.C. Sec. 136-136 y); codified regulations at 40 CFR 162–180.
6. FD&C Act, Section 201 (p) (definitions, "new drug").
7. a) Liquid soap category will reach $250 million by 1985. In: The Rose Sheet (June 29, 1981), p. 3. b) SoftSoap expected to add $65 million to Colgate-Palmolive's, ibid, August 17, 1987: 2–3.
8. a) Antiseptic wash monograph directions with manufacturer reference suggested. In: The Rose Sheet. February 10, 1997, p. 6–7. b) Fischler G., Shaffer M. Healthcare continuum: a model for the classification and regulation of topical antimicrobial wash products. The Healthcare Continuum Model Symposium, Washington, D.C., June 2–3, 1997.
9. (a) FD&C Act, Section 601 (a). (b) Hair-dye products. In: FDA's Cosmetics Handbook. Wash-

ington, D.C.: U.S. Government Printing Office, 1992, pp. 11–12; (c) 21 CFR 70.3 (u); (d) 21 CFR 73.2150; (e) 21 CFR 70.5(a).

10. a) Nitrosamine-contaminated cosmetics; call for industry action; request for data; notice, 44 FR 21365-21367, April 10, 1979. b) *FDA's Cosmetics Handbook*. Washington, D.C.: U.S. Government Printing Office, 1992, p. 8–9. c) Greif M, Wenninger JA, Yess N. Cosmetic regulation: an overview of FDA's role. Cosmetic Technology, 1980:43–44. d) Chou HJ. Determination of diethanolamine and N-nitrosodiethanolamine in fatty acid diethanolamines. J. of AOAC International. 1998:81(5), 943–947. e) Havery DC, Chou HJ. N-nitrosamines in cosmetic products: an overview. Cosmetics and Toiletries 1994:109(5), 53–58, 61–62.

11. Ref. 10 b., loc cit., p. 9.

12. a) Ref. 10, p. 9, *loc cit.*; b) RE Black, FJ Hurley, and DC Havery, ''Determination of 1,4-Dioxane in Ethoxylated Cosmetic Raw Materials and in Cosmetic Finished Products,'' *J of AOAC International*, 84 (2001), accepted for publication (in press).

13. a) 21 CFR 110.3–110.93. b) Cosmetic good manufacturing practice guidelines. In: FDA's Cosmetics Handbook. Washington, D.C.: U.S. Government Printing Office, 1992, p. 4–6.

14. a) Halper AR to Milstein SR, personal communication, February 1, 2000. b) Food and Drug Administration Recall Policies. Informational flier. U.S. Department of Health and Human Services, Public Health Service, Food and Drug Administration, Center for Food Safety and Applied Nutrition, Washington, D.C.

15. Calogero C. Regulatory review, Cosmetics and Toiletries, 2000; 115(7):26.

16. a) Duffy DT. Classification and regulation of cosmetics and drugs: a legal overview and alternatives for legislative change,'' American Law Division, Congressional Research Service, The Library of Congress, Washington, D.C., May 4, 1990, p. CRS-16. b) Yingling GL, Onel S. Cosmetic regulation revisited. In: Brady RP, Cooper RM, Silverman RS, eds. Fundamentals of Law and Regulation. Vol. 1. Washington, D.C.: Food and Drug Law Institute (FDLI), 1997: 315–346. c) Bass IS. Enforcement powers of the Food and Drug Administration: foods, dietary supplements, and cosmetics'', *ibid*, 55–90; d) E.G. Murphy and P.J. Wilson, Regulation of cosmetic products. In Williams DF and Schmitt WH, eds., Chemistry and Technology of the Cosmetics and Toiletries Industry, 2nd Edition, London: Blackie Academic & Professional, 1996:344–361.

17. Rumore MM, Strauss S, Kothari AB. Regulatory aspects of color additives. Pharmaceutical Technology. 68, 70, 72, 74, 76, 78, 80, 82. March 1992.

18. FDA's Cosmetics Handbook. Washington, D.C.: U.S. Government Printing Office, 1992, p. 2.

19. Wenninger JA, Canterbery RC, McEwen GN. International Cosmetic Ingredient Dictionary and Handbook, 8th Edition. Washington, D.C.: The Cosmetic, Toiletry, and Fragrance Association, (CTFA), 1999.

20. Permanent Listing of Color Additive Lakes; Proposed Rule, 61 FR 8372–8417, March 4, 1996.

21. 21 CFR 70.5 (a).

22. 21 CFR 73.1150; 21 CFR 73.2150.

23. 21 CFR 70.5 (b).

24. a) The Federal Fair Packaging and Labeling Act, 15 U.S.C. Sec. 1451 et. seq. b) 15 U.S.C. Sec. 1459 a (definitions).

25. Cosmetic Ingredient Labeling and Voluntary Filing of Cosmetic Product Experiences. Regulations for the Enforcement of the Federal Food, Drug and Cosmetic Act and the Fair Packaging Labeling Act. Cosmetic Ingredient Labeling. 38 FR 28912-28917 @28912, October 17, 1973.

26. a) The American Technology Preeminence Act of 1991 [Pub. L. 102–245, Section 107], February 14, 1992. b) Pub. L. 102–329, August 3, 1992. c) Metric Labeling; Quantity of Contents Labeling Requirements for Foods, Human and Animal Drugs, Animal Foods, Cosmetics, and Medical Devices; Proposed Rule. 58 FR 67444-67464, December 21, 1993.

27. Council Directive 76/768/EEC on the Approximation of the Member States Relating to Cos-

metic Products, OJECNI, 169, 262 (July 27, 1976) (hereinafter referred to as the Cosmetic Directive).

28. Council Directive 93/35/EEC (June 14, 1993) (hereinafter, referred to as the Sixth Amendment to the Cosmetic Directive).

29. Bailey JE to McEwen GN, personal communication June 1, 1995. b) Citizen Petition [Docket No. 96P-0347], September 20, 1996; c) *ibid*, personal communication, January 17, 1996.

30. Tamper-Resistant Packaging Requirements; Certain Over-the-Counter Human Drugs and Cosmetic Products; Contact Lens Solutions and Tablets; Final Rules. 47 FR 50442-50456 @ 50447, November 5, 1982.

31. a) FDA Office of Regulatory Affairs. FDA Investigations Operations Manual. Washington, D.C., January 2000, Chapter 10—reference materials, subchapter 1020—guidelines and other guidance materials, Section 1023—cosmetics. b) Guide to Inspections of Cosmetic Product Manufacturers. FDA/ORA Web site address: http://www.fda.gpv/ora/inspect_ref/igs/cosmet.html.

32. a) Beyond approval: drug manufacturer regulatory responsibilities. In: Mathieu M. New Drug Development: A Regulatory Overivew, 4th Ed. Waltham, MA: PAREXEL International Corporation, 1997:272–279. b) 21 CFR. 211 (Current Good Manufacturing Practice for Finished Pharmaceuticals), April 1, 2000.

33. a) Subchapter G—Cosmetics. Reorganization and Republication. 39 FR 10054-10064 @ 1059-10062, March 15, 1974. b) Modification in Voluntary Registration of Cosmetic Industry Data. Final Rule. 46 FR 38073-38074, July 24, 1981. c) Modification of Voluntary Filing of Cosmetic Product Experiences. Final Rule. 51 FR 25687, July 16, 1986.

34. Modification in Voluntary Filing of Cosmetic Product Ingredient and Cosmetic Raw Material Composition Statements. Final Rule, 57 FR 3128-3130, January 28, 1992.

35. Food and Cosmetic Labeling; Revocation of Certain Regulations. Final Rule. 62 FR 43071-43075 @ 43073, August 12, 1997.

36. a) Voluntary Cosmetics Registration Program: Suspension of Activity—March 30, 1998. (Letter to Industry Participants, Department of Health and Human Services, Public Health Service, Food and Drug Administration). b) FDA Cosmetics Office registration program suspended. The Rose Sheet, April 6, 1998, p. 1.

37. Voluntary cosmetics registration program reinstated with no changes. The Rose Sheet, January 11, 1999, p. 3.

38. VCRP reporting incentives to boost industry participation considered. The Rose Sheet, November 15, 1999, pp. 8–9.

39. Bergfeld WF, Elder RL, Schroeter AL. The cosmetic ingredient review self-regulatory safety program. Dermatologic Clinics 1991; 9(1):105–122.

40. Ford RA. The toxicology and safety of fragrances. In: Muller PM, Lamparsky D, eds. Perfumes, Art, Science, and Technology, London and New York: Elsevier Applied Science, 1991: 441–463.

41. a) Morrison T. Using the Lanham Act to achieve truth in advertising. Drug & Cosmetic Industry (DCI), 24, 26, 28, 30, 32, 81–83, April 1989. b) Donegan TJ. Section 43 (a) of the Lanham Trademark Act as a private remedy for false advertising. Food Drug Cosmetic Law Journal 1982; 37:264–288.

42. a) Government regulation of competition and pricing. In: Anderson RA, Fox I, Twomey DP. Business Law & The Legal Environment. Comprehensive Volume (16th Edition). Cincinnati, OH: South-Western College Publishing, 1996, pp. 60–68. b) Antitrust issues and pricing strategy (discriminatory pricing). In: Stern LW, Eovaldi TL. Legal Aspects of Marketing Strategy: Antitrust and Consumer Protection Issues. Englewood Cliffs, NJ: Prentice-Hall, 1984, pp. 263–279.

43. a) National Advertising Division, Children's Advertising Review Unit, & National Advertising Review Board Procedures (June 10, 1993). New York: Council of Better Business Bureaus, 1996. b) Smithies RH. Substantiating performance claims. Cosmetics and Toiletries 1984; 99(3):79–81, 84.

44. a) The social and legal impact of advertising. In: Bovee CL, Arens WF. Contemporary Advertising. Homewood, IL: Richard D. Irwin, 1982, pp. 60–86. b) Handler J. The self-regulatory system—an advertiser's viewpoint. Food Drug Cosmetic Law Journal 1982; 37:257–263.

45. McNamara SH. The 'C' in the FDC Act. FDA CONSUMER 1981; 15(5):62–63.

46. a) Steinberg DC. Compliance with self-regulation. Cosmetics and Toiletries, 2000; 115(4): 37–40.

47. Hendrick BS, Horton LR. International harmonization of cosmetic regulation. In: Brady RP, Cooper RM, Silverman RS, eds. Fundamentals of Law and Regulation. Vol. 1. Washington, D.C. Food, Drug, and Law Institute (FDLI), 1997:485–505.

48. Ibid, p. 488.

49. a) Sunscreen Drug Products for Over-the-Counter Human Use; Final Monograph. Final Rule. 64 FR 27666-27693, May 21, 1999. b) Skin Bleaching Drug Products for Over-the-Counter Human Use; Tentative Final Monograph; Notice of Proposed Rulemaking. 47 FR 39108-39117, September 3, 1982. c) Antiperspirant Drug Products for Over-the-Counter Human Use; Tentative Final Monograph; Proposed Rule. 47 FR 36492-36505, August 20, 1982. d) Dandruff, Sebborheic Dermatitis, and Psoriasis Drug Products for Over-the-Counter Human Use; Final Rule. 56 FR 63554-63569, December 4, 1991 (as amended as 59 FR 4000, January 28, 1994).

50. a) Santucci LG, Rempe JM. Legislation and safety regulations for cosmetics in the United States, Europe, and Japan. In: Butler H, ed. Poucher's Perfumes, Cosmetics, and Soaps, 9th Edition. Vol. 3. London: Chapman & Hall, 1993:566–571. b) Steinberg DC. Global understanding 2000. Toward global harmonization of cosmetic regulation. Cosmetics and Toiletries, 2000; 115 (8):27. c) Ref. 47, op. cit., p. 496–498. d) Anon., Minutes of the Third Summit of the Public Health Authorities of the Americas, Lima, Peru, June 15–16, 2000. e) Ref. 47, op. cit., p. 498–501.

51. Ref. 47, op. cit., p. 504.

52. a) International Harmonization; Draft Policy on Standards; Availability; Notice. 59 FR 60870-60874 (November 28, 1994). b) International Harmonization; Policy on Standards; Notice. 60 FR 53078-53084 (October 11, 1995); c) Food and Drug Administration Modernization Act of 1997 (Pub. L. No. 105–115, November 15, 1997).

62

Legislation in Japan

Mitsuteru Masuda
Lion Corporation, Tokyo, Japan

REGULATORY ENVIRONMENT

The cosmetic regulations in Japan are extensive and complex [1]. The legal classification of topically applied products is different from the United States and the European Union, where they are divided into only two categories: drugs and cosmetics. In Japan, there are additional regulations covering cosmetic products with pharmacological action, called quasidrugs, which are ranked between cosmetics and drugs [2]. Under the Pharmaceutical Affairs Law, cosmetics, as well as drugs and quasidrugs, are also subject to premarket clearance by the Ministry of Health and Welfare (MHW) [1]. The definitions of drugs, cosmetics, and quasidrugs in the regulations [3] read as follows:

Drugs are defined as:

1. Articles recognized in the official Japanese Pharmacopoeia.
2. Articles (other than quasidrugs) that are intended for use in the diagnosis, cure, or prevention of disease in man or animals, and that are not equipment or instruments (including dental materials, medical supplies, and sanitary materials).
3. Articles (other than quasidrugs and cosmetics) that are intended to affect the structure or any function of the body of man or animals, and that are not equipment or instruments (Paragraph 1, Article 2 of the Law).

Quasidrugs are articles that have the purposes given as follows and exert mild actions on the human body, or similar articles designated by the Minister of Health and Welfare. They exclude not only equipment and instruments, but also any article intended, in addition to the following purposes, for the use of drugs previously described in (2) and (3).

1. Prevention of nausea or other discomfort, foul breath, or body odor.
2. Prevention of prickly heat, sores, and the like.
3. Prevention of hair loss, restoration of hair, or depilation of unwanted hair.
4. Killing or prevention of rats, flies, mosquitoes, fleas, etc. for maintaining the health of man or animals (Paragraph 2, Article 2 of the Law).

Quasidrugs designated by the Minister of Health and Welfare (Notification No. 14, 1961), include cotton products intended for sanitary purposes (including paper cotton), as well as the following products with a mild action on the human body:

1. Hair dyes
2. Agents for permanent waving
3. Products that combine the purposes of use as stipulated in Paragraph 3, Article 2 of the Law (on cosmetics), with the purposes of prevention of acne, chapping, itchy skin rash, chilblain, etc., as well as disinfection of the skin and mouth
4. Bath preparations

Among the products just described, the third category comprises the so-called medicated cosmetics.

The term ''cosmetics'' means any article intended to be used by means of rubbing, sprinkling, or by similar application to the human body for cleaning, beautifying, promoting attractiveness, altering the appearance of the human body, and for keeping the skin and hair healthy, provided that the action of the article on the human body is mild. Such articles exclude the articles intended, besides the aforementioned purposes, for the use of drugs previously described in (2) or (3), and quasidrugs (Paragraph 3, Article 2 of the Law).

COSMETICS

At each stage of development, manufacture/import, distribution, and use, the prescribed regulations are put into practice, including systems of the examination for approval, manufacture/importation, distribution control, and postmarketing surveillance, respectively [3].

Procedures for premarket clearance have been simplified. As a series of steps for streamlining the cosmetic approval and licensing system, cosmetics using ingredients listed in the Comprehensive Licensing Standard of Cosmetics by Category (CLS) and that are in compliance with the Standards established, do not require approval but require a license by category (Table 1) [4–6]. Licensing will be granted by category according to the CLS [7]. As for the cosmetic product category, there were 35 separate categories at one time. These were reduced to 25 in 1994 and integrated into 11 in 1997 (Table 1) [6]. Additions to and review of the cosmetic ingredients list have recently been made almost at annual intervals. On the other hand, cosmetics using ingredients that are not in compliance with the CLS require approval by category, and a prior evaluation is conducted of the particulars indicated in the application filed for approval [4,5]. The following cosmetics are included in this group [7]:

- Cosmetics containing new ingredient or ingredient not listed in the CLS.
- Cosmetics containing ingredient in a larger quantity exceeding the upper limit specified in the CLS.
- Cosmetics containing ingredient not listed in the intended category of the CLS, but in another category of the CLS.
- Cosmetics whose method of use, etc., are clearly different from the cosmetics defined in the CLS.
- Cosmetics containing hormones; these products are not included in the CLS, and an application for approval must be made.

The following data must be attached to the application where appropriate (these are especially required for cosmetics containing a new ingredient):

TABLE 1 The Categories of Cosmetic Products

Categories	Definition of the products
Cleansing preparations	Exclusively used for cleansing
Haircare preparations	Exclusively used on the hair and scalp
Treatment preparations	Used for keeping the skin healthy
Makeup preparations	Mainly used for makeup effect
Fragrant preparations	Liquid, powdered, and other fragrance products aimed at providing scent; fall under the classification of "perfumes"
Suntan and sunscreen preparations	Exclusively used for tanning or sunscreening
Nail makeup preparations	Exclusively used for protecting nails, makeup effect on the nail, or are used for removing nail enamel
Eyeliner preparations	Used for makeup effect on the eyelids by using them along the hairline of eyelashes
Lip preparations	Exclusively used for makeup effect on the lips or are used for protecting lips
Oral preparations	Used for cleansing the mouth or preventing halitosis
Bath preparations	Used to cleanse the body and to enjoy the fragrance; used by placing them into a bathtub or by other similar action

Source: Ref. 6.

- Origin and background of discovery
- Previous use in foreign countries
- Characteristics and comparison with other cosmetics
- Determination of chemical structure
- Physicochemical properties
- Safety

In the case of cosmetics containing liposomes, the data attached to the application should include the stability of the liposome during product distribution and safety.

QUASIDRUGS

In the Pharmaceutical Affairs Law, quasidrugs are defined as articles having "fixed purpose of use" and "mild action on the body," or similar articles designated by the Minister of Health and Welfare. Most of the products in this category are what we call "pseudodrugs" or "cosmeceuticals," a current definition of which would be "those products that will achieve cosmetic results by means of some degree of physiological action" [8]. The defined quasidrug products include mouth refreshers, body deodorants, talcum powders, hair growers, depilatories, hair dyes, permanent waving products, bath preparations, medical cosmetics (including medical soaps), medicated dentifrices, and so on [3,9].

At each stage of development, manufacture/import, distribution, and use, the prescribed regulations are enforced [3]. Manufacturers of quasidrugs are required to obtain government approval before marketing. Approval of a product under an application for manufacturing/importing is the responsibility of the MHW. Is it adequate as a quasidrug in view of its efficacy, safety, etc.? Therefore, the examination procedures for approval as well as the data and documentation required to be submitted for filing an application differ with the indications and effects of each product [3]. The following data must be attached according to the kind of ingredients employed, and so on:

- Origin, background of discovery, use in foreign countries, etc.
- Physicochemical properties, specifications, testing methods, etc.
- Stability
- Safety
- Indications or effects

The scope of the data to be attached to the application depends on the type of quasidrug; (1) new quasidrugs that obviously differ from any previously approved products with respect to active ingredients, usage and dosage, and/or indications or effects; (2) quasidrugs identical with previously approved quasidrug(s); or (3) other quasidrugs that are other than those specified in (1) and (2) [3].

All products for approval as a quasidrug must be within the scope stipulated by the Pharmaceutical Affairs Law. Thus, approval of a product as a quasidrug is determined by an integrated judgement of various factors such as its ingredients, quantity (composition), indications and effects, usage and dosage, and dosage form. For example, those products whose effects are not mild—hence, coming under the category of poisons or deleterious drugs—are not approved even if their indications and effects and dosage forms are within the scope of the quasidrugs legislation. Likewise, products for which the intended use deviates from the scope of quasidrug are also not approved even if their effects are mild [3].

COSMETICS IN THE FUTURE

The Japanese Government sets objectives to relax or abolish many of the current regulatory items in various industries. As a part of these plans, cosmetic deregulation has been progressing based on the government's policy to review current licensing systems and ingredient labeling controls [10]. A committee, which was organized on the basis of a plan drafted by the government, was commissioned in order to figure out how to bring about a deregulated domestic market and a harmonized international market [11]. On March 31, 1997 the future direction and issues to be addressed in connection with cosmetic regulations were set out by the committee in the form of an interim report [4]. The following is an outline that indicates the shift of the regulatory system to one based on the manufacturers' self-responsibility, basically similar to that of the European Union and the United States [4,10].

1. Ingredient substance controls: Recompilation of the Negative List, the Positive List, and the Existing List of Ingredient Substances in order to abolish the current premarketing licensing systems.
2. Licensing systems for companies manufacturing and importing cosmetics: Maintenance of current systems in principle, while establishing new quality-control systems and simplifying requirements for license approval.
3. Ingredients labeling control: Creation of regulations that force cosmetic manufactures and importing companies to include all ingredients on the label in order to give consumers sufficient information to help them evaluate and select the cosmetics.
4. Promotion of the appropriate uses of cosmetics, and collecting and releasing to the public information on the safety of cosmetics.

After investigation by the working group on the specific issues indicated by the interim report, the committee has issued a final report. The report is entitled "How cosmetic regulations should be in the future" and consists of three parts [4,5]; 1) background of discussions on cosmetic regulation, 2) desired future regulations and specific handling procedure, and 3) issues remaining to be addressed.

The main points of the second part (desired future regulations and specific handling procedure) are as follows:

(1) Ingredient Control. It is appropriate to control the use of the ingredients through a list of prohibited and restricted ingredients (Negative List), and by doing so to abolish the approval system by category, as well as to control specific ingre-

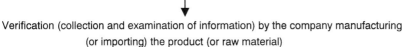

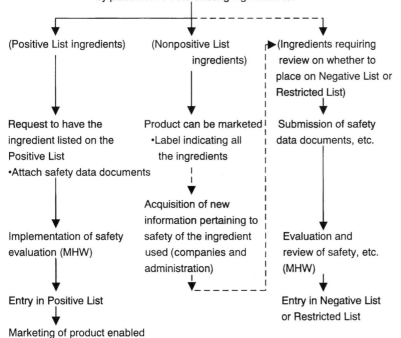

FIGURE 1   Flow chart of the procedure for treating new ingredients for cosmetics. (From Refs. 4 and 5.)

dient groups (preservatives, UV absorbents, coal tar colors) that require cautious handling under appropriate safety evaluation, by drawing up a list of ingredients that may be used in formulations (Positive List). As for the new ingredients, the procedure for introducing them shall be as indicated on the flow chart shown in Figure 1 [4,5].

(2) Licensing System. A manufacturing or importing licensing system should be maintained.

(3) Regulations on Ingredient Labeling. As it is important to provide adequate information to consumers to facilitate their selection and verification of a product, in principle an "all-ingredient labeling system" shall be adopted for ingredients used in formulations.

(4) Cosmetic information, etc.

The MHW is now studying the possibility of amending the law and regulations in order to implement the new system by fiscal year 2000 according to the final report.

QUASIDRUGS IN THE FUTURE

There has been a great demand by consumers for innovative cosmetic products with pharmacological action, i.e., pseudodrugs or cosmeceuticals such as skin antiaging products. To satisfy their demands, research on the skin has been undertaken to develop new active ingredients for skin antiaging products. How should those products be legally categorized? Quasidrugs would seem to be suitable for such products to be categorized. However, all of the products have not always been approved as quasidrugs to date. Taking antiwrinkle products, for example, no new products have been approved under the existing quasidrug specifications.

Generally, topically applied quasidrugs are intended to mollify unwanted aspects of the skin and have a mild action on the human body, whereas medical drugs are intended to treat specific diseases. Therefore, hair-growth products with a mild action on male-pattern baldness, which is not a disease [2], are quasidrugs. On the other hand, products intended for alopecia areata, which is a disease, are regarded as drugs. The natural aging of skin, like wrinkling, is not a disease, for example. We should also keep in mind that "high efficacy" should not always involve "strong action." There will be many pseudodrugs or cosmeceutical products with mild actions showing good efficacy.

Legally, the Minister of Health and Welfare can add new, novel types of products to the current list of types of quasidrugs [12]. Therefore, we hope that before long the aforementioned new products will be listed as quasidrugs.

REFERENCES

1. Schmitt WH, Murphy EG. An overview of worldwide regulatory programs. In: Estrin NF, ed. The Cosmetic Industry: Scientific and Regulatory Foundations. New York: Marcel Dekker, 1984:133–159.
2. Vermeer BJ, Gilchrest BA. Cosmeceuticals: Proposal for rational definition, evaluation, and regulation. Arch Dermatol 1996; 132:337–340.
3. Editorial supervision by Pharmaceuticals and Cosmetics Division, Pharmaceutical Affairs Bureau, Ministry of Health and Welfare. Guide to Quasi-drug and Cosmetic Regulations in Japan. Tokyo: Yakuji Nippo, 1992.

4. Committee on Cosmetic Regulations. Final report on How Cosmetic Regulations Should Be in the Future. Tokyo, Japan, July 23, 1998.

5. Uemura N. Final report on how cosmetic regulations should be in the future (review). Fragrance J 1998; 9:79–85.

6. Preface. In: The Comprehensive Licensing Standards Of Cosmetics By Category. Tokyo: Yakuji Nippo, 1998:13–14.

7. Supplement. In: Pharmaceuticals and Cosmetics Division, Pharmaceutical Affairs Bureau, Ministry of Health and Welfare, ed. Guide to Quasi-drug and Cosmetic Regulations in Japan. Tokyo: Yakuji Nippo, 1994.

8. Stimson N. Cosmeceuticals: realising the reality of the 21st century. SÖFW 1994; 120:631–641.

9. Society of Japanese Pharmacopoeia. Guide to Quasi-drug and Cosmetic Regulations in Japan. (Japanese ed.) 3d ed. Tokyo: Yakuji Nippo, 1996.

10. Arimoto T. The Current State of Japan's Cosmetic Regulatory System Liberalization. International Regulatory Congress, Florence, Italy, Apr. 22–23, 1998.

11. Deregulation of the Cosmetics Sector in Japan. In: CTFA/TRN Vol. 11. No. 5. 1997:28.

12. Komiya H. Regulatory frame and problems related to quasi-drug. J Japanese Cosmet Sci Soc 1991; 15:37–40.

63

Stability Testing of Cosmetic Products

Perry Romanowski and Randy Schueller
Alberto Culver Company, Melrose Park, Illinois

INTRODUCTION

Products formulated by cosmetic chemists are intended to perform a variety of ''miracle'' functions, such as reshaping hair, delivering fragrance, smoothing and softening skin, imparting color to the face, and cleansing the entire body. Chemists can deliver many of these miracles by using the variety of technologies described elsewhere in this book. In using these technologies to develop products, chemists must be aware of formulation issues that might prevent the product from performing optimally. Assessing product stability is a critical part of this formulation process. This chapter discusses the basic principles of stability testing of cosmetic delivery systems. We will begin with a general definition of stability testing and move on to problems encountered by specific formula types. We will conclude this section with a discussion of stability issues that are not necessarily directly related to the formulation, such as processing and packaging.

A PRACTICAL DEFINITION OF STABILITY TESTING

Stability testing may be defined as the process of evaluating a product to ensure that key attributes stay within acceptable guidelines. In order to make this testing meaningful, it is important to accurately establish the nature of these critical product attributes, to measure how they change over time, and to define what degree of change is considered acceptable. Defining which parameters are crucial requires a combination of chemical knowledge about the formula and common sense about product usage. The chemist should be aware that cosmetic products must not only continue to function over time but must also look, feel, and smell the same each time the consumer uses them. Therefore, testing must evaluate esthetic characteristics in addition to functional properties. This is an important consideration because cosmetic products can change in a number of different ways, which may affect consumer perception. For example, fragrances become distorted, colors may fade or darken, and consistency may change, resulting in a thicker or thinner product. Chemists must determine which of these product characteristics will change over time and design appropriate testing to measure the extent of the changes. Nacht cites several technical issues to be considered, including compatibility between the delivery system and the active ingredient, compatibility with the overall formula, appropriate mechanism of release for the particular application, the rate of release of the active ingredient, and overall safety for the user [1]. This chapter discusses some of the key tests that the chemist can use to measure the changes in these characteristics. An important fact to remember is that no product remains unchanged forever. Depending on the intended use of the product and its anticipated shelf life, a small change over time may be inconsequential or devastatingly detrimental. In general, if a change is consumer-perceptible, the product may not be considered stable.

USEFUL INFORMATION PROVIDED BY STABILITY TESTING

Stability data are useful as an "early warning system" that can alert the chemist to potential formulation/package-related problems. Such advance information can be helpful in many ways.

Guiding the Chemist During Product Development

While you are formulating a product, preliminary testing of its stability can guide you in making modifications to ensure that it is stable. If you determine, for example, that an emulsion shows separation after exposure to freeze/thaw conditions, you may elect to modify the surfactant system to correct the problem and then repeat the test on the modified formula to determine whether it performs better or worse. Preliminary stability test data are an important parts of the trial-and-error development process.

Ensuring That the Product Will Continue to Be Esthetically Acceptable to the Consumer

More than other products, cosmetics are intended to be esthetically pleasing to the consumer. For this reason consumers are likely to notice subtle changes in the odor or appearance of their favorite products. Since no product remains 100% unchanged as it ages, it is critical that the chemist anticipate the changes that may occur and make sure that they stay within limits that are not consumer-perceptible. Stability testing allows you to see how the product will behave over time.

Determining That the Product Will Perform as Intended and Remain Safe to Use

Studying the performance of samples that are exposed to accelerated aging lets you assess how the product will function over time. This is particularly important for cosmetic products that use the technologies described in this book to deliver "active" ingredients. If the formula is not stable, the delivery of the active ingredient may be impaired. Take, for example, the case of an antiperspirant stick with an encapsulated fragrance that is released upon exposure to moisture and heat. If the delivery system is poorly designed, the fragrance may be released too soon or not at all. Properly designed stability testing can reveal such problems so that corrective action can be taken.

Forewarning the Company About Problems That Might Occur After Consumer Purchase

For example, testing can show that the product may thicken somewhat over time and may be difficult to dispense from the package. Realizing this beforehand is important to the company because it will allow the company to anticipate consumer reaction.

Even though stability testing provides much useful information, it is not an exact science and will not guarantee a trouble-free product, but it can give an idea of the risks involved and help provide a solid scientific foundation for evaluation of future problems.

STABILITY TEST DESIGN

When faced with a situation where testing might be appropriate, ask some basic questions about the task ahead.

Why Is Testing Being Done?

Why is testing necessary? Are you concerned with product appearance or do you want to determine if specific performance characteristics change over time? The reasons for doing the tests will determine what kind of tests are required. Therefore it is critically important to approach this testing with a scientific mind set and to have a clearly defined hypothesis to be tested. Take, for example, the case of a skin lotion formula that develops an unpleasant odor. The reason for the test is to determine what is causing the odor. Your hypothesis may be that the fragrance you have selected is reacting with the formula ingredients to cause this problem. To test this hypothesis appropriately, you will need to assess the odor of the unfragranced base to determine how the fragrance affects the overall smell of the product. In this example, the unfragranced samples are the controls because the fragrance, which is the scientific variable, has been removed. Evaluation of appropriate control samples can prove or disprove the hypothesis—i.e., that the fragrance is causing the problem.

Another example illustrating the importance of conducting a properly controlled study is the case of an emulsion that separates after prolonged storage in its plastic bottle. In this case the reason for the test is to determine what is causing the separation. One hypothesis may be that the package is allowing water vapor to escape, thus leading to emulsion instability. To test this hypothesis, you will need to screen out the variable of concern: the packaging. Therefore, control samples could be packaged in glass to eliminate the possibility of moisture loss. If the control samples do not show the same instability that the packaged samples show, you have demonstrated that the packaging material is indeed having a negative effect on the product.

Finally, consider a case where the variable of interest is the viscosity of the product. If you are concerned that the product may become too thick over time and will not dispense properly, you could design a study to track product batches with varying initial viscosity. Suppose the target viscosity is 20,000 cps. You could monitor the viscosity of a series of batches with viscosities ranging from low to high. You may make batches which are initially at 5000, 10,000, 15,000, and 20,000 cps, respectively. You would then monitor the viscosity of these batches as a function of time and temperature. You may learn that viscosity does not change significantly from the initial value, which means that a very narrow specification will be required. In other words, the product must be very close to its final viscosity when it is produced. On the other hand, you may discover that as long as the initial viscosity is between 5000 and 15,000 cps, the product will build to 20,000 cps within 2 weeks and stay at that level for 2–3 years. In this case your specification can be rather broad, since—regardless of the initial value—the consumer will only be exposed to product that is 20,000 cps. In all these cases, understanding why the test needs to be done helps you establish appropriate controls, which are essential if meaningful test results are to be obtained.

What Is Being Tested?

Another important factor to understand is the status of the formula being tested. Is it a developmental prototype or the final production material? Consider a situation, as in the example provided above, where you are primarily concerned with the change in product viscosity. Furthermore, consider that the final color and fragrance of the product have not yet been firmly established, although there are several candidates under evaluation. You could prepare samples with every possible color/fragrance combination and measure their viscosity over time. This could involve thousands of samples and tens of thousands of measurements, which are both costly and time-consuming. So, bearing in mind that you are testing a prototype and not a finished product, you may instead opt to test the uncolored, unfragranced base formulation first. In this way you can expeditiously get data on the parameter of interest—in this case viscosity. By evaluating prototypes early on, you have given yourself more time to react to problems. Of course, the testing may have to be repeated once the final formula is established because the fragrance may affect viscosity. Similarly, if the final production package is not yet available, you may choose to evaluate formula stability in a packaging material that approximates the characteristics of the final container. Here too, the final formula and package combination must eventually be tested together, because the formula may interact unfavorably with the package. Asking the ''what'' question will help make your testing meaningful without forcing you to go to excessive lengths.

Where Will Test Samples Be Stored and How Many Are Necessary?

Ideally, you could gain information on formula stability by performing exhaustive tests on every variable involved in every formulation you work with, but this is not always feasible, because proper testing requires a significant commitment of time and resources. Therefore, most companies have standardized test procedures for the storage of stability samples which depend on the objective of the study. Such procedures involve evaluations of samples stored at a variety of conditions and include enough samples to be statistically significant. Usually sample storage is done at elevated temperatures, under freeze and/or freeze thaw conditions, and with exposure to various types of light. Elevated temperature storage is critical, since the rate of chemical reactions roughly doubles for every 10°C increase in temperature. Storage at higher temperatures allows you to accelerate the aging process and to see certain problems much sooner than they would appear at room temperature. Of course, the potential drawback is that, at high temperatures, you may be forcing reactions to occur that would not happen at all at lower temperatures. Cold storage evaluates conditions that may negatively affect the solubility of ingredients or stability of emulsions. Sunlight and ultraviolet (UV) light exposure can reveal problems with ingredients that are reactive to the respective wavelengths; fragrances and colors are particularly sensitive in this regard. The most common storage conditions used in this industry are 54°C or 50°C, 45°C, 37°C or 35°C, room temperature (25°C), 4°C, freeze/thaw, and exposure to fluorescent and natural light.

Since many of the tests that must be conducted to evaluate product performance will affect the sample physically (e.g., spraying an aerosol can), multiple samples are required at each storage condition to ensure there will be enough samples left for evaluation at the end of the test period. Depending on the protocol set by your organization, as many as one hundred or more samples may be required for a complete study. Again, you should follow your corporate guidelines to make sure that sample quantities will be enough for a thorough evaluation of all necessary conditions.

How Samples Are Evaluated and What to Look for—Identification of Instability

How samples are evaluated depends entirely on the type of product and the nature of the problems that might occur. Instability is typically identified by evaluating various product characteristics either by subjective observation of properties—such as color, odor and appearance—or by objective instrumental evaluation of pH, viscosity, particle size, and electrical conductivity. For instance, simply looking at a sample that has been stored at accelerated temperatures can often reveal significant changes such as color changes, emulsion separation, or rheological changes. Similarly, a quick olfactory evaluation can uncover major flaws in fragrance stability. More rigorous characterization of product attributes can be obtained instrumentally—for example, with a viscometer or pH meter. These instruments are highly sensitive and can distinguish small changes in products. Such changes are important to note since, as in the case of a change in pH, they may represent chemical reactions that are occurring in the formula.

Other specialized testing can be performed to quantify specific changes in formulated systems. For example, microscopic evaluation and light scattering are used to appraise changes in particle size and distribution of emulsions. A Coulter counter is also used for these determinations [2], as are conductivity measurements [3]. Nuclear magnetic resonance (NMR) and x-ray crystallography can also be used to reveal additional information regarding emulsion structure. In certain systems, specific assays are performed to measure the activity of functional ingredients. These types of tests are tailored for the compound in question. For instance, the bactericidal efficacy of preservatives or other antimicrobial compounds may be measured over the course of a stability test. In addition, chromatographic tests, spectroscopic measurements, titrametric evaluations, and other wet chemical methods can be used to detect signs of instability. Other indications of instability include incompatibility of product and package, which can lead to weight loss and package degradation (such as softening or cracking of container walls, clogging of orifices, corrosion of metal parts, etc. [4]). But perhaps the most important question to ask in assessing instability is to determine how much change is acceptable. Knowlton and Pearce have stated that a useful rule of thumb is to consider product rejection if the attributes being measured deviate by more than 20% of their original value [4]. This value is an interesting reference point; however, for some formulations, much smaller deviations may be critical. The impact of such changes must be assessed on a case-by-case basis.

SITUATIONS THAT REQUIRE STABILITY TESTING

A good chemist should have an understanding of factors that are critical to product stability, so that appropriate testing can be conducted when necessary. Situations in which stability testing is generally necessary include but are not limited to the following situations: consideration of a new formulation, qualification of new raw materials, evaluation of new manufacturing processes, and testing of different packaging components. As you will see, stability testing is not a finite, one-time task; instead, it is an ongoing, dynamic process that begins when the product is being developed and continues to evolve as the formula, packaging, or manufacturing processes change.

FORMULA-RELATED REASONS TO STABILITY TEST

Specific Considerations Related to Development of Particular Formula Types

The process of stability testing a product is closely tied to the process of creating the formulation. As you develop formulations, you should always screen stability samples early in the process to make sure that your efforts are headed in the direction that will lead to a stable product. Every formula will have slightly different stability testing requirements, but for the sake of this discussion, we will give primary consideration to the types of cosmetic delivery systems detailed in this text.

Emulsions

Emulsions are among the most common types of delivery systems used for cosmetic products. They enable a wide variety of ingredients to be quickly and conveniently delivered to hair and skin. While many definitions of emulsions have been proposed, we will define them as heterogeneous systems in which at least one immiscible or barely miscible liquid is dispersed in another liquid in the form of tiny droplets of various sizes [5]. Consequently, these systems are inherently unstable and eventually, given enough time or energy, will separate into separate phases.

Emulsions used for cosmetic products are typically semisolid materials composed of an oil (hydrophobic) phase and a water (hydrophilic) phase. These phases are characterized as either the internal phase or external phase, depending on the overall composition of the emulsion. The internal phase is that which is contained inside separate discrete particles surrounded by surfactants; these particles are known as micelles. The external phase is the "solvent" or diluent, which surrounds the micelles. Usually, the external phase is the more abundant one. Depending on the composition of each phase, simple emulsions can be either oil in water or water in oil, the type of which depends specifically on what emulsifier is used.

Although the internal-phase particles of an emulsion are polydisperse (meaning they have various sizes), their average size is often used for emulsion classification [6]. When the average diameter of internal particles is less than 100 Å, the system is called a *micellar emulsion*. A particle diameter of 2000 to 100 Å is called a *microemulsion*. Larger particles produce macroemulsions, which are the most common types found in cosmetic formulations. More complex emulsions can have multiple internal phases. These emulsions, called *multiple emulsions*, can be oil in water in oil or some combination. For cosmetic applications, they are formed by first making a water-in-oil emulsion and then mixing that emulsion with a water phase. These types are particularly useful for encapsulating materials giving prolonged release when applied to a surface such as skin [7].

Stability Considerations

Since emulsions represent a mixture of two or more materials that are not miscible in each other, they are, according to the second law of thermodynamics, inherently unstable. This means that eventually the two phases will separate. The degree and speed of instability are quite variable. For example, a mixture of mineral oil and water when shaken will form a macroemulsion, which immediately separates upon standing. Other emulsions can remain stable for years, but eventually all emulsions will separate. While the second law of thermodynamics suggests that emulsions will separate over time, it does not provide a mechanism of this destabilization. Investigation into how emulsions destabilize has revealed three primary processes leading to instability: flocculation, creaming, and coalescence [8].

Flocculation

This process is characterized by a weak, reversible association between droplets of the emulsion's internal phase. Each individual droplet maintains its own identity; thus there is no change in the basic droplet size [8]. Flocculation represents a less serious sign of instability, which can be reversed by shaking the system [9].

Creaming

When particles of an emulsion aggregate, there is a tendency for upward sedimentation. This causes a partial separation of the emulsion into two emulsions, one of which is richer in the internal phase and the other richer in the external phase [9]. As in the case of flocculation, this stability problem can be reversed by agitation.

Coalescence

An aggregation between two particles can, if the two particles combine, lead to the formation of one larger particle. This process, known as coalescence, represents a more serious stability problem. A related phenomenon is that of Ostwald ripening, in which the particles all tend to become the same size. Both of these processes are irreversible and can eventually lead to complete separation of the internal and external phases of the emulsion [10]. An alternative consequence of these forms of instability is phase inversion, in which the internal phase becomes the external phase and vice versa [9]. For stability considerations, this change is typically undesirable, since it will change the physical properties of the product.

All emulsions are potentially subject to all of these destabilizing processes simultaneously, and the resulting effects on any given emulsion will vary. For example, microemulsions and micellar emulsions are initially transparent. Over time, the size of their internal-phase particles may increase, and they will develop translucent appearance. Since macroemulsions are opaque, a similar change in appearance will not be notable; however, there may be changes in viscosity and measurable separation. Multiple emulsions are typically less stable than monoemulsions. Over a short period of time, the number of multiple emulsion particles tend to be reduced. This results in the "leaking out" of some of the encapsulated material and reduces the duration of prolonged release.

In addition to the inherent processes that destabilize emulsions, other factors may be involved. Storage temperature has been shown to affect emulsion product stability. Generally, elevated temperatures result in destabilization, while reduced temperatures improve emulsion stability. Aqueous-phase evaporation may also contribute to instability over the life of a product. Microbial contamination can also cause a breakdown of emulsion stability. Finally, chemical reactions within the emulsion can lead to a change in the stability of the emulsion. While these types of reactions can be initiated by temperature increases, they can also be prompted by UV light or other types of electromagnetic radiation.

VESICULAR SYSTEMS—LIPOSOMES AND NIOSOMES

Definition/Description

Vesicular systems encompass a number of delivery technologies, including liposomes and niosomes. Both of these systems employ a "vessel" to contain active ingredients within a formula and to provide controlled delivery of these ingredients. Nacht defines controlled delivery as a "system that would result in a predictable rate of delivery of its active ingredients to the skin" [1]. Liposomes are a classic example of this technology, in which phospholipids are used to create lipid "capsules" that can be loaded with various ingredients. Although liposomes are enjoying tremendous popularity in cosmetics today, they have their roots back in the early 1960s. At that time Professor Bangham, at the Institute for Animal Physiology in Cambridge, U.K., was one of the first to speculate that lipids such as phosphatidyl choline could be used to create sealed vesicles with bilayer membranes similar to cell membranes [1]. Niosomes are another delivery technology related to liposomes; the difference is that, unlike liposomes, niosomes are based on nonionic surfactants. L'Oréal pioneered the development of nonionic liposomes using nonionic surfactants such as polyoxyethylene alkyl ethers combined with fatty alcohols or fatty acids [1].

Stability Considerations

Liposome and niosome stability may be referred to in terms of leakage of contents, presence of oxidation products, or changing particle size due to aggregation formation and fusion. They are rather fragile capsules, and certain precautions must be taken to make sure that they remain intact and are able to deliver their contents. Leakage can be caused by mechanical forces like high-shear processing, which should be avoided. Similarly, excessive heat, which may destabilize the lipid bilayers, should be avoided. Perhaps most notably, liposomes may be solubilized by surfactants that may be present, and therefore they are not suitable for use in detergent systems. This is particularly true of systems such as shampoos and body washes, which contain strong anionic surfactants that can dissolve the lipid walls. In fact, even though liposomes are often used in creams and lotions, the emulsifiers used in these formulas may also be enough to disrupt the fragile walls. For these reasons, many formulators believe that gels are the ideal vehicle for liposomes because they lack the high HLB (hydrophilic lipophilic balance) surfactants present in many conventional emulsions, which might disrupt the lipid bilayers [10]. There is hope for using liposomes in emulsion. K. Uji et al. report that stable liposome suspensions can be prepared by using a cross-linked acrylic acid/alkyl acrylate copolymer at very low concentrations, because it can effectively stabilize lecithin liposomes in o/w emulsions [11]. Furthermore, there is some evidence in the patent literature that the addition of collagen, albumin, or gamma globulin to the liposomes can decrease the harmful effects of detergents [10].

In addition to leakage, vesicle systems may fuse together and no longer be available as discrete units for the delivery of active agents. According to Weiner, such fusion can occur for several reasons, including preparation below their transition temperature, the presence of contaminants such as fatty acids and divalent cations, changes in pH, or the addition of nonelectrolyte hydrophobic molecules [12]. Furthermore, phase separation of bilayer components can occur upon extended storage. In an excellent review on the subject, Fox refers to an article by Crommelin et al., that reports on preserving the long-term stability of liposomes. Crommelin discusses the chemical pathways by which phospholipids can degrade: by hydrolysis of the ester groups or oxidation of the unsaturated acyl chains. This research points to an optimal pH for liposome stability. For phosphotidylcholine liposomes, the pH for the lowest hydrolysis rate was found to be 6.5. The stability of liposomes was further enhanced by using phospholipids with fully saturated acyl chains (like those made from hydrogenated soybeans, so the opportunity for oxidation is reduced) [10]. Similarly, liposomes may be stabilized by sugar esters, for example, maltopentose monopalmitate have been used to improve stability of cosmetic systems [13].

For a more detailed discussion of the morphology of liposomal bilayers, we refer the reader to Liposomes: From Biophysics to Therapeutics [12]. The author provides an excellent discussion of the elastic properties and tensile strength of liposomes as well as the effect of solvents and osmotic effects on liposomal structures.

MOLECULAR CARRIERS
Definition / Description

Molecular carriers represent a delivery system in which one compound is used to bind another compound to a substrate, thereby changing the former's characteristics. This allows the bound material to be delivered to a surface and released when conditions are appropriate. One example of this type of technology is cyclodextrin chemistry. Cyclodextrins are created from starch-derived glucopyranose units and are classified as cyclic oligosaccharides. When formed, they contain a hydrophobic cavity capable of entrapping molecules of different sizes, shapes, and polarities. Molecules entrapped as such are found to be more resistant to environmental stresses and therefore more stable [14]. They can be used to entrap various types of compounds such as fragrances, vitamins, pigments, and dyes. Cyclodextrins have been used in cosmetic products for a variety of reasons, such as to reduce odor in mercaptan-containing systems [15], improve the stability of hair dyes [16], and as an active ingredient to treat acne [17].

Stability Issues

The complex of the cyclodextrin with a guest molecule is typically quite stable under ambient temperatures and dry conditions. However, in the presence of certain materials the guest molecule can be prematurely displaced thereby reducing the effectiveness of the delivery system [18]. This factor is of major concern when developing and particularly when assessing the stability of a formula.

PARTICULATE SYSTEMS—MICROCAPSULES, BEADS, AND MICROSPHERES
Definition / Description

Microcapsules are one of the oldest controlled release technologies. They were developed to produce carbonless carbon paper and are composed of a core with the active ingredient surrounded by a shell, analogous to an egg. Microcapsules may have a multilayer construction with multiple cores containing the active. The active ingredients are released either by rupture of the capsule walls or by diffusion/permeation of the contents [1]. Fairhurst and Mitchnick list a range of materials that are typically used in this regard including adhesives, drugs, colors, fragrances, flavors, agricultural chemicals, solvents and oils. Classic shell materials include gelatin or gum arabic, cellulosic polymers, or synthetic polymers [19]. Starch based capsules are often used to deliver fragrance and cosmetic ingredients.

Beads and microspheres are small solid particles onto which other ingredients can be adsorbed for later delivery. Nylon particles, for example, are useful for delivery of certain active ingredients. Antiperspirant salts are said to be more efficacious when delivered via nylon spheres, and the esthetics of the product are said to be improved. Coloring agents may be delivered in this manner as well; Schlossman discloses a patented method (U.S. patent 5,314,683) of coupling cosmetic pigments to microspheres to provide uniform reflectivity, improved dispersion, and superior viscosity characteristics [10]. Tokubo et al. describe a process for preparing spherical hectorite particles, with a diameter of about 100 Å, which can be used to deliver glycerin and solid pigments such as titanium dioxide, zinc oxide, and ferric oxide.

Stability Considerations

Microcapsules are somewhat fragile physically and care must be taken to avoid premature rupture and release of the contents. Excessive temperature should be avoided by adding microencapsulated ingredients late in the manufacturing process. Likewise, refrain from formulating with materials that may act as solvents on the capsules walls. Finally, avoid high-shear processing, such as milling and homogenizing, which can physically disrupt the capsules. Additional techniques for enhancing the stability of microcapsules can be found in the technical literature. Fox refers to an interesting Shiseido patent for improving the stability of gelatin microcapsules by coating the surface of the capsule with a basic amino acid or its polymer [10]. In general, microcapsules are a stable, efficacious method of delivering chemicals in cosmetics. In fact, when properly formulated, microcapsules can actually enhance stability of systems by protecting the ingredients they carry from external forces. For instance, in an example provided by the Mono-Cosmetic Company, ascorbic acid particles are coated with silicone or a polymer—e.g., ethyl cellulose, to protect the ascorbic acid against oxidation [10]. Similarly, in delivering cosmetic materials via beads and microspheres, care must be taken not to disturb the matrices physically. As with microcapsules, excessive shear can be a problem, for if the capsules are broken, their ability to retain the ingredient to be delivered will be impaired.

GENERAL CONSIDERATIONS RELATED TO FORMULA MODIFICATION

Regardless of which delivery technology you choose to utilize in a formulation, there are certain fundamental stability considerations that you must deal with. For each of the technologies discussed above, factors such as raw material sources, manufacturing process, and packaging composition all play a role in product stability.

Raw Material Substitution

Often it becomes necessary to substitute one raw material for another similar material. This frequently occurs because a supplier discontinues one of the raw materials used in your formula. In exchange, a different, yet supposedly "identical," material may be offered. Depending on the chemistry of the materials involved, there is no way to anticipate if such a change will affect formula stability. Therefore, in such situations you must conduct testing to ensure your formula will remain stable. Similarly, you may wish to substitute another material that is cheaper but is not anticipated to function differently. For example, in a shampoo formula, you may substitute sodium lauryl sulfate for ammonium lauryl sulfate. Given the functional similarities between the two, you would not anticipate significant problems; nonetheless, some degree of stability testing would be prudent.

Alternate Vendor Qualification

You may also elect to qualify alternate raw material suppliers for ingredients in the formula. It is desirable to have secondary sources for most raw materials to ensure a steady supply and competitive pricing. Unfortunately, even though raw materials from different suppliers may have the same CTFA (Cosmetics, Toiletries, and Fragrance Association) designation, they may not be chemically identical, because chemical feedstocks and processing conditions vary between suppliers. Therefore, a raw material from one supplier cannot always be automatically inserted into a formula developed with a different supplier's raw material. The impact of even seemingly inconsequential change in raw materials must be established by stability testing.

NON–FORMULA-RELATED REASONS

Processing Issues

In addition to the formulation and raw material issues described above, there are processing issues that can affect product stability. For example, stability testing is typically required the first time a new formulation is made on a large scale. This is because the way in which the product is made on a large scale can have a dramatic effect on its stability. This is particularly true of emulsions, because the energy used in processing determines particle size and distribution, which helps determine product stability. The only way to fully assess the impact of the chosen manufacturing method on product stability is to evaluate samples made under actual production conditions. This may require that a trial production batch be made prior to commercialization of the formula. At the very least, stability testing should be done on the first production batch of any new product, so that the impact of actual production processing conditions may be evaluated.

Once a manufacturing process has been shown to be successful, any changes to that process may require additional testing. Alterations in the order of raw material addition may be necessary to reduce processing time; changes in heating and cooling rates may occur due to differences in heat transfer in large batches; and different mixing conditions will all affect the amount of shear the product experiences. Any one of these changes will cause stability problems.

Packaging Issues

Even with the formulation and manufacturing processes held constant, variations in packaging material can cause problems that require stability testing. Not all packages are created equal: glass and plastic behave differently, and different kinds of plastic vary in properties such as oxygen permeability, color fastness, and thermal resistance. Certainly a new combination of formula and package should be tested, and even a change in an existing packaging material or the supplier of that material merits evaluation. The stability of aerosol systems, for example, is extremely package-dependent, since the package composition will help to determine how resistant the final product is to corrosion. The overall objective is to be alert for changes to the formulation/manufacturing/packaging system that may necessitate additional testing, so that you can be confident that your product will remain stable. Of course, your observations should not be limited to the formula itself. Changes that result from formulation and packaging interaction may be critical to total product integrity. To this end, weight loss, changes in plastic color and odor, and other package-related observations are important. The objective is to gain as much knowledge as possible regarding the behavior of the product over time.

CONCLUSION

This chapter is intended to provide insight into the issues associated with the stability testing of cosmetic products. For the beginning chemist, we stress the importance of careful, methodical observation to ensure that as many stability problems as possible are identified. For the veteran formulator, we urge periodic review of the latest technical literature so that it will be possible to keep pace with new developments in stabilizing the specific delivery systems discussed in this book. Hopefully the references we have provided will be helpful in this regard.

REFERENCES

1. Nacht S. Encapsulation and other topical delivery systems. Cosmet Toilet 1995; 110(9):25–30.
2. Rieger M. Stability testing of macroemulsions. Cosmet Toilet 1991; 106(5):59–66.
3. Jayakrishnan A. Microemulsions: evolving technology for cosmetic applications. J Soc Cosmet Chem 1983; 34:343.
4. Knowlton J, Pearce S. The Handbook of Cosmetic Science and Technology. Oxford, England: Elsevier Advanced Technology, 1993:436–439.
5. Becher P. Emulsions: Theory and Practice. New York: Reinhold, 1965:2.
6. Prince L. Microemulsions: Theory and Practice. New York: Academic Press, 1977:1–2.
7. Fox C. An introduction to multiple emulsions. Cosmet Toilet 1986; 101(11):101–102.
8. Becher P. Encyclopedia of Emulsion Technology. New York: Marcel Dekker, 1983:133–134.
9. Eccleston GM. Application of emulsion stability theories to mobile and semisolid O/W emulsions. Cosmet Toilet 1986; 101(11):73–135.
10. Fox C. Advances in cosmetic science and technology: IV. Cosmetic vehicles. Cosmet Toilet 1995; 110(9):59–68.
11. K Uji K et al. J Soc Cosmet Chem Jpn 1993; 27:206–215.
12. Ostro MJ, ed. Liposomes: From Biophysics to Therapeutics. New York: Marcel Dekker, 1987: 343.
13. Fox C. Cosmetic raw materials literature and patent review. Cosmet Toilet 1991; 106(8):78.
14. Dalbe B. Use of cyclodextrins in cosmetics. 16th IFSCC Meeting, New York, 1991. pp. 635–639.
15. Kubo S, Fumiaki N. US patent 4,548,811. Shiseido Company Ltd.
16. Oishi T et al. US patent 4,808,189, Hoyu Co.
17. Koch J. US patent 4,352,749.
18. Duchene D. New Trends in Cyclodextrins and Derivatives. Dermal Uses of Cyclodextrins and Derivatives. Paris: 1991:473–474.
19. Fairhurst D, Mitchnik M. Submicron encapsulation of organic sunscreens. Cosmet Toilet 1995; 110(9):47.

64

Stability Control: Microbiological Tests

Michel J. Devleeschouwer
Free University of Brussels, Brussels, Belgium

Françoise Siquet
Colgate-Palmolive Technology Center, Milmort, Belgium

MICROBIOLOGICAL CONTROL OF RAW MATERIALS

Microbial Health Hazards by Contaminated Products

The microbial spoilage of cosmetics has been reported in the literature for many years [1–3]. One of the first reported incidents [4] is the death by tetanus of four babies in New Zealand in 1946, the vector being a contaminated talcum powder. The same vector was the source of two other cases of tetanus in an English hospital [5]. Since the 1960s, cases of cosmetic-induced infections were described in parallel with the awareness of the problem for topical drugs [6–12]. The isolated organisms were Gram-negative bacteria from the genus *Klebsiella*, *Enterobacter*, *Serratia*, and *Pseudomonas* [13,14]. The organism *Pseudomonas aeruginosa*, a particularly virulent hospital pathogen transmitted by eye cosmetics, led to cases of infections and even blindness [15–20], or folliculitis from sponges [21]. Studies were then conducted to evaluate the importance of the problem [22–29] and to investigate the primary contaminating sources such as raw materials, personnel, water, and packaging, as well as secondary sources, such as the consumer [30].

Sources of Contamination

These can be divided into three groups [11,28,31,32]:

1. The microbiological quality of raw materials, including water;
2. The manufacturing process; and
3. The galenical form (which is made with vegetable and/or animal extracts) of the product.

Microbiological Quality of Raw Materials, Including Water

Their quality depends upon their origin. Raw materials from animal or vegetable origin can be heavily contaminated with 10^6 or even more organisms per gram or milliliter [33–35]. Fecal bacteria are regularly identified. In contrast, synthetic raw materials are relatively free from contamination, with the exception made for some that have steps in their manufacture, such as kaolin, some sugars and vitamins, some synthetic surfactants (e.g., sodium lauryl ether sulfate [SLES]), or partially hydrated salts. A recent study in our laboratory (Boussard et al., unpublished data) showed that out of 188 different synthetic tested raw materials, only 48, or 25.5%, gave results higher than 100 organisms per gram or milliliter. The recovered organisms were bacilli or Gram-positive cocci. A microbiological testing program of the raw materials must be set up.

Water remains one of the most important contamination factors of a product. Species like *Pseudomonas*, *Achromobacter*, *Aeromonas*, or *Flavobacterium* are recovered from natural waters [36]. Softening or deionization treatments frequently alter the microbiological water quality. These systems must be well maintained and the water microbiologically treated, using, e.g., ultraviolet (UV) lamps or/and bacterial filtration to ensure optimal quality. Microbiological control of production water should be made at least each working day, and a validation program of the water quality set up.

Manufacturing Process

During the manufacturing process, contamination can occur through contact by the operators, the manufacturing equipment, and the air. The micro-organisms capable of contaminating a cosmetic from human sources are part of the rhinopharyngal, buccal skin, hair, hand skin, and, in some circumstances, intestinal floras. Among these, fecal streptococci, staphylococci, enterobacteria, and *Pseudomonas* have sufficient vitality to survive and even to multiply in a product.

The manufacturing equipment is also an important source of contamination, coming from maintenance materials (oils, greases), from poor cleaning and/or disinfection on a regular basis, and from product changeover. The design of the equipment is also participating in this process: a piece of equipment that cannot be totally emptied is critical; the equipment storage conditions must also be optimized to avoid product residues stagnant in the system. The design of cleaning in place (CIP) systems must be carefully evaluated: a CIP that leaves a small quantity of stagnant water together with diluted product will have a negative effect instead of a beneficial one.

Attention must be paid to the air quality of the manufacturing rooms. The number of workers and the importance of their movements contributes to 80% of aerial contamination [37]. Air conditioning contributes to 15% of this contamination, and the room structure (materials used) to 5%. It is thus necessary to fix acceptable levels for the biocontamination of the air and to control the air quality. According to the European Good Manufacturing Practices (GMPs) [38], the limits of the class D rooms should be used (200 organisms/m^3).

Galenical Form of the Product

A parameter of crucial importance in the microbiological stability of a formulation is its water availability, or a_w. This aspect will be discussed at the end of this chapter. Some processes, such as manufacturing at high temperature (e.g., lipsticks) can help to reduce or avoid bacterial contamination. Thus high-risk products are aqueous-based products containing raw materials from biological origin such as lotions, suspensions, creams, gels, and emulsions, especially if they are manufactured at room temperature.

Establishment of Microbial Limits

For many years there have been discussions on whether total count would be sufficient to guarantee the microbiological quality of a cosmetic, or if the exclusion of specified microorganisms, pathogens, or potential pathogens would also be required. The current trend is to require quantitative and qualitative microbial limits. Acceptance criteria for cosmetics and control methods will be issued in the Seventh Amendment of the European Cosmetic Directive. Nevertheless, the acceptance criteria will be minimal criteria that fulfill the public health expectations, such as:

1. *Microbial limits for finished products.* Maximum 1000 organisms/g or mL, and absence of *Staphylococcus aureus, Candida albicans*, enterobacteria, and *Pseudomonas aeruginosa* in one gram or milliliter of the product. Exceptions are baby-care products, eye products, and products for intimate hygiene—maximum 100 organisms/g or mL, and absence of *Staphylococus aureus, Candida albicans*, enterobacteria, and *Pseudomonas aeruginosa* in one gram or milliliter of the product.

2. *Microbial limits for raw materials.* Maximum 100 organisms/g or mL, and absence of *Staphylococcus aureus, Candida albicans*, enterobacteria, and *Pseudomonas aeruginosa* in one gram or milliliter. Limits for water as raw material could be fixed at maximum 100 organisms/mL and absence of coliforms and *Pseudomonas aeruginosa* in 100 mL.

However, what must be the attitude of a manufacturer if one of the following germs is identified in a product: Gram-negative bacilli other than enterobacteria and *Pseudomonas aeruginosa*, staphylococci different from *Staphylococcus aureus*, or fecal streptococci? What is the significance of this regarding manufacturing hygiene? Are these organisms harmless? Furthermore, in addition to the human safety, it must be emphasized that contamination of products with nonharmful organisms can partially or totally destroy the product aesthetic (e.g., perfume, color) and can alter the product performance. The rise of these questions emphasizes the need of internal quantitative and qualitative microbiological safety margins and of a quality-assurance system.

Use of Validated Methods to Control Products and Water

Microbiological Control of Finished Products and Raw Materials

The method described here is based on the method for microbiological analysis of nonsterile pharmaceuticals in the 3rd edition of the *European Pharmacopeia* [39,40] and from a publication of a working party of the "Fédération Internationale Pharmaceutique" [41].

Sample Preparation. A 10% homogeneous solution or suspension of the product is prepared with a sterile neutralizing solution or a sterile buffered peptone saline solution at pH 7. The neutralizing solution is used in case of the presence of known or suspected antimicrobial substances in the product. The pH 7 solution is used in case of preservative-free raw materials. For nonsoluble products, 0.1% of tween 80 or heating at a temperature not higher than 40°C for half an hour maximum can help in the homogenization. The neutralizing solution is basically letheen broth (Difco) supplemented with various inhibitors of the preservatives or disinfectants. The 10% homogenate is then used to perform the bacterial and fungal counts and to investigate the presence of specified microorganisms. If, for technical reasons, the use of 10 g sample is not possible, 5, 2.5, or even 1 g can be mixed for a total suspension of 100 mL.

Validation of the Preservative's Inactivation. The efficacy of the neutralizing solution must be validated in order to avoid false-negative results. For this purpose, 1 mL of the preserved sample or 1 mL sterile normal saline is added to 9 mL neutralizing solution. The two tubes are mixed well and let to rest for 10 minutes. 0.1 mL of a mixed suspension of *Staphylococcus aureus* ATCC 6538 and *Pseudomonas aeruginosa* ATCC 9027 at 10^4 bacteria/mL are then added to the tubes, which are mixed again. The colony-forming units in each tube are estimated. The difference in the results must be lower than $\frac{1}{2}$ log between the tubes.

Bacterial and Fungal Counts. From the 10% homogenate, an appropriate number of successive tenfold dilutions in the sterile buffered peptone saline at pH 7 are carried out. A plate count is then made by transferring duplicates of 1 mL of the dilutions in sterile Petri dishes, followed by the addition of 15 mL melted agar. Tryptic Soy agar is used for the bacteria and Sabouraud Chloramphenicol agar for yeast and moulds. For the bacterial counts the dishes are incubated at 30 to 35°C for 5 days, and for the yeast and moulds, 20 to 25°C for 5 to 7 days. The Petri dishes used for the fungal counts are also used to check the presence of *Candida albicans*.

Investigations for the Presence of Specific Microorganisms
   1. Enterobacteria and other gram-negative organisms. One milliliter or 1 g of the 10% homogenate is mixed with 100 mL enterobacteria enrichment broth (EEB) and incubated at 35 to 37°C for 24 to 48 hours. Subcultures are then carried out on violet red bile dextrose VRBG agar dishes and incubated at 35 to 37°C for 18 to 24 hours. The colonies of presumptive Gram-negative organisms are then identified.
   2. *Escherichia coli.* One milliliter or 1 g of the 10% homogenate is mixed with 100 mL Mac Conkey broth and incubated at 43 to 45°C for 18 to 24 hours. Subcultures are carried out on Mac Conkey agar dishes incubated at 43 to 45°C for 18 to 24 hours. The colonies of lactose-fermenting gram-negative organisms are then identified.
   3. *Pseudomonas aeruginosa* and other gram-negative organisms growing on Cetrimide agar. One milliliter or 1 g of the 10% homogenate is mixed with 100 mL Tryptic Soy broth (TSB) and incubated at 35 to 37°C for 24 to 48 hours. Subcultures are carried out on Cetrimide agar dishes incubated at 35 to 37°C for 18 to 24 hours. The colonies are then identified.
   4. *Staphylococcus aureus.* One milliliter or 1 g of the 10% homogenate is mixed with 100 mL TSB and incubated at 35 to 37°C for 24 to 48 hours. Subcultures are carried out on Baird Parker agar dishes incubated at 35 to 37°C for 18 to 24 hours. The black colonies are then identified.

Validation of the Sterility of the Media. Sterility of all the media must be checked. For example, sterile saline is used instead of the sample and the bacterial counts and the appropriate investigations for specific organisms are performed. No microbial growth must be recorded in this assay.

Validation of the Growth-Promoting Properties of the Selective Media. The following reference strains are incubated separately in TSB at 30 to 35°C for 18 to 24 hours: *Staphylococcus aureus* ATCC 6538, *Pseudomonas aeruginosa* ATCC 9027, and, *Escherichia coli* ATCC 8739. Each bacterial suspension is diluted to obtain around 1000 organisms per milliliter. The three suspensions are equally mixed together and 0.3 mL of the mixture (containing about 100 organisms of each strain) are used as the inoculum to perform the investigations for the specific micro-organisms. The organisms must be detected in the media used for this assay.

Microbiological Control of Water

The microbiological quality of water is of particular importance and can be checked quantitatively and qualitatively. For the quantitative determinations of a potential water contamination, 100 mL or 10 mL of water are filtered through bacteriological filters (porosity of 0.45 μm). After filtration, the filters are deposited on the surface of Tryptic Soy agar Petri dishes. Amounts of 1 mL and 0.1 mL of water are also incorporated in two melted tryptic soy agar for a plate count in duplicate. All the dishes are incubated at 30 to 35°C for 3 to 5 days. For the qualitative determinations, 100 mL of water are filtered through 0.45 μm sterile filters. The filters are laid down on sterile Mac Conkey Petri dishes for the coliform bacteria and on Cetrimide agar Petri dishes for *Pseudomonas*. These are incubated at 30 to 35°C for 3 to 5 days. Questionable colonies are identified.

CHALLENGE TEST FOR THE EFFICACY OF PRESERVATION

Aim of Preservation

It is generally accepted that adequate preservation of a finished product, with preservatives or based on active preservation of a formulation, implies that the product remains stable and safe during storage (shelf-life) and consumer use [1,42–46]. From a public-health point of view, preservation must avoid infection of the consumer, and for product-quality reasons it must prevent a deterioration of the preparation. It is especially important to point out that the use of preservatives must not mask a lack of hygiene during manufacture. It is thus imperious to manufacture any cosmetic product according to Good Manufacturing Practices (GMPs) [34] such as imposed by the 6th Amendment of the European Directive 76/768/CEE [47], and to reach at the end of the manufacture the microbiological quality level discussed earlier in this chapter. Furthermore, the challenge test to evaluate the efficacy of preservation must not be simply performed on a lot-per-lot basis. The test has to be essentially connected with each development phase of the preparation [48]. It must be as simplified as possible for routine use, easy to standardize, and reproducible. Moreover, the test method must be able to show the potential intrinsic antibacterial efficacy of a formulation and should thus be performed on each finished product in its intact original container as well. Indeed, changes in the composition of the preparation have a tremendous influence on preservation [49,50]. Even minor changes in perfumes or dyes can affect the global behavior of the product [2,51,52]. Moreover, the material of the container and its type of closure influences the efficacy of the preservation and the protection of the product during use [45,53–55]. Rubber closures are, for example, known to absorb some amount of preservative from a solution [56,57]. Shave foams are often presented in containers under pressure with a propeller gaze such as butane. These storage conditions can widely influence the survival of some aerobic contaminants. Moreover, refrigeration can alter the preservative efficacy [58]. The preservatives may be inactivated by the components of the product [59].

Activity Spectrum of a Preservative

The use of the word ''antimicrobial'' preservative raises the need to define exactly what kind of activity is needed for a preservative. What are the organisms of concern: bacteria, fungi, viruses, or even spores? The scale of the activity spectrum is based on almost three parameters: (1) the survival, or even multiplication, of particular organisms in a wide range of products; (2) the pathogenicity of these organisms by the route of administration; and (3) the possibility to find effective chemicals at nontoxic concentrations.

Sporicidal action must not be considered because sporicidal chemicals are very rare (e.g., aldehydes are too toxic to be used in a cosmetic product at effective concentrations). Moreover, infectious problems induced by spore formers are very seldom, as previously discussed for the talcum powder in this chapter. Even if aerobic spore formers are often found in raw materials and finished products, according to Davis [13] they should not be a hazard to human health.

Virucidal action is not considered for cosmetics. These facts restrict the spectrum of a cosmetic preservative to bacteria and fungi. According to the most widespread opinion, a bactericidal and a fungicidal effect is needed so that the contaminating organisms accidentally introduced in the preparation will be killed. A bacteriostatic or fungistatic action could eventually be accepted to stabilize a preparation during the shelf-life of a unidose, nonsterile product. For the fungicidal and bactericidal actions, the concentration of the preservative must be toxicologicaly acceptable.

Test Organisms

As previously discussed, the range of organisms must contain bacteria and fungi. Within these we must find Gram-positive and Gram-negative bacteria because the structure of the bacterial wall influences the penetration and thus the efficacy of the preservating agent. For the fungi, representatives of the two fungal forms must be used, namely the vegetative yeast cell and the mould spore. The choice of species is directed by their skin and mucosal pathogenicity for cosmetics. Product degradation capabilities are also taken into account to choose the species. So among the Gram-positive species, *Staphylococcus aureus* is an important skin pathogen, as is *Pseudomonas aeruginosa* for the Gram-negative bacteria. This latter organism is also able to use many compounds, such as preservatives or even disinfectants, as a carbon source and is very adaptative in adverse environmental conditions even in pure water [60,61]. For the yeast, *Candida albicans* is a skin pathogen and *Aspergillus niger* is a representative of the degradation flora. The choice of strains for a standardized assay must be guided by the need to compare results obtained in different laboratories, and in this way culture-collection strains are chosen coming from the American Type Culture Collection (ATCC). The strains normally used are as follows: (1) *Staphylococcus aureus* ATCC 6538, (2) *Pseudomonas aeruginosa* ATCC 9027, (3) *Candida albicans* ATCC 10231, and (4) *Aspergillus niger* ATCC 16404. These strains are to some extent resistant to the antimicrobials, and some are also used for testing disinfectants or antibiotics. For a representative preservation-efficacy test, it is also recommended to add strains isolated from the environment, water, or contaminated products. These strains live in the vicinity of or even inside the product, are well adapted to adverse conditions, and are often resistant to preservatives or even disinfectants [62–64]. Nevertheless, after a few passages in culture media, this particular resistance can disappear. Precautions must be taken to avoid this, such as immediate storage in appropriate medium by deep freezing or in liquid nitrogen.

Test Conditions and Validations

The challenge test consists in an artificial contamination of the tested sample and counting of the survivors during a period of 4 weeks maximum. Even if several preservative efficacy tests exist as described in the USP23 [65], the Japanese Pharmacopeia [66], or the CTFA test [67–74], the general conditions of the test described here are those of the European Pharmacopeia [43], adapted from a Federation Internationale Pharmaceutique (FIP) working party publication [44]. Several points, such as validations and strain maintenance, are described here in more detail.

Maintenance of Microbial Strains

The cultures can be maintained as described in the CEN 216 PrEN 12353 document [75]. Stock cultures are maintained at a temperature below $-18°C$. To prepare the working culture, subcultures are originated from the culture stock by streaking onto adequate agar medium slopes. The second and/or third subcultures can be used as the working cultures.

Preparation of the Inoculum

The subcultures to be used in the test are plated on Petri dishes of suitable media, e.g., Tryptic Soy Agar (TSA) for the bacteria and Sabouraud Dextrose Agar (SDA) for the fungi. After adequate incubation—18 to 24 hours for the bacteria, 48 hours for the yeast, and 3 to 5 days for the mould—the cultures are collected with sterile, normal saline. The suspensions are then calibrated against a Mac Farland scale or by using any suitable calibration system. This calibrated suspension homogenized at a maximum ratio of $1:100$ (0.2 mL in 20 µg or mL, for example) of the tested sample must give between 5.10^5 and 5.10^6 organisms per millilitre or gram. Such a high inoculum density is imposed not only by the counting technique of the survivors, or the "plate count," but also by the importance of the logarithmic reduction asked for the products.

Test Conditions

The first day of the challenge test, the product and two controls—one comprising the tested product without preservatives and one of normal saline with 1% peptone—are inoculated with each microbial strain. A microbial count is immediately performed after homogeneization on this group of three vials. Counts are performed after dilution of 1 g or mL of the sample, with 9 mL of neutralizer. The neutralizing solution used is the same as in the first part of this chapter. Further dilutions are made in normal saline in order to perform a plate-count technique according to the estimate contamination. Sampling is performed in the same way for the preserved samples, after 2, 7, 14, and 28 days of storage of the inoculated product kept at room temperature in the dark or in its normal storage conditions.

To estimate the starting value 100%, the product effect must be evaluated on the inoculum. So, the inoculum level is estimated in a nonpreserved test product, if available, and compared with the level measured into normal saline containing 1% of peptone. If the following occur: (1) data obtained in the nonpreserved product are equivalent to those obtained in saline, and this value is chosen as the starting level (100%); (2) the data obtained in the product is < or = 1 log from the saline data, the value obtained in the saline control is chosen as the starting value; and (3) if the product data are > 1 log from the saline control, this is an indication of product contamination and the test is invalid. The results of the test are expressed as logarithmic reduction versus time of the value taken as 100%.

Validation of the Contamination of the Sample

The contamination of the sample consists of a homogeneous incorporation into the sample of a single strain at a maximum ratio of 1% of calibrated suspension. Most of the time, the inoculum is aqueous and dispersed in an aqueous phase; for some products, addition of tween 80 ou isopropylic myristate could be useful to homogenize the inoculum. In some cases, a dried inoculum suspended in isododecane is used to contaminate fatty products. It is indispensable to ascertain that the inoculum can homogeneously be dispersed through the product. This is nearly immediate for liquids but much more difficult for oily products such as creams or mascaras. A validation is thus performed using a nonpreserved product that is inoculated with the calibrated suspension and homogenized. At least three different samples are taken from the product and the results of the counts obtained for these samples are compared. The difference between samples must be less than 1 log.

Validation of the Neutralizing Solution

Because a neutralizing solution is used as first dilutant when counting the survivors, the efficacy of the neutralizing solution must be validated in order to avoid false-negative results. For this purpose, 1 mL of the preserved sample or 1 mL sterile normal saline are added to 9 mL neutralizing solution. The two tubes are well mixed and let at rest for 10 minutes. 0.1 mL of a 10^{-3} dilution of the calibrated suspension are then added and mixed to both tubes. The colony-forming units in each tube are estimated, and the difference in results between the tubes must be less than 1 log.

Interpretation of the Results

The criteria taken by the European Pharmacopeia for the topically applied product are a good base of discussion [43]. For bacteria, the recommended criteria (level A) are a 2 log reduction after 2 days, 3 log after 7 days, and no increase in the recovered bacteria after 28 days. For fungi, a 2 log reduction is requested after 14 days with no increase of the counts after 28 days. This requirement of no increase of the counts at the end of the test period is of particular importance. Indeed, even if the logarithmic reduction attained by a product is greater than the requirement, a regrowth of the organisms during the examination period is unacceptable. This would indicate that the micro-organisms are able to adapt their metabolic capacities to use the product, and its preservative in particular, as carbon source. In the European Pharmacopeia, it is also stated that, in justified cases, e.g., when adverse reactions could occur, level B criteria can be used to interpret the results. These are: for bacteria, a 3 log reduction after 14 days and no increase of the counts after 28 days; and for fungi, 1 log reduction after 14 days and no increase of the counts after 28 days.

DETERMINATION OF WATER AVAILABILITY OR a_w

Water availability (a_w) is defined as the water available for bacterial metabolism and is evaluated by measurement of the water vapor pressure at the surface of a product or a raw material. It can be defined as the following ratio:

$$A_w = \frac{\text{water vapor pressure over substance at } t°}{\text{water vapor pressure over pure water at } t°}$$

It depends on temperature and on formulations. It is not correlated with the total water content of a formula but depends of the quantity of water "trapped" into the formula chemicals. Ingredients such as humectants, gums, or others, use the water to swell and so this water is no longer available for bacterial growth. As water is a critical growth factor for micro-organisms, one of the means to preserve a formula is to decrease the level of water availability, optimizing a formula by the inclusion of ingredients that fix the water. Most *Pseudomonas* cannot grow if the a_w is less than 90%, and under 70% the probability of microorganism growth in the product is lowered [76].

The a_w of a product is evaluated through the use of a moisture-sensing device that measures the head space relative humidity on the top of the product surface contained in a closed jar or dish after equilibration. This device must first be calibrated, using calibration standards. The standards are selected to represent low, medium, and high value operation or to bracket the area of interest. In general, the standards are saturated salt solutions such as NaCl ($a_w = 0.75$), $BaCl_2$ ($a_w = 0.90$), and LiCl ($a_w = 0.11$). As the a_w measurement is temperature dependent, it is recommended to perform the calibrations and measures at controlled room temperature. Table of commonly used standards and their temperature variations can be found in Ref. 77.

CULTURE MEDIA, NEUTRALIZING SOLUTION, AND BUFFERS

TABLE 1 Sterile Neutralizing Solution

Lecithin	4.0 g
Polysorbate 80	30.0 g
Peptamin	10.0 g
Beef extract	5.0 g
Histidine	1.0 g
Sodium laurylsulfate	4.0 g
Sodium chloride	5.0 g
Distilled water	1000 mL

TABLE 2 Sterile Buffered Peptone Saline at pH 7

Monopotassium phosphate	3.56 g
Dihydrated disodium phosphate	7.23 g (equivalent to 0.067 M)
Sodium chloride	4.30 g
Meat or casein peptone	1.0 g
Purified water	1000 mL

Note: 1 g/L or 10 g/L of polysorbate 20 or 80 can be added to the solution. Sterilize in the autoclave at 121°C for 15 minutes.

TABLE 3 Tryptic Soy Agar

Tryptone	15.0 g
Soya peptone	5.0 g
Sodium chloride	5.0 g
Agar	15.0 g
Purified water	1000 mL

Note: Sterilize in the autoclave at 121°C for 15 minutes. pH must be 7.3 ± 0.2.

TABLE 4 Sabouraud Chloramphenicol Agar

Meat and casein peptone	10 g
Dextrose	40 g
Chloramphenicol	0.05 g
Agar	15 g
Purified water	1000 mL

Note: Sterilize in the autoclave at 121°C for 15 minutes.

TABLE 5 Enterobacteria Enrichment Broth (EEB Mossel)

Tryptose	10.0 g
Dextrose	5.0 g
Disodium phosphate	8.0 g
Monopotassium phosphate	2.0 g
Oxgall	20.0 g
Brilliant green	0.0135 g
Purified water	1000 mL

Note: Heat to 100°C for 30 minutes, cool immediately. pH 7.2 ± 0.2.

TABLE 6 Agar with Crystal Violet, Neutral Red, Bile Salts, and VRBG Agar with Glucose

Yeast extract	3.0 g
Peptone	7.0 g
Bile salts	1.5 g
Lactose	10.0 g
Sodium chloride	5.0 g
Agar	15.0 g
Neutral red	0.03 g
Crystal violet	0.002 g
Dextrose	10.0 g
Purified water	1000 mL

Note: Heat to boil, do not autoclave. pH 7.4 ± 0.2.

TABLE 7 Mac Conkey Broth

Peptone	20.0 g
Lactose	10.0 g
Oxgall	5.0 g
Brom cresol purple	0.01 g
Purified water	1000 mL

Note: Sterilize by autoclave at 121°C for 15 minutes. pH 7.3 ± 0.2.

TABLE 8 Mac Conkey Agar

Casein peptone	17.0 g
Meat peptone	3.0 g
Lactose	10.0 g
Sodium chloride	5.0 g
Bile salts	1.5 g
Agar	13.5 g
Neutral red	0.03 g
Crystal violet	0.001 g
Purified water	1000 mL

Note: Sterilize by autoclave at 121°C for 15 minutes. pH 7.1 ± 0.2.

TABLE 9 Tryptic Soy Broth

Casein peptone	17.0 g
Soja peptone	3.0 g
Sodium chloride	5.0 g
Dipotassium phosphate	2.5 g
Dextrose	2.5 g
Purified water	1000 mL

Note: Sterilize by autoclave at 121°C for 15 minutes. pH 7.3 ± 0.2.

TABLE 10 Cetrimide Agar

Peptone	20.0 g
Magnesium chloride	1.4 g
Dipotassium sulfate	10.0 g
Cetrimide	0.3 g
Agar	13.6 g
Glycerol	10.0 mL
Purified water	1000 mL

Note: Sterilize by autoclave at 121°C for 15 minutes. pH 7.2 ± 0.2.

TABLE 11 Baird Parker Agar

Peptone	20.0 g
Beef meat extract	5.0 g
Yeast extract	1.0 g
Lithium chloride	5.0 g
Agar	20.0 g
Glycine	12.0 g
Sodium pyruvate	10.0 g

Note: Sterilize by autoclave at 121°C for 15 minutes. Cool to 45–50°C and add 10 mL of a sterile potassium tellurite solution at 10 g/L and 50 mL of an egg yolk emulsion.

TABLE 12 Sabouraud Dextrose Agar

Peptone	10.0 g
Dextrose	40.0 g
Agar	15.0 g

Note: Sterilize by autoclave at 121°C for 15 minutes.

REFERENCES

1. Hugo WB. Antimicrobial agents as preservatives in pharmaceutical and cosmetic products. Introduction: the scope of the problem. J Appl Bacteriol 1978; 44:Siii–Sv.
2. Orth DS, Lutes CM. Adaptation of bacteria to cosmetic preservatives. Cosm Toil 1985; 100(2): 57–59.
3. Anelich LE, Korsten L. Survey of micro-organism associated with spoilage of cosmetic creams manufactured in South Africa. Int J Cosm Science 1996; 18:25–40.
4. Tremewan HC. Tetanus neonatorium in New Zealand. N Z Med J 1946; 45:312–313.
5. Sevitt S. Source of two hospital infected case of tetanus. Lancet 1949; 2:1075–1077.
6. Noble WC, Savin JA. Steroid cream contaminated with *Pseudomonas aeruginosa*. Lancet 1966; 1:347–349.
7. Morse LJ, Williams HL, Grenn FP Jr, Eldridge EE, Rotta JR. Septicemia due to *Klebsiella pneumoniae* originating from a hand cream dispenser. New Engl J Med 1967; 277:472–473.
8. Morse LJ, Schonbeck LE. Hand lotions a potential nosocomial hazard. New Engl J Med 1968; 278:364–369.
9. Wilson LA, Keuhne JW, Hall SW, Ahearn DGH. Microbial contamination in ocular cosmetics. Am J Ophtalmol 1971; 71:1298–1302.
10. Smart R, Spooner DF. Microbiological spoilage in pharmaceuticals and cosmetics. J Soc Cosmet Chem 1972; 23:721–737.
11. Dony J. Problèmes microbiologiques posés par les cosmétiques. J Pharm Belg 1975; 30:223–238.
12. Wilson LA, Julian AJ, Ahearn DG. The survival and growth of microorganisms in mascara during use. Am J Ophthalmol 1975; 79:596–601.
13. Davis JG. The microbial stability of cosmetics and toilet preparations. Soap Perfum Cosmet 1973; 46:409–418.
14. Goldman CL. Microorganisms isolated from cosmetics. D&CI July 1975:40–41.

15. Marzulli FN, Evans JR, Yoder PD. Induced pseudomonas keratitis as related to cosmetics. J Soc Cosmet Chem 1972; 23:89–97.

16. Chowchuvech E, Sawicki L, Tenenbaum S, Galin MA. Effect of various microorganisms found in cosmetics on the normal and injured eye of the rabbit. Am J Ophthalmol 1973; 75:1004–1009.

17. Wilson LA, Ahearn DG. Pseudomonas induced corneal ulcers associated with contaminated eye mascaras. Am J Ophthalmol 1977; 54:112–119.

18. Ahearn DG, Sanghvi J, Haller GJ, Wilson LA. Mascara contamination: in use laboratory studies. J Soc Cosmet Chem 1978; 29:127–131.

19. Reid FR, Wood TO. Pseudomonas corneal ulcer: the causative role of eye cosmetics. Arch Ophthalmol 1979; 97:1640–1641.

20. Brannan DK. Cosmetic preservation. Cosm Toil 1996; 111:69–83.

21. Frenkel LM. Pseudomonas folliculitis from sponges promoted as beauty aids. J Clin Microbiol 1993; 31:2838.

22. Jarvis B, Reynolds AJ, Rhodes AC, Armstrong M. A survey of microbiological contamination in cosmetics and toiletries in the UK (1971). J Soc Cosm Chem 1974; 25:563–575.

23. Dawson NL, Reinhardt DJ. Microbial flora of in-use, display eye shadow testers and bacterial challenges of unused eye shadows. Appl Environ Microbiol 1981; 42:297–302.

24. Economou-Stamatelopoulou C, Chitiroglou-Lada A, Papavassiliou J. Contamination microbienne de savons. Pharm Acta Helv 1982; 57:298–300.

25. Baird RM. Bacteriological contamination of products used for skin care in babies. Int J Cosmet Sci 1984; 6:85–90.

26. Ashour MSE, Hefani H, El-Tayeb OM, Abdelaziz AA. Microbial contamination of cosmetics and personal care items in Egypt 1. Cosm Toil 1987; 102:61–68.

27. Abdelaziz AA, Alkofahi A. Microbiological profile of selected samples of ⟨⟨Al-Kohl⟩⟩ eye cosmetics in northern Jordanian provinces before and after use. Zentralbl Bakteriol Mikrobiol Hyg B 1989; 187:244–253.

28. Dony J, Devleeschouwer MJ. Contamination microbienne des produits bruts d'origine végétale: incidence pour les préparations cosmétiques. J Pharm Belg 1989; 44:411–419.

29. Misclivec PB, Bandler R, Allen G. Incidence of fungi in shared-use cosmetics available in the public. J AOAC Int 1993; 76:430–436.

30. Hingst V. The importance of contaminated dental care commodities results of field research. Zentralbl Bakteriol Mikrobiol Hyg B 1989; 187:337–364.

31. FIP 1972: pureté microbiologique des formes pharmaceutiques non obligatoirement stériles. Rapport commun du Comité des laboratoireset des services officiels de contrôle des médicaments et de la section des pharmaciens de l'industrie de la FIP. J Mond Pharm 1972; 15:88–100.

32. Devleeschouwer MJ. Flore microbienne des médicaments. Espèces opportunistes et antibiorésistance. Ph.D. thesis, Université Libre de Bruxelles, Bruxelles, Belgium, 1980.

33. Schiller I, Kuntscher H, Wolff A, Nekola M. Microbial content of nonsterile therapeutic agents containing natural or seminatural active ingredients. Appl Microbiol 1968; 16:1924–1928.

34. Pedersen EA, Ulrich K. Microbial contents in nonsterile pharmaceuticals III raw materials. Dansk Tideskr Farm 1968; 42:71–83.

35. Steinberg D. Botanical extracts and preservation issues. Cosm Toil 1991; 106:73–74.

36. Wallhausser KH. Sterilisation-Desinfektion-Konservierung-Keimidentifizierung-Betriebshygiene. Stuttgart: Georg Thieme Verlag, 1978.

37. Agnew B. The Laminar Flow Clean Room Handbook. 3rd ed. California: Agnews Higgins, 1968.

38. European Commission, Directorate General III, working party on ⟨control of medicines and inspections⟩. Revision of the annex 1 of the EU guide to Good Manufacturing Practice. Manufacturing of sterile medicinal products, 1 January 1997.

39. Contrôle de la contamination microbienne dans des produits non obligatoirement stériles, dé-

nombrement des germes viables totaux; 2.6.12. Pharmacopée européenne IIIed, Conseil de l'Europe, Strasbourg 1997:83–87.

40. Contrôle de la contamination microbienne dans des produits non obligatoirement stériles, recherche des microorganismes spécifiés. Pharmacopée européenne IIIed, Conseil de l'Europe, Strasbourg 1997:87–89.

41. FIP 1975: Pureté microbiologique des formes pharmaceutiques non obligatoirement stériles: méthodes d'examen. 2ème rapport commun du Comité des laboratoires et Services Officiels de contrôle des médicaments et de la section des Pharmaciens de l'industrie. Pharm Acta Helv 1976; 51:33–40.

42. Baird RM. The occurrence of pathogens in cosmetics and toiletries. J Soc Cosm Chem 1977; 28:17–20.

43. Efficacité de la conservation antimicrobienne 5.1.3. Pharmacopée européenne IIIed, Conseil de l'Europe Strasbourg, 1997:296–298.

44. FIP 1980. Essai d'efficacité de la conservation antimicrobienne des préparations pharmaceutiques. 3ème rapport commun du Comité des Laboratories et Services offciels de cobntrôle des médicaments et de la section des pharmaciens de l'industrie de la FIP. Pharm Acta Helv 1980; 55:40–49.

45. FIP 1984. The test for efficacy of antimicrobial preservatives of pharmaceuticals. 3rd joint report of the Committee of Official laboratories and drug control services and the section of industrial pharmacists. FIP. In: Kabara JJ, ed. New York: Marcel Dekker, 1984:423–440.

46. Lorenzoitti OJ. A preservative evaluation program for dermatological and cosmetic preparation. In: Kabara JJ, ed., New York: Marcel Dekker, 1984:441–463.

47. 6th amendment (93/35/EEC) of the Council Directive of 27 July 1976 on the approximation of the laws of the Member States relating to cosmetic products (76/768/EEC). Official Journal n°L 151, June 23, 1993.

48. Moore KE. Evaluating preservative efficacy by challenge testing during the development stage of pharmaceutical products. J Appl Bacteriol 1978; 44:SXLIII-SLV.

49. Wan LS, Kurup TRR, Chan LW. Partition of preservatives in oil/water systems. Pharm Acta Helv 1986; 61:308–313.

50. Kurup TR, Wan LSC, Chan LW. Availability and activity of preservatives in emulsified systems. Pharm Acta Helv 1991; 66:76–82.

51. Sakamoto T, Yanagi M; Fukushima S, Mitsui T. Effect of some cosmetic pigments on the bactericidal activities of preservatives. J Soc Cosm Chem 1987; 38:83–98.

52. Steinberg DC. Preserving foundations. Cosm Toil 1995; 110:71–74.

53. McCarthy TJ. Interaction between aqueous preservative solutions and their plastic containers. Pharm Weekbld 1970; 105:557–563, 1139–1146.

54. Melichar M, Podstatova H, Pokorny J, Hybasek P, Pokorna M. Mikrobiologische reinheit der arzneizubereitungen Teil 1: Externa: der einfluss von cremetyp, behälter, aufbewahrung, temperatur und applikation. Pharmazie 1980; 35:484–488.

55. Brannan DK, Dille JC. Type of closure prevents microbial contamination of cosmetics during consumer use. Appl Environ Microbiol 1990; 56:1476–1479.

56. Lachamn L, Weinstein S, Hopkins G, Slack S, Eisman P, Cooper J. Stability of antibacterial preservatives in parenteral solutions I. Factors influencing the loss of antimicrobial agents from solutions in rubber-stopped containers. J Pharm Sci 1962; 51:224–232.

57. Lachman L, Urbanyl T, Weinstein S. Stability of antibacterial preservatives in parenteral solutions IV. Contribution of rubber closure composition on preservative loss. J Pharm Sci 1963; 52:244–249.

58. Lehmann CR. Effect on refrigeration on bactericidal activity of four preserved multiple-dose injectable drug products. Am J Hosp Pharm 1977; 34:1196–1200.

59. Grigo J. Microorganisms in drugs and cosmetics—occurrence, harms and consequences in hygienic manufacturing. Zentralbl Bakteriol [Orig B] 1976; 162:233–287.

60. Yanagi M, Onishi G. Assimilation of selected cosmetic ingredients by microorganisms. J Soc Cosmet Chem 1971; 22:851–865.

61. Levy E. Insights into microbial adaptation to cosmetic and pharmaceutical products. Cosm Toil 1987; 102:69–74.

62. Decicco BT, Lee EC, Sorrentino JV. Factors affecting survival of *Pseudomonas cepacia* in decongestant nasal sprays containing thimerosal as preservative. J Pharm Sci 1982; 71:1231–1234.

63. Bosi C, Davin-Regli A, Charrel R, Rocca B, Monnet D, Bollet C. Serratia marcescens nosocomial outbreak due to contaminated hexetidine solution. J Hosp Infect 1996; 33:217–224.

64. Zani F, Minutello A, Maggi L, Santi P, Mazza P. Evaluation of preservative efficacy in pharmaceutical products: the use of a wild strain of *Pseudomonas cepacia*. J Appl Microbiol 1997; 83:322–326.

65. Antimicrobial preservatives efficacy. ⟨51⟩, United States Pharmacopeia 23, United States Pharmacopeial Convention, Rockwell, MD, 1994: 1681.

66. Preservatives—efficacy test. Japanese Pharmacopeial Forums, 1995; 4:664–668.

67. McEwen GN, Curry AS. Determination of the adequacy of preservation testing of aqueous liquid and semi-liquid eye cosmetics (1975). Cosmetic Toiletry and Fragance Association Guidelines, Washington, D.C.: CFFA, 1983.

68. Brannan DK, Dille JC, Kaufman DJ. Correlation of in vitro challenge testing with consumer use testing for cosmetic products. Appl Environ Microbiol 1987; 53:1827–1832.

69. Connolly P, Bloomfield SF, Benyer SP. A study of the use of rapid methods for preservative efficacy testing of pharmaceuticals and cosmetics. J Appl Bacteriol 1993; 75:456–462.

70. Connolly P, Bloomfield SF, Denyer SP. The use of impedance for preservative efficacy testing of pharmaceuticals and cosmetic products. J Appl Bacteriol 1994; 76:68–74.

71. Farrington JK, Martz EL, Wells SJ, Ennis CC, Holder J, Levchuk JW, Avis KE, Hoffman PS, Hitchins AD, Madden JM. Ability of laboratory methods to predict in-use efficacy of antimicrobial preservatives in an experimental cosmetic. Appl Environ Microbiol 1994; 60:4553–4558.

72. Hodges NA, Denyer SP, Hanlon GW, Reynolds JP. Preservative efficacy tests in formulated nasal products: reproducibility and factors affecting preservative activity. J Pharm Pharmacol 1996; 48:1237–1242.

73. Lenczewski ME, McGavin ST, Vandyke K. Comparison of automated and traditional minimum inhibitory concentration procedures for microbiological cosmetic preservatives. J AOAC Int 1996; 79:1294–1299.

74. Lenczewski ME, Kananen LL. Automated screening method for determining optimum preservative systems for personal and home care products. J AOAC Int 1998; 81:534–539.

75. PrEN12353. Chemical disinfectants and antiseptics. Preservation of microbial strains used for the determination of bactericidal and fungicidal activity. CEN/TC 216 HWG N114, 18/02/1998.

76. Legenhausen R. Water activity measurements. Microbiological quality of water-based product. Center for Professional Advancement Course, Amsterdam, 1989.

77. Greenspan M. Humidity fixed points of binary saturated aqueous solutions. J Res Nat Bureau Standards, 1977; 81a:89–96.

65

Introduction to the Proof of Claims

Marc Paye
Colgate-Palmolive Research and Development, Inc., Milmort, Belgium

André O. Barel
Free University of Brussels, Brussels, Belgium

With the continuous increase in the variety of cosmetic products proposed to consumers over these last decades, it has become more and more difficult for them to decide what the most appropriate products are for their needs. Aware of such difficulties, cosmetic manufacturers have understood that the success of a product today is not only a question of performance, but also a question of how it is promoted to the potential buyer. Progressively, product promotion took more importance and advertising claims became more aggressive and closer to the limit of what could be scientifically shown and consumer-perceived. In order to monitor the claims made about cosmetic products and protect the consumer against misleading advertisement, several national/federal agencies have issued rules under the form of laws, or directives, to ensure that proper substantiation of claims exists. Furthermore, relying on such rules, competitors always remain ready to challenge unfair or doubtful claims. Last but not least, the consumers themselves have become more critical and, when they feel that their product does not provide the properties that it claims, do not hesitate to stop buying the product as well as the other products of the same brand. It has thus become a priority for the cosmetic chemist to be able to show and substantiate the properties that are claimed for his or her product.

The objectives of this introduction to the proof of claims are as follows:

1. To briefly describe the regional requirements related to the proof of claims.
2. To explain the different existing categories of claims.
3. To review the types of support that can be made.

REGIONAL REQUIREMENTS

Although all over the world the motivation exists to protect the consumer against misleading claims, the current situation is quite different between Europe, the United States, and Japan regarding claim substantiation requirements and the limit of definitions of a cosmetic product. This latter point has been discussed in previous sections (see Part 7 of this book). Specific regulations are summarized hereafter.

The United States

The U.S. federal law does not require premarketing proof of claims but prohibits false advertisement. In the case of a challenge (e.g., by a competitor, a consumer association, a government agency), the manufacturer must be prepared to defend the claims made on the product. However, the challenger has to first provide arguments questioning the validity of the claim. It is quite frequent in the United States for claims to be challenged, and most companies preferably develop scientifically valid claims support strategies and dossiers before marketing their new product.

Several federal authorities controlling cosmetic claims exist. The U.S. Food and Drug Administration (FDA), through the Federal Food, Drug and Cosmetic Act (FDC Act) and the Fair Packaging and Labeling Act (FPL Act), has the main jurisdiction and responsibility on claims made on the labeling of the products. The Federal Trade Commission (FTC) monitors product advertising (e.g., television, radio, magazine). When a claim is related to both advertising and labeling, the two agencies usually collaborate with each other. However, even if both agencies condemn in their respective Acts consumer misleading, neither clearly defines the legal standard for illegality. The manufacturer will thus rely upon a "reasonable" basis to support its claims, and most challenges will be treated on a case-by-case basis.

Another significant control of advertising is performed by the National Advertising Division (NAD) of the Council of Better Business Bureaus, which is a self-regulatory, nongovernmental body evaluating the truth and accuracy of challenged advertising. NAD is usually the first body to receive complaints about claims from competing companies or consumer associations. Through several control and communication steps between the two challengers, NAD may decide to involve the appropriate government Agency (FDA or FTC). Several examples of challenged claims have been summarized by Davis and McNamara [1] and Friedel [2], that can help in understanding the U.S. situation.

The European Union

In the European Union, cosmetic claims substantiation is regulated by the 6th Amendment to the Cosmetic Directive, effective since January 1, 1997. In that amendment, it is stated that cosmetics and toiletries manufacturers making claims for their products have to demonstrate the proof of their claims. The dossier containing these proofs has to be readily available if requested by the competent authority. The dossier may be written in English or in the language of the country where it is deposited. More details on the Cosmetic Directive can be obtained in Chapter 60.

As in the United States, no clear definition about the meaning of proof of claims has been given, so manufacturers have to define by themselves what they consider to be a "reasonable" and "acceptable" proof for their claim. Such a consideration will often depend on the type and originality of the claim, the type of product and the market in which it will compete, the consequences and benefits that the consumer can expect from the claimed effect, and the image, scientific honesty, and competency of the manufacturer.

Although the 6th Amendment to the Directive aimed at uniformizing the differences between countries, big differences still exist regarding how to monitor the proof of claims dossiers, which is basically subject to the interpretation of the Directive within individual state laws. In most countries, such monitoring will essentially be postmarketing in the case of a challenge, but in some countries a premarketing review of the claims can be requested by a National Review Board (e.g., Greece). Some types of claims are also not uniformly accepted for cosmetic products by all E.U. members; this is, for instance, the case of claims that can be overlooked as "medically oriented" such as "dermatologically tested" or "hypoallergenic" (e.g., not allowed in Denmark for cosmetics). The decision for acceptable claims and reasonable supporting dossier should thus always be reviewed in line with the individual national laws, if any, of the country where marketing is intended.

Japan

In Japan, the situation is different in the sense that claims are reviewed before marketing of the cosmetic product. The Ministry of Health and Welfare (MHW) has to provide a license to the product to allow its marketing. The limit of the definition of purely cosmetic products is also different in Japan than in the European Union and United States, with the existence of "quasi-drugs" classified between cosmetics and drugs. This has been reviewed in Chapter 62.

CATEGORIES OF CLAIMS

However they are used (e.g., label, television, or magazine advertising), claims related to cosmetic products can be subdivided into several categories. Table 1 summarizes these categories and provides some examples for each. As previously explained, all claims are not applicable everywhere in the world for cosmetic products and can fall under different regulations in some places.

TABLE 1 Categories of Claims

Categories of Claims	Examples
Claims related to physical and chemical properties	Contains x% of an active
	Neutral pH
	20% more in the bottle
	More concentrated
Claims related to the test procedure or to an endorsement	Dermatologist, dermatologically tested
	Tested under the Good Clinical Practices Principles
	Tested and approved by an institute
Safety-related claims	Mild, gentle on the skin
	For sensitive skin
	Skin-repair properties
	Hypoallergenic
Objective efficacy claims	Moisturizing, hydrating
	Improves elasticity, firmness of skin
	Skin-whitening effect
	Sunscreen effect
	Antiperspirant, deodorant
Subjective claims	Skin will feel softer; more hydrated
	With a pleasant feel, texture
	Smells fresher
Cultural claims	Contains 100% natural ingredients
	Not tested on animals
Juxtaposition claims	Contains an ingredient known for such a property

1.   Claims related to physical and chemical properties of the product can be substantiated by measuring directly the claimed characteristic in the product by an analytical method. The measurement methodology has, however, to be well established and validated.

2.   Claims related to the test procedure or to an endorsement by an outside authority simply describe the way, person/title, or place where the product has been tested. They are usually perceived by the consumer as proof of a well-tested, quality product. It is essential for such claims to show the property that the consumer can expect from the product, even if it is not directly advertised. For example, the claim "dermatologist tested" means that the product has been tested by a dermatologist, but also implies that the results of the test were good and that the product is, e.g., mild on the skin, or has a skin-beneficial property shown by the dermatologist.

3.   Safety-related claims make the consumer confident about the innocuousness of the product and the benefits to their body. These claims usually require clinical tests on human volunteers according to protocols published in the scientific literature and performed under high-quality standards. In some cases, in vitro tests can also be accepted if it can be shown that they are able to prove the claimed property for the type of product in test.

4.   Objective efficacy claims are probably the most frequent, and those inducing the highest expectation from consumers. This is why they require solid efficacy data dossiers. Many biometric methodologies currently allow getting a direct measurement of the skin properties [3] that are expected to be respected or modified by the cosmetic product. In vivo tests with human volunteers are often recommended or even the only possibility offered to the cosmetic chemist, but other types of tests can also be used in some cases, such as cell-culture tests [4–6].

5.   Subjective claims are related to a property or function of the product that is perceived by the consumer. The property does not necessarily have to be objectively substantiated by direct measurement. Only tests on human volunteers can be performed, such as sensory tests (Chap. 71) or well-designed consumer tests.

6.   Cultural claims are usually related to the composition of the product and take advantage of the current trends. Their value to the consumer is often dependent on the education, country, or environment. They link the composition of the product to ecological, ethical, or moral considerations (e.g., naturality of ingredients, absence of tests on animals).

7.   Juxtaposition claims refer to the presence of an ingredient in a product and to the known property of the ingredient, without claiming that the complete product has the property. This type of claim can be supported by proving the presence of the ingredient in the product (analytical methods) and relating the claimed property to that ingredient through literature data or any type of appropriate test on the pure ingredient.

Several of these categories can be further subdivided in terms of absolute or comparative claims. The following four subcategories can be described as follows:

(a)   Noncomparative claims: they simply refer to a property of the product without any direct comparison to another product. However, it is obvious that even if not classified as such, all claims contain a comparative connotation. For instance, claiming that a product is mild means that this is not the case for all other products. Similarly, claiming that a product is hydrating for the skin refers to the hypothesis that some other products are not. Examples include claims that a product is mild, hydrating, protects the skin, and softens the skin.

(b)   Claims comparing a new product to the one it replaces in the market place: in the proof of claim dossier, a direct comparison between the two products will be required. The kind of test depends on the claim. Examples include x% more efficacy, milder than ever, and even milder than before.

(c)   Purely comparative claims comparing the new product to competitive ones for the claimed property: this kind of claim is likely to be challenged by competitors and requires a solid supporting dossier where direct comparison between the products is made. The test methodology has to be well justified and validated for the objective. Such comparative claims are quite usual in the United States; in Europe they are allowed only under restricted and severe conditions. Examples include milder than product x and y, and more hydrating than product z.

(d)   Absolute claims: the comparison is not limited to a few mentioned products as previously discussed, but the product claims to be the best in the market for a given property or to completely fulfill a specific function. Such claims require very solid dossier and can be invalidated if even one competitive product can be shown to be superior on this property. Examples include the mildest, nothing more hydrating, total protection, and complete diet for the skin.

TYPE OF SUPPORT

Whenever the nature of the effect or the product justifies it, the claims on cosmetic products must be shown. However, the type of support has never been clearly and officially defined, so that any kind of support could be acceptable at the condition it can be scientifically and reasonably justified. Different ways to support cosmetic claims [7] are reviewed hereafter; some have already been briefly discussed earlier in this chapter.

Comparison to a Similar Formula

If the product is derived from another formula by a minor modification, it is not always necessary to repeat the claim-supporting test for the new product. In such a case, it has however to be clearly justified that the change is not to affect the claimed property. Depending on the claims, certain modifications can be considered minor or not. Similarly, for a line of products with minor differences between individual products, some claims can often be shown on only a few products of the line and then extended to the other products.

Literature Search

For some types of claims, literature data can be considered as effective claim-support dossier. This is, for instance, the case of claims on ingredients entering into the composition of the cosmetic product; often, the proof of the ingredient property can be found into the scientific literature. It should be noticed, however, that peer-reviewed literature usually has more credit than supplier literature in the case of a challenge, although the latter can also be used if supported by well-controlled tests.

In Vitro Tests

In vitro tests never have the same value as in vivo data obtained from clinical tests run on human volunteers. This is why they are mostly used in combination with other types of data. However, in some cases (depending on the claim or the availability of alternative tests), in vitro tests can be used on their own to support claims, provided that the test is proven to be scientifically valid for the intended objective. From the most promising and usual in vitro tests, 3-D cell-culture methodologies probably receive the most credit for investigating many cosmetic product properties, from skin mildness to more specific properties like sun protection [4–6].

For special dermatocosmetic claims, such as fat reduction and anticellulites effects, in vitro data are mostly presented as direct support. However, in such cases, scientifically valid in vivo testing about the efficacy of these treatments is not always available, and often cumbersome, difficult, and of long duration. Extrapolation of in vitro data or even of supplier literature on the efficacy of the actives is often used, without really proving the claims.

In Vivo Tests on Human Volunteers: Clinical Studies

The most direct proof of a claim is to show the product effect directly on the human volunteers using the product. Many test protocols may be used depending on the objective. Most protocols have been published in scientific literature and are well-established tests. They go from very exaggerated application conditions [8–11] to normal usage of the product by the subjects in the laboratory or at home [12,13]. It is obvious that the more realistic the application condition, the more powerful the demonstration of the effect. Besides the application procedure, these protocols can also differ by the assessment technique of the claimed effect: scoring of the effect by an expert evaluator, objective measurement of the property by a biometric technique, or self-assessment of the subjective effect by the user.

Assessment by an Expert Evaluator

This type of evaluation concerns a cosmetic effect that can be determined by visual, tactile, or olfactive assessment. Examples of scoring scales for the assessment of dry skin have been given by Serup [14]. The evaluator is trained to make such an assessment, reliable and fully independent of the product manufacturer. In some cases, the evaluator will be a dermatologist, an ophthalmologist, or a dentist, but this is not mandatory provided that the evaluator can justify his/her qualification. When the test protocol is appropriate, expert evaluations are frequently combined with other assessment methods. Examples of claims easily supported by expert evaluation are: skin whitening, antiwrinkle, hair shine, and deodorancy. Safety claims are also appropriate for such an assessment to check the absence of erythema or dryness after product application.

Measurement by Means of Biometric Methodologies

A huge amount of biometric methods have developed over the two last decades, which now allow objective and quantitative measurement of most skin properties, such as elasticity, firmness, color, barrier properties, moisture content, relief, and blood flow [3,15,16]. This kind of evaluation is highly valuable thanks to its objectivity and sensitivity, and can identify small differences between products to support comparative claims. Those biometric measurements must however take into account several key rules: 1) many external factors can affect the measurements that have to be made according to specific guidelines [17–20]; 2) the interpretation of the data has to be done by an expert in the field able to relate the collected data to physiological parameters; and 3) the instruments must be highly reliable. Under such conditions, instrumental measurements are highly valuable and have revolutionized the way of supporting cosmetic claims. However, instrumental methodologies have nowadays become so sensitive that questions can sometimes be raised about the relevancy of such small differences between products for consumers who are not always able to detect them.

Self-Assessment of the Effect by the Volunteers

When used in clinical tests, this type of evaluation is usually combined with other assessments. It is, however, not applicable to all test procedures, and requires that the product has been placed in contact with a sufficiently large area of the body to provide an effect that can be self-perceived. When confirming objective measurements of the property, this self-evaluation is extremely powerful because it expresses that the measured effect is really meaningful to the consumer.

Sensory Tests with Human Volunteers

The self-perception of the product effect by the volunteers can be obtained independently of a clinical test; in such a case a specific test procedure has to be designed. Sensory tests are limited to the so-called sensory claims, which clearly state that the product modifies the perception of a property of the skin or hair (e.g., you can feel your skin ''softer'' or ''more hydrated''). When the sensory effect of the product is obvious and can be easily perceived by a large majority of people, the test can be performed on a panel of regular (or ''naïve'') volunteers, without any specific selection criteria regarding their capability to feel differences. However, the self-perception of stimuli or of a skin feel is very variable between subjects and, often, differences between products are not so obvious for a ''naïve'' user; it is then necessary to run the sensory test either on a very large panel (sometimes several hundreds of volunteers) or to use a panel of volunteers specifically selected and trained to perceive small differences for the kind of product in test. (For more details on sensory tests, the reader is referred to Chapter 71.)

Consumer Tests

These tests are performed at the end of the development phase of the product, and consist in providing consumers with the product to use at home for a certain period of time, according to their usual habits and practice. Expected sensory/efficacy properties of the product can be checked from these tests by means of a questionnaire filled out by the users.

The information collected from consumer tests are very helpful in supporting cosmetic claims, as it will reassure the manufacturer that its product is not misleading the user about the claimed property. Consumer tests, like sensory tests, are mostly used to support claims such as those related to odor perception, skin sensation, tactile or visible properties of skin or hairs, and taste of oral-care products. However, because of the subjectivity of the data, such tests, to be valuable, must be performed very carefully. The questionnaire has to be prepared by a specialist on this kind of test, and cannot be oriented toward the answers of the users. For more details, the reader is referred to specific guidelines for consumer testing [21].

Multiapproach for Claim Support

As previously shown, all the approaches described for supporting claims on cosmetic products have own advantages as well as weaknesses. In order to combine the strengths of several, a multitest or multievaluation approach, combining expert assessments, instrumental measurements, and subjective data from the user, is often considered to be an ideal support for a claim. However, depending on the type of claim, for cost and time reasons, it is not always necessary to go so far in the dossier if one test obviously and undoubtly provides the proof of the claimed effect.

CONCLUSION

Claims on cosmetic products are extremely varied and often depend on the product, the market, and the current trends. However, several claims have been used on different product types for many years. Testing strategy for some is described in the following chapters. They cover some safety-related claims (e.g., mildness, sensitive skin–designed products, noncomedogenicity claims), some efficacy claims (e.g., skin-hydration effect, smoothing and antiwrinkle effect) and sensory claims. The proposed tests especially aim at guiding the skin scientists to design their own protocols based on reasonable scientific considerations, and do not intend to impose strict testing procedures.

REFERENCES

1. Davis JB, McNamara SH. Regulatory aspects of cosmetic claims substantiation. In: Aust LB, ed. Cosmetic Claims Substantiation. Vol. 18. New York: Marcel Dekker, 1998:1–20.
2. Friedel SL. Technical support for advertising claims. J Toxicol-Cutan Ocular Toxicol 1992; 11:199–204.
3. Willoughby M, Maibach HI. Cutaneous biometrics and claims support. In: Aust LB, ed. Cosmetic Claims Substantiation. Vol. 18. New York: Marcel Dekker, 1998:69–86.
4. Jackson EM. Supporting advertising claims. Reviewing a three-dimensional in vitro human cell test. Cosmet Toilet 1993; 108:41–42.
5. Majmudar G, Smith M. In vitro screening techniques in dermatology. A review of the tests, models and markers. Cosmet Toilet 1998; 113:69–76.
6. Roguet R. Intérêt des modèles de peaux reconstruites en cosmétologie. Cosmétologie 1997; 13:38–43.
7. DGCCRF-D'UMA Commission 30. Evaluation de l'efficacité des produits cosmétiques. Les recommandations de la DGCCRF. Cosmétologie 1997; 15:44–46.
8. Frosch PJ, Kligman AM. The soap chamber test: a new method for assessing the irritancy potential of soaps. J Am Acad Dermatol 1979; 1:35–41.
9. Sharko PT, Murahata RI, Leyden JJ, Grove GL. Arm wash with instrumental evaluation—a sensitive technique for differentiating the irritation potential of personal washing products. J Derm Clin Eval Soc 1991; 2:19–27.
10. Clarys P, Manou I, Barel AO. Influence of temperature on irritation of the hand/forearm immersion test. Contact Dermatitis 1997; 36:240–243.
11. Charbonnier V, Morrison BM Jr, Paye M, Maibach HI. Open application assay in investigation of subclinical irritant dermatitis induced by sodium lauryl sulfate (SLS) in man: advantage of squamometry. Skin Res Technol 1998; 4:244–250.
12. Jackson EM, Robillard NF. The controlled use test in a cosmetic product safety substantiation program. J Toxicol-Cutan Ocular Toxicol 1982; 1:117–132.
13. Paye M, Gomes G, Zerweg Ch, Piérard GE, Grove GG. A hand immersion test in laboratory-controlled usage conditions: a need for sensitive and controlled assessment methods. Contact Dermatitis 1999; 40:133–138.
14. Serup J. EEMCO guidance for the assessment of dry skin (xerosis) and ichtyosis: clinical scoring systems. Skin Res Technol 1995; 1:109–114.

15. Wiechers JW, Barlow T. Skin bioengineering techniques for substantiating cosmetics claims. Cosmet Toilet 1998; 113:81–83.

16. Kajs TM, Gartstein V. Review of the instrumental assessment of skin: effects of cleansing products. J Soc Cosmet Chem 1991; 42:249–271.

17. Rogiers V, Derde MP, Verleye G, Roseeuw D. Standardized conditions needed for skin surface hydration measurements. Cosmet Toilet 1990; 105:73–82.

18. Berardesca E. EEMCO guidance for the assessment of stratum corneum hydration: electrical methods. Skin Res Technol 1997; 3:126–132.

19. Piérard GE. EEMCO guidance for the assessment of skin colour. J Am Acad Derm Venereol 1998; 10:1–11.

20. Morrison BM Jr. ServoMed evaporimeter: precautions when evaluating the effect of skin care products on barrier function. J Soc Cosmet Chem 1992; 43:161–167.

21. The Advertising Research Foundation. Guidelines for the public use of market and opinion research. New York, NY, 1981.

66

Tests for Sensitive Skin

Alessandra Pelosi, Sabrina Lazzerini, and Enzo Berardesca
University of Pavia, Pavia, Italy

Howard I. Maibach
University of California at San Francisco School of Medicine,
San Francisco, California

INTRODUCTION

Sensitive skin is a condition of subjective cutaneous hyperreactivity to environmental factors. Subjects experiencing this condition report exaggerated reactions when their skin is in contact with cosmetics, soaps, and sunscreens, and they often report worsening after exposure to dry and cold climate.

Although no sign of irritation is commonly detected, itching, burning, stinging, and a tight sensation are constantly present. Generally, substances that are not commonly considered irritants are involved in this abnormal response. They include many cosmetic ingredients such as dimethyl sulfoxide, benzoyl peroxide preparations, salicylic acid, propylene glycol, amyldimethylaminobenzoic acid, and 2-ethoxyethyl methoxycinnamate [1].

Sensitive skin and subjective irritation are widespread but still far from being completely defined and understood. Burckhardt [2] hypothesized a correlation between sensitive skin and constitutional anomalies and/or other triggering factors such as occupational skin diseases or chronic exposure to irritants. On the other hand, Bjornberg [3] proposed that no constitutional factors play a role in the pathogenesis of sensitive skin, although the presence of dermatitis shows a general increase in skin reactivity to primary irritants lasting months.

EPIDEMIOLOGICAL STUDIES

Recent findings suggest that higher sensitivity can be attributable to different mechanisms. Hyperreactors may have a thinner stratum corneum with a reduced corneocyte area, causing a higher transcutaneous penetration of water-soluble chemicals [4]. In 1977, Frosch and Kligman [5], by testing different irritants, showed a 14% incidence of sensitive skin in the normal population, likely correlated to a thin permeable stratum corneum, which make these subjects more susceptible to chemical irritation.

Many epidemiological studies have been carried out to assess whether or not a correlation with sex, skin type, or age could be found. Contradictory findings have been reported. Some investigators [6,7] documented a higher reactivity to irritants mostly in females, but other experimental studies did not confirm this observation. Bjornberg [8], using six different irritants by patch-test application, found no sex-related differences. Moreover Lammintausta [9], studying the response to open and patch-test application of sodium lauryl sulphate (SLS), found mild interindividual variations in transepidermal water loss (TEWL) and dielectric water content (DWC) values, but no sex-related differences in the reaction pattern.

In 1982, Frosch [10], using dimethylsulfoxide, show a correlation between the minimal erythema dose (MED) and the response to irritants; the higher the inflammation, the lower the MED. Subsequently, a correlation between skin reactivity and skin type was reported; higher reactions were detected in subjects with skin type I [11]. Moreover, in eczema skin reactivity is enhanced [12]. Studies performed on animal models showed that strong irritant reactions in guinea pigs significantly reduced the threshold of skin irritation [13]. On the other hand, hyporeactive states may be induced by skin treatment. Subclinical dermatitis, after repeated cutaneous irritation by open application, may induce skin hyporeactivity [14]. This can also be one of the mechanisms of false-negative patch test.

Skin reactivity seems also to change depending on age. The literature is contradictory. For example, Nilzen and Voss Lagerlung [15] reported higher reactivity patch-test reactions to soaps and detergents in the elderly, whereas Bettley and Donoghue [16] reported a lower reactivity in the same group.

Coenraads et al. [17] showed a higher skin reactivity to croton oil in the older patient group, but no differences by testing thimochinone or croton aldehyde. Recently, Grove [18], by testing croton oil, cationic and anionic surfactants, weak acids, and solvents, reported a lower susceptibility in older subjects in terms of less-severe skin reactions. Aged skin seems to have a reduced inflammatory response either to irritants or to irritation induced by UV light [19]. On the other hand, after irritating the skin, increased TEWL values were recorded in the older subjects compared with the young. This finding could be related to a deficient "early warning detection system" in the elderly. The lack of any visible response can lead to continued exposure to external irritants and higher risk of damage to skin-barrier function.

CLINICAL PARAMETERS

Because of the lack of clinical signs, the phenomenon of sensitive skin is difficult to document. Attempts to identify clinical parameters in subjects with subjective irritation indicate that these individuals tend to have a less hydrated, less supple, more erythematous, and more teleangiectatic skin compared with the normal population. In particular, significant differences were found for erythema and hydration/dryness [20].

TESTS FOR SENSITIVE SKIN

Recently, because no visible clinical signs of irritation are detected in sensitive skin, new methods of sensory testing have been increasingly used to provide definite information.

QUANTITATION OF CUTANEOUS THERMAL SENSATION

The superficial skin layer includes sensory nerve fibers connected to specialized receptors such as corpuscles or naked nerve endings. A Beta fibers, myelinated (conduction velocity of 2–30m/sec), mediate the touch, vibration, and pressure sensation. A Delta fibers, smaller and myelinated (conduction velocity of >30m/sec), mediate cold and pain sensation. C fibers, small and nonmyelinated, mediate warm and itching sensation. Quantitative sensory testing (QST) methods have been used mainly to study the impairment of somatosensory function in neurological diseases; particularly in dermatology, thermal sensation testing analysis is becoming the most used QST technique [21]. It assessed function in free nerve endings and their associated small myelinated and nonmyelinated fibres. This method is able to measure the threshold of warm and cold sensation as well as hot and cold pain.

All modern automated thermal testing instruments include a thermode (Poltrier device) with semiconductor junctions made of different metals. Depending on the polarity of the electric current, the skin is heated or cooled; different thermic sensations are reproduced on the different sides of the junctions.

In the center of the thermode, a thermocouple records the temperature. TSA 2001 (Medoc Company, Ramat Yshai, Israel) is considered one of the most advanced portable thermal sensory-testing devices. Basically, its measures the hot or cold threshold and the suprathreshold pain magnitude. It operates between 0°C and 54°C.

The thermode in contact with the skin produces a stimulus whose intensity increases or decreases until the subject feels the sensation. As the sensation is felt, the subject is asked to press a button. The test is then repeated two more times in order to get a mean value. Using this method, artefacts can occur because of the lag time the stimulus needs to reach the brain. This inconvenience can be avoided by using relatively slow rates of increasing stimuli. The stimulus can also be increased stepwise and the subject is told to say whether or not the sensation is felt. When a positive answer is given, the stimulus is decreased by one-half the initial step and so on, until no sensation is felt. The subject's response determines the intensity of the next stimulus. The limitation of this second method is that a longer performance time is required.

STINGING TEST

Stinging seems to be a variant of pain that develops rapidly and fades quickly any time the appropriate sensory nerve is stimulated. Although this method lacks objective criteria, it is widely accepted as a marker of sensitivity and has often been used in skin-irritation studies [5]. It provides information to establish those subjects experiencing invisible cutaneous irritation.

It is performed by applying to the skin hydrosoluble substances such as lactic acid or capsaicin. The test is usually carried out on the nasolabial fold, a site richly innervated with sensory fibers. Subjects first undergo a facial sauna for 5 to 10 minutes, then an aqueous lactic acid solution (5–10% according to different methods] is rubbed with a cotton swab on the test site. In order to have a more reliable response, it is recommended to apply an inert control substance, such as saline solution, to the contralateral test site. After application, within a few minutes a moderate to severe stinging sensation occurs for the ''stingers group.'' These subjects are then asked to describe the intensity of the sensation using a point scale. Hyperreactors, particularly those with a positive dermatological history, have higher scores. An alternative test involves the application of 2 mL of 90% aqueous dimethylsulfoxide (DMSO) in a small glass cup on the cheek for 5 minutes. This procedure causes intense burning in stingers and, after application, tender wheal and persistent erythema often occur. By contrast, lactic acid produces no visible changes. Using this screening procedure, 20% of the subjects exposed to 5% lactic acid in a hot, humid environment were found to develop a stinging response [5]. Lammintausta et al. confirmed these observations [22]. In this study, 18% of subjects were identified as stingers. In addition, stingers were found to develop stronger reactions to materials causing nonimmunological contact urticaria, to have increased values of TEWL and increased blood-flow velocimetry values after application of an irritant under patch test.

EVALUATION OF ITCHING RESPONSE

Recent studies show that a new class of C fibers with an exceptionally lower conduction velocity and insensitivity to mechanical stimuli can likely be considered as afferent units that mediate the itchy sensation [23]. Indeed, this subjective feeling has been extensively investigated but no explanation of the individual susceptibility to the itching sensation, without any sign of coexisting dermatitis, has been found. Laboratory investigation of the itch response has also been limited.

An itch response can be experimentally induced by topical or intradermal injections of various substances such as proteolytic enzymes, mast cell degranulators, and vasoactive agents. Histamine injection is one of the more common procedures: histamine dihydrochloride (100 μg in 1 mL of normal saline) is injected intradermally in one forearm. Then, after different time intervals, the subject is asked to indicate the intensity of the sensation using a predetermined scale and the duration of itch is recorded. Information is always gained by the subject's self-assessment.

A correlation between whealing and itching response, produced by applying a topical 4% histamine base in a group of healthy young females, has been investigated by Grove. The itching response was graded by the subjects using the following scale: none, slight, moderate, and intense. The data showed that, despite the fact that 90% of the wheals were greater than 8 mm in diameter, only 50% of the subjects experienced pruritus; patients with large wheals often had no complaints of itching, suggesting that the dimensions of the wheals do not correlate well with pruritus. In addition, itch and sting perception seem to be poorly correlated. Grove [18] compared the cumulative lactic acid sting scores with the histamine itch scores in 32 young subjects; all the subjects who were stingers were also moderate to intense itchers, while 50% of the moderate itchers showed little or no stinging response.

Yosipovitch [24], studying the effects of drugs on C fibers during experimentally induced itch, showed that topically applied aspirin rapidly decreases histamine-induced itch. This result can be attributed to the role that prostaglandines play in pain and itch sensation [25]. Localized itching, burning, and stinging can also be a feature of nonimmunological contact urticaria. This condition, still not completely defined, is characterized by a local wheal and flare after exposure of the skin to certain agents. Different combinations of mediators such as non–antibody-mediated release of histamine, prostaglandins, leukotriens, substance P, and other inflammatory mediators may likely be involved in the pathogenesis of this disorder [26]. The fact that prostaglandins and leukotriens may play a role in the inflammatory response is supported by the inhibition of the common urticants by both oral acetylsalicylic acid and indomethacin and by topical diclofenac and naproxen gel [1]. Several substances, such as benzoic acid, cinnamic acid, cinnamic aldehyde, and nicotinic acid esters, are capable of producing contact nonimmunological urticaria, eliciting local edema and erythematous reactions in half of the individuals. Provocative tests are usually used to identify subjects experiencing this condition: benzoic acid, sorbic acid, or sodium benzoate in open application well reproduce the typical symptoms in subjects suspected of contact nonimmunological urticaria.

WASHING AND EXAGGERATED IMMERSION TESTS

The aim of these tests is to identify a subpopulation with an increased tendency to produce a skin response. In the washing test [27], subjects are asked to wash their face with a specific soap or detergent. After washing, individual sensation for tightness, burning, itching, and stinging is evaluated using a point scale previously determined. The exaggerated immersion test is based on soaking the hands and forearms of the subjects in a solution of anionic surfactants (such as 0.35% paraffine sulfonate, 0.05% sodium laureth sulfate-2EO) at 40°C for 20 minutes. After soaking, hands and forearms are rinsed under tap water and patted dry with a paper towel. This procedure is repeated two more times, with a 2-hour period between each soaking, for 2 consecutive days. Before the procedure, baseline skin parameters are evaluated. The other evaluations are taken 2 hours after the third and sixth soakings and 18 hours after the last soaking (recovery assessment). All of the skin parameters are performed after the subjects have rested at least 30 minutes at 21 ± 1°C.

CORNEOSURFAMETRY

This method, recently described [28], investigates the interaction of surfactants with the human stratum corneum. It is performed as follows: cyanoacrylate skin-surface stripping (CSSS) is taken from the volar aspect of the forearm and sprayed with the surfactant to be tested. After 2 hours, the sample is rinsed with tap water and stained with basic fuchsin and toluidine blue dyes for 3 minutes. After rinsing and drying, the sample is placed on a white reference plate and measured by reflectance colorimetry (Chroma Meter® CR200; Minolta, Osaka, Japan).

The index of mildness (CIM = luminacy L*-chroma C*) is taken as a parameter of the irritation caused by the surfactant. This index has a value of 68 ± 4 when water alone is sprayed on the sample and decreases when surfactant is tested, with stronger surfactants lowering the values. Piérard et al. [29], testing different shampoo formulations in volunteers with sensitive skin, showed that corneosurfametry correlates well with in vivo testing. A significant negative correlation ($p < 0.001$) was found between values of colorimetric index of mildness (CIM) and the skin compatibility parameters (SCP) that include a global evaluation of the colorimetric erythemal index (CEI) and the TEWL differential, both expressed in the same order of magnitude.

In the same study, corneosurfametry showed less interindividual variability than in vivo testing, allowing a better discrimination among mild products. An interesting finding showed that sensitive skin is not a single condition. Goffin et al. [30] hypothesized that the response of the stratum corneum to an environmental threat might be impaired in different groups of subjects experiencing sensitive skin. Data of the corneosurfametry, performed after testing eight different house-cleaning products, showed that the overall stratum corneum reactivity, as calculated by the average values of the corneosurfametry index (CSMI) and the CIM, is significantly different ($p < 0.01$) between detergent-sensitive skin and both nonsensitive and climate/fabric sensitive skin as well.

CONCLUSIONS

Sensitive skin represents a widespread condition of susceptibility to exogenous factors. The reason why some subjects react with subjective symptoms like itching, burning, stinging, prickling, or tingling is unclear. However, a correlation of increased reactivity in subjects with a history of dermatitis and the association of increased reactivity with skin type I has been reported. Noninvasive evaluation of sensitive skin may successfully predict individual susceptibility to cosmetic-related adverse reactions. All of the efforts in this direction appear undoubtedly important to improve tolerance to the majority of cosmetic products.

REFERENCES

1. Amin S, Engasser PG, Maibach HI. Side-effects and social aspect of cosmetology. In: Baran R, Maibach HI, eds. Textbook of Cosmetic Dermatology. 2d ed. 1998; 60:709–746.
2. Burckhardt W. Praktische und theoretische bedeutung der alkalineutralisation und alkaliresistenzproben. Arch Klin Exp Derm 1964; 219:600–603.
3. Bjornberg A. Skin Reactions to Primary Irritants in Patients with Hand Eczema. Goteborg: Isaccsons, 1968.
4. Berardesca E, Cespa M, Farinelli N, Rabbiosi G, Maibach HI. In vivo transcutaneous penetration of nicotinates and sensitive skin. Contact Dermatitis 1991; 25:35–38.
5. Frosch PJ, Kligman AM. A method for appraising the stinging capacity of topically applied substances. J Soc Cosmet Chemist 1977; 28:197–209.
6. Agrup G. Hand eczema and other hand dermatoses in South Sweden. Academic dissertation. Acta Dermato Venereol 1969; 49(suppl. 161).
7. Fregert S. Occupational dermatitis in 10 years material. Contact Dermatitis 1975; 1:96–107.
8. Bjornberg A. Skin reactions to primary irritants in men and women. Acta Dermatol Venereol 1975; 55:191–194.
9. Lammintausta K, Maibach HI, Wilson D. Irritant reactivity in males and females. Contact Dermatitis 1987; 17:276–280.
10. Frosch P, Wissing C. Cutaneous sensivity to ultraviolet light and chemical irritants. Arch Derm Res 1982; 272:269–278.
11. Lammintausta K, Maibach HI, Wilson D. Susceptibility to cumulative and acute irritant dermatitis. An experimental approach in human volunteers. Contact Dermatitis 1988; 19:84–90.
12. Bettley FR. Non specific irritant reactions in eczematous subjects. Br J Dermatol 1964; 76:116–121.
13. Roper SS, Jones EH. An animal model for altering the irritability threshold of normal skin. Contact Dermatitis 1985; 13:91–97.
14. Lammintausta K, Maibach HI, Wilson D. Human cutaneous irritation: induced hyporeactivity. Contact Dermatitis 1987; 17:193–198.
15. Nilzen A, Voss Lagerlund K. Epicutaneous tests with detergents and a number of other common allergens. Dermatologica 1962; 124:42–52.
16. Bettley FR, Donoghue E. The irritant effect of soap upon the normal skin. Br J Dermatol 1960; 72:67–76.
17. Coenraads PJ, Bleumink E, Nofer JP. Susceptibility to primary irritants. Age dependence. Contact Dermatitis 1975; 1:377–381.
18. Grove GL. Age-associated changes in integumental reactivity. In: Léveque JL, Agache PG, eds. Aging Skin. Properties and Functional Changes. New York: XX, 1993; 16:227–237.
19. Gilchrest BA, Stoff JS, Soter NA. Chronologic aging alters the response to ultraviolet-induced inflammation in human skin. J Invest Dermatol 1982; 79:11–15.

20. Seidenari S, Francomano M, Mantovani L. Baseline biophysical parameters in subjects with sensitive skin. Contact Dermatitis 1998; 38:311–315.
21. Yosipovitch G, Yarnitsky D. Quantitative sensory testing. In: Maibach HI, Marzulli FN, eds. Dermotoxicology Methods: The Laboratory Worker's Vade Mecum. New York: Taylor & Francis, 1997; pp 315–320.
22. Lammintausta K, Maibach HI, Wilson D. Mechanisms of subjective (sensory) irritation: propensity of nonimmunologic contact urticaria and objective irritation in stingers. Dermatosen in Beruf und Umwelt 1988; 36(2):45–49.
23. Schmelz M, Schmidt R, Bichel A, Handwerker HO, Torebjörk HE. Specific C-receptors for itch in human skin. J Neurosci 1997; 17(20):8003–8008.
24. Yosipovitch G, Ademola J, Ping Lui, Amin S, Maibach HI. Topically applied aspirin rapidly decreases histamine-induced itch. Acta Demato Venereol (Stockh) 1977; 77:46–48.
25. Lovell CR, Burton PA, Duncan EH, Burton JL. Prostaglandins and pruritus. Br J Dermatol 1976; 94:273–275.
26. Lahti A, Maibach HI. Species specificity of nonimmmunologic contact urticaria: guinea pig, rat and mouse. J Am Acad 1985; 13:66–69.
27. Hannuksela A, Hannuksela M. Irritant effects of a detergent in wash and chamber tests. Contact Dermatitis 1995; 32:163–166.
28. Piérard GE, Goffin V, Piérard Franchimont C. Corneosurfametry: a predictive assessment of the interaction of personal care cleansing products with human stratum corneum. Dermatology 1994; 189:152–156.
29. Piérard GE, Goffin V, Hermanns-Le T, Arrese JE, Piérard Franchimont C. Surfactant-induced dermatitis: comparison of corneosulfametry with predictive testing on human and reconstructed skin. J Am Acad Dermatol 1995; 33:462–469.
30. Goffin V, Piérard Franchimont C, Piérard GE. Sensitive skin and stratum corneum reactivity to household cleaning products. Contact Dermatitis 1996; 34:81–85.

67

Tests for Skin Hydration

Bernard Gabard

Spirig Pharma Ltd., Egerkingen, Switzerland

INTRODUCTION

Writing about skin hydration means simultaneously writing about dry skin and its treatment by moisturizers. Dry skin has never really been defined in a repeatable way. In fact, this expression prejudices into believing that the skin does have a reduced water content, although this was never confirmed or denied. Generally speaking, dry skin signifies that the skin surface looks as though it is lacking in water, this being reinforced by the pharmacological effect of hydrating the skin surface by appropriate treatments.

Experimental models used for measuring skin hydration are basically clinical models incorporating or not noninvasive bioengineering measurements. To ensure meaningful results, the outlines of the intended studies should be of modern design incorporating blinding, randomization, and a suitable statistical control (particularly if different products are to be compared). This last point means including a predetermined adequate number of subjects in the study. The general ethical and legal frames of such clinical studies required for claim support are well defined in corresponding monographs or publications covering extensively the general procedures to be followed and the prerequisite information needed about the products to be tested [1–3].

Regardless of the method used, a further important point concerns standardization of the experimental conditions. To obtain acceptable and reproducible results, measurements should be performed with relaxed patients and/or volunteers already acclimatized for at least 20 minutes to controlled ambient temperature and relative humidity conditions. Both factors mainly affect sweat-gland activity, but other parameters should equally be considered with attention to, e.g., anatomical skin site, test products remaining or not on the skin, and correct handling of the measuring equipment if any. All these possible influences on measurement outcome have been discussed in detail in recent guidelines and in pertinent reviews [4–6].

A CLINICAL EVALUATION: THE REGRESSION METHOD

The dermatologist is perfectly able to clinically grade a given state of skin dryness (e.g., surface roughness, squames, and fissures). Clinical evaluation and grading of skin hydration is based on visual and tactile evaluation of clinical signs. There are numerous possibilities of testing, but basically they rely on the regression method, published in 1978 by Kligman [7], which is still used as an industry standard. Briefly, female subjects with moderate to severe xerosis of the legs are selected following strict criteria. The test products are applied under controlled conditions by trained employees twice daily 5 days a week for 3 weeks. Three days after treatment ends, the follow-up period begins. Scoring is also completed 3 and 7 days later. Treatment period may be shortened to 2 weeks if necessary. A recent guideline ensures that clinical scoring of the hydration state of the skin surface will be conducted based on the same definitions [4]. Caution is given upon scoring by the subjects themselves, as their perception of their skin condition may not be the same as the dermatologist's [4,8].

INCORPORATING BIOENGINEERING METHODS

A large number of bioengineering methods are now available to evaluate hydration (or dryness) of the skin directly or indirectly. Inclusion of these methods in the study protocol opens many possibilities for getting meaningful results such as design variations, optimization of the claim support, and also, most importantly, improvement of cost effectiveness by shortening the duration of experiment, using a lower number of subjects, and strengthening the statistical evaluation.

Concerning the numerous techniques available for the evaluation of skin hydration, the reader is referred to very recent monographs describing these methods in a detailed fashion [8–13]. They mainly include measurements of electrical properties, spectroscopic methods such as infrared absorption spectroscopy and emission, evaluation of the barrier function of the stratum corneum (SC), measurement of mechanical properties, nuclear magnetic resonance imaging, skin-surface topography, and scaling evaluation. However, in this short review, examples of possible designs will be given that use bioengineering techniques based only on the electrical properties of the SC or on measurement of transepidermal water loss (TEWL) (for a review of modern suitable measuring equipment see Refs. 8, 12, 13).

Static Measurements

Short-Term Tests/Single Application

The tests are conducted on the forearm of healthy subjects and allow a randomized side-to-side comparison of test products with a placebo or vehicle, a known active product, and untreated control skin. Four to six products may be simultaneously tested. The products are applied at the rate of 2 mg/cm². Two different experimental designs may be used.

1. The test products are left in place for 1 hour (or another suitable duration, e.g., 3 h [14]). Measurements are conducted at different times thereafter. Removal of excess or nonpenetrated product is preferable before measuring, especially if the preparation contains a high proportion of lipids. Most moisturizers show a rapid increase of measured hydration values (Fig. 1).
2. The test products may be applied on similar areas at the same rate but under occlusion with a standard occluding patch overnight for 16 hours. The next morning, measurements are conducted in the same way as in part 1 beginning 1 hour after removal of the occlusion patch (Fig. 2). This last procedure better picks up the activity of a humectant contained in the test preparation, whereas

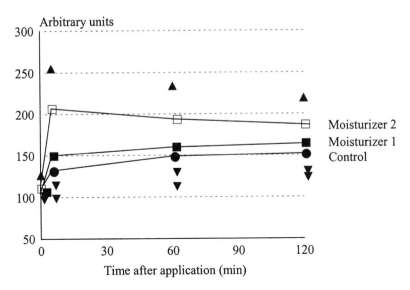

FIGURE 1   Example of hydration changes after 1 h application of two different o/w moisturizers containing both 2% urea as humectant. Hydration evaluation: NOVA DPM 9003; Means + or − half SD: ▲ ▼; Moisturizer 1: ■; Moisturizer 2: □; Control (untreated skin): ○. Start values (Time 0) measured before application of the products.

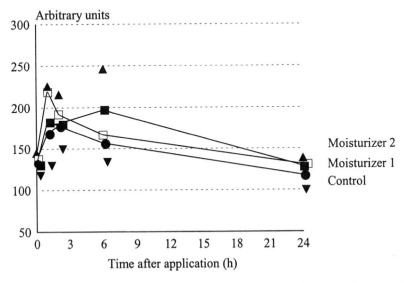

FIGURE 2   Example of hydration changes after 16 h occlusive application of two different o/w moisturizers containing both 2% urea as humectant (same products as in Figure 1). Start values (Time 0) measured before the occlusive application of the products. (For further details, see legend of Figure 1.)

the vehicle effect is strongly attenuated by the uniform conditions encountered under the occlusion patch.

Long-Term Tests/Multiple Applications

The design of these tests and selection of subjects is similar to the regression method previously described but with a modified and shortened regression protocol [15]. The treatment period extends over 1 week only, and the regression phase takes place over the following week. Bioengineering measurements are conducted 12 to 16 hours after the treatment or moisturizer application, and for the last time on the Monday following the regression week. Inclusion of these noninvasive measurements allowed rapid and reliable product-performance evaluation.

Dynamic Measurements

These tests, in addition to the classic evaluation of skin hydration, provide information on some dynamic properties of the SC [16–18]. These properties are likely to be modified by the humectants (e.g., glycerol, urea, and alpha-hydroxy acids) incorporated in the moisturizers used for treatment. Generally speaking, dynamic function tests are characterized by the assessment of the skin response to a given external stimulus that can be of physical (e.g., water, occlusion, stretch, heat) or chemical (e.g., drugs, irritants) nature. These dynamic tests may be used either during short-term or long-term product testing, and will usually be performed before and at different time points after treatment.

The Sorption-Desorption Test (SDT)

This test gives information about the water-binding capacity of the uppermost layers of the SC [16,18]. It is best conducted using measurement devices that are able to measure hydration on a wet surface and that give instantaneous readings on contact with the skin. This first value represents the hydration state of the SC. Then 50 µl of distilled water are pipetted onto the skin, left in place for exactly 10 seconds, wiped with a soft paper towel, and then hydration is immediately measured. This value represents the hygroscopicity of the superficial SC. Further measurements are taken at 0.5, 1, 1.5, and 2 minutes. The area under the curve from 0.5 minutes onwards represents the water-holding capacity of the superficial SC (Fig. 3).

The Moisture-Accumulation Test (MAT)

This test gives information about the quantity of moisture the SC may accumulate during a given time [17,18]. This test is conducted with a device able to measure continuously after bringing the probe in contact with the skin surface. The probe then remains on the skin for 3 minutes, thereby creating occlusive conditions. The MAT measures the accumulation of water under the probe every 0.5 minutes. Water accumulation is evaluated by calculating the area under the time curve until 3 minutes (Fig. 4).

The Plastic Occlusion Stress Test (POST)

The POST may also be considered a dynamic test and gives information about SC hydration, integrity of the barrier function, and SC water-holding capacity [19,20]. It consists of occluding the skin with a plastic chamber (e.g., Hilltop chamber or a similar occlusive device) for 24 hours. Then the occlusion is removed and the evaporation of the accumulated water is measured each minute for 30 minutes as TEWL. This technique has been

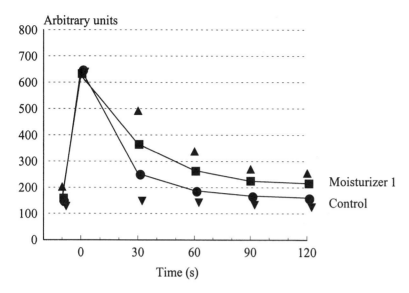

FIGURE 3   Time course of hydration changes during a sorption-desorption test (SDT) performed 60 min after a single 1 h short-term application of moisturizer 1. (For further details, see legend of Figure 1.)

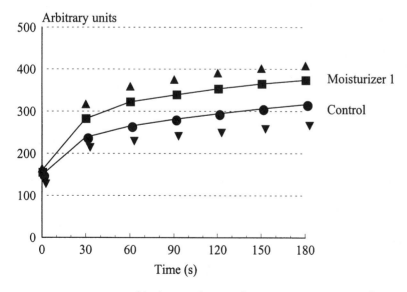

FIGURE 4   Time course of hydration changes during a moisture accumulation test (MAT) performed 60 min after a single 1 h short-term application of moisturizer 1. (For further details, see legend of Figure 1.)

thoroughly described in recent guidelines [21,22]. The measurement is called skin surface water loss (SSWL) and not TEWL, because it does not represent the true TEWL but the sum of the TEWL and the evaporation of water trapped within and over the SC under the occlusive equipment, at least at the beginning of the measurement period. During these first minutes of evaporation, the SSWL is proportional to SC hydration. At the end of the dehydration time, SSWL is greatly reduced and mainly TEWL is measured. Therefore, changes induced in the last part of the curve reflects the barrier function of SC.

Other Suitable Tests

Some well-defined properties of the skin are more or less dependent on SC hydration and may be evaluated with the following bioengineering methods:

- Mechanical or viscoelastic properties (elasticity, extensibility) [23]
- Skin-surface roughness [24]
- Skin-surface scaling [25]

Some other techniques are also indicated for evaluating SC hydration, but they are not available for routine experimentation at the present moment. They have been critically reviewed and evaluated in a recent publication to which the reader is referred [8].

CONCLUSION

During the evaluation of SC hydration in vivo, it must be kept in mind that no absolute determination of a water content or concentration is possible. This holds for clinical evaluation and for bioengineering measurements as well. For this reason, several measurement techniques should be used simultaneously during a study. Not only is the information gained from these different experimental approaches complementary, and of great benefit if they are integrated in a clinical evaluation, but one should remember that moisturizers may influence skin hydration in different ways. Thus, different aspects of hydration changes need to be investigated, such as water binding, water retention, or emolliency, which is also a further part of a moisturizer's action. Last, it should be remembered that, in order to obtain meaningful results, proper design of the study, inclusion of a suitable number of subjects, strict standardization of measurement conditions, and all other relevant factors need to be tightly controlled. Only by assuring the best quality level will results be obtained that will help to design and use optimal moisturizers.

REFERENCES

1. Seidenschnur EK. FDA and EEC regulations related to skin: documentation and measuring devices. In: Serup J, Jemec GBE, eds. Handbook of Non-Invasive Methods and the Skin. Boca Raton: CRC Press, 1995:653–665.
2. COLIPA (The European Cosmetic, Toiletry and Perfumery Association). Guidelines for the evaluation of the efficacy of cosmetic products, 1997.
3. Davis JB, McNamara SH. Regulatory aspects of cosmetic claims substantiation. In: Aust LB, ed. Cosmetic Claims Substantiation. New York: Marcel Dekker, 1998:1–20.
4. Serup J. EEMCO guidance for the assessment of dry skin (xerosis) and ichthyosis: clinical scoring systems. Skin Res Technol 1995; 1:109–114.
5. Berardesca E. EEMCO guidance for the assessment of stratum corneum hydration: electrical methods. Skin Res Technol 1997; 3:126–132.

6. Wilhelm KP. Possible pitfalls in hydration measurements. In: Elsner P, Barel AO, Berardesca E, Gabard B, Serup J, eds. Skin Bioengineering: Techniques and Applications in Dermatology and Cosmetology. Current Problems in Dermatology, Vol. 26. Basel: Karger, 1998:223–234.

7. Kligman AM. Regression method for assessing the efficacy of moisturizers. Cosmet & Toilet 1978; 93:27–35.

8. Barel AO, Clarys P, Gabard B. In vivo evaluation of the hydration state of the skin: measurements and methods for claim support. In: Elsner P, Merk HF, Maibach HI, eds. In: Cosmetics: Controlled Efficacy Studies and Regulations. Berlin: Springer, 1999:57–80.

9. Tagami H, Ohi M, Iwatsuki K, Kanamaru Y, Yamada M, Ichijo B. Evaluation of the skin surface hydration in vivo by electrical measurements. J Invest Dermatol 1980; 75:500–507.

10. Levêque JL, De Rigal J. Impedance methods for studying skin moisturization. J Soc Cosmet Chem 1983; 34:419–428.

11. Levêque JL. Cutaneous Investigation in Health and Disease: Noninvasive Methods and Instrumentation. New York: Marcel Dekker, 1989.

12. Elsner P, Berardesca E, Maibach HI. Bioengineering of the Skin: Water and the Stratum Corneum. Boca Raton: CRC Press, 1994.

13. Serup J, Jemec GBE. (1995) Handbook of Non-Invasive Methods and the Skin. Boca Raton: CRC Press, 1995:159–170.

14. Serup J. A three-hour test for rapid comparison of effects of moisturizers and active constituents (urea). Acta Derm Venereol (Stockh) 1992; (suppl. 177):29–33.

15. Grove G. Skin surface hydration changes during a mini-regression test as measured in vivo by electrical conductivity. Curr Therap Res 1992; 52:1–6.

16. Tagami H, Kanamaru Y, Inoue K, Suehisa S, Inoue F, Iwatsuki K, Yoshikuni K, Yamada M. Water sorption-desorption test of the skin in vivo for functional assessment of the stratum corneum. J Invest Dermatol 1982; 78:425–428.

17. Van Neste D. In vivo evaluation of unbound water accumulation in stratum corneum. Dermatologica 1990; 181:197–201.

18. Treffel P, Gabard B. Stratum corneum dynamic function measurements after moisturizer or irritant application. Arch Dermatol Res 1995; 287:474–479.

19. Berardesca E, Maibach HI. Effect of nonvisible damage on the water-holding capacity of the stratum corneum, utilizing the plastic occlusion stress test (POST). In: Frosch PJ, Doom-Goossens A, Lachapelle JM, Rycroft RJG, Scheper RJ, eds. Current Topics in Contact Dermatitis. Berlin: Springer, 1989:554–559.

20. Berardesca E, Elsner P. Dynamic measurements: the plastic occlusion stress test (POST) and the moisture accumulation test (MAT). In: Elsner P, Berardesca E, Maibach HI, eds. Bioengineering of the Skin: Water and the Stratum Corneum. Boca Raton: CRC Press, 1994:97–102.

21. Pinnagoda J. Hardware and measuring principles: evaporimeter. In: Elsner P, Berardesca E, Maibach HI, eds. Bioengineering of the Skin: Water and the Stratum Corneum. Boca Raton: CRC Press, 1994:51–58.

22. Pinnagoda J, Tupker RA, Agner T, Serup J. Guidelines for transepidermal water loss measurement: a report from the standardization group of the European Society of Contact Dermatitis. Contact Dermatitis 1990; 22:164–168.

23. Barel AO, Lambrecht R, Clarys P. Mechanical function of the skin: state of the art. In: Elsner P, Barel AO, Berardesca E, Gabard B, Serup J, eds. Skin Bioengineering: Techniques and Applications in Dermatology and Cosmetology. Current Problems in Dermatology, Vol. 26. Basel: Karger, 1998:69–83.

24. Marks R. How to measure the effects of emollients. J Dermatol Treat 1997; 8:S15–S18.

25. Schatz H, Altmeyer PJ. Dry skin and scaling evaluated by D-Squames and image analysis. In: Serup J, Jemec GBE, eds. Handbook of Non-Invasive Methods and the Skin. Boca Raton: CRC Press, 1995:153–157.

68

Tests for Skin Protection: Barrier Effect

Hongbo Zhai and Howard I. Maibach
*University of California at San Francisco School of Medicine,
San Francisco, California*

Barrier creams (BC) may play an important role in the prevention of contact dermatitis [1–6], and various in vitro and in vivo methods have been developed to evaluate their efficacy. In practice, their use remains the subject of lively debate; some reports suggest that inappropriate BC application may exacerbate, rather than prevent, irritation [1–3, 6–9]. The accuracy of measurements depends on the use of proper methodology. This chapter reviews the investigative details of pertinent scientific literature, and summarizes the methodology and efficacy of BC.

IN VITRO METHODS

In 1946, Sadler and Marriott [10] introduced some facile tests to evaluate the efficiency of BC. One method used the fluorescence of a dyestuff and eosin as an indicator to measure penetration and the rates of penetration of water through BC; this is rapid and simple, but provides only a qualitative estimate.

Suskind [11] used a simple method to measure the relative efficacy or repellency of several formulations with film-immersion tests in a specific exposure. Results showed two formulations (containing 52.5% silicone in bentonite and 30% silicone in petrolatum) were both effective against a range of aqueous irritants or sensitizers.

Langford [12] conducted in vitro studies to determine the efficacy of the formulated fluorochemical (FC)–resin complex included against solvent penetration through treated filter paper, solvent repellency on treated pigskin, and penetration of radio-tagged sodium lauryl sulfate through treated hairless mouse skin. He also conducted an in vivo study on 75 persons who had all previously experienced irritation on their hands because of continued contact with solvents. Eighty-three percent of the panelists stated the cream was effective in protecting their hands.

Reiner et al. [13] examined the protective effect of ointments both on guinea pig skin in vitro and on guinea pigs in vivo. The permeation values of a toxic agent through unprotected and protected skin within 10 h as a function of time was determined radiologically and enzymatically. Permeation of the toxic agent was markedly reduced by polyethylene-glycol ointment base and ointments containing active substances. In in vivo experiments on guinea pigs, mortality was greater after applying the toxic agent to unprotected skin. All formulations with nucleophilic substances markedly reduced the mortality rate.

Loden [14] evaluated the effect of BC on the absorption of (^{3}H)-water, (^{14}C)-benzene, and (^{14}C)-formaldehyde into excised human skin. The control and BC-treated skins were exposed to the test substance for 0.5 hours, whereupon absorption was determined. The experimental cream ''water barrier'' reduced the absorption of water and benzene but not formaldehyde. One cream slightly reduced benzene and formaldehyde absorption. The other two creams did not affect the absorption of any of the substances studied.

Treffel et al. [15] measured in vitro on human skin the effectiveness of BC against three dyes (eosin, methylviolet, and oil red O) with varying n-octanol/water partition coefficients (0.19, 29.8, and 165, respectively). BC efficacy was assayed by measurements of the dyes in the epidermis of protected skin samples after 30 minutes of application. The efficacy of BC against the three dyes showed in several cases data contrary to manufacturer's information. There was no correlation between the galenic parameters of the assayed products and the protection level, indicating that neither water content nor consistency of the formulations influenced the protection effectiveness.

Fullerton and Menne [16] tested that the protective effect of various ethylenediaminetetraacetate (EDTA) barrier gels against nickel contact allergy using in vitro and in vivo methods. In an in vitro study, about 30 mg of barrier gel were applied on the epidermal side of the skin and a nickel disc was applied above the gel. After 24-hours application, the nickel disc was removed and the epidermis separated from the dermis. Nickel content in epidermis and dermis was quantified by absorption differential pulse voltammetry (ADPV). The amount of nickel in the epidermal skin layer on barrier gel–treated skin was significantly reduced compared with the untreated control. In vivo patch testing of nickel-sensitive patients was performed using nickel discs with and without barrier gels. Test preparations and nickel discs were removed 1 day after application, and the test sites were evaluated. Reduction in positive test reactions was highly significant on barrier gel–treated sites.

Zhai et al. [17] used an in vitro diffusion system to measure the protective efficacy of Quaternium-18 bentonite (Q18B) gels to prevent 1% concentration of [^{35}S] sodium lauryl sulfate (SLS) penetration on human cadaver skin. The accumulated amount of [^{35}S]-SLS in receptor-cell fluid were counted to evaluate the efficacy of the Q-18B gels over a 24-hour period. These test gels significantly decreased SLS absorption when compared with unprotected-skin control samples. The percent protection effect of three test gels against SLS percutaneous absorption was 88%, 81%, and 65%, respectively.

IN VIVO METHODS

In 1940, Schwartz et al. [18] introduced an in vivo method to evaluate the efficacy of a vanishing cream against poison ivy extract using visual erythema on human skin. The test cream was an effective prophylaxis against poison ivy dermatitis when compared with unprotected skin.

Lupulescu and Birmingham [19] observed the ultrastructural and relief changes of human epidermis after exposure to a protective gel, acetone, and kerosene on humans. Unprotected skin produced cell damage and a disorganized pattern in the upper layers of epidermis. Application of a protective agent before to solvent exposure substantially reduced the ultrastructural and relief changes of epidermis cells.

Lachapelle and co-workers [3, 20–23] used a guinea pig model to evaluate the protective value of BC and/or gels by laser Doppler flowmetry and histological assessment. The histopathological damage after 10 minutes of contact to toluene was mostly confined to the epidermis, whereas the dermis was almost normal. The dermal blood-flow changes were relatively high on the control site compared with the gel-pretreated sites.

Frosch et al. [1, 8, 9, 24, 25] developed the repetitive irritation test (RIT) in the guinea pig and in humans to evaluate the efficacy of BC by using a series of bioengineering techniques. The cream-pretreated and -untreated test skin (guinea pig or humans) was exposed daily to the irritants for 2 weeks. The resulting irritation was scored on a clinical scale and assessed by biophysical techniques' parameters. Some test creams suppressed irritation with all test parameters, some failed to show such an effect, and some even exacerbated the irritation [9].

Zhai [2] used an in vivo human model to measure the effectiveness of BC against dye-indicator solutions: methylene blue in water and oil red O in ethanol, which are representative of model hydrophilic and lipophilic compounds. Solutions of 5% methylene blue and 5% oil red O were applied to untreated and BC-pretreated skin with the aid of aluminum occlusive chambers for 0 and 4 hours. At the end of the application time, the materials were removed, and consecutive skin-surface biopsies (SSB) obtained. The amount of dye penetrating into each strip was determined by colorimetry. Two creams exhibited effectiveness, but one cream enhanced the cumulative amount of dye.

Zhai et al. [5] introduced a facile approach to screening protectants in vivo in human subjects. Two acute irritants and 1 allergen were selected: 1) sodium lauryl sulfate (SLS), representative of irritant household and occupational contact dermatitis, 2) the combination of ammonium hydroxide (NH_4OH) and urea to simulate diaper dermatitis, and 3) Rhus to evaluate the effect of model protective materials. Test materials were spread onto test area, massaged, allowed to dry for 30 minutes, and reapplied with another 30-minute drying period. The model irritants and allergen were applied with an occlusive patch for 24 hours. Inflammation was scored with an expanded 10-point scale at 72 hours after application. Most test materials statistically suppressed the SLS irritation and Rhus allergic reaction rather than NH_4OH and urea-induced irritation.

Wigger-Alberti et al. [26] determined which areas of the hands were likely to be skipped on self-application of BC by fluorescence technique at the workplace. Results showed the application of BC was incomplete, especially on the dorsal aspects of the hands. Brief data of recent experiments of BC are summarized in Table 1.

CONCLUSIONS

Some BC reduce CD under experimental conditions. But, inappropriate BC application may enhance irritation rather than benefit. To achieve the optimal protective effects, BC should be used with careful consideration based on specific exposure conditions; also, the proper use of BC should be instructed.

In vitro methods are simple, rapid, safe, and are recommended in the screening procedure for BC candidates. With radiolabeled methods, we may determine the accurate protective and penetration results even in the lower levels of chemicals because of the sensitive radiolabeled counting when BCs are to be evaluated. Animal experiments may be used to generate kinetic data because of a closer similarity between humans and some animals (e.g., pigs and monkeys) in percutaneous absorption and penetration for some compounds. But no one animal, with its complex anatomy and biology, will simulate the penetration in humans for all compounds. Therefore, the best estimate of human percutane-

TABLE 1 Brief Data from Recent Experiments of BC

Models		Irritants or allergens	Barrier creams	Evaluations by	Efficacy	Authors and Refs.
In vitro	In vivo animals or humans					
Human skin		Dyes (eosin, methylviolet, oil red O)	16 Barrier creams	Amount of dyes in the epidermis	Various % protection effects	Treffel et al. [15]
Human skin	Nickel-sensitive patients	Nickel disc	Ethylenediaminetetraacetate (EDTA) gels	Nickel content	Significantly reduced the amount of nickel in the epidermis in vitro, and significantly reduced positive reactions in vivo	Fullerton and Menne [16]
Human skin		[^{35}S]-SLS	3 Quaternium-18 bentonite (Q-18B) gels	Amount of [^{35}S]-SLS	% protection effect was 88%, 81%, and 65%, respectively	Zhai et al. [17]
	Guinea pigs	n-Hexane, trichlorethylene, toluene	3 water-miscible crams	Morphological assessment	Limited protective effects	Lachapelle et al. [23]
	Guinea pigs and humans	SLS, sodium hydroxide, toluene, lactic acid	Several barrier creams	Various bioengineering techniques	Some of them suppressed irritation, some failed	Frosch et al. [1, 8, 24, 25]
	Humans	Dyes (methylene blue and oil red O)	Three barrier creams	Amount of dye penetrating into strips	Two of them exhibited effectiveness, one enhanced cumulative amount of dye	Zhai and Maibach [2]
	Humans	SLS, ammonium hydroxide (NH$^+$OH) and urea, Rhus	Several protectants	Clinical scores	Most suppressed the SLS irritation and Rhus allergic reaction, failed to NH$^+$OH and urea irritation	Zhai et al. [5]
	Humans	Self-application of BC	An oil-in-water emulsion	Fluorescence technique	Self-application of BC was incomplete	Wigger-Alberti et al. [26]

ous absorption is determined by in vivo studies in humans. The histological assessments may define what layers of skin are damaged or protected, and may provide the insight mechanism of BC. Noninvasive bioengineering techniques may provide accurate, highly reproducible, and objective observations in quantifying the inflammation response to various irritants and allergens when BC are to be evaluated that could assess subtle differences to supplement traditional clinical studies.

To validate these models, well-controlled field trials are required to define the relationship of the model to the occupational setting. Finally, the clinical efficacy of BC should be assessed in the workplace rather than in experimental circumstances.

REFERENCES

1. Frosch PJ, Schulze-Dirks A, Hoffmann M, Axthelm I, Kurte A. Efficacy of skin barrier creams. (I). The repetitive irritation test (RIT) in the guinea pig. *Contact Dermatitis 28*:94, 193.
2. Zhai H, Maibach, HI. Effect of barrier creams: human skin in vivo. *Contact Dermatitis 35*: 92, 1996.
3. Lachapelle JM. Efficacy of protective creams and/or gels. In: Elsner P, Lachapelle JM, Wahlberg JE, Maibach HI, eds. *Prevention of Contact Dermatitis, Current Problems in Dermatology*. Basel: Karger, 1996; 182.
4. Zhai H, Maibach HI. Percutaneous penetration (Dermatopharmacokinetics) in evaluating barrier creams. In: Elsner P, Lachapelle JM, Wahlberg JE, Maibach HI. eds. *Prevention of Contact Dermatitis, Current Problems in Dermatology*. Basel: Karger, 1996; 193.
5. Zhai H, Willard P, Maibach HI. Evaluating skin-protective materials against contact irritants and allergens. An in vivo screening human model. *Contact Dermatitis 38*:155, 1998.
6. Wigger-Alberti W, Elsner P. Do barrier creams and gloves prevent or provoke contact dermatitis? *Am J Contact Dermatitis 9*:100, 1998.
7. Goh CL. Cutting oil dermatitis on guinea pig skin. (I). Cutting oil dermatitis and barrier cream. *Contact Dermatitis 24*:16, 1991.
8. Frosch PJ, Schulze-Dirks A, Hoffmann M, Axthelm I. Efficacy of skin barrier creams. (II). Ineffectiveness of a popular ''skin protector'' against various irritants in the repetitive irritation test in the guinea pig. *Contact Dermatitis 29*:74, 1993.
9. Frosch PJ, Kurte A, Pilz B. Biophysical techniques for the evaluation of skin protective creams. In: Frosch PJ, Kligman AM, eds. *Noninvasive Methods for the Quantification of Skin Functions*. Berlin: Springer-Verlag, 1993; 214.
10. Sadler CGA, Marriott RH. The evaluation of barrier creams. *Br Med J 23*:769, 1946.
11. Suskind RR. The present status of silicone protective creams. *Ind Med Surg 24*:413, 1955.
12. Langford NP. Fluorochemical resin complexes for use in solvent repellent hand creams. *Am Ind Hyg Assoc J 39*:33, 1978.
13. Reiner R, Roßmann K, Hooidonk CV, Ceulen BI, Bock J. Ointments for the protection against organophosphate poisoning. *Arzneim-Forsch/Drug Res 32*:630, 1982.
14. Loden M. The effect of 4 barrier creams on the absorption of water, benzene, and formaldehyde into excised human skin. *Contact Dermatitis 14*:292, 1986.
15. Treffel P, Gabard B, Juch R. Evaluation of barrier creams: an in vitro technique on human skin. *Acta Derm Venereol 74*:7, 1994.
16. Fullerton A, Menne T. In vitro and in vivo evaluation of the effect of barrier gels in nickel contact allergy. *Contact Dermatitis 32*:100, 1995.
17. Zhai H, Buddrus DJ, Schulz AA, Wester RC, Hartway T, Serranzana S, Maibach HI. In vitro percutaneous absorption of sodium lauryl sulfate (SLS) in human skin decreased by Quaternium-18 bentonite gels. In vitro & Molecular Toxicol 12:11, 1999.
18. Schwartz L, Warren LH, Goldman FH. Protective ointment for the prevention of poison ivy dermatitis. *Public Health Rep 55*:1327, 1940.

19. Lupulescu AP, Birmingham DJ. Effect of protective agent against lipid-solvent–induced damages. Ultrastructural and scanning electron microscopical study of human epidermis. *Arch Environ Health 31*:29, 1976.
20. Mahmoud G, Lachapelle JM, Neste DV. Histological assessment of skin damage by irritants: its possible use in the evaluation of a 'barrier cream'. *Contact Dermatitis 11*:179, 1984.
21. Mahmoud G, Lachapelle JM. Evaluation of the protective value of an antisolvent gel by laser Doppler flowmetry and histology. *Contact Dermatitis 13*:14, 1985.
22. Mahmoud G, Lachapelle J. Uses of a guinea pig model to evaluate the protective value of barrier creams and/or gels. In: Maibach HI, Lowe NJ, eds. *Models of Dermatology*. Basel: Karger, 1987; 112.
23. Lachapelle JM, Nouaigui H, Marot L. Experimental study of the effects of a new protective cream against skin irritation provoked by the organic solvents n-hexane, trichlorethylene and toluene. *Dermatosen 38*:19, 1990.
24. Frosch PJ, Kurte A, Pilz B. Efficacy of skin barrier creams. (III). The repetitive irritation test (RIT) in humans. *Contact Dermatitis 29*:113, 1993.
25. Frosch PJ, Kurte A. Efficacy of skin barrier creams. (IV). The repetitive irritation test (RIT) with a set of 4 standard irritants. *Contact Dermatitis 31*:161, 1994.
26. Wigger-Alberti W, Maraffio B, Wernli M, Elsner P. Self-application of a protective cream. Pitfalls of occupational skin protection. *Arch Dermatol 133*:861, 1997.

69

Objective Methods for Assessment of Human Facial Wrinkles

Gary Grove and Mary Jo Grove
KGL's Skin Study Center, Broomall, and cyberDERM, inc., Media, Pennsylvania

INTRODUCTION

The skin, especially that of the face, undergoes very characteristic changes with advancing age. Although there are other overt morphological changes that can be considered as markers of cutaneous aging, the degree of wrinkling in the "crow's feet" area seems to have the greatest impact. Thus, it is not surprising that considerable effort has been expanded to develop skincare products and cosmetic surgical procedures that can effectively restore a more youthful appearance.

Wrinkles can be easily visualized and many clinical studies have involved the use of ranking scales that rely on subjective assessments by expert graders. To improve the validity and reproducibility of this approach, more complex ordinal scales with semiquantive word descriptors and reference photographs have been devised by several investigators [1–3]. For example, Daniell [1] devised a set of reference photographs that illustrates his six-point grading scheme for evaluating crow's-feet wrinkles in the lateral periorbital area. Such reference photographs can be used to train inexperienced graders and periodically review the competency of all evaluators. Nevertheless, the major drawback to this type of approach is that it provides no permanent records that fully describe the skin-surface features or allow retrospective analysis. Instead, we must rely on the subjective judgements of trained graders and their ability to recall from memory the full range of changes in skin-surface features that might occur in each situation.

This problem can be overcome by taking standardized photographs before treatment and at various intervals during the treatment period. This provides a series of photographs that not only documents the study but can also be used to quantify the therapeutic response. This can be done by a panel of blinded, independent readers who are remote from the study environment as was done for photodamaged skin treated with isotretinoin [4] or alpha-hydroxy acids [5]. Although clinical assessments and photography are useful methods for assessing such changes in photodamaged skin, we are concerned that they might not be appropriate for studying wrinkles. This is especially true for photography in which changes in lighting or facial expression can greatly influence the appearance of lines and wrinkles. We are also concerned that concurrent improvements in other facial features, such as a decrease in mottled pigmentation or increased dermal blood flow, might partially unblind or unduly influence the investigator while judging the drug's impact on wrinkles. Thus, there is clearly a need for a more objective method to evaluate the effects of various treatments on facial lines and wrinkles.

CHAPTER OBJECTIVE

In this chapter, we will describe how optical profilometry [6] can provide an objective measure of wrinkling that can complement clinical assessment of various agents and procedures that might be useful in the therapy of photodamaged skin. Our approach is a variant of the skin-surface replica approach first described by Corcuff and colleagues [7–10]. Silicon rubber impression materials can be used to make a mold of the skin surface that faithfully captures its fine facial lines and wrinkles [11]. Such samples provide a permanent topographic record and can easily be taken serially from the same site with extended periods between each sample. By using image-analysis techniques similar to those used by NASA to map the lunar landscape during the Ranger missions [12], we can extract numeric information that describes the microtopographic features of the skin in the same way. Instead of using the sun to sidelight the moon's craters and crevices, we use a fiberoptic illuminator set at an appropriate angle to bring out the skin-surface details of interest.

BASIC METHODOLOGY
Skin-Surface Impressions

The site to be sampled should be delineated by affixing adhesive paper rings with orientation tabs such as those manufactured by CuDerm (Dallas, TX). Because the crow's feet furrows taper and become less pronounced as you move away from the periorbital area, it is extremely important that the site be located precisely. To facilitate relocating this site for subsequent serial samples, close-up photographs can be taken of the region with the adhesive rings properly placed for each panelist, as shown in Figure 1 for the crow's foot region.

Of the dental-impression materials that have been used, Silflo from Flexico Develop-

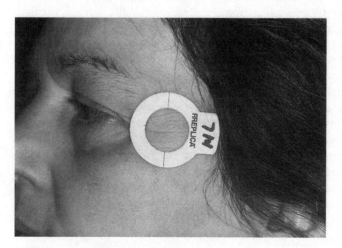

FIGURE 1   Placement of CuDerm Replica Locator Ring for obtaining silicone rubber impression from the crow's feet region.

ments Ltd. (Potters Bar, UK) is the best choice for skin-surface replicas. It not only offers a very high degree of fidelity, but the white opaque surface is ideal for viewing under reflected light used in image analysis. Moreover, these types of samples could be stored for at least 2 years without any fear of alteration in microtopography.

To make a impression, a thin layer of freshly prepared Silflo is gently spread over the bounded area of the ring and allowed to flow into the various furrows, creases, and fine lines that mark the surface. Within a few minutes, the material will polymerize and the replica is removed by gently lifting away from the skin using the orientation tab of the paper ring. It is important that the panelist remains calm with eyes closed and face relaxed during the polymerization phase. Because of the hydrophobic properties of silicon rubber, holes will form if the panelist is sweating from being too warm or emotionally stressed. Other artifacts such as bubbles can be created if the mixture is stirred too vigorously, causing it to froth. Alternatively, if the resin is not adequately mixed with the hardener or the mixture is allowed to partially polymerize before application, the specimens will lack detail.

Image Analysis

The general principles of image analysis for measuring the microtopography of the skin surface as captured in replica specimens have been previously described [6,7]. Briefly, these instruments consist of a high-resolution, black-and-white digital camera that is interfaced into a computer that contains specially designed image-processing hardware and software. The resulting image consists of a 640×480 pixel matrix with 256 gray levels. By selecting proper thresholds based on gray-level values, the image can be segmented into features of interest, such as wrinkles, and subsequently analyzed. One of the advantages of using replicas over photographs is that only topographic features are captured in the white replicas, which can be studied in all three dimensions by taking lighting angles into consideration. In striking contrast, not only are the photographs limited to two dimensions, but color variations attributable to mottled pigmentation greatly complicate the analysis.

In this application, the replica specimen is sidelighted using a fiberoptic illuminator set at a precisely defined angle to bring out the surface details of interest. In general, the lower the light source the greater the detail will be. In the case of a child, an angle of 15° to 20° will enable the observer to see a large number of fine lines, whereas for deeper furrows and creases such as crow's feet in an adult, an angle of 38° to 45° is optimal. In both cases, lines and wrinkles will cast shadows that are contrasted against the white background of the replica. Figure 2 illustrates that differences in the degree of wrinkling in the crow's foot region can be readily appreciated in this manner.

Because of the extreme anisotrophy of the skin, it is extremely important to take note of the position of the light source relative to the orientation of the specimen. Indeed, the major furrows and lines that are recognized as crow's feet are highly directional with 180° symmetry. For technical reasons, it is far simpler to rotate the sample than to have the lighting system revolve to simulate the movement of the sun. This is accomplished by a using a lazy Susan as a revolving sample holder, and great care is taken to ensure that the replica is held perfectly flat and centered with regard to both the light source and video camera during this movement. In the automated system of Corcuff and Leveque [10], the specimen is rotated at 9° steps through 360°, giving a series of 40 values. When plotted as polar coordinates according to the angle of rotation, one obtains a "rose of direction." A min-max at 180° is readily apparent, and taking measurements in both orien-

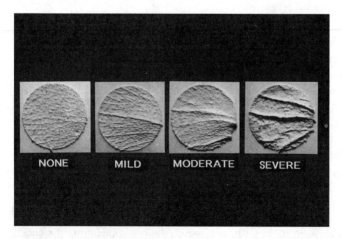

FIGURE 2 Representative silicone rubber impressions cast from the crow's foot region showing different degrees of wrinkling.

tations is sufficient for most applications. In our convention, the north-south axis is when the orientation of the lighting is perpendicular to the major furrows, whereas with the east-west it is parallel.

In addition to the angle of lighting, the uniformity of the incident light is critical. Interfering lights and changes in ambient lighting will influence the reproducibility of the measurements; it is best to work in total darkness. Fluctuations in the electronic circuits of the digitizing camera must also be minimized. As a rule, all these types of errors can be controlled by routinely using a series replicas as reference standards to ensure the analysis is being properly conducted.

The digitized image can be mathematically represented as a three-dimensional matrix of numbers. The x and y values are polar coordinates that provide the location of the pixel whereas the z value represents the brightness of the pixel in terms of its gray level. In one analytical approach, the digitized image is segmented into a binary image consisting of shadows and background by choosing an appropriate gray-level threshold. The percentage of the surface area occupied by shadows in a standard field of view is directly related to its topography. Obviously, if the surface is rather smooth and flat, there will be few shadows and this value will be small. On the other hand, if the skin is wrinkled and rough, the shadowed areas will be correspondingly larger. Moreover, because the angle of illumination is known, the horizontal projection of these shadows can be used to estimate their mean depth. Indeed, more sophisticated analyses such as the coefficient of developed skin surface (CDSS), which is a mathematical expression of true-versus-apparent surface area as pioneered by Corcuff's group [7–10], are possible.

In optical profilometry, a profile that represents the surface features at that specific location is created by plotting the gray-level values across a horizontal segment of this digitized image. This graphic display (Fig. 3) is similar to that achieved through mechanical profilometry with stylus devices, and we can extract numeric information that describes the microtopographic attributes in much the same way. Of the many parameters available for assessing skin-surface topography, both Rz and Ra have proved to be the most useful. To compute Rz, the profile is first divided into five equal segments along the x-axis. The minimum–maximum differences within each of the five segments are then determined,

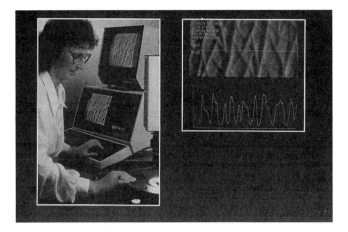

FIGURE 3   Basic set-up and profile of skin surface topography generated by image analysis of side-illuminated silicone rubber impressions.

and Rz is calculated as the average of these five local values. To compute Ra, an average line is generated to run through the center of the profile, and the area that the profile describes above and below this reference line is determined.

REPRESENTATIVE RESULTS

Photodamaged Skin with Topical Tretinoin

Computerized image analysis of silicone rubber impressions of the skin surface has been used to document the effects of topically applied tretinoin cream on photodamaged facial skin in several multicenter clinical trials [6, 12–15]. Although coarse wrinkles have been diminished, it is clear that the primary effect is on superficial, fine lines, as shown in Figure 4.

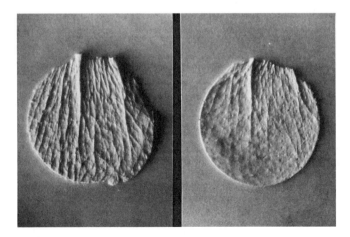

FIGURE 4   Representative silicone rubber impressions from the crow's foot region of a patient before and after 6 months of treatment with 0.05% tretinoin emollient cream.

Cutaneous Resurfacing Using High-Energy, Pulsed CO₂ Lasers

Although cutaneous resurfacing with CO_2 lasers is not a new technique, the older systems were not well suited for the delicate areas around the eyes and mouth. The newest generation of high-energy pulsed ("ultrapulse") CO_2 lasers produces high-energy bursts that allow maximal lesional ablation with minimal heat conduction to uninvolved skin which greatly reduces the risks of scarring. Alster [16] has shown that although both the surgipulse and ultrapulse high-energy CO_2 lasers are effective in reducing the appearance of periorbital rhytides, computer analysis of skin-surface impressions shows a more substantial improvement after ultrapulse laser treatment. Indeed, the skin-surface texture was found to be comparable to normal. Alster [17] has also used optical profilometry to document that laser resurfacing can also effectively improve or even eliminate atrophic facial acne scars.

CONCLUDING REMARKS

The use of silicon rubber impressions allows one to capture the microtopographic features of the skin surface that can be subsequently measured using well-established image-analysis techniques. These samples are durable, easy to store, and can be readily transported from the clinical center to a remote site for objective measurements in a truly blinded manner. Moreover, these samples allow one to obtain serial samples of the same skin surface over prolonged periods of time. As pointed out by Leveque [18], numerous factors can alter the appearance or actual dimensions of wrinkles. It is extremely important to understand that extreme care must be taken to ensure that the impression be artifact free and truly the skin surface being studied. The before- and after-treatment comparisons must be based on identical areas and use the same conditions of analysis.

REFERENCES

1. Daniell HW. Smoker's wrinkles: a study in the epidemiology of "crow's feet." Ann Intern Med 1971; 75:873–880.
2. Griffiths CEM, Wang TS, Hamilton TA, Voorhees JJ, Ellis CN. A photonumeric scale for the assessment of cutaneous photodamage. Arch Dermatol 1992; 128:347–351.
3. Larnier C, Ortonne JP, Venot A, Faivre B, Beani JC, Thomas P, Brown T, Sendagorta E. Evaluation of cutaneous photodamage using a photographic scale. Br J Dermatol 1994; 130:167–173.
4. Armstrong RB, Lesiewicz G, Harvey G, Lee LF, Spoehr KT, Zultak M. Clinical panel assessment of photodamaged skin treated with isotretinoin using photographs. Arch Dermatol 1992; 128:352–356.
5. Stiller MJ, Bartolone J, Stern R, Smith S, Kollias N, Gillies R, Drake LA. Topical 8% glycolic acid and 8% l-lactic acid creams for treatment of photodamaged skin. Arch Dermatol 1996; 132:631–636.
6. Grove GL, Grove MJ, Leyden JJ. Optical profilometry: an objective method for quantification of facial wrinkles. J Am Acad Derm 1989; 21:631–637.
7. Corcuff P, Chatenay F, Leveque JL. A fully automated system to study skin surface patterns. Int J Cosmet Sci 1984; 6:167–176.
8. Corcuff P, deRigal J, Leveque JL, Makki S, Agache P. Skin relief and aging. J Soc Cosmet Chem 1983; 34:177–190.
9. Corcuff P, Leveque JL, Grove GL, Kligman AM. The impact of aging on the microrelief of perio-orbital and leg skin. J Soc Cosmet Chem 1987; 82:145–152.

10. Corcuff P, Leveque JL. Skin surface replica image analysis of furrows and wrinkles. In: Scrup J and Jemec GBE, eds. *Handbook of Non-invasive Methods and the Skin.* Boca Raton: CRC, 1995:89–96.
11. Grove GL, Grove MJ. Objective methods for assessing skin surface topography noninvasively. In: Leveque JL, ed. Cutaneous Investigations in Health and Disease. New York: Marcel Dekker, 1989: 1–32.
12. Grove GL, Grove MJ, Leyden JJ, Lufrano L, Schwab B, Perry BH, Thorne EG. Skin replica analysis of photodamaged skin after therapy with tretinoin emollient cream. J Am Acad Dermatol 1991; 25:231–237.
13. Olsen EA, Katz HI, Levine N, et al. Tretinoin emollient cream: a new therapy for photodamaged skin. J Am Acad Dermatol 1992; 26:215–224.
14. Weinstein GD, Migra TP, Poch PE, et al. Topical tretinoin for treatment of photodamaged skin. A multicenter study. Arch Dermatol 1991; 127(5):659–665.
15. Gilchrest BA. Treatment of photodamage with topical tretinoin: an overview. J Am Acad Dermatol 1997; 36(?)S27- 36.
16. Alster TS. Comparison of two high-energy, pulsed carbon dioxide lasers in the treatment of periorbital rhytides. Dermatol Surg 1996; 22:541–545.
17. Alster TS, West TB. Resurfacing of atrophic facial acne scars with a high-energy, pulsed carbon dioxide laser. Dermatol Surg 1996; 22:151–155.
18. Leveque JL, EEMCO guidance for the assessment of skin topography. J Eur Acad Dermatol Venereol 1999; 12(2):103–114.

70

Acnegenicity and Comedogenicity Testing for Cosmetics

F. Anthony Simion
The Andrew Jergens Company, Cincinnati, Ohio

INTRODUCTION

Many people experience facial acne, especially in their teens and early 20s. It typically causes distress, and in some individuals contributes to a lowered self-image [1]. As consumers age the prevalence of acne decreases, although it can be triggered by factors such as stress, medications, and the use of cosmetics [2–4]. Indeed, there are many reports of cosmetics causing comedones, or acneform eruptions. These adverse reactions are of great concern to consumers, many of whom look for products that will not cause such problems. Hence, cosmetics manufacturers strive to develop products that do not cause comedones or acne. Products are frequently labeled noncomedogenic and/or nonacnegenic. Consumers use these terms interchangeably, although comedone formation and acnegenicity are not the same. To consumers, the key issue is that the cosmetics they use do not cause breakouts.

COMEDOGENICITY

Comedone formation occurs when the pattern of keratinization inside the sebaceous follicle changes. Within the keratinocytes, these changes include the production of different keratins and a reduction in the number of lamellar granules [5]. There is also an increase in mitotic activity [6]. As a result the keratinocytes do not desquamate properly and the follicular duct is blocked. It is not known what causes these changes, but the result is a microcomedone. As further keratinized material accumulates, the follicle becomes visible from the surface as a closed comedone, or whitehead (Fig. 1). As more material accumulates, the follicle distends and open comedones, also know as blackheads are formed. The black color is attributable to the oxidation of lipids as they reach the skin's surface. The test methods to assess comedogenesis are designed to quantify the hyperkeratotic plugs.

ACNEGENICITY

The hyperkeratotic plug results in sebum accumulating in the follicilar duct and the sebaceous gland. This enables the anaerobic bacteria, *P. acnes*, to proliferate. The follicular

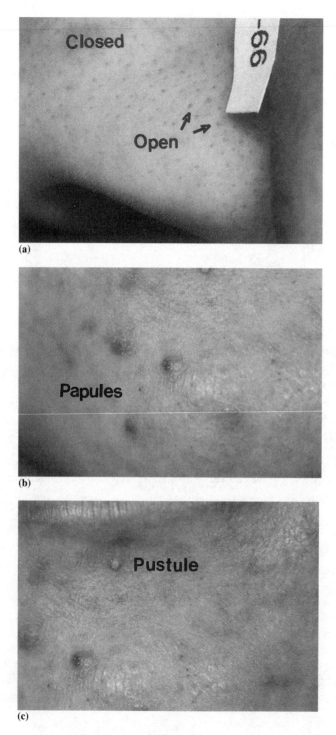

FIGURE 1 Examples of the different forms of comedones and acneform eruptions. (a) Closed and open comedones. (b) Papules. (c) Pustules.

duct will expand until it ruptures, releasing the bacteria and their metabolic products into the surrounding dermis. Both immunological and irritant reactions occur. In severe acne, elevated levels of anti–*P. acnes* antibodies are detected. Irritation may come from the fatty acids that are the result of sebaceous triglyceride digestion by bacteria. Certainly at the histological level, the classic signs of inflammation such as a neutrophilic infiltrate are observed. The consumer recognizes this as acne pustules and papules.

PUSTULOGENIC POTENTIAL

Upon first using a new cosmetic, papules and pustules are sometimes observed after a few days. To the consumer this is acne, although this type of papulopustular reaction may be a form of follicular irritation. Certainly, as Mills and Berger pointed out, it occurs more quickly than can be accounted for by the formation of hyperkeratotic plugs and its sequalae [7]. Thus, Mills and Berger suggested that pustulogenic potential—the ability to cause inflammatory lesions—should be differentiated from comedogenic potential—the ability to cause the formation of hyperkeratotic plugs.

TEST METHODS

Human and animal models have been used to assess the comedogenic potential of cosmetic products and their ingredients. Both models require repeated applications of the materials to the skin for 2 to 4 weeks. The number of hyperkeratotic impactions produced is compared with positive and negative controls.

Animal Models

The rabbit ear is the most commonly used animal model. The rabbit's ear follicle has many structural similarities to the human sebaceous follicle. In 1941, Adams et al. [8] showed that the rabbit ear would respond similarly to human skin when exposed to chlorinated hydrocarbons, the most common cause of acne in industrial accidents. Until the rise of the animal rights movement in the late 1980s, cosmetic products were routinely screened using rabbits. Briefly, the method entails that the test product or ingredient is applied daily to the inner surface of one ear. This site is left open. The other ear is used as the negative control. At the end of either 2 or 4 weeks, the animal was sacrificed, and the degree of follicular hyperkeratinization is assessed. Frequently this was done by taking histological sections and giving an overall score based on the number and degrees of compacted follicles. Occasionally the impactions were removed from the ear using cyanoacrylate glue on a glass slide. This method is now frequently used in human testing.

The results from the rabbit-ear studies show that some cosmetic ingredients have comedogenic potential. These include branched chain esters and compounds that have solubility in both oil and water (hydrophile-lipophile balance (HLB) of 10–12) [9]. However, if these materials are chemically modified, or included at low levels with other ingredients in cosmetics, then their comedogenic potential is nullified. This was shown by Fulton [9] as well as Kligman and Mills [2]. Fulton showed that chemically modifying cosmetic ingredients can greatly effect their comedogenic potential. For instance, PEG-16 Lanolin gives a severe comedogenicity score of 4 on a 0 to 5 scale, whereas the higher–molecular weight and more water-soluble PEG-75 Lanolin yields a score of 0 under the same test conditions (Table 1). Furthermore, Fulton showed that the comedogenic potential of fatty acid solutions was greatly reduced by replacing sunflower oil with acetone or ether as the solvent. Kligman and Mills reported that the comedogenic potential of vegetable oils is dose dependent, being abolished by diluting to 25% with mineral oil. From these observations, it appears vital to assess the comedogenic potential of the final product [7]. Additionally, Fulton and his colleagues screened the comedogenic potential of many ingredients and products [9,10]. Some of these results are included in Table 1.

It is interesting to note that the primary irritation potential does not correlate with comedogenic potential. For instance, sodium lauryl sulfate, which is frequently used as a model irritant, is noncomedogenic [11]. Conversely, many esters—such as isopropyl isostearate—that are highly comedogenic are relatively nonirritating.

To detect weak comedogens, the rabbit-ear assay was modified. Product applications were increased from 2 to 4 weeks, enabling the assay to detect products that cause comedones in a small but sensitive groups of consumers. The method may be overly sensitive for the average consumer, so there is a risk of false positives. Conversely, products that are noncomedogenic in the 4-week rabbit ear test are unlikely to cause comedone formation even in acne-prone consumers.

Many adverse reactions that consumers describe as breakouts or blemishes are not attributable to comedone formation. This is readily appreciated from the rapid onset of the blemish (a few days), which is too rapid for the formation of hyperkeratotic plugs in the follicular ducts. Furthermore, the formation of open or closed comedones frequently occurs without skin redness, whereas breakouts and blemishes described by consumers do have an inflammatory component. To better understand pustule formation, Wahlberg and Maibach developed a model to assess pustulogenic potential [12]. The test materials were placed on rabbits' backs and occluded for 24 hours. For some ingredients, the skin had to be abraded with a sterile needle to produce pustules. Pustule formation is dose dependent. Irritants such as sodium lauryl sulfate can elicit pustules even though they are noncomedogenic.

Human Models

Human models have been developed for looking at both acnegenic and comedogenic potential. Mills and Kligman first described the human comedogenic model in 1982 [13]. It is becoming more extensively used in the cosmetics industry as companies continue to avoid animal testing. In the human procedure, up to six test materials are applied to the upper back for 48 to 72 hours under an occlusive or, if necessary, a semiocclusive patch. Patches are applied three times a week for 4 weeks to give the 28 days of continuous exposure.

After induction, the test sites are sampled using an epidermal biopsy. A glass slide coated with cyanoacrylate (e.g., Crazy Glue®) is briefly applied to the skin for 1 minute. After it has dried the slide is removed, taking the follicular plugs and much of the stratum corneum with it. The size and number of follicular impactions are assessed using a 0-to-3 scale and compared with positive and negative controls. Positive controls include acetylated lanolin and coal tar. Mills and Kligman showed that the human model gave similar results to the 2-week rabbit-ear method (Pearson r = 0.944, n = 32 cosmetic ingredients or products). However, the rabbit-ear model appears to be somewhat more sensitive than the human assay (Table 2).

Recently, a new method for epidermal biopsies has been validated. The method uses

TABLE 1 Comedogenicity and Irritation Potential of Cosmetic Ingredients in the Rabbit-Ear Model

Ingredient	Comedogenicity	Irritation
Oils		
Cocoa butter	4	0
Coconut butter	4	0
Evening primrose oil	3	2
Soyabean oil	3	0
Peanut oil	2	0
Castor oil	1	0
Sunflower oil	0	0
Mineral oil	0–2	0
Lanolin and derivatives		
Acetylated lanolin	0	0
Acetylated lanolin alcohol	4	2
Anhydrous lanolin	0–1	0
Lanolin alcohol	0–2	0
PEG-16 Lanolin	4	3
PEG-75 Lanolin	0	0
Fatty acids and esters		
Lauric acid	4	1
Myristic acid	3	0
Palmatic acid	2	0
Stearic acid	2–3	0
Butyl stearate	3	0
Cetyl acetate	4	2
Cetyl ester NF	1	1
Isopropyl isostearte	5	0
Isopropyl lineolate	4	2
Isopropyl myristate	5	3
Alcohols, sugars, and their derivatives		
Isopropyl alcohol	0	0
Cetyl alcohol	2	2
Isocetyl alcohol	4	4
Oleyl alcohol	4	2
Stearyl alcohol	2	2
Sorbitol	0	0
Sorbitan laurate	1–2	1–2
Sorbitan oelate	3	0
Sorbitan stearate	0	0
Oleth-3	5	2
Oleth-5	3	2
Oleth-10	2	1
Oleth-20	1	0

Source: Ref. 9.

TABLE 2 Comparison of Human-Back and Rabbit-Ear Comedogenicity Scores

Material	Mean comedogenicity score	
	Rabbit*	Human
Acetylated lanolin alcohol	3	2
Cocoa butter	3	2
5% crude coal tar**	3	3
Isopropyl myristate	1	0.4
Safflower oil	1	0
5 or 8% sulfur**	3	2
2.5% sulfur**	2	1.2
Hydrophilic ointment	0	0

* Comedogenicity scored on a 0–3 scale, n = 3 rabbits and 5 humans.
** These test material were diluted with hydrophilic ointment. All other test materials used at full strength.
Source: Ref. 13.

commercially available cosmetic strips that are designed to remove impactions from the face without damaging the skin [14]. The bioré pore strip®, which uses a cationic polymer, preferentially interacts with the proteins of the hyperkeratotic plugs but not the stratum corneum. The plugs have more acidic amino acids and are therefore more negatively charged than the surrounding stratum corneum. An example of the bioré pore strip removing impactions from the nose is shown in Figure 2. Rizer et al. showed that the bioré pore strip® removed over 70% of the impactions that cyanoacrylate removes, but without the damage of the latter. The bioré pore strip is more effective than other cosmetic strips in removing plugs from the follicles. The other strips use nonionic polymers, which are not able to preferentially interact with the follicular plugs.

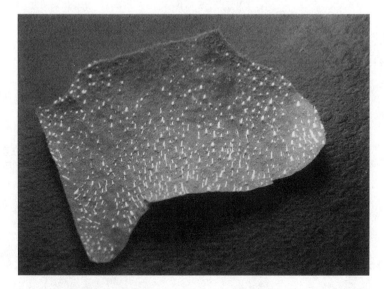

FIGURE 2 Half a bioré pore strip under UV light. The hyperkeratotic impactions on the strip fluoresce due to the *P. acnes.*

One advantage that the bioré strips have over the cyanoacrylate glue is that it is far less damaging and irritating to the skin. Therefore, it can be used to measure comedone formation on the face at the end of usage studies. Cyanoacrylate is too damaging to be acceptable to most test panelists for use on their face. The bioré pore strip has been shown to be acceptable to panelists; indeed, this is its intended use.

Human Usage Tests

Ultimately, all predictive models must be related to back to the consumers' experience in the marketplace. Consumers who experience an adverse reaction will report it in terms most familiar to them. Most consumers do not differentiate between acne and comedone formation, or blemishes and breakouts.

One approach to assessing the rate of adverse reactions is to have a group of consumers use a product for several weeks [15–18]. Test subjects should be evaluated for comedones, pustules and papules at the beginning of the study, and then at set intervals. A 1-week evaluation will reveal any propensity to cause irritation, including follicular irritation that panelists may recognize as breakouts. Any sensory irritation will become evident during the first week. Three and six-week evaluations are used to detect comedogenicity and acnegenicity. This design is consistent with the recommendation of the American Academy of Dermatology's consensus panel on acnegenicity testing [19].

A sizable proportion of adverse reactions is experienced by vulnerable subgroups. A subgroup for irritation may include panelists whose skin is readily irritated by surfactants. Another subgroup will include panelists with acne-prone skin. Both subgroups should be identified and form a significant part of the test panel. This will enable the investigator to identify potential problems before the product reaches the marketplace.

SUMMARY

The induction of comedones and acneform eruptions is a significant concern to many consumers, especially those with acne-prone skin. Any product that has a propensity to produce these eruptions will be unsuccessful in the marketplace. Indeed, many consumers expressly look for products that are labeled noncomedogenic and/or nonacnegenic.

Cosmetics manufacturers are meeting this consumer demand by showing that their products do not cause comedones and/or acne breakouts, and label their products accordingly. Consumers judge a facial cosmetic on whether it causes breakouts, blemishes, bumps, or blackheads. There are multiple causes for the reaction, including comedone formation and follicular irritation. Consumers do not differentiate between the biological mechanisms; they are only concerned with the results they produce.

Today, human models have replaced animals for testing both comedogenicity and acnegenicity. Comedone formation is determined by continuously patching the material on the human back for 28 consecutive days. Comedones are quantified by extracting the plugs from the follicle using cyanoacrylate glue on a glass slide or a bioré pore strip® containing cationic polymers. The degree of the impactions is compared with positive and negative controls.

Acnegenicity is assessed by human-use testing, where a panel of consumers uses the product under normal conditions. The skin is evaluated by a trained observer for comedones, papules, and pustules at the beginning of the study, and then after 1, 3, and 6 weeks of usage. Cosmetic pore strips such as bioré® can be used to assess comedone formation.

These can remove follicular plugs from the face without the skin damage associated with cyanoacrylate.

REFERENCES

1. S MacDonald Hull, WJ Cunliffe, BR Hughes. Treatment of the depressed and dysmorphopho-bic acne patient. Clin Exp Dermatol 16: 210–211, 1991.
2. AM Kligman, OH Jr Mills. Acne Cosmetica. Arch Dermatol 106: 843–850, 1972.
3. G Plewig, JE Jr Fulton, AM Kligman. Pomade Acne. Arch Dermatol 101: 580–584, 1970.
4. C Berlin. Acne comedo in children due to paraffin oil applied on the head. Arch Dermatol 69: 683–687, 1954.
5. JS Strauss. Sebaceous Glands in 'Dermatology in General Medicine' Eds. Fitzpatrick TB, Eisen AZ. Wolff K. et al., 4th Edition vol 1, p 709–726 (1993).
6. G Plewig, JE Jr Fulton, AM Kligman. Cellular dynamics of comedo formation in acne vulgaris. Arch Dermatol 102: 12–29, 1971.
7. OH Jr Mills, RS Berger. Defining the susceptibility of acne-prone and sensitive skin popula-tions to extrinsic factors. Dermatol Clinics 9: 93–98, 1991.
8. EH Adams, DD Irish, HC Spencer, et al. The reponse of rabbit skin to compounds reported to have caused anceform dermatitis Ind Med 2: 1–4, 1941.
9. JE Jr Fulton, Comedogenicity and irritancy of commonly used ingredients in skin care prod-ucts. J Soc Cosmet Chem 40: 321–333, 1989.
10. JE Jr Fulton, SR Pay, JE III Fulton. Comedogenicity of current therapeutic products, cosmetics, and ingredients in the rabbit ear. J Amer Acad Dermatol 10: 96–105, 1984.
11. WE Morris, SC Kwan. Use of the rabbit ear model in evaluating the comedogenic potential of cosmetic ingredients. J Soc Cosmet Chem 34: 215–225, 1983.
12. JE Walhberg, HI Maibach. Sterile Cutaneous Pustules: a manifestation of primary irritancy? In: Models in Dermatology 2: 297–302 Maibach HI and Lowe N, eds. Pub Krager (1985).
13. OH Jr Mills, AM Kligman. A human model for assessing comedogenic substances. Arch Der-matol 118: 903–905, 1982.
14. RL Rizer, JK Woodford, FA Simion et al. 'The follicular bioposy for assessing comedo-genicity: a comparison of a pore strip and cyanoacrylate.' Poster at the International Society of Bioengineering and the Skin, June 1998.
15. EM Jackson, NF Robillard. The controlled use test in a cosmetic product safety substantiation program. J Toxicol Cut & Ocular Toxicol 1: 117–132, 1982.
16. OH Jr Mills, RS Berger, TJ Stephens et al. Assessing acnegenic and acne aggravating potential. J Toxicol Cut & Ocular Toxical 8: 353–360, 1989.
17. EM Jackson. Clinical assessments of acnegenicity. J Toxicol Cut & Ocular Toxicol 8: 389–393, 1989.
18. A Ghassemi, R Osborne, KA Korman, et al. Demonstrating the ocular safety of an eye cosmetic product using alternatives to animal eye irritation tests. Poster at the Society of Toxicology Meeting in Cincinnati, OH, March 1997.
19. JS Strauss, EM Jackson et al. American Academy of Dermatology Invitational Symposium on Comedogenicity, J Amer Acad Dermatol 20: 272–277, 1989.

71

Sensory Testing

Linda P. Oddo and Kathy Shannon
Hill Top Research, Inc., Scottsdale, Arizona

Although most individuals don't realize it, they conduct sensory tests on a daily basis. Throughout the day, personal sensory assessments are made about the taste acceptability or liking for different foods for many different attributes. Individuals evaluate haircare products for various properties, not only while using the product but also for feel of the hair after shampooing. Every time a cosmetic product, moisturizer, or any other skincare product is applied to the skin, sensory assessments are made.

In very simple terms, the field of sensory testing applies controls, data-collection skills, and reproducible methodology to these types of assessments for the purpose of collecting not only viable but valuable information about the test materials. Civille [1] states that ''[t]he primary function of sensory testing is to conduct valid and reliable tests, which provide data on which sound decisions can be made.''

Although the roots of sensory testing as a discipline exist in the food industry, its applications have steadily earned respect in the consumer and pharmaceutical industries. Science now plays an important role in the field of cosmetology by providing guidance to the product formulator in predicting consumer response and by supporting or defining product claims.

Currently, trained sensory judges are routinely used in the development of many cosmetic products. Trained panels are used to evaluate the skin-feel properties of not only topical cosmetic products but any product that is applied to the skin. Trained judges are used to evaluate haircare products, and sensory judges are critical to determining oral and axillary malodor.

Using carefully controlled sensory applications, sensitive-skin subjects can be identified and selected. The response of these subjects can then be trusted to aid in the development of and/or to identify acceptable sensitive-skin cosmetic products. Finally, by applying sensory scaling techniques and controls to the design of self-assessment questionnaires, they are often added to clinical studies to provide a potential insight to consumer response. The primary focus of this chapter is to describe some of the sensory methods and tools that are currently being applied in these areas.

AXILLARY MALODOR EFFICACY

Generally, axillary malodor efficacy tests are conducted on three product types: antiperspirants, deodorants, and soaps. Although antiperspirants are primarily designed to inhibit sweat production, they are also considered deodorants because they inhibit sweat, which acts as a culture medium for bacteria to produce, degrade, and form malodor. Deodorants are formulated to control malodor only, through absorption, fragrance masking, and/or by reducing antibacterial activity. Some soap products may also reduce axillary malodor by fragrance masking and/or inhibiting bacterial growth.

The use of sensory testing applications is the primary methodology used to establish deodorant efficacy. In 1987, the sensory testing division of The American Society for Testing and Materials (ASTM) published the Standard Practice for the Sensory Evaluation of Axillary Deodorancy [2]. This document recommends that a product meet the criteria presented in the standard in order for it to qualify as an effective deodorant.

The basic design for conducting a deodorant study consists of selecting subjects with high axillary malodor, applying or using the test material at selected intervals, and then measuring the level of axillary malodor using a panel of trained odor judges. The test material is considered effective if there is a statistical difference between it and a placebo or untreated control. Factors that are critical to the test design and consequently a successful study are the subject selection, subject restrictions, odor-judge selection and training, selection of a suitable test location, and using appropriate scaling techniques.

Subjects should be selected from the user population and have a distinct axillary odor. Those with extremely high or low odor and those with large differences in odor level between the right and left axillae are usually disqualified. It is important that potential subjects participate in a washout or conditioning period before selection to prevent a carryover effect from the use of other products. For a minimum of 7 days, subjects are not allowed to use any axillary products and are instructed to wash the axillae only with a mild, nondeodorant soap. Other restrictions that are known to interfere with sensory odor assessments require the subjects to abstain from swimming, excessive exercise, and from using any fragranced products. They must also avoid spicy foods, and before an odor evaluation they are restricted from smoking.

Perhaps the most crucial factor in a well-executed malodor efficacy test is the selection and training of qualified odor judges. This process requires management support and commitment, a sensory staff or analyst to conduct the training, and a pool of available and interested candidates. Other factors to consider are the time commitments to not only select and train the judges but to continually maintain and validate their performance. The odor–judge selection and training process involves four basic steps: 1) interviewing candidates, 2) conducting screening tests, 3) training, and 4) validating performance.

During the interviewing process, candidates who have conflicting commitments or interfering health problems should be discontinued. A description of the test and the odor-judge process must be explained to each individual. If possible, because of the unusual nature of the intended task—sniffing the axillary region of subjects—a video of the process should be shown. Through interaction and discussion, those candidates who show a sincere interest and are willing to commit to the program are identified.

In vitro screening tests are administered to the potential odor judges to determine their olfactory acuity and ability to discriminate and reproduce results. Because it is possible for some individuals to be insensitive to some of the odors generated by the human body, potential judges should also be screened for this inherent lack of sensitivity.

An inability to recognize some body odors is commonly referred to as ''specific anosmia.'' The anosmias that have been identified in axillary odor include sweaty, urinous, musky, and hircine odors, with the primary anosmia being a urinous smell. It has been reported that as many as 46 to 50% of the population are insensitive to the urinous odor [3]. Because of this high percentage, judges should be screened for the insensitivity using the odorant androstenone. Individuals who can smell this compound will rate it extremely strong and often find it offensive, whereas those who are anosmic will rate it low or may not smell it at all.

The odorant used most often to represent a sweaty smell is isovaleric acid. It is therefore often used in odor, judge acuity screening tests. Potential judges are often given a series of paired comparisons and at least one ranking test of the five established levels of isovaleric acid (Table 1) [4].

For the paired comparison tests, potential judges are given at least eight different combinations of concentrations. The pairs should represent different levels of difficulty between samples, e.g., 0.013 versus 0.87 and 0.053 versus 0.22. In the ranking test, a sample of each concentration is presented. Before administering the tests, the samples should be placed in identical bottles or jars. Each bottle is identified by a unique three-digit number. The pairs and ranking test should be randomly presented to the candidates with a distinct rest period between each test. When presented with each pair, the odor-judge trainee is asked to identify which sample has the stronger or more intense odor. For the ranking test, they rank the samples from the least to the most intense odor. It is always very important to control the conditions of the test area when administering any sensory test [5].

In addition to determining acuity, reproducibility should also be considered. This can be accomplished by administering the same tests one or two more times on separate days. The order of set presentation, bottle order, and coding system must be changed between days.

Training is initiated once individuals who show a high olfactory acuity and consistency are identified. Several steps are involved in the training process, including establishing a standard method for evaluating, identifying judge restrictions, providing reference standards that represent the scale, and conducting training sessions.

The method frequently used to evaluate the axillary region involves placing the nose near the surface of the skin located in the center of the axilla and taking several short bunny sniffs. Judges clear the sinuses by breathing into a cotton material or toweling between evaluations. The evaluation method should also include an established rest period between evaluations and/or subjects (e.g., 30 or 60 sec). The judges must also avoid touching the subject with either their nose or hands. In addition to avoiding contact, the

TABLE 1 Five Established Levels of Isovaleric Acid

Odor level	Concentration of aqueous solution of isovaleric acid (mL/L)
Slight	0.013
Definite	0.053
Moderate	0.22
Strong	0.87
Very strong	3.57

judges are restricted from wearing any personal products with a distinct fragrance. They should also be restricted from eating certain foods before evaluating.

Critical in the evaluation process is identifying a scale. To evaluate the intensity or express the degree to which axillary odor is present, two types of scales are usually considered. One is a line scale, which consists of a standard-length line on which the judge makes a mark. The primary disadvantage to this approach is that judges may have difficulty establishing consistency without a number to remember [6]. Category scale methods are perhaps the most frequently used. This type of scale involves using sets of words and/or numbers to identify established intervals on the scale.

Among the available category scales, a 0-to-10 numerical scale has been used to evaluate or score malodor intensity. Although some descriptive language may vary slightly, the zero on this scale consistently represents no malodor while the 10 represents extremely strong malodor. Table 2 is a complete example of a 0-to-10 numerical scale.

In addition to being used in judge-acuity screening tests, isovaleric acid is often used as a reference standard when training judges to use malodor intensity scales. The five concentrations previously identified can be used to represent various points on the selected scale or other concentrations can be used. After introducing the reference points, the judges should practice until they can repeatedly assign the correct score to each reference under blind conditions.

New judges being introduced to human axillary odors should, if available, train with an experienced judge. The new judge observes the score given to a certain subject then evaluates the same subject. After participating in this capacity for a period, the judge in training evaluates the subject first and then observes the scores given by the established judge. Finally, the judge trainee evaluates independently until statistical analyses of his/her data correlates with the established judges.

Training new judges without the benefit of established judges can be accomplished by using a couple of different approaches. In one approach, the sensory scientist training the group can determine the odor level of selected subjects then introduce the new judges to these odor levels using the previously discussed techniques. Another approach allows the new group of judges to standardize their scores through consensus. After each evaluation, the group discusses their scores, and repeats the process until they agree on the odor level for that subject. This process is repeated until independent evaluations correlate.

TABLE 2 A 0-to-10 Numerical Scale

Numerical value	Description of malodor
0	None, no malodor
1	Threshold malodor
2	Very slight malodor
3	Slight malodor
4	Slight to moderate malodor
5	Moderate malodor
6	Slightly strong malodor
7	Moderately strong malodor
8	Strong malodor
9	Very strong malodor
10	Extremely strong malodor

Although this approach is more time consuming, it often establishes a strong sense of commitment and involvement in the process for the new judges.

Once established, odor judges can be used to evaluate any personal-care product used in the axillae to control malodor. By using combinations of subject selection, product-treatment techniques, post-treatment evaluation times, and controlling environmental conditions, an almost endless number of possibilities can be evaluated by the judges. In addition to directly evaluating human subjects, odor judges can also be used to evaluate axillary odor that has been transferred to some other medium such as a t-shirt or a cloth worn against the axilla.

ORAL MALODOR EFFICACY

Currently, oral malodor efficacy studies are conducted with toothpastes, cleansers, powders, mouth rinses, toothbrushes, breath mints, tongue scrapers, and any oral treatment whose primary or secondary function is to reduce or control halitosis. Oral treatments are designed to control, mask, or eliminate sulfur-producing bacteria, the primary component of bad breath.

To accommodate the large variety of consumer products currently available for treating halitosis, clinical studies vary in their design. Variables include the profile of the target population in their medical and dental history, current health conditions, and personal practices. Other elements considered when designing oral-malodor clinical studies include the number of treatments, evaluations, and post-treatment evaluation intervals. Evaluations may include any combination of professional examinations, microbiology sampling, oral-malodor assessments, and instrumental measurements.

Instruments that have been used to measure levels of malodor include gas chromatograph (GC), which has been used to analyze oral volatile sulfur compounds. In a clinical study comparing the GC with sensory odor judges, the instrumental measurements showed good correlation with the organoleptic assessments. The GC, however, is considered large, cumbersome, and difficult to use in a clinical setting [7]. A portable sulfide monitor, easier to use in a clinical environment, has also been investigated and found to fall within the range observed with the GC. When compared with odor judges, the Halimeter® also significantly correlated ($p < 0.001$) with sensory ratings [8].

Although good correlation has been established, the manufacturer of the Halimeter® states that the data independently cannot confirm the existence of oral malodor because volatile sulfur compounds are not constant in any one person. They recommend using the instrument with other procedures, such as bacterial cultures and organoleptic measurements to assess levels of oral malodor.

Organoleptic measurements or assessments are generally conducted by judges specifically trained to evaluate oral malodor. The selection and training of these judges is similar to the techniques used to select and train axillary malodor judges. Differences include the use of reference standards more appropriate to oral malodor and training the judges in a different process of evaluation. In the oral-malodor evaluation process, the judge and subject are separated by a solid partition. The partition has a small circular opening in which the subject inserts a glass rod. During the actual assessment, the subject places his/her mouth around the end of the glass rod and either holds his/her breath or exhales into the tube while the judge places his/her nose near the other end of the tube.

Currently, two very different types of sensory scales are being used to measure oral malodor. One applies hedonic measurements whereas the other approach uses category

TABLE 3 The Peryam and Pilgrim Scale

Numerical value	Hedonic description
1	Most pleasant
2	Very pleasant
3	Moderately pleasant
4	Slightly pleasant
5	Neutral (not bad/no odor/not good)
6	Slightly unpleasant
7	Moderately unpleasant
8	Very unpleasant
9	Most unpleasant

scaling. Typically, hedonic measurements are used by untrained consumers to indicate a level of liking for the material in question. For example, Tonzetich used a panel of eight ''observers'' to rate their responses to different oral-cleansing treatments on a 0-to 6-point hedonic scale. On this scale, 0 represents an absence of odor, while 6 represents a strongly objectionable odor [9]. By using the term ''objectionable,'' the scale becomes a measure of displeasure or disliking for the odor.

Hedonic measurements have been successfully used by a smaller group of judges who have been trained to score the presence of oral malodor as unpleasant and the absence of malodor as pleasant. These judges use the 9-point hedonic scale developed by Peryam and Pilgrim (Table 3) [10]. This scale has a neutral midpoint with degrees of pleasant or unpleasant increasing in opposite directions.

Judges trained to use a category scale are instructed to rate the intensity of the odor present. The pleasantness of the smell is not considered. Various lengths or sizes of the scales can be used if the judges are trained to identify the different intensities, and if they not only correlate to each other but are also reproducible. Examples include a 0-to-3 numerical scale, in which each score represents a range of odor (Table 4) [11].

Each point on the following 0-to-5 scale (Table 5) is designed to represent one level or intensity of oral malodor.

In a paper presented at the 4th International Conference on Breath Odor (IADR), intensity judges using the 0-to-5 category scale were compared with hedonic judges who applied the 9-point hedonic Peryam and Pilgrim scale. The purpose of the research was to determine if both types of judges were able to assess oral malodor under an identical clinical setting. Results found a positive treatment effect from baseline compared with the control when either the hedonic scale or intensity scale was used ($p = 0.0001$), with similar percent reductions for each set of judges. The intensity scores had a reduction

TABLE 4 An Example of the 0-to-3 Numerical Scale

Numerical value	Description of malodor
0	None to low odor
1	Low to moderate
2	Moderate to high
3	High malodor

TABLE 5   An Example of the 0-to-5 Scale

Numerical value	Description of malodor
0	No odor
1	Questionable odor
2	Faint odor
3	Moderate odor
4	Strong odor
5	Very strong odor

from baseline of -4.51, -2.32, -1.19, and -0.23 (for immediate, 30-, 60-, and 90-min post-treatment respectively) as compared with the hedonic scores which had a reduction of -4.29, -2.49, -1.65, and $-.88$ [12].

Frascella also used both types of judges to compare the effect of a chlorine dioxide treatment on mouth odor. In this research, the intensity judges used a 0-to-4 category scale and the hedonic judges used a 7-point bidirectional scale. In this research, both judges showed significant treatment effects at the 2- and 4-hour evaluation intervals [13].

In addition to using trained-judge assessments and instrumental measurements to determine levels of oral malodor, some work has been done to better understand the role of self-perception or self-assessment of oral-care treatments. Most agree that individuals have trouble detecting their own halitosis because of adaptation or dulling of sensations that result from continued exposure [14,15]. Because of this, adaptation attempts to accurately conduct self-evaluations using methods such as cupping the hand over the mouth, licking the hand, smelling dental floss, and breathing into fabric have not correlated well with more objective assessments [16]. Regardless, there still remains a potential value to understanding when and how individuals perceive their breath as offensive. This may be better understood by focusing on other self-perceptions rather than self-assessments.

Recently, a self-perception questionnaire was administered to 32 subjects participating in an oral-malodor study that included hedonic and intensity organoleptic evaluations. In addition to assigning a breath-odor score, subjects were asked to rate other experiences. These perceptions included current pleasantness of taste, freshness of the mouth, clean mouth feel, general feeling of offensiveness, a bitter taste, and feel of teeth. Finally, subjects were asked to rate the overall effectiveness of the product. At each post-treatment interval, responses to each question showed statistically significant differences among treatments favoring the positive control ($p < 0.001$). These findings supported the trained-judge assessments [17]. This is an area of thought that deserves further exploration and understanding. As individuals or consumers ultimately decide when they need to freshen their breath and their subjective evaluation that often determines the effectiveness of the treatment when used in a personal setting.

DESCRIPTIVE SKIN FEEL

Skin feel is an important sensory area for bodycare and cosmetic products. These sensations directly affect the consumer's perception about the efficacy of the product. Products that are efficacious may not be successful when marketed because of negative reactions to how quickly they absorb, smell, feel during application, or feel and look on the skin after use. Whereas a clinical study can show that a lotion or cream can alter the surface of the skin, only a sensory test can predict if this alteration will be perceptible to the consumer and give dimension and value to these perceptions.

These studies are conducted using descriptive sensory analysis. Descriptive analysis is perhaps one of the most sophisticated techniques used in the field of sensory testing. With this approach, participants or panel members describe the perceived characteristics of a material and then measure the strength of selected attributes on a scale. Formal descriptive analysis started in the food industry in the 1950s with Flavor Profile, which is a process for describing the aroma and flavor of various food products. A Texture Profile method was later developed in the 1960s to focus on the textural aspects of foods that were omitted in Flavor Profile [18]. Although this method was eventually expanded by Schwartz to include terminology specific to the skin feel of products, it remained based on the underlying principles of the original Texture Profile method [19].

Quantitative Descriptive Analysis (QDA) was perhaps one of the first descriptive approaches developed to investigate both foods and other consumer products. This method uses panel members who are users of the specific product being evaluated. Unlike other methods, these panelists spend only 5 to 6 hours in training sessions during which they develop a language for the product. According to Stone, there is ''no attempt to standardize responses, scores or train to score a particular attribute to some standard.'' Products are tested over several days using a repeated trials design collecting at least three responses from each participant for each parameter. Supporters believe this approach frees the methodology from dependence on the same panel and allows the language to be dynamic [20].

To capture the effect of time on the release of various attributes, time-intensity descriptive analysis was developed. This approach provides information on the dynamic nature of the response by monitoring the intensity of specific attributes over time. For example, the panel member may be asked to rate the intensity of several attributes every 10 to 15 seconds after use. With products that have a tendency to noticeably change over time, this technique has the potential to provide significantly more information than the more traditional sensory methods that measure attributes at specific intervals [21].

In the Spectrum descriptive analysis method, panel members rate the intensity of a product in relation to absolute or universal scales that are constant for all product types. This approach provides tools to custom design a panel for a specific product category and can be applied to a variety of product areas, including personal care. The final panel of approximately 15 members is carefully selected from a large group of individuals who participate in two screening phases. Once screened, the identified candidates then participated in at least 3 months of training during which they review samples that represent the product category, review references, define terminology, evaluate products, and discuss results. The performance of the panel must be established before they evaluate unknown test materials [22].

The DermatoSensory Profile approach to descriptive skin-feel analysis was introduced in 1986. Originally this panel was trained to evaluate only lotions and creams, but was expanded to other products that affect the feel of the skin, e.g., soaps, facial cleansers, antiperspirants, powders, and shaving products. The original panel of judges was carefully screened and selected before spending approximately 6 months in training. During this training period, under the guidance of a moderator, the group worked with a wide variety of marketed products to establish key attributes, agree on definitions, determine evaluation procedures, and select reproducible reference standards. The outcome involves a process of applying a standard amount of the test sample to a circle marked on the inner arm. Most of the attributes are evaluated independently with appropriate reference products continually used to anchor the 0- to 10-point intensity scales [23]. Some of the lotion and cream attributes selected by the panel include the rate of absorption, shine, greasy oily, drag, stickiness, ease of spread, and residue at several intervals after application. When five marketed products described as four oil-in-water (o/w) formulations and one water-in-oil (w/o) formulation were evaluated, the panel was capable of showing significant differences among all of the products for different attributes [24].

In 1992, the ASTM published the Standard Practice for Descriptive Analysis of Creams and Lotions [25]. This practice identifies the elements of and the process for training a skin-feel panel. In addition to identifying the needed equipment, it presents a process for screening and selecting panel members. One section describes an evaluation procedure that, in addition to explaining an application process, also discusses sample preconditioning, conditioning aspects of the skin including skin temperature, and environmental conditions of the test area. Evaluation intervals, definitions, and suggested references are included for each listed attribute. The practice does state, however, that it should be used by individuals who have become familiar with the process and have previous experience with sensory testing.

Descriptive skin panels fill the gap between clinical and marketing data by providing information that can help predict or better understand consumer needs. It has been used develop a master profile of a product that is later used for quality-control purposes or to improve the product. Panel information has also been frequently used to determine differences in currently marketed products whereas the descriptive terms and results are often used to promote or market the product.

There were a number of product-performance trends in the skincare industry during the past decade that may have benefited from a descriptive profile, in either the product-development stage or in better understanding the competition. For example, hydrating agents were added to increase skin moisturization. Although the physiological improvement of these agents is established in clinical studies, descriptive sensory data is essential to identifying potential consumer perceptibility. The move to silicone emulsion systems to decrease the heavy, greasier feel created with oil systems was a natural application for descriptive skin-feel data. Finally, industry responded to the increase in consumer awareness of the cumulative effect of sun exposure on the skin by adding sunscreens to many bodycare and cosmetic products. However, the addition of sunscreens often affects the skin-feel properties of the product. For example, they can increase the rate of absorption, add a greasy feeling, and create a heavier texture to the product. Descriptive skin-feel analysis was and continues to be an appropriate tool to address and minimize the effect of these changes on consumer perception.

DESCRIPTIVE HAIRCARE

The competitive world of haircare products is very dependent on consumer perception. The success of a product often depends on whether the user perceives a positive change or believes the claims being presented. Regardless of what can be shown clinically, it is ultimately the consumer who decides if his/her hair is shinier, easier to comb, has more body, or holds a curl longer. For these reasons, descriptive sensory analysis plays an essential role in the product-development stage. When appropriate sensory tools are used, these characteristics can be confidently assessed in a controlled environment. Formula changes as well as new ingredients and ideas can be screened before substantiating product-performance claims with large-scale consumer studies.

Currently, the majority of descriptive sensory analysis with haircare products is being conducted internally. Most manufacturers use licensed cosmetologists, trained panels, or groups of semitrained consumers. Some companies will use each of these tools depending on the stage of development or the product type.

Cosmetologists are perhaps the most sophisticated tool used, and sometimes the most challenging to the sensory scientist. Regardless of experience, these individuals must be screened and carefully selected. Once selected they must be trained to follow established procedures such as those for washing the hair, combing the hair, and touching the hair. They are also trained in what characteristics or attributes to evaluate and when. Because these individuals often have many years of experience working in a salon environment, they are often faced with the challenge of changing old habits. At the same time, the cosmetologist typically provides a certain level of knowledge or experience that even well-trained consumers don't possess.

Panelists for a descriptive haircare panel are selected and trained using techniques similar to those identified for developing skin-feel panels. However, these panelists are trained to evaluate hair rather than their own skin. Consequently, providing samples during the training process becomes perhaps the biggest challenge to developing the panel. Hair swatches are often used during the training process because using actual subjects can become costly and burdensome. They also provide a distinct advantage because the type and condition of the hair can be carefully controlled. This introduces one of the primary considerations of evaluating haircare products; subject selection. Because products will react differently on different hair types, subjects must be carefully screened and selected based on the type of hair they have. Some of the things that must be considered are hair texture, thickness, length, color, and amount of natural curl. The condition of the hair (e.g., dry or oily) and pretreatments, (e.g., permed or colored) must also be considered. A well-defined profile of the subject should be established before testing, and a method for selecting subjects using the trained panel, cosmetologist, or an independent person should be built into the program.

Depending on local laws and regulations, unlicensed trained panelists may not be allowed to handle the subjects. Because they may be restricted from shampooing, they are often only used to evaluate the feel or appearance of the hair. Some panels are trained only to evaluate hair swatches or a combination of both.

As mentioned earlier, because the majority of descriptive sensory analyses with haircare products is conducted internally, very little has been published in this area. To provide the industry with information, ASTM committee E18.0 on sensory testing is in the process of finalizing a standard practice for the descriptive analysis of shampoo performance [26]. This practice will present an overview of several options, some of which were previously described, that the sensory associate can follow to develop a hair descriptive program. Similar to the skin-feel standard practice, it will identify necessary equipment, a process for screening panel members and/or cosmetologist(s), as well as evaluation and application procedures. Although this document will focus on shampoo performance, it has the potential to provide an excellent panel foundation that can be expanded to the other haircare products.

ANTI-IRRITANT APPLICATIONS

Manufacturers fully understand the necessity of thorough safety testing before introducing a topically applied product. A battery of standard safety tests to determine the irritancy potential of the product to contact sensitization and photosensitization are routinely conducted. However, often missing are tests to determine potential subjective discomfort to the product, such as stinging, burning, and itching. In 1977, Frosch acknowledged that products that meet standard safety parameters may still be rejected by the consumer if disagreeable subjective discomfort develops after application [27].

Early work in this area investigated subjective response to substances applied to skin that had been damaged by either blisters [28] or scotch tape–stripped skin [29]. However, these were considered measurements of pain rather than measurements of more transient subjective discomfort. In response to concerns that some substances, such as sunscreens, may cause delayed stinging, Frosch and Kligman developed a method for identifying potential ''stingers.'' This method involved applying lactic acid to the nasolabial fold and cheek area of subjects brought to a profuse state of sweating. The intensity of stinging was then measured by the subject using a 4-point scale at 2.5, 5.0, and 8.0 minutes after application. It was also established that a stinging response could be induced in nonsweating subjects by increasing the concentration of lactic acid. An arbitrary method for classifying the irritancy potential of substances was also developed that identifies if the substance has a slight, moderate, or severe potential to cause stinging [27]. Although this method was established over 20 years ago, modified versions of it remain the basis for identifying subjects that are unusually sensitivity to stinging.

Grove improved the method by defining the demographic profile of the subjects and recommending the exclusion of males and older individuals. He also established criteria limiting the frequency of use and determined that sensitive subjects often reported a history of problems with soaps, cosmetics, and other personal-care products. Subjects who repeatedly reported a stinging response to lactic acid applied under ambient conditions were also tested for a burning and itching response. A method for evaluating burning sensations using a 20:80 mixture of chloroform:methanol pipetted into a greased aluminum cylinder covered and placed against the skin was used. To elicit itching, a 4% histamine base was also loaded into a grease-ringed cylinder and placed against the skin. Results found good correlation between burning and stinging, but individual response variability was rather high. A distinct correlation between itching and stinging was not observed [30].

A new interest in subjective sensory responses was renewed with the impact of alpha-hydroxy acids (AHAs) in the marketplace. When applied to the skin, these acids often cause a burning, stinging, and/or itching response, often without a visible sign of typical irritation. Draelos states that users have been conditioned to believe that stinging or burning sensations are an indication that the product is working, whereas ''in fact, they feel pain because the acid has penetrated the dermis and is interacting with the dermal nerve endings [31].'' Manufacturers have responded to these concerns by introducing a second generation of AHAs that do not penetrate the skin to the same degree. Although the FDA has found AHAs safe at low concentrations, the need to routinely include independent sensory assessments in the standard battery of safety studies is apparent.

Obviously missing from the available literature is a clear understanding of the sensory principles that were followed, which opens the door to certain questions that need to be addressed. Were the testing environments controlled? How were the unknown materials presented to the subjects? Were different scales explored? How was the scale that was used presented to the subjects?

For example, it may be advantageous to screen individuals for current use of certain medications that may affect their response, such as cortisones and other anti-inflammatory medications. Subjects should be screened for obvious skin pathology or irritation as well as a history of allergic reactions. When conducting the screening test or evaluating unknowns, the subjects should be preconditioned for several days. During this period, they should be provided with instructions informing them of, e.g., which cleanser to use, when males can or can't shave, what cosmetics are acceptable the day of the study, and when to cleanse the face. If the test is to be conducted at ambient conditions, the subjects should be preconditioned in a quiet, climate-controlled room. If the subjects will be brought to a "profuse" state of sweating, this state should be carefully defined to ensure that all are brought to the same level.

The actual screening probe should be administered in isolated areas to avoid subject interaction and influence. The subjects should not be told what the appropriate response is. For that reason, it would be wise to either eliminate the word "stinging" from the scale or not let the subject see the scale and ask them to verbalize their response. The "purest" way to approach it would be to administer the test and ask the subject to report any sensation they experienced. To increase the sensitivity of the results and decrease variability it may be worthwhile to explore a 0- to 7-point scale. Finally, the frequency of subject use should be limited with a distinct rest period (~48 hours) between evaluations. With these considerations incorporated with the methods previously developed, it would be possible to quantitatively assess the intensity of facial stinging. Once a reliable method is established, a database of responses to known ingredients can be collected that will allow unknown substances to be tested for subjective discomfort with confidence.

REFERENCES

1. Meilgaared M, Civille G, Carr B. Sensory Evaluation Techniques. Vol. 1. Boca Raton: CRC Press, Inc., 1987:1.
2. American Society for Testing and Materials. ASTM Designation E1207-87, ASTM Annual Book of Standards, Vol. 15.07. Standard Practice for the Sensory Evaluation of Axillary Deodorancy. 1987.
3. Labows J, Leyden J, Preti G. Axillary Odor Determination, Formation, and Control. Cosmetic Science and Technology. Vol. 20, 71
4. Wild J, Bowman J, Oddo L. Clinical Evaluation of Antiperspirants and Deodorants. Cosmetic Science and Technology. Vol. 20, 1999:318.
5. Chambers E, Wolf M. Sensory Testing Methods. ASTM Manual: MNL 26. General Requirements for Sensory Testing. 1996:3–5.
6. Meilgaared M, Civille G, Carr B. Sensory Evaluation Techniques. Vol. 2. Boca Raton: CRC Press, Inc., 1987:3.
7. Niles H, Gaffer A. Relationship between sensory and instrumental evaluations of mouth odor. J Soc Cosmet Chem 1993; 44:101–107.
8. Rosenberg M, Kulkarni G, Bosy A, McCulloch C. Reproducibility and sensitivity of oral malodor measurements with a portable sulphide monitor. J Dental Res 1991; 70(11):1436–1440.
9. Tonzetich J, Ng SK. Reduction of malodor by oral cleansing procedures. Oral Surg 1976; 42:172–181.
10. Peryam D, Pilgrim F. Food Technol 1957; 11:9–14.
11. Schmidt N, Tarbet W. The effect of oral rinses on organoleptic mouth odor rating and levels of volatile sulfur compounds. Oral Surg 1978; 45:876–882.
12. Borden L, Oddo L, Bowman J. Correlation between Hedonic and Intensity Measurements for the Evaluation of Oral Malodor. Presented at 4th International Conference on Breath Odor, UCLA, Los Angeles, CA, Aug. 1999.

13. Frascella J, Gilbert R, Femandex P, Gorden J. Effect on oral malodor of chlorine dioxide assessed by a hedonic panel. TKL Research Abstract.
14. Rosenberg M. Clinical assessment of bad breath: current concepts. JADA 1996; 127:475–481.
15. Tonzetich J. Production and origin of oral malodor: a review of mechanisms and methods of analysis. J Peridontal 1977; 48:13–20.
16. Rosenberg M, Kozlovsky A, Gelemter L, Cheriak O, Gabbay J, Baht, R, Eli I. Self-estimation of oral malodor. J Dental Res, 1995; pp. 1577–1582.
17. Oddo L, Borden L, Bowman J. Comparison of trained judge measurements to self-perception of oral malodor. Abstract, 4th, International Conference on Breath Odor, UCLA, Aug. 1999.
18. Chambers E, Wolf M. Sensory Testing Methods, ASTM Manual: MNL, General Requirements for Sensory Testing. 1996; 26:58–63.
19. Schwartz N. Method to skin care products. J Texture Studies, 1975; 6:33.
20. Stone H, Side J. Sensory evaluation for skin care products. Cosmet Toilet.
21. Lee W. Single-point versus time-intensity sensory measurements. J Sensory Studies 1989; 4:19–30.
22. Meilgaard C. Descriptive Analysis Techniques, Designing a Descriptive Procedure: The Spectrum Method. Boca Raton CRC Press, 1991: 196–199.
23. Oddo L, Aust L. Applications of sensory science within the personal care business, J Sensory Studies 1989; 3:187–191.
24. Aust L, Oddo L, Wild J, Mills O. The descriptive analysis of skin care products by a trained panel of Judges. J Soc Cosmet Chem 1987; 38:443–449.
25. Standard Practice for Descriptive Analysis of Creams and Lotions, ASTM E1490, Annual Book of ASTM Standards, Vol. 15.07.
26. Standard practice for descriptive analysis of shampoo performance. ASTM Committee E18.0, publication pending.
27. Frosch P, Kligman A. A method for appraising the stinging capacity of topically applied substances. J Soc Cosmet Chem 1977: 197–209.
28. Armstrong D, Dry M, Keele C, Markham J. Methods for studying chemical excitants of cutaneous pain in man. J Physiol 1951; 115:59.
29. Laden K, Studies on irritancy and stinging potential. J Soc Cosmet Chem 1973; 24:385–383.
30. Grove G, Soschin D, Kligman A. Adverse Subjective Reactions to Topical Agents, Cutaneous Toxicity. New York: Raven Press 1984, pp. 203–211.
31. Brewster B. MD's address sensory irritation from AHA's. Cosmet Toilet 1998; 113:9–10.

Index